HANDBOOK OF ANALYTIC PHILOSOPHY OF MEDICINE

Philosophy and Medicine

VOLUME 113

For further volumes:
http://www.springer.com/series/6414

HANDBOOK OF ANALYTIC PHILOSOPHY OF MEDICINE

by
KAZEM SADEGH-ZADEH
University of Münster, Münster, Germany

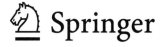

Kazem Sadegh-Zadeh
University of Münster
Theory of Medicine Department
48149 Münster
Germany
kazem@sadegh-zadeh.de

ISSN 0376-7418
ISBN 978-94-007-2259-0   e-ISBN 978-94-007-2260-6
DOI 10.1007/978-94-007-2260-6
Springer Dordrecht Heidelberg London New York

Library of Congress Control Number: 2011936738

Printed on acid-free paper

Springer is part of Springer Science+Business Media (www.springer.com)

To

Maria, David, and Manuel

Foreword

This work will shape the philosophy of medicine for years to come. There are very few scholarly endeavors that truly encompass a field while also having the promise of shaping and changing that field. Kazem Sadegh-Zadeh has produced such a volume for the philosophy of medicine. This is a foundational work of amazing depth and scope, which is also user-friendly. No one engaged in the philosophy of medicine will in the future be able to proceed, save in the light of and in response to the analyses, arguments, and reflections Sadegh-Zadeh has compassed in this extraordinarily rich and important study. He has succeeded in bringing together in an integrated vision an exploration of the epistemological, practical, and logical frameworks that sustain the engagement of physicians, as well as define the place of patients in medicine. This opus magnum provides remarkably careful explorations of the concept of disease, as well as of the diagnosis and treatment of patients in the acts of medical knowing and treatment. It situates the intertwining of diagnoses, the appreciation of therapy warrants, and the engagement of physicians in treating patients within the complex phenomenon of medicine. This work even has what is tantamount to an appendix that shows the bearing of logic on medicine.

The work begins with a careful exploration of the language of medicine, attending to its epistemic impact, its syntax, semantics, and pragmatics, including the various ways in which medical concepts are framed and engaged. Sadegh-Zadeh then examines medicine's encounter with the patient as a bio-psycho-social reality caught up in the drama of health, illness, and disease. In this study of medical practice, Sadegh-Zadeh creatively attends to the interaction of patient and physician in clinical practice. His analysis of the interconnection of anamnesis, diagnosis, prognosis, therapy, and prevention in the clinical context is innovative, displaying a remarkable depth of understanding that constitutes not just a foundational contribution to the literature, but a reframing of the field. It offers a comprehensive perspective, which is a tour de force. Drawing on a nuanced and subtle appreciation of epistemology in general and an account of the character of medicine in particular, Sadegh-

Zadeh explores the semantics and pragmatics of medical knowledge. He then relates these reflections to the intertwining of moral concerns, the character of logic in medicine, and a consideration of medical ontology within which, among other things, he provides a careful analysis of medical reality and the character of medical truth. He ties all of this to what can only be described as a powerful vision of the conceptual fundamentals that constitute the scope of the philosophy of medicine. Sadegh-Zadeh offers what will without doubt for the foreseeable future be the most widely influential and comprehensive account of the philosophy of medicine.

This impressively nuanced work bears the mark of a lifetime of research, reflections, and publications on the philosophy of medicine. While others were engaged in the birth of bioethics, Sadegh-Zadeh was focusing with critical energy on the philosophy of medicine. As a result, he became one of the central figures driving the re-emergence of the philosophy of medicine as a scholarly field. Early on, he helped to establish and then expand the scope and depth of philosophical medicine. One must note in particular that he aided in supporting scholarship in the philosophy of medicine through his pioneering work with his journal *Metamed* which was established in 1977, and which then later took the name *Metamedicine* and which finally became *Theoretical Medicine*. He has also been involved from the early years in *The Journal of Medicine and Philosophy*. Both through his own scholarly articles, as well as through creating vehicles for the publication of scholarly articles, his work in the philosophy of medicine has helped locate bioethics within the broader geography of the foundational explanation and therapeutic concerns that define medicine. As a physician and philosopher, Sadegh-Zadeh has without flinching addressed the conceptually challenging issues that lie at the basis of a philosophical appreciation of contemporary medicine. The result is that Kazem Sadegh-Zadeh has come to have a command of the philosophy of medicine possessed by no other scholar.

Drawing on a rich lifetime of scholarship, Sadegh-Zadeh has been able to integrate recent work in epistemology, the philosophy of science, and logic in a work in the philosophy of medicine. Because of his disciplined and innovative eye, this volume sheds a bright analytic light on the character of contemporary medicine and charts the future of the philosophy of medicine. It is marked both by creativity and an encyclopedic scope, and will establish itself as the standard for the field. It is likely that no one could have accomplished such a substantial exploration of the nature of medicine, other than Kazem Sadegh-Zadeh. He has produced an indispensable resource for scholars in the philosophy of medicine, including those working in bioethics. This work surely secures Kazem Sadegh-Zadeh's place as a cardinal founder of the contemporary field of the philosophy of medicine.

H. Tristram Engelhardt, Jr.
Professor, Rice University
Professor Emeritus, Baylor College of Medicine

Houston, TX
April 23, 2011

Preface

Medicine is a science and practice of intervention, manipulation, and control concerned with curing sick people, caring for sick people, preventing maladies, and promoting health. What necessitates this task, is the human suffering that results from maladies, and the desire for remedy and relief. Medicine serves this human need by attempting to lessen suffering that human beings evaluate as *bad,* and to restore and augment well-being that human beings evaluate as *good.* On this account, medicine as health care is *practiced morality* insofar as it acts against what is bad, and promotes what is good, for human beings. And insofar as it seeks rules of action toward achieving those goals and strives continually to improve the quality and efficacy of these rules, i.e., as clinical research, it belongs to *normative ethics.* Medicine is not human biology, biophysics, biochemistry, or biopathology. Nor is it any sum of these and similar biomedical and natural sciences. To view it as such, would shift medicine toward bio- and anthropotechnology where morality and ethics would lose their meaning and significance. As an aid in preventing such an autolysis of medicine, the present book elucidates and advances the view sketched above by:

- analyzing the structure of medical language, knowledge, and theories,
- inquiring into the foundations of the clinical encounter,
- introducing the logic and methodology of clinical decision-making,
- suggesting comprehensive theories of organism, life, and psyche; of health, illness, and disease; and of etiology, diagnosis, prognosis, prevention, and therapy,
- investigating the moral and metaphysical issues central to medical practice and research.

To this end, the book offers in its final Part VIII, as an appendix so to speak, a concise introduction to some focal systems and methods of logic that are needed and used throughout. Each line, paragraph, and page of its remaining seven parts relies upon what precedes it and what has been said in Part VIII.

The readers, therefore, should study the book systematically following the instructions given in Figure 1 on page 8. In that case, it will prove absolutely self-contained. It does not require any special knowledge and is easily accessible to all interested students. By virtue of its didactic style, the book is also usable in graduate courses in the philosophy of medicine, bioethics, medical ethics, philosophy, medical artificial intelligence, and clinical decision-making.

My thanks are due to H. Tristram Engelhardt, Jr., from whom I have learned, among many other things, that the concept of disease *says what ought not to be* (Engelhardt, 1975, 127). It is thus a deontic concept (from the Greek δέον, *deon,* for "what is binding", "duty") which obliges us to act. Since this normative aspect is dismissed by most physicians and philosophers of medicine alike, initially I wanted to analyze and demonstrate it in what eventually became the present handbook, HAPM, by means of deontic logic. In the process of writing, however, my thoughts extended beyond the concept of disease to the entire field of medicine when I fully recognized the deonticity of the field as a whole in the early 1980s (Sadegh-Zadeh, 1983). Although it is a fascinating feature of medicine that places the institution of health care in the same category as charity, it seems to have been overlooked by philosophers of medicine and medical ethicists until now. I hope they will concern themselves with this issue and discover additional facts about it when they read HAPM.

Also, my intellectual debt is to four scholars whose works greatly impacted my way of thinking and my life: Karl Eduard Rothschuh (1908–1984), one of my teachers at the University of Münster in Germany, ignited my love for the philosophy of medicine in 1964 when I was a graduate student of medicine and philosophy; Patrick Suppes's precision in philosophizing taught me analytic philosophy in the late 1960s; Newton C.A. da Costa's paraconsistent logic changed my view of logic and my Weltanschauung in the late 1970s; and Lotfi A. Zadeh's fuzzy logic changed everything anew and inspired me to initiate fuzzy analytic philosophy and methodology of medicine in the early 1980s.

I am particularly grateful to my wife, Maria, for surrounding me with so much love and support over the long period of creating HAPM; and to my sons, David and Manuel, for their assistance. Manuel drew the figures. David did extensive LATEX work (references, indexes) and produced, with the aid of Matlab®, the 3D representation of high blood pressure on page 672.

I would also like to extend special thanks to the editors of the *Philosophy and Medicine* for including HAPM in their highly respectable book series, and for excellent supervision, advice, and support; to Mr. Richard Preville in Charlotte, North Carolina, for carefully transforming my imperfect 'German English' into well-readable English; and to Springer for their outstanding production process management. But without the patient and competent work of three anonymous reviewers, none of us would be reading this line right now. I wholeheartedly thank all of them for their thoughtful comments and valuable suggestions.

Some of the ideas in this handbook present a further development of their seeds and preliminary forms that have appeared in my previous publications.

Specifically, my theories of health and disease in Section 6.3, of etiology in Section 6.5, and of diagnosis in Section 8.2 are based on my "Fundamentals of clinical methodology", 1-4, in *Artificial Intelligence in Medicine* (1994-2000); on my theory of fuzzy health, illness, and disease in *The Journal of Medicine and Philosophy* (2000, 2008); and on my "The logic of diagnosis" in *Handbook of the Philosophy of Science,* Vol. 16 (2011). Section 16.5.4 relies on my previous articles "Fuzzy genomes" and "The fuzzy polynucleotide space revisited" in *Artificial Intelligence in Medicine* (2000, 2007). Although during the process of writing the handbook, I have drawn on this previously published work, most of this material has been substantially revised, rewritten, and supplemented.

One of the reviewers proposed that I create a companion website for HAPM, which could provide a glossary and additional resources online. I welcomed the proposal, as I have already been offering a website on philosophy of medicine in German for many years. This website has now been internationalized to facilitate studies in the analytic philosophy of medicine, including HAPM. You may take a look at it here ⇒   http://www.philmed-online.net

Tecklenburg,   *Kazem Sadegh-Zadeh*
Germany 49545   Emeritus Professor of Philosophy of Medicine
Summer 2010   University of Münster, Germany

Contents

Part II Medical Praxiology

Part III Medical Epistemology

Part VI Medical Metaphysics

Part VII Epilog

Part VIII Logical Fundamentals

0

Introduction

> In a pain there is always more knowledge about the truth than in all wise men's serenity. All I know I have learned from the unfortunates, and what I recognized I saw through the look of the pained (Stefan Zweig, 1993, 56, translated by the present author).

0.1 A Fresh Start

Errors of diagnosis and treatment are major problems in health care, despite recent advances in biomedical and clinical sciences and technology. They are due to physician fallibility, on the one hand; and medical imperfection, on the other, raising the question of how the failures emerge and whether it is possible to prevent them. To evaluate this question and to understand its far-reaching implications, we may first briefly consider the following five examples:[1]

A 42-year-old female teacher consulted her family physician because of diarrhea that had lasted for five days. The doctor diagnosed enteritis and administered antibiotics. The patient died the next week. An autopsy revealed that she had a stomach cancer.

A 49-year-old male physiologist had been suffering from some malaise for several weeks. Based on his own expert knowledge, he convinced himself that he had exocrine pancreatic insufficiency, i.e., lowered production of digestive enzymes by pancreas. He visited an internist to have his suspicion examined. The doctor took some blood tests. A few days later, she calmed the patient down assuring him he did not have an exocrine pancreatic insufficiency. Since his health didn't improve, in the years that followed he successively consulted five additional doctors, to receive additional, conflicting diagnoses. It was only the last, sixth, doctor who was able to confirm his own, initial suspicion of suffering from exocrine pancreatic insufficiency, and to help him.

A 56-year-old housewife complained of being poisoned by her neighbors, and was hospitalized in a psychiatric institution. Paranoid schizophrenia was diagnosed. In the third year of her hospital life, a new, young doctor at the ward discovered that the patient had cancer of the esophagus. He concluded the cancer had certainly existed, at least as a precancer, prior to the patient's hospitalization three years earlier, and had caused her gastro-esophageal dis-

---

[1] Two of these examples, the second and third one, are real patient histories encountered by the author himself. The other three are based on (Cutler, 1998).

tress that she had interpreted as a symptom of being poisoned by her neighbors. But it was now too late to correct the past. She died shortly after the diagnosis was made.

A 22-year-old female student was diagnosed of having multiple sclerosis because of her complaints of permanent, unbearable headaches, and of some sensory and muscular problems. She was treated for multiple sclerosis over the next eight years. After she moved to another city and changed her apartment, her health problems disappeared immediately. No further treatment was needed. She was able to continue her university studies. Her new doctor speculated that effluents from the furniture in her previous apartment might have been the cause of her health problems.

A 39-year-old male engineer had several episodes of sharp, stabbing left chest pain. The pain lasted only a few minutes each time, did not radiate, and was not related to physical activity. The physician whom he visited, found that his ECG was normal and all blood parameters, including blood lipids, were also normal. No risk factors were present. The patient had no history of any disease. X-rays of thoracic organs displayed no abnormalities. The doctor diagnosed Tietze's syndrome and sent the patient home, assuring him that he had no serious health problem. He was asked to return in six weeks. Two weeks later the physician read his obituary notice in the local newspaper. He had not survived a second heart attack.

There are still many more misdiagnoses, wrong treatments, and physician-caused misfortunes, pains, and deaths. Why and how do they arise? I have tried to understand this phenomenon since my clinical training at the end of the 1960s. Living in West Berlin then, i.e., the free sector of then divided Berlin, Germany, I regularly witnessed at clinical rounds the debates between our chief and senior officers about their conflicting bedside diagnoses and treatment recommendations. It was surprising and even disturbing to me as a young physician to encounter such differences among their clinical judgments. This observation made me aware of an issue for the first time that our teachers had not taught us during our medical education, i.e., methods of clinical reasoning. Clinical reasoning, also called clinical decision-making, diagnostic-therapeutic decision-making, and clinical judgment, lies at the heart of clinical practice and thus medicine. Although as students of medicine we had learned large parts of natural sciences, anatomy, physiology, biochemistry, pathology, pathophysiology, and many clinical disciplines, diseases, therapies, and methods of diagnosing and treating individual, *specific* diseases such as gastritis, leukemia, schizophrenia, etc., we had learned nothing about how to search for a diagnosis and treatment *in general,* i.e., how to arrive at a clinical judgment. I asked myself whether there was a scientific methodology of clinical judgment that our teachers had withheld from us, and if so, what did it look like? My extensive search was disappointing. It revealed that there was no such methodology. I have since been concerned with this topic, and have found that a variety of highly intriguing logical, linguistic, methodological, epistemological, moral, and metaphysical issues and problems are involved. The present book addresses these issues and problems, many of which have either been overlooked or neglected until now by both medicine and its philosophers. Their analysis will not only enrich medical practice, research, and philosophy, but may also stimulate interest in the other areas involved.

0.2 The Objective

Medicine constitutes one of the major and most influential social institutions, including religion, law, education, and government, that interpret, rule, and shape our lives. It is therefore desirable to examine the adequacy and quality of its methods, means, practices, and perspectives. The present book undertakes such an examination by inquiring into the structure, nature, and goals of medicine. Our aim is to clarify the conceptual, methodological, epistemological, moral, logical, and metaphysical foundations of medicine in order to understand what occurs in the doctor-patient clinical encounter; what factors, forces, and sciences determine the dynamics and products of this interaction system; and how to best organize it.

0.3 The Subject

To attain our above-mentioned goals, we shall do analytic philosophy of medicine. But what is analytic philosophy of medicine?

Analytic philosophy that has emerged at the turn of the 20th century, is a well-established method of philosophical inquiry by means of logical and conceptual analysis. It was founded by the German mathematician and logician Friedrich Ludwig Gottlob Frege (1848–1925), and the British mathematician and logician Bertrand Arthur William Russell (1872–1970).[2] It attempts to clarify the structure and meaning of concepts, conceptual systems, knowledge, and action, and to analyze and improve methods of scientific investigation and reasoning. Accordingly, *analytic philosophy of medicine* is philosophy of medicine by means of logical and conceptual analysis (Sadegh-Zadeh, 1970a–c, 1977c).

My basic motive for analyzing medicine logically is my long-standing interest in the sources and conundrums of physician fallibility and medical imperfection; my desire to contribute to enhanced physician performance; and my

---

[2] It is sometimes maintained in the literature that analytic philosophy was founded by the British philosopher George Edward Moore (1873–1958) and the Austrian-British philosopher Ludwig Wittgenstein (1889–1951). However, it began earlier in Gottlob Frege's works on the philosophy of mathematics and language (Frege, 1884, 1891, 1892a, 1892b, 1893, 1904; Kenny, 2000), which caused Bertrand Russell to change his previous, Hegelian perspective (Russell, 1969) and initiate the logical phase of his philosophical inquiries as of 1900 (Russell, 1903, 1905, 1914, 1919; Whitehead and Russell, 1910).

conviction that such enhancement is feasible by employing logic in medicine. A measure of physician performance is provided by the quality of diagnostic-therapeutic decisions. Since these decisions are the obvious outcome of clinical reasoning, their quality mirrors the quality of that reasoning. It is well known, however, that despite the advances in medical science and technology, many clinical decisions turn out wrong, leading to malpractice suits. As some statistic report, there are 30–38% misdiagnoses (Gross and Löffler, 1997; Sadegh-Zadeh, 1981c). At first glance, these errors call into question the clinical competence of the physicians involved. Viewed from a practical perspective, this deficiency in physician performance may appear as a failure that in principle is avoidable by improving the diagnostic-therapeutic methodology, say for example, using 'medical expert systems'. However, there are also scholars who interpret it as an inevitable physician fallibility due to the peculiarity of clinical practice as "a science of particulars" (Gorovitz and MacIntyre, 1976).

I have been concerned with the issues surrounding clinical reasoning and its imperfection for about forty years. In the present book, some of the main results of this endeavor are discussed. They reveal the deeply philosophical-metaphysical character of medicine, the realization of which is likely to exert far-reaching impacts on both medicine and philosophy of medicine. The discovery that was briefly mentioned on page IX in the Preface, represents one of them. That is, (i) medicine as health care consists of obligatory well-doings and avoiding prohibited wrong-doings, and is thus *practiced morality*; and (ii) as clinical research, it seeks, justifies, and establishes rules of that practice, and thus, belongs to *normative ethics* (Sadegh-Zadeh, 1983). In contrast to the philosophically and methodologically sterile debate about whether medicine is a science or an art (Montgomery, 2006; Munson, 1981), the above thesis asserts that medicine is a deontic, i.e., duty-driven and normative, discipline. (The adjective "deontic" originates from the Greek term δέον, *deon,* for "what is binding", "duty".) I am convinced that philosophers of medicine, as well as medical professionals, will welcome this surprising finding. As we shall see later, its recognition and understanding requires minutely detailed logical analyses of medical language, concepts, knowledge, and decisions. The logic primer provided in the final part of the book is meant to make such illuminating analyses possible. Apart from its philosophical-metaphysical fertility, the finding will also stimulate medical informaticians and expert system researchers to customize their clinical decision-support programs and hospital information systems accordingly, and to base them on deontic logic. (For deontic logic, see Section 27.2 on page 927.)

The book is divided into eight parts, Parts I–VIII, which comprise 30 chapters. The starting-point is *the patient,* examined in Part II, since the philosophy of medicine that I shall develop will be tailored to her/his needs and interests. To this end, in the opening Part I preceding it, the language of medicine is carefully analyzed and enriched with methods of scientific concept formation, to contribute to its improved use in clinical practice, medical research, and philosophy of medicine.

In Part II, the patient is interpreted as a bio-psycho-social and moral agent in order to propose a theory of organism, an emergentist theory of psyche, and a concept of sociosomatics that substitutes for psychosomatics. This interpretation will help to provide an understanding of what it means to say that such an agent may feel ill, or be categorized as diseased. In the pursuit of this understanding, the concepts of health, illness, disease, diagnosis, prognosis, therapy, and prevention are logically analyzed, and a number of novel conceptual frameworks are advanced. These include *the prototype resemblance theory of disease,* according to which a few prototype diseases determine, by similarity relationships, the whole category of diseases; a *probabilistic theory of etiology,* which reconstructs medical causality as probabilistic-causal associations between cause and effect; and a *theory of relativity of clinical judgment,* according to which diagnostic-therapeutic decisions and preventive measures are relative to a number of parameters. The aim is to inquire into how medicine is engaged in shaping the human world, by deciding who is a patient to be subjected to diagnostics and therapy, and who is a non-patient. In this way, nosology, pathology, etiology, diagnostics, prognostics, therapy, and prevention are understood as conceptual and methodological endeavors that serve as means of medical worldmaking. All necessary logical tools are provided in our logic primer in Part VIII.

Part III is devoted to medical knowledge. In it, we analyze the concept and types of medical knowledge to expose the relationships of this knowledge to what it talks about. It is shown that medical knowledge consists of norms, hypotheses, and theories. While for syntactic reasons medical norms and most types of medical hypotheses are unverifiable, theories are empirically not testable at all because, like norms, they do not consist of statements of facts. They are conceptual structures, just like buildings are architectural structures. Several example theories are reconstructed according to this *non-statement view* of theories, to discuss its medical-epistemological consequences. An important question in this context is from where medical theories and knowledge arise. It is shown that, in contrast to our received views, the sources of medical knowledge and theories are medical-scientific communities and not individual scientists. Pronouncements such as "Robert Koch discovered the bacillus of tuberculosis" are inappropriate because underlying such a discovery are groups of scientists and technical assistants, research funding agencies, and a number of social and political-historical factors. This social-constructivist idea was first developed by Ludwik Fleck and adopted later by Thomas Kuhn. It is of particular significance in medicine because it implies that, by and large, medical-scientific communities determine the nature of medical truth and the way how to act. We even go one step further to suggest a theory of *technoconstructivism,* according to which scientific research today is in transition to engineering; and scientific knowledge is increasingly being constructed as a technical product and commodity by technology.

In Part IV, the concept of medical deontics is introduced to include under this umbrella term all medical research, on the one hand, whose outcome is formulated by deontic sentences, namely ought-to-do rules; and all medical practices that obey such deontic rules, on the other. Thus, medical deontics not only covers normative medical ethics and law, but also diagnostic-therapeutic research as well as clinical practice. This momentous *deonticity* of medicine also includes the concept of disease, that is argued to be a deontic concept created by the minimal common morality in the human society. As was already pointed out above, the deontic character of medicine has been ignored until now. I hope that philosophers of medicine, and medical ethicists as well, will concern themselves with this intriguing feature of health care in order to open new fields of research and to enlarge our understanding of how maladies and healing are intertwined with morality and charity.

Part V deals with the roles that systems of logic play *in* medicine, and with the question whether there is an inherent logic *of* medicine. It is shown that, due to the syntactic richness of medical language, different types of logic are required to cope with it in medical research and practice, because it transcends the scope and capabilities of individual logic systems. In this plurality of logics in medicine, an exception is provided by fuzzy logic. Fuzzy logic, also briefly introduced in our logic primer in the final Part VIII, is a logic of vagueness, and therefore highly suitable for use in medicine. It is a general enough logic to satisfy almost all logical needs of medicine, and moreover, to serve as an outstanding methodological tool for constructing innovative techniques of problem solving in research and practice. This has been demonstrated by an extensive application of fuzzy logic to clinical, biomedical, conceptual, medical-deontic, and metaphysical issues. By virtue of its wide applicability, strength, and elegance, it is likely to become the leading logic in medicine in the not-too-distant future. Besides the logical pluralism referred to above, no other logical peculiarity of medicine is observed that would require a specific *medical logic*. However, that does not mean that there is no *rationale* behind medical thinking and acting.

Medical metaphysics is the subject of Part VI. It is primarily concerned with medical ontology, medical truth, and the nature of medicine. Ontology is divided into pure ontology, applied ontology, and formal ontology. In these three areas, novel suggestions have been made by using fuzzy logic. Specifically, we have introduced a fuzzy ontology that seems to be auspicious for both medicine and philosophy. It not only determines degrees of being by means of a fuzzy existence operator, that we have dubbed the *Heraclitean operator*, but also makes it possible to construct a fuzzy mereology, by means of which vague part-whole relationships become tractable. Of particular importance is our distinction between *de re* and *de dicto* ontology, that is based on a syntactic criterion, and enables differentiation between fictional entities such as Sherlock Holmes, and real ones. The salient advantage of this approach is that it allows precise analyses of controversial questions like "are diseases fictitious or real?". Using this approach, we have extensively examined the ontological problems associated with nosology, psychiatry, and psychosomatics, and have also critically explored the so-called biomedical ontology engineering that is expanding today. Regarding medical truth, it has been shown that there is sufficient evidence to support the assertion that medical truths are system-relative, and are formed within the respective health care systems themselves. They do not report scientifically discovered facts 'in the world out there'. Particular emphasis has been placed on the analysis of medicine as a scientific field. Abandoning widespread, exclusive mono-categorizations such as "medicine is a science" versus "medicine is an art", we have demonstrated that in declarations of the type "medicine is such and such", the global term "medicine" should be differentiated to recognize that medicine, comprising many heterogeneous disciplines, belongs to a large number of categories. For example, without doubt biomedicine is natural science; clinical research, however, is practical science; it is also normative ethics; clinical practice is practiced morality; and so on. What is worth noting, is that medicine is also a *poietic* science that invents, designs, and produces medical devices in the widest sense of this term, from drugs to prosthetics to brain chips to artificial organs to artificial babies. Medicine is thus on its way to become an engineering science, conducted as health engineering and anthropotechnology.

Part VII of the book attempts to clarify some epistemological and metaphysical issues that our preceding analyses of medicine have revealed. First, taking into account the peculiarities of medicine, the concept of science is explicated to demonstrate why the traditional understanding of this concept in the general philosophy of science is terribly one-sided. The yield is a tripartite concept of science that, in contrast to the traditional mono-scientism, suggests three different types of science: theoretical science, practical science, and deontic science. Medicine comprises all three types of science. Second, it is shown that rationality cannot be a criterion of the scientificity of medicine, because rationality is something relative, and depends on the perspective from which it is judged. Third, it is argued that this dependence on perspective is an inescapable property of views, rendering *perspectivism* an interesting approach to epistemology and ontology both in medicine and elsewhere.

To conduct the studies sketched above, we must first assemble the logical and conceptual tools that we shall use. This task is accomplished in Part VIII of the book as a sort of appendix. It provides the logical fundamentals comprising a brief outline of the relevant fields from classical set theory and logic, to modal logics, non-classical logics and probability logic, and further on to fuzzy set theory and logic. For readers not acquainted with logic and its terminology, Part VIII is the prerequisite for understanding the medical-philosophical frameworks and theories developed in the book.

0.4 Methods of Inquiry

It is a truism that a tool for analyzing a particular object should be sufficiently sensitive to the subtleties of that object. Otherwise, the details and peculiarities of the analysandum will be lost. For example, it would be fatuous if someone tried to examine a biological cell by employing a pneumatic hammer, since such a brute-force approach only destroys the cell. The ingenious apparatus of a microscope and thin light waves will be necessary to discern what is before one's eyes. The same holds for analyzing a scientific enterprise itself. Medicine as a scientific enterprise is too complex an area to be amenable to coarse and crude tools and techniques of inquiry.

My interest in the subject addressed in this book goes back to my youth when, in the early 1960s, I was a graduate student of medicine and philosophy at the University of Münster in Germany. Initially, I was an adherent to phenomenologic and hermeneutic approaches, until analytic philosophy persuaded me in the late 1960s that it was a more adequate and superior method of philosophical analysis in medicine. I had the good fortune to realize early on that in philosophizing on topics such as diagnostic-therapeutic reasoning or the conceptual structure of medical theories, well-developed, sensitive, and precise tools and techniques such as logic are required. The reason why logic is needed rather than a pneumatic hammer for such an inquiry, is simply that both diagnostic-therapeutic reasoning and the-

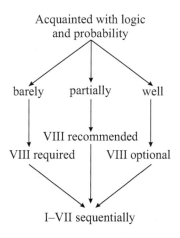

Fig. 1. How to read this book

ory structures have some logical characteristics, which are not adequately analyzable by tools other than logic. Accordingly, my approach to philosophy of medicine in this book takes an analytic route. It is my conviction that medicine will only benefit from logical self-analysis.

0.5 How to Read this Book

As a consequence of using logic as our method of inquiry, the book is not light reading like a traditional medical-philosophical treatise. Some knowledge of logic is required to understand the analyses, reconstructions, and constructions involved. For those readers who are not acquainted with logic, a logic primer is provided in the final part of the book, Part VIII, that they may consult before or while reading chapters of the book. In that case, the book will be self-contained and easily accessible to any interested student. The author recommends that you study the logic primer first, and then proceed sequentially through Parts I–VII and not skip anything. The book has been organized systematically and should be read accordingly (Figure 1).

Part I

The Language of Medicine

1

The Epistemic Impact of Medical Language

1.0 Introduction

"I feel really embarrassed about this, but I have this sudden burning and pressing in the left side of my chest", the patient Dorothy McNeil said. "You know, doctor, my daughter's pregnant. She's not married, just 17 years old. My husband had an accident a few years back and can't work. He's been sitting at home ever since. My baby boy is disabled. I have to bear the burden for all of them. I also have to take care of my parents who live with us in our apartment. You know, doctor, having to deal with all of that, without a job and without help, this chest pain just isn't fair. And to make things worse, we're in the process of getting evicted. Where am I supposed to go with a disabled little boy, a pregnant teenager, a husband who can't work, elderly parents to care for, and no money? It's no wonder I have chest pain. I can't sleep. I'm awake all night worrying about what's going to happen to us. This is my life. I feel lost ... "

Patients give their doctors similar reports about their illness experience every day. The melodramatic language and idioms they use, the putative-causal connections they suppose, and the folk explanation of their altered state of health they directly or indirectly suggest, all form a narrative artwork, a *story,* that the physician has to listen to, interpret, and evaluate by means of her own language. What she has to accomplish in this process, is to identify and decipher the actual problem of a *wounded storyteller* (Frank, 1997).

The illness narrative of the wounded storyteller is part of her life history. So, several questions arise. How is the physician to appropriately interpret and understand the patient's stories if she cannot disentangle the intricate network of the patient's life history to see things the way the patient sees them? What's more, is the question as to which one of the patient's stories is true, a mere interpretation, a confabulation, a complaining expression of her current dejection, or conveys some causally relevant information. How on this uncertain ground may she assist the patient to regain the meaning of her life

K. Sadegh-Zadeh, *Handbook of Analytic Philosophy of Medicine,*
Philosophy and Medicine 113, DOI 10.1007/978-94-007-2260-6_1,
© Springer Science+Business Media B.V. 2012

she feels she's lost? Virginia Woolf (1882–1941) in her novel *The Waves* put it excellently:

'Now to sum up', said Bernard. 'Now to explain to you the meaning of my life. Since we do not know each other (though I met you once, I think, on board of a ship going to Africa), we can talk freely. The illusion is upon me that something adheres for a moment, has roundness, weight, depth, is completed. This, for the moment, seems to be my life. If it were possible, I would hand it to you entire. I would break it off as one breaks a bunch of grapes. I would say, "Take it. This is my life".

But unfortunately, what I see (this globe, full of figures) you do not see. You see me, sitting at a table opposite you, a rather heavy, elderly man, grey at the temples. You see me take my napkin and unfold it. You see me pour myself out of a glass of wine. And you see behind me the door opening, and people passing. But in order to make you understand, to give you my life, I must tell you a story – and there are so many, and so many – stories of childhood, stories of school, love, marriage, death, and so on; and none of them are true. Yet like children we tell each other stories, and to decorate them we make up these ridiculous, flamboyant, beautiful phrases ...' (Woolf, 1977, 187–188).

Does any of the factors reported in the wounded storyteller's story above play any causative role in the genesis of her health problems, for example, the pregnancy of her teenaged daughter, the incapacitation of her husband, the disability of her boy, or the notice to quit their apartment? Is it possible that her chest pain only coincides by chance with her family situation and history, and she is merely making up 'flamboyant, beautiful phrases' about her life because she is suffering and narrates from this aching perspective? Is it imaginable that she will see things and herself otherwise, and will narrate cheerful stories tomorrow when she feels better?

Will the physician's language, replete with anatomical and biochemical vocabulary, disease and syndrome labels, and diagnostic-therapeutic termi-nology, enable her to decipher the actual problem of the wounded storyteller? Will it help her appropriately categorize the information she receives, and identify in the story any causally relevant factors that might be responsible for Mrs. Dorothy McNeil's ill health?

What do such critical terms as "suffering", "illness", "disease", "syn-drome", "causative role", "causally relevant", and "coincidence by chance" mean? Depending on how the physician's language is structured and whether it contains useful definitions of these and related terms that are important in eliciting information about the patient's problems, her diagnostic-therapeutic assumptions and strategies will vary. The concepts that a doctor literally *possesses,* determine how and what she sees. They direct and govern her per-ceptions and observations, her reasoning and decision-making. Her response to the wounded storyteller's voice will therefore be shaped by her medical language and the philosophy behind it. So, before we start looking into our medical-philosophical issues proper, we shall take a look at the role the lan-guage of medicine plays in the conditioning and structuring of a physician's medical knowledge, beliefs, conjectures, decisions, and actions.

Knowledge, belief, and conjecture play a fundamental role in medical practice and research. Almost everything that a physician qua physician, and a medical researcher qua researcher, says or does, has to do with what she knows, believes, or conjectures. In later chapters, we shall be concerned, among other issues, with logical, methodological, and philosophical problems of medical knowledge, belief, and hypotheses, as well as with their acquisition and application in medical research and practice. Here as elsewhere, however, there are intimate relationships between language and knowledge. Medicine is no exception. Medical language structures medical knowledge. Medical concepts and the ways they are introduced and used, shape both the process and content of medical thinking, as well as shape the way medical issues are represented and dealt with, i.e., health, illness, disease, remedy, life, and death. Therefore, we must first inquire into the nature of medical language in order to make clear how it impinges on medical knowing, believing, and practicing. After taking some preparatory steps toward this goal in this chapter, we shall discuss the syntax, semantics, and pragmatics of medical language and the varieties of medical concepts. These preliminaries will enable us to present a methodology of scientific concept formation in medicine in the closing chapter of Part I. Thus, our studies divide into these five chapters:

1   The Epistemic Impact of Medical Language
2   The Syntax and Semantics of Medical Language
3   The Pragmatics of Medical Language
4   Varieties of Medical Concepts
5   Fundamentals of Medical Concept Formation.

As was mentioned above, medical research, knowledge, and practice are not independent of the structure, quality, and logic of medical language. For example, it makes a difference whether we define our medical concepts clearly or leave them undefined to be arbitrarily interpreted by their users. To elucidate the significance that medical language has both inside and outside of medicine, we will in this chapter analyze the following issues:

1.1   Types of Knowledge
1.2   Propositional Knowledge
1.3   Propositions and Facts
1.4   Medical Sentences and Statements
1.5   Medical Concepts
1.6   How to Care About our Medical Concepts?

1.1 Types of Knowledge

Medical language has an ineluctable, substantial impact on the nature, content, and reliability of medical knowledge, and thus on the quality of medical research and practice. In what follows, we will study the reasons why the structure of medical language and the way concepts are introduced, interrelated with one another, and used in medicine, do matter practically, epistemically, and epistemologically. Consider the following few examples and the roles they play in medical practice and research:

- the concepts of *health, illness,* and *disease;*
- individual disease names such as *myocardial infarction, hepatitis, drug addiction, multiple sclerosis, schizophrenia, alcoholism,* and the like;
- seemingly solid conceptual ingredients such as *organism, cell, the genetic code, gene, nerve membrane potential, immunity, autoimmune disease,* etc.; and
- practical or metapractical concepts like *diagnosis, diagnostic accuracy, prognosis, treatment, treatment efficacy, etiology, cause, multifactorial genesis, risk, risk factor, prevention, evidence-based medicine,* and so on.

The problems and methods of concept formation in medicine will be discussed in detail in Chapter 5 below. In the present context, however, it goes without saying that if terms like those above are introduced into medical language in a way that allows individual doctors too much latitude in interpretation, the doctors are likely to have no common knowledge about the entities, processes, or actions the terms are supposed to designate. There would be no way to know whether occurrences that are diagnosed and treated by individual doctors as, for example, *myocardial infarction,* are 'the same thing'. What is even worse, these doctors will not be aware that their common knowledge is semantically blurred, and thus, while communicating with each other about 'the same thing', they may actually be talking about completely different things. To get a rough sense of the impact that the meaning and use of such terms as above in particular, and of medical language in general, exert on *medical knowledge,* let us take a provisional look at the word "know" and at how we usually talk about knowledge.

First of all, we must distinguish between *tacit* knowledge and *explicit* knowledge. Tacit knowledge is hidden from the awareness of the knower and cannot be, or cannot be easily, communicated to another person. An example is one's ability to intuitively read facial expressions and to understand the body language of others. By contrast, whoever possesses some explicit knowledge is also aware of, and in principle capable of verbalizing, it. The focus of our interest will be the explicit knowledge.

We usually talk about explicit knowledge in different ways. (i) Someone can know a particular object, place, or individual in the sense of being acquainted with that object, place, or individual. For example, "you know your next-door neighbor". This sort of knowledge is termed *knowledge by acquaintance.* (ii) Someone can, by a direct perception, become aware of something. For instance, during an appendectomy a surgeon may notice that the patient is bleeding from an artery, and may immediately act to repair the artery and stop the bleeding. This kind of knowledge, "the patient is bleeding from an artery", is referred to as *perceptual knowledge*. (iii) Some scholars argue that human beings are in principle capable of discerning the moral good. Individuals with this capability would be in possession of *moral knowledge*. (iv) Someone may know how to act in a particular situation in terms of having a specific skill and practical proficiency. For example, the above-mentioned surgeon may know how to repair a damaged artery and may do so successfully in the situation described above. Practical competence of this type may be called *practical knowledge*. Practical knowledge is a particular subtype of *procedural knowledge* or *know-how* that is used to perform some task and to attain a goal, e.g., to diagnose or treat a particular disease state, to play chess, to construct a radio, to go from the train station to the center of the city, etc. Below, we shall distinguish from know-how the so-called *know-that*.

In explaining the influence of medical language on medical knowledge, a fifth type of knowledge termed *propositional knowledge* will play a predominant role. But what is propositional knowledge? The expression of propositional knowledge in scientific areas, including medicine, is what is publicly available in printed or electronic media such as textbooks and journals, and is communicated in medical education, continuing education, conferences, etc. To avoid any speculation, we will approach this type of knowledge by looking briefly at the concepts of a *propositional attitude* and *proposition* in the next two sections.

1.2 Propositional Knowledge

Concisely, propositional knowledge is an individual's mental state of *knowing that* something is the case. To bring the term more sharply into focus, we will first consider as an example the following sentences and will compare them with one another:

    a. I *know that* Mr. Elroy Fox has angina pectoris,

    b. Elroy Fox *believes that* he has angina pectoris,

    c. His wife *doubts that* he has angina pectoris,   (1)

    d. His daughter *fears that* he has angina pectoris,

    e. His landlord *hopes that* he has angina pectoris.[3]

Verbs such as "to know", "to believe", and others whose derivatives are used in the example group (1) above, are called *intentional* verbs, and the derived predicates "knows that", "believes that", and others are referred to as intentional predicates. There are different types of intentional predicates, for example, (i) epistemic-doxastic ones such as "knows that", "is convinced that", "believes that", "conjectures that", "considers it possible that", "doubts that";

---

[3] Mr. Elroy Fox will serve as our example patient throughout. His patient history is briefly described in Section 8.1.1.

(ii) emotive or boulomaic ones such as "fears that", "hopes that", "desires that"; and ('₁i) others. When discussing modalities in Section 27.0 and epistemic logic in Section 27.3, we shall deal with these binary predicates which belong to the class of modal operators. (The Greek terms ἐπιστήμη (epistēmē) and δόξα (doxa) mean, respectively, "knowledge" and "belief, opinion". The adjective "boulomaic" derives from the Greek verb βούλομαι (boulomai) meaning "to wish", "to desire", and "to will".)

What the phrase "intentional predicate" used above means, may be briefly explained. The technical term "intentional", already employed in a related sense by the scholastics in the Middle Ages, derives from the Latin verb "intendere" which is composed of the preposition *in* and the verb *tendere* for "to direct, to aim, to extend". It has been re-introduced into the modern philosophy by the German-Austrian philosopher and psychologist Franz Clemens Brentano (1838–1917). His first concern in psychology was to find a feature that characterizes mental states and acts, and distinguishes them from other entities. He thought that he had found such a characteristic in the *intentionality*, i.e., directedness, of mental states and acts:

Some things, e.g., a picture or some sentences, are *about,* or *represent,* or are *directed toward* other things. For instance, the statement "I know that Mr. Elroy Fox has angina pectoris" is *about* Mr. Elroy Fox. A picture of you on the desk of your beloved is *about* you. But "?§xa]" is not about anything. The desk of your beloved is not about anything either. The *aboutness* or directedness briefly characterized in the preceding sentences is the *intentionality* mentioned above. Something that is about, or represents, or is directed toward some other thing is said to have intentionality. According to Brentano, (i) all and only mental states and acts are intentional states and acts, they have intentionality; and (ii) no physical object or phenomenon has intentionality. Thus, mental states or acts such as *knowing, believing, hoping, thinking,* and so on are intentional states or acts. That means that whenever someone knows or believes or loves … or thinks, then she knows or believes or … thinks *something.* Her knowing, believing, hoping, loving, or thinking is *directed toward* that something. The object that a mental state or act is about, or is directed toward, or represents, is called the *intentional object* of that state or act (Brentano, 1874).

The intentional object of an intentional state need not necessarily exist. For example, when I believe that there are gold mountains on the moon, then I have a belief and it has an intentional object, i.e., the state of affairs that there are gold mountains on the moon. But this intentional object does not exist. The aboutness and directedness of a mental state is a relation, referred to as an *intentional relation,* between the state and its intentional object. The above-mentioned predicates such as "knows that" and "believes that" are intentional predicates because they denote such intentional relations. We shall observe below that what they are directed toward, i.e., their intentional object, is a *proposition*. Therefore, mental states and acts of the type above portraying a person who stands in an intentional relation to something, are called *propositional attitudes*. Thus, knowing, or believing, or hoping, or fearing that something is the case, are propositional attitudes.

A propositional attitude of the form "someone knows that something is the case" is referred to as an *epistemic propositional attitude,* i.e., if and only if its intentional predicate is an epistemic predicate such as "knows that" in the first example in (1) above. What is usually called *propositional knowledge* is an epistemic propositional attitude. We shall study it in what follows.[4]

1.3 Propositions and Facts

In a propositional attitude of the form *someone Xs that something is the case,* with '*Xs*' being any intentional predicate such as "knows", "fears", or "desires", we distinguish two parts: (i) the initial segment "someone *Xs* that" includes an intentional predicate such as "knows" or "fears"; and (ii) the second part embedded in the that-clause, i.e., "something is the case", to which the predicate is applied, constitutes the content or object of the attitude, and is referred to as a *proposition.* A proposition is what a person *x* knows, believes, doubts, fears, hopes, etc. Knowing, believing, doubting, fearing, and hoping in the example group (1) on page 15 above are five different attitudes toward one and the same proposition that *Elroy Fox has angina pectoris.* Obviously, a propositional attitude is a relational mental state or act associating a person, *x*, with a proposition, *p.* Thus, it is a binary relation between a person *x* and a proposition *p.* (What is a binary relation? Readers not acquainted with logic and its terminology, are requested to study Part VIII first.) The label "propositional attitude" derives from this object of the attitude, i.e., the proposition. We shall in the present context be concerned only with epistemic propositional attitudes, i.e., *knowing that.* Given an epistemic propositional attitude of the form:

Someone *knows that* something is the case,

the proposition of the attitude is represented by the expression "something is the case" following the phrase "that", be it an elementary one like in the first two examples, or a compound one like in the third example in (2):

a. You *know that* Hippocrates was a Greek physician,

b. I *know that* the patient Elroy Fox has angina pectoris, (2)

c. Dr. Robert Gallo *knows that* AIDS is caused by HIV

and HIV is a retrovirus.

In these three examples, we have three different knowers and three different propositions that they know, i.e., *Hippocrates was a Greek physician, the patient Elroy Fox has angina pectoris,* and *AIDS is caused by HIV and HIV is a*

---

[4] What we have referred to as 'intentional verbs' above, are also called 'propositional verbs' after Bertrand Russell (Russell, 1918).

retrovirus, respectively. A known proposition may be of arbitrary complexity comprising a simple proposition or a compound one that may also amount to a big scientific theory or library. Let us therefore express the wording (2) above by the following general formula (3):

$$x \; knows \; that \; p \qquad\qquad (3)$$

or $K(x,p)$ for short, such that K is the epistemic predicate "knows that", x is the knower, and p is the proposition she knows. This binary epistemic predicate, K, is exactly the modal operator of epistemic logic discussed in Section 27.3.

Now the question arises what in an epistemic propositional attitude $K(x,p)$ the proposition p is that the person x knows. We must first convince ourselves that it is not a sentence. You may, without uttering any sentence, know that something is the case, for example, that *Hippocrates was a Greek physician.* Sentences are written or spoken strings of linguistic signs, and thus, linguistic entities. But a proposition is a non-linguistic entity and constitutes the object and *content* of a propositional attitude. What you know, is not the sentence "Hippocrates was a Greek physician", but *what is said thereby.* Otherwise put, a proposition is what is asserted when an 'inner' propositional attitude is disclosed. A proposition itself is not an assertion. Like a headache or desire that you may tacitly have, you may hide your epistemic propositional attitude as your inner mental state when you know that *Hippocrates was a Greek physician.* Arguably, you *can* assert what you know if you utter *Hippocrates was a Greek physician.*

A proposition a person knows is thus a linguistically assertable, non-linguistic entity. It may be asserted by statement-making about it, as when a person utters or inscribes a sentence. The sentence is of course a linguistic entity. Once asserted, the non-linguistic proposition one knows becomes the message conveyed by the sentence as a linguistic medium. It is now the content of the sentence, i.e., what the sentence means and says. Obviously, the same content may be expressed with different words and in different languages.

For instance, you may also utter the assertable proposition that *Hippocrates was a Greek physician* in German, i.e., *Hippokrates war ein griechischer Arzt,* and even in Chinese, Hebrew, Papiamentu, or in any other language you are conversant with. Although you are using different words and are emitting incommensurable sounds and melodies in those distinct languages, or are inscribing different characters, all of your distinct sentences have the same content that says, in English, that Hippocrates was a Greek physician. This trans-language content of your multilingual sentences is the *proposition* you know.

Conversely, one and the same sentence may have different meanings depending on who utters it when and where, for instance, the sentence "I am 68 years old". This sentence may be true of a given person at some time, but false of another person, and also false of the same person at another time. That is, one and the same sentence may express different propositions depending on the speaker, time, and place. Therefore, we must clearly distinguish between proposition and sentence. They are by no means identical. For the reasons sketched thus far, a proposition must be viewed as a non-linguistic, abstract entity. It is the mental representation, or rather the idea, of a *state of affairs,* be it a concrete or abstract one, real or unreal, existent or non-existent. The state of affairs is described by the sentence uttered or inscribed. Figure 2 illustrates the relationships discussed above.

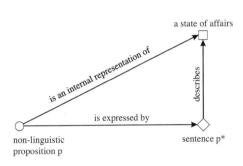

Fig. 2. The triangular relationships between propositions, sentences, and states of affairs

Many philosophers and scientists are wont to refer to a proposition p as a 'fact'. According to this view, an individual x who believes or fears that p, would believe or fear a fact. This view is hopelessly wrong. While the term "fact" implies or insinuates uncontested truth inviting or committing one to trust in what the person x believes or fears, she may believe or fear something in vain like a mentally ill patient believes or fears all manner of possible and impossible things. Factual and possible states of affairs are therefore to be distinguished. A proposition represents a possible state of affairs. Some, but not all, possible states of affairs are also factual ones. For our future purposes, a notion of 'fact' may be provisionally introduced right now. It will be revised in a later chapter. A state of affairs is a fact with respect to a particular language if there is a statement in this language that describes that state of affairs and is considered true. For example, the state of affairs that the Eiffel Tower is in Paris is a fact with respect to English because there exists a statement in English that describes it and is considered true, i.e., "the Eiffel Tower is in Paris". Thus, only some propositions represent facts, some other ones do not. For instance, the state of affairs that man is mortal is not a fact because we do not know whether the statement "man is mortal" is true. That man is immortal is not a fact either. We shall therefore prefer to employ the more general label "state of affairs".

1.4 Medical Sentences and Statements

Since the focus of our interest in the present context is only propositional knowledge, henceforth we will omit the qualification "propositional" and use the shorter term "knowledge" to mean just propositional knowledge. Our cursory discussion above of the general form of an epistemic propositional attitude, "x knows that p" or $K(x, p)$, demonstrated that knowledge is a two-place relation between a knower and a proposition. It is the intentional relation of knowing discussed in Section 1.2.

What is known by a knower x, i.e., her *knowledge*, is a proposition p. The proposition p need not be known by another person y because $K(x, p)$ may be true, while $K(y, p)$ is false. The relational nature of knowledge reveals the truism that without knowers there can be no knowledge even if in the absence of all knowers the countless textbooks, documents, and databases in libraries, computers, and elsewhere may not cease to exist in 'the world out there'. That means that knowledge is not the content of books, journals, and other containers that will never be read and known by any knower. Otherwise put, knowledge per se and apart from all knowers does not exist. Knowledge *is a part of the knower* and consists of her hidden, epistemic mental state when she knows that p. But there is a method to get rid of this tiresome subject-dependence of knowledge. We shall introduce it in Definition 117 on page 387.

Suppose that a medical researcher has discovered and learned something in her laboratory, and thus knows something new that other people don't know yet. Now the question arises how this knower may disclose that hidden 'part of herself' termed *knowledge* to render it accessible to other persons so as to communicate with them about it. That is, how does personal knowledge of a knower become a publicly perceptible entity to enter 'the public domain', so to speak, enabling other individuals to learn about 'that hidden part' of her? It is not difficult to recognize that such publicization of personal knowledge requires some kind of communication between the knower and others. The device enabling the communication that mediates epistemic relations between them is what we usually call 'language', be it a phonetic or script system of signs, a transmission method of another type such as Morse Code, or beating a drum in the bush. An individual's knowledge hidden from the awareness of other persons would remain hidden forever if there were no language. It must be linguistically disclosed. From this second truism it is clear that the manner of how language is used in communicating knowledge, i.e., the words and sentences that an agent chooses to express her inner knowledge, will shape the item of knowledge that is being communicated. Knowledge is constructed both while and by communicating about it because what transports it to other minds is the *expression* of knowledge.

That means in our present context that we shall have to pay particular attention to medical language, for it plays a fundamental role in acquiring, formulating, justifying, maintaining, communicating, and applying medical knowledge in research and practice. Medical language is the interface between medical knowers and the known, and as such, it contributes significantly to both the success and the failure of their interactions with the known and with one another. It is my conviction based on my clinical and methodological experience since my early youth that physician fallibility, in general, and all unfortunate failures of the type reported in the opening Section 0.1 on page 1, in particular, are considerably due to serious deficiencies of medical language.

Philosophy of medicine should therefore foster the interest in searching for methods of how they can be reduced. In dealing with seemingly remote subjects such as intentional objects and propositions we are following exactly that interest.

Propositions known by a particular knower refer to or represent actual, possible, imaginary, or fictitious ways the world is, will, or could be. As was pointed out above, as objects of intentional, mental relations of the knower to them, they are hidden from the awareness of other persons. Fortunately, however, the knower may disclose them by *statement-making through sentences* that she utters to talk and communicate about them, and thereby to transmit or transport her knowledge, whereas mental states and propositions themselves cannot be transmitted and transported to others. For example, we express the proposition that the patient Elroy Fox has angina pectoris, by the sentence:

The patient Elroy Fox has angina pectoris.   (4)

It is obvious that in contrast to the abstract, *non-linguistic* proposition that is known by a knower, sentence (4) expressing it is a *linguistic* entity uttered orally or written on paper. For this reason, a sentence must not be confused with the proposition expressed thereby. To elucidate, take a look at page 21 of ten copies of this handbook. You will encounter there sentence (4) above ten times. Being ten distinct objects in distinct locations, placed on different shelves, and read by different persons at different times, all of them say one and the same thing nonetheless, i.e., *the patient Elroy Fox has angina pectoris.* Thus, all of them report only one and the same proposition that represents only one and the same state of affairs. You will not be faced with ten distinct states of affairs expressed by ten distinct utterances. Here is another example. When I state in writing that I admire Sister Teresa, and my wife says orally that her husband admires Sister Teresa, we both are producing two different *sentences,* whereas we are making one and the same *statement* that refers to one and the same proposition. It is therefore advisable to clearly differentiate between three distinct entities:

sentence	is:	linguistic
statement	is:	linguistic
proposition	is:	non-linguistic, i.e., the content of a propositional attitude.

There are two categories of sentences, token sentence and type sentence. The sequence (4) above is a *token sentence,* and you encounter ten additional token sentences of the same type on page 21 of ten copies of this book. As a physical object consisting of a sequence of signs, each of these token sentences is an individual instance of a *type sentence* consisting of seven words that is represented by all of them.

Some, not all, sentences convey statements. A *statement* is a type sentence of a particular kind. To obtain this notion, we must first observe that in our communications and interactions, we use a variety of sentences, for example, the following ones:

- interrogatives: e.g., "Do you have headaches?";
- requests: e.g., "Tell me more about that, please!";
- imperatives: e.g., "Don't smoke!";
- expressives: e.g., "Oh, what fun it is to read in this book";
- declaratives: e.g., "Elroy Fox has angina pectoris".

Important in our present discussion is the latter category of sentences known as declarative sentences.[5] Traditionally, they are considered to be descriptions of states of affairs asserting that something is the case. We shall see below that this view is not quite correct. To differentiate, we therefore distinguish between two subclasses of declarative sentences:

- *constatives,* also called assertives or assertions such as "Elroy Fox has angina pectoris" and "The Eiffel Tower is in Paris"; $\qquad$ (5)
- *performatives* such as "I promise to visit you tomorrow" (see Section 3.3 on page 53).

A *statement* is a constative, specifically a constative type sentence. Such a sentence is an assertion and states that something is, was, or will be the case, e.g., "Elroy Fox has angina pectoris". Statements too are linguistic entities.

A constative token sentence will simply be referred to as a *sentence.* Note that sentences are used, whereas statements are made. A sentence is made *up of* words, a statement is made *in* words. The same sentence may be used to make different statements. For instance, when I now say "I am 68 years old" and you also now say "I am 68 years old", we are using one and the same sentence to make two different statements which need not have the same truth value. While my sentence makes a true statement, your sentence probably does not do so. For more details on this topic, see (Grayling, 2004).

In our logic primer in Part VIII, the question will arise as to what the bearers of truth values, *true* and *false,* are. This issue can be clarified here: The genuine truth bearers are statements because they assert something, they claim that something is the case. Bearing this in mind, in some particular context it may appear permissible for stylistic reasons to talk of a true or false sentence. Note, however, that interrogatives, requests, imperatives, and expressives mentioned above are not susceptible of being true or false. Although they are sentences, they are not statements because they are not constatives.

---

[5] In this book, the term "category" is used as a synonym of the terms "class" and "set". While usually the latter two terms are employed in formal contexts, e.g. 'the set of prime numbers' in mathematics, we shall refer to real-world classes as categories. Examples are the category of birds, the category of diabetics, the category of Gothic cathedrals, the category of diseases, and the category of declarative sentences. We use the term in its natural language sense that is to be distinguished from the formal concept of category which is the subject of the mathematical *Category Theory,* a branch of abstract algebra (Awodey, 2006).

Due to carelessness, usually no distinction is made in philosophical and even logical literature between the three different categories listed above. It is the unique statement that asserts the proposition someone knows, e.g., the proposition that *Elroy Fox has angina pectoris,* whereas the multiple, isomorphic sentences as concrete tokens, broadcast the same statement at different times and locations. The statement is an abstract entity.

Recall now our medical researcher x above who knows that p. Suppose that she is about to share her knowledge with other members of the medical community and tries to put it into words, to publicize it so to speak. In so doing she will face a difficult epistemological problem. How is she to form her statement, to find the 'right words' to verbalize the proposition she knows? She has a boundless language with a huge number of words, labels, and modes of expression at her disposal. How should she choose from among them particular terms to say what she knows? Should she say that the patient Elroy Fox has angina pectoris, or should she prefer to say that the patient Elroy Fox has precordial chest pain? What is it that she actually knows?

To assess the medical significance of these questions, we must consider the roles both of these competing terms, "angina pectoris" and "precordial chest pain", play. The concept of *angina pectoris* referred to in the former utterance, "the patient Elroy Fox has angina pectoris", lends to the statement a causally explaining flavor because this assertion draws the attention of the hearer to Elroy Fox's coronary arteries which, as the hearer correctly interprets, may have some atherosclerotic lesions engendering myocardial ischemia that causes angina pectoris. By contrast, the latter, alternative utterance "the patient Elroy Fox has precordial chest pain" employing the concept of *precordial chest pain* is merely descriptive and confined to the surface of the body. Precordial chest pain, i.e., chest pain felt before the heart, has other possible sources unrelated to heart and its arteries. So, the hearer will in this case think of numerous, divergent diagnostic hypotheses ranging from angina pectoris to esophagitis to skeletal-neural afflictions to pancreatitis, and so on. Obviously, the way we select the words that we deem to be the right labels to denote the constituents of our 'inner' knowledge we want to assert, does indeed matter.

1.5 Medical Concepts

We have just arrived at a critical point of our inquiry where we face the problem of how a medical knower should use the language of medicine to put into words what she actually *knows*. In order for her not to be categorized as a parrot or a compulsive, neurobiological speech robot, the way she selects the words to express her knowledge, must be viewed as her voluntary decision act (see the problem of free will on page 144).

If it is true that we are not neurobiological speech robots and the expression of what we claim to know originates from our own well-thought and voluntary linguistic decision-making in selecting particular words as the 'right' ones, while disregarding other ones, then the question arises what relation there exists between the words we choose, on the one hand; and the propositions we know, on the other. What in a proposition do our words relate or refer to? For example, when by using the word "angina pectoris" I make the statement "Elroy Fox has angina pectoris", what part of my knowledge that *Elroy Fox has angina pectoris* does my word "angina pectoris" express in my statement? One should be aware that the relation asked for is something to be invented and constructed and not to be discovered. It would be a futile task to search for 'the true relation' in the real world out there between words and their referents supposing that the reference relation was independent of our constructing act because such a search for 'the true relation' would require there being a *natural* or god-given and objective relation between a word and its referent. However, the historical change of languages and of relations between their terms and what they denote demonstrates that such a realistic position is unjustified.

The relation in question we conceive as one between words or *terms* as linguistic particles, on the one hand; and *concepts* as propositional particles, on the other. Stated succinctly, terms correspond to concepts. For instance, the term "angina pectoris" expresses, names, or denotes *the concept of* angina pectoris; and the *term* "precordial chest pain" expresses, names, or denotes *the concept of* precordial chest pain.

What is a concept and what is the difference between terms and concepts? The two preliminary examples above demonstrate that a *concept* is not a *term* and a term is not a concept. A concept is expressed by a term. The term "angina pectoris", a word consisting of 14 letters and used in uttering the diagnosis "Elroy Fox has angina pectoris", is not *the concept of* angina pectoris since this concept, like any other one, does not consist of letters. If it were so, we would have ten separate concepts of angina pectoris in ten distinct exemplars of the sentence "Elroy Fox has angina pectoris" printed in ten copies of the present book. However, we don't. All ten terms in those ten sentences refer to one and the same concept of angina pectoris. The concept is not the term. Rather, it embraces all that we have to answer when the question is posed: What does "angina pectoris" mean? Let us consider a tentative and informal answer to this question:

> *Someone has angina pectoris when:* she has precordial chest pain brought on by stress or exertion and relieved by rest or nitrates, and presents electrocardiographic or scintigraphic evidence of is- (6)
> chemia during pain or exercise.

The term "angina pectoris" expresses the entirety of what is described in the text block in (6) above following the "when" phrase. And this whole is, according to the present answer, *the concept* of angina pectoris. Obviously, it does not consist of 14 letters arranged like in the *term* "angina pectoris". It does not consist of letters at all.

Similarly, *the concept* of precordial chest pain that was considered a potential alternative in the quest above is not the *term* "precordial chest pain".

Terms are labels and belong to language, concepts do not. For instance, an English speaking person ignorant of German may possess the concept of angina pectoris, i.e., know what angina pectoris is, yet not know that the German term "Engegefühl in der Brust" denotes just that concept. This latter remark should suffice to illustrate the unbridgeable ontological gap between terms and concepts.

To summarize, the gap has two aspects. First, concepts are contents of mental acts of *conception,* and as such, non-linguistic entities, whereas terms are linguistic ones. Therefore, second, one person may express a particular concept by the term "ABC", whereas another person expresses it by the term "XYZ". For example, someone may express the concept of *chest* by the term "pectus", another by the term "Brust", still another by the term "poitrine" or "pecho", "petto", and so on. That means that one and the same concept may be named by a variety of terms. What complicates matters is that a particular term may in different contexts express different concepts. For instance, the term "pain" in "chest pain" means a physical suffering and discomfort, whereas in a context such as "you are forbidden to escape under pain of death" it indicates a threat. These brief notes demonstrate that the term-to-concept relation is not one-to-one, i.e., one term to one concept, but many-to-many (Figure 3).

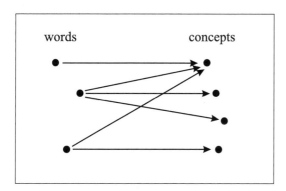

Fig. 3. A concept may be termed differently. Conversely, a term may name different concepts. Thus, we are faced with a many-to-many relation. And this *fact* is sufficient evidence of the non-naturalness of the term-to-concept relation pointed out above. We shall come back to this issue later on

Specifically, as contents of acts of conception, concepts are the constituents of propositions just like terms are the constituents of sentences that describe propositions. For instance, the constituents of the proposition that *Elroy Fox has angina pectoris* are, first, the individual concept of being a male named *Elroy Fox,* and second, the general concept of having angina pectoris, i.e., the concept that applies to every individual who *has angina pectoris.* See sentence (6) above.

In our statements, we use terms as linguistic means to denote concepts as the non-linguistic entities that we are talking about by those statements. At the same time, by virtue of being the name of a concept, a term refers to what that concept represents or creates. These relationships are illustrated in Figure 4.

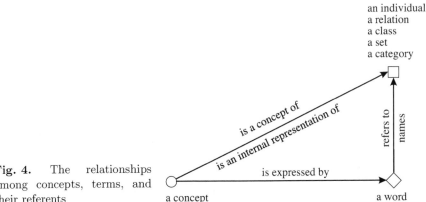

Fig. 4. The relationships among concepts, terms, and their referents

Based on the above considerations, we may *talk* about a concept in an intersubjectively controllable, 'objective', manner by referring to what it supposedly represents, that is, by talking about the entity outside the concept being conceptualized thereby. For example, an objective analysis of the concept of angina pectoris would be an inquiry into the syntax, semantics, and pragmatics of the term "angina pectoris".

1.6 How to Care About our Medical Concepts?

So far our discussion about the relationships between medical language and knowledge has brought in the following result.

Medical knowledge is based on propositions. As contents of mental acts and states, propositions are composed of concepts that mentally represent or create more or less complex structures. The simple example (6) above demonstrates that we express concepts by shorthands usually called words or *terms*. We use such terms in making statements about what we know, in order to communicate our knowledge, e.g., "*angina pectoris* is caused by myocardial ischemia". In this way, medical knowledge becomes the seeming content of sentences that we exchange by talking, listening, writing, and reading as if sentences actually contain and carry knowledge. The phrase "seeming" in the latter suggestion alludes to what has already been said earlier, i.e., without knowers there is no knowledge even though stored sentences may survive the mortal knowers. Sentences are and remain mere sequences of lifeless letters or sounds.

If it is true that without knowers there is no knowledge, then we ourselves are the agents whose minds on the basis of what we already know, transform a new sequence of lifeless letters or sounds into knowledge when receiving it from any source, be it a person, a book, a radio, or something else. The transformation of such a sterile sequence of letters or sounds into knowledge is accomplished by evoking or producing propositions in the receiver's mind. Suppose, for example, that I tell you "Elroy Fox has angina pectoris". It goes without saying that, first, if you do not possess a concept of angina pectoris, you will not understand my sentence at all. And, second, if you possess a concept of angina pectoris that differs from mine, you will understand my sentence differently than I do, and possibly, misunderstand it. That means that you will ascribe to Elroy Fox a set of features that differs from the set I ascribe to him. We shall see the world differently, so to speak. To elucidate, let us further assume that I possess a concept of angina pectoris along the lines presented in (6) above, whereas your concept may be the following one:

Someone has angina pectoris when: she has precordial chest pain radiating to the left shoulder and upper arm.

It is obvious that for two very different concepts both of us use one and the same term as its name, i.e., "angina pectoris". Therefore, the surface identity of our knowledge about Elroy Fox consisting in the isomorphism of the following two sentences (a) and (b):

a. "Elroy Fox has angina pectoris"   committed by me, and
b. "Elroy Fox has angina pectoris"   committed by you

will conceal both the background conceptual differences between us and the following one-to-many relation:

The same term "angina pectoris"   is assigned to: my concept
                                   and to: your concept.

One-to-many assignments of this type have a very broad spectrum among the users of medical language. It would not be an exaggeration even to say that every user of a particular medical term such as "angina pectoris", "multiple sclerosis", "schizophrenia", and the like has her private, idiosyncratic concept to which she assigns that term. No doubt, the ensuing semantic chaos is detrimental to medical knowledge and can only lead to misunderstandings, fruitless debates, and unsolvable disagreements. The chaos is mainly due to the following circumstance: Terms and concepts are not cared about to the effect that medical language, especially the clinical sublanguage, is in a disastrous state. To confirm this, have a look at the exposition of individual disease terms and concepts in clinical textbooks and journals. No book or journal article dealing with a particular disease such as angina pectoris agrees with another one on the concept they term "angina pectoris".

Now the question arises, how are we to care about our medical terms and concepts to avoid or reduce such semantic chaos? The remainder of Part I is devoted to this fundamental issue.

1.7 Summary

To examine how medical language impinges on medical knowledge, we have distinguished between several types of knowledge and have decided to concern ourselves only with propositional medical knowledge. Propositional knowledge is a subjective, epistemic state of a human being that can be uttered by an assertion of the form "I know that p". The terminal segment of such an epistemic utterance, i.e., p, is a proposition. For example, the epistemic utterance "I know that AIDS is caused by HIV" refers to the proposition that *AIDS is caused by HIV*. Propositions are non-linguistic entities. They are asserted by statements, which, in turn, are represented by constative type sentences. Propositions, statements, and sentences are three different categories of entities. In talking about propositions, we use sentences to make statements. Concepts are parts of propositions. They are referred to by words in our sentences. A central issue in the philosophy of medical knowledge concerns the problem of how to use the language in order that the right words are chosen to appropriately denote the concepts and represent the propositions. A prerequisite for an ideal use and performance of medical language is to sufficiently care about our terms and concepts.

2

The Syntax and Semantics of Medical Language

2.0 Introduction

When did you last say to someone that you had a headache? Did the listener understand what you meant? If you now reply "yes", how do you know that? Perhaps she usually means by the term "headache" something different than you do. How can we find out whether or not this assumption is true?

When did you last say that someone, for example, a patient or a relative, had jaundice? Did you mean that her skin and the whites of her eyes looked yellow? Do you say "yellow"? What does this term mean? Try to explain it to me and to yourself. After having explained it, consider the following, additional question. Under what light condition did you look at her skin and the whites of her eyes? Try to look at them under another light condition and to describe what you see then.

"Language is the source of misunderstandings", the Little Prince said to the fox. Language is the source of misunderstandings and errors not only because we often don't know whether our listener correctly understands what we say, but also because we ourselves often cannot exactly explain what we really mean by what we say. For example, try to explain to your listener what you mean when you say that you have a 'headache', are 'depressed', or that your patient has 'multiple sclerosis', 'delusions', an 'illness', or a 'disease'. These examples demonstrate that especially in medicine, the language we use often leaves us in the lurch because it is semantically underdeveloped and does not accord with ideal, scientific standards. In the current section, we will try to understand this *fact* in order to find out whether it is possible to ameliorate it by using sophisticated methods of concept formation that are unknown or neglected in medicine. Our discussion divides into the following six parts:

K. Sadegh-Zadeh, *Handbook of Analytic Philosophy of Medicine,*
Philosophy and Medicine 113, DOI 10.1007/978-94-007-2260-6_2,
© Springer Science+Business Media B.V. 2012

2.1 Medical Language is an Extended Natural Language

Although medical technology has developed breathtaking techniques and devices in many areas, e.g., in surgery, cardiology, clinical chemistry, etc., medical language is still light years away from similar achievements. To understand the reasons for this linguistic stunting, we must first distinguish between *natural* languages such as English and German, on the one hand; and *formal* languages, on the other. The former ones emerge and evolve naturally in the communities employing them, whereas the latter ones are artificially constructed for use in disciplines such as mathematics, logic, and computer programming (see Part VIII).

Formal languages are characterized by a precise syntax and semantics. By contrast, a natural language has a fairly vague syntax known as its grammar, and lacks any explicit semantics. Its semantics is implicitly determined by a dynamic group decision-making in the process of its use in communities. How people use a term determines what it means. Its use varies over time.

To explain, note that every scientific branch has its own scientific language. Examples are the languages of physics, chemistry, theology, and medicine. Unlike the formal languages of mathematics, logic, and computer programming that are artificial systems of signs with precise syntactic and semantic rules, most scientific languages develop as mere expansions of natural language by adding technical terms to it. Medical language belongs to this category. It emerges from natural, workaday language by adding terms such as "angina pectoris", "appendicitis", "nerve membrane potential", "immunocytoma", etc. This is the reason why it has no specific syntax and semantics. To give an example, consider the term "disease" that denotes the fundamental concept of medicine, i.e., the concept of disease, underlying nosology and clinical research and practice. Although one would expect it to be a well-defined term, it is as yet an undefined one. Nobody knows what it exactly means, and apart from some philosophers of medicine, nobody is interested in its exact meaning. The term languishes without any semantics as if it were an irrelevant or gratuitous one. Its derivatives share with it the same semantic obscurity. For instance, it is unclear what the adjective "diseased" means and what its application domain might be. To which one of the following classes are we allowed to apply it?

Human beings, organisms, minds, organs, tissues, cells, molecules, genes, animals, plants, societies, buildings, machines, planets.

Although all of us will agree that human beings may be diseased, questions of the following type will give rise to fruitless debates: Can an organism be diseased? Can a human mind be diseased? Can an organ be diseased? Can there be diseased tissues, cells, genes, molecules, etc.? These brief notes demonstrate how the inexactitudes and peculiarities of natural language enter into medicine. In the next sections, we shall be concerned with some of these peculiarities. However, it may be useful first to consider the general semantics of medical terms.

2.2 What a Medical Term Means

It may seem natural to suppose that the meaning of a word is something that enables it to play the role it plays in human language and communication. For example, nobody is surprised at experiencing that in response to the request "Doctor, please measure my *blood pressure!*" the doctor measures one's *blood pressure* instead of taking an X-ray photograph of the stomach. Otherwise put, the meaning of a word such as "blood pressure" is what transforms it from being an empty sound or inscription, into an effective and useful device in human communication. As plain as this seems, there is as yet no commonly accepted answer to the question "what does 'meaning' mean?". A variety of controversial theories of meaning have been put forward until now each of them having its own advantages and shortcomings. See, for example (Frege, 1892a, 1892b; Quine, 1960; Grice, 1989; Dummett, 1993).

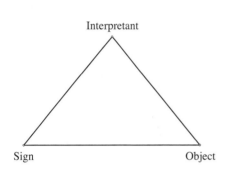

Fig. 5. The semiotic triangle

Traditionally, a term is viewed as a linguistic label that signifies (denotes, designates) an object in the world, be it a concrete or an abstract one. The term is thought to stand in the language as a representer for that object, e.g., "apple" for the fruit *apple*; "belief" for the propositional attitude *belief*; "cirrhosis" for the liver disease *cirrhosis*; "David" for my son *David*; and so on. According to this traditional conception, for the user of a term as its interpretant, the term's meaning comes from this term-to-object correlation. The well-known semiotic triangle reflects this signification idea (Figure 5). It appears at first sight that there is some evidence in favor of this traditional view. For example, from the difference in the veracity of the following two statements, we must conclude that each of the two terms "The Eiffel Tower" and "The World Trade Center" signifies a corresponding object in the world:

1. The Eiffel Tower was destroyed on September 11, 2001, by terrorist attacks;

2. The World Trade Center in New York was destroyed on September 11, 2001, by terrorist attacks.

Nevertheless, the conception of "meaning as signification" is not convincing. The reason is that from the huge ocean of linguistic expressions only individual constants, i.e., proper names, may be considered as signifiers such as, for example, "Albet Einstein", your and my name, "The Eiffel Tower", "The World Trade Center", and others. We shall see below that the remainder of the ocean has nothing to do with signifying and representing any object in the world. For instance, what object in the world does a term such as "love", "schizophrenia", "sin", "electron", or "my death" signify? Such expressions do not derive their meaning from signifying anything in the world out there, but from the way they are related with other expressions within the language itself. We will therefore suggest a suitable, practical frame to guide our discussions in what follows.

The tradition of the modern meaning philosophy started with Gottlob Frege's conception of meaning as a compound of a term's *extension* and *intension* (Frege, 1892a, 1892b; Carnap, 1947). First, the denotation or *extension* of a linguistic expression, relative to a particular language, is the single object or the set of objects to which the expression refers. For example, the extension of the term "Albert Einstein" is, relative to the English language, the famous physicist Albert Einstein, and the extension of the term "has angina pectoris" comprises, relative to the same language, the set of all patients who have angina pectoris. Second, the connotation or *intension* of an expression is, relative to a particular language, the informational content of the expression consisting of the set of all features an object must possess to belong to its extension. For instance, the intension of the term "has angina pectoris" is, relative to the English language, the property of having angina pectoris, i.e., a set of features such as precordial chest pain brought on by stress or exertion, electrocardiographic or scintigraphic signs of myocardial ischemia during pain or exercise, etc. Thus, we may conveniently say that the meaning of a term t relative to a particular language $\mathcal{L}$ is an ordered pair consisting of its extension and intension. That is: the meaning of t relative to language $\mathcal{L} = \langle$extension of t relative to $\mathcal{L}$, intension of t relative to $\mathcal{L}\rangle$.

The extension of a term is also called its referent. The term-to-referent relation is named *reference*. For example, the referent of "has angina pectoris" is, relative to the English language, the set of all patients who have angina pectoris. The intension of a term is also called its *sense*. So, one could also say that the meaning of a term relative to a particular language consists of its referent and sense relative to that language. Thus, meaning is language relative.

Note the following two important principles: (i) 'same extension, different intension' is possible; (ii) 'same intension, different extension' is impossible. The first principle means that two terms may be *coextensive* in that they refer to the same object or set of objects, while having different senses nonetheless.

For example, the terms "equilateral triangle" and "equiangular triangle" are coextensive. Both of them refer to one and the same set of triangles. However, they don't have the same sense because a triangle's having three equal sides is a different feature than its having three equal angles. That means that two coextensive terms are not in general interchangeable if they are not *cointensive*, i.e., if they have not the same intension. Consider, for instance, the predicates "is a female" and "has two X chromosomes". They are coextensive because the set of females is exactly the set of those human beings who have two X chromosomes. Suppose now that the following sentence is true:

Hippocrates knows that his patient *Alcestis* is a female.

Surprisingly, this sentence will become false if we replace the term "is a female" with "has two X chromosomes":

Hippocrates knows that his patient *Alcestis* has two X chromosomes.

The reason is that the two terms are not cointensive. They have different senses. Two millennia ago Hippocrates couldn't know anything about his patient's chromosomes. By contrast, 'same intension, different extension' can never occur. Cointensive terms are necessarily also coextensive and may always be substituted for one another.

In closing this section, we will now utilize the terminology above for medical terms. To this end, the following types of medical terms are to be distinguished (readers not acquainted with logic and its terminology should study Part VIII first):

1. Individual constants (proper names) such as "the patient Elroy Fox", "Albert Einstein", "Elroy Fox's heart".
2. m-place predicates with $m \geq 1$ such as the unary predicate "has angina pectoris"; the binary predicate "... is lateral from ..."; the ternary predicate "... is located between ... and ..."; and so on. An example may illustrate the latter predicate: "The forefinger is located between the thumb and the middle finger", formalizable by $Pxyz$.
3. n-place function symbols with $n \geq 1$ such as the unary function symbol "the heart rate of" in the following statement: "The heart rate of Elroy Fox is 76", i.e., $hr(\text{Elroy Fox}) = 76$.

Since an n-ary function is an $(n+1)$-ary relation, an n-ary function symbol may be reconstructed as an $(n+1)$-ary predicate. For instance, the unary function symbol 'hr' in group 3 above may be rewritten as a binary predicate of the following form: $HR(\text{Elroy Fox}, 76)$. For this reason, function symbols need not always be considered separately and are included as predicates in group 2 above.

We can now inquire into the meaning of such terms. The meaning of a medical term in a particular language consists of its extension and intension relative to this language, i.e., its referent and sense. First, the extension of a proper name is the individual person or object the name refers to; its intension is the property of being that individual or object. Second, the extension of an n-ary predicate is the set of all objects the predicate applies to; its intension comprises all features an object must have to be a member of that extension. For instance, the unary predicate "has Alzheimer's disease" has all human beings as its extension who suffer from Alzheimer's disease. Its intension is the state of having this disease, that is, a set of defining symptoms and signs such as memory impairment, apraxia, agnosia, etc.

Since meaning is language relative, it does not *reside* in a term itself. One will not be able to uncover it by inspecting or analyzing the printed or spoken word. The meaning of a term manifests itself in the manner of how the users of a language use the term in their communications, including writings. That is, it manifests itself in their linguistic behavior. For instance, if the members of a community currently *employ* in their utterances the term "fever" to talk about the state of elevated body temperature of a patient, then in this community the term "fever" presently means elevated body temperature. Maybe after a few months, years, or decades they will use it in other circumstances, for example, to refer to flying saucers. It will in that case be true to say that in this language community *the meaning of the term "fever" has changed*, i.e., both its extension and intension. But what is it that has changed? It is the behavior of the members of the community in using, and in reacting to, particular utterances that has changed, i.e., the modes of their language use as Ludwig Wittgenstein would say.[6]

Although Wittgenstein's conception of 'meaning as use' may appear to be at variance with the Fregean conception of meaning as 'extension and intension', they are compatible. Fregean meaning is in fact determined by how people use the elements of language.

2.3 Ambiguity

In addition to its language dependence, meaning is also context-dependent. An instance to support this thesis is the ambiguity, or polysemy, of terms. A term is called *ambiguous*, or polysemous, if it has more than one meaning. Such a term is differently used and understood in different contexts. For example, the term "bank" has at least three different meanings: financial institution, the ground near a river, a supply such as a sperm bank. This type of ambiguity cannot be avoided and is harmless. But there is also another type of ambiguity that is not harmless. Although it could in principle be avoided, it is scarcely noticed in medical community. It dominates the language of medicine, especially the clinical sublanguage. We have already referred to it on page 27 as a one-to-many assignment of words to concepts such that one

---

[6] The idea of *meaning as use* has been developed by Ludwig Wittgenstein in his posthumously published work *Philosophical Investigations* (1953). See below.

and the same word is used as a name for different concepts possessed by different individuals. For example, if the word:

"schizophrenia"   names: (a) my concept of schizophrenia,
                             (b) your concept of schizophrenia, and
                             (c) the concept of any other person,

whereas the concept of schizophrenia everyone of us possesses is *a private one* different from the others, and there is no public, agreed-upon concept of schizophrenia shared by all of us, then our communication about schizophrenia will suffer from an *inter-user ambiguity* of the term. As a consequence, we shall talk past each other. For this reason, the inter-user ambiguity is semantic-pragmatically malignant. The only cause of this widespread disease of medicine is that most medical terms are not defined, a circumstance that in clinical domains gives rise to misdiagnoses because it prevents the emergence of a reliable and useful knowledge. It can easily be remedied by teaching medical students, scientists, and authors how to *define* terms so that in their publications they could clearly define a new term that they introduce. The acquisition of this basic skill is sorely needed in medicine. We shall come back to this issue in Chapter 5.

2.4 Vagueness

Another ubiquitous phenomenon in medicine and its language is *vagueness*. It is something different than ambiguity. Since it is of paramount importance in medicine and medical ethics, and may be regarded a reason to revise the fundaments of medical sciences, practice, and reasoning, it merits particular attention and appropriate evaluation and treatment. We shall touch on only a few aspects of this comprehensive topic in the following three sections:

2.4.1   The Nature of Vagueness
2.4.2   The Sorites Paradox
2.4.3   Varieties of Vagueness

to suggest a solution. For a comprehensive account, see (Graff and Williamson, 2002; Hyde, 2008; Keefe, 2007; Sorensen, 2004; Williamson, 1994).

2.4.1 The Nature of Vagueness

In this book we are concerned, among other things, with the philosophy, methodology, and logic of clinical judgment. Central to clinical judgment in the clinical encounter and the diagnostic-therapeutic process is the question whether or not the health condition of a patient is an instance of a particular symptom, syndrome, disease, allergy, impairment, and the like. The result of such categorization is usually expressed by declarative sentences of the form "the patient is an X, she is not a Y". For example, "the patient has angina pectoris, she does not have pneumonia". The physician will encounter many problems in her decision-making when the labels of the respective categories, i.e., the terms "angina pectoris" and "pneumonia" in the present example, are *vague*. The logical, epistemological, and practical aspects of this issue are examined in what follows. First, the nature of vagueness will be analyzed in these two sections:

▶ Vagueness described
▶ Vagueness defined.

To understand our analyses requires acquaintance with logic, especially fuzzy logic, discussed in Part VIII.

Vagueness described

To begin with, we distinguish between clear-cut terms and vague terms. A *clear-cut* term has an extension with sharp, abrupt boundaries. An example is the term "even number". Its potential application domain is the set of integers, with its extension being the set of even numbers $\{\ldots, -4, -2, 0, 2, 4, \ldots\}$. Given any member, e.g., 275 or 276, the term either definitely applies or definitely does not apply to that number. There is no third possibility and no reason for uncertainty whether the number is even or not. The term is not tolerant, so to speak. Otherwise put, the application of the term to a number such as 276 generates a bivalent statement that is either true or false, i.e., the statement "276 is an even number" in the present case. By contrast, an expression is *vague* if it behaves according to the following tolerance principle, TP. See also (Forbes, 1985, 161):

> A term t is tolerant iff an object to which it applies, a t-object,   (TP)
> is allowed to be slightly different from what it is to remain still
> a t-object.

The shorthand "iff" stands for "if and only if" throughout. For example, a young man would still be considered young even if he were a few days younger or older than he actually is. In other words, adding a few days to, or subtracting a few days from, his age does not make him abruptly *non-young*. This tolerance of the term "young" brings with it a continuousness of its extension such that it contains borderline cases of which it is not definitely decidable whether or not the expression applies. This indeterminacy and undecidability is not caused by a lack of information about the term or the objects. For instance, the term "young" has borderline cases such as 42-year-old human beings. Although an individual of this age qualifies as a borderline 'young' human being, no empirical, conceptual, or logical analysis will enable us to decide whether she is definitely young or definitely not young. The set of young people as the referent of the term "young" has a broad grey area, and the people who are 42 years old reside in that area (see Figure 100 on page 1002).

Most medical terms, e.g., "icteric", "angina pectoris", "inflammation", "pneumonia", "Alzheimer's disease", and "schizophrenia" resemble our example "young" and are vague because they are tolerant according to TP above. Before inquiring into the nature and consequences of their vagueness, we will take a look at a short text on *pneumonia* quoted from a clinical textbook to see why vague terms are both unavoidable and desirable in medicine. As a technical term, "vague" is by no means pejorative:

In adolescents and adults the onset is sudden and may come 'out of the blue'; but often the patient has indeed a cold or other respiratory infection and rapidly becomes much more ill, perhaps with an initial rigor but always with a sharp rise in temperature, usually to 101–103 °F. Pleuritic pain usually develops over the affected lobe. The patient may become aware that he is breathing rapidly and certainly feels ill. Initially there may be a dry, painful cough but soon the cough becomes productive of sputum which is characteristically 'rusty' due to its content of altered blood from the foci of red hepatization; quite commonly, however, it is purulent or slightly bloodstained. It is often viscid and difficult to expectorate and this adds to the patient's pain.

In infants the clinical features are less constant and often misleading. Pneumonia in the newborn may present as pyrexia or tachypnoea with hyperthermia or as a feeding problem. In older children, signs of meningeal irritation and complaints of upper abdominal pain commonly dominate the clinical picture, while the initial pyrexia may cause convulsions or vomiting in children aged 1–5 years. Children under 7 years seldom spit (Passmore and Robson, 1975, 18.28).

A closer look at the text above shows that a variety of vague notions are involved in presenting and conveying medical knowledge. First of all, we encounter four types as described in Table 1.

Table 1: Some types of vague or fuzzy terms in medical language

Type of terms:	Examples:
1. Vague predicates:	child, adolescent, adult, cold, ill, pneumonia, rigor, viscid, purulent, pyrexia, tachypnoea, hyperthermia, rusty, cyanosis, icterus, red, yellow, pain, headache, malaise, hepatomegalia, tender, polyuria, oliguria, sub-clinical, etc.
2. vague quantifiers:	few, many, most, almost all.
3. vague temporal notions:	acute, chronic, sudden, rapidly, soon.
4. vague frequency notions:	almost always, commonly, usually, often, quite often, very often, seldom, quite seldom, very seldom, etc.

We will here concentrate on vague predicates only. Let us use the first term as an example. It is true that a 1-year-old human being is a child. 2-year-olds,

3-year-olds, and 16-year-olds are also children. However, is someone who is seventeen, eighteen, or nineteen years of age a child? Yes or no? We cannot definitely reply *yes* or *no* because people of these ages are borderline cases of the term "child". We will study this phenomenon below.

Let us distinguish between the extension of a predicate and the complement of its extension. Its extension is given by the set of those objects to which the predicate applies. The complement of its extension is given by those objects to which it does not apply. Those objects of which it is not certain whether or not the predicate applies, constitute its borderline cases called its grey area or *penumbra*. A clear-cut predicate such as "even number" does not have a penumbra. By contrast, it is characteristic of a vague predicate such as "child" to have a more or less broad penumbra, and thus, to lack a sharp dividing line between its extension and the complement of its extension. Its penumbra is due to its tolerance according to the tolerance principle, TP, above. That we have difficulty in deciding whether seventeen-, eighteen- or nineteen-year-olds are children, indicates that they reside in the predicate's penumbra. Figure 6 illustrates this circumstance.

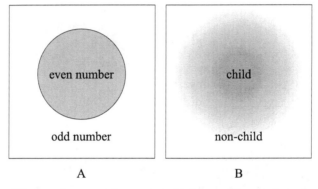

Fig. 6. The difference between clear-cut and vague predicates metaphorically visualized. A: The extension of a clear-cut predicate and its complement are separated from one another by a clear-cut line. B: By contrast, a vague predicate has borderline cases that form a penumbra around the predicate's extension blending it as a fuzzy domain into the complement of its extension

Vagueness defined

A slight formalization may reveal why it is impossible to eliminate, or resist, the semantic tolerance, elasticity, and permissiveness of vague terms like "young", "ill", "icterus", etc. To this end, let us introduce the operator "definitely", symbolized by Δ, such that if α is a statement, $\Delta(\alpha)$ says "definitely α". For example, if we are directly standing in front of the Eiffel Tower in

Paris, we may justifiably maintain that Δ(this building is the Eiffel Tower), i.e., "this building is definitely the Eiffel Tower".[7]

We will first define what it means to say that a predicate is vague: A predicate is vague if it denotes a vague class. But what is a vague class?

Definition 1 (Vagueness). *A class C is vague iff $\exists x \neg \Delta(x \in C) \wedge \neg \Delta(x \notin C)$.*

That means that a class is vague if and only if there are some objects which neither definitely belong to it nor definitely do not belong to it. It is exactly these objects that form, or reside in, the penumbra of the vague class. For example, the individual Pablo Picasso shows that the class of bald people is vague because:

$\neg\Delta$(Picasso is bald) $\wedge \neg\Delta$(Picasso is not bald).

It is indefinite whether Picasso is bald and it is indefinite as well whether he is not bald. Let α be any statement, the following sentence:

$\neg\Delta(\alpha) \wedge \neg\Delta(\neg\alpha)$

says that we neither know whether α is true nor know whether $\neg\alpha$ is true. This is equivalent to the following statement:

$\neg\big(\Delta(\alpha) \vee \Delta\neg(\alpha)\big).$

From this we can conclude that:

$\neg\Delta(\alpha \vee \neg\alpha).$

And that means that in the following disjunction contained in it:

$\alpha \vee \neg\alpha$

neither α has a truth value nor its negation $\neg\alpha$. But this sentence is exactly the Law or *Principle of Excluded Middle* of classical logic that is extensively discussed in Part VIII and will be referred to on several occasions in future chapters. Although the disjunction ought to be definitely true, it is not. Obviously, there is a conflict between vague terms and classical logic. Their tolerant behavior is not covered by classical-logical laws. Otherwise put, classical logic is not reasonably applicable to bald men, young people, icteric patients, and similar things. The only conclusion we can draw from this finding is that classical logic is not the appropriate logic for dealing with vagueness. This fact has already been observed by one of the prominent founders and pioneers of the modern classical logic, Bertrand Russell, as early as 1923 (Russell, 1923).

Due to their penumbra, vague terms generate logical, epistemological, and practical problems which are best demonstrated by the paradoxes of vagueness

---

[7] The definiteness operator Δ as well as the approach to vagueness using it I owe to Timothy Williamson (2005, 695 ff.).

they give rise to. The prototypical one is the paradox of the heap termed the *Sorites* paradox. This paradox will be sketched below to better understand the nature of, and to ask whether there are any remedies for, vagueness in medicine. For details on the philosophy of Sorites, see (Keefe, 2007).

2.4.2 The Sorites Paradox

A paradox (from Lat. "para" = *beyond*; Gr. "δοξα" = *belief, opinion*) is a correct logical argument that leads from apparently true premises to a false conclusion. The Sorites paradox that will be briefly outlined in this section, emerges from applying classical logic to statements that contain vague terms. It demonstrates how one may classical-logically fall from apparent truth into obvious untruth, an awkward situation we may get in when we unavoidably use in our statements vague terms such as "child", "bald", "heap", "young", "pneumonia", "icterus", "cyanosis", and the like. First consider the following simple example.

Would you say that a one-day-old human being was a child? Yes. Would you say that a two-day-old human being was a child? Yes. Would you say that a three-day-old ...? Yes ..., and so on. But if we continue this question-answering game, you cannot reasonably maintain, for example, that a 36,500-day-old human being was a child. So, where would you draw the line? That is, how would you precisely define the term "child" by fixing a definite age? You will not be able to do so.

One can try to get rid of this annoying and seemingly unsolvable dilemma by a legal decision to entitle a citizen "mature" when she becomes 18 years old, and by issuing the edict "A mature person is not a child any more". This possibility of legal intervention in the semantics of vague terms demonstrates that with regard to a vague term two types of borderline cases must be distinguished: *spurious* and *genuine* ones. Obviously, the borderline cases of the predicate "child" are spurious ones. They disappear by a legal settlement of the issue and transforming the vague term "child" into a clear-cut one. However, not all problematic terms can be defined by legal authorities without engendering absurdities. There are genuine borderline cases that are clearly not legal issues. For instance, would you say that a man with one hair on his head was a bald man? Yes. Would you say that a man with two hairs on his head was a bald man? Yes ..., and so on. But again, if we continue our question-answering game, you cannot reasonably maintain, for example, that a man with 200,000 hairs on his head was a bald man. So, where would you draw the line for baldness?

There is no doubt that drawing any sharp demarcation line in the following fashion to resolve the bald-man dilemma would be absurd: "A man with less than x hairs on his head is bald" where one may substitute for x any favorite number, e.g., 5273 or any other one. The dilemma is known as the bald man or *falakros* puzzle, from the Greek φαλκρος (falakros) meaning "bald"; and belongs to a group of related, ancient puzzles attributed to the logician Eubulides of Megara, a contemporary of Aristotle (Kneale and Kneale, 1968, 114). All of them have the same logical structure. They provoke paradoxical arguments known as little-by-little arguments, and are subsumed under the umbrella label *Sorites* paradox. The term "sorites" derives from the Greek σωρειτης (soreites) meaning "in heaps". Stated semiformally, the paradox emerges from an argument of the following type with a basis step and an induction step being its premises (readers not acquainted with logic are requested to study Part VIII first):

BASIS STEP: A single grain of sand does not make a heap;
INDUCTION STEP: Adding one grain of sand to something that is
       not a heap, does not turn it into a heap.
THEREFORE: 100,000 grains of sand do not make a heap.[8]

This is a valid deductive argument by mathematical induction (for the notion of mathematical induction, see footnote 194 on page 985). It leads from apparently true premises to a false conclusion nonetheless. To understand and analyze the problem, let us rewrite the argument in a somewhat more precise fashion. Henceforth, the phrase "therefore" will be symbolized by a straight line between the premises and their consequence:

1. 1 grain of sand does not make a heap;
2. If n grains of sand do not make a heap, then $n + 1$ grains of sand do not make a heap;

---

3. 100,000 grains of sand do not make a heap.

The first premise, *the basis step*, of the argument is true. Its second premise, *the induction step*, is seemingly true. The deduction is correct. But the conclusion is false. Where lies the problem? To elucidate the issue without complicated proofs, the argument can be reformulated by splitting up the premise used in the induction step as follows:

1. 1 grain of sand does not make a heap;
2. If 1 grain of sand does not make a heap, then 2 grains of sand do not make a heap;
3. If 2 grains of sand do not make a heap, then 3 grains of sand do not make a heap;
 ⋮
n. If 99,999 grains of sand do not make a heap, then 100,000 grains of sand do not make a heap;

100,000 grains of sand do not make a heap.

---

[8] An alternative formulation is the following, reverse argument by gradual decrease: 100,000 grains of sand constitute a heap. Removing a single grain of sand from a heap results in a heap. Hence, null grains of sand constitute a heap.

Each one of the premises is based on the understanding that heaphood does not depend on a single grain of sand. All of them, taken separately, are true. The reasoning step from premises to conclusion indicated by the phrase "therefore" is based on the Chain Rule of deduction presented in Table 36 on page 895. So, it is correct. Nevertheless, the conclusion is false. Why?

Since according to Metatheorem 1 on page 900 the deduction rules of classical logic are considered to be sound and truth preserving, whereas the conclusion of the argument above is obviously false, the question arises where this falsehood comes from. Vagueness philosophers concerned with the paradox are still puzzled about its genesis. However, most of their explanations are not convincing. The least plausible one is the so-called epistemicism that holds the view that vagueness is a kind of ignorance. It says, in essence, that the paradox reflects our ignorance of the location of the 'real borderline' between what is a heap and what is not a heap. That is, there really exists a non-heap which by adding a single grain of sand turns into a heap, but we do not know which one it is (Keefe and Smith, 1999; Sorensen, 2004; Williamson, 1994, 2005).

But this view is mistaken. A closer look at the induction premises 2 through n shows that by the Chain Rule they imply the following claim: "If 1 grain of sand does not make a heap, then 99,999 grains of sand do not make a heap". This, however, is an obvious untruth. It is hidden in the whole of the *premises* of the argument. Thus, the Sorites paradox is in fact no paradox, but a logically sound argument with false premises. Their falsehood is caused, and concealed, by little-by-little steps that according to the above-mentioned tolerance principle, TP, *all vague terms* allow. This is the well-known *slippery slope*.

The predicate "heap" is such a vague term. This is unveiled by the operator Δ introduced on page 38. It shows that with respect to many different collections of sand grains, the term gives rise to a statement of the form $\neg\Delta$(this collection of sand grains is a heap) $\wedge$ $\neg\Delta$(this collection of sand grains is not a heap). That is, $\neg\Delta(\alpha) \wedge \neg\Delta(\neg\alpha)$ if α is a shorthand for the sentence "this collection of sand grains is a heap". A finding of the form $\neg\Delta(\alpha) \wedge \neg\Delta(\neg\alpha)$ exactly characterizes the penumbra of a vague predicate. Every predicate that generates a penumbra is vague and denotes a class without sharp boundaries.

In Section 30.1 on page 995, we distinguish between classical or crisp sets, on the one hand; and fuzzy sets, on the other. In contrast to a crisp set, a fuzzy set does not have sharp boundaries. The solution to the Sorites paradox is this: A vague predicate refers to a fuzzy set and not to a crisp set. In other words, the extension of a vague predicate is a fuzzy set. Therefore, a vague or fuzzy predicate such as "is bald" or "is a heap" is not two-valued. Thus, it is not the case that such a predicate either applies to an object or not. A man is not simply either bald or not bald, but bald to a particular extent and not bald to another extent. Likewise, a collection of sand grains is not simply either a heap or not a heap, but a heap to a particular extent and not a heap to another extent. In fuzzy logic, the Sorites paradox cannot arise because arguments such as above are simply not possible. Moreover, the Principle of Excluded Middle cannot be violated because this law is not valid in fuzzy logic. See Section 30.2.5 on page 1010.

2.4.3 Varieties of Vagueness

So far we have not touched the question of where to locate vagueness. We must take a cursory glance at this issue because we shall need some clarity about it in later chapters. Is vagueness something merely linguistic? Is it something epistemic? Does it concern the semantic relation of reference? Or is it something ontic, i.e., inherent in the things themselves? We will briefly discuss the above questions in the following four sections:

▶ Linguistic vagueness
▶ Epistemic vagueness
▶ Semantic vagueness
▶ Ontic vagueness.

Linguistic vagueness

If vagueness were merely a linguistic property of expressions, it could always be removed by making precise the respective terms. The definition of the vague term "child" by the precise concept of maturity on page 40 was such an example. But whenever the attempt to make an expression percise generates absurdity or impracticality, as is the case with terms such as "bald", then non-linguistic vagueness outside language is involved. For instance, try to introduce a precise concept of baldness by, say, defining that a person with less than 5273 hairs on her head was bald. In contrast to the vague notion of baldness, this new, precise concept is both bizarre and impractical. Baldness is too complex a property to be captured by a simple numerical term. A more adequate method is required, e.g., by reconstructing the fuzzy set of bald people by means of its membership function. We shall come back to this issue in Section 18.3.

Epistemic vagueness

What is usually viewed as epistemic vagueness, is nothing different than epistemic uncertainty, i.e., uncertain knowledge. For example, we don't know yet whether myocardial infarction is a genetic disease or not. Any assertion on the genetic origin of the patient Elroy Fox's myocardial infarction will therefore be something uncertain, something hypothetical and conjectural, i.e., it will have an indeterminate truth value. This kind of truth-value indeterminacy of statements is obviously due to a lack of information and would be removed if a sufficient amount of information were available. Therefore, it is not advisable to refer to it as vagueness. The vagueness we have been talking

about in previous sections concerns conceptual vagueness such as the features
heap, bald, tall, red, icteric, and the like, but not propositional aspects and
qualities mirrored as epistemic uncertainty. Conceptual vagueness does indeed
cause epistemic uncertainty, but such an uncertainty per se is not vagueness.

Semantic vagueness

As far as linguistic expressions, pictures, or perceptions represent something,
for example, picture x representing person y, such a binary representational
relation may be expressed by "$Repr(x, y)$" to say that x *represents* y. The
relation *Repr* may of course be vague if x does not represent y isomorphically.
For there may be a better representation that displays more details of y than
x does. Thus, a representation as a semantic relation of reference may be more
or less vague. It is a *vague relation.*

Ontic vagueness

The adjective "ontic" means "concerning the being". It originates from the
Greek term $o\nu$ (on) that derives from the present participle of the Greek verb
$\varepsilon\iota\nu\alpha\iota$ (einai) for "to be".

Ontic vagueness is the prototypical vagueness and the source of all other
types of genuine vagueness. It concerns the vagueness of individual objects,
classes, relations, and states of affairs in 'the world out there'. Are there such
vague entities? And what does their vagueness look like?

Concisely, we cannot know how things are 'in themselves' irrespective of
whether or how they are perceived, recognized, or represented. As we shall see
in Chapter 23 on page 807, the world looks different depending on what glasses
we put on. We may therefore be tempted to take the position that "we shall
never know whether there is vagueness in the world out there and whether
objects or states of affairs can be vague". To assert or to deny vagueness in
the world, will remain an ontological postulate in any case. From a practical
perspective, however, it appears reasonable to prefer the affirmative. That
means that it is more reasonable than not to suppose that there are vague
individual objects, vague sets, including relations, and vague states of affairs.
To give three corresponding examples, (i) a frog is a vague animal, i.e., an object with indeterminate spatio-temporal boundaries, because it is impossible
to determine when it emerges from a tadpole. There is no abrupt end of being
a tadpole and no abrupt start of being a frog. The transition is continuous.
Similarly, (ii) the class of bald human beings has no sharp boundaries. It has a
penumbral region of genuine borderline cases that imperceptibly vanishes into
the set of non-bald people. Finally, (iii) there are also vague states of affairs.
For a state of affairs amounts to the belonging of an object to a class. For
example, the state of affairs that *Picasso is bald* entails Picasso's membership
in the class of bald people. If the class an object belongs to is a vague set,
such as *bald,* and the object resides in its penumbra, the state of affairs turns

out to be something indefinite. That means, according to the terminology we have introduced on page 38, $\neg\Delta$(Picasso is bald) $\wedge$ $\neg\Delta$(Picasso is not bald). That Picasso is not definitely bald and not definitely not bald is an ontically indefinite, i.e., *vague,* state of affairs.

When we apply these consideration to medicine, we shall easily recognize that many medical objects and subjects, e.g., cells, tissues, organs, organisms, persons, patients, symptoms, diseases, individual disease states of patients, and recovery processes are ontically vague to the effect that their vagueness is principally not eliminable. We shall come back to this issue in Chapter 19 on page 711. Fuzzy set theory is a conceptualization and precise theory of ontic vagueness (see Section 30.1 on page 995).

2.5 Clarity and Precision

"Clarity" is the antonym of vagueness. For instance, "living thing" and "ill" are vague terms, whereas "brother" and "Aspirin" are clear. Precision, however, is something more than mere clarity. A term is precise if it is a clear-cut one due to its numerical nature. A numerical term measures a property such as age, or weight, or intelligence by assigning numbers to it (see Section 4.1.4 on page 70). For example, the term "17 years old" in the statement "Amy is 17 years old" is a numerical, and thus a *precise,* term.

Usually, precision is viewed as an ideal in science. Vagueness is frowned upon, especially in natural sciences. It is generally recommended to make precise or sharpen vague terms. To implement this recommendation radically, however, would mean to give up the tolerance principle TP mentioned on page 36 and to eliminate vague terms from the language of medicine. The idea is based on a misunderstanding and is neither beneficial nor practicable for following reasons:

First, it is not reasonable to sharpen or make precise every vague term because this would severely change natural languages and thereby damage their expressive power. To vaguely say that a patient is icteric is much more informative than to precisely say that the light reflected by her skin has a wavelength of 570 nanometers. Second, it would become almost impossible to learn and to employ precise terms in everyday life. For instance, before asserting anything about the color of an object, we would have to measure the wavelength of the light it reflects. Third, medicine is concerned with highly complex systems and issues such as the human organism, suffering persons, and their treatment. By increasing the precision of their analysis, the relevance of the information obtained is not necessarily increased. This has been well expressed by the inventor of fuzzy logic, Lotfi A. Zadeh, whose *Principle of Incompatibility* reminds us to prefer relevance to precision: "Stated informally, the essence of this principle is that as the complexity of a system increases, our ability to make precise and yet significant statements about its behavior diminishes until a threshold is reached beyond which precision and significance (or relevance) become almost mutually exclusive characteristics" (Zadeh, 1973, 28). We shall come back to this issue on page 607.

2.6 Semantic Nihilism

Our philosophizing on medical language aims at practical goals. One of these goals is to explore whether and how medical language is tied to the real world of suffering human beings and their affairs. We must pay attention to this problem again and again in order to reduce and neutralize the influence that unworldly scientific ambitions and speculations exert on medical knowledge and action by deforming medical language and its semantics. To assess the importance of the issue, we may ask ourselves whether there are any methods of scientific concept formation on which the introduction of terms such as, for example, "schizophrenia", "membrane channels", or "autoimmunity" is based. To this problem area belongs first of all the inquiry into the nature of the meaning of medical terms, i.e., into the medical word-to-world relationship:

Does a medical term *refer* to something in the world? Does it have a *meaning?* The immediate answer to this question will in general be 'yes' because, it will be argued, "otherwise our medical theorizing and practicing would be in vain". We have shared this traditional view until now and have argued above that medical terms indeed have a meaning, e.g., the terms "heart" and "angina pectoris". For instance, everybody knows that the term "heart" refers to the central organ of the circulatory system beating in one's chest. It would therefore be strange if someone tried to deny that "heart" refers to, and *means*, just that central organ. However, it is exactly this denial that is the claim of Ludwig Wittgenstein's later philosophy. Words don't mean anything, he says. They refer to nothing. They are only used as a ball is used in a ball game. The use of a word is its meaning and vice versa. In the present section, we will take a brief look at this disturbing semantic nihilism that was developed by Ludwig Wittgenstein in his *Philosophical Investigations* (Wittgenstein, 1953).

Our aim here is to present Wittgenstein's alternative view that has significant consequences for our understanding of medical semantics and for the analysis and evaluation of medical knowledge and action. Our discussion is based on, and will draw and benefit from, Saul Kripke's interpretation of Wittgenstein's view (Kripke, 1982).

Ludwig Wittgenstein (1889–1951) was a Vienna-born philosopher who taught philosophy at the University of Cambridge from 1939 to 1947. He is viewed as the most influential analytic philosopher of the twentieth century. His work is commonly divided into an early period, culminating in his epoch-making booklet *Tractatus Logico-Philosophicus* (first published in 1921), and a later period from 1929 until his death, culminating in his eminent, posthumously published *Philosophical Investigations* (1953). Both periods are dominated by a concern with the nature of language and the impact it has on mathematics, logic, philosophy, and psychology. In the early work, *Tractatus*, language is treated in a syntactic, semantic, and logical way abstracting from the language user. In the later, pragmatic period, however, the language users, their linguistic activities, and their *form of life* are considered to be the determinants of almost everything. (For the concepts of syntax, semantics, and pragmatics, see Section 26.1.4 in Part VIII.)

Between his earlier and later writings lies the dramatic change of his philosophy around 1929. His theory of language presented in the later period is practically the repudiation of *Tractatus*. We shall here touch on only one aspect of his new philosophy, i.e., his pragmatic view of semantics expressed by the slogan that *use exhausts meaning*. He begins this philosophy with a criticism of the traditional conception of meaning according to which "Every word has a meaning. This meaning is correlated with the word. It is the object for which the word stands" (Wittgenstein, 1953, section 1).

Usually we believe in this doctrine. We believe, for example, that the word "angina pectoris" stands for a malady consisting of a group of symptoms such as precordial chest pain radiating to the left shoulder and upper arm. Accordingly, we also believe that grasping an expression, or meaning something by an expression such as "angina pectoris", is a mental state or act. Wittgenstein, however, says that there is no such mental state or act. There is no such 'meaning something' by an expression. A word does not stand for something that might be its meaning. To understand a word is not to know what it means, but to know how to use it.

How does Wittgenstein substantiate this view? His reasoning is based on the notion of *following a rule* that we will briefly sketch in order to evaluate his insight and his alternative proposal. To this end, we will understand by the term "linguistic rule", or "rule" for short, a standard method or procedure prescribing how a particular term is to be used. Examples are the definition of a term, grammatical rules, and algorithms.[9] Since the consistent application of a term such as "angina pectoris" may be construed as following a rule, i.e., following its definition, we may choose any term such as, for instance, "angina pectoris", "democracy", "minus", or "plus" to study Wittgenstein's argument. For the sake of convenience and transparency, however, we will use the latter term as an example.

Suppose you have examined a patient, and on the basis of your final diagnosis you have administered her a particular drug. The maximum dose per day one is allowed to take of this drug, is 120 milligrams. The first portion that you gave her about midday was 80 mg. You advise her to take a second

---

[9] An *algorithm* is a well-defined, finite sequence of instructions for solving a specified problem. It belongs to the category of *procedural knowledge* (see pages 15 and 451). The execution of an algorithm is thus a finite procedure and terminates at some point with a definite result. Examples are the rules of basic arithmetical operations (addition, subtraction, multiplication, division). The term "algorithm" derives from the italicized surname of the medieval Iranian mathematician Abu Abdullah Mohammed ibn Musa *al-Khwarizmi* (around 800–845). He is viewed as 'the father of algebra'.

portion in the evening. The tablets you prescribe for her are 40 mg each. How many tablets is she allowed to take in the evening? One tablet or two or more? You are computing the total amount for current day in case she takes a single tablet in the evening: $80 + 40 = ?$ You perform the computation and straightforwardly obtain "120", the maximum admissible dose. However, your patient is a well-known skeptic and claims that your calculation was wrong. "$80 + 40 = 150$", she says, "so I must not take the whole tablet in the evening". It is true that you have computed only finitely many sums in the past. Let us suppose that you have never performed a computation such as '$80 + 40$'. The largest number involved in your exercises may have been 40 (or any other number you like provided you adapt the example accordingly). Nevertheless, you are absolutely sure that your answer "120" for "$80 + 40 = ?$" is the only right one, and that you must give it if you want to accord with what you have meant by the sign '$+$' in the past. Therefore, you defend your current computation and try to convince your patient that she has made a mistake. "I have always *meant* the function 'sum' when I have used '$+$' in the past", you say. "And $80 + 40$ is 120".

Your patient stresses that she is not questioning the accuracy of your computation. Nor are your cognitive power and your memory of your computations in the past under dispute. However, you are asked to prove that you have *meant* by "$+$" the function "sum" in the past and not another function, say "qusum", that may be symbolized by "$\oplus$" and defined as follows:

$$x \oplus y = \begin{cases} x + y & \text{if } x, y \leq 40 \\ \\ 150 & \text{otherwise.} \end{cases} \tag{7}$$

Your patient urges you to demonstrate in the details of your past applications of "$+$" a *fact* in support of your claim that you have meant the function "sum" rather than "qusum" as in (7) above. It will not be difficult for you to recognize that there exists no such fact constitutive of your *having meant* "sum" rather than "qusum" by "$+$" because all of your past applications of "$+$" are in complete accord with *qusum*. So, you ought seriously consider the question what rule you have followed until now, the rule for *sum* or the one for *qusum?* Since this question is undecidable, nothing can justify your belief that the answer "120" to the query "$80 + 40 = ?$" is the right one. You are allowed to do otherwise: Do what you like! There is no such behavior as *following a rule*.

We could of course add to the rule *qusum* a large number of different, other rules all of which would share the past history of your sum rule for "$+$" in the same fashion as *qusum* does (see Figure 7). Since your past computation behavior has been finite, and as such, is compatible with all of these distinct rules, the nagging question you will face is this: Which one of these distinct rules did you follow in the past when performing a computation, for example, "$80 + 39 = ?$". Be it as it may, you could now go in the same or another direction according to how you choose to act. Thus, there is always a large, practically infinite number of divergent and incompatible ways to perform a computation such as "80 + 40 = ?". Therefore, your claim that you mean the *sum* rule by "+" needs to be acknowledged by the community depending on your observable responses to additional problems indicating how you *use* "+". The supposed mental fact constituting your meaning *sum* rather than *qusum* by "+" has thus been replaced with a social fact. Otherwise put, to obey a rule, be it a rule of science or a rule of a game such as chess, is a practice, a custom, an *institution* (Wittgenstein, 1953, sections 199 and 202).

From what has been said above it should be clear that this conclusion does not only concern you or the expression "+". It applies to all users of medical language and all terms.

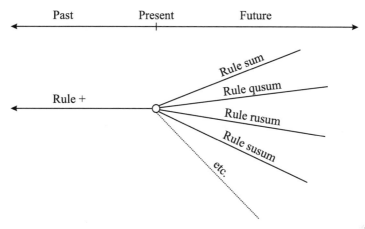

Fig. 7. The compatibility with our *past* behavior of a variety of "possible" and "impossible" rules each of which we may choose to apply in the future

2.7 Summary

Medical language is an expansion of natural, everyday language by adding technical terms. It lacks specific syntax and semantics. Most of its terms are either undefined or not satisfactorily defined. This deficiency is disadvantageous both in medical research and practice and may be responsible for many misdiagnoses. In addition, medical terms are ambiguous and vague. We have shed some light on the nature of vagueness and have distinguished between spurious and genuine vagueness. In contrast to spurious vagueness, genuine vagueness cannot be eliminated. Moreover, it is a desirable property because the precision of scientific investigations decreases the relevance of their results.

The best method of dealing with vagueness is fuzzy logic discussed in Chapter 30 on page 993. We shall see in later chapters that its application may also advance medical semantics by improving methods of concept formation in medicine. We have determined the meaning of a medical term to be its extension and intension. A different view has been held by the late Ludwig Wittgenstein who has rejected all theories of meaning to suggest his semantic nihilism instead according to which a term has no meaning per se. Its meaning is the manner of its use by members of a community. We shall try to utilize this pragmatic view in our philosophy of medicine in the next chapters.

3

The Pragmatics of Medical Language

3.0 Introduction

Our brief sketch of the problematic character of the traditional semantic conception of meaning has demonstrated that meaning cannot be separated from the role the users of a language play in their communication with one another. One of the features of this role is the control of the language use and verbal behavior of individuals by the community. It is thus the community that determines and judges what words and sentences 'mean'. This is just indicative of the pragmatic dimension of language. Consequently, what medical terms and sentences 'mean', and what someone 'means' by using a particular medical term or sentence, also depends on pragmatic contexts and circumstances. To understand the importance and practical consequences of this pragmatic perspective, we will now consider the following three central aspects:

  3.1 The So-Called Language Games
  3.2 Assertion, Acceptance, and Rejection
  3.3 Speech Acts in Medicine.

3.1 The So-Called Language Games

Sometimes it is said that a particular word used or an assertion made by someone, 'is a mere language game'. For example, some social scientists and health care critics consider medical diagnoses to be 'language games'. But what does the term "language game" mean in such judgments?

The phrase "language game" is not a technical term with a strict meaning. It was employed by Ludwig Wittgenstein in the second period of his philosophy after 1929 to prompt us into seeing a similarity between language use and games. In his later years, he himself didn't believe in this conception any more. When introducing it he was, as a semantic nihilist, of the opinion that understanding a word is not an inner process of grasping its meaning. The

K. Sadegh-Zadeh, *Handbook of Analytic Philosophy of Medicine,*
Philosophy and Medicine 113, DOI 10.1007/978-94-007-2260-6_3,
© Springer Science+Business Media B.V. 2012

only important measure is the observable behavior of the user of the word. For example, when we want to know whether someone can play chess, we shall not be interested in anything that goes on inside him, but we shall have to ask him to demonstrate his capacity by *playing* chess. Like any game, playing chess is governed by a set of rules that one must learn. By analogy, he considered linguistic competence something observable and governed by rules of using elements of language. These rules are learned by a child like she learns to play a game. "I shall in the future again and again draw your attention to what I shall call language games. These are ways of using signs simpler than those in which we use the signs of our highly complicated everyday language. Language games are the forms of language with which a child begins to make use of words" (Wittgenstein, 1958, 17).

As we have seen in the preceding section, Wittgenstein more and more grew skeptical of his above idea and lost his belief in the rule-governedness of language and in the rule-following by language users. It turned out to be impossible to confirm or disconfirm that an individual correctly applies a rule 'because she has grasped it'. Correctness in applying a rule is adjudicated by the community and is thus a social judgment and decision.

Regarding a specialty such as medicine and its language, 'community' means primarily the scientific and professional medical community. But is it really this community which determines whether a physician does or does not 'understand' medical language correctly, for example, whether she does or does not understand the term "angina pectoris"? There is sufficient evidence for the belief that the answer to this question is 'yes'. There is no other way to confirm or disconfirm whether a particular physician 'correctly' understands the meaning of the term "angina pectoris" than by examining the correctness of her diagnoses and treatment decisions. That is, analogous to the chess player above, the observable behavior of the medical language user provides the only decisive criteria to review her medical-linguistic competence. We should be aware that only the professional community has the capability and authority to conduct such a review. We shall come back to this important issue in later sections (8.2.9; 8.2.12; 11.5.4; 20.3).

3.2 Assertion, Acceptance, and Rejection

The fact that it is the medical-professional community that adjudicates and regulates the use of medical language, has significant theoretical and practical consequences. They concern medical truth and falsehood first of all. The reason is that whenever you put forward a new general medical statement such as "angina pectoris is caused by coronary artery obstruction", or a singular medical statement such as "Elroy Fox has angina pectoris", you can always be asked the question *how do you know that?* Regardless of how you justify your assertion, the skeptic may retort, analogous to the case of 'sum' and 'qusum' in Section 2.6 on page 46, that you have applied the term "angina pectoris" incorrectly and, therefore, you have said something false. As shown in the preceding section, you cannot defend the truth of your claims in such circumstances. If the community does not approve your truths, you are left alone with all of them (see Section 20.4).

The only solution to the dilemma is to give up the adherence to merely semantic concepts of truth and falsehood, and to search for pragmatic, i.e., intersubjective, substitutes which would enable us to examine whether a particular statement satisfies certain criteria of *assertability* and *acceptability*, instead of asking whether it is true or false. The community would of course have to set up such criteria so as to inform its members on what conditions an assertion is justified and on what conditions it will be considered acceptable. There are as yet no explicitly formulated criteria of this type, however. Asserting, accepting, and rejecting is something unconstrained in medicine. The reasons for this laissez-faire circumstance we shall discuss in Chapter 12 on technoconstructivism.

3.3 Speech Acts in Medicine

The lack of assertability criteria is particularly deleterious in clinical practice since it contributes to idiosyncrasies in knowledge production, and thus, to unreliable knowledge and inefficacious rules of action. This, in turn, increases physician fallibility. We will now throw some light on the linguistic causes of this situation to search for remedies.

Traditionally, clinical practice is viewed as an application to patients of biomedical sciences, supposing that like scientific activities, clinical practice searches for truth, e.g., true diagnoses and prognoses about patients. In a later chapter, we shall demonstrate that by contrast, clinical practice is a source of *facts* in that the practicing physician *produces* facts by uttering diagnoses and prognoses and by extending treatment recommendations. She produces these facts by employing medical language and performing speech acts. To explain this account, a brief sketch is given below of the concept of a *speech act*. This will play an important role in our future discussions (see also Sections 8.2.9; 8.3.4; and 8.4.4).

It is usually believed that as human beings, we perform actions only by our extremities and sense organs in that, for example, we enter our study by using our legs, take a book from the shelf by using our arms, read it by using our eyes, and so on. Surprisingly, the Oxford philosopher John Langshaw Austin (1911–1960) presented in a paper in 1946 and in his lectures during the 1950s an intriguing theory built around his discovery which holds that by speaking we can also perform actions. The actions we may perform in this way he called *speech acts*. So, his theory has come to be known as *speech act theory* (Austin 1946, 1956, 1962, 1979; Searle, 1969).

In the context of discussions on speech act theory, it has become common to use the term "act" instead of "action". A simple example of speech acts is the act that one performs when one says "I promise", e.g., when I say to a severely ill patient "I promise to visit you at home". By uttering this sentence, I do not describe anything existent or non-existent. I do not make a statement about myself and my behavior. I do not say that I was making a promise. Rather, I am actually *making* a promise. Thus, I do not pronounce, or report on, the act of my doing. I just *do it*. I perform the action, specifically the act of promising. My utterance is my promise that I make. Our discussion of this focal issue will demonstrate that not only are the core accomplishments of clinical practice in diagnosis, prognosis, and therapy the doctor's speech acts, which she performs by using the language of medicine, but also even medical knowledge itself originates from particular types of speech act (see Sections 11.5.3 and 14.4).

As was pointed out on page 22, we must distinguish between different types of sentences, e.g., interrogatives, requests, imperatives, and declaratives. Most important for our present discussion are declarative sentences. We divided in (5) on page 22 declarative sentences into *constatives* and *performatives*:

As far as a declarative sentence such as "The Eiffel Tower is in Paris" states that something is, was, or will be the case, it is called a claim-making sentence, a statement, assertion, or *constative* (from the Latin "constare" meaning "to stand firm, to be fixed"). In contrast to interrogatives, requests, and imperatives, a constative makes a validity claim and may therefore turn out true or false. For example, the constative "you have a coronary heart disease" that is told to the patient Elroy Fox, may turn out to be true if a coronary angiography reveals that at least one of his coronary arteries is atherosclerotically narrowed. However, it is also possible that the constative will turn out false.

Austin discovered that although a majority of declarative sentences we speak look like constatives, they state nothing. For instance, it was already noted above that the declarative sentence "I promise to visit you at home" that I utter to the patient Elroy Fox, is not a description of something in my mind or in the world out there. It is an act of promising that I *perform* by my very utterance itself. Thus, it is a performative utterance, or simply a *performative*. While the patient Elroy Fox can reasonably tell me "you said that you promised", his claim "you stated that you promised" would be self-defeating.

A performative is a first person declarative sentence in the singular or plural, present indicative tense, e.g., "I promise to visit you at home" or "we promise to operate on your heart tomorrow". There is a fundamental difference between such a performative and a constative. In contrast to constatives, a performative does not communicate truth or falsehood. It is an action performed by the speaker or speakers. So, it cannot be true or false, but only successful or unsuccessful.

It is worth noting that a performative is a self-referring and self-verifying sentence. First, a performative utterance such as "I promise to visit you at home" refers to itself and to nothing else in the world insofar as the speaker announces what she does, i.e., promising; it shows that the speaker is doing the promising by using the phrase "I promise ...". Second, it verifies itself; although it is not true of an antecedent fact prior to the utterance, it becomes true of the fact that it creates itself, i.e., the fact of promising (see also Section 11.5.3 on page 512).

A speech act thus comprises three partial actions called locution, illocution, and perlocution. The *locutionary act* is the phonetic act of saying something, e.g., the speaking of the seven-word sentence ⟨I, promise, to, visit, you, at, home⟩. This act is only a physical occurrence and serves as a means of performing the mission of the speech act, i.e., the *illocutionary act*. The illocutionary act is the performative speech act proper, e.g., the act of promising, welcoming, apologizing, and the like:

I promise to visit you at home	≡	promising
I welcome you	≡	welcoming
I apologize	≡	apologizing
I swear	≡	swearing
we name this newborn 'David'	≡	naming, baptizing, christening.

The two acts mentioned always develop some side-effects 'in the world out there'. For example, my act of promising may please, disappoint, annoy, or frighten other people and make them take any action. This impact of a speech act on others constitutes the *perlocutionary act*.

In Section 8.2.9 on page 335, we shall interpret clinical judgments as speech acts. At this time, we only briefly illustrate this idea by means of the notion of diagnosis. When I say to my patient Elroy Fox "I hereby diagnose you as having acute appendicitis", then I *make* a diagnosis. This diagnosis is a speech act with its locution being the phonetic utterance of the eight-word sentence mentioned. Its illocution is the making of a diagnosis. If on the basis of my diagnosis the patient now decides to undergo a surgical operation, his decision will be the perlocutionary act or effect that I also have caused by my utterance.

To summarize, in a speech act the locutionary act is the act *of* saying something. The illocutionary act is the act of performance *in* saying something. The perlocutionary act is an act done *through* the former two acts. Illocutionary acts constitute the core of speech acts. Just as we do things by using our hands and feet, we do other things by using our mouth in that we utter performative sentences and thereby do illocutionary acts.

A *performative verb* is a verb that in a performative names its illocutionary act, e.g., the verb "to promise" in the performative "I promise to examine you tomorrow". Other examples are: to welcome, to apologize, to swear, to request, to warn. We may thus distinguish between explicit and implicit performatives. An *explicit* performative explicitly contains a performative verb, e.g., "I promise to examine you tomorrow". In an *implicit* performative the verb is omitted. For example, a sentence such as "you have acute appendicitis" may at first glance appear as a constative. However, it is an implicit performative. It can be revealed as an explicit performative by inserting the missing performative verb: "*I assert that* you have acute appendicitis". This example shows that there is really no sharp dividing line between performatives and constatives because almost all constatives can be revealed to be performatives pruned of their performative verbs. This finding has important philosophical consequences both in general, and particularly in medicine (see Section 11.5.3 on page 512).

3.4 Summary

The question of whether a physician understands and uses medical language properly, is adjudicated by medical-professional communities and authorities. Her clinical judgments are thus subject to social control. However, the ultimate measure of approval is not their truth, but their assertability according to some agreed-upon standards. In making clinical judgments, the physician acts by speaking in that she performs speech acts. Thus, an important class of medical actions and attitudes turn out to be such speech acts, e.g., clinical diagnoses and medical knowledge in general that is "declared to be knowledge" (see Section 11.5.3).

4

Varieties of Medical Concepts

4.0 Introduction

As a science and practice of health care with responsibilities for individual and social health affairs, medicine has many objectives including the following ones: (1) to analyze and describe the human body and soul in order to obtain knowledge about human health, illness, and diseases as well as therapy and prevention; and (2) to build general theories on health, illness, diseases, therapy, and prevention. These tasks comprise the following groups of activities that characterize medicine as research and practice: etiology, diagnosis, prognosis, therapy, and prevention of maladies. We shall be concerned with the analysis and philosophy of these activities in the next chapters. To prepare our inquiries and discussions, we must be aware that in fulfilling the tasks above, medicine uses a particular language that we have referred to as *medical language* in preceding chapters. It goes beyond the everyday language and is based on a specific vocabulary consisting of technical terms such as "cell membrane", "myeloblastoma", "angina pectoris", "genetic disease", "leucocytosis", and so on. On the one hand, every day new terms are added to this vocabulary, e.g., "immune assay", "dissociative identity disorder", and "AIDS". On the other hand, some other terms of the language sink into oblivion because they are not used any more, for example, "hysteria", "chlorosis", "leucophlegmatia", and "dysautonomia". Such medical-linguistic dynamics brings with it a continuous change of medical expressiveness and knowledge to the effect that new diseases are diagnosed in clinical practice, new therapies against these diseases are introduced, and new preventions and interventions are undertaken. To name all these new items, new terms have to be introduced into medical language. We must therefore ask ourselves by what methods the new *terms* are best introduced to ensure that they work in medical research and practice. To answer these questions, first we will undertake a typology of medical terms in the following four sections. To understand them will require acquaintance with logic and its terminology (see Part VIII):

K. Sadegh-Zadeh, *Handbook of Analytic Philosophy of Medicine*,
Philosophy and Medicine 113, DOI 10.1007/978-94-007-2260-6_4,
© Springer Science+Business Media B.V. 2012

4.1 Qualitative, Comparative, and Quantitative Concepts

As was emphasized in Section 1.5 on page 23, terms represent concepts. For instance, the term "angina pectoris" represents the concept of angina pectoris. By introducing a new term, a new concept is introduced. We may therefore use in the present context the notions "term" and "concept" interchangeably. Accordingly, we call the methods of introducing new scientific terms *methods of scientific concept formation*. Before we proceed to discuss these methods, four main classes of medical concepts are distinguished, i.e., individual, qualitative, comparative, and quantitative concepts. Examples are:

- individual: William Osler, The Hastings Center
- qualitative: systole, icteric
- comparative: higher systolic blood pressure than ... ,
- quantitative: systolic blood pressure.

These four main types of concepts play different roles in medical language, and also their theoretical and practical potential is different. We will now take a brief look at them in turn. For details, see (Carnap, 1962, 1966; Hempel, 1952; Krantz et al., 2007; Luce et al., 2007; Suppes et al., 2007).

4.1.1 Individual Concepts

Individual concepts denote individual objects. For instance, "William Osler" refers to the famous Canadian internist Sir William Osler (1849–1919), whereas "The Eiffel Tower" denotes the well-known building in Paris. These two examples demonstrate that when the referent of an individual concept is a determinate, individual object, the concept is a proper name or *individual constant*. If the referent is not a particular individual, but an indeterminate and unknown one, the concept is called an *individual variable* such as "someone", "a", and "an" in statements like "if someone has bronchitis, then she coughs".[10]

---

[10] The term "variable" is ambiguous and plays different roles in different contexts and disciplines. It means, in general, something that varies or is prone to variation, be it an object, an attribute, or a relation. (i) In mathematics and logic, a *variable* is a symbol that acts as a placeholder for some other, specified entity. For instance, in an arithmetical formula such as $x + y = z$, the symbols "x", "y", and "z" are placeholders for any numbers, e.g., $5 + 7 = 12$. They are not variables for everything, for example, for people or for cities. Thus, "Amy + Beth = siblings"

An individual variable may be symbolized by "x", or "y", or similar, un-interpreted signs. For instance, we may formalize our last example by the statement "if x has bronchitis, then x coughs", or formally "$\forall x(Bx \rightarrow Cx)$. Thus, an individual variable such as "x" is a place-holder for any individual, consequently for William Osler too. So, our example statement implies that "if William Osler has bronchitis, then he coughs".

The question of what counts as an individual object, depends on the perspective from where objects are viewed. For instance, in a clinical textbook that deals with human diseases, human beings are individuals. In a textbook of biochemistry, on the other hand, where the same human beings are broken down, the individuals now are the ingredients obtained, i.e., the molecules, each of which could be referred to by a proper name. The 'container' of these new individual objects, formerly an individual itself, has now turned out a huge *set* of individuals. In a nutshell, the term "individual" does not denote an ontological, but a perspectival category of objects.

4.1.2 Qualitative Concepts

What we shall need in the following sections, are the terms "extension", "intension", "extensional", and "intensional". They can be found on pages 32 and 823.

Qualitative or classificatory concepts are either unary predicates or non-comparative, many-place predicates. It has already been outlined on the above-mentioned pages that from the intensional point of view they denote attributes, also called features, traits, characteristics, and criteria such as "is red", "has angina pectoris", "is healthy", "is icteric", "is an ape", "is beautiful", "loves" in statements like "x loves y", etc. Viewed from the extensional perspective, they signify classes, i.e., sets, also called categories. Examples are italicized terms in the following statements:

This rose *is red*,
Elroy Fox *has angina pectoris*,
Jesus *loves* his mother.

---

turns out meaningless; (ii) in all other branches, a variable is a qualitative or quantitative attribute (feature, trait, characteristic, etc.) that may take any of a set of different, 'variable', values. For example, *the color* of an object is a qualitative variable that may take one of the values *white, yellow, red,* etc. Its *temperature* is another, quantitative variable that may take a value on a specified scale such as Celsius or Fahrenheit (see quantitative concepts on page 70); (iii) also the so-called *random variables* in probability theory and statistics are variables in the latter sense. In tossing a dice, for example, the sentence "the dice will fall up with the face X" uses the variable X, referred to as a random variable, which may take one of the values 1, 2, 3, 4, 5 or 6 (see footnote 190 on page 977); and (iv) see also linguistic and numerical variables in fuzzy logic (pp. 78 and 1018).

They denote, respectively, the class of red objects, the class of those patients who have angina pectoris, and the class of those people some of whom love some other ones. Formalized, the above examples mean:

Pa

Qb

Rcd

In these examples, the first two predicates, P and Q, are unary, while the third one, R, is binary. They stand for the classificatory concepts of being *red*, having *angina pectoris*, and *loving* someone, respectively. We have emphasized on several occasions that in this book we have chosen the extensional perspective. Classificatory concepts emerge by *taxonomy*. We will introduce this term in the following three sections:

▶ Classification
▶ Ordinary or crisp taxonomy
▶ Fuzzy taxonomy

to distinguish between different types of taxonomy each of which yields classificatory concepts of a particular type.

Classification

In everyday life and science, we divide the world of our experience as well as abstraction into individual objects such as things, events, processes, etc., and classes thereof. The latter ones are usually called kinds. Examples are human beings, apes, trees, bushes, diseases, patients with hepatitis A, B, C, D, ..., etc. *Classificatory concepts* referred to above are labels that we attach to such *classes* as their names in order to be able to talk about them by using these names.

We must distinguish between (i) classification of particulars, i.e., individual objects, e.g. "Elroy Fox is a diabetic", and (ii) classification of classes such as "diabetics have a metabolic disease". For the sake of uniformity, classification is performed by means of the subsumption relation "*is_a*". The classification of particulars is the same as the membership of an object x in a set A, i.e., $x \in A$ such as "Elroy_Fox $\in$ dabetics", and is referred to as *predication*. But the classification of classes, called *taxonomy*, is much more complicated. It will be considered in some detail below.

Ordinary or crisp taxonomy

The term "taxonomy" comes from the Latin term "taxon" that originates from the Greek τάξις (taxis) for "order". Taxonomy is the theory as well as the practice of classification. The term "classification" is ambiguous, for a classification can be (i) ascending or (ii) descending. In the former case (i), a particular class of objects is said to be a subclass of a superclass, e.g.:

1. homo sapiens is a primate,
2. hepatitis is an infectious disease,
3. an insulin pump is a machine.

In the second case, (ii), a given universe of discourse Ω, i.e., a category of objects under consideration, is partitioned into two or more subclasses $A, B, C, \ldots$ For the term "universe of discourse", see Section 25.2.4 on page 829. For example, we may divide the class of:

4. human beings into diabetics and non-diabetics,
5. viruses into DNA viruses and RNA viruses,
6. human beings into females, males, and hermaphrodites,
7. physicians into internists, surgeons, pediatricians, and so forth,
8. numbers into natural, rational, real, complex numbers, and so on.

Taxonomy comprises both, ascending classification as well as partitioning. The result of a taxonomy is a particular system, or family, of $n > 1$ classes. In our fifth example above this family of classes consists of two classes, the class of DNA viruses and the class of RNA viruses.

Unfortunately, *the result* of the taxonomy of a universe of discourse is also called a taxonomy. It is said, for example, that "the taxonomy of viruses comprises the class of DNA viruses and the class of RNA viruses", or "the taxonomy of human beings comprises the class of females, the class of males, and the class of hermaphrodites". A nosological system is such a taxonomy of diseases. Thus, the term "taxonomy" is ambiguous like the term "terminology" that is used as the name of an activity as well as its result, e.g., "the terminology of pediatrics".[11]

Suppose that our universe of discourse, Ω, is the set of all patients who have any skin disease, i.e.:

$$\Omega = \{x \mid x \text{ has a skin disease}\}. \tag{8}$$

If we now partition this class into subclasses such that we obtain:

the class of those who have melanoma $= \{x \mid x \text{ has melanoma}\} = A_1$
the class of those who have psoriasis $= \{x \mid x \text{ has psoriasis}\} = A_2$
the class of those who have eczema $= \{x \mid x \text{ has eczema}\} = A_3$

and so on, then what arises is a family of $n > 1$ classes, $\{A_1, A_2, \ldots, A_n\}$, with each member A_i being a proper subset of the universe of discourse (8):

---

[11] Other classification systems that are also considered taxonomies in medicine are ICD and SNOMED. ICD is the *I*nternational *C*lassification of *D*iseases and constitutes a coded system of names of diseases and of a number of complaints, symptoms, signs, and findings. Its current label is "International Statistical Classification of Diseases and Related Health Problems". SNOMED, i.e., *S*ystematized *N*omenclature of *Med*icine, is a comprehensive and multidimensional medical vocabulary covering clinical and non-clinical areas.

$A_1 \subset \Omega,$
$A_2 \subset \Omega,$

$\vdots$

$A_n \subset \Omega.$

In natural medical language, the subclasses are labeled:

melanoma $\equiv A_1$
psoriasis $\equiv A_2$
eczema $\equiv A_3$

such that it is said:

melanoma, psoriasis, eczema, basal cell carcinoma, ... are skin diseases

with:

melanoma *is_a* skin disease,
psoriasis *is_a* skin disease,
eczema *is_a* skin disease,

and so on. As outlined on page 105, due to the polysemy of the word "is" in natural languages, the subsumption predicate "*is_a*" is easily mistakable because it seems to stand in all contexts for the membership predicate "$\in$" to assert that:

melanoma $\in \Omega$ i.e., $A_1 \in \Omega$ $\equiv A_1$ *is_a* Ω,
psoriasis $\in \Omega$ $A_2 \in \Omega$ $\equiv A_2$ *is_a* Ω,
eczma $\in \Omega$ $A_3 \in \Omega$ $\equiv A_3$ *is_a* Ω,

etc. But this is *not* the case. Ex hypothesi, the class Ω given in (8) above is divided into $n > 1$ subclasses $A_1, A_2, \ldots, A_n$ to the effect that the relation between a subclass A_i and the base class Ω is not elementhood $\in$, but proper subsethood $\subset$ such that:

$\Omega = A_1 \cup A_2 \cup \ldots \cup A_n$

and thus:

$A_i \subset \Omega$ for $1 \leq i \leq n$
$\Omega \neq \{A_1, A_2, \ldots, A_n\}$
$A_i \in \{A_1, A_2, \ldots, A_n\}$
$A_i \notin \Omega.$

According to the definition of proper subsethood $\subset$ on page 829, we have that every *member* of a subclass A_i is a member of the class Ω, but not vice versa. That means in our present example that (i) every patient with melanoma is a skin disease patient; (ii) every patient with psoriasis is a skin disease patient; (iii) every patient with eczema is a skin disease patient, and so forth. Otherwise put, whoever has melanoma has a skin disease; whoever has psoriasis has a skin disease, and so on to the effect that we have:

melanoma patients $\subset$ skin disease patients,

psoriasis patients $\subset$ skin disease patients,

etc. Formally, $\forall x(A_i x \rightarrow \Omega x)$ and $\neg \forall x(\Omega x \rightarrow A_i x)$. Thus, descending taxonomy is the partitioning of a given universe of discourse Ω into two or more subclasses. We are here concerned with classical, ordinary, or *crisp* taxonomy and shall discuss *fuzzy* taxonomy in the next section.

After the preliminaries above, we define a descending crisp taxonomy, i.e. partitioning, of a universe of discourse Ω to be a collection $\pi = \{A_1, \ldots, A_n\}$ of ≥ 2 non-empty subclasses $A_1, A_2, \ldots, A_n$ such that these subclasses are pairwise disjoint and their union equals Ω. That is:

1. $A_i \cap A_j = \varnothing$ for all $i \neq j$,
2. $A_1 \cup \ldots \cup A_n = \Omega$.

The names of the subclasses yield a system of $n \geq 2$ classificatory or qualitative concepts. For example, the partitioning of viruses into {DNA viruses, RNA viruses} is a crisp, *dichotomous* classification by introducing 2 classificatory concepts. The partitioning of blood cells into {erythrocytes, leucocytes, thrombocytes} is a crisp, *trichotomous* classification by introducing 3 classificatory concepts. The current partitioning of viral hepatitis into {hepatitis A, hepatitis B, ..., hepatitis G, hepatitis non-A-to-non-G} is a crisp, *octotomous* classification by introducing 8 classificatory concepts.

Taxonomy through classificatory concepts yields hierarchical systems of the type "P *is_a* Q", "Q *is_an* R", "R *is_an* S", and so forth such that subtype-supertype relationships between classes emerge. For instance, hepatitis A and hepatitis B are subtypes of hepatitis; hepatitis is a liver disease; a liver disease is an accessory digestive glands disease; and so on. Such classifications by introducing classificatory concepts are ubiquitous in medicine, for example, in histology where tissues are divided into muscle tissue, nervous tissue, connective tissue, epithelial tissue, and so on; or in nosology where diseases are divided into infectious diseases, genetic diseases, mental diseases, etc. In any event, a classification will not 'naturally' end at a particular, ultimate level. It can always and arbitrarily be continued. For instance, infectious diseases are further partitioned into viral infections, bacterial infections, helminthic infections, etc. Viral infections are still partitioned into infections by DNA viruses and infections by RNA viruses. The partitioning process will never come to an end because no such end can be postulated to exist in advance. Maybe one will go round in circles. That is why there is no 'natural' classification of a domain. Every classification, including the classification of natural objects into so-called 'natural kinds', e.g., animals into different animal species, is artificial. As a result, there is also no natural system of diseases to the effect that diseases are not 'natural kinds'. See Section 6.4.2.

It is worth noting that when partitioning a given class Ω into subclasses such as $A_1, A_2, \ldots, A_n$, crisp classification is based on the belief that the members of each of these subclasses have some features *in common* by virtue of which they belong to the same class A_i. The features may be symptoms or any other properties. This is the doctrine of classical concept formation that we shall discuss on pages 79 and 158–162. Fuzzy classification is conducted whenever there are no such common features shared by members of a subclass. In this case, *similarity* between objects is the only taxonomic criterion. The two approaches thus produce classificatory concepts of completely different type. We shall elaborate on this distinction in Sections 4.4 and 6.3.1.

Fuzzy taxonomy

In fuzzy taxonomy, a universe of discourse Ω is partitioned into a number of fuzzy subclasses $A_1, A_2, \ldots, A_n$. In contrast to crisp taxonomy, in this case there is no disjointness between the emerging subclasses $A_1, A_2, \ldots, A_n$ because, as fuzzy sets over Ω, they have no sharp boundaries. As a result, their union does not in general equal the base class Ω. That is, the requirements 1–2 above are not satisfied. For example, the partitioning of human beings into the subclasses {healthy, ill} is a *fuzzy*, dichotomous classification by introducing two fuzzy classificatory concepts, "healthy" and "ill", such that:

healthy $\cap$ ill $\neq \varnothing$
healthy $\cup$ ill $\neq \Omega$.

See Section 6.3.4 on page 192. To illustrate the difference between the two types of taxonomy, suppose we divide a given class of objets, Ω, into several fuzzy subclasses referred to as $A_1, A_2, \ldots, A_n$. For example, we conduct in the class of human beings a tetratomous fuzzy partitioning into the classes of people who have *no* angina pectoris (A_1), *mild* angina pectoris (A_2), *moderate* angina pectoris (A_3), and *severe* angina pectoris (A_4). Depending on the degree of clarity of the four concepts {no angina pectoris, mild angina pectoris, moderate angina pectoris, severe angina pectoris}, the borderline between each two of the emerging four classes $A_1, \ldots, A_4$ will have a particular degree of *sharpness* ranging from the maximum 1 to the minimum 0. That is, only to a particular extent between 0 and 1 will the borderline be discriminant to separate the four patient types from one another. The broader the concepts' penumbras, the more members from neighboring fuzzy subclasses will reside in each of them. Otherwise put, the resulting subclasses will have borderline cases. Fuzzy taxonomy produces such fuzzy subclasses. It represents one of the most advanced branches of fuzzy research with a wide range of application, and has come to be known as fuzzy clustering, fuzzy cluster analysis, or fuzzy pattern recognition. Because of the complexity of the methods involved, they cannot be discussed here. For details, see (Bezdek, 1981; Bezdek et al., 1999; Höppner et al., 2000; Miamoto et al., 2008).

Fuzzy taxonomy yields fuzzy classificatory concepts referred to as fuzzy predicates. When dealing with vagueness in Section 2.4, we subsumed them under *vague* terms. The vast majority of classificatory concepts in medicine belong to this category. Examples are all disease and symptom names, e.g., *angina pectoris, multiple sclerosis, gastritis, depression, schizophrenia, cough, fever, pain, tired, sleepless*, etc. It is impossible to exactly separate the class of people who have any of these diseases or symptoms, from those who don't have it. The borderline is blurred.

On the other hand, a classificatory concept such as "even number" that denotes a class with sharp boundaries, we call a *crisp* classificatory concept or predicate. Such terms are found only in formal sciences such as mathematics and logics. Presumably there is no single medical concept of this type. That means that *all medicine is fuzzy*. This is the main reason why fuzzy logic is indispensable both in medicine and its philosophy (see Chapter 30).

4.1.3 Comparative Concepts

Since most or all classificatory concepts in medicine are fuzzy, the question of whether a particular object either falls into a given class or outside of it, can only seldom be categorically answered Yes or No. Does, for instance, Elroy Fox have myocardial infarction? He indeed presents some of the defining features of this class, but not all of them with certainty. Maybe he doesn't have myocardial infarction?

Like Elroy Fox, in most cases objects present the defining criteria of a class only *more or less* markedly. This ubiquitous circumstance brings with it the possibility of comparing two members of a fuzzy class A, such as the class of anxious patients, with respect to their class membership, e.g., the members Elroy Fox and John Davey. After a thorough comparison, one may eventually come to the conclusion that "Elroy Fox is more A than John Davey is". For instance, Elroy Fox *is more anxious than* John Davey. The predicate just used, i.e., "is more anxious than", represents a comparative concept. Comparative concepts stand between classificatory and quantitative ones and are of paramount importance in advancing medical sciences and philosophy. We will therefore consider them briefly in the following two sections:

▶ Comparative concepts are many-place predicates
▶ Some properties of relations.

Comparative concepts are many-place predicates

A predicate that expresses a relation between two or more objects is a many-place predicate. The following anatomical examples demonstrate two binary predicates and a ternary one:

The mouth is caudal from the nose,
The forefinger is longer than the thumb,
The heart lies between the left and the right lung.

Put formally, that means:

x is caudal from y	$\equiv Axy$
x is longer than y	$\equiv Bxy$
x lies between y and z	$\equiv Cxyz.$

While the first and third predicate, A and C, are classificatory concepts, the second predicate, B, is a comparative one. Thus, comparative concepts are a subgroup of many-place predicates and represent a particular type of relations. Specifically, they express *comparisons* between objects. For instance, by comparing the length of the forefinger with the length of the thumb we were able to state in the second example above that the forefinger is *longer than* the thumb. We could do so because our language provides us with the comparative concept of is "longer than". Other comparative examples are: more than, less than, shorter than, smaller than, older than, warmer than, faster than.

Statements that use comparative concepts convey more information about their objects than classificatory ones do. For example, although these two classificatory statements "Elroy Fox is schizophrenic" and "John Davey is schizophrenic" say something about two patients, we would obtain more information about their state of health if we had a comparative concept of schizophrenia at our disposal that would reveal whether one of them is *more schizophrenic than* the other. While a qualitative concept P such as "is schizophrenic" merely enables classificatory categorization judgments like "x_1 is P", "x_2 is P", and the like; a comparative concept over the same class, say "is more P than", lends an order to the class such that the individual x_1 is more P than x_2 is more P than x_3 is more P than x_4 and so forth. Consider for instance the statements:

x_1 is more schizophrenic than x_2
x_2 is more schizophrenic than x_3
x_3 is more schizophrenic than x_4

and so on. This order is formally analogous to other, well-known orders like, for example, the following one regarding the lengths of objects:

x is longer than y
y is longer than z.

By inventing and employing creative methods, numbers can be unambiguously assigned to the links of an order of this kind to state, for example, that the length of x is 5; the length of y is 3; the difference between them is $5 - 3 = 2$; their total length is $5 + 3 = 8$; etc. Thus, classes denoted and ordered by comparative concepts are easily amenable to numerical operations. To this end, it is useful to introduce a comparative concept of P not in the simple, customary form as above expressing a strict 'more P than' or 'less P than' relation, but to complement it by an equality component such that the predicate assumes the following structure:

is as P as or more P than

conveniently representable by:

is at least as P as.

Now our example predicate used above would look like this:

is at least as schizophrenic as

that is an abbreviation of "is as schizophrenic as or more schizophrenic than". For instance, the sentence "Elroy Fox is at least as schizophrenic as John Davey" abbreviates the longer sentence "Elroy Fox is as schizophrenic as or more schizophrenic than John Davey". From a concept of this basic design, it is easily possible by simple definitions to obtain directly the three concepts below. When for the sake of convenience we symbolize the binary predicate "is at least as schizophrenic as" by "$\succeq$", then the sentence "x is at least as schizophrenic as y" becomes easily representable by "$x \succeq y$". We may now define three derived concepts "$\approx$", "$\succ$" and "$\prec$" in the following way:

1. $x \approx y$ iff $x \succeq y$ and $y \succeq x$
2. $x \succ y$ iff $x \succeq y$ and not $y \succeq x$
3. $x \prec y$ iff $y \succ x$.

That reads:

1'. x is *as schizophrenic as* y iff x is at least as schizophrenic as y and y is at least as schizophrenic as x,
2'. x is *more schizophrenic than* y iff x is at least as schizophrenic as y and y is not at least as schizophrenic as x,
3'. x is *less schizophrenic than* y iff y is more schizophrenic than x.

As before, the shorthand "iff" reads "if and only if". We have here presented only the syntax of the comparative predicate "is at least as schizophrenic as". We have not lent a semantics to it because our aim is not to construct a theory of schizophrenia. To semantically define it is the task of those scientists who wish to incorporate into their theories such a concept. They could do so, for instance, by constructing a scoring system that (i) is based, say, on 100 features like symptoms, signs, and findings that schizophrenic patients may present; and (ii) enables comparison of the scores of two or more schizophrenic patients; or in any other way. The term is used here only as a formal example and as a proxy for all comparative concepts one applies or needs in medicine. We could also have chosen any other comparative disease phrase as well, e.g., "*x has at least as severe a myocardial infarction as y*" or "*x is at least as diabetic as y*". We have deliberately preferred the nebulous term "schizophrenia" to show that even arcane elements of medical language can be made precise to enhance the efficiency of their use. A couple of methods for defining such terms will be introduced below. In laying the groundwork, however, our goal is to discuss formal aspects of how comparative concepts as intermediates between qualitative and quantitative concepts lead us directly from 'qualities' to 'quantities'. First we consider a few interesting properties of our example comparative predicate $\succeq$ ("is at least as schizophrenic as").

It is obvious that any schizophrenic individual x is at least as schizophrenic as herself, i.e., $x \succeq x$. Thus, $\succeq$ is a reflexive relation. If x and y are two schizophrenics, then either $x \succeq y$ or $y \succeq x$. That means that the relation $\succeq$ strongly connects all members of the class of schizophrenic patients because given any two such individuals, one of them is at least as schizophrenic as the other. Thus, the relation $\succeq$ is strongly connected. By virtue of these two capacities, *reflexivity* and *strong connectedness*, the relation "is at least as schizophrenic as" induces an *order* in the class of schizophrenics. To understand the nature of this order, and to recognize how it easily lends itself to numerical operations to yield a quantitative concept, i.e., a quantitative concept of schizophrenia in the present example, we will discuss below some basic vocabulary for use here and in later chapters.

Some properties of relations

In the following multiple definition, the predicate variable "R" serves as a place-holder for any binary relation. For the sake of readability, we use it in infix notation like in the sentence "x loves y" such that the expression "xRy" reads "x stands in the relation R to y". For the term "structure" that we use, see paragraph *Structures* on page 877.

Definition 2 (Properties of relations). *If $\langle \Omega, R \rangle$ is a structure with R being a binary relation on the domain Ω, then R is:*

1. reflexive *in Ω iff for all x in Ω, xRx,*
2. irreflexive *in Ω iff for all x in Ω, $\neg xRx$,*
3. symmetric *in Ω iff for all x and y in Ω, if xRy, then yRx,*
4. asymmetric *in Ω iff for all x and y in Ω, if xRy, then $\neg yRx$,*
5. antisymmetric *in Ω iff for all x and y in Ω, if xRy and yRx, then* $x = y$,
6. transitive *in Ω iff for all x, y, and z in Ω, if xRy and yRz, then xRz,*
7. connected *in Ω iff for all x and y in Ω, if $x \neq y$, then xRy or yRx,*
8. strongly connected *in Ω iff for all x and y in Ω, either xRy or yRx.*

For example, we have seen above that our example relation $\succeq$ ('is at least as schizophrenic as') is reflexive in the set of human beings because it is true of every human being x that $x \succeq x$. Also the equality component of the relation, i.e., $\approx$ ('is as schizophrenic as'), is reflexive because $x \approx x$ holds true for all individuals. However, the inequality component of the relation, i.e., $\succ$ ('is more schizophrenic than'), is irreflexive because $\neg(x \succ x)$ for all x. In addition, it is asymmetric since it is true that if $x \succ y$, then $\neg(y \succ x)$.

Definition 3 (Equivalence relation). *If* $\langle \Omega, R \rangle$ *is a structure with R being a binary relation on* Ω, *then R is an* equivalence relation *on* Ω *iff R is reflexive, symmetric, and transitive in* Ω.

The equality component $\approx$ of our example relation $\succcurlyeq$ is an equivalence relation on the set of schizophrenics because it is reflexive, symmetric, and transitive. However, its more-than component $\succ$ is irreflexive, asymmetric, and transitive and, thus, no equivalence relation.

An equivalence relation R on a universe of discourse Ω partitions Ω into a possibly infinite number of subsets such that the relation R holds among all members of each of these subsets. The subsets are therefore referred to as *equivalence classes* with respect to R, or R-equivalence classes for short. If x is any element of Ω, the R-equivalence class containing x is denoted by $[x]$. For example, in the set of all schizophrenic patients, Elroy Fox is in a particular equivalence class with respect to the relation "is as schizophrenic as". Thus, "[Elroy Fox]" represents just this equivalence class.

As an equivalence relation, the equality component $\approx$ of our comparative concept $\succcurlyeq$ ('is at least as schizophrenic as') lends a *quasi-order* to the class of schizophrenics. However, if $\approx$ is supplemented with the more-than component $\succ$, the ensuing relation $\succcurlyeq$ renders the whole class a *linearly ordered* entity like a string of pearls with $[x] \succ [y]$ such that an equivalence class $[x]$ as a pearl succeeds another pearl $[y]$ if $x \succ y$.

As was stated above, of any two schizophrenics x and y, it is true that either $x \succcurlyeq y$ or $y \succcurlyeq x$ to the effect that $\succcurlyeq$ is strongly connected as defined in clause 8 of Definition 2 above. A relation of this type is called a *linear ordering*. Here are a few ordering relations we shall refer to below:

Definition 4 (Ordering relations). *If* $\langle \Omega, R \rangle$ *is a structure with R being a binary relation on* Ω, *then R is:*

1. *a* quasi-ordering (or pre-ordering) *of* Ω *iff R is reflexive and transitive in* Ω,
2. *a* weak ordering *of* Ω *iff R is transitive and strongly connected in* Ω,
3. *a* partial ordering *of* Ω *iff R is reflexive, transitive, and antisymmetric in* Ω,
4. *a* linear (or total, complete, simple) ordering *of* Ω *iff R is reflexive, transitive, antisymmetric, and connected in* Ω.

For instance, our example relation $\succcurlyeq$ ('is at least as schizophrenic as') is a linear ordering of the set of schizophrenics because it is reflexive, transitive, antisymmetric, and connected in this set. Its latter property according to clause 7 of Definition 2 follows from its strong connectedness outlined above. On the basis of Definition 4, some additional useful notions are introduced:

Definition 5 (Orders). *A structure* $\langle \Omega, R \rangle$ *with R being a binary relation on* Ω *is:*

1. *a* quasi-order *iff R is a quasi-ordering of* Ω,

2. *a weak order* iff *R is a weak ordering of* Ω,
3. *a partial order* iff *R is a partial ordering of* Ω,
4. *a linear order* iff *R is a linear ordering of* Ω.

The considerations above demonstrate that a comparative concept such as "is at least as schizophrenic as" will render the class of schizophrenic patients a *linear order* in which every two patients can be exactly compared with, and distinguished from, one another. Note that the concept does in no way touch or damage the psychic, subjective, societal, human, moral, or metaphysical aspects, the 'nature' so to speak, of a patient's schizophrenia. It is only a new and instrumental mode of speaking about the afflicted that enables useful research and practice.

4.1.4 Quantitative Concepts

Usually quantification is equated, not quite correctly, with measurement and measuring. Since these terms are ambiguous and easily misunderstood, there is some opposition to "measuring things" in medicine as well as philosophy of medicine. Measurement and measuring are viewed as something anti-humanistic. This is, of course, not true. Suppose, for example, that someone is trying to render *pain, schizophrenia, depression,* or even *illness* and *disease* measurable. She will be reproached by the humanist for "disregarding, distorting, and destroying the nature of pain, schizophrenia, depression, illness and disease, and thereby dehumanizing medicine". This critique stems from the belief that the qualities of the measured entity are damaged in some way by measuring them. By explaining the nature of quantitative concepts in the present section, we shall try to reconcile the humanist and the quantification-ist. Our discussion divides into the following four parts:

▶ Quantitative concepts are functions
▶ Homomorphism
▶ How to construct a quantitative concept
▶ Some properties of quantitative concepts.

Quantitative concepts are functions

In natural languages, the denotations of classificatory concepts such as the attributes *red, good, bad, long, beautiful, warm, pain, ill, angina pectoris, delusion, schizophrenia,* and the like are usually considered from the intensional point of view, and are therefore referred to as qualities. We have seen in the preceding section that it is also possible to talk about 'qualities' by using comparative concepts. In addition to comparative concepts, there is yet another mode of representing qualities in our languages that consists in assigning them numerals according to a rule. The concepts obtained in this way are called *quantitative* concepts since they specify the magnitude of an attribute when,

for example, we say that Elroy Fox is 49 years old or that he is 180 centimeters tall. These statements say, in other words, that *the age of* Elroy Fox is
49 years and *the height of* Elroy Fox is 180 centimeters. The italicized terms
in these two examples, i.e., "the age of" and "the height of", denote quantitative concepts. They are quantifying, respectively, the qualities *age* and
height. Roughly, the *quantification* of a quality (attribute, property, feature,
trait, characteristic) means to translate it into the language of quantities, i.e.,
numbers, so as to allow use of the entire corpus of mathematics in dealing
with it. This is the only mission of quantitative concepts. (Readers not sufficiently acquainted with logic are reminded for the last time to study Part
VIII because it will be impossible to understand the following analyses and
discussions without sufficient knowledge of logic.)

The two simple examples above demonstrate that, while classificatory and
comparative concepts are predicates, quantitative concepts belong to the class
of functions and are represented by function symbols such as "the age of" and
"the height of". Consider, for instance, a function such as fatherhood. This
function maps the set of human beings into the set of males such that the
term "the father of" assigns to a human being such as Jesus a unique male
as his function value: *The father of Jesus is Joseph.* That means, formally,
that $father(Jesus) = Joseph$, i.e., $f(x) = y$. Since the values of the function
'father' are not numbers, it is called a non-numerical function. However, there
are also functions that take numbers as their values and are therefore referred
to as *numerical* functions. Examples are:

the age of Elroy Fox is 49	$\equiv age(\text{Elroy Fox}) = 49$
the height of Elroy Fox is 180	$\equiv height(\text{Elroy Fox}) = 180$
the sum of 5 and 3 is 8	$\equiv +(5, 3) = 8$
the heart rate of Elroy Fox is 76	$\equiv hr(\text{Elroy Fox}) = 76$
his systolic blood pressure is 130	$\equiv sbp(\text{Elroy Fox}) = 130$
his blood sugar concentration is 90	$\equiv bsc(\text{Elroy Fox}) = 90$
his blood cholesterol concentration is 195	$\equiv bcc(\text{Elroy Fox}) = 195.$

In these examples, we have the following numerical functions: *age, height, sum,
heart rate, systolic blood pressure, blood sugar concentration,* and *blood cholesterol concentration.* A quantitative concept is just such a numerical function
and nothing more. Contrary to what some may believe, it does not damage
the quality that it quantifies. Moreover, it is an inconsistent behavior to talk
about one's age, height, heart rate, blood pressure, blood sugar concentration,
etc., but to condemn quantitative concepts in the same breath.

A quantitative concept as a numerical function is introduced by means of
an *operational definition* discussed on page 91 below. This method of definition represents the best suited technique to disambiguate existing vague terms
or to construct new, precise terms by connecting their application to human
actions. By standardizing their meaning this way and by enabling us to apply
mathematical methods to their referents, quantitative terms are highly instrumental. A quick look at the plain and lucid logic behind them will reveal

their basic structure, and will demonstrate why they are so useful. As outlined above, we must first of all realize that a quantitative concept *quantifies* some attribute of a class of objects or phenomena. It does so by assigning numbers to them such that the structure of these objects and phenomena, and the relationships between them under certain empirical operations, are *mirrored* by the structure of the assigned numbers and the relationships between them under corresponding arithmetical operations. To clarify what this means, we need the technical term *homomorphism*, which is introduced below.

Homomorphism

A homomorphism is a special type of mapping from one set to another set. Let us take a look at a simple example. Let A be a set of inhabitants of the city Berlin consisting of married couples. We thus have an ordered pair $\langle A, is\_married\_to \rangle$ such that A is a set of Berliners and *is_married_to* is a binary relation thereon to the effect that any Berliner, $a \in A$, *is_married_to* another Berliner, $b \in A$. And let B be a set of inhabitants of the city Paris who are neighbors of one another such that any of its members *is_a_neighbor_of* another member thereof. Thus, we have a second ordered pair $\langle B, is\_a\_neighbor\_of \rangle$ consisting of a set of Parisians and the binary relation *is_a_neighbor_of* thereon. Now, people of set A from Berlin are invited to visit Paris. Parisian people from set B will be hosting them individually. Let *host_of* be a function from set A to set B which assigns to each Berliner a Parisian host. If a is a Berliner, her Parisian host, a', is written $host\_of(a) = a'$. The function *host_of* may have the following property:

> **host_of:** If any two Berliners, a and b, are married to each other, then their Parisian hosts are neighbors of each other. That is: If $a \in A$ *is_married_to* $b \in A$, then $host\_of(a)$ *is_a_neighbor_of* $host\_of(b)$. (9)

That is, married couples from Berlin will stay in Paris as neighbors of each other. Obviously, the function *host_of* maps the structure $\langle A, is\_married\_to \rangle$ to the structure $\langle B, is\_a\_neighbor\_of \rangle$ in such a way that it sends set A into set B, and the relation *is_married_to* into the relation *is_a_neighbor_of*. Otherwise put, it is a *relation preserving function* from set A to set B in that the A-relation "*is_married_to*" between A-members is preserved in the B-relation "*is_a_neighbor_of*" between B-members. Such a relation preserving function is called a homomorphism.

To be more precise, we will first recall the notion of a relational structure that is introduced on page 877. A relational system, relational structure, or simply a *structure* is a set together with one or more relations on that set. That means that if Ω is any set of objects, and $R_1, \ldots, R_n$ are $n \geq 1$ relations thereon, then the $(n + 1)$-tuple $\langle \Omega, R_1, \ldots, R_n \rangle$ is a structure. For instance, the ordered pair $\langle \{x \mid x$ is a human being$\}, loves \rangle$ with *loves* being a binary relation on the set of human beings, is a structure since the relation of loving structures the base set $\{x \,|\, x$ is a human being$\}$ of human beings. For some member a of this set, there is another member b such that a *loves* b. Note that in a structure $\langle \Omega, R_1, \ldots, R_n \rangle$, some or all of the relations $R_1, \ldots, R_n$ may be *functions* since a function is a single-valued relation.

More generally, the universe Ω of a structure $\langle \Omega, R_1, \ldots, R_n \rangle$ may consist of $m \geq 1$ sets $\Omega_1, \ldots, \Omega_m$ such that $R_1, \ldots, R_n$ are relations on any combination of them or any Cartesian product of them. If $\langle \Omega, R_1, \ldots, R_n \rangle$ with $n \geq 1$ is a structure, its *type* is the sequence $\langle r_1, \ldots, r_n \rangle$ of arities of the relations $R_1, \ldots, R_n$, i.e., a sequence $\langle r_1, \ldots, r_n \rangle$ of length n such that an r_i is the arity of the relation R_i. Thus, $r_i = k$ if R_i is a k-place relation. For instance, the type of the structure $\langle \{x \,|\, x$ is a human being$\}, resides\_between, loves \rangle$ is $\langle 3, 2 \rangle$ because 'resides_between' is a ternary relation, and 'loves' is a binary relation. Examples are *"a resides_between b and c"* and *"a loves b"*.

Definition 6 (Homomorphism). *Let $\mathcal{A}$ and $\mathcal{B}$ be two structures of the same type such that:*

$$\mathcal{A} = \langle A, R_1, \ldots, R_n \rangle$$
$$\mathcal{B} = \langle B, R'_1, \ldots, R'_n \rangle.$$

A function f from set A to set B is a homomorphism *from the structure $\mathcal{A}$ into the structure $\mathcal{B}$ iff it is relation preserving, that is, iff:*

$$f : A \longmapsto B$$

such that for all $x_1, x_2, \ldots, x_m \in A$ with $m \geq 1$ we have that:

If $R_i(x_1, x_2, \ldots, x_m)$, then $R'_i\big(f(x_1), f(x_2), \ldots, f(x_m)\big)$

for $i = 1, \ldots, n$.

The last clause means that if any objects in set A stand in a relation R_i to each other, then their f-images in set B stand in the relation R'_i to each other. Otherwise put, the function f sends set A into set B, relation R_1 into relation R'_1, and so on, eventually sending relation R_n into relation R'_n. In this way, it accomplishes a specific mapping from the whole structure $\mathcal{A}$ to the whole structure $\mathcal{B}$ such that the relations $R_1, \ldots, R_n$ are mapped to the relations $R'_1, \ldots, R'_n$, respectively, and thus each relation R_i from the structure $\mathcal{A} = \langle A, R_1, \ldots, R_n \rangle$ is *preserved* in the structure $\mathcal{B} = \langle B, R'_1, \ldots, R'_n \rangle$.

For instance, let R_X and R_Y be two not necessarily distinct relations on sets X and Y, respectively. They structure these sets, X and Y, yielding the structures $\langle X, R_X \rangle$ and $\langle Y, R_Y \rangle$. The example given above consists of two such structures:

$$\langle X, R_X \rangle \quad \equiv \quad \langle \text{some inhabitants of Berlin, } is\_married\_to \rangle$$
$$\langle Y, R_Y \rangle \quad \equiv \quad \langle \text{some inhabitants of Paris, } is\_a\_neighbor\_of \rangle.$$

The function *host_of* described in (9) above is a homomorphism from the structure $\langle X, R_X \rangle$ into the structure $\langle Y, R_Y \rangle$ because it maps X to Y:

$$host\_of : X \mapsto Y$$

and has the following property: If any two members, a and b, of the domain X stand in the relation R_X to each other, then their images in the range Y of the function, i.e., $host\_of(a)$ and $host\_of(b)$, stand in the relation R_Y of neighborhood to each other. That is:

IF:	$R_X(a, b)$	i.e.,	*a is married to b*
	$host\_of(a) = a'$		*host_of(a) is a'*
	$host\_of(b) = b'$		*host_of(b) is b'*
THEN:	$R_Y(a', b')$		*a' is_a_neighbor_ of b'.*

How to construct a quantitative concept?

We can now define what a quantitative concept is. Roughly, a *quantitative concept* is a homomorphism f from a relational empirical, i.e., experiential, structure $\langle \Omega, R \rangle$ consisting of a domain Ω and an ordering relation R thereon, into a relational, numerical structure $\langle \mathbb{R}, \geq \rangle$ such that $\mathbb{R}$ is, usually, the set $\mathbb{R}^+$ of positive real numbers, and $\geq$ is the 'is greater than or equals' relation thereon. Thus, a quantitative concept is simply *a real-valued homomorphic function f*, i.e., it takes real numbers as its values.[12]

For example, let Ω be the set of human beings suffering from a particular disease, say schizophrenia; and suppose this domain has been linearly ordered by a comparative relation $\succcurlyeq$ such as 'is at least as schizophrenic as'. We have in this case the relational, empirical structure $\langle \Omega, \succcurlyeq \rangle$ such that Ω is the set of schizophrenics and $\succcurlyeq$ is a binary ordering relation thereon, specifically, a linear ordering. Now the quantification, also called *measurement*, of schizophrenia consists in finding a function f that homomorphically maps the structure $\langle \Omega, \succcurlyeq \rangle$ to the structure $\langle \mathbb{R}^+, \geq \rangle$ of positive real numbers. According to our definition above, f must be a function such that:

$$f : \Omega \mapsto \mathbb{R}^+$$

and:

If $x \succcurlyeq y$, then $f(x) \geq f(y)$ \qquad for all $x, y \in \Omega$.

---

[12] The set of real numbers, simply called the 'reals' or 'the real line', and written $\mathbb{R}$, consists of the union of *rational* and *irrational* numbers. A rational number, e.g., 5 or 0.4, is a number that can be expressed as a fraction $\frac{x}{y}$ where the numerator x and the denominator y are integers. A number that is not rational is called an irrational number. Such a number cannot be expressed as a fraction $\frac{x}{y}$ for any integers x and y. A famous example is the square root of 2, i.e., $\sqrt{2}$. It has a decimal expansion that neither terminates nor becomes periodic. The set of real numbers is *uncountable* because there is always a number between a real number x, e.g., 3.14, and its supposed successor.

The latter clause says that under the function f the relation $\geq$ between numbers preserves the properties of the relation $\succeq$ between schizophrenics. That means that whenever two members, x and y, of the domain Ω stand in the relation $\succeq$, i.e., 'x is at least as schizophrenic as y', then their images $f(x)$ and $f(y)$ in the range of the function, i.e., their scores in $\mathbb{R}^+$, stand in the relation $\geq$ such that $f(x) \geq f(y)$. This requirement entails:

1. If $x \approx y$, then $f(x) = f(y)$
2. If $x \succ y$, then $f(x) > f(y)$.

Suppose the individual a is said to suffer from schizophrenia, and there is a schizophrenia test such that the score patient a receives on this test, e.g., a score of 238, is referred to as her "schizophrenia index", $SI(a)$ for short. Then the above results 1 and 2 say, first, that if individual a is as schizophrenic as individual b, then the SI of a equals the SI of b; and, second, that if a is more schizophrenic than b, then the SI of a is greater than the SI of b:

1'. If a is as schizophrenic as b, then $SI(a) = SI(b)$,
2'. If a is more schizophrenic than b, then $SI(a) > SI(b)$.

The construction of such a homomorphic function SI as a *schizophrenia test* yields a quantitative concept of schizophrenia. It renders the class of schizophrenics a linear order because $\langle \mathbb{R}^+, \geq \rangle$ is a linear order. For the notion of a linear order, see Definition 5 on page 69.

To summarize, the logic behind quantitative concepts and measurement is this simple idea: A quantitative concept is *a homomorphism from an attribute into real numbers*. Well-known examples are the quantitative concepts of length, weight, height, age, temperature, and all measurements of the parameters of an organism such as heart rate, blood pressure, blood sugar, cholesterol, uric acid, and the like. Once a homomorphism f from a structure $\mathcal{A} = \langle \Omega, R_1, \ldots, R_n \rangle$ into the structure of positive real numbers $\mathcal{B} = \langle \mathbb{R}^+, R'_1, \ldots, R'_n \rangle$ has been established, f is said to give a *representation* that provides a correspondence between both structures, $\mathcal{A}$ and $\mathcal{B}$, and the triple $\langle \mathcal{A}, \mathcal{B}, f \rangle$ is called a *scale*, for example, $\langle$Physical objects, Positive real numbers, length in meter$\rangle$. Often the homomorphism f alone is referred to as a scale. For instance, 'length in meter' and the above-mentioned 'schizophrenia test' are considered scales.

Note, however, that the term "measurement" is ambiguous. On the one hand, it means the concrete process of measuring some attribute of a particular object or of an n-tuple of objects, e.g., the measuring of Elroy Fox's blood pressure. On the other hand, the procedure of introducing a new quantitative concept such as a "schizophrenia index" by constructing an appropriate schizophrenia test is also called measurement. In the present context the term is used in the latter sense, i.e., quantification of an attribute.

Some properties of quantitative concepts

Two types of measurement must be distinguished, a *fundamental* measurement and a *derived* measurement. A derived measurement is one which presupposes another, antecedently available measurement on which it is based. For instance, the quantification of *erythrocyte sedimentation* by introducing the concept of erythrocyte sedimentation rate yields a test by which to measure the distance red blood cells fall in a test tube in one hour. The unit is mm/h. Obviously, the test is based on the quantitative concepts of length and time interval, i.e., measurement of length and time. Thus, it is a derived measurement. By contrast, the quantification of the attributes "long" and "short" by the concept of *length* is a fundamental measurement because it does not presuppose the use of any other, prior measurement. Presumably, all measurements in medicine are derived ones.

Two additional types of measurement are to be distinguished, *extensive measurement* and *intensive measurement*. To this end, we differentiate between additive and non-additive attributes, also called extensive and intensive attributes, respectively. Let x and y be two rods, e.g., two pencils. Their combination through their concatenation yields a new object, say $x \circ y$, where 'o' is the operation of combination. We know that the length of this new object $x \circ y$ is the arithmetical sum of the lenghts of its two constituents, that is:

$$length(x \circ y) = length(x) + length(y).$$

Due to the general validity of this relationship, length is an additive or extensive attribute. By contrast, temperature is a non-extensive, i.e., intensive, attribute. When you mix two liquids, the temperature of the resulting liquid does not equal the sum of the temperatures of its constituent liquids. The same is true of human intelligence. The joint IQ of two persons does not equal the arithmetical sum of their individual IQs. So, intelligence is an intensive attribute.

A measurement f is called an extensive measurement if there is an operation of combination, written $\circ$, such that for any two objects x and y we have $f(x \circ y) = f(x) + f(y)$. It is called an intensive measurement, otherwise. Accordingly, symptoms, signs, and diseases turn out to be non-additive attributes like *temperature* and *intelligence*. Their quantification will yield an intensive measurement. You cannot add, for instance, the patient Elroy Fox's heart rate to his wife's and obtain their joint heart rate, whereas you can do so regarding their weights, ages, and heights.

4.2 Dispositional Terms in Medicine

Sugar is *soluble* in water. The patient Elroy Fox is *allergic* to penicillin. Terms such as "soluble in water" and "allergic to penicillin" do not denote observable attributes of objects. Although we can see that a particular, little object is white and cube-shaped, we cannot see whether it is soluble in water. Likewise, we can see that Elroy Fox is blonde and has blue eyes. But we cannot see whether he is allergic to penicillin. What, then, do the two terms "soluble in water" and "allergic to penicillin" refer to if they do not denote manifest attributes? They mean that sugar has the *tendency* to dissolve when it is put into water, and that Elroy Fox has the *tendency* to show allergic reactions when he takes penicillin.

The examples above demonstrate that two types of attributes are to be distinguished. On the one hand, there are permanently present, so-called *categorical*, attributes such as eye color. On the other hand, there are hidden, *dispositional* attributes or dispositions that may become manifest only under certain circumstances, e.g., water solubility and penicillin allergy. Tendencies, capacities, and potentialities are dispositions. In order to see whether an object is soluble in water, it must be put into water; in order to see whether an individual is allergic to penicillin, she must be given penicillin; and so on. A disposition manifests itself only in a certain, specified condition. Thus, it is a conditional attribute. Many attributes dealt with in medicine are dispositions. Examples are pathogenicity of micro-organisms, virulence, pathibility of human beings, and mental traits or features such as anxiety and intelligence.

Terms that denote dispositions are aptly referred to as *dispositional terms*. They constitute a subcategory of classificatory concepts. Examples are predicates such as "is allergic" and "is pathogenic", and mental terms such as "is anxious" and "is intelligent", whereas terms such as "is icteric", "coughs", and "is cyanotic" are not dispositional, but categorical ones. According to Gilbert Ryle, most mental terms are dispositional terms and denote conditional behavior (Ryle, 1949).

The semantic nature of dispositional terms is not yet well understood. Introducing them into scientific languages is, therefore, difficult and controversial. This may explain why most or even all dispositional-medical terms lack a clear meaning. We shall come back to this issue in Section 5.3.3 on page 91 where we shall suggest introducing them by exploiting the method of operational definition.

It is worth noting that the classes of categorical and dispositional attributes are fuzzy sets in that there is no sharp dividing line between them. Sometimes it is difficult and even impossible to say whether a particular attribute is definitely categorical or definitely dispositional. Examples are diseases such as AIDS, leukemia, diabetes, and others. On the one hand, one is inclined to assume that a disease state such as AIDS is permanently present in a patient, and thus a categorical attribute. On the other hand, in order to determine whether an individual has AIDS, she must be examined under specified conditions, e.g., by performing an HIV test. However, we know that most diseases can only be diagnosed under such specified diagnostic conditions. Thus, they may be viewed as dispositions. As a result, not every term can be said to be definitely categorical or definitely dispositional.

4.3 Linguistic and Numerical Variables in Medicine

As was noted in Section 4.1.4 above, the nature of quantities and qualities is often misunderstood in medicine. On the one hand, there are some humanists who grumble about quantification and measurement because they believe that by measuring magnitudes, qualities are lost. On the other hand, there are some quantificationists who share David Hume and Lord Kelvin's naive view that numbers are the best, or even only, source of knowledge.[13] However, keen perception will reveal that whether something appears as *quality* or *quantity* is not an ontic feature of 'the thing' itself. It depends on whether in describing 'the thing' one employs a qualitative or a quantitative language. As a result, both types of concepts are useful and both are needed in medical language. In Section 30.4.1 on page 1018, a sketch is given of the *theory of linguistic variables* constructed by Lotfi A. Zadeh which (i) treats qualitative concepts as linguistic variables and quantitative concepts as numerical variables, and (ii) convincingly demonstrates that the two concept types are not alternatives, but complementary (Zadeh, 1973, 1975b–c, 1976a–b, 1979).

The language of medicine is replete with so-called *soft* terms that we have called qualitative or classificatory concepts in Section 4.1.2 above. Examples are names of symptoms and diseases such as "icterus", "cyanosis", "headache", "anxiety", "hypertension", "Alzheimer's disease", and others. One need not abandon such terms on the grounds that they are soft. Most of them may either be precisely reconstructed and treated as linguistic variables, or as linguistic values of such variables to make them amenable to methods of fuzzy logic. We shall extensively use this technique in future chapters by reconstructing terms such as "body temperature", "heart rate", and "hypertension" as triangular and trapezoidal linguistic variables, respectively. (For the notion of a variable, see footnote 10 on page 58.)

---

[13] According to his famous, empiricist stance, the Scottish philosopher David Hume (1711–1776) said: "When we run over our libraries, persuaded of these principles, what havoc must we make? If we take in our hand any volume of divinity or school metaphysics, for instance, let us ask, *Does it contain any abstract reasoning concerning quantity and number? No. Does it contain any experimental reasoning concerning matter of fact and existence? No.* Commit it then to the flames, for it can contain nothing but sophistry and illusion" (Hume, 1748, quoted from [1894], 165). Another famous Scottish scholar, the mathematician and physicist Lord William Thomson alias Baron Kelvin of Largs (1824–1907), argued in the same vein in 1883: "In physical science a first essential step in the direction of learning any subject is to find principles of numerical reckoning and practicable methods for measuring some quality connected with it. I often say that when you can measure what you are speaking about and express it in numbers, you know something about it; but when you cannot measure it, when you cannot express it in numbers, your knowledge is of a meager and unsatisfactory kind: it may be the beginning of knowledge, but you have scarcely, in your thoughts, advanced to the state of science, whatever the matter may be" (Thomson, 1891), quoted from (Zadeh, 1975c).

4.4 Non-Classical *vs.* Classical Concepts

In Part VIII and in serveral other places in this book we have emphasized that the basic logic and methodology of reasoning operative in Western science we have inherited from the ancient Greek philosophers, particularly from Aristotle. It is a two-valued system in which among some additional principles, the truth values "true" and "false" play the governing role. We have termed this bivalent system the *Aristotelean worldview*. What the current revolution by fuzzy logic discussed in Chapter 30 is bringing about, is the displacement of this time-honored, bivalent worldview (see footnote 163 on page 875).

The Aristotelean worldview also includes an idea of *concept* and concept formation that, though unworldly and inadequate, has reigned over the past two millennia. It goes back to Plato's dialogue Meno, written around 380 BC. In this dialogue, Meno asks Socrates to tell him whether virtue is acquired by teaching or by practice. Since their conversation is very instructive, so let us listen to a little bit:

Socrates replies: "Meno, be generous, and tell me what you say that virtue is". Meno then says that there are many virtues, but Socrates asks him to define what all virtues have in common.

Meno: There will be no difficulty, Socrates, in answering your question. Let us take first the virtue of a man – he should know how to administer the state, and in the administration of it to benefit his friends and harm his enemies; and he must also be careful not to suffer harm himself. A woman's virtue, if you wish to know about that, may also be easily described: her duty is to order her house, and keep what is indoors, and obey her husband. Every age, every condition of life, young or old, male or female, bond or free, has a different virtue: there are virtues numberless, and no lack of definitions of them; for virtue is relative to the actions and ages of each of us in all that we do. And the same may be said of vice, Socrates.

Socrates: How fortunate I am, Meno! When I ask you for one virtue, you present me with a swarm of them, which are in your keeping. Suppose that I carry on the figure of the swarm, and ask of you, What is the nature of the bee? and you answer that there are many kinds of bees, and I reply: But do bees differ as bees, because there are many and different kinds of them; or are they not rather to be distinguished by some other quality, as for example beauty, size, or shape? How would you answer me?

Meno: I should answer that bees do not differ from one another, as bees.

Socrates: And if I went on to say: That is what I desire to know, Meno; tell me what is the quality in which they do not differ, but are all alike; – would you be able to answer?

Meno: I should.

Socrates: And so of the virtues, however many and different they may be, *they have all a common nature* which makes them virtues; and on this he who would answer the question, "What is virtue?" would do well to have his eye fixed: Do you understand? (Plato, 2008, 1–3. Emphasis added by the present author).

According to this ancient construal, it is generally supposed that every category of objects, i.e., every set and class, is characterized by the 'common nature' of its members, that is, by a number of properties that are *common to all* of them. We shall refer to this construal as the classical *common-to-all postulate*:

Common-to-all postulate: A concept is defined by indicating some features that are common to *all* members of the category represented by that concept.

Correspondingly, a concept will be referred to as a *classical* one if it obeys the ancient common-to-all postulate above. An example is the concept of *square*. The category of squares is characterized by the following four properties of its members: closed figure, four straight sides, all sides equal in length, equal angles.

It is generally believed since Socrates, Meno, Plato, and Aristotle that all concepts in science and everyday life are classical concepts in the above sense. We shall convincingly demonstrate on page 158 ff., however, that this belief is untenable. It is responsible for much syntactic, semantic, and philosophical confusion and fruitless debate in all of the scientific branches, especially medicine and its philosophy. For example, the concept of disease as the basic concept of medicine does not denote a category whose members obey the common-to-all postulate. Diseases do not have a number of properties in common like squares do. We shall call a concept of this type a *non-classical* one if its denotation violates the common-to-all postulate. The concept of disease is an example par excellence which we shall come back to in Section 6.3.1 where we take up the issue of non-classical versus classical concepts in medicine.

4.5 Summary

A variety of medical concepts have been outlined. Particular attention has been paid to the structure and logic of classificatory, comparative, and quantitative concepts. All of them are important and useful constituents of medical language. In addition, we have also briefly introduced the class of dispositional terms, emphasizing that the names of many diseases may be conceived of as such terms and handled accordingly. Linguistic and numerical variables have also been briefly mentioned. They will be thoroughly discussed in Section 30.4.1 in Part VIII. Finally, we have introduced a novel distinction between classical and non-classical concepts in medicine. This issue will be developed in Section 6.3.1. We will now turn to the question of how the concept types discussed above may be defined.

Fundamentals of Medical Concept Formation

5.0 Introduction

The remarkable skill with which children intuitiviely use spoken language demonstrates that knowledge of semantics is not a necessary condition for fluently speaking a language. However, the sensible and responsible use of language in a science such as medicine requires more than intuitive linguistic behavior. The application of terms, especially of disease terms to patients in diagnoses such as "Elroy Fox has angina pectoris", often has many serious consequences. In light of this, one ought to be well acquainted with the syntax and semantics of one's terms, so that one may choose the 'right words' in communicating one's observations and experiences. Maybe Elroy Fox does not have angina pectoris, but pneumonia? How will one differentiate between a situation where one term is appropriate and the other not, and another where the reverse is true? Technical problems of this type amount to asking the semantic question: "What does the term such-and-such mean?", or equivalently, "how is the term such-and-such *defined* in medicine?". We are seldom able to answer such questions in medicine with certainty. The reason is that in medicine and many other fields alike, the term "definition" itself is used so loosely that it is often confused with:

- *meaning analysis:* What do people understand by the term X? It is said, for example, "by the term 'disease' one understands this and that";
- *description:* The enumeration of some of the properties an entity has and some of the relations in which it stands.

As a result, in most texts and contexts definitions are not provided where they are necessary. The introduction of a new term in a publication is scarcely accompanied by its definition. Instead of presenting a definition, either a meaning analysis of the term is given, or a description is given of its referent, i.e., of its denotation. And since meaning analyses and descriptions are relative to perspectives and contexts, we encounter the same term used in various

K. Sadegh-Zadeh, *Handbook of Analytic Philosophy of Medicine,*
Philosophy and Medicine 113, DOI 10.1007/978-94-007-2260-6_5,
© Springer Science+Business Media B.V. 2012

ways, without its users possessing a common concept. It is no exaggeration to characterize this situation in medicine as semantic chaos. The chaos would not deserve any attention, however, if it were not practically detrimental in research and practice. The best way to prevent the damage it causes is to learn something about methods of scientific concept formation. The present chapter provides a brief introduction to such a methodology. In what follows, we shall discuss the main methods of scientific concept formation, i.e., *definition* and *explication*. Our discussion divides into the following four sections and is based on, and extends, the most valuable pioneering studies by Carl Gustav Hempel, and especially, Patrick Suppes (Hempel, 1952; Suppes, 1957, 151–173, 246–260):

5.1   What a Definition is
5.2   What Role a Definition Plays
5.3   Methods of Definition
5.4   What an Explication is.

5.1 What a Definition is

Two types of definitions have been distinguished since Aristotle, *real* definitions and *nominal* definitions. However, we consider only nominal definitions proper definitions. Ironically, so-called real definitions do not exist. This is explained below.

Part of the widespread Aristotelean worldview is a concept of definition that is still used in almost all disciplines outside logic and mathematics. But the concept's vagueness allows that even taxonomy and empirical analysis are mistaken for definition. Specifically, the relation of proper subsethood between a subset B and a superset A, i.e., $B \subset A$, is erroneously called a 'definition' of B by A. A simple example is the subcategory-category relation "a woman is a female, adult human being". In this example, *adult human being* is an antecedently available category. A subcategory of it is formed, and referred to as *woman*, whose members have the property of being *female*. Thus, in Aristotelean terminology a definition is considered to be an act of the following type:

- within a base category A such as *adult human being*, called the genus,
- a subcategory (subclass, subset) B such as *woman*, called a species, is delimited
- by indicating $n \geq 1$ features such as *female*, referred to as differentia specifica, that the species B has. They distinguish it from other subcategories of the genus A.

That is simply $B \subset A$. In our example above, *female* is the differentia specifica of the species *woman* in the genus *adult human being*, whereas in the same genus the differentia specifica of the species *man* would be *male*. This famous

Aristotelean type of definition by *genus et differentiam specificam* is traditionally called a *real definition* because it allegedly identifies the 'real characteristics' or 'the essence' of an entity like being female as the real characteristic or essence of being a woman. This essentialistic terminology is the source of the afore-mentioned, traditional confusion of definition with fact-stating description. We therefore abandon both the construal as well as the terminology. There are no such things as 'real definitions'. What is called "real definition" is in fact either ascending taxonomy or empirical analysis. For the notion of ascending taxonomy, see the concept of ordinary taxonomy on page 60.

We understand by "definition" a *sentence* that standardizes and regulates *how a particular term is to be used*, i.e., a sentence that fixes and establishes both the meaning of an expression and the syntax of its use. For instance, the sentence "Someone has ARDS if and only if she has an acute respiratory distress syndrome" is a definition of the new term "ARDS". It introduces this term as a short *name* for the longer sequence "acute respiratory distress syndrome" and establishes the syntax of its use ('x has ARDS') in order that one avoids to say, for example, "x bears ARDS". Thus, a definition is always a *nominal* definition (nomen = name), and as such, it is a stipulative sentence and never a constative or descriptive one. For instance, the term "ARDS" describes or reports nothing. Definitions are uninformative. They are only useful.

According to the brief characterization above, the term "definition" and its derivatives belong to metalanguage. With only one exception, the so-called ostensive definition discussed on page 101, a definition is a stipulative sentence suggesting that a new term τ, called the *definiendum*, be considered as synonymous with another, already known expression δ, referred to as the *definiens*, that defines the definiendum. Plainly expressed, it says "let the term τ be synonymous with the expression δ". For example:[14]

Let "ARDS" be synonymous with "acute respiratory distress syndrome".

Other linguistic conventions are of course admissible to present such a definition, for instance:

"ARDS" $\equiv$ "acute respiratory distress syndrome",
"ARDS" $=_{\text{Def}}$ "acute respiratory distress syndrome",
"ARDS" $=:$ "acute respiratory distress syndrome".

However, when syntactically unusual and incomplete sentences of this or similar type are contained in the premises of any argument, no system of logic can draw any conclusions from them. So, it is recommended not to formulate a definition in a manner such as above, which is not amenable to reasoning

---

[14] For the terms "metalanguage" and "object language", see page 852. What is said in the present section and the next, does not pertain to so-called ostensive definitions. This type of definition is actually not a definition, but an *interpretation*. See Section 5.3.7 on page 101.

and logic. A definition ought always to be a syntactically complete, correct, and definite sentence that is easily amenable to logical operations. For these reasons, a correct definition is not formulated at the *metalinguistic level* as above. Rather, it is fetched down to the level of object-language by avoiding metalinguistic quotation marks. We may therefore suggest the following definition of "ARDS" as an example to illustrate:

Definition 7 (ARDS). *Someone* has ARDS *if and only if she has an acute respiratory distress syndrome.*

The defining connective "if and only if", i.e., the biconditional '↔', serves the purpose of establishing a complete synonymy between the definiendum and definiens.

5.2 What Role a Definition Plays

Definitions are the basic building blocks of a language. A definition introduces into a language a new symbol or term as a synonym for some already available and known expressions to represent them as a shorthand. For this reason, it is *not creative*. That means that it is not a statement about any fact or state of affairs, and does not carry or produce any information or content. Therefore, it is neither true nor false. For example, the definition of "ARDS" above does not add any information to medical language or knowledge, and is void of any truth or untruth. However, as a shorthand, the acronym "ARDS" may facilitate communication in many situations and respects. Note that we could also have chosen the new term "XYZ" instead of "ARDS". The choice of definienda is arbitrary. The same applies to definientia. Thus, definitions are arbitrary and do not represent any 'reality'. To repeat, there are no 'real definitions'. All correctly conducted defintions are nominal ones.

Since a definition is not creative, a term that has been introduced as the definiendum of a definition, may in any context be replaced with its definiens. That is, all definitionally introduced expressions are *eliminable* from language. For instance, instead of saying that the patient Elroy Fox has ARDS, we may also omit this term and say that he has an acute respiratory distress syndrome. The term "ARDS" we have defined above is not really needed.

However, by introducing new expressions into a language, definitions enhance its formal-expressive power. In this way, they facilitate the investigations and actions which one may undertake by using that language. They may help systematize knowledge or reformulate it, may contribute to knowledge-based computations, and accelerate both the application and the production of knowledge and information. Seen from this perspective, definitions have an instrumental value. They may forge links between different sublanguages or theories, for instance, between neurophysiology, on the one hand; and mathematics and physics, on the other. Examples are definitions in neurophysiology which introduce quantitative concepts of membrane depolarization, and thereby connect these different disciplines with one another resulting in a mathematical-physical theory of nerve membrane potential ('Hodgkin and Huxley'). As this example demonstrates, there are no sharp boundaries between concept formation and theory construction. Sometimes the definition of a concept leads to a more or less magnificent theory and even a scientific revolution. For instance, fuzzy logic and technology have emerged from a single definition, i.e., the definition of the term "fuzzy set" (Sadegh-Zadeh, 2001a).

As an example, the term "ARDS" was defined above by the terms "acute", "respiratory", "distress", and "syndrome". If in this manner, a term A is defined by $m \geq 1$ terms $B_1, \ldots, B_m$, and each part of this definiens, a B_i, is defined by $n \geq 1$ other terms $C_1, \ldots, C_n$, and so on, we eventually obtain chains of definitions of which a language in general, and medical language in particular, consists. The definition chains in a scientific language must satisfy the following two requirements. In natural language they fail to do so:

First, in order for a language not to be semantically circular and thus vacuous, no member in a definition chain is allowed to be circular. A definition is *circular* if its definiendum is completely defined by itself or has already been used in the definiens of a prior definition. For instance, "ARDS" must not be defined by itself and must not be used directly or indirectly in the definition of any part of its definiens ("acute", "respiratory", "distress", and "syndrome").

Second, since the definition chains in a language cannot be infinite, they will originate from initial, basic definitions which are not preceded by other definitions. That means that the primary terms used in the definientia of the basic definitions cannot have been defined themselves by other terms. They are usually referred to as the *undefined terms* of a language, or *its primitives* for short. But how do primitives themselves get their meaning to render the language something meaningful, i.e., tied to 'reality'? The answer suggests itself: The primitives are *interpreted* by extra-linguistic entities. We shall be concerned with this problem when discussing the method of ostensive definition on page 101.

5.3 Methods of Definition

In a thorough analysis of the literature in logic and mathematics – and only in these two disciplines – one encounters six practically applied methods of definition. We shall reconstruct and discuss them in this section. Although a seventh one is commonly used as well, there are only a few people who are aware of it. In what follows, we will show that these seven methods are instrumental for use in medicine and may enhance its scientificity. For obvious reasons, we shall try to be sufficiently clear and shall therefore employ techniques of formalization. All logic tools needed are to be found in the logic primer in Part VIII.

First recall the notion of *universal closure*, introduced on page 869 and in Definition 210: Let α be a first-order formula of any complexity with $n \geq 1$

free individual variables $x_1, \ldots, x_n$. Its universal closure is the closed general-ization $\forall x_1 \ldots \forall x_n \alpha$ that does not contain free individual variables any more. A simple example is the following sentence:

$$\forall x \forall y \forall z (Fxy \wedge Fyz \rightarrow Gxz) \tag{10}$$

that is the universal closure of $Fxy \wedge Fyz \rightarrow Gxz$. A possible interpretation is the following statement: For all x, for all y and for all z, if x is the father of y and y is the father of z, then x is the grandfather of z. All variables in the core formula "$Fxy \wedge Fyz \rightarrow Gxz$" of (10) are bound by the quantifier prefix $\forall x \forall y \forall z$. The whole sentence is closed. We shall see that a definition must be such a closed universal sentence and is not allowed to contain free variables. For the sake of convenience, a universal closure of the form:

$$\forall x_1 \ldots \forall x_n \alpha$$

will sometimes be abbreviated to the handy sequence:

$$\mathcal{Q} \alpha$$

where the prefix $\mathcal{Q}$ stands for the entire quantifier prefix $\forall x_1 \ldots \forall x_n$ of the sentence with $n \geq 1$. For instance, the universal closure 10 above is $\mathcal{Q}(Fxy \wedge Fyz \rightarrow Gxz)$.

Note that in medicine two types of terms are subject to definition, i.e., (i) m-ary predicates with $m \geq 1$ such as *has ARDS, is a diabetic, is more schizophrenic than*, etc., symbolized by $P, Q, R, \ldots$; and (ii) n-ary function symbols with $n \geq 1$ such as *the white blood cell count of, the heart rate of*, etc., symbolized by $f, g, h, \ldots$ As in these examples, we shall for simplicity's sake use predicates and function symbols autonymously. That is, each symbol will metalinguistically serve as its own name so as to omit quotation marks to enhance readability. See page 853. To the same end, within formalized sentences such as above we shall omit brackets if they are dispensable according to the rules of parsimony given on page 866. For reasons to be explained below, we shall confine ourselves to definitions in languages of the first order. But our methods of definition are also applicable in higher-order languages. We will now introduce the following seven methods of definition in turn some of which have been reconstructed, made explicit, and formalized for the first time by Patrick Suppes on whose work our discussion is based (Suppes, 1957, 151–173, 246–260):

5.3.1 Explicit Definition

The elementary type of definition is the so-called *explicit definition*. It has the structure of a biconditional and is therefore deductively the most productive one. A biconditional constitutes the main building block of all types of definition. As an opening example, consider a simple explicit definition of a unary predicate, i.e., the predicate "has leucocytosis".

Definition 8 (Leucocytosis: 1). *An individual* has leucocytosis *iff her white blood cell count per cubic millimeter of blood exceeds 9000.*

To study its logical structure, this definition will be formalized. To this end, let us symbolize the predicate "has leucocytosis" by LEU, and the function symbol "white blood cell count per cubic millimeter of blood" by $wbcc$ such that:

$LEU x$	reads:	x has leucocytosis
$a > b$		a exceeds b
$wbcc(x)$		the white blood cell count of x
		per cubic millimeter of blood.

Now, the following Definition 9 reveals the logical structure of Definition 8 above:

Definition 9 (Leucocytosis: 2). $\forall x \big(LEU x \leftrightarrow wbcc(x) > 9000 \big).$

That reads: For all x, x has leucocytosis if and only if the white blood cell count of x per cubic millimeter of blood exceeds 9000. The definiendum, $LEU x$, is written on the left-hand side of the biconditional. It introduces the new, unary predicate "has leucocytosis". The definiens that defines this new predicate appears on the right-hand side of the biconditional.

After this guiding exercise, we will now formulate the general rule for explicitly defining predicates. In all of the following rules, the symbol δ is used as a general sentence variable to connote "*definition*".

Rule 1: Explicit definition of predicates. A sentence δ is an explicit definition of an n-ary predicate P in a language $\mathcal{L}$ iff:

1. δ is a universal closure in $\mathcal{L}$ of the form $\forall x_1 \ldots \forall x_n (P x_1 \ldots x_n \leftrightarrow \beta)$,
2. $x_1, \ldots, x_n$ are $n \geq 1$ distinct individual variables,
3. β is a sentence that does not contain the predicate P,
4. β has no free individual variables other than $x_1, \ldots, x_n$.

An example was presented in Definition 9 above. In that definition, the term "9000" in the definiens was not an individual variable, but an individual constant. Our next example concerns the definition of function symbols. A simple exercise is the function symbol "heart rate". Informally, *the heart rate of a human being is the number of her heart beats per minute.* To formalize this definition, let us fix the symbols we need:

$hr(x)$ reads: the heart rate of x
Hzx z is the heart of x
Bzy z beats y times per minute.

Definition 10 (Heart rate: 1). $\forall x \forall y \forall z (hr(x) = y \leftrightarrow Hzx \land Bzy)$.

According to the symbols above, this definition reads: For all x, for all y and for all z, the heart rate of x equals y if and only if x's heart beats y times per minute. Here is the general rule for defining function symbols:

Rule 2: Explicit definition of function symbols. A sentence δ is an explicit definition of an n-ary function symbol f in a language $\mathcal{L}$ iff:

1. δ is a universal closure in $\mathcal{L}$ of the form $\forall x_1 \ldots \forall x_n \forall y (f x_1 \ldots x_n = y \leftrightarrow \beta)$,
2. $x_1, \ldots, x_n, y$ are $n + 1$ distinct individual variables with $n \geq 1$,
3. β is a sentence that does not contain the function symbol f,
4. β has no free individual variables other than $x_1, \ldots, x_n, y$.

Rules 1 and 2 show this important characteristic of a definition: The definiendum in the definition of a symbol *is always the atomic sentence of that symbol*. That is, the definiendum in the definition of an m-place predicate P is the predication $P x_1 \ldots x_m$; and the definiendum in the definition of an n-place function symbol f is the equality $f x_1 \ldots x_n = y$. Thus, a definiendum is never a negation or a compound sentence. Negative symbols such as in "$\neg P x_1 \ldots x_m$" and "$\neg (f x_1 \ldots x_n = y)$ are not defined, but only positive ones. We shall encounter this basic requirement in all methods discussed below.

The method of explicit definition and the examples presented above show in addition that one never defines a predicate P or a function symbol f as an isolated symbol such as, for example, "*has leucocytosis* means such-and-such" or "*heart rate* means such and such". Rather, one introduces a new concept by means of its atomic sentence as the definiendum. In this way, the definition becomes amenable to logical operations. Moreover, the complete syntax of the new term is fixed by the definiendum and will prevent idiosyncratic linguistic usages.

Very often a function symbol is defined by other function symbols. To demonstrate, suppose we already have the following function symbol "nhb" at our disposal:

$nhb(x)$ $\equiv$ the number of heart beats of x per minute.

The above term "heart rate" in Definition 10 could then be introduced as follows:

Definition 11 (Heart rate: 2). $\forall x \forall y (hr(x) = y \leftrightarrow nhb(x) = y)$.

In defining a function by other functions like in the last definition, Rule 2 may be simplified as follows: We need not use a biconditional as required in Rule 2; for the sake of convenience, a biconditional may be replaced with an identity as the following alternative definition demonstrates:

Definition 12 (Heart rate: 3). $\forall x\big(hr(x) = nhb(x)\big)$.

It reads that the heart rate is the number of heart beats per minute. Both definitions, 11 and 12, are equivalent. The simplified method of defining function symbols is fixed by the following additional rule:

Rule 3: Explicit definition of function symbols by other function symbols. A sentence δ is an explicit definition of an n-ary function symbol f in a language $\mathcal{L}$ iff:

1. δ is a universal closure in $\mathcal{L}$ of the form $\forall x_1 \ldots \forall x_n (f x_1 \ldots x_n = t)$,
2. $x_1, \ldots, x_n$ are $n \geq 1$ distinct individual variables,
3. t is a term (in logical sense, see page 861) that does not contain the function symbol f,
4. t has no individual variables other than $x_1, \ldots, x_n$.

This useful method may be exemplified by an additional definition. We define the function symbol "maternal grandfather" by the two function symbols "father" and "mother":

$$\forall x \Big(maternal\_grandfather(x) = father\big(mother(x)\big)\Big).$$

The definition says that the maternal grandfather of x is the father of the mother of x, that is, $f(x) = g\big(h(x)\big)$. Written as a biconditional, it would take the following, more complicated form:

$$\forall x \forall y \Big(maternal\_grandfather(x) = y \leftrightarrow father\big(mother(x)\big) = y\Big).$$

In rounding out our discussion of explicit definitions, we will formulate a rule for defining individual constants, although unlike the logical-mathematical sciences there is no need in medicine to define any individual constant, e.g., *Rudolf Virchow, William Osler, 7,* and the like. For this reason, we shall in general omit rules for defining individual constants for the remaining methods of definition discussed below.

Rule 4: Explicit definition of individual constants. A sentence δ is an explicit definition of an individual constant a in a language $\mathcal{L}$ iff:

1. δ is a universal closure in $\mathcal{L}$ of the form $\forall x(a = x \leftrightarrow \beta)$,
2. x is an individual variable,
3. β is a sentence that does not contain the individual constant a,
4. β has no free individual variables other than x.

5.3.2 Conditional Definition

In many cases, the application of a new concept introduced by a definition is confined to particular circumstances or domains, or requires other specific preconditions. Such a precondition may be placed, as a conditional, before an explicit definition to obtain a so-called *conditional definition*. Consider the following, alternative Definition 13 of the predicate "has leucocytosis" that was tentatively introduced by Definition 9 above. Our terminology is:

Hx	reads:	x is a human being
$LEUx$		x has leucocytosis
$a > b$		a exceeds b
$wbcc(x)$		the white blood cell count of x
		per cubic millimeter of blood.

Definition 13 (Leucocytosis: 3). $\forall x \Big(Hx \rightarrow \big(LEUx \leftrightarrow wbcc(x) > 9000 \big) \Big)$.

That reads: For all x, if x is a human being, then x has leucocytosis if and only if the white blood cell count of x per cubic millimeter of blood exceeds 9000. This simple example demonstrates that many definitions in medicine, especially in clinical medicine, are, or can only be reconstructed as, conditional definitions. Compare Definition 13 with Definition 9 of the same term in the preceding section. It is obvious that the definition of the predicate "has leucocytosis" in Definition 9 is not adequate. A closer look reveals that it says "a thing x has leucocytosis iff ...". However, it is preferable not to speak of arbitrary "*things* x which have leucocytosis", but to attach the new term in the definiendum to a variable that ranges over the domain of its proper application instead, to human beings in the present example. This is made possible by the condition "if x is a human being" prefixed to the biconditional "$LEUx \leftrightarrow wbcc(x) > 9000$" in the definition above. A veterinarian will need and use other concepts of leucocytosis, for example, for horses, dogs, mice, and other animal species because the normal white blood cell count in distinct species varies. She will thus need to prefix to an appropriate, defining biconditional another precondition, e.g., "if x is a horse, then ..."; "if x is a dog, then ..."; and so on. The precondition represents the phrase "in" used in expressions such as "*in* human beings, leucocytosis is such and such ...", or "*in* male human beings, leucocytosis is...", etc.

Below are the general rules for conditional definitions of predicates and function symbols. From now on, we shall for the sake of convenience abbreviate a universal closure $\forall x_1 \ldots \forall x_n \alpha$ simply to $\mathcal{Q}\alpha$ where $\mathcal{Q}$ represents the whole quantifier prefix $\forall x_1 \ldots \forall x_n$.

Rule 5: Conditional definition of predicates. A sentence δ is a conditional definition of an n-ary predicate P in a language $\mathcal{L}$ iff:

1. δ is a universal closure in $\mathcal{L}$ of the form $\mathcal{Q}(\alpha \rightarrow (Px_1 \ldots x_n \leftrightarrow \beta))$,
2. $x_1, \ldots, x_n$ are $n \geq 1$ distinct individual variables,
3. α and β are sentences that do not contain the predicate P,
4. β has no free individual variables other than $x_1, \ldots, x_n$.

Rule 6: Conditional definition of function symbols. A sentence δ is a conditional definition of an n-ary function symbol f in a language $\mathcal{L}$ iff:

1. δ is a universal closure in $\mathcal{L}$ of the form $\mathcal{Q}(\alpha \rightarrow (fx_1 \ldots x_n = y \leftrightarrow \beta))$,
2. $x_1, \ldots, x_n, y$ are $n + 1$ distinct individual variables with $n \geq 1$,
3. α and β are sentences that do not contain the function symbol f,
4. the variable y is not free in α,
5. β has no free individual variables other than $x_1, \ldots, x_n, y$.

The method of conditional definition will be frequently used in later chapters of this book. In this section, our final example illustrates Rule 6 above for conditionally defining a function symbol. The definition of the term "heart rate" in the explicit Definitions 10–12 could be improved by replacing them with a conditional definition that bears the precondition "x is a human being". Again, our terminology is:

Hx reads: x is a human being
$hr(x)$ the heart rate of x
$nhb(x)$ the number of heart beats of x per minute.

Definition 14 (Heart rate: 4). $\forall x \forall y \Big(Hx \rightarrow \big(hr(x) = y \leftrightarrow nhb(x) = y \big) \Big).$

With reference to Rule 3 in the preceding section, we may again simplify Definition 14 by the following equivalent definition:

Definition 15 (Heart rate: 5). $\forall x \Big(Hx \rightarrow \big(hr(x) = nhb(x) \big) \Big).$

In contrast to explicitly defined terms, a term introduced by a conditional definition cannot in general be eliminated in all contexts by its definiens. This is only possible in cases where the precondition of the definition is satisfied. For example, if we are told that the heart rate of a particular creature is 76, we cannot deduce from this information and Definition 14 or 15 that "the number of heart beats of that creature per minute is 76". However, we can do so if in addition we know that the creature is a human being.

5.3.3 Operational Definition

Although in some scientific areas, especially in social sciences, there is much vague talk against and criticism of 'operationalization' and 'operationalism', these two notions are in fact very fruitful. We will explain them in this section in order to show in Part II that most of what clinical medicine accomplishes, is based on, and would be impossible without, operationalization.

The terms "operationalization" and "operational definition" came into being by the U.S.-American physicist Percy Williams Bridgman (1882–1961). Based on his philosophizing about Einstein's concept of simultaneity, he introduced the idea that a scientific concept must be defined in terms of the *operations* by which its referent is measured, or by which the question is examined whether it can be applied to a particular object (Bridgman, 1927, 1936). He even went so far as to maintain that "the concept is synonymous with the corresponding set of operations" (Bridgman, 1927, 5). This represents the legendary doctrine of operationalism. Only on the basis of such an exaggeration could the well-known behavioristic slogan emerge which says that "intelligence is what an intelligence test measures".

Operationalization is simply the introduction of a term by an operational definition. An operational definition is a conditional definition of the form $\mathcal{Q}(\alpha \rightarrow (\gamma \leftrightarrow \beta))$ whose precondition α indicates some human operations, i.e., actions, and its component β, the definiens, indicates some results of those operations such that the definiendum γ applies to the respective object or situation only if the results β are obtained. To illustrate, let the definiendum γ be the sentence "Px" containing the unary predicate "P". Then the definition says: If you do α, then object x is P if and only if β obtains. Here is a simple example definition introducing the clinical notion of acute gastritis:

Definition 16 (Acute gastritis: 1). *If an individual is gastroscopically examined, then she* has acute gastritis *iff her gastric mucosa shows subepithelial hemorrhages, petechiae, and erosions.*

This is an operational definition because it requires us to perform an operation, i.e., gastroscopy in an individual, to bring about a condition that makes it possible to decide whether the predicate "has acute gastritis" does or does not apply to that individual. From the consideration above it is easy to see that one's prejudiced criticism of operationalism may be misguided. Whoever agrees to be examined by her doctor according to the operationally defined concept of acute gastritis above, while criticizing and opposing 'operationalism' and 'operationalization', is confused about the nature of operationalism and operationalization. Below, Definition 17 formalizes the definition above to reveal its logical structure. For this purpose, we will use the following symbols:

GEx	reads:	x is gastroscopically examined
AGx		x has acute gastritis
$GMyx$		y is the gastric mucosa of x
SHy		y shows subepithelial hemorrhages
PEy		y shows petechiae
ERy		y shows erosions.

Definition 17 (Acute gastritis: 2). $\forall x \forall y (GEx \wedge GMyx \rightarrow (AGx \leftrightarrow SHy \wedge PEy \wedge ERy))$.

Rule 7: Operational definition of predicates. A sentence δ is an operational definition of an n-ary predicate P in a language $\mathcal{L}$ iff:

1. δ is a universal closure in $\mathcal{L}$ of the form $\mathcal{Q}(\alpha \rightarrow (Px_1 \ldots x_n \leftrightarrow \beta))$,
2. $x_1, \ldots, x_n$ are $n \geq 1$ distinct individual variables,
3. α and β are sentences that do not contain the predicate P,
4. sentence α describes $m \geq 1$ actions,
5. β has no free individual variables other than $x_1, \ldots, x_n$.

Rules for defining function symbols will be omitted since they resemble the pattern we have already dealt with in preceding sections. Instead, we will now come back to the definition of *dispositional terms* that we postponed in Section 4.2.

Recall our discussion of dispositional attributes and terms on page 76. A dispositional attribute, such as penicillin allergy, is not a categorical attribute to be permanently present. It manifests itself only under a certain circumstance C, and so it is a conditional attribute, i.e., conditional on the circumstance C. Therefore, operational definitions are appropriate tools for introducing dispositional-medical terms. By operationally defining a dispositional term, some actions can be specified in the precondition clause of the definition that may bring about the circumstance C under which the dispositional attribute will manifest itself if it is present. This, in turn, enables a decision about whether the term may or may not be applied to the respective object or situation. Here are two simple examples:

- If penicillin is administered to someone, then she has a *penicillin allergy* iff she shows allergic reactions.

Allergic reactions are symptoms such as hives, rash, itchy skin, wheezing, swollen lips, tongue or face, and others. "She has a penicillin allergy" does not merely mean that the individual shows allergic reactions right now. Rather, she is assumed to have a hidden disposition that manifests itself under the influence of the administered penicillin. Another simple example is this:

- If an object is struck, then it is *fragile* iff it breaks.

Like a penicillin allergy, fragility is not a categorical attribute, but a disposition that manifests itself under certain circumstances. Such a circumstance is specified by the precondition clause of the operational definition above, i.e., "if an object is struck". Fragility is ascribed to the object under this circumstance, when we see it breaking.

In the empiricist philosophy of science, an operational definition of the form $\mathcal{Q}(\alpha \to (\gamma \leftrightarrow \beta))$ above whose definiens β indicates *observable* phenomena or events such as allergic reactions or breaking, has come to be termed a *reduction sentence* because it reduces the meaning of the definiendum γ to observables. For instance, someone may operationally define "anxiety" by a definiens β that refers not to hidden inner feelings of the individual, but to public parameters of the organism, e.g., flight behavior and increased heart and breathing rates. Such a definition is a reduction sentence. Reduction sentences have been proposed in the empiricist philosophy as a method of defining dispositional terms (Carnap, 1936; Hempel, 1954).

We have already pointed out on page 77 that most diseases may be viewed as dispositional attributes. On this account, reduction sentences seem to provide an excellent device for defining the names of diseases, as in Definitions 16 and 17 above introducing the notion of acute gastritis. But it has been shown in the literature that the definition of a term by a reduction sentence may lead to epistemological problems if there are additional reduction sentences about the same term. We shall come back to this issue in Section 6.4.3 on page 202. For a detailed discussion of the problem, see (Stegmüller 1970, 213–238).

It has also been proposed to conceive dispositional terms as modal concepts by way of attaching to definiens β the possibility operator "it is possible that" in the following fashion (for the possibility operator, see Section 27.1.1 on page 913):

$$\mathcal{Q}\big(\alpha \to (\gamma \leftrightarrow \Diamond\beta)\big).$$

For example, the modal re-definition of the dispositional term "penicillin allergy" defined above would read: If penicillin is administered to someone, then she has a penicillin allergy if and only if she *can show* allergic reactions. It is not yet clear, however, whether this modal proposal is acceptable. It doesn't seem to be so.

Our considerations above demonstrate that the *operationalization* of an attribute is characterized by indicating some operation(s) through which a condition is produced that enables one to decide whether the attribute is present or absent. There is a widespread belief according to which the operationalization of an attribute consists in its quantification, e.g., the quantification of time. But this view is grossly wrong. See, for example, the operational definitions of the terms "has a penicillin allergy", "is fragile", and "has acute gastritis" above. None of them is a quantitative term. Obviously, qualitative terms can also be operationalized.

5.3.4 Definition by Cases

Sometimes it is desirable to have a concept that acts as a function over a universe of discourse Ω, and is capable of assigning to an object in Ω different values depending on what condition the object satisfies from among a variety of alternative conditions. Such case-differentiating concepts are exclusively functions, not predicates. For instance, consider the binary functions *max* and *min* which we shall frequently employ to determine, respectively, *the greater* and *the smaller* of two numbers (x, y). We have, for example, $max(7, 5) = 7$ and $min(8, 4) = 4$. The two functions are commonly defined as follows:

Definition 18 (Maximum and minimum of two numbers: 1).

$$max(x, y) = \begin{cases} x & \textit{iff } x \geq y \\ y & \textit{otherwise.} \end{cases}$$

$$min(x, y) = \begin{cases} x & \textit{iff } y \geq x \\ y & \textit{otherwise.} \end{cases}$$

Although the scheme above is commonly used in the literature, it is an intuitive illustration, but not a formally correct definition. A formally correct version has to take into account that both the definiendum and the definiens must be sentences and, in addition, the definiendum must be the atomic sentence of the term to be introduced. That means in the present case that our definiendum ought to have the following, atomic structure: $max(x, y) = z$. The scheme above may now be rewritten as a correct definition thus:

Definition 19 (Maximum and minimum of two numbers: 2).

a) $\forall x \forall y \forall z \Big(max(x, y) = z \leftrightarrow \big((x \geq y \to z = x) \land (y > x \to z = y) \big) \Big).$

b) $\forall x \forall y \forall z \Big(min(x, y) = z \leftrightarrow \big((y \geq x \to z = x) \land (x > y \to z = y) \big) \Big).$

Each of these biconditionals is obviously an explicit definition. Consider the first one that defines *"max"*. Its definiens on the right-hand side of the biconditional sign is a conjunction of two conditionals. These conditionals cover two mutually exclusive cases. The first case on the left-hand side of the conjunction is when x exceeds or equals y. In this case, $max(x, y)$ is taken to be $x \in \{x, y\}$. The second possible case on the right-hand side of the conjunction is when y exceeds x. In this case, $max(x, y)$ is taken to be $y \in \{x, y\}$. Thus, depending on which one of the two disjoint cases obtains, $x \geq y$ or rather $y > x$, the function $max(x, y)$ computes a corresponding value. Such a definition is therefore referred to as a *definition by cases*. It is worth noting that the number of the defining cases is not limited to 2 as in definitions above. It may be more than 2 and even infinite. This is captured by the following rule:

Rule 8: Explicit definition by cases. A sentence δ is an explicit definition by cases of an n-ary function symbol f in a language $\mathcal{L}$ iff:

1. δ is a universal closure in $\mathcal{L}$ of the form $\mathcal{Q}(fx_1 \ldots x_n = y \leftrightarrow \beta_1 \land \ldots \land \beta_m)$,
2. $x_1, \ldots, x_n, y$ are $n + 1$ distinct individual variables with $n \geq 1$,
3. $\beta_1, \ldots, \beta_m$ are $m > 1$ mutually exclusive sentences, preferably conditionals, fixing the value y of the function f for $m > 1$ mutually exclusive cases. They do not contain the function symbol f,
4. $\beta_1, \ldots, \beta_m$ have no free individual variables other than $x_1, \ldots, x_n, y$.

Supposing that a new n-ary function f for multiple, i.e. $m > 1$, cases is definable according to Rule 8, one may present the definition in the following, general, schematic fashion that we are already familiar with:

$$f(x_1, \ldots, x_n) = \begin{cases} y_1 & \text{iff condition } C_1 \text{ is satisfied,} \\ y_2 & \text{iff condition } C_2 \text{ is satisfied,} \\ \vdots \\ y_m & \text{iff condition } C_m \text{ is satisfied.} \end{cases}$$

Due to the simplicity and clarity of such schemes, definitions by cases are always presented in this form. We shall make use of this technique on several occasions in later chapters. According to the concept of conditional definition of function symbols given in Rule 6 on page 90, a definition by cases of a function need not necessarily be an explicit definition like above-mentioned examples. It may also be a conditional, including operational, definition by cases with a precondition α as shown by the following example that defines a quaternary function f:

$$\text{If } \alpha, \text{ then } f(x_1, x_2, x_3, x_4) = \begin{cases} y_1 & \text{iff condition } C_1 \text{ is satisfied,} \\ y_2 & \text{iff condition } C_2 \text{ is satisfied,} \\ \vdots & \\ y_m & \text{iff condition } C_m \text{ is satisfied.} \end{cases}$$

This option is cast in the following rule that in contradistinction to Rule 8 allows sentence δ to be a conditional definition:

Rule 9: Conditional definition by cases. A sentence δ is a conditional definition by cases of an n-ary function symbol f in a language $\mathcal{L}$ iff:

1. δ is a universal closure in $\mathcal{L}$ of the form $\mathcal{Q}(\alpha \rightarrow (fx_1 \ldots x_n = y \leftrightarrow \beta_1 \wedge \ldots \wedge \beta_m))$,
2. $x_1, \ldots, x_n, y$ are $n + 1$ distinct individual variables with $n \geq 1$,
3. α is a sentence that does not contain the function symbol f,
4. $\beta_1, \ldots, \beta_m$ are $m > 1$ mutually exclusive sentences, preferably conditionals, fixing the value y of the function f for $m > 1$ mutually exclusive cases. They do not contain the function symbol f,
5. the variable y is not free in α,
6. $\beta_1, \ldots, \beta_m$ have no free individual variables other than $x_1, \ldots, x_n, y$.

5.3.5 Recursive Definition

The question "what is disease?" remains open and constitutes a fundamental puzzle in medicine. We shall suggest a theory of disease in Section 6.3 that promises a solution. In that theory, and in other contexts, we shall make use of a method of concept formation that has come to be termed *recursive definition*. The Latin word "recursion" means "backward movement" and "turning back". A recursive definition, also infelicitously called an *inductive definition*, aptly defines a term by backward movement within the definition itself. Since the method is highly important as well as demanding, we ought to have it firmly in hand before moving on. To understand it properly, we will illustrate the technique by analyzing the example below. Consider the following definition of the term "descendant":

- A descendant of a person is a child of that person or a child of a descendant of that person.

This is a recursive definition. It defines "descendant" in terms of other descendants by using a recurrence relation called recursion. We will semi-formalize it in order to elucidate its logical structure and the method of recursive definition:

Definition 20 (Descendant: 1). $\forall x \forall y \forall z \big(x$ *is a* descendant *of y* $\leftrightarrow$
$\quad x$ *is a child of y* $\vee$ $(z$ *is a descendant of y* $\wedge$ x *is a child of z)\big)$.

This sentence defines by a biconditional the binary predicate "is a descendant of" and thereby determines a potentially infinite set of descendants of y, e.g., of Adam or James Joyce. Because of its biconditional form, it seems prima facie to be an explicit definition, but it is not. It violates clause 3 of Rule 1 for explicit definitions stated on page 87 in that it defines the definiendum "descendant" by using this term itself in its definiens. That is, the definiendum *recurs* in its own definiens on the right-hand side of the biconditional sign. However, we will now convince ourselves that this recurrence does not cause any circularity of the definition.

The definiens of our definition above at the right-hand side of the biconditional is a disjunction of two components. First, on the left-hand side of the disjunction sign "$\vee$", the initial element of the set of descendants is defined by the term "is a child of". Thus, the new term "descendant" is now available and can be applied to at least one object. Second, with the aid of this locally *available* term "descendant", an arbitrary number of descendants are produced on the right-hand side of the disjunction sign. For each time when we are asked whether someone is a descendant of y, we need only examine whether she is a child of y. If so, then she is a descendant of y. Otherwise, we ask whether she is a child of a descendant, z, of y. To determine whether z is a descendant of y, we go back to the first step and ask whether z is a child of y, and so on. This repeated backward movement eventually enables a decision whether someone is a descendant of y or not.

Like definition by cases discussed in the preceding section, the recursive definition has traditionally got a much simpler form of presentation than our example Definition 20 above. Written in an abridged form that is commonly used in the literature, our example would be split into two sentences and would look as follows:

1. A child of a person is a descendant of that person;
2. Also a child of a descendant of a person is a descendant of that person.

These two sentences constitute a conjunction. The first sentence is termed the initial step or the *basis step*, and the second sentence is referred to as the induction step, or more appropriately, the *recursion step*. They proceed by first specifying in sentence 1 the initial member of the set to which the new term "descendant" may be applied, and then, by turning back in sentence 2 to what has already been specified. These two steps jointly *constitute a recursive definition* and suffice to determine the potentially infinite set of all descendants of an individual.

The simplified definition above is a classical-logical consequence of a complete and correct definition such as Definition 20. It is thus a legitimate short form. To demonstrate this, the definition above will be formalized:

1. If x is a child of y, then x is a descendant of y;   (Basis step)
2. If z is a descendant of y and x is a child of z,   (Recursion step)
   then x is a descendant of y.

Further formalized, we obtain a recursive definition in the standard, simplified form:

Definition 21 (Descendant: 2).

1. $\forall x \forall y (Cxy \rightarrow \boldsymbol{D}xy)$
2. $\forall x \forall y \forall z (Dzy \wedge Cxz \rightarrow \boldsymbol{D}xy)$.

Here the symbol:

C stands for the binary predicate: is a *child* of
D stands for the binary predicate: is a *descendant* of.

Definition 21 consists of two conditionals. The antecedents of both conditionals constitute the definiens, whereas their uniform consequent is the definiendum, i.e., the term "descendant" written as bold $\boldsymbol{D}$. This term has been defined by a pair of sentences. The places where it is a definiendum, have been boldfaced. However, the term appears in the definition an additional time, this time as part of the *definiens* in the antecedent of the recursion step. Thus, it has first been defined by the term "child" in the basis step, and then, by the terms "child" and the already available term "descendant" in the recursion step. The use of antecedently available information, generated by iterated application of the definition itself, gives the method of recursive definition a fundamental and most fruitful role in mathematics, logic, and informatics. The invention of the method in 1931 by Kurt Gödel gave rise to the theory of *recursive functions and computability*, and critically contributed to the emergence of theoretical informatics and artificial intelligence research and technology (Gödel, 1931; Rogers, 1987).

To demonstrate that a standard, pruned recursive definition such as Definition 21 is implied by a complete definition such as Definition 20, we will formalize the latter according to the terminology introduced above:

Definition 22 (Descendant: 1′). $\forall x \forall y \forall z (Dxy \leftrightarrow Cxy \vee (Dzy \wedge Cxz))$.

Assertion 1. *Definition 22* $\vdash$ *Definition 21.*

Proof 1:

1. *Definition 22*   Premise
2. $Dxy \leftrightarrow Cxy \vee (Dzy \wedge Cxz)$ Iterated $\forall$-Elimination: 1
3. $Cxy \vee (Dzy \wedge Cxz) \rightarrow Dxy$ $\leftrightarrow$-Elimination: 2

4. $(Cxy \to Dxy) \land (Dzy \land Cxz \to Dxy)$ Antecedent Split: 3
5. $Cxy \to Dxy$ $\land$-Elimination: 4
6. $Dzy \land Cxz \to Dxy$ $\land$-Elimination: 4
7. $\forall x \forall y (Cxy \to Dxy)$ Iterated $\forall$-Introduction: 5
8. $\forall x \forall y \forall z (Dzy \land Cxz \to Dxy)$ Iterated $\forall$-Introduction: 6
9. *Definition* 21 $\equiv$ 7, 8. QED[15]

For the deduction rules applied in Proof 1, see Tables 36 and 37 on pages 895 and 898, respectively.

Our discussion above concerned the recursive definition of predicates only. The recursive definition of functions is the main domain of application of the recursive technique. However, since the recursive definition of functions is more or less analogous to the above procedure, we shall not concern ourselves with this aspect.

Rule 10: Recursive definition of predicates. A sentence δ is a recursive definition of an n-ary predicate symbol P in a language $\mathcal{L}$ iff:

1. δ is a universal closure in $\mathcal{L}$ of the form $\mathcal{Q}((\alpha \to Px_1 \ldots x_n) \land (\beta \to Px_1 \ldots x_n))$,
2. $x_1, \ldots, x_n$ are $n \geq 1$ distinct individual variables,
3. α and β are sentences,
4. while sentence α does not contain the predicate P, sentence β does,
5. α has no free individual variables other than $x_1, \ldots, x_n$.

It is both possible and admissible to combine a recursive definition with other types such as conditional definitions, operational definitions, and definition by cases. We will not go into details here. But the combination of a recursive definition with a definition by cases may be illustrated to obtain a *recursive definition by cases*. As an example, consider the following recursive definition by cases of a function symbol, i.e., the function $\hat{s}$ for "substitution of terms" that should now be added to Definitions 212 and 213 on pages 870 and 871. See footnote 161 on page 870.

Definition 23 (Substitution of terms).

$$\hat{s}(t_\circ, x, t) = \begin{cases} t & \text{if } x \equiv t_\circ \\ x & \text{if } \exists y (t_\circ \equiv y \text{ and not } x \equiv y) \\ f\big(\hat{s}(t_1, x, t), \ldots, \hat{s}(t_n, x, t)\big) & \text{if } t_\circ \equiv f(t_1, \ldots, t_n). \end{cases}$$

---

[15] Traditionally, the acronym "QED" marks the end of a proof. It abbreviates the scholastic dictum "quod erat demonstrandum" meaning "the thing that was to prove".

5.3.6 Set-Theoretical Definition

There is a limitation to the methods of definition that we sketched in the preceding sections. The Rules 1–10 are restricted to first-order languages, i.e., languages in which quantifiers range over individual variables only (see page 873 in Part VIII). To define terms that require a higher-order language, the rules would have to be adapted accordingly. For example, the famous *definition of identity* by the so-called Leibniz's Law is an explicit definition in a language of the second order. It stipulates that an object x is identical to an object y if and only if it has every property P that object y has:

Definition 24 (Leibniz's Law). $\forall x \forall y (x = y \leftrightarrow \forall P(Px \leftrightarrow Py))$.[16]

The method of concept formation by set-theoretical definition is the most general, inventive, and powerful one not affected by language restriction. It is at once the least complicated and most transparent one available to us, and we shall use it throughout. With it we can employ all the techniques of the formal sciences as well as their theories. It allows us not only to introduce new concepts and to formulate new theories, but also to reconstruct available scientific concepts, theories and theory nets, and to analyze and systematize them. It was invented by the so-called Bourbaki Group of mostly French mathematicians in the 1950s (Bourbaki, 1950, 1958), and was further developed by the Stanford mathematician and philosopher of science Patrick Suppes, born in 1922 in Tulsa, Oklahoma. Its core device is "to define a predicate in terms of notions of set theory. A predicate so defined is called a *set-theoretical* predicate" (Suppes, 1957, 249).[17]

A very simple example may serve as an illustration. We shall encounter additional, more complex examples in later chapters. The predicate we want to define set-theoretically is the predicate "is an immunity structure". It delineates systems which are composed of organisms infected with some infectious material that causes particular processes in them. We shall come back to this predicate on page 421.

Definition 25 (Immunity structure). *For every ξ, ξ is an* immunity structure *iff there are Ω and X such that:*

> *1. $\xi = \langle \Omega, X \rangle$;*
> *2. Ω is a non-empty set of living organisms;*

---

[16] The reason why Definition 24 is called *Leinbiz's Law*, is this. The so-called principle of the *identity of indiscernibles*, i.e., $\forall x \forall y (\forall P(Px \leftrightarrow Py) \rightarrow x = y)$, is a principle of formal ontology that was first formulated in 1686 by Gottfried Wilhelm Leibniz in his *Discourse on Metaphysics* (Leibniz 2006). It says that no two distinct objects have exactly the same properties. The converse of the principle, i.e., $\forall x \forall y (x = y \rightarrow \forall P(Px \leftrightarrow Py))$, expresses the *indiscernibility of identicals*. Definition 24 above is the conjunction of these two principles that yields a biconditional.

[17] See footnote 73 on page 405

3. X is a non-empty set of harmful organisms, viruses, or substances, re-ferred to as agents;

4. If some elements of X invade or attack any members of Ω, then these members destroy or render them harmless.

This predicate signifies a set whose members are organisms which are immune against invading agents. It will serve as a point of departure in our epistemological studies about theories in medicine in Part III. An additional example may be briefly presented to explain some useful terminology of concept formation by set-theoretical tools that we shall need later on. When introducing the concept of probability by Definition 237 on page 975 of our logic primer in Part VIII, we have used the method of set-theoretical definition implicitly. To make it explicit, we will redefine the notion of "is a probability space", this time as a set-theoretical predicate:

Definition 26 (Probability space). *x is a* (finitely additive) *probability space iff there are Ω, $\mathcal{E}$, and p such that:*

1. *$x = \langle \Omega, \mathcal{E}, p \rangle$;*
2. *Ω is a non-empty set referred to as the sample space;*
3. *$\mathcal{E}$ is an algebra of sets on Ω referred to as the event algebra;*
4. *p is a function such that $p : \mathcal{E} \mapsto [0,1]$;*
5. *For every A, $B \in \mathcal{E}$:*

   5.1. $p(A) \geq 0$
   5.2. $p(\Omega) = 1$
   5.3. If $A \cap B = \varnothing$, then $p(A \cup B) = p(A) + p(B)$.

The two examples above demonstrate that a set-theoretical definition is formulated completely by means of set-theoretical terminology. The clauses of such a definition are referred to as its *axioms*. The term "axiom" originates from the Greek $\alpha\xi\iota\omega\mu\alpha$ (axioma) meaning "the required" or "requirement". Two types of axioms are distinguished, *structural* axioms and *substantial* axioms. Structural axioms characterize the structure of the predicate. In Definition 26, sentences 1–4 are structural axioms. The first one specifies the structure and the other three characterize it. Substantial axioms *describe* the structure. The present example has only one substantial axiom comprising three parts, i.e., axiom 5 including the three Kolmogorov Axioms (see page 975).

5.3.7 Ostensive Definition

What is called 'ostensive definition', is the least known method of concept formation. However, it is one of the most important ones for the functioning of our languages because, like operational definition, it imports *meaning* into the otherwise empty web of words. It will become clear below that ostensive definition is in fact not a method of definition, but of semantic interpretation. As we shall demonstrate later on, it plays a fundamental role in the genesis of the concept of disease and nosological systems.

Except for operational definition, all other methods of definition discussed thus far are verbal ones in the sense that each of them defines a word by other words. Verbal methods alone are not able to relate a language with the outside world, and to pervade it with meaning. As was emphasized on page 85, the chains of verbal definitions in a language come eventually to an end. The definientia of their basic definitions from where the chains start, i.e., the primary terms or primitives of the language, are not defined by any other terms. So, from where does meaning flow into the semantically lifeless definition chains?

The primitives receive their meaning not from verbal definitions, but from another source: They are directly *interpreted* by extra-linguistic entities. The interpretation consists in establishing a denotative word-to-world link by performing a more or less complex, behavioral-social act of pointing to an object such as a newborn, dog, ship, street, building, and the like, and assigning to it the word in question, e.g., "XYZ", *as its name* by exclaiming:

"You will be called XYZ !"   (11)

The ceremony is well-known in everyday life as naming, baptizing, or christening, and has been termed *ostensive definition* in philosophy. The adjective "ostensive" derives from the passive, past participle "ostensivum" (i.e., pointed to with a finger, shown, demonstrated) of the Latin verb "ostendere" meaning "to point to", "to show", "to demonstrate". For example, when the man, who would later invent the general and special theories of relativity, came into being in the southern German city Ulm, his parents and relatives presented him to city authorities, pointed to him, and exclaimed: "This newborn human being we call *Albert Einstein*". By so doing, the hitherto meaningless word "Albert Einstein" was *interpreted* by that newborn human being.

With the social act of baptizing, a word – term or name – that was meaningless before, acquires meaning. It is ostensively defined in that it is *interpreted* by pointing to an object and exclaiming the baptism formula 11. Similarly, many classificatory primitives such as "red", "yellow", "pain", and the like are learned by the developing child during a process of repeatedly pointing to objects by her educators, and exclaiming "this ball is *red*", "this rose is *red*", "this candy is *red*", etc. Nobody teaches the child the word "red" by presenting her a verbal definition of the term, be it an explicit, conditional, operational, set-theoretical one, or the like. The skeptic may try to define the term "red" of our perceptual language, not that of the physics, verbally.[18]

---

[18] Sometimes we encounter in the literature also the term "contextual definition", as if there were such a method of definition. But this is not the case. People who use the term maintain that "the contextual definition of an expression is a definition in which the term is embedded in a context that explains it. For example, a contextual definition of the term "bradycardia" might be: 'Someone has bradycardia' means that 'her heart rate is below 50'". A closer look shows that their wording only clumsily recapitulates what we have considered a prerequisite

5.4 What an Explication is

From defining we must distinguish another important method of concept formation that has come to be termed *explication*. It is a technique of conceptual analysis. With it one doesn't introduce a completely new concept. Explication is the transformation of an already existing, unclear concept, called *explicandum*, into a new, clear concept, referred to as explicans or *explicatum* (Carnap, 1947, 1962). Suppose, for instance, that someone justifiably criticizes the ill-defined notion of "heart attack" and undertakes a more or less painstaking conceptual analysis of this term. She eventually shows that the class of people with so-called 'heart attack' is fuzzy, and in addition, consists of different fuzzy subclasses. She performs a fuzzy taxonomy and delineates the emerging fuzzy subclasses, names them "angina pectoris", "myocardial infarction", "atrial fibrillation", "ventricular fibrillation" and "sudden cardiac arrest", and clearly *defines* all these terms. By this endeavor, she has replaced the ill-defined explicandum "heart attack" with several, distinct, and well-defined explicata. The endeavor is called an *explication* of the term "heart attack".

An explication may include syntactic, semantic, pragmatic, logical, and empirical analyses as well as definitions. Sometimes it may even lead to the construction of a theory, or to large-scale research programs and traditions. It may take years, decades, centuries, or even millennia. For instance, the explication of the concepts "therefore" and "hence" took more than two millennia, from Aristotle to Gottlob Frege (1848–1925), and eventually brought about what is called logic and artificial intelligence today, with their central concepts being *logical inference* and *computability*. To give another example, the explication of the concept of disease by the present author that has led to the *prototype resemblance theory of disease,* took 30 years (see page 174).

We stated previously in Section 2.1 that medical language is an extended natural language, specifically an outgrowth of everyday language. For this reason, it is prone to, and contains plenty of, ambiguity and inexactitude. Among the inexact and vague concepts are not only many clinical terms such as names of symptoms and diseases, but also fundamental concepts of medicine such as *disease, cause of disease, diagnosis, prognosis, treatment efficacy, risk,* and others. We shall be concerned with the explication of these concepts in Part II. In view of the abundant imprecision in medical language, it is a moral task of medical professionals and philosophers of medicine as well to try to reduce imprecision by clarifying unclear concepts, i.e., by explicating them. In so doing one must be cautious of the pitfalls of one's own language, especially of the following deadly ambiguity.

When explicating a concept X, the initial, motivating question that is usually asked is "what is X?". For example, "what is self-consciousness?" or

---

for any definition to fix, in the definiendum, the *syntax of the use of the new term* that is to be defined. See Section 5.1 on page 82. Thus, the phrase "contextual definition" is gratuitous and does not designate an additional, specific method of definition.

"what is disease?". The goal of such a question is to analyze the meaning of the term "X" and to explicate or even to define it. Unfortunately, the question is almost always misunderstood and inadequately handled because both words, "what" and "is", as well as their combination are vague. This will be explained in the following two sections:

    5.4.1   What: Quod *vs.* Quid
    5.4.2   Is.

5.4.1 What: Quod *vs.* Quid

The word "what" has at least two different meanings that correspond to the Latin *quod* and *quid*. Thus, a what-is-X question may be asked in one of the following two modes:

- quod mode
- quid mode.

Depending on which one of these modes is meant by the question, the answer is completely different. To demonstrate, let us ask a what-is-X question: What is disease? Asked in the *quod mode*, the question means:

> What is really a *thing that* (quod) we call disease? Is it a   (quod)
> natural phenomenon, or an artifact, or a functional disabil-
> ity, or ... or ... what else?

In this question, it is antecedently clear what things are called disease. That is, the meaning of the term "disease", and thus, the class of diseases is known to the questioner. The goal of the inquiry is only to learn something more about the thing that is already known, and to find out to which other classes it belongs. Thus, what is *unknown* is whether what is *known* belongs to some other classes *A, B, C,* ... The question asks to which one of the classes *A, B, C,* ... does disease belong? Is it a natural phenomenon, or an artifact, or a functional disability, or ... or ...? Possible answers are, for example, "disease is a bodily disorder", "disease is a functional disability ...", or something like that. In a nutshell, a what-is-X question in quod mode is not an explicative, but a *taxonomic query*. By contrast, ask the question now in the *quid mode*:

> Of all things in the world, *what* (quid) thing is disease? This   (quid)
> thing, or that thing, or ... or ... what else?

In this case, the meaning of the word "disease", and thus, the class of diseases is unknown to the questioner. The goal of the inquiry is an explication of the vague term "disease" in order to find out how it is defined, or even to define it in the context of a new theory. The confusion of the two completely different meanings of the "what is X?" question, quod versus quid, is the source of a *fundamental catastrophe* in medicine where pointless taxonomic subsumption debates about whether "disease is this thing" or "disease is that thing" are mistaken for philosophy of disease. We shall come back to this issue in Section "Petitio principii" on page 156.

5.4.2 Is

Even more difficult to understand is the particle "is" of a what-is-X question because it has many meanings in natural languages. This was recognized for the first time by the logicians Augustus De Morgan (1806–1871) and Bertrand Russell (1872–1970). See (Russell, 1903, 64). It is the most perilous term of human languages and plays at least seven logically different roles two of which will be discussed in Chapter 18 on page 685, and five of which indicate:

membership, predication	e.g.:	Elroy Fox is ill	$a \in X, \quad Xa$
subsethood		man is a mammal	man $\subseteq$ mammal
equality		two and three is five	$(2+3) = 5$
conditional		man is mortal	x is a man $\rightarrow x$ is mortal
biconditional		false is not true	α is false $\leftrightarrow \alpha$ is not true.

Membership and subsethood constitute what we have called a subsumption relation, "is_a", in Section 4.1.2 on page 60. For all these reasons, a what-is-X question is by no means clear. Even the questioner is not always fully aware what she is really asking.

5.5 Summary

There is as yet no methodology of scientific concept formation as an established discipline. As a result, there exists no logic and methodology of definition, even though it is the core technique of concept formation. Only logicians, mathematicians, and analytic philosophers practice in their publications a variety of specific methods of definition that propagate by internal tradition. From this literature we have assembled the following seven techniques, and guided by Patrick Suppes's outstanding work (1957, 151–173, 246–260), have formally reconstructed: explicit definition, conditional definition, operational definition, definition by cases, recursive definition, set-theoretical definition, and ostensive definition. We have also briefly outlined the valuable technique of explication proposed by Rudolf Carnap (1947, 1962). Each of these methods has its own domain of application and usability. Their use in medicine may reduce the semantic chaos that characterizes medical language and theorizing.

In introducing the above-mentioned methods, we have deliberately confined ourselves to a language of the first order. As outlined on page 873, the only variables contained in an elementary language of this type are individual variables over which quantifiers range. The aim of our restriction has been to avoid complicating the issue by considering higher-order languages. A methodology of definition in higher-order languages is beyond the scope of the present book. We must emphasize, however, that our approach needs to be extended to also cover higher-order and even many-sorted languages because it is in these languages that concept formation in real-world scientific practice is actually conducted. To give an example that at the same time explains the notion of a *many-sorted language*, consider Definitions 151–153 on pages 563–564. To keep the definitions easily readable, we have in those and many other definitions in the book omitted an explicit display of universal closures. One should be aware, however, that the omitted universal quantifiers in some of these definitions range not only over a single sort of individual variables, e.g., variables for human beings or natural numbers, but also over other sorts of variables, and even over predicates, i.e., sets of such variables, and additional sorts of objects such as operators, sentences α, β, γ, and others. Thus, *many sorts* of objects are involved in a language that is used in real-world concept formation. To appropriately manage reasoning in such an inhomogeneous language requires, correspondingly, a *many-sorted logic* that is not covered in this book.

Part II

Medical Praxiology

6

The Patient

6.0 Introduction

Medicine is concerned with the treatment of sick people, the promotion and protection of health, and the prevention of maladies and human suffering. This wide-ranging task is accomplished through medical practice and medical research, though no sharp boundary between them can be drawn. For the purposes of our discussion in the present Part II, we shall focus on medical practice. The term "practice" derives from the Greek word $\pi\rho\alpha\xi\iota\varsigma$ (praxis) that means "doing", "acting", and "action". Thus, by the term "medical praxiology" we understand the *theory of medical practice*, i.e., the philosophy, methodology, and logic of medical doing and acting (Sadegh-Zadeh, 1981d, 183).

The core subject of medical praxiology is clinical practice. As mentioned above, clinical practice overlaps clinical research. Investigations into the causation of maladies and course of diseases, the reliability of diagnostic techniques, and the efficacy of treatments are all activities that cannot be separated from clinical practice. Since these and related activities produce medical knowledge, medical praxiology will also touch on issues of medical knowledge gained by clinical practice. For this reason, there is no sharp division between medical praxiology and medical epistemology. The latter will be the subject of our discussion in Part III.

Clinical practice is centered on (i) the *patient*. Its main active agent is (ii) the *physician*, or more generally, the diagnostic and therapeutic group or team. Their actions, constituting (iii) the *clinical practice*, deal with what is traditionally called patient history or anamnesis, diagnosis, prognosis, therapy, and prevention. We shall therefore focus on the philosophy, methodology, and logic of these three subjects in the following chapters:

6 The Patient
7 The Physician
8 Clinical Practice.

K. Sadegh-Zadeh, *Handbook of Analytic Philosophy of Medicine*,
Philosophy and Medicine 113, DOI 10.1007/978-94-007-2260-6_6,
© Springer Science+Business Media B.V. 2012

In philosophical and methodological inquiries into medicine, three approaches may be clearly distinguished: (a) a descriptive, (b) a normative, and (c) a reconstructive-constructive approach. A *descriptive* approach is concerned with how things are in order to understand how medicine works, e.g., 'how doctors think' (Montgomery, 2006; Groopman, 2007) when making diagnostic-therapeutic decisions; what they understand by the term "diagnosis"; how they actually perform diagnostics; and so on. Such an approach requires empirical studies and belongs to empirical linguistics, behavior analysis, psychology, and sociology (Elstein et al., 1978). A *normative* approach is prescriptive and articulates how the physician or medical researcher ought to reason, diagnose, treat the patient, etc. By contrast, a *reconstructive-constructive* approach analyzes the existing concepts, methods, knowledge, and theories metatheoretically, e.g., the concepts of disease, diagnosis, therapy, etc. The aim is to improve them by detecting their shortcomings and by advancing new ideas and tools for use in enhancing the quality of clinical decision-making, medical research, and health care. As we are conducting analytic philosophy of medicine, our approach falls under the third, reconstructive-constructive category. We shall neither conduct empirical surveys about how physicians actually think, nor put forward normative requirements. We shall only advance suggestions which the reader may evaluate, and decide to accept or reject.

In the passage above, the terms "diagnostics" and "diagnosis" distinguish between two completely different issues. This distinction will be maintained and play an important role throughout. While diagnostics is an *investigation* into the patient's health condition to gather information about her suffering and to explain, for example, why she has fever and shortness of breath, diagnosis represents the *outcome* of that investigation. An example is the statement "Elroy Fox has pneumonia" that a doctor makes as a result of subjecting Mr. Elroy Fox to diagnostics. It is misleading to call both of them, the investigation and its result, "diagnosis", as is regrettably often done in the English language.

A widespread misconception about medicine has it that medicine is concerned with illness and disease. However, the subject of medicine is *the patient* with the ends being directed toward the relief, prevention of human suffering, and saving human life. Accordingly, medicine needs a *theory of the patient* first of all. Nosology and pathology as studies of illness and disease may be viewed as elements of such a theory. Seen from this perspective, clinical research and practice are to be based on the question: What is a patient? That is, what characteristics distinguish a patient from a non-patient? The present Chapter 6 is concerned with this question.

The inquiry into what a patient is, intersects with medical anthropology that is concerned with the question of *what is a human being?* This is the fundamental philosophical question of medicine because, as an experimental and diagnostic-therapeutic discipline, it undertakes momentous interventions in human life. It therefore needs an image of the human being so as to examine whether medical interventions are in accord with, or contravene, that image.

For example, it is a legitimate question to ask whether the transplantation of animal cells, tissues, and organs into humans, i.e., xenotransplantation, or whether the designing of offspring by genetic engineering, is morally permissible. Since anthropology is basically a philosophical endeavor, medicine at its foundations turns out to intersect with philosophy.

We shall consider the patient as a bio-psycho-social agent who is suffering or whose life is threatened by some occurrences inside or outside of her body, usually called diseases, pathogenic environments, etc. Our aim is to understand what these occurrences may look like and how they may be conceptualized, systematized, recognized, causally analyzed, and controlled. Thus, our discussion consists of the following five sections:

6.1   The Suffering Individual
6.2   The Bio-Psycho-Social Agent
6.3   Health, Illness, and Disease
6.4   Systems of Disease
6.5   Etiology.

6.1 The Suffering Individual

As stated above, prevention and relief of human suffering is one of the primary ends of medicine. We must therefore understand what the pursuit of this goal requires and implies.

There are two common-sense postulates which say that, first, if a particular state of affairs is to be prevented or altered, one must know its cause, and second, one must manipulate or eliminate that cause. Although these postulates are not quite true, they underlie medicine and almost all other areas of deliberate human action. Accordingly, knowledge about the causes of suffering is considered a prerequisite of its prevention and relief. That means that if a particular type of suffering is caused by an event E, call it damage, the prevention or amelioration of that type of suffering requires that you be aware of the causative role of event E and try to prevent, manipulate, or even eliminate E. The prevailing view in medicine about where in a human being suffering occurs, is that it occurs in the body. A minority locates suffering in the mind, psyche, soul, or spirit. However, as Eric Cassell rightly points out, the attempt to understand the nature and the sources of suffering, will require that medicine overcome the traditional dichotomy between body and mind. For suffering is not identical with pain. It is also not identical with distress or grief. The locus of suffering is the metaphysical person (Cassell 2004, 29 ff.):

Suffering occurs when an impending destruction of the person is perceived; it continues until the threat of disintegration has passed or until the integrity of the person can be restored in some other manner. It follows, then, that although it often occurs in the presence of acute pain, shortness of breath, or other bodily symptoms, suffering extends beyond the physical. Most generally, suffering can be defined as the state of severe distress associated with events that threaten the intactness of person (ibid., 32).

Thus, we are led to the question of what a person is and what the preconditions of her suffering are. In what follows, we shall be concerned with this basic element of our theory of the patient.

6.2 The Bio-Psycho-Social Agent

6.2.0 Introduction

It is widely lamented that since René Descartes the human being is partitioned into two parts, body and mind, or organism and psyche, and that this dualism is the cause of many aberrations and mistakes in medical thinking and practice. We shall not join in with this lament and criticism. Instead, we shall develop our own anthropology that overcomes the traditional mind-body dualism and has its roots in (Engel, 1977; Rothschuh, 1963; Sadegh-Zadeh, 1970a–b, 2000d).

To begin with, a patient is a living body whether she be a fetus or newborn, a child, adult, or elderly. A living body may also develop a psyche as it grows. For our purposes, we shall consider the terms "mind" and "psyche" as synonyms and will use them interchangeably. The psyche is both a product and part of the organism. In addition, as a living body the patient is inevitably a member of a family, a community, and a larger society. Below, we shall study these three aspects of a patient as a *bio-psycho-social* agent in order to understand the nature of health and disease, suffering and recovering:

    6.2.1   The Living Body
    6.2.2   The Psyche
    6.2.3   The Social Agent.

6.2.1 The Living Body

A living human body is not a mere assemblage of things such as arms, legs, stomach, brain, and other parts. It has an organized structure that we call an *organism*. In this section, we will look at a theory of organism that will play a basic role in the integrated, triadic system of the patient as a bio-psycho-social agent. The term "system" will be used not as a stopgap, but as a key technical term throughout. It will therefore be introduced first in order to aid in our understanding of the following terms: causal system, cyclic-causal system, distributed system, poietic system, endopoietic system.

Our aim is to show that the patient as a living body may be viewed as an *endopoietic system*, i.e., a system that builds interior worlds within itself, one of which is traditionally called the psyche or mind. The phrase "poiesis" derives from the Greek term ποιέω (poieo) meaning "to make, to produce, to create". The novel concept of *endopoiesis*, "making inner worlds", will provide our solution to the age-old mind-body problem. To this end, we will clarify our basic terminology in the following sections:

▶ What a system is
▶ The graph of a system
▶ The organism is a cyclic-causal system
▶ The organism is a distributed system
▶ The organism is a source of emergence
▶ The organism is a poietic system
▶ The organism is an endopoietic system
▶ The organism is a fuzzy causal system
▶ Is the organism a machine?

What a system is

For the sake of convenience, a crisp notion of a system will be introduced first. It will be specialized to the notion of a fuzzy system on page 126 below.

A mere assemblage is a collection of any objects without any bonds or relationships between them. For example, a pencil, a book, and a photograph of my family on the desk in front of me is an assemblage. It is simply an unstructured set. No relationships between its members have been specified yet. Since the behavior of an object in the collection is independent of the behavior of the others, an assemblage does not constitute a whole, 'it is not greater than the sum of its parts'. However, as the well-known postulate of the holistic metaphysics states, *the whole is greater than the sum of its parts*. This is so because the whole is a system.[19]

A *system*, from the Greek term σύστημα (sistema) meaning "standing together", is an entity composed of interrelated parts. Hence, it consists of:

- a set of objects,
- a set of relationships between these objects.

The objects are called its *components*, constituent parts, or elements. The relationships between them are referred to as its *relations*. Thus, a system may be defined as an ordered pair $\langle C, R \rangle$ of two sets, C and R, such that C is a set of components and R is a set of relations between them:

system = $\langle$Components, Relations between components$\rangle = \langle C, R \rangle$.

For instance, a family consisting of the mother Ada, the father Bert, and the daughter Carol constitutes a system whose components are these three

---

[19] The holistic postulate is generally attributed to Aristotle (Metaphysics, 1045 a 10). But the alleged source does not contain the apodictic wording of the postulate. It may have arisen from the Euclidean axiom "The whole is greater than the part". See also footnote 20 on page 121.

individuals and whose relations include, for example, spousehood, parenthood, and love. That is:

a family system $= \langle\{\text{Ada, Bert, Carol}\}, \{\text{spousehood, parenthood, love}\}\rangle$

such that we have:

$$\mathcal{C} = \{\text{Ada, Bert, Carol}\} \qquad \equiv \{a, b, c\}$$
$$\mathcal{R} = \{\text{spousehood, parenthood, love}\} \qquad \equiv \{R_1, R_2, R_3\}$$

and thus:

a family system $= \langle\{a, b, c\}, \{R_1, R_2, R_3\}\rangle$

with:

$$R_1 \equiv aR_1b \ \& \ bR_1a \qquad \equiv a \text{ is married to } b;\ b \text{ is married to } a,$$
$$R_2 \equiv aR_2c \ \& \ bR_2c \qquad \equiv a \text{ is } c\text{'s parent};\ b \text{ is } c\text{'s parent},$$
$$R_3 \equiv aR_3b \ \& \ bR_3a \ \& \qquad \equiv a \text{ loves } b;\ b \text{ loves } a;\ a \text{ loves } c;\ b \text{ loves } c.$$
$$\quad\ aR_3c \ \& \ bR_3c$$

A democratic state is also a system. Its components are the population, the parliament, the government, the ministries, and many other things. And between them hold relations such as electing, governing, commanding, and the like. An organism is a system as well. Its components are its cells, tissues, organs, and organ systems. And there is a huge set of relations between them such as the anatomical relation of parthood; the metabolic-biochemical relation of delivering a material from one component to another; the bioelectric relation of producing an electrical impulse that excites another component; etc. Later in this chapter, we shall demonstrate that clinical reasoning, too, may be interpreted as a system. Its components are agents and their actions with some particular epistemic, moral, and logical relations between them.

The graph of a system

Systems may be formally reconstructed and studied by representing them as graphs. To use this technique, we need to understand a few elementary terms, i.e., "directed graph", "cyclic graph", "path", and "tree".

Informally, a *graph* is a collection of dots connected to each other by lines (see Figure 8). A dot is called a vertex or *node*, and the connection between two nodes is referred to as an arc or *edge*. Thus, we may formalize a graph as an ordered pair $\langle N, E \rangle$ consisting of two sets, N and E, such that N is the set of nodes, E is the set of edges, and an edge $e \in E$ joins two nodes $x_1, x_2 \in N$:

graph $= \langle\text{Nodes, Edges}\rangle = \langle N, E \rangle.$

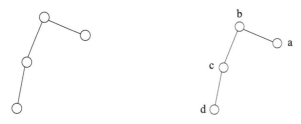

Fig. 8. Left: A simple graph with 4 nodes and 3 edges connecting them

Fig. 9. Right: The same graph as in Figure 8. The set of its nodes is $N = \{a, b, c, d\}$. An edge connects two nodes x_1 and x_2 and may therefore be written as the pair $\{x_1, x_2\}$. In the present graph, the set of edges is $E = \{\{a, b\}, \{b, c\}, \{c, d\}\}$. Thus, the graph may be formally represented as the ordered pair $\langle \{a, b, c, d\}, \{\{a, b\}, \{b, c\}, \{c, d\}\} \rangle$ with 4 nodes and 3 edges. The edges, representing a relation defined on set N, are formally displayed as the pairs of nodes they join

An edge joining two nodes x_1 and x_2 is written $\{x_1, x_2\}$. See Figure 9. A *system* may be represented as a graph of the form $\langle N, E \rangle$ such that the system's components constitute the nodes, N, and its relations are the edges, E, between the nodes (Figure 10). Two nodes in a graph are called *adjacent* if there is an edge connecting them. For instance, in Figure 10 two adjacent nodes are the cities Hamburg and Berlin, whereas Frankfurt and Berlin are not adjacent.

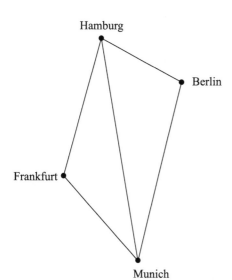

Fig. 10. The graph of the highway system connecting the cities Hamburg, Berlin, Munich, and Frankfurt in Germany. Two adjacent nodes are joined by an edge. An additional edge joins Hamburg and Munich directly. Thus, the system is the following structure: $\langle \{$Hamburg, Berlin, Munich, Frankfurt$\}$, $\{\{$Hamburg, Berlin$\},\{$Hamburg, Munich$\}$, $\{$Hamburg, Frankfurt$\}$, $\{$Berlin, Munich$\}$, $\{$Frankfurt, Munich$\}\} \rangle$

In the graphs presented above an edge is pointing to both directions between two adjacent nodes. For example, the Hamburg-Berlin highway goes from Hamburg to Berlin and vice versa. However, there are also graphs in which an edge is pointing to one direction only like a one-way street, so to speak. Such a directed edge is aptly represented by an arrow. A graph with directed edges is called a *directed* graph (see Figure 11).

For our purposes, we shall be concerned with directed graphs only. If a directed graph includes at least two adjacent nodes with more than one edge between them, it is called a directed multigraph (Figure 12). As the figure demonstrates, there is no limit to the number of relations in a system. A multigraph of a system with many types of relations between its nodes may become too complex to manage. It is therefore typical to simplify the study of systems by concentrating on only one type of relation joining the nodes, and neglecting for a time the remaining relations. We shall take advantage of this approach, using simplified graphs with only one type of edges representing only one type of relation (Figure 13).

A graph $G' = \langle N', E' \rangle$ is a subgraph of a graph $G = \langle N, E \rangle$ if its nodes N' are a subset of N, and its edges E' are a subset of E. This notion renders system-subsystem relationships easily analyzable. For instance, system A in Figure 13 is a subsystem of both B and C, and system B is a subsystem of C.

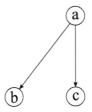

Fig. 11. A directed graph. It shows a small family consisting of father a and his two children b and c. A directed edge "→" represents the asymmetric relation "is the father of". a is the father of b (left arrow) and a is the father of c (right arrow)

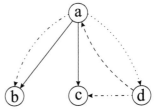

Fig. 12. A directed multigraph of a family with four types of relations: Father-of, wife-of, husband-of, and educating. a is the father of b. a is the father of c. a is the husband of d. d is the wife of a. Father a educates child b. Mother d educates child c

A *path* in a graph is a route that connects one node to another node along edges. Thus, it is a sequence of concatenated edges leading from one particular node to another node in the graph. The number of edges in a path is called the *length* of the path. Formally, a path of length $n \geq 1$ from a node x_0 to a node x_n in a directed graph $G = \langle N, E \rangle$ is an ordered tuple $\langle x_0, \ldots, x_n \rangle$ of distinct nodes such that any pair $\langle x_{i-1}, x_i \rangle$ in the tuple is an edge, where $1 \leq i \leq n$. For instance, in graph C in Figure 13 the quadruple $\langle d, a, b, c \rangle$ is a path of length 3 from node d to node c, that is, the path $d \to a \to b \to c$.

A *cycle* of length $n \geq 1$ is a path $\langle x_0, \ldots, x_{n-1}, x_0 \rangle$ which begins and ends on the same node. For example, in graph C in Figure 13 the path $\langle b, c, a, b \rangle$ is a cycle of length 3. A graph that has at least one cycle, is called a *cyclic*

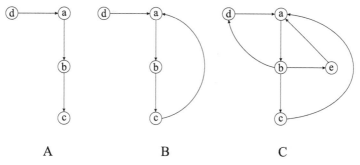

Fig. 13. Three directed graphs. In classical set theory, a relation R is a subset of a Cartesian product. Thus, $R \subseteq X \times X$ is a relation on set X. Accordingly, a graph may be viewed as a pair $\langle N, E \rangle$ where E is a relation on set N. On this account, a *directed graph* is easily representable as the ordered pair $\langle N, E \rangle$ of its nodes and edges such that the set of its edges, E, is a set of *ordered pairs* of nodes. For example, the graph A in the present figure is $\langle \{a, b, c, d\}, \{\langle a, b \rangle, \langle b, c \rangle, \langle d, a \rangle\} \rangle$ such that an ordered pair such as $\langle a, b \rangle$ in its E component represents the directed edge with the arrow from node a to node b. Thus, the set of edges, E, of a directed graph $\langle N, E \rangle$ is a subset of the Cartesian product $N \times N$. In other words, the edge set E is a binary relation on the node set N, called the *adjacency relation*. Thanks to this set-theoretical method of representing *systems* as directed graphs, they may be formally compared with each other by comparing their set-theoretical representations

graph. A graph with no cycles is referred to as an *acyclic* one. A system whose graph is a cyclic graph is a *cyclic system*. Otherwise, it is an acyclic system.

Let $G = \langle N, E \rangle$ be a directed graph and $x, y \in N$ be two nodes, then node x is called a predecessor or *parent* of node y, and y is called a successor or *child* of x, if there is an edge $\langle x, y \rangle \in E$. A node with no parents is called a *root*. If there is a path from a node x to a node y, then x is an ancestor of y and y is a descendant of x. A directed acyclic graph is called a *forest* if every node $x \in N$ has at most one parent. A forest with exactly one root is a *tree*. See Figure 14.

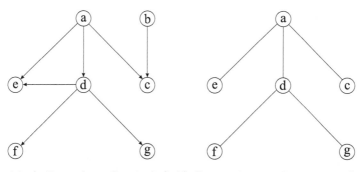

Fig. 14. A directed acyclic graph (left). By pruning we obtain a tree (right)

The organism is a cyclic-causal system

A *causal system* is a system whose components are connected with one another by a causal relation. Otherwise put, a system $\langle C, \mathcal{R} \rangle$ is a causal system if the set of its relations, $\mathcal{R}$, contains a causal relation. A causal relation between a component x and another component y of a system means that x causes something in y. For example, there is a causal relation between the sinus node of the heart and myocardium (= heart muscle) because the former produces electrical signals that cause the contraction of the latter. We shall explicate the notion of a *cause* in Section 6.5 on page 219. In the present context, we may provisionally use the following simplified notion.

We shall consider an event A to be a (positive or negative) cause of an event B if (i) A occurs earlier than B and changes (increases or decreases) the probability of B occurring; and (ii) there is no other event C preceding A such that C is also a cause of B, whereas the later event A doesn't alter C's causal influence on B. For example, at first glance a falling barometer reading seems to be the cause of a storm because it always precedes the latter and increases the probability of its occurrence. The decrease in air pressure that occurs before the barometer reading falls, also seems to be a cause of the storm. However, the falling barometer reading does not affect the causal influence of decreasing air pressure. So, the barometer reading is merely a spurious cause of the storm.

The organism is a causal system. Each one of its components is causally related with a myriad of other components, e.g., via blood, nerves, muscles, etc. If $\langle N, E \rangle$ is the graph of a causal system, we may interpret the edges, E, as the causal relation between the system's nodes N. We may in this way distinguish between linear-causal systems and cyclic-causal systems. A causal system is a linear-causal system if its graph is acyclic. By contrast, a causal system is a cyclic-causal system if it has a cyclic graph. See Figures 15–16.

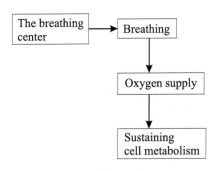

Fig. 15. The graph of a linear causal system. Compare with the naked graph A in Figure 13

The human organism is too complex a system to be representable in one single directed graph. Only partial graphs are feasible. Most of these graphs contain, as in Figure 16, causal cycles demonstrating that the organism is a *cyclic-causal system*.

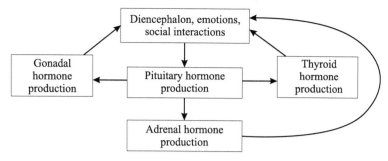

Fig. 16. The graph of production and regulation of some hormones. It represents a cyclic-causal system. Compare with the naked graph C in Figure 13

The organism is a distributed system

A system whose components are themselves systems is referred to as a distributed system. In the graph of a distributed system, all nodes are systems. The system emerges from their collaborative activity.

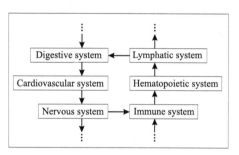

Fig. 17. Human organism as a distributed system. Each node is a system itself. The arrows are causal edges

The human organism is a distributed system. It is made up of numerous subsystems such as the cardiovascular system, respiratory system, nervous system, digestive system, immune system, endocrine system, and so on (see Figure 17). Each of these subsystems consists of even deeper subsystems such as different organs, tissues, and cells. For instance, the central nervous system is composed of the cerebrum, cerebellum, spinal cord, and autonomic nervous system. Again, each of these components is a distributed system and so forth (Figure 16 above). The subsystems of a distributed system, i.e., the nodes of its graph, may be arbitrarily distant from one another. In any event, through their inter-subsystem connectedness at different levels they bring about a complicated network with hierarchical and heterarchical levels of interaction to the effect that a living whole emerges, i.e., the living body (Figure 18).

The organism is a source of emergence

The concept of emergence will play a central role in our theory of the nature and origin of the psyche. It will therefore be introduced in some detail below.

Like any other object, a component or part of a system has a number of properties. For example, in the human organism as a system the part *pancreas* lies on the posterior wall of the omental bursa, weighs about 80 grams, produces hormones, digestive enzymes, bicarbonate, and so on. Assemble *all* such properties of *all parts* of the organism and call the collection ALL-PARTS'-PROPERTIES. Surprisingly, the organism as a *whole* has properties that are not contained in ALL-PARTS'-PROPERTIES. Otherwise put, the organism as a whole is not identical with the sum of its parts.

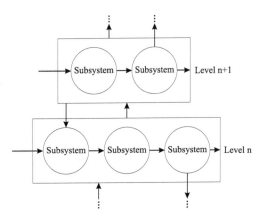

Fig. 18. Cyclic-causal relationships at different levels between the organism as a supersystem and its subsystems

It is something else. It has properties which none of its parts has. We call them systemic properties, i.e., properties of the system itself as a whole. For instance, the organism walks, eats, sleeps, dreams, thinks, loves, believes, etc. But neither the pancreas nor any other part of the organism walks, eats, sleeps, dreams, thinks, loves, or believes. The systemic properties that the organism has and that its parts lack, are *new*, or novel, with respect to ALL-PARTS'-PROPERTIES. That means:

There are properties that obtain of a system as a whole and do not obtain of its lower-level parts. A property of this type is new with respect to lower-level parts and properties in the system. It is caused by the *interaction* of all lower-level parts of the system and cannot be reduced to these parts as separate entities. This novelty and non-reducibility may be understood by way of a contrasting example:

The patient Elroy Fox does not feel well and shows a bronze skin color. The examination reveals that he has hepatitis that usually causes icterus, and in addition, he has myelodysplastic syndrome that causes increased melanin deposition in the skin. He is hospitalized and treated accordingly. After a few weeks his hepatitis is cured. His skin color now turns from bronze to grey. It takes a few additional weeks until his myelodysplastic syndrome is also cured. As a consequence, the grey coloration of his skin also disappears.

The example above shows that the patient's property *bronze skin color* is separable into two partial properties, i.e., yellow and grey skin coloration, each of which is attributable to a separate part or disordered function of the organism, i.e., yellow to hepatitis associated with the liver, and grey to myelodysplastic syndrome associated with bone marrow. A separable property $P = P_1 \cup P_2$ of this type is obviously compositional such that it is reducible to its constituent causes, i.e., hepatitis and myelodysplastic syndrome in the present example. It is a *resultant* of these causes. That is, hepatitis ∪ myelodysplastic syndrome → yellow ∪ grey, while yellow ∪ grey = bronze coloration of the skin. Thus, resultant properties in the organism are separable and reducible. By contrast, a systemic property such as loving or believing is non-separable and non-reducible. As mentioned above, such a property is called *emergent* as opposed to *resultant* (Lewes 1874, vol. II, 412).

Emergence is a phenomenon peculiar to the whole of a system as compared to its components. It is due simply to the fact that a system is an ordered pair ⟨Components, Relations between components⟩ which on logical grounds is different from its components:

$$\langle \text{Components, Relations between components} \rangle \neq \{ \text{Components} \}.$$

Thanks to the existing web of relations between them, the components bring about the system as a whole by their interaction, call this synergism. This is why any systemic property at a particular level of the organization of a system is an emergent property with respect to its lower level components' properties. The most interesting emergent systemic property of the organism is the *psyche*, which we shall study below. For a precise concept of emergence, see Definition 176 on page 729.[20]

The organism is a poietic system

To demonstrate that what is called the psyche is an emergent systemic feature of the organism, we shall first introduce a few conceptual tools. To begin with, it will be shown that the organism is a poietic system.

A *poietic system*, or a production system, is a system that makes, produces, or creates something. Examples are bakeries, brickyards, factories, bacteria, the stomach, the liver, etc. The latter one, for instance, receives blood and produces from it a large number of substances, e.g., bile, cholesterol, prothrombin, etc. Formally, a production system consists of:

---

[20] An elementary example of emergent properties is the sweet taste of sugar. It is an emergent property with respect to all the properties of carbon, hydrogen, and oxygen of which sugar is composed. A property P of a system $S = \langle \{C_1, \ldots, C_m\}, \{R_1, \ldots, R_n\} \rangle$ is an emergent property if (i) there is a general statement, say 'law', which states that all *systems* of the type S have that property; and (ii) the existing knowledge about the components $C_1, \ldots, C_m$ does not imply that they will produce the property P. That is, P cannot be explained or predicted by, and thus is not reducible to, the behavior of system components. This is the reason why "the whole is greater than the sum of its parts". The history of the concept of emergence begins with the British philosopher John Stuart Mill (1806–1873). In his *A System of Logic* (1843, 8th edition 1874), he anticipated what would later be called *resultant* and *emergent* effects by the British philosopher and literary critic George Henry Lewes (1817–1878) in his *Problems of Life and Mind* (1874, vol. II, 412).

- a set of *materials*,   such as: flour and water from which
- a set of *products*,   such as: bread is made by employing
- a set of *production operations*.

Thus, a production system is a system of the following form:

$$\langle \{\text{materials, products}\}, \{\text{production operations}\} \rangle$$

whose components are the set of *materials* and *products*, and whose relations are the set of its *production operations*. A production operation is a relation in the formal sense of the term and relates some material with some product produced therefrom. That is:

Operation O produces from material m the product p

such that we have $O(m, p)$. For instance, a metabolic operation in the organism relates a set of particular molecules with another such set in that it produces from the former ones the latter ones.

The organism is a poietic system of the type just defined in that it receives or takes from its environment materials from which it produces some products by employing a variety of production operations, be they of metabolic, mental, behavioral, or another type. Among its products are entities like physical energy, sweat, urine, feces, hairs, children, novels, poems, scientific theories, books, music, emotions, ideas, thoughts, political systems, love, peace, war, religious belief, etc.

Many causal cycles in the organism are well known as feedback loops. They may be negative or positive. Negative feedback enables regulatory mechanisms in the system to maintain equilibrium, e.g., the level of blood sugar concentration, blood pressure, heart rate, etc. Positive feedback amplifies deviation from equilibrium, and is thus a precondition of change, growth, and evolution.[21] Various products of the organism are catalyzers, e.g., enzymes and hormones. They catalyze biochemical processes. The production of many catalyzers is regulated in feedback loops to the effect that the process of catalysis, the loop, becomes an autocatalytic one. Regulatory mechanisms and autocatalysis render the organism an *autonomous system*.

---

[21] 'Positive' and 'negative' do not mean desirability or undesirability. When any change (increase or decrease) of the activity of a component occurs in a feedback loop, i.e., causal cycle, a *negative* feedback means that the cycle reverses the direction of change. For example, in the causal loop in Figure 16, hyperactivity of the thyroid gland will cause the hypophysis to reduce its thyroid-stimulating hormone, TSH, to the effect that the thyroidal hyperactivity stops. In a *positive* feedback loop, however, the response of the intervening component increases the deviation in the same direction. While negative feedback loops sustain stability of the system, positive feedback loops may run out of control and are thus destabilizing.

The organism is an endopoietic system

The prefix "endo" means *in, inner, interior*. The neologism "endopoiesis" is used as a shorthand for "the making of inner worlds" or *inner worldmaking* (Sadegh-Zadeh, 1970a–b, 2000d).

According to the theory of organism being outlined here the organism, as a poietic system, is in particular an *endopoietic system* bringing about many inner parts of itself, inner worlds so to speak. Examples are specific, acquired immunities against infectious diseases. Another one is what is usually called the psyche. We will clarify this idea by introducing the following three interdependent terms:

a. endomorphism,
b. endomorphosis,
c. fuzzy endomorphosis.

With the aid of these new concepts, an *endomorphosis theory of mind* will be proposed which says that the human mind, or psyche, is a fuzzy endomorphosis of the organism. Let us first recall the basis of our concepts, the term "homomorphism" introduced by Definition 6 on page 73:

Let $\mathcal{A} = \langle A, R_1, \ldots, R_n \rangle$ and $\mathcal{B} = \langle B, R'_1, \ldots, R'_n \rangle$ be two structures of the same type consisting of the base sets A and B, and the relations $R_1, \ldots, R_n$ and $R'_1, \ldots, R'_n$ thereon, respectively. A homomorphism from the structure $\mathcal{A}$ into the structure $\mathcal{B}$ is simply a relation preserving function h that maps the base set A of the first structure to the base set B of the second structure, $h : A \mapsto B$, in such a way that each relation $R_i \in \{R_1, \ldots, R_n\}$ between R_i-relata in set A is preserved in the relation $R'_i \in \{R'_1, \ldots, R'_n\}$ on set B. Our aim in introducing these tools is to show that the psyche may be conceived of as an emergent product of the organism under particular types of homomorphism from some states of the organism into other ones. They map the states of the organism to some of their own subsets to yield something that is referred to as the 'psyche'. To understand the nature of this mapping, we introduce below a special type of homomorphism called an *endomorphism*.

Definition 27 (Endomorphism). *If a function h is a homomorphism from a structure $\langle A, R_1, \ldots, R_n \rangle$ into another structure $\langle B, R'_1, \ldots, R'_n \rangle$, then it is an* endomorphism *on A iff $A = B$. That is, an endomorphism maps a set homomorphically to itself.*

For example, let $\langle \mathbb{R}^+, \geq \rangle$ be a structure consisting of the set of positive real numbers, $\mathbb{R}^+$, and the usual 'is greater than or equals' relation thereon. And let h be a mapping from $\mathbb{R}^+$ to $\mathbb{R}^+$:

$$h : \mathbb{R}^+ \mapsto \mathbb{R}^+$$

such that:

$$h(x) = x^2 \qquad \text{for all } x \in \mathbb{R}^+ \text{ where } x^2 \text{ is the square of } x,$$

then h is a homomorphism from $\langle \mathbb{R}^+, \geq \rangle$ into $\langle \mathbb{R}^+, \geq \rangle$ on the grounds that h is relation preserving. Whenever $x \in \mathbb{R}^+ \geq y \in \mathbb{R}^+$, then $h(x) \geq h(y)$, i.e., $x^2 \geq y^2$. Due to the self-mapping $h \colon \mathbb{R}^+ \mapsto \mathbb{R}^+$, the homomorphism h that in the present example signifies the squaring function $x^2 = x \cdot x$, is an endomorphism on $\mathbb{R}^+$.

According to our terminology, a set A may be simultaneously structured by many relations $R_1, \ldots, R_n$ yielding the structure $\langle A, R_1, \ldots, R_n \rangle$. The number n of relations on a set A is not limited. The inhabitants of a city as a base set A, for instance, are structured by neighborhood, spouse-hood, employer-employee relationship, teacher-pupil relationship, etc. Such a structure $\langle A, R_1, \ldots, R_n \rangle$ entails the individually discernible substructures $\langle A, R_1 \rangle$, $\langle A, R_2 \rangle$, ..., and $\langle A, R_n \rangle$. Depending on specific self-mappings of set A with respect to any of the relations $R_1 \ldots, R_n$ thereon, such a multi-ply structured set A may have a variety of endomorphisms constituting *the set of its endomorphisms*. We symbolize this set of endomorphisms of a set X by '$endo(X)$'. To give an example, consider the above set $\mathbb{R}^+$ of positive real numbers. The above-mentioned endomorphism by the squaring function $h(x) = x^2$ is only one single member of the huge set $endo(\mathbb{R}^+)$.

With the aid of the terminology above, we shall try to understand the nature and origin of mental states. To this end, the notion of endomorphism will be further specialized to the notion of a partial endomorphism.

Definition 28 (Partial endomorphism). *An endomorphism h from a structure $\langle A, R_1, \ldots, R_n \rangle$ into another structure $\langle B, R'_1, \ldots, R'_n \rangle$ is a partial endomorphism on A iff B is a subset of A, i.e., iff h maps A to a subset of itself. Otherwise put, an endomorphism h is a partial endomorphism iff $range(h) \subseteq domain(h)$. See Figure 19.*

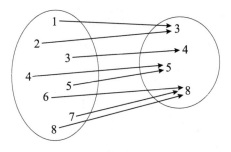

Fig. 19. A partial endomorphism. The set $\{1, 2, 3, 4, 5, 6, 7, 8\}$ is mapped to its subset $\{3, 4, 5, 8\}$ with respect to the relation "is greater than or equals" ($\geq$). If an element of the domain of the function is greater than or equals another element y, then its image is greater than or equals the image of y

Partial endomorphisms provide a basis for what we shall refer to as *endomorphosis* in the organism, a process that brings about the psyche. This idea may be illustrated by a simple example. When afflicted with an infectious disease such as measles, an organism's immune system begins producing antibodies and other forms of immunity against that disease. Specifically, the organism acts as a production system of the form $\langle \{antigens, antibodies\}, \{f\} \rangle$ that by a production operation, denoted "f", produces antibodies against anti-gens. That means that during the disease phase of the organism, its states map to states of its own immune system:

f: *states of the organism* $\mapsto$ *states of the immune system,*

symbolized by:

$f : A \mapsto B$

where $B \subseteq A$. The mapping is accomplished by states of the organism, i.e., set A, through exerting *causal influence* on the states of the immune system, set B, to produce a specific immunity. There are two aspects to be mentioned here:

First, the causal mapping of the organism to the immune system, denoted by the production operation "f" above, is a homomorphism. The reason is that if x and y are two antigens of the same type that cause the organism's immune system to produce two antibodies, $f(x)$ and $f(y)$, these antibodies are also of the same type in that they are directed against the same class of antigens. Thus, the homomorphism f is one from the structure $\langle A, R \rangle$ into the structure $\langle B, R \rangle$ where:

A is the set 'states of the organism'
B is the set 'states of the immune system'
R is the relation 'x is of the same type as y', and
$B \subseteq A$.

Second, the states of the immune system as the range of the homomorphism f are a subset of the domain A of f, that is, a subset of the states of the organism. Hence, the homomorphism f is a partial endomorphism. That means that the organism produces the immunity against a particular disease, such as measles, by a partial endomorphism. One may also concisely state that the organism produces an inner part of itself to act as a measles immune system.

A partial endomorphism as a whole is a function, $f : A \mapsto B$. Its range B is also called the *image* of the function. The domain of an endomorphism, A, may be a time-varying, dynamic set that grows or shrinks. An example is provided by the states of an infected organism that endomorphically map to a subset of themselves to produce immunity. In such cases with a dynamic domain, the image of the function f will also be subject to change. The process of acquiring immunity against a disease is such a change. A partial endomorphism of this type with a dynamic image we call a *dynamic partial endomorphism*. The acquisition of specific immunity against an infectious disease is an example.

Dynamic partial endomorphisms have a peculiarity that renders them out-standing processes to bring about emergent phenomena such as the psyche. To explain, suppose f and g are two dynamic partial endomorphisms of the form $f : A \mapsto B$ and $g : C \mapsto D$. They may also be one and the same dynamic en-domorphism at two successive points in time. Their dynamic character brings

with it that the image B of the first endomorphism, f, may become totally
or partially included in the domain C of the second endomorphism, g, to be
mapped to its image D. In such a case, we say that the first endomorphism
is totally or partially *embedded* in the second one. See Figure 20.

Fig. 20. The total embedding of the dynamic partial endomorphism f in the dynamic partial endomorphism g. A bold
arrow symbolizes a partial-endomorphic
mapping. The thin arrow from the image of the function f to the image of
the function g means that the image of
f is part of the domain of g, and thus
mapped by g to its image. Note that a
total embedding of an endomorphism f
in an endomorphism g is in fact a composition $g \circ f$ of the two functions. For composition of functions, see Section 25.4.2
on page 841

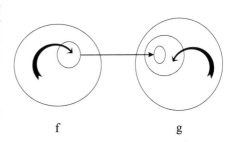

The embedding of a dynamic partial endomorphism in another one strings
them together to yield chains of arbitrary length. A chain of length $n \geq 1$
emerging in this way we refer to as a causal endomorphism or *endomorphosis*
of length n, or an *n*-ary endomorphosis for short, if each endomorphism in
the chain is a *causal relation*. This is the case when in an endomorphism
$f : A \mapsto B$ the function f is a causal relationship between A and B such
that A has a causal impact on B, for example, in the acquisition of immunity
when states of an infected organism cause the production of antibodies in the
immune system.

Our concept of endomorphosis is based on the idea that, in the organism, the image B in a dynamic partial endomorphism $f : A \mapsto B$ is a dynamic
entity that is produced by the organism itself, and therefore, subject to change
depending on all other changes occurring in the organism. Below we shall ask
whether the psyche and mental phenomena such as perception and consciousness may be understood as endomorphoses of the organism. To this end, we
will first fuzzify our terminology to build an instrumental framework.

The organism is a fuzzy causal system

In preceding sections, the organism has been characterized as a distributed,
cyclic-causal, autonomous, and endopoietic system capable of endomorphosis.
This conception will now be fuzzified because in reality the organism is a
fuzzy system rather than a crisp one. Its states, such as 'high blood pressure',
that exert causal influence on other states or processes, such as 'myocardial

blood flow' and 'cerebral blood flow', are vague to the effect that their causal influences also are vague occurrences. As a result, an n-ary endomorphosis in the organism must be viewed as a fuzzy process. To introduce such a concept of an *n-ary fuzzy endomorphosis*, we will start with fuzzifying the notion of a system itself. Concisely, a system S of the form:

$$S = \langle \text{Components, Relations between components} \rangle$$

is a *fuzzy system* if the relations between its components are fuzzy relations. For the notion of a *fuzzy relation*, see Section 30.3 on page 1011.

A more precise concept of a fuzzy system is obtained by fuzzifying the notion of a graph because a system is represented by a graph. A system is fuzzy if it has a *fuzzy graph*. But what is a fuzzy graph? It is simply a graph $\langle N, E \rangle$ whose nodes and edges are fuzzy sets. The most obvious case is when in a graph $\langle N, E \rangle$ the set of edges, E, is mapped to the unit interval $[0, 1]$ to yield a fuzzy set, and thus a fuzzy graph. This will now be explained.

Usually, the components of a system are connected to each other in varying degrees. Accordingly, the graph of a system may have information attached to each edge expressing some knowledge about the local strength of the relationship between its nodes. Well-known examples are road maps in which the distances between cities, as the graph's nodes, are indicated along the roads. Any such graph is called *weighted* if each edge is assigned some specific number. The number reflects the weight attached to the respective edge. Viewed from the formal perspective, that means that if $G = \langle N, E \rangle$ is a graph, then the set E of its edges as a subset of the Cartesian product $N \times N$ of its nodes is mapped to a set of numbers such that a number r can be attached to an edge $\langle a, b \rangle \in E$ as its value to obtain the triple $\langle a, b, r \rangle$. For instance, the set of cities on a road map is pairwise mapped to the set of positive real numbers such that a real number r is assigned to a pair of cities, $\langle a, b \rangle$, as their distance to yield the weighted edge $\langle a, b, r \rangle$, e.g., $\langle Hamburg, Berlin, 244 \rangle$ where the number 244 means "244 kilometers". See Figure 21 A.

Analogously, those parts of the human organism which are causally connected to each other, may do so with varying causal strength. For example, the anterior lobe of the pituitary gland exerts a greater causal influence on the thyroid gland than the posterior pituitary lobe. That means that in the causal graph of the human organism, the anterior lobe of the pituitary gland is causally *more strongly* connected to the thyroid gland than the posterior pituitary lobe. Generalizing this observation, we may state that the strength of causal relationship between the nodes of a graph may vary among its edges. A particular pair of nodes, $\langle a, b \rangle$, may be causally more strongly connected than another pair $\langle c, d \rangle$. That would mean that the extent of causal influence of a on b is greater than that of c on d. It is possible to express the strength of connection between two such nodes numerically (see Figure 21 B).

If in a weighted graph the weights of edges range over the unit interval $[0, 1]$ only, like in Figure 21 B, then obviously the set of edges, E, is mapped to the unit interval $[0, 1]$, and thus, we have a fuzzy set of edges to the effect that

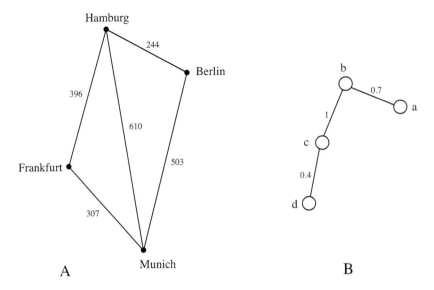

Fig. 21. Two weighted graphs. A: The beeline graph of four German cities. Compare with Figure 10 on page 115. B: A fuzzy graph. The graph is B = ⟨{a, b, c, d}, {⟨b, a, 0.7 ⟩, ⟨b, c, 1 ⟩, ⟨c, d, 0.4 ⟩}⟩. Obviously, the first component of B is a set of nodes, and its second component is a fuzzy relation on that set comprising the fuzzy edges of the graph. Compare with Figures 9–10 on page 115

the graph becomes a *fuzzy graph*. In a fuzzy graph, any edge ⟨x, y⟩ that joins the two nodes x and y with weight w may be formally represented by ⟨x, y, w⟩, for example, ⟨x, y, 0.7⟩. Thus, a fuzzy graph is a graph with weighted edges of the form ⟨x, y, w⟩ such that $w \in [0, 1]$.

When discussing etiology in Section 6.5, we shall see that in a causal system such as the human body the strength of the causal relationship between two nodes may be measured over the unit interval [0, 1]. For instance, in the example above the causal influence of the anterior lobe of the pituitary gland on the thyroid gland may amount to 0.7. If we similarly supplement the edges in the graph of the causal system *human body* with the weights of their causal strength, we obtain a fuzzy graph revealing that the human organism is a *fuzzy system* (Sadegh-Zadeh, 1982d).

To summarize as well as generalize the illustration above, we saw on page 114 that a graph is an ordered pair ⟨N, E⟩ with N being a set of nodes and E a relation on N. Similarly, a fuzzy graph is an ordered triple $G = ⟨N, \widetilde{N}, \widetilde{E}⟩$ with $\widetilde{N}$ being a fuzzy subset of N, called the *fuzzy node set* of G, and $\widetilde{E}$ being a fuzzy relation on $\widetilde{N}$ referred to as the *fuzzy edge set* of G. Note that in a fuzzy graph the set of nodes is also fuzzified yielding the fuzzy node set $\widetilde{N}$. For the sake of notational convenience, a fuzzy graph is also written as an ordered pair $\langle \widetilde{N}, \widetilde{E} \rangle$. However, in the special case where all elements of $\widetilde{N}$ have the value 1, i.e., are crisp, the fuzzy graph is written $\langle N, \widetilde{E} \rangle$ like in Figure 21 B.

A fuzzy graph represents a fuzzy system. The organism is a fuzzy system of this type, whose components are fuzzy entities and the causal relationships between them are fuzzy causal relations. A fuzzy system of this type we call a *fuzzy causal system*. Thus, the organism is a fuzzy causal system. See also Section 6.5.

Is the organism a machine?

Since René Descartes there has been an ongoing debate about whether the human organism is a machine or not. We will not participate in this debate, as it is exclusively due to confusions about the concepts of organism and machine. Our aim here is to help settle the controversy in the philosophy of medicine between the so-called mechanists and humanists by concisely presenting the general, formal concept of machine, which was developed in the sciences of logic and mathematics during the last century. We shall also need the concept of machine in Chapter 12 to demonstrate that a medical experiment is a machine, specifically a knowledge machine.

There are two main types of machines, crisp and fuzzy ones. We shall first outline the crisp concept of a machine, followed by its fuzzy counterpart. In both cases, we shall confine ourselves to *deterministic, finite-state* machines. There are also indeterministic and infinite-sate machines. We will not go into details here, however. For details on the theory of machines, see (Anderson, 2006).

A deterministic, finite-state or sequential machine, usually called an input-output machine or automaton, is a dynamic system comprising (a) a finite number of *internal states*; (b) a *state-transition relation*, S, that upon receiving some *input stimuli* transforms some current internal states to new ones; and (c) an *output relation*, OR, that associates a sequence of internal states with a sequence of *output states* called responses, actions, or products. A pretty simple example is a flower vending automaton. It contains flowers as its internal states, and you input money into it to get some flowers as output. This brief sketch may be precisely represented by the following set-theoretical predicate:

Definition 29 (Finite-state machine). *An object x is a finite-state machine iff there are I, Z, O, S, and OR such that:*

1. *$x = \langle I, Z, O, S, OR \rangle$;*
2. *$I = \{i_1, i_2, \ldots\}$ is a non-empty, finite set referred to as input states or stimuli;*
3. *$Z = \{z_0, z_1, z_2, \ldots\}$ is a non-empty, finite set called internal states of the machine with z_0 being its initial state in order that it can start;*
4. *$O = \{o_1, o_2, \ldots\}$ is a non-empty, finite set called output states, responses, actions, or products;*

5. S is a ternary relation on the Cartesian product $I \times Z \times Z$ called state-transition relation. It associates elements of set I with elements of set Z to generate new elements in set Z. Otherwise put, when an input $i_k \in I$ comes in and the machine is in the internal state $z_i \in Z$, then on this basis the state transition relation S produces the next internal state $z_{i+1} \in Z$, i.e., $S(i_k, z_i, z_{i+1})$. For instance, $S(i_6, z_4, z_5)$. In this example, S produces from the sixth input and fourth internal state the fifth internal state;

6. OR is a binary relation on the Cartesian product $Z \times O$ referred to as response or output relation. It associates sequences of set Z with sequences of set O. That is, it produces from an internal state $z_i \in Z$ an output state $o_j \in O$ such that $OR(z_i, o_j)$. For instance, $OR(z_5, o_3)$. In this example, OR produces from the fifth internal state the third output. See Figure 22.

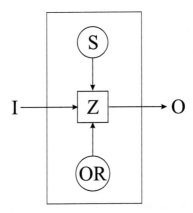

Fig. 22. The basic scheme of a deterministic, finite-state or sequential machine

A concept of *fuzzy machine* is easily obtained from the crisp concept above by fuzzifying its constituents. A machine is simply a fuzzy one if (a) its input, internal, and output states are fuzzy sets; and (b) its state-transition relation and output relation are fuzzy relations on those sets. For details on fuzzy machines, see (Klir and Yuan, 1995; Mordeson and Malik, 2002).

Definition 30 (Finite-sate fuzzy machine). *An object x is a* finite-state fuzzy machine *iff there are I, Z, O, S, and OR such that:*

1. $x = \langle I, Z, O, S, OR \rangle$;
2. $I = \{I_1, I_2, \ldots\}$ *is a non-empty, finite set of fuzzy sets (input states);*
3. $Z = \{Z_0, Z_1, Z_2, \ldots\}$ *is a non-empty, finite set of fuzzy sets (internal states);*
4. $O = \{O_1, O_2, \ldots\}$ *is a non-empty, finite set of fuzzy sets (output states);*
5. S *is a ternary fuzzy relation on $I \times Z \times Z$ (state-transition relation);*
6. OR *is a binary fuzzy relation on the Cartesian product $Z \times O$ (output relation).*

For instance, radios, windmills, computers, and as we shall demonstrate in Chapter 12, scientific experiments are all finite-state, fuzzy machines. Plants and animals fit the concept of fuzzy machine as well. For example, a cat receives a fuzzy set of optical stimuli as input. This input excites a number of its retinal and brain cells (transition of internal states), and it sees a dog approaching and runs away (output, product, response, action). The internal states subject to transition constitute a fuzzy set in that there are no sharp boundaries between those retinal and brain cells which participate in the cat's optical perception, and those which do not. The state-transition relation, i.e., the neuronal excitation in the present example, is also a fuzzy relation because it relates a fuzzy set of input stimuli with a fuzzy set of internal states to produce a new fuzzy set of internal states. Thus, the cat referred to is a fuzzy machine. To justify this claim, let there be a cat with following characteristics:

I_1 $\equiv$ a fuzzy set of optical stimuli that meets the cat's eyes;

Z_0 $\equiv$ a fuzzy set of initial states of some retinal and brain cells of the cat, i.e., their states before they are affected by I_1;

Z_1 $\equiv$ another fuzzy set of internal states of some retinal and brain cells of the cat, i.e., their states after they are affected by I_1;

Z_2 $\equiv$ a fuzzy set of states of some motoneurons and muscles of the cat;

O_1 $\equiv$ a fuzzy set of motor reactions of the cat called "running away";

S $\equiv$ a fuzzy state-transition relation such that $S(I_1, Z_0, Z_1 \cup Z_2)$;

OR $\equiv$ a fuzzy output relation such that $OR(Z_2, O_1)$.

Our claim that the cat above is a fuzzy machine means that its following subsystem is a finite-state, fuzzy machine according to Definition 30:

$$\langle \{I_1\}, \{Z_0, Z_1, Z_2\}, \{O_1\}, S, OR \rangle.$$

Many other features of the same cat characterize it as a fuzzy machine in the same fashion, e.g., its reproductive faculty and its nutrition, digestion, and metabolism. Roughly, our example cat is a *model for* the set-theoretical predicate "is a finite-state, fuzzy machine" introduced by Definition 30. For the notion of a "model for a set-theoretical predicate", see page 408. The general notion of a model has been introduced on page 886 in Part VIII.

6.2.2 The Psyche

As was emphasized previously, there is no mind-body dualism in our theory of the patient. Rather, the organism and mind, i.e., psyche, constitute a unity in that the psyche is produced, like disease-specific immunity, by the organism as one of its subsystems. This *endopoietic* whole-part relationship between the organism and its psyche will be outlined in what follows.

We should be aware at the outset that the doctrine of mind-body dualism arises from obscuring the nature of mental states (events, processes, properties, features, attributes, traits, faculties) such as intelligence, memory, thoughts, emotions, feelings, sensations, perceptions, and the like. To clarify the issue, we shall first differentiate between two types of mental states, objective and subjective ones, and shall argue that what is usually called the *psyche*, is characterized by subjective mental states.

In addition to the term "psyche", there are two other umbrella terms under which human subjective mental states are subsumed, i.e., "consciousness" and "self-consciousness". An individual who manifests a subjective mental state by reporting, for example, "I am *happy*", "I am in *pain*", or "I *believe* that AIDS is caused by HIV", indicates thereby that she is conscious, or aware, of herself. To explain the nature and origin of the human psyche, the terms "consciousness" and "self-consciousness" are better candidates because in each case they refer to a particular, existent individual, whereas the term "psyche" merely nominalizes something too obscure to be sensibly analyzable. For this reason, it is both convenient and sufficient to explain what consciousness and self-consciousness are and where they come from. To this end, we shall advance an emergentist theory of consciousness and self-consciousness to argue that they originate from the organism by fuzzy endomorphosis. Our analysis is thus concerned with:

▶ Mental states and terms
▶ The concepts of consciousness and self-consciousness
▶ Cerebral representation of the organism
▶ The origin of consciousness and self-consciousness.

Mental states and terms

To understand consciousness and self-consciousness, we must first understand the nature of mental states and the terms that denote them. We distinguish the following two types of mental states:

a) *subjective* mental states: A subjective mental state is one whose presence or absence in an individual can only be determined by the individual herself. Examples are properties such as *pain, sadness, pleasure, anxiety, hope, belief, conviction,* and other propositional attitudes. Only an individual herself has the so-called privileged access to her subjective mental states and can recognize that she feels pain, is sad, is pleased, believes that the Eiffel Tower stands in Tokyo, etc.

b) *objective* mental states: An objective, or intersubjective, mental state is one whose presence or absence in an individual can also be determined by persons other than the individual herself. For example, a statement such as "Elroy Fox is intelligent" or "Elroy Fox has a good memory" can be verified or falsified by a psychologist who is different from Elroy Fox.

Terms denoting such mental states are referred to as subjective mental terms and objective mental terms, respectively. It is worth noting that there is no sharp division between objective mental terms and behavioral ones, i.e., terms that refer to observable, public behavior such as *hyperactivity*. Thus, objective mental terms do not give rise to metaphysical debates in the philosophy of mind. The main source of controversies is the class of subjective mental terms. Therefore, only terms of this type will be considered here. They describe self-consciousness proper. For this reason, the question of what self-consciousness is, reduces to what subjective mental terms refer to. There are competing answers to this question that have come to be called "theories of mind". We shall consider them in Section 19.3.1.

The concepts of consciousness and self-consciousness

To explicate the concept of self-consciousness, we shall start with the basic attribute *consciousness*, which some living creatures possess. The self-consciousness of a creature is an attribute of this creature that refers to its own consciousness. Contemporary neurosciences and neurophilosophy have caused much conceptual confusion by ceaselessly propagating the thesis that the brain is the source and seat of consciousness and self-consciousness. However, we shall see below that this thesis is grossly wrong. Consciousness and self-consciousness are features of the whole organism brought about by the synergism, i.e., collaboration, of its subsystems. They are not faculties of the single organ *brain* because, like any other organ, the brain is not self-sustaining. Rather, it is dependent on the rest of the organism, and its functioning is conditioned and influenced thereby. This fundamentally important fact will be demonstrated by differentiating between consciousness and self-consciousness in the following two sections.

Consciousness

Consciousness, or awareness, is a systemic property of human beings and some animals. The qualification "systemic" means that it is the whole organism as a system that is aware of something, but none of its proper parts such as the liver, the big toe, or the brain. Otherwise put, the correct syntax of the two-place predicate "is aware of" is the sentence "x is aware of y" such that x is an organism. And "awareness" means the state or process of recognizing by the organism that there is something, y, in the outer world or in its own inner world, e.g., perceiving a bird in a garden, smelling a flower in a vase, having a stomachache, or feeling sad. These examples show that what we shall be considering here is the so-called *phenomenal consciousness*.[22]

According to the considerations above, awareness has two integral aspects. On the one hand, an organism may be aware of something in the external

---

[22] Some philosophers of mind also debate additional types of consciousness that we shall not consider here, e.g., monitoring consciousness, access consciousness, transitive and intransitive consciousness, etc. (Block, 1997, 213 ff.)

world. On the other hand, it may be aware of something in its internal world. These two capabilities may be referred to as exo-cognition and endo-cognition, respectively. For instance, a cat that sees a dog or a mouse nearby is aware of something in the external world. This exemplifies exo-cognition. And when she feels hungry or is in pain, then she is perceiving some states of her own organism. In this case, she is aware of something in her internal world. This exemplifies endo-cognition. The consciousness of an organism comprises its exo-cognition and endo-cognition (Sadegh-Zadeh, 1970b).

The awareness sketched thus far may be termed awareness or consciousness of the first order, denoted C_1. The subject of C_1 comprises entities and processes in the external and internal world of the organism. Self-consciousness is something different. We shall conceive it as an awareness of the second order, C_2, whose subject is the consciousness of the first order itself, C_1. Thus, it is an awareness of one's own awareness, i.e., a meta-awareness in the following sense.

Self-consciousness

Not every conscious organism is self-conscious, be it an animal or a human being, e.g., a newborn or a severely brain-damaged patient. A conscious creature that is aware of something is self-conscious if she is, in addition, *aware of the fact that* she herself is the agent of that first-order awareness. Otherwise put, self-consciousness is self-referential consciousness. For example, a cat that *feels a pain* in her paw is in fact aware of that pain. But this conscious cat is not aware that it is she who feels pain. She lacks the self-reference of her consciousness, i.e., the awareness that she herself is the subject of her awareness of the pain. The same holds true for a severely brain-damaged patient in the vegetative state. Although she may experience pain or high body temperature, she will *not know* that she is experiencing pain or high body temperature. By contrast, a healthy, adult human being knows that her consciousness concerns herself. She is aware that it is she who is perceiving a bird in a garden, is smelling a flower in a vase, or feels sad or hungry. Thus, in addition to being conscious, a healthy, adult human being is self-conscious. What is this self-consciousness and how does it arise?

The prefix "self" plays a fundamental role in the terms "self-conscious" and "self-consciousness". It is an analog of the prefix found in well-known concepts such as "self-control", "self-determination", "self-organization", and others (see also Sommerhoff, 2000, 48). It does not designate an invisible, incorporeal entity, instance, agent, or power hidden somewhere in the human organism as its "self" of which one is aware when one is self-conscious. It only means that in being self-conscious, an organism refers to it*self*. This self-reference is usually communicated by first-person sentences of the form "I am such and such", for example, "I am hungry", "I see a bird in the garden", or "I feel sad". By demonstrating that such first person sentences are gratuitous, we will shed some light on the prefix "self", and thus on self-reference and self-consciousness.

A first-person sentence is the expression of an organism's self-ascription "I am such and such" that is based on its *self-monitoring* (Baars, 1988), traditionally termed "introspection". It is always of the form "I X". Representing the perspective of the experiencing agent, it is composed of the first-person pronoun "I" and at least one verb X, e.g., "feel sad" or "am hungry". By means of the pronoun "I", a first-person sentence "I X" points to the producer of the sentence and is, therefore, called an indexical behavior or indexical utterance. Particularly important for understanding self-reference and self-consciousness, then, is understanding the nature and role of the indexical "I".

An *indexical* is a referring term that picks a particular object out from among a myriad of objects. Examples are expressions such as "here", "now", "this", "I", and "you". Which particular thing an indexical picks out, depends on the context of its utterance. For instance, the indexical "here" refers to the place of utterance, and the indexical "now" refers to the time of utterance. Likewise, the pronoun "I" is simply an indexical that refers to whoever is speaking. Thus, it represents an expression of self-reference. So, the sentence "I am happy" uttered by you means something different than when I use the same sentence. For details on indexicals, see (Brinck, 1997; Perry, 2000).

Whether loudly spoken, written, or silently thought, by conveying the self-reference of the speaker, the use of the indexical "I" indicates her self-monitoring. Despite widespread and diverse psychological theories on the opaque Ego, e.g., the Freudian psychoanalysis, it is sobering to recognize that like any other indexical, "I" is a gratuitous phrase. It can completely be omitted. Any first-person report of the form "I am such and such" may be replaced without loss by the declarative utterance "the organism that is speaking to you is such and such", e.g., "the organism that is speaking to you feels happy", or "the organism that is speaking to you has a stomachache". For details of this *redundancy theory of "I"*, see (Sadegh-Zadeh, 2000d).

According to the redundancy theory of "I", the indexical "I" plays only a social role to directly announce or indicate the author of a message to the recipients of the message. There are no such instances as *the Ego, the I*, or *the Self* in the human psyche having the gratuitous phrase "I" as their voice. This pragmatic indexical merely represents the self-reference of a self-monitoring organism. Therefore, to be an indexically self-referential organism capable of self-monitoring is simply to be self-conscious.[23]

---

[23] There is obviously a considerable difference between our concept of self-consciousness and that of some other authors such as Ned Block who says: "Self-consciousness is the possession of the concept of the S E L F and the ability to use this concept in thinking about oneself" (Block, 1997, 213). We do not postulate the existence of a *Self* in the organism (Sadegh-Zadeh, 1970a–b, 2000d). The idea of conceiving instances such as *I, Ego*, and *Self* in the human psyche has originated with René Descartes. He was the first in the history of Western philosophy to nominalize the pronoun "I" by the subject "I" (ego) in the following way: "I

Thus far we have arrived at the conclusion that a first-person, mental statement made by an agent is a self-monitoring, or introspective, self-ascription or *self-diagnosis*. If the agent's name is "a", then a first-person sentence such as "I am sad" uttered by a is the same as "a is sad" diagnosed by a. Like any other diagnosis, a mental self-diagnosis may of course be a misdiagnosis. A hearer cannot discern whether a mental, first-person self-diagnosis made by a speaker is right or wrong. When someone says "I am sad", the hearer is always entitled to ask, for example, "is she really sad, as she says, or maybe she is in pain? Does she possibly confuse sadness and pain?". That is, the self-consciousness of an individual is prone to error and even illusion and delusion. Its reliability depends, among other things, on the semantic quality of the language an agent uses in her first-person sentences. Misunderstandings will arise when she understands, for example, by "feeling hungry" or "feeling sad" something different than other people do. Unfortunately, however, a semantic consensus about subjective mental terms will never be reached because all subjective mental states are fuzzy. No sharp division exists, for example, between anxiety, sadness, and pain. Moreover, due to the social origin and character of language, an individual's use of mental vocabulary to describe her mental states is socially shaped. As a result, self-consciousness as the self-diagnostic capacity of the individual is society-dependent (see Section 6.2.2).

Let α be a mental self-diagnosis by an individual. The state of affairs diagnosed by α is denoted $\hat{s}(\alpha)$. For instance, given a mental predicate P, then the state of affairs referred to by the self-diagnosis "I am P" is $\hat{s}(I$ am $P)$. A simple example is $\hat{s}(I$ am sad), i.e., a speaker's self-reported *sadness* communicated by her introspective first-person sentence "I am sad". Now, the central question regarding the nature of self-consciousness is this:

- What kind of an entity is a state of affairs of the type $\hat{s}(I$ am $P)$, and how is it diagnosed by an agent who reports "I am P"?

To answer this question, we will first introduce the notion of a cognitive system by distinguishing between *explorative* systems and *cognitive* systems.

An explorative system is one that by exploring the external world is capable of finding and localizing objects. For example, a radar can find out the position and trajectory of moving objects, e.g., flying aircrafts. Thus, it is an explorative system. Likewise, bats and whales are explorative systems. They use ultrasound to localize distant objects. A specialized explorative system

---

know that I exist, and ask myself, what *this I* is whom I know" ("Novi me existere; quaero quis sim ego ille quem novi" (Descartes, 1986, 84) (emphasis added). Following Descartes, John Locke committed a similar mistake by nominalizing the particle "self" occurring in phrases such as "oneself", "myself", and "itself" in the following way: "*Self* is that conscious thinking thing, (whatever Substance, made up of whether Spiritual, or Material, Simple, or Compounded, it matters not) which is sensible, or conscious of Pleasure and Pain, capable of Happiness or Misery, and so is concern'd for it *self*, as far as that consciousness extends" (Locke, 2008, Book II, section xxvii, § 17, p. 214).

may also possess internal representations of the objects that it explores. For example, a particular, sophisticated radar may be an expert device for recognizing specific types of aircrafts, say Boeing aircrafts. The representation of the object in the explorative system may be something physical, chemical, graphical, or otherwise. In any event, the device compares with its internal representation the reflected signals received from the external object, and is able to categorize it in this way. An explorative system with such additional, diagnostic capability is referred to as a *cognitive* system. Human beings and higher animals are cognitive systems. They not only explore, but also recognize objects in their surroundings.

What if a cognitive system possesses internal representations not only of external objects, but also of its own constituent parts, for example, when a radar entails internal representations of its own screws, or an organism houses internal representations of its stomach, gallbladder, and fingers? This unsurprising question suggests that we distinguish between exo-cognitive and endo-cognitive systems depending on whether the objects recognized are in the external or in the internal world of the cognitive system. The cognitive systems discussed above, e.g., the expert radar, are only exo-cognitive systems. Human beings and higher animals, however, are in addition capable of endo-cognition. They possess internal representations of their constituent parts and are thus capable of recognizing processes occurring in themselves, for example, a stomachache (see below).

The above self-diagnosis of the form "I am P" is based on exo-cognition *and* endo-cognition. The subject of this cognition is the state of affairs $\hat{s}(\text{I am } P)$. A prerequisite is an internal representation of $\hat{s}(\text{I am } P)$. This prerequisite is fulfilled in human beings and higher animals by the representation of the organism in the brain that will be outlined in the next section.

Cerebral representation of the organism

Consciousness includes awareness of the surrounding world (exo-cognition) and of one's own body, feelings, and thoughts (endo-cognition). Endo-cognition and exo-cognition become possible only because the human brain houses an extensive internal representation of the body, the so-called *body schema,* on the one hand; and of the external world, on the other. The former is innate, while the latter is acquired by experience. The causal relevance of these two cerebral representations to the emergence of consciousness and self-consciousness will be discussed in what follows. Our discussion relies upon (Sadegh-Zadeh, 1970b, 2000d; Sommerhoff, 2000).

By stimulating the cerebral cortex, i.e., the outer layer of the brain, of awake epileptic patients during operations, the Canadian neurosurgeon Wilder Graves Penfield (1891–1976) and his team discovered in the 1950s that the human body was relatively extensively represented in different cortical areas (Penfield and Jasper, 1954). There are two major representations that have come to be known as Penfiled's homunculi or the body scheme, a primary *somatosensory* and a primary *somatomotor* one (Figure 23).

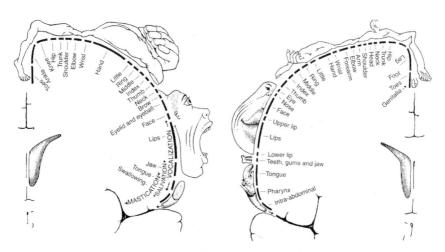

Fig. 23. Drawings of somatosensory (left-hand side) and somatomotor (right-hand side) representations of the human body in the cerebral cortex (Standring, 2005). Note that some body parts such as the face and the hand have a disproportionately larger representation than other areas. This is the reason why regions such as finger-tips and lips (in the left-hand side representation) are much more sensitive to touch, temperature, pressure, and pain than, say, the heels. The primary somatomotor representation (right-hand side) from where motor impulses to skeletal muscle groups originate, is located in the cortex of frontal lobe of the brain. It is responsible for intentional actions. The Latin term "cortex" means the outer layer of an organ, and "cortical" is its adjective

We shall here be concerned with the somatosensory representation only. The primary somatosensory representation is located in the cortex of the parietal lobe. Neurons of this area receive signals from the receptors of peripheral senses (touch, temperature, pressure, pain) in the skin, muscles, joints, and upper parts of the digestive and respiratory systems, i.e., mouth, pharynx, and larynx. So, this somatosensory representation in the parietal lobe is the cerebral center of information for an organism about its own somatosensory state. For example, when there is an injury to the right middle finger, this peripheral damage will excite via neural pathways the cortical neurons in the right parietal lobe where the right middle finger is represented, and the individual will experience *pain* in that finger. We shall discuss below how this awareness of pain may be understood as an endo-cognition. A second important aspect of the cerebral representation of the body is the origin, or 'seat', of basic emotions such as fear and pleasure in the *limbic system*. This system consists primarily of the hypothalamus, amygdala, hippocampus, parahippocampal cortex, and nucleus accumbens, the so-called pleasure center. It is densely connected with the neocortex in the prefrontal lobe and is therefore nicknamed *the feeling part of the thinking brain*.[24] In addition to the cerebral representation of the body (CRB) sketched above, there is also a cerebral representation of the external world (CREW) as it is presented to us by our tactile, visual, auditory, olfactory, and other sensory subsystems. For example, sensory pathways for vision and hearing reach their primary *projection areas* in the occipital cortex and superior temporal gyrus, respectively. There is a hierarchy of such sensory projection areas with primary, secondary, and higher areas representing the visual and auditory inputs in increasingly abstract ways. Also note that the CREW is actually a representation of the current state of body parts, e.g., retina, ear, and nose, as stimuli from the external world affect their excitable receptors. For this reason, we consider the CRB and CREW jointly as a *cerebral representation of the organism* (CRO). On the basis of the CRO, consciousness and self-consciousness emerge in the following way:

The origin of consciousness and self-consciousness

Almost all sensory occurrences in body parts are signalled to, and causally influence the neural processes in, the CRO. The first result is a body sense, i.e., a subverbal awareness about the body and its location and movement in the external world. We consider the processes in the CRO to be the *primary consciousness* because by these processes the organism demonstrates that it is aware of the occurrences from which they originate (Sadegh-Zadeh, 1970b; Sommerhoff, 2000, 62). For instance, an injury in the right middle finger causes some neural changes in that finger's map in the somatosensory homunculus. These cerebral-neural changes together with the peripheral injury itself and all other bodily reactions to the injury are subjectively experienced as pain. This subjective experience, referred to in the philosophy of mind as a "quale" (in the singular, and "qualia" in the plural), is a new, emergent feature of the whole organism brought about by its collaborating subsystems. It is not produced by a single body part, is not identical with the neural processes in the CRO, and cannot be reduced to them. (For the concept of emergence, see footnote 20 on page 121, as well as page 728.)

The occurrences in the primary representation areas of CRO are re-represented, or *metarepresented*, in higher-order regions of the brain, i.e., in

---

[24] Roughly, the human brain consists of three layers. The oldest layer is called the *reptilian brain* that mainly consists of the brainstem (medulla oblongata, pons, cerebellum, etc.). It controls survival activities such as breathing, heart rate, and balance. The *mammalian brain* is layered over the reptilian brain. It consists primarily of the *limbic system* (from the Latin term "limbus" meaning "border") and controls the autonomic nervous system and the endocrine system. The most recent layer is the *primate brain* or *neocortex* mainly consisting of the wrinkled covering of the brain hemispheres (Standring, 2005).

secondary and tertiary projection and association areas where different sensory modalities are associated with one another, e.g., touch with hearing and seeing. These higher-order regions also include the two speech centers, i.e., Broca's and Wernicke's areas (see page 727). The speech centers 'read' the metarepresentations and describe them, implicitly or explicitly, by first-person sentences of the form "I see a bird in the garden" or "I feel pain in my right middle finger". These self-reported metarepresentations are endo-cognitions. They constitute the self-consciousness of the organism, which self-referentially monitors and diagnoses the processes occurring within itself by using the pronoun "I". As was outlined on page 135, the first-person pronoun "I" should not give rise to the variegated issues of "self" in the philosophy of mind. It is a gratuitous indexical and may be replaced with a definite descriptor such as "the organism that is speaking to you now". Its origin and function are to be sought in the social sphere, which thereby plays a major role in the genesis and development of self-consciousness, i.e., mind (see Section 6.2.2).[25]

The stream of consciousness and self-consciousness is involuntarily stored in memory in terms of episodes. These episodes are also subject to metarepresentation, reflection, re-interpretation, and reorganization by higher regions of the brain. The edifice of these unceasingly reshaped episodes includes a self-image of the individual, on the one hand; and a world-image or worldview, on the other. It entails a past, a present, and a future. The meaning as well as the time order of a past or present experience may change upon reflection and in light of new experiences. The past may change the present and the present may change the past. Parts of the edifice may actively or passively sink into oblivion and become unconscious or be lost forever. What is usually called mind, essentially involves this dynamic construct that may best be characterized as a *palimpsest*. The palimpsest is self-referential in that it is more or less accessible to current self-consciousness and amenable to being processed thereby (Sadegh-Zadeh, 1970b).[26]

The palimpsest theory of mind above implies that without memory there is no mind. The primary consciousness may remain intact nonetheless because the CRO still works, and it is independent of memory. For instance, a patient with advanced Alzheimer's disease has lost her memory and consequently also

---

[25] The gratuitousness of "I" is reflected in every scientific publication whose author says "the present author found in her research that such and such is the case" rather than "I found in my research that such and such is the case".

[26] A palimpsest is a written page that has been frequently re-used by scraping off, or writing over, the original writing. The term derives from the Greek πάλιν (palin) for "again", and ψάειν (psaein) for "to scrape". It has first been used by Cicero (106–43 BC) to refer to the Roman practice of scraping and reusing waxen tablets. An allusion to memory as a palimpsest was made for the first time in 1828 by the English poet Samuel Taylor Coleridge (1772–1834) who in a prefatory note to his fragmentary poem "The Wanderings of Cain" wrote "I have in vain tried to recover the lines from the palimpsest tablet of my memory ..." (Reisner, 1982, 93).

her mind, whereas she is still capable of feeling pain in her right middle finger. This example convincingly demonstrates that the absence of self-consciousness is compatible with the presence of consciousness, but not vice versa. This is why consciousness is legally and morally significant in deciding life and death questions. For from both a legal and moral point of view it is the presence of consciousness that brings an agent's interests to bear.

On the considerations above, we suppose that like specific immunity against a particular infectious disease, also consciousness, self-consciousness, and mind emerge as inner worlds of the organism by the process of fuzzy endomorphosis. To explain, we need to take two minor steps. First, we will extend the basic notion of endomorphosis, which was introduced on page 126, to obtain the notion of fuzzy endomorphosis. Second, we will be more explicit about what is represented by the CRO.

An endomorphism f from a structure $\mathcal{A} = \langle A, \mathcal{R} \rangle$ into another structure $\mathcal{B} = \langle B, \mathcal{R}' \rangle$ is referred to as a fuzzy endomorphism if A and B comprise fuzzy sets and the homomorphism $f \colon A \mapsto B$ maps fuzzy sets in A to fuzzy sets in B. An n-ary fuzzy endomorphosis is a chain of $n \geq 1$ dynamic, causal, fuzzy endomorphisms such that each of them is embedded in the succeeding one. For the basic notions of dynamic and causal endomorphism, see page 126.

We will now briefly explain what is represented by the CRO in the brain and how the representation works. Single states of an individual organism at a particular time are physiological features such as blood pressure, blood sugar level, heart rate, the number of excited retinal neurons, the magnitude of excitation of cutaneous pain receptors, and so on. Let the set of *all* such states in an individual at a particular time t be denoted by Ω, referred to as the state space of the organism at that time. This state space Ω may be fuzzified by taking into account that an individual may have, for example, *high* blood pressure, *low* blood sugar level, *medium* heart rate, *a few* excited retinal neurons, etc. The collection of these single states is a fuzzy set of states over Ω. There are a practically infinite number of such fuzzy sets over the state space Ω any one of which the individual may present at time t, referred to as the *current state of the organism*. The set comprising all fuzzy sets over Ω constitutes the fuzzy powerset of the state space Ω, i.e., $F(2^{\Omega})$. The current state of the organism is thus an element of $F(2^{\Omega})$, i.e., a fuzzy set of states. (For the concept of fuzzy powerset, see Section 30.2.3 on page 1007.)

The CRO provides a representation of the *current state* of the organism. Represented in the proper sense of this term are those body parts which are connected with the somatosensory homunculus and primary sensory projection areas via neural pathways. Almost all sensory occurrences in those body parts are signalled to, and causally influence the neural processes in, the CRO. In addition to this direct causal impact via neural pathways, however, a large number of other states of the organism are *humorally* mediated to the somatosensory homunculus and primary sensory projection areas via blood circulation. In this way, neurophysiologically relevant chemical and biochemical substances in the blood originating from all body cells exert significant causal impact on neural processes in the cerebral representation areas. Examples are not only substances such as oxygen, carbon dioxide, electrolytes, trace elements, glucose, hormones, and toxic material, but also non-chemical factors such as heart rate and blood pressure. All such substances and factors and their increase and decrease maintain and influence the metabolism in, and the excitability of, neurons in the CRO. We are emphasizing this non-neural control of the CRO because it is generally overlooked in the neurophysiology, psychology, and philosophy of mind. We are therefore suggesting a holistic theory of mind according to which the mind does not depend on the brain alone and is not just in the head. It is produced *by the whole organism* in the following way (Sadegh-Zadeh, 1970b, 2000d):

Let $A \in F(2^\Omega)$ be the current state of an organism, i.e., the fuzzy set of *all* states of the organism at a particular time t. The causal impact of the organism on its CRO is an endomorphism of the organism on the grounds that A is homomorphically mapped to some brain cell states, i.e., to a subset of A itself in the somatosensory homunculus and primary projection areas. The homomorphic character of the mapping consists in the fact that via neural pathways, (i) spatially close body areas in the periphery map to spatially close brain cells, and (ii) temporally close states of body parts cause temporally close states of brain cells. That is, topographic closeness between body parts and temporal closeness between their states are the relations that are preserved in the CRO. Thus, CRO as an endomorphism is in fact a fuzzy endomorphism since the organisms's current state, A, is a fuzzy set and maps to one of its own subsets.

As pointed out above, the CRO is metarepresented in higher-order brain areas. This metarepresentation is also a fuzzy endomorphism in the same fashion as above. In this way, the primary CRO becomes embedded in a succeeding fuzzy endomorphism. These concatenated fuzzy endomorphisms are causal relations since the CRO is caused by the periphery and causes the metarepresentation. Thus, they bring about an n-ary *fuzzy endomorphosis* called self-consciousness.

6.2.3 The Social Agent

As human beings, we are unable to live as monads. Everyone of us is a member of one or more groups and a larger society. Anything we do or achieve is largely dependent on the co-operation of others. This is the spirit of Aristotle's famous dictum "man by nature is a social animal" (Aristotle, 2009, Book One, Part II). It is not our aim here to discuss the sociology of the patient as a 'social animal'. Instead, to round off our medical anthropology, we will briefly touch on the following three aspects in order to show that the patient's health, illness, and recovery are subject to the consequences of her unavoidable interactions: the social construction of the patient's self-consciousness, the pathogenicity of interactions, and morality. The consideration of morality will directly lead us to the question of what it means to say that the patient ought to be treated as a person. Thus, our discussion divides into the following four sections:

- ▶ Sociosomatics
- ▶ The moral agent
- ▶ Free will
- ▶ The patient as a person.

Sociosomatics

Living in a society brings with it many consequences, such as exposure to contagious diseases. However, contagious diseases are not the only effects of social interactions. In general, an individual's interactions with others will have a causal impact on almost all areas of her development and life. For instance, there are theories according to which even mental states are socially constructed by a growing individual's interactions (Wittgenstein, 1953, sections 243–317; Bloor, 1983, ch. 4). When some observable behavior of a child is interpreted as an indicator of pain by adults, and the child is told "you're in pain" instead of "you are under demonic attack", then the child learns to label her similar sensations as "pain" instead of "demonic attack". In other circumstances, she is told that she's *afraid, sad, unjust,* or something of the like. And again, she learns new words to categorize her behavior in the future. That means that the discourses an individual is involved in during her growth, provide her with her conceptual repertoires. It is through these that she learns to categorize, label, and describe objects and processes in her internal and external worlds. The linguistic practices embedded in a culture structure the subjectivity and experience of the individual and thereby shape her exo-cognition and endo-cognition, i.e., consciousness and self-consciousness. The self-image that an individual forms by her self-monitoring and self-diagnoses as well as her worldview, or world-image, are thus socially grounded and conditioned.

Stressful social interactions affect the emotional sphere of an individual by causing specific neurophysiological processes in her limbic system. Since this system is directly involved in the regulation of the endocrine and immune systems (Ader, 2007; Wolkowitz and Rotschild, 2003), illness experiences, disorders, and diseases may be caused and recovery processes may be supported or delayed by specific modes of interaction. Although such experiences, disorders, and diseases have traditionally come to be termed *psychosomatic*, they obviously originate from the individual's social sphere. Therefore, their categorization as sociosomatic disorders and diseases is preferable (see page 733).

The moral agent

Society functions by virtue of the legal and moral rules that regulate the coexistence of its members. Of particular importance among moral rules are the basic ones that constitute the *common morality* (see page 567). According to these rules a patient, as a member of the society, has some moral responsibilities and claims. It is these basic moral responsibilities and claims that render her a moral agent. In her capacity as a moral agent, she makes decisions whose consequences affect her life and interactions significantly. Thus, the *sociosomatic* processes she is involved in are set in motion by herself. That means that as a moral agent, the patient is responsible for any change in her health condition insofar as the change has been directly caused by her own deliberate action. To give a familiar example, an individual who has been a smoker for thirty years and now suffers from lung cancer, is responsible for the genesis of this disease state. Such responsibility presupposes that the individual has, or has had, free will to choose among alternative possibilities, e.g., smoking and not smoking. This presupposition holds in any circumstances in which the individual is to be considered a moral agent. Additionally, a libertarian society and health care system cannot deny the adult patient's right to refuse any diagnostic examination and treatment provided that the refusal does not endanger public health. This very right of refusal also presupposes that the patient has free will and does not stand under any coercion to refuse medical intervention (Sadegh-Zadeh, 1981b).

The supposition that human beings have free will, we refer to as the *axiom* of free will. A libertarian society must endorse this axiom because (i) without the moral and legal responsibility of individuals no humane society can exist; and (ii) free will is a necessary condition of moral and legal responsibility. Surprisingly, however, nowadays there is a vociferous opposition to this axiom in neurosciences and neurophilosophy. Since both the acceptance as well as rejection of the axiom affect the concept of patient and thereby shape the foundations of the clinical encounter, we will discuss in the next section why its rejection is self-defeating.

Free will

If we are to consider the patient as a person, we must address the issue of free will, for traditionally free will is considered a condition of personhood. But although it has been debated over the last two millennia, there is as yet no general agreement on whether human beings have free will or not (Kane, 2002, 2003; O'Connor, 2000; Walter, 2001; Watson, 2003). There are those who argue that free will is incompatible with the natural laws governing human biology, known as incompatiblilists; and there are those who view the two as compatible, known as compatibilists. We will not participate in this debate, as it is an outgrowth of mind-body dualism that we do not endorse. Instead, our aim here is, first, to briefly present an argument that demonstrates the meaninglessness of the prevailing doctrine of those neuroscientists and neurophilosophers who, for reasons other than those of the incompatibalists, deny the existence of free will; and second, to suggest a concept of autonomy.

The U.S.-American neurophysiologist Benjamin Libet and his collaborators conducted a series of experiments in the 1980s to analyze the relationships between the activity of cerebral neurons and voluntary acts. Among other things, they found that "Freely voluntary acts are preceded by a specific electrical charge in the brain (the 'readiness potential', RP) that begins 550 milliseconds before the motor act. Human subjects become aware of intention to act 350–400 ms after RP starts, but 200 ms before the motor act" (Libet et al., 1982, 1983; Libet, 1985, 1999, 2004). These authors didn't conclude from their finding that there was no free will. But they triggered the emergence of a neuroscience-based doctrine of the unfree will in neurophilosophy which says that the subjective feeling of free choice is an illusion. There is no free will. Decisions and actions are caused by natural laws operative in the brain (Libet et al., 1999; Roth and Vollmer, 2002; Roth, 2003; Singer and Metzinger, 2002; Singer, 2003).

No neurophysiological counter experiments are required to show, however, that at least some human beings do in fact have free will. This is easily demonstrated by the self-defeat of the doctrine of the unfree will above:

Whoever subscribes to the doctrine must suppose that, in contrast to her belief, she herself has free will. Otherwise, the meaningfulness of her whole theory collapses. Were her theory meaningful, she would be held to the following absurd self-description: "I have no free will. I am solely caused by natural laws in my brain to do the things I do. This brings with it that it is not my will to tell you what I am telling you right now. I am forced to do so by natural laws operating in my brain. What you are hearing right now is in fact those laws speaking to you. Needless to say, therefore, that also the theory of unfree will is their theory, not mine, so that I am not responsible for advancing their theory. Nor can I make any claim regarding its truth or untruth. Any epistemological questions regarding their theory must be directed to the natural laws themselves residing in my brain" (see also Engelhardt, 1986, 106).

The stubborn problem of free will may be resolved by taking into account that the first person pronoun "I" is an indexical, as was discussed on page 135. Let a statement of the form "I now want to X" be an utterance made by an agent who is going to X where the phrase "to X" refers to an action such as "to sing", "to open the window", or something like that. In such an utterance, the indexical "I" stands for the self-reference of the system, which is able to monitor itself and put forward the self-diagnosis "I now want to X". This self-diagnosis does not entail anything indicative of an immaterial *will* that might or might not be independent of neurophysiological processes in the brain. It is merely a report on the biological state *of* the organism by the organism itself that is about to X. Interpreted in the terminology of the Libet experiments referred to above, the self-diagnosis "I now want to X" announces in a subjective language the readiness potential, RP, that is underway to produce a motor act and has just been mapped to the CRO, i.e., the cerebral representation of the organism, discussed in Section 6.2.2 on page 137. Whether the readiness potential is allowed to propagate to the periphery and to trigger a motor act or not, is under the complete control of those regions of the brain which produce the self-consciousness. "But the conscious function could still control the outcome; it can veto the act. Free will is therefore not excluded" (Libet, 1999, 47, 51–52).

An agent who is capable of reflective evaluation of possible alternatives of her impending action, is also capable of vetoing and stopping the propagation of the readiness potential to the muscles by choosing from among alternative actions $A_1, \ldots, A_n$ the action A_i instead of another action A_j with $i \neq j$. For example, she stops the decision "I now want to open the window" and chooses the alternative action "I now want not to open the window" in that she stops the readiness potential in order not to open the window, although she wanted to do so 50 milliseconds ago. She thereby has control over her behavior, which through the following chain of reasoning leads us to conclude she has autonomy:

Control of the behavior of a system by the system itself is self-control. A system that is capable of both setting its goals and self-control is capable of self-determination. A self-determined system is said to have autonomy. We suppose that an adult individual has autonomy. Call it "free will" if you so wish.

Autonomy is neutral with regard to determinism and indeterminism. Even in a deterministic world autonomous systems are possible. Many human beings are such autonomous systems. However, autonomy is not a global capability that encompasses all the decisions that an agent makes. There are decisions and actions that an agent cannot control. That is, with respect to such decisions and actions she has no free will. For example, she is forced by nature to satisfy her primary biological needs, and thus, she *cannot* want not to eat, not to drink water, or not to sleep; she *must* want to do so. But there are also decisions with respect to which she is self-determined, e.g., whether to consult Dr. *A* or to prefer Dr. *B* when she needs medical assistance. In a nutshell, some human beings are able to freely make some of their decisions.[27]

The patient as a person

In modern medicine, the physician is required to treat the patient as a person. There is as yet no common concept of a person, however. On the one hand,

---

[27] The most interesting theory of free will in the history of this problem has been presented by the U.S.-American philosopher Harry Gordon Frankfurt (1971). He differentiates between first-order and second-order volitions. A volition of the first order is described by usual sentences of the type "I want to X" where "to X" refers to a̱ action. The object of a second-order volition, however, is not an action, but a volition of the first order. Thus, an alcohol addict may entertain the second-order volition "I want to want not to drink alcohol". Should she succeed in bringing about the efficacious first-order *will* not to drink alcohol any more, then she has herself generated the will she wants to have. Since the action, or behavior, not to drink alcohol any more is freely wanted, the agent *has* free will. Frankfurt's theory may be viewed as a mentalistic concept of what we have called *autonomy* (see Sadegh-Zadeh, 1981b).

a person is obviously not simply identical with a human being; and person-hood is not considered identical with consciousness, self-consciousness, psyche, or mind. On the other hand, fetuses, infants, and severely brain-damaged patients are not categorized as persons. That means that persons are a sub-category of human beings. This brings with it two problems, a moral problem and a semantic problem.

Usually, a person is said to be *a self-conscious and rational being with free will and a sense of moral concern*. If we take this definition seriously, we face the question whether it is meaningful to require that the patient be treated as a person. If so, then pediatric as well as severely brain-damaged patients could not be treated as persons; the definition excludes them. We would thus obtain a two-class system of health care where some patients are treated as persons and others as non-persons. How could we morally justify putting a particular type of patient at a disadvantage because they are not considered persons?

Apart from this moral problem, the semantic vagueness of the above-mentioned concept of a person indicates that the category of persons cannot be sharply delimited. The category is not a natural kind. It is something artificial that emerges by introducing the new term "person" into the language. The category depends on how one defines the term, and it is unquestionably too complex a category to be conceived as crisp. As a result, it will not be possible to delimit personhood according to the classical type of concept above:

An individual is a person iff she has the properties $A, B, C, \ldots$ (12)

that reduces the category to a limited number of necessary and sufficient fea-tures $A, B, C, \ldots$ common to all of its instances. What that means, will be discussed in detail later on page 162 because it requires the notion of a non-classical concept that we have only lightly touched on pages 79–80. At this juncture, we may state that the category of persons can best be conceived as irreducible and established by reconstructing the concept as a *prototype resemblance predicate* (see page 183). To help us understand the notion, con-sider that the question "what is a person?" may adequately be answered by a sentence such as (i) "persons are Albert Schweitzer and similar beings", or (ii) "persons are Jesus Christ and similar beings", or (iii) "persons are the present reader and similar beings". Each of these possible and admissible definitions introduces the concept of a person as a prototype resemblance predicate where Albert Schweitzer, Jesus, and the present reader are the prototypes *ostensively defining* the concept (for the method of ostensive definition, see page 101). All three definitions are equivalent. But the advantage of a definition like (i) and (ii) is that Albert Schweitzer and Jesus are well-known to the effect that the definition is generally understood. Unfortunately, a detailed explication of the concept of a person is beyond the scope of this book; it would in fact deserve a separate volume.

Nevertheless, any adequate concept of a person will be inevitably vague. However, as we have seen in other vague concepts, this does not mean that we cannot sensibly talk about it and its properties, but only that the category of persons lacks sharp boundaries. Eric Cassell has proposed a conception that is in complete accord with such vagueness. He calls his conception a "description of the person" (Cassell, 2004, 36–41). We will introduce the descriptors of his proposal as tags only, call them features, properties, or attributes, and their specification will be omitted. According to Cassell, a person (1) has personality and character; (2) has a past; (3) has a family; (4) has a cultural background; (5) has roles; (6) has relationships and interactions with others; (7) has relationships with herself; (8) is a political being; (9) does things; (10) is often unaware of much that happens to her and why; (11) has regular behaviors; (12) has a secret life; (13) has a perceived future; and (14) has a transcendent dimension. Cassell shows how the suffering of a patient depends on these aspects such that by considering them the physician may relieve her suffering to better effect. Thus, suffering is not mere pain and discomfort; the entirety of the individual in space, time, and beyond is involved.

Since each of the 14 Cassellian features above may be present in different individuals to different extents, they result in a *fuzzy concept of person*. That is, the category of persons is a fuzzy set, and for that reason, irreducible to a limited number of features $A, B, C, \ldots$ as in (12) above. Personhood, then, is not a crisp, all-or-nothing property that one definitely has or definitely lacks. Individuals possess it to one degree or another. This is also true of a single individual at different periods of her life; her degree of personhood varies over time. The idea of *degrees of personhood*, then, seems to be a legitimate idea for analysis. Thus, among the most profound questions of medicine and philosophy is: When do we gain personhood and when do we lose it? From our considerations above it follows that personhood commences and ceases gradually, and thus, is an episode in the life of an individual. We shall come back to this issue in Section 18.2 on page 698.

6.2.4 Summary

Medicine is not concerned with illness and disease, but with suffering human beings called patients. For this reason, a theory of the patient ought to constitute its basis. Theories of health, illness, and disease are parts of such a theory of the patient. In the preceding sections, we have considered the patient from a limited perspective as a bio-psycho-social agent and have tried to explicate the three aspects of this concept. First, we discussed the question of what it means to say that the patient is a living body. The living body was interpreted as an organism. The organism, in turn, is a causal system and source of emergent properties. Two central characteristics of this causal system are that it is a fuzzy causal system and an endopoietic system. As an endopoietic system, it is capable of building inner worlds as its subsystems. Second, the psyche was interpreted as one of these subsystems of the organism that emerges by fuzzy endomorphosis of the whole organism. It is not a product, property, or faculty of the brain. The current neurocentrism in deciphering mental phenomena is misguided. Third, as a social agent, a human being is subject to the consequences of her interactions. Through the perceptual system of the social agent, the interactions affect her emotional, cognitive, endocrine, and immune subsystems in the cerebral representation of the organism. Therefore, the concept of sociosomatics was suggested as a means of understanding the genesis of the so-called psychosomatic disorders and diseases.

6.3 Health, Illness, and Disease

6.3.0 Introduction

As a bio-psycho-social agent, an individual may transition from the state of *health* to the state of *illness* on account of *disease*. But what do these three categories mean exactly: health, illness, and disease? How are they conceptualized in medicine? As they stand now, are they fruitful concepts or do they need improvement? Why does medicine categorize some human conditions as diseases? Is this categorization based on explicit and intelligible rules? In this section, we shall address these questions and related issues.

Health, illness, and disease are central themes of not only medicine, but of human existence. Although philosophical inquiry into these themes constitutes a long-standing and significant part of the philosophy of medicine, there is as yet no general agreement on what health, illness, and disease are.[28] The inquiry seems to have reached an impasse. What we have received so far may be summarized by a few labels (Sadegh-Zadeh, 2000c, 2008):

- naive normalism,
- descriptivism,
- normativism,
- fictionalism,
- metaphorism, and
- philistinism.

Naive normalism is the view upon which the standard health care in university hospitals is based. It says that health is normality and diseases are abnormalities. Normality, according to this view, is the range of statistical values that occurs with the most frequency. If the statistics reveal that 95% of the adult population has a blood cholesterol level of 160 to 200 mg%, then this is the 'normal' range of blood cholesterol in adults. Any deviation from this range is 'abnormal' and thus a disease. Philosophically embellished versions of this mathematical and conceptual naivety are to be found in (Christopher Boorse, 1975, 1977, 1997).

Descriptivism, also called "the biostatistical theory", says that "health and disease are value-free scientific concepts. Health [...] is the absence of disease;

---

[28] See, for example (Caplan et al., 1981; Caplan et al., 2004; Humber and Almeder, 1997; Rothschuh, 1975).

disease is only statistically species-subnormal biological part-function; therefore, the classification of human states as healthy or diseased is an objective matter, to be read off the biological facts of nature without need of value judgments" (Humber and Almeder, 1997, 4; Boorse, 1997). This view is also labeled *naturalism* since its advocates consider diseases natural phenomena to be encountered, *qua diseases*, in the real world out there.

Normativism is the opposite standpoint and suggests that the classification of certain groups of phenomena as illnesses or diseases is based on value judgments (Engelhardt, 1975, 1976, 1986; Margolis, 1969, 1976). According to Engelhardt, the concept of disease is not merely descriptive, but also normative. It says what ought not to be (1975, 127). "As a zoologist one may have an interest in determining what levels of function characterize a particular species. One may in addition be interested in discovering the evolutionary processes that led to these circumstances. But such are not the interests of physicians or patients who have nonepistemic goals such as the relief of pain, the preservation of function, the achievement of desirable human form and grace, and the postponement of death" (Engelhardt, 1986, 171).

In contrast to the three views above, *fictionalism* denies the very existence of disease. "Disease is a genuine fiction" (Koch, 1920, 130–131). "There are no diseases, there are only sick people" (Armand Trousseau 1801–1867). Thomas Szasz's *metaphorism*, confined to psychiatry only, denies the existence of mental illnesses and diseases. According to him, such illnesses and diseases are mere myths and metaphors (Szasz, 1960, 1970, 1984).

Finally, there is a view advanced by the Swedish philosopher Germund Hesslow that may aptly be referred to as *philistinism* because Hesslow terms himself a *philistine* (["GH, a philistine"], Hesslow, 1993, 2). He maintains that the three notions of health, illness, and disease are superfluous in medicine and irrelevant to clinicians and medical scientists on the grounds that "There is no biomedical theory in which disease appears as a theoretical entity and there are no laws or generalizations linking disease to other important variables" (ibid., 5). However, a cursory glance at clinical literature, medical education, physician-patient interaction, and the place of health care in society reveals that his view is fundamentally wrong. Hesslow unfortunately mistakes biomedicine for medicine. The term "biomedicine" denotes the so-called medical biosciences such as anatomy, biochemistry, cytology, physiology, etc. It is true that all these disciplines are natural-scientific endeavors because researchers in these disciplines concentrate on the biology of mice, rats, rabbits, and other animals. And since they are not concerned with the population of suffering human beings, they are in fact doing zoology. However, it is the suffering human being, the *Homo patiens*, that constitutes the subject of clinical medicine. Clinical knowledge as well as relevant patient documents are replete with disease names and disease classifications and descriptions.

Missing from the ongoing controversial debate on health and disease is the logical analysis of these notions. In what follows we shall undertake, by way of logic, an explication of the concepts of health, illness, and disease, and shall put forward a novel theory of these three subjects, which may stimulate further research and discussion.

We will start with the conceptual and philosophical problems of what is called disease. Our approach will bring with it some methodological innovations that can be used in the subsequent analyses and discussions on health and illness. Specifically, a theory of non-classical concepts will be presented to show that the concept of disease is a non-classical one. On the basis of prototype theory and fuzzy logic, a *prototype resemblance theory of disease* will be proposed. Similarly, the concepts of health and illness will be fuzzy-logically reconstructed. We shall see that if approached this way, many philosophical problems traditionally associated with these basic concepts of medicine will turn out pseudo-problems. Our analyses divide into the following four sections:

6.3.1   Disease
6.3.2   Health
6.3.3   Illness
6.3.4   Disease, Health, and Illness Violate Classical Logic.

6.3.1 Disease

Suffering abounds in the human world. But not all types of suffering fall within the responsibility of medicine. For instance, people who suffer from poverty, loneliness, or political repression would be misguided to seek the advice of physicians. Medicine is concerned with human suffering only if it is a facet of *illness*. Illness, also called *sickness* from the perspective of an observer, may be engendered by a variety of causes. Among them is a cause of a particular type called *disease*. For medicine to help someone who is ill on account of a disease, there must be reliable knowledge about that disease. The field of *nosology* is responsible for gathering such knowledge.

Derived from the Greek term νόσος (nosos) meaning "illness" and "disease", nosology is a basic clinical inquiry into illness and disease, a *science of the patient* so to speak. As a basic clinical science, nosology is not a domain-confined specialty like cardiology or orthopedics, but a transdisciplinary endeavor undertaken in all clinical fields. It should be carefully distinguished from diagnostics. The purpose of the latter is to acquire specific knowledge about an *individual* patient's health condition, whereas nosology is concerned with the *class* of suffering individuals, i.e., with all patients, in order to gather general knowledge on the nature of human suffering.

A physician or clinical scientist as a nosologist subdivides the class of human beings, separating health from non-health, illness from non-illness, disease from non-disease. She describes states and types of human suffering, and categorizes them as individual diseases such as *diabetes mellitus, AIDS,* and *Alzheimer's disease,* also called disease entities, clinical entities, and nosological entities. She groups them, according to some criteria, in a system to build a *nosological system.* In such a system, related diseases are collected in more or less coherent groups, or subcategories, to enable systematic studies as well as efficient work in diagnostics, therapeutics, epidemiology, and preventive care. Familiar nosological subcategories are, for instance, infectious diseases, heart diseases, metabolic diseases, genetic diseases, mental diseases, and others that include individual diseases such as diabetes mellitus, measles, pneumonia, multiple sclerosis, myocardial infarction, etc. See Figure 24.

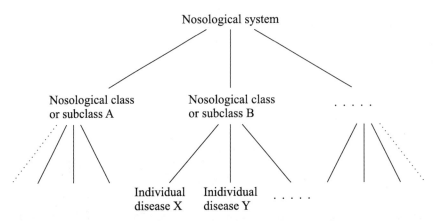

Fig. 24. A nosological system is a classification system of individual diseases based on the taxonomic *is_a* relation (see page 60) such as "diabetes mellitus is a metabolic disease". Many individual diseases are grouped in a disease category or subcategory such as *metabolic diseases, infectious diseases,* or others

Nosology is concerned with:

- symptoms and signs (≡ symptomatology),
- causes (≡ etiology),
- development (≡ pathogenesis),
- social dimensions (≡ epidemiology)

and additional aspects of individual diseases. As a scientific activity, nosology is methodologically and epistemologically underdeveloped and in need of improvement in both its foundations and performance. To this end, it will constitute the subject of our analysis and discussion in the present section. What we are doing here may therefore be termed theoretical nosology or metanosology.

For the difference between nosology and pathology, see Section 6.4.3 on page 202. To begin with, we shall first briefly explain why disease should not be considered the opposite of health. We shall then carefully distinguish between *disease* (in the singular) as a general category, on the one hand; and *individual diseases* (in the plural) such as measles, AIDS, myocardial infarction, and pneumonia as its subcategories or members, on the other (see Figure 25).

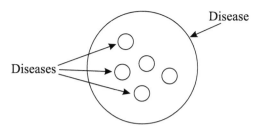

Fig. 25. Category-subcategory relationship. "Disease" (in the singular) is the general category, while "diseases" (in the plural) are its subcategories or members

The *concept of disease* does not denote the individual diseases. Its referent is the general category, disease. It will be reconstructed as a non-classical concept and explicated by our *prototype resemblance theory of disease*. Our analysis thus divides into the following ten sections:

▶ Malady
▶ 'The' disease *vs.* 'a' disease
▶ Type disease *vs.* token disease
▶ Petitio principii
▶ Classical concepts
▶ Non-classical concepts
▶ Resemblance structures
▶ Human conditions
▶ Similarity
▶ The prototype resemblance theory of disease.

Malady

Usually, health and disease are construed as conceptual opposites in that health is defined as the absence of disease and vice versa. However, it has been argued that the opposite of health, i.e., 'unhealth', is not disease, but *malady* (Clouser et al., 1997; Gert et al., 2006; Sadegh-Zadeh, 1982d, 2000c). Malady is a broader category than disease.[29] It comprises, besides disease as one of its subcategories, many others such as injury, wound, lesion, defect, deformity, disorder, disability, and the like. An individual need not have a disease to lack health. Disciplines such as trauma surgery and reconstructive orthopedics demonstrate that a malady such as injury or deformity that is something different than disease, will suffice to impair an individual's health and to render her in need of medical assistance and care. Therefore, we may metalinguistically state that the antonym of the term "health" is the term "malady" and not the term "disease". Every disease is a malady, but not vice versa (Figure 26).

While a non-disease term that denotes a malady, e.g., "injury", may be explicated plainly, the question of "what is disease?" presents recalcitrant problems both to medicine and its philosophy. As a result, there is as yet

---

[29] For the term "category", see footnote 5 on page 22.

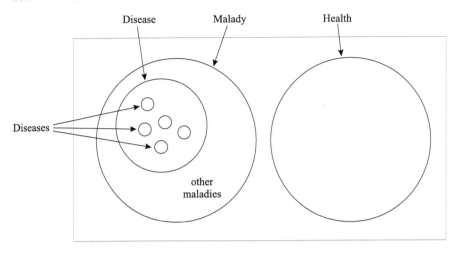

Fig. 26. Human conditions unsharply divide into two categories, *malady* and *health*. The former category comprises subcategories such as diseases, injuries, wounds, etc.

no generally accepted concept of disease. Instead, almost every physician and every philosopher of medicine has her own notion of what disease might be. In what follows, we shall explain how this situation arose and suggest remedial measures. To aid in our discussion, we will first differentiate between several usages of the term "disease".

'The' disease *vs.* 'a' disease

Besides the one mentioned above, there are other semantic problems in the philosophy of disease. They include the following two basic misunderstandings: (1) the confusion of (i) disease as a general category with (ii) individual diseases; and (2) the confusion of a patient's disease state with (i) or (ii).

All of us are familiar with clinical terms such as "pulmonary tuberculosis", "myocardial infarction", "gastric ulcer", "diabetes mellitus", and "AIDS". They denote individual diseases, also called clinical entities, disease entities, or nosological entities, i.e., *diseases* in the plural. We are told that currently the approximate number of these individual diseases amounts to 50,000. Each one of them is *a* disease. To contribute to the eradication of the above-mentioned, pernicious confusion of (i) with (ii), we will call any phrase that denotes *a* disease, i.e., any of the 50,000 individual diseases, a *nosological predicate*. By using a nosological predicate in a statement like "Mr. Elroy Fox has pulmonary tuberculosis", an individual disease is predicated, i.e., ascribed to a person.

Therefore, there are currently about 50,000 nosological predicates in medical language. No doubt, a nosological predicate is clearly definable by a set of necessary and sufficient features, e.g., "someone has pulmonary tuberculosis if and only if she has pneumonia caused by Koch's bacillus". However, this definition defines what pulmonary tuberculosis is. It does not define *what disease is*. The definition of none of the 50,000 nosological predicates defines the term "disease". To be distiguished from *a* disease is the general category, or class, *the disease* that comprises all of these individual diseases and is thus something different from each one of its 50,000 members. The general category of birds as a class is not identical with particular bird species such as robin, sparrow, crow, ostrich, and so on. It includes all of these species. Likewise, the general term "bird" is not identical with specific terms such as "robin", "sparrow", etc. We must therefore not confuse a category with its members. *Disease* is the category. Individual diseases, or *diseases* for short, are its members (Sadegh-Zadeh, 1977a). To summarize, distinguisch between:

- the concept of disease, on the one hand, and
- nosological predicates, on the other.

A *nosological predicate* such as "Alzheimer's disease", "multiple sclerosis", "AIDS", and the like denotes an individual disease, while disease as a general category, or disease_in_general, is the denotation of the *concept of disease*. What is almost never noticed in medicine and its philosophy, *nosological predicates are not concepts of disease*. They are concepts of disease just as little as the proper names "The Himalaya" or "The Alps" are concepts of mountain. Thus, there are fundamental semantic differences between these two types of notions and between what they denote. Due to these differences they require distinct methods of inquiry. Otherwise put, we must differentiate between disease_in_general as a general category, on the one hand, and the 50,000 individual diseases as its subcategories or members, on the other. The confusion of these two different ontological levels is a typical category mistake and a main source of misunderstandings in the philosophy of disease. Our focus is the general category *disease* denoted by the concept of disease.[30]

Type disease *vs.* token disease

We must be aware that the *disease state of a patient* is also something different from both an individual disease and the general category. To this end, we differentiate between token disease and type disease.

---

[30] Surprisingly, there are still philosophers who do not understand the distinction between the general concept of disease and nosological predicates, and are therefore incapable of recognizing that the former one is a prerequisite for constructing the latter ones. Worall and Worall, for example, suggest that we should concentrate on individual diseases to evade a general concept of disease. The rationale behind their suggestion is the value-ladenness of the concept of disease, while they want to keep medicine a purely scientific, non-evaluative enterprise: "How could medicine be scientific, if its central notion – that of disease – is shot through with values?" (Worall and Worall, 2001). It is recommended that before doing philosophy of medicine, philosophers inform themselves a little bit about medicine to get an idea of what they are philosophizing about.

A *token disease* is simply the spatio-temporally localized disease state of a patient as the manifestation of *a* disease in an individual. For example, if the patient Elroy Fox has diabetes mellitus, then his disease state, which may be described by the statement "Elroy Fox has hyperglycemia and glucosuria and polydipsia" and categorized by the diagnosis "Elroy Fox has diabetes", is a token disease. The class, or the category, of all patients whose disease state is described by the same nosological predicate *"P"*, e.g., "has diabetes", represents *the type disease P*, i.e., diabetes in the present example. Thus, token disease pertains to an individual, while type disease is a category. Put in scholastic terms, token disease is a particular; type disease is a universal. (For the terms "particular" and "universal", see Section 18.1.1 on page 694.)

The distinction above will prove of paramount importance in debates between descriptivists and normativists about whether disease is something value neutral or value-laden because more often than not both parties are victims of a confusion. The question of whether the categorization of something as a disease is a value judgment or not, does not concern the token disease, but the type disease. No doctor diagnoses an individual patient as being in a particular disease state, say diabetes, on the basis of a value judgment. By contrast, it is a legitimate question to ask whether the decision to categorize a particular cluster of features, say {blue-eyed, thin-lipped, long-eared}, as a type disease is based on a value judgment or not.

The confusion of token disease with type disease can be avoided by distinguishing between nosology and diagnostics. Nosology is concerned with the clinical investigation into, and classification of, type diseases. By contrast, diagnostics is concerned, among other things, with the token disease identified on the basis of an antecedently available nosological system and vocabulary. We are concerned here with metanosology and not metadiagnostics.

Petitio principii

In the preceding section, we have called the class that contains all individual diseases, the category of diseases or simply the category *disease*. Specialists assert that this category currently comprises about 50,000 members. Everyday new ones are added, e.g., alcoholism, computer-game addiction, and attention-deficit hyperactivity disorder, while others are removed, e.g., homosexuality, hysteria, and drapetomania.[31] The category is thus dynamic, which leads us to ask questions such as, "How can this nosological dynamics be explained

---

[31] *Drapetomania* was considered a disease by the racist, U.S.-American physician Samuel Adolphus Cartwright (1793–1863). In a paper entitled "Report on the diseases and physical peculiarities of the Negro race" and published on May 7, 1851 in *New Orleans Medical and Surgical Journal* (Cartwright, 2004, 33), he claimed that the black slaves who run away have a mental disease that causes them to flee captivity, and called this imaginary disease "drapetomania". This phrase derives from the Greek terms δραπετης (drapetes) and μανια (mania) meaning, respectively, "runaway slave" and "overwhelming desire and urge".

and justified?", and "Are there any principles governing it?". We must answer these to understand why the category *disease* includes phenomena such as alcoholism, computer-game addiction, and attention-deficit hyperactivity disorder, while excluding other phenomena such as drapetomania, hysteria, and chlorosis, or even lying, shareholding, tax evasion, and dictatorship.

A nosologist wields vast power since *diseases* come primarily from nosology, which in turn drives the machinery of the health care industry. The categorization of a new phenomenon X as a disease stands at the end of a more or less long-term process of investigation and discussion which we view as a nosological decision or act of the medical community. In performing such an act, physicians or clinical scientists, as nosologists, partition the population of human beings into two categories, the category of those who have the new disease, X, and the category of those who don't have it. From the methodological point of view, the nosologists' act comprises two steps. First, they introduce, usually by poor definitions or no definitions, new nosological predicates such as "diabetes mellitus" into the language of medicine. They suggest, for example, that "diabetes mellitus is the state of having insulin deficiency, hyperglycemia, and glucosuria", or more generally, "X is the state of having the features A, B, C". Second, they assert that "X is a disease". They may say, for instance, "diabetes is a disease". Now our basic question is this: When asserting that the new class X is a disease, how do or could they justify this categorization? Could it be that X was not a disease and they have erred?

We have a new class X, e.g., diabetes, on the one hand, and the category *disease* already containing 49,999 members, on the other. What is the rationale behind the 50,000th categorization statement "X is a disease"? Why isn't it asserted that "X is not a disease" instead? Is there a reason for preferring affirmation to denial? If medicine had a *concept of disease*, we could answer these questions by simply examining whether the new phenomenon X matches our concept of disease to become a new member of the category *disease*. However, there is unfortunately no such concept. The result of lacking such a measure is that every nosologist implicitly or explicitly obeys an idiosyncratic concept of disease. The present author once recorded 14 different such concepts used in 14 medical textbooks (Sadegh-Zadeh, 1977a, 11).

Consequently, the question of "what is disease?" constitutes an ongoing subject of debate. However, as outlined on page 104, the polysemy inherent in the particles "what" and "is" causes the question to be almost always improperly interpreted and handled. Although it is meant to be a question in the *quid mode* and thus in pursuit of an explication or definition of the term "disease", it is persistently handled as if it were in the *quod mode*, and as such, a taxonomic question. Subsequently, a fruitless search ensues for a set of 'essential features common to all diseases' that are presupposed by the questioner to be diseases *a priori*, i.e., before she has a concept of disease she is searching for. Thus, one looks at 'known diseases' to abstract from them features that define the unknown term "disease". For example:

A disease is a type of internal state which is either an impairment of normal functional ability or a limitation on functional   (13)
ability caused by environmental agents (Boorse, 1997, 9).

However, this method of concept formation by abstracting features 'common
to all diseases' is a petitio principii on the grounds that 'diseases' will come
into being qua diseases only a posteriori, i.e., after a concept of disease has
been defined, but not before. Consider that prior to defining a concept of
tree there are no such things as 'trees'. Analogously, a concept of disease has
to precede the inclusion of some phenomena as its individual instances, and
the exclusion of other phenomena as its non-instances. That means that the
quid mode question "what is disease?" (what is a tree? what is a mountain?
what is love?) can only be decided prescriptively, not descriptively. It must
be tackled axiomatically and cannot be answered empirically. It would be
bizarre to believe that the conceptual boundary between tree and bush could
be determined by empirical examination of trees and bushes before there exist
any concepts of *tree* and *bush*. The same is true of the boundary between
disease and non-disease. The concept of disease in medicine is an analog of
the concept of right in the theory and practice of jurisdiction. Nobody will be
able to find out "what is right?" by inspecting the real-world human behavior
or existing laws and legal literature. This is so because it is a normative
concept, and as such, it can only prescriptively be established (Sadegh-Zadeh,
1980c, 408).

The lack of a concept of disease and the petitio principii above result from
the fact that it is impossible to arrive at a concept of disease using traditional
methods of concept formation. There is a pervasive, but wrong, belief that
every category is characterized by a finite number of essential features common
to all of its instances and can be represented by a concept that indicates
those features "common to all". This belief, which we identified on pages 79–
80 and termed the *common-to-all postulate* on page 80, originates from the
ancient Greeks, especially Plato and Aristotle. However, the former Berkeley
experimental psychologist Eleanor Rosch and others in the last quarter of the
20th century have presented extensive evidence against this classical doctrine
(Rosch, 1973, 1975, 1978, 1988; Rosch and Mervis, 1975; Smith and Medin,
1981). Below we shall sketch the evidence to demonstrate why the deeply
entrenched doctrine is methodologically untenable and needs to be replaced
with a non-classical conception.

Classical concepts

As was pointed out on pages 79–80, we distinguish between classical and non-
classical concepts. In this section and the next, we shall explain the difference
between them to argue that the concept of disease is non-classical and should
be treated accordingly. We may provisionally state that a concept is classical
in the manner of Plato and Aristotle if it denotes a category whose members

have a number of identical properties, or a 'common nature'. Otherwise, it is said to be non-classical. We shall be more precise below.

To begin with, an object should not be confused with its name. Here the term "object" is a general phrase like "entity", denoting everything, be it existent or non-existent. We have already emphasized previously that all definitions are *nominal* definitions. That is, when defining something, it is always the *name* (= nomen) of an object that is defined and never the object itself. An object is not defined, it is demarcated, described, characterized, analyzed, and the like. The term "definition" is a metalinguistic one, and as such, applies to elements of language only.

In what follows, we shall be concerned with categories as our objects. Their names are known as classificatory or qualitative concepts, terms, or predicates dealth with in Section 4.1.2. For example, the term "bird" is the name of the category of birds; the term "fruit" is the name of the category of fruits; likewise, the term "disease" is the name of the category of diseases. Thus, it is terms like "bird", "fruit", and "disease" as elements of language that are defined, not the categories that they denote as their referents in 'the world out there'. By defining its name, a category is demarcated or delimited. Before being delimited, there is no such category with the specific boundaries given thereby. Having said that, for the sake of convenience, and when the context is unambiguous, the wording "we will now define the category X" may be preferred to the cumbersome formulation "we will now define the predicate 'X' that denotes the category X". Let C be such a category. Consider now a sentence of the form "x is a C" stating that the object x belongs to that category, e.g., "Figure 27 is a square" (see Figure 27).

Fig. 27

In this example, Figure 27 is our object x, and *square* is the category C to which it belongs. We use this simple example rather than medical examples, which would be too complex and unnecessarily difficult. Suppose now that someone points to Figure 27, declaring that "Figure 27 is a square". When asked "how do you know that? Is it possible that it isn't?", she will try to justify her claim by explaining that the figure has a set of features (or synonymously: properties, attributes, characteristics, criteria, traits) that define the 'nature' or 'essence' of a square. For instance, she will say that "it is a closed figure, it has four straight sides, its sides are equal in length, and it has equal angles". If our question was not about a square, but about something else, e.g., "why do you categorize diabetes as a disease? Is it possible that it isn't?", we would get an analogous answer. She may reply, à la Christopher Boorse (see his definition of the term "disease" presented in (13) on page 158 above), "because diabetes impairs the normal functional ability, and the impairment of normal functional ability is the essential feature of a disease".

As these examples demonstrate, it is customarily assumed that for a given category there are a number of 'essential' features defining it. This assumption implies that in order for something, such as Figure 27 or diabetes, to be a member of a particular category C, *it must possess a set of defining features* to meet the nature or essence of C-hood. This is the classical, essentialist reduction of a category and concept to a finite number of defining features. It will therefore be referred to as the view of *reductive definability* of concepts. Accordingly, a category is said to be a *reducible category* if its name is reductively definable, an *irreducible category*, otherwise. We may now define what we mean by the term "classical concept":

Definition 31 (Classical and non-classical concepts). *A concept C is:*
1. *a reducible or classical one iff it denotes a reducible category, e.g., the concept of square in the example above;*
2. *an irreducible or non-classical one iff it denotes an irreducible category, e.g., our concept of disease (see below).*

The doctrine of reductive definability has been so influential throughout history that it has left no room for alternative perspectives. It is no surprise, then, that the concept of disease has been subjected to this doctrine. It has been erroneously considered reductively definable and therefore denoting a reducible category. Accordingly, it is supposed that for an entity to be a member of this category, i.e., *a* disease, "it must possess a set of defining features" to meet the nature of diseasehood. It is said, for example by Boorse in (13) above, that it must bear the feature "impairment of normal functional ability or a limitation on functional ability caused by environmental agents" and the like. We shall demonstrate why this essentialist approach is inadequate and unacceptable. To this end, we must take a few preliminary steps.

A reducible category, denoted by a concept C, is a class whose members share $n \geq 1$ *common* features, say $F_1, \ldots, F_n$, such that these features are individually necessary and jointly sufficient to define the concept C. In this way, the category is reduced to the common possession of the features $F_1, \ldots, F_n$, that is, to $F_1 \& \cdots \& F_n$. In our present example, we would obtain the following definition of our concept where x is any object:

$$x \text{ is } C \text{ iff } x \text{ is } F_1 \text{ and } \ldots \text{ and } x \text{ is } F_n. \tag{14}$$

For instance, the concept of "square" denoting the category of square objects may be defined by the above-mentioned features "closed figure, four straight sides, sides equal in length, equal angles" as follows:

x is a square iff   1. x is a closed figure and   (15)

2. x has four straight sides and

3. x's sides are equal in length and

4. x has equal angles.

The feature set $F = \{F_1, \ldots, F_n\}$ with $n \geq 1$ used in the present example is $F = \{$closed figure, four straight sides, sides equal in length, equal angles$\}$ with $n = 4$. For a feature F_i from among the feature set $\{F_1, \ldots, F_n\}$ to be individually necessary, each instance of the category must have it. For a set of features $\{F_1, \ldots, F_n\}$ to be jointly sufficient, each entity having that feature set must be an instance of the category. Thus, the feature set is a defining one for the concept C.

Apparently, this reductive view of concepts is based on, and reflects, the ancient view that we have termed the *common-to-all* postulate on page 80. The view is generally held in medicine, in all other disciplines, and in everyday life. It says that for any concept signifying a corresponding category there are a limited number of defining features *common to all* of its instances. For example, in order for something to be a square, it must have the features such and such; in order for something to be a bird, it must have the features such and such; likewise, in order for something to be a disease, it must have the features such and such; and so on. From a logical point of view, this position requires that any concept C be defined by a biconditional of the form (14) above that has the structure of an explicit definition. The biconditional (14) is equivalent to the conjunction of the following two conditionals:

1. If x is C, then x is F_1 and ... and x is F_n
2. If x is F_1 and ... and x is F_n, then x is C.

Sentence 2 expresses the joint sufficiency of the features. Sentence 1 states the individual necessity of the features since it is, according to the rule 'Consequent Split' mentioned in Table 37 on page 898, equivalent to the following set of sentences:

If x is C, then x is F_1
If x is C, then x is F_2
$\vdots$
If x is C, then x is F_n

each of which requires the individual presence of a feature, F_i. (In a conditional of the form "if α, then β", the antecedent α is said to be *sufficient* for the consequent β. And the consequent β is said to be *necessary* for the antecedent α since the conditional is equivalent to its contraposition "if not β, then not α". If β is not true, then α is not true. So, β is necessary for the truth of α.)

Since Plato and Aristotle, it has been believed that *all* categories are of the reducible type characterized above. Accordingly, in nosology and metanosology one tries to define the concept of disease similarly to how a square is defined, i.e., as if there existed a finite number of features $F_1, \ldots, F_n$ *common to all* diseases such that "something is a disease if and only if it has the features $F_1, \ldots, F_n$". Only from such beliefs can feature-enumerating ambitions emerge like the one cited in (13) on page 158: "A disease is a type of internal state which is either an impairment of normal functional ability, i.e., a reduction of one or more functional abilities below typical efficiency, or a limitation on functional ability caused by environmental agents" (Boorse, 1997, 7 f.). As a result, no consensus will ever be reached on the concept of disease, since different scholars have different tastes and choose to enumerate different sets of features. This continuing disagreement and debate may come to an end only by recognizing that the category of diseases is irreducible, as we shall demonstrate in what follows.

Non-classical concepts[32]

In contrast to the traditional view sketched in the preceding section, nearly all real-world categories are irreducible, and according to our terminology introduced in Definition 31 above, all concepts denoting such categories are non-classical concepts. In most cases, the instances of a real-world category do not possess a set of common features as square figures do. Examples are birds, fruits, vegetables, furniture, and as we shall see below, diseases. For example, try to propose a set of defining features that are common to all members of the category *bird* embracing such diverse subcategories as robin, sparrow, nightingale, crow, bird of paradise, bird of prey, albatross, ostrich, emu, penguin, etc. You will not succeed, as these innumerable bird types do not share a set of birdhood-establishing features such as, for instance, {has feathers, has a beak, flies, chirps, lays eggs, ... } that would define the 'nature' of birdhood. Rather, they are characterized by only *partially overlapping* feature sets such as {A, B, C}, {B, C, D}, {C, D, E}, {D, E, F}, {E, F, G}, and others as follows:

Robin:	ABC	(16)
crow:	BCD	
eagle:	CDE	
ostrich:	DEF	
penguin:	EFG	
...	...	

Although neighboring bird types in this chain have something in common, two distant ones such as robin and penguin evidently have nothing in common. And most interestingly, there is nothing common to all. All of them are birds nonetheless because, due to the adjacent members' *resemblance* with respect to two features, the birdhood of only one member in the chain causes

---

[32] The idea of non-classical concepts outlined in this section is based on the theory of categorization that has originated with the former Berkeley psychologist Eleanor Rosch (1973, 1975, 1978). About the issues discussed in the current sections I have learned a lot from (Reed, 1972; Rosch, 1973, 1975, 1978, 1988; Smith and Medin, 1981; Lakoff, 1987; Andersen, 2000). All constructions, conceptualizations, and errors are my own responsibility, however.

the birdhood of the rest. We may now realize how distorted an image of 'the world out there' we have got from classical-style thinking. Such a way of seeing the world prompts us to look for features *common-to-all* entities that we subsume, or want to subsume, under a general label such as "bird", "fruit", "vegetable", "furniture", or "disease". And wherever we fail to identify such common features, we are prone to suppose or even to insist that the entities possess them nevertheless, as we are unable to imagine that it could be otherwise.

One encounters similar frustration in searching for a set of defining features that might be *common-to-all* instances of the category *disease*. But there are simply no diseasehood-establishing properties uniformly recurring in all individual diseases which could be represented by a reductively defined, unobjectionable concept of disease. To put it concisely, there is no such thing as 'the nature of disease'. For instance, in medicine human conditions such as myocardial infarction, acute hearing loss, alopecia areata, and abnormal prognathism are considered diseases. However, they have nothing in common that would justify their uniform categorization as diseases, e.g., no electrocardiogram abnormalities, no enzyme increase or decrease, no infection or inflammation, no swelling or pain, no impairment of functional ability, no sleeplessness, and nothing else. (The term "alopecia areata", from the Greek word $\alpha\lambda\omega\pi\varepsilon\kappa\iota\alpha$ (alopekia) for "mange in foxes", means circumscribed hair loss on the scalp or elsewhere on the body such that hairs fall out in small patches. The term "prognathism" is a compound of the Latin preposition *pro* and the Greek noun $\gamma\nu\dot{\alpha}\theta o\varsigma$, *gnathos*, meaning "jaw".)

Note that our denial of 'the nature of disease' above concerns only the general category *disease*. We are here not talking about 'the nature of individual clinical entities'. An individual clinical entity may of course have defining features to enable the formation of a nosological predicate in classical fashion as a classical concept. For instance, we have seen previously that the nosological predicate "pulmonary tuberculosis" may be introduced by an explicit definition of the following form: "A person has pulmonary tuberculosis if and only if she has pneumonia caused by Koch's bacillus". The definiens of this definition fixes the features "has pneumonia" and "is caused by Koch's bacillus" as sufficient and necessary conditions of pulmonary tuberculosis. This example underscores once again the difference between *nosological predicates* and the *concept of disease* discussed in Section 6.3.1 on page 154. But a nosological predicate is not a concept of disease. While it may denote a reducible category, the denotation of the concept of disease is an irreducible category.

A category such as *bird, fruit, vegetable, furniture,* and *disease* is irreducible if, like (16) above, there is no defining set of necessary and sufficient features common to all of its instances. An irreducible category does not satisfy the common-to-all postulate of reducible categories. This curious finding does not mean or imply that terms denoting irreducible categories such as *bird, fruit, vegetable, furniture,* and *disease* are undefinable, rendering the construction and maintenance of scientific languages impossible. On the contrary, it only disproves the universality of the classical doctrine of reductive definability based on the ancient common-to-all postulate. We have therefore to abandon this doctrine and search for another principle of categorization that works. The solution we are seeking lies in the relationship of *similarity* between the instances of an irreducible category. Their mutual similarity welds them together to constitute the category independently of how different they may be. We will now sketch this idea to explore whether we can use it in our metanosology.

Resemblance structures

The category of diseases will be reconstructed as a structure in which the relation of similarity between its members and some prototypes plays a basic role. It will therefore be referred to as a *prototype resemblance category*. The construction of this concept takes the following two steps:

▷ Wittgensteinian family resemblance
▷ Prototype resemblance categories.

Wittgensteinian family resemblance

Ludwig Wittgenstein's famous concept of family resemblance will serve as a heuristic tool, though, it is both defective and not directly useful to us. This will be briefly explained.

In the early twentieth century, there emerged a discussion on the vagueness of statements and concepts (Peirce, 1902; Russell, 1923; Black, 1937, 1963), which eventually led to the genesis of many-valued logics, on the one hand (Post, 1921; Łukasiewicz, 1930; Reichenbach, 1944; Kleene, 1952); and of fuzzy logic, on the other (Zadeh, 1965a–b). Although Ludwig Wittgenstein did not publicly participate in this discussion, in the second, post-Tractarian phase of his philosophizing as of 1929 (see Section 2.6 on page 46) he was also concerned with the vagueness of concepts. In his posthumously published *Philosophical Investigations* (Wittgenstein, 1953), he discovered the limitation and inadequacy of the reductive common-to-all postulate. In a context analyzing issues related to language, meaning, reference, and vagueness, he introduced the legendary notion of a *language-game* (ibid., section 7) that paved the way for a new direction in the philosophy of language. To explain this novel term he referred to *games,* and by reflecting on their category, he destroyed the time-honored common-to-all postulate thus:

Consider for example the proceedings that we call "games". I mean board-games, card-games, ball-games, Olympic games, and so on. What is common to them all? – Don't say: "There must be something common, or they would not be called 'games'" – but *look and see* whether there is anything common to all. – For if you look at them you will not see something that is common to *all*, but similarities, relationships, and a whole series of them at that. To repeat: don't think, but look! – Look for example at board-games, with their multifarious relationships. Now pass to card-games; here you find many correspondences with the first group, but many common features drop out, and others appear. When we pass next to ball-games, much that is common is retained, but much is lost. – Are they all 'amusing'? Compare chess with noughts and crosses. Or is there always winning and losing, or competition between players? Think of patience. In ball-games there is winning and losing; but when a child throws his ball at the wall and catches it again, this feature has disappeared. Look at the parts played by skill and luck; and at the difference between skill in chess and skill in tennis. Think now of games like ring-a-ring-a-roses; here is the element of amusement, but how many other characteristic features have disappeared! And we can go through the many, many other groups of games in the same way; can see how similarities crop up and disappear.

And the result of this examination is: we see a complicated network of similarities overlapping and criss-crossing: sometimes overall similarities, sometimes similarities of detail (Wittgenstein, 1953, section 66).

I can think of no better expression to characterize these similarities than "family resemblances;" for the various resemblances between members of a family: build, features, colour of eyes, gait, temperament, etc. etc. overlap and criss-cross in the same way. – And I shall say: 'games' form a family ... (ibid., section 67).

The central idea that Wittgenstein has suggested loosely in the context quoted above, is the replacement of the common-to-all postulate with *family resemblance*.[33] A vast amount of thought has been devoted to this proposal in philosophy and social sciences ever since. However, it remains a mere metaphor yet. Notwithstanding the prominence it has gained in the literature in the meantime, we shall refrain from using it in our metanosology to explain why 50,000 heterogeneous human conditions such as myocardial infarction and alopecia areata are deemed to form, like Wittgenstein's 'games', a coherent category called the category of 'diseases'. Our reason for refraining is that Wittgenstein's conception of family resemblance is philosophically defective. This may be easily demonstrated in the following way:

The resemblances between members of a family are causally due to the members' origin from the same germ line. So, we may state: "The origin of the members a and b from the same family is the cause of their resemblance". However, Wittgenstein reverses this causal order in that he metaphorically explains, or justifies, the belonging of some members to the same family by resemblances between them: "The resemblance between the members a and b is the cause, or reason, of their belonging to the same family". That is, Wittgenstein's idea around resemblance as a basis of categorization carries something innovative and interesting, though, we must give up its constituent term "family" to prevent misconceptions. By so doing we may forge a link

---

[33] It is said that Wittgenstein might have adopted the idea of family resemblance from Friedrich Nietzsche. Nietzsche in his *Beyond Good and Evil* (first published in 1886) is speculating about the "family resemblance of all Indian, Greek, and German philosophizing", which he attributes to the "affinity" of their languages (Nietzsche, 1955, section 20).

between his insights and Eleanor Rosch's aforementioned experimental studies on categorization to construct in the next section a new concept that we term *"prototype resemblance category"*. It will constitute one of the basic tools in our philosophy of disease.

Prototype resemblance categories

A reducible category such as the category of even numbers or square figures is a sharply bound collection of homogeneous objects all of which to the same extent share, due to their ('common to all') uniformity, a number of common-to-all features. For example, there is no even number that is more even or less even than another even number. The number 18 is as even as the number 332. All even numbers are equally even.

In contrast to this, there are no common-to-all features in an irreducible category. Both regarding their number as well as their intensity, the features are unequally distributed over the category members to the effect that some members appear *more typical* of the category than other ones. In the category of birds, for instance, a robin seems to be a more birdlike, typical bird than a penguin. This was convincingly demonstrated by Eleanor Rosch who in experimental studies asked the subjects to rate on a scale from 1 to 7 the typicality of different kinds of birds. Robins were considered the best examples followed by doves, sparrows, and canaries. Owls, parrots, and toucans occupied a medium position. Ducks and peacocks were considered less good examples. Penguins and ostrichs ranked lowest. Similar experiments were carried out for the categories furniture, fruit, and clothing (Rosch, 1975).

On the basis of the findings reported by Eleanor Rosch and others, a *non-classical theory of concepts* is emerging according to which a concept determines a category not by identifying necessary and sufficient features of its members, but by exhibiting the *relational structure* of the category that is characterized by best examples, called prototypes, such that other category members resemble them to different extents. In the category of birds, for instance, a robin *has feathers, has a beak, lays eggs, chirps, flies,* and so on. Penguins, however, do not possess all of these features. They cannot chirp and fly. They only resemble robins to the extent that they *have feathers, have a beak, and lay eggs.* This partial similarity to robins renders them less typical examples of birds than robins are, though, they are considered birds nonetheless. Thus, defining features of robins such as *has feathers, has a beak, lays eggs, chirps, flies,* and the like are not necessary conditions for an entity to count as a member of the category.

Related examples are the category of fruits with, for instance, an orange being a more typical fruit than a coconut; the category of vegetables with spinach being a more typical vegetable than melon; and furniture with chair and sofa being more typical instances than picture and radio.

The variance of typicality among the instances of an irreducible category lends to the category an internal structure with a central tendency such that some members are more central to the category than other ones at its periphery, giving rise to gradients of category membership. The most central members, let us call them foci or cores, may be viewed as the category's prototypes.

It is interesting to observe that a member's being a *more-typical-instance-than* another member is obviously a *relational feature,* specifically a comparative one in the form of *"x is a C more than y is",* where C is the category. For example, "a sparrow is more birdlike than a penguin". The comparative feature, *"more birdlike than"* in the present example, induces some kind of gradedness of membership in the category. This gradedness is best reconstructible as degrees of feature matching, i.e., similarity between less typical members of the category and its prototypes. Such a category we therefore call a *prototype resemblance category,* in contrast to the defective Wittgensteinian family resemblances. Below we shall introduce this novel concept to interpret the category of diseases as an instance thereof.[34]

Human conditions

The concept of fuzzy set discussed in Chapter 30 will be used as a tool to introduce both the notion of disease and the notion of similarity that we need in analyzing the resemblance of what is called *a* disease with prototypes. In this section, we will prepare the conceptual basis of our task.

Our aim is to clarify the term "disease" and to develop a precise concept of disease. To do so we must forget the 'disease' paradigm that we have inherited from our ancestors, and begin anew. Our first axiom is that the potential domain of application of our term "disease" should not consist of objects such as bookshelves, cars, planets, ants, or organs, tissues and cells, but of complex *human conditions* such as heart attack, stroke, breast cancer, love, believing, happiness, tax evasion, and many other possible and impossible things insofar as they are *human conditions.* Thus, the general and basic term we will use before we have a concept of disease, is the phrase "human condition". In the present section, this concept will be introduced to delimit the category of human conditions as the universe of our discourse. Later on the term "disease" will be ostensively interpreted over this general universe of our discourse to constitute a subcategory thereof.

A human condition such as heart attack, love, or happiness is conceived of as a set of $n \geq 1$ states in which a human being may be at a particular instant of time. A simple example is the following set of states we encounter in the individual Elroy Fox: {Elroy Fox is old, Elroy Fox has grey hair, Elroy

---

[34] When a preliminary version of our theory of disease was published in the Journal of Medicine and Philosophy in 2008 (Sadegh-Zadeh, 2008), the journal issue editor wrote in his prefatory comments: "The notion of a family resemblance concept is used by Sadegh-Zadeh in contrast to the classical understanding of a concept, ..." (Hinkley, 2008, 101). Our outline above shows that Hinkley's judgment and comment is incorrect. It has been made sufficiently clear that prototype resemblance is not family resemblance.

Fox is a Catholic, Elroy Fox is happy, Elroy Fox has a headache, Elroy Fox has a fever, Elroy Fox coughs, ... etc. ... }. To simplify the handling of such data, we represent a human condition not as a set of states as above, but as a *set of features* that characterize those states. Our last example now presents itself as the following set of features:

{old, grey hair, Catholic, happy, headache, fever, cough, ... etc. ... }

that the patient Elroy Fox has. This example demonstrates that human conditions are not, and should not be, confined to biological or biomedical states of the organism. They may be conceived as entities that also refer to subjective, religious, moral, social, and transcendental worlds of a *person* such as, for example, intelligence, love, pain, distress, feelings of loneliness, beliefs, desires, behavioral disorders, etc. We have thus freed ourselves from the biased notions of "symptom", "sign", and the like to prevent nosological prejudices. By assigning names to human conditions it becomes possible to identify them as specific feature sets by using their names such as, for example:

- heart_attack = {chest_pain, elevated_CK_concentration, tachycardia, ... etc. ... },
- measles = {rash, Koplik's_spots, cough, fever, ... etc. ... },
- gastric_ulcer = {epigastric_pain, anorexia, vomiting, ... etc. ... },
- alopecia_areata = {hair_loss_on_the_scalp, ... etc. ... },
- being_in_love = {happy, sleepless, longing_for_the_lover, ... etc. ... }.

For instance, the term "heart attack" above denotes a human condition that consists of the features chest pain, elevated concentration in blood of creatine kinase (CK) enzyme, tachycardia, etc. In our pursuit of a concept of disease, it would be useful to be able to compare such human conditions with one another and to examine the similarity and dissimilarity between them. This requires a powerful concept of similarity. We shall introduce such a concept below. To this end, human conditions will be conceived as partial manifestations of a *standardized and agreed-upon*, global feature space $\mathcal{F}$ such as, for example:

$\mathcal{F}$ = {chest pain, elevated CK concentration, tachycardia, vomiting, anorexia, epigastric pain, rash, Koplik's spots, cough, fever, increased white blood count, bodily lesion, distress, discomfort, incapacity, dependency, premature death, dyspepsia, coma, bradycardia, elevated LDH, delusion, fear, ... etc. ... etc. ... }.

For simplicity's sake, let us symbolize this global feature space, $\mathcal{F}$, in the following fashion:

$$\mathcal{F} = \{F_1, F_2, F_3, \ldots, F_n\}$$

where each F_i with $1 \leq i \leq n$ is a feature such as chest pain, elevated CK, tachycardia, and the like. We can now represent a human condition such as heart attack, measles, gastric ulcer, and so on as a fuzzy set over the feature space $\mathcal{F}$ in the following way. A feature F_i from the standardized feature set $\mathcal{F}$ that is present in a human condition, is written $(F_i, 1)$, whereas a feature F_j that is not present, is written $(F_j, 0)$. Two example are:

$$\text{heart\_attack} = \{(F_1, 1), (F_2, 1), (F_3, 1), \ldots, (F_i, 0), (F_j, 0), (F_k, 0), \ldots\}$$
$$\text{measles} \quad\; = \{(F_1, 0), (F_2, 0), (F_3, 0), \ldots, (F_i, 1), (F_j, 1), (F_k, 1), \ldots\}.$$

More specifically:

$$\text{heart\_attack} = \{(\text{chest\_pain}, 1), (\text{elevated\_CK}, 1), \ldots, (\text{rash}, 0),$$
$$(\text{Koplik's\_spots}, 0), \ldots \text{ etc.}\}$$
$$\text{measles} \quad\; = \{(\text{chest\_pain}, 0), (\text{elevated\_CK}, 0), \ldots, (\text{rash}, 1),$$
$$(\text{Koplik's\_spots}, 1), \ldots \text{ etc.}\}.$$

In these fuzzy sets, a value such as 1 or 0 is the degree of membership of the respective feature F_i and indicates its presence or absence in the respective human condition as a fuzzy set. In a real-world human condition, however, a feature may not be definitely present or absent, but present to a particular extent different than 1 and 0. For instance, someone may have:

{mild chest pain, highly elevated CK, severe tachycardia, ...},

whereas someone else has:

{severe chest pain, slightly elevated CK, moderate tachycardia, ...},

and still another person has:

{very severe chest pain, slightly elevated CK, mild tachycardia, ...}.

That means that a feature such as *chest pain* may be considered a linguistic variable as discussed on pages 78 and 1019. As a linguistic variable, it may assume from among its term set any value such as mild, severe, very severe, and the like. This option calls for representing a feature as an ordered pair of attribute-value type, i.e., ⟨attribute, value⟩ consisting of a feature and its value such as, for example:

{(chest pain, severe), (CK, highly elevated), (tachycardia, moderate), ...},
{(chest pain, very severe), (CK, highly elevated), (tachycardia, mild), ...},
{(chest pain, mild), (CK, slightly elevated), (tachycardia, severe), ...}.

Idealizing these considerations, we may also adopt the more general view that a human being presents with a particular *fuzzy subset* of the feature space $\mathcal{F} = \{F_1, F_2, F_3, \ldots, F_n\}$ above, for example, with the following one:

{(chest_pain, 1), (elevated_CK, 0.4), (tachycardia, 0.9), ...},

or with this one:

{(chest_pain, 0), (elevated_CK, 0), (tachycardia, 0), ...}.

These two fuzzy sets are fuzzified human conditions, or *fuzzy human conditions* for short. The first one says that chest pain is present to the extent 1, elevated creatine kinase enzyme is present to the extent 0.4, and tachycardia is present to the extent 0.9. The second one means that each feature is present to the extent 0. Note that these numbers do not represent measurement results indicating measured intensity, concentration, frequency, weight, height or other quantities. They are fuzzy set membership degrees representing the extent to which a respective feature such as chest pain is a member of the fuzzy set. The answer to the important question as to the origin of such feature weights may be found at the end of Section 30.1 on page 1003.

Based on the view sketched thus far, 'diseases' will be construed as fuzzy human conditions. To this end, the feature space $\mathcal{F} = \{F_1, F_2, F_3, \ldots, F_n\}$ will be mapped to the unit interval $[0, 1]$ to obtain all possible fuzzy human conditions. Since we shall talk about a myriad of fuzzy human conditions, let us symbolize individual, fuzzy human conditions by $H_1, H_2, H_3, \ldots$ and so on. Correspondingly, their membership functions may be denoted by $\mu_{H_1}, \mu_{H_2}, \mu_{H_3}, \ldots$, and generally, by μ_{H_i} as the membership function of any human condition H_i with $i \geq 1$. Each of them specifically maps $\mathcal{F}$ to $[0, 1]$:

$$\mu_{H_i} : \mathcal{F} \mapsto [0, 1] \qquad \text{for } i \geq 1.$$

In this way, we obtain an infinite number of different fuzzy human conditions $H_1, H_2, H_3, \ldots$ over the feature space $\mathcal{F}$ such as, for instance:

$H_1 = \{(\text{chest\_pain}, 1), (\text{elevated\_CK}, 0.4), (\text{tachycardia}, 0.9), \ldots\}$,
$H_2 = \{(\text{chest\_pain}, 0), (\text{elevated\_CK}, 1), (\text{tachycardia}, 0), \ldots\}$,
$H_3 = \{(\text{chest\_pain}, 0), (\text{elevated\_CK}, 0), (\text{tachycardia}, 0), \ldots\}$,

and so on. A particular individual such as Elroy Fox may have H_1, whereas another individual such as Dirk Fox has H_2, still another individual such as Carla Fox has H_3, and so on. Interestingly enough, what is usually called an individual disease, will turn out to be such a fuzzy set. As we shall see later on, once individual diseases are represented in this way, they become precisely comparable with one another, although they may have nothing in common in the ordinary sense. Examples are H_1 and H_3 above. Elroy Fox (H_1) has chest pain, Carla Fox (H_3) has no chest pain. Elroy Fox has considerably elevated CK, Carla's CK is not elevated, and so on. We shall introduce a concept of similarity that enables us to measure the similarity and dissimilarity between such human conditions, although they have nothing in common.

Summarizing, we may state that the infinite set of all fuzzy sets over the feature space $\mathcal{F} = \{F_1, F_2, F_3, \ldots, F_n\}$, i.e., the fuzzy powerset of $\mathcal{F}$, constitutes the category of fuzzy human conditions. Let this category be denoted by $\mathcal{H}$. Each of its members is a fuzzy human condition of the form:

$$H = \left\{ \left(F_1, \mu_H(F_1)\right), \left(F_2, \mu_H(F_2)\right), \ldots, \left(F_n, \mu_H(F_n)\right) \right\} \tag{17}$$

over the feature space $\mathcal{F} = \{F_1, F_2, F_3, \ldots, F_n\}$, where an F_i is a feature such as chest pain, elevated CK, etc., and $\mu_H(F_i)$ is a real number in the unit interval $[0, 1]$ indicating the degree of its membership in the human condition H. The heart attack of a particular patient may be described, for example, by the fuzzy set $\{$(chest_pain, 1), (elevated_CK, 0.4), (tachycardia, 0.9), $\ldots$ etc.$\}$.

Similarity

The irreducible category of diseases will be construed as a set of human conditions whose members are individual diseases. The latter will be compared with one another to analyze similarities and dissimilarities between them. To this end, a concept of similarity is briefly introduced below.

The most interesting and best-known concept of similarity outside fuzzy logic is the one suggested by Amos Tversky (1977). However, viewed from the perspective of fuzzy logic it is too coarse, and thus, not good enough. We shall therefore replace it with one constructed by means of our fuzzy-logical terminology.

Let Ω be a universe of discourse, e.g., the above-mentioned feature space $\mathcal{F}$. Its fuzzy powerset is $F(2^{\mathcal{F}})$, i.e., *the set of all fuzzy sets* over $\mathcal{F}$ comprising all fuzzy human conditions. Similarity will be conceived as a quantitative relation between each two members, A and B, of such a fuzzy powerset. It will be represented by a binary function with the syntax "fuzzy set A is similar to fuzzy set B to the extent r", symbolized by $simil(A, B) = r$. This new concept will enable us to measure how similar, for example, the following two fuzzy sets are:

$\{$(chest_pain, 1), (elevated_CK, 0.4)$\}$,
$\{$(chest_pain, 0.7), (elevated_CK, 0.8)$\}$.

An inverse semantic relationship ties the terms "different" and "similar". It says that the less different two objects, the more similar they are, and vice versa. This implies that the less different two fuzzy sets, the more similar they are. In complete accord with this precept, we shall construct our fuzzy set similarity relation as the inverse of *fuzzy set difference*. So, we need to introduce a notion of fuzzy set difference as our basic term first.

The difference between two fuzzy sets, A and B, will be defined as a quantitative relation of the form "fuzzy set A differs from fuzzy set B to the extent r", symbolized by $diff(A, B) = r$. The value r is a real number in the unit interval $[0, 1]$. In defining the basic notion $diff(A, B)$ we shall need the following three auxiliary notions, introduced in turn: collective summation symbol $\sum$, fuzzy set count, the absolute value of a real number.

If $r_1, \ldots, r_n$ are any real numbers, for instance 5, 18, -2, then their sum is conveniently written by using the summation symbol sigma, $\sum$, thus:

$$\sum r_i \qquad \qquad for\ 1 \leq i \leq n$$

in place of the familiar notation $r_1 + \cdots + r_n$. That is, the collective summation symbol is defined by:

$$\sum r_i = r_1 + \cdots + r_n \qquad for\ 1 \le i \le n.$$

For example, if our numbers $r_1, \ldots, r_n$ are 5, 18, -2; then we have $\sum r_i = 5 + 18 + (-2) = 21$. As a first application of $\sum$, we may demonstrate how the *count* of a fuzzy set A, denoted by $c(A)$, is obtained.

Definition 32 (Fuzzy set count). *If $A = \{(x_1, \mu_A(x_1)), \ldots, (x_n, \mu_A(x_n))\}$ is a fuzzy set, then its* size *or* count *is simply the sum of its membership degrees, that is:*

$$c(A) = \sum \mu_A(x_i) \qquad for\ 1 \le i \le n$$
$$= \mu_A(x_1) + \cdots + \mu_A(x_n).$$

For instance, regarding our fuzzy set $A = \{(x,\ 1),\ (y,\ 0.4),\ (z,\ 0.9)\}$ we have $c(A) = 1 + 0.4 + 0.9 = 2.3$.

The final auxiliary notion we need is the term "the absolute value of a real number". The absolute value of a real number r, represented by $|r|$, is its size without regard to its sign. For instance, $|-5| = 5$ and also $|5| = 5$. Thus we have $|-7 + 3| = 4$ and $|-0.2 - 0.8| = 0.6$. The precise definition of the term $|r|$ is as follows:

Definition 33 (Absolute value). *For all r, if r is a real number, then:*

$$|r| = \begin{cases} r & if\ r \ge 0 \\ -r & if\ r < 0. \end{cases}$$

In the above example, we have $|-5| = -(-5) = 5$. Thus, $|-5| = |5| = 5$. The notion of absolute value is useful in situations where it is not desirable to obtain a negative number as the outcome of a calculation. A negative outcome $-r$ is converted to a positive one by $|-r|$. Such is the case, as we soon shall see, when we want to determine the degree of difference between two fuzzy sets. This notion will now be introduced. To this end, let Ω be a universe of discourse and let A and B be two fuzzy sets in Ω such that:

$$A = \{(x_1, a_1), \ldots, (x_n, a_n)\}, \tag{18}$$
$$B = \{(x_1, b_1), \ldots, (x_n, b_n)\},$$

where an a_i is the degree of membership of x_i in set A, and a b_i is the degree of membership of the same object x_i in set B. The difference between such fuzzy sets is defined as follows:

Definition 34 (Fuzzy set difference). *If A and B are two fuzzy sets of the form above, then:*

$$diff(A,\ B) = \frac{\sum_i |a_i - b_i|}{c(A \cup B)}.$$

Expressed in plain words, the function *diff* measures the difference between two fuzzy sets A and B in the following way:

a) For each object x_i in both sets A and B:
b) from the degree of its membership in set A we subtract its degree of membership in set B,
c) we add up the absolute values of all differences thus obtained (the numerator of the fraction above), and
d) average the outcome over the size of both sets, that is, over the count $c(A \cup B)$ of their union (the denominator of the fraction above).

For example, if our fuzzy sets are:

$$X = \{(x, 1), (y, 0.4)\},$$
$$Y = \{(x, 0.8), (y, 0.6)\}.$$

then we have:

$$
\begin{aligned}
diff(X, Y) &= \frac{|1 - 0.8| + |0.4 - 0.6|}{1 + 0.6} \\
&= \frac{0.4}{1.6} \\
&= 0.25.
\end{aligned}
$$

This calculation shows that set X differs from set Y to the extent 0.25. With the above in mind, we may now introduce fuzzy *similarity* as the additive inverse of fuzzy set difference in the following way (adapted from Lin, 1997):

Definition 35 (Fuzzy [set] similarity). $simil(A, B) = 1 - diff(A, B)$.

For instance, our two example fuzzy sets X and Y above with the difference 0.25 between them are *similar* to the extent $1 - 0.25 = 0.75$. A convenient method of computing similarities is provided by the Similarity Theorem that is implied by Definitions 34 and 35. We shall use it for our computations below. For the proof of the theorem, see (Lin, 1997):

Theorem 1 (Similarity Theorem).

$$simil(A, B) = \frac{c(A \cap B)}{c(A \cup B)}.$$

Regarding our two example fuzzy sets X and Y above, we have according to this theorem: $simil(X, Y) = \frac{0.8 + 0.4}{1 + 0.6} = \frac{1.2}{1.6} = 0.75$.

Similarity as defined above, is a relationship between fuzzy sets. According to Definition 35, its extent is a real number in the unit interval $[0, 1]$. The concept introduced is applicable to fuzzy human conditions, and consequently, to diseases. Summarizing, we may state that both *diff* and *simil* are binary numerical functions that map the Cartesian product of the fuzzy powerset of a universe of discourse, Ω, to the unit interval:

$$diff: F(2^\Omega) \times F(2^\Omega) \mapsto [0, 1]$$
$$simil: F(2^\Omega) \times F(2^\Omega) \mapsto [0, 1].$$

In closing this section, it is worth noting that the *dissimilarity* between two fuzzy sets A and B is the inverse of their similarity and is, therefore, straight-forwardly definable in the following way:

Definition 36 (Fuzzy [set] dissimilarity). $dissimil(A, B) = 1 - simil(A, B)$.

This together with Definition 35 above implies: $dissimil(A, B) = diff(A, B)$. Thus, dissimilarity and difference are identical.

The prototype resemblance theory of disease

How can we exploit the constructs provided in the preceding sections to clarify and understand the category of diseases? How can we ascertain a difference in the typicality of diseases such that, for example, myocardial infarction may bear a greater diseasehood than alopecia areata, while another phenomenon such as homosexuality or the running away of slaves may turn out a non-disease? Where do diseases come from? Are they value-free, natural phenomena to be discovered in the world out there, or are they man-made, value-laden artifacts? In the present section, we shall put forward a conceptual framework capable of resolving problems of just this type. Our first step in this direction is the construction of the concept of a *prototype resemblance category*. It will be instrumental in demonstrating that diseases, in the plural, are members of a prototype resemblance category that is an irreducible category constituted by some prototypes to which the remaining members of the category, 'the diseases', are similar to different extents.

In our analyses, the notions of "resemblance" and "similarity" will be considered synonyms. But for the sake of mnemonic convenience, they will play distinct contextual roles. The term "resemblance" is preferred for use only in the proper name "resemblance category". In all other contexts the term "similarity" and its derivatives are used.

It was noted above that the current nosological system of medicine allegedly comprises about 50,000 individual diseases. Examples are myocardial infarction, gastric ulcer, breast cancer, alcoholism, schizophrenia, alopecia areata, etc. A fundamental problem of metanosology neglected in medicine is the question *why* these human conditions are categorized as 'diseases' and others are excluded, e.g., menstruation, pregnancy, tax evasion, smoking, love, torture, terrorism, and so on. Of course, we do not mean that the latter examples are, or have to be categorized as, diseases. We only ask for what reason they are *not* categorized as diseases.

What is called *a* disease in medicine, is representable as a fuzzy human condition of the form $H = \{(F_1, \mu_H(F_1)), (F_2, \mu_H(F_2)), \ldots, (F_n, \mu_H(F_n))\}$. In this fuzzy set, each F_i is a feature from the standardized, agreed-upon feature space $\mathcal{F} = \{F_1, F_2, F_3, \ldots, F_n\}$ mentioned on page 168 above. It may be a symptom, complaint, problem, sign, or finding; and $\mu_H(F_i)$ is the degree of its membership in fuzzy set H. Formal examples are:

$$\text{myocardial\_infarction} = \{(F_1,1),(F_2,1),(F_3,1),\ldots,$$
$$(F_i,0),(F_j,0),(F_k,0),\ldots \text{ etc. } \ldots\}$$
$$\text{gastric\_ulcer} \qquad = \{(F_1,0),(F_2,0),(F_3,0),\ldots,$$
$$(F_i,0.8),(F_j,0.7),(F_k,1),\ldots \text{ etc. } \ldots\}$$
$$\text{alopecia\_areata} \qquad = \{(F_1,0),(F_2,0),(F_3,0),\ldots,$$
$$(F_i,0),(F_j,0),(F_k,0.2),\ldots \text{ etc. } \ldots\}.$$

For instance, myocardial infarction may be something like the following fuzzy set:[35]

$$\{(\text{chest\_pain, 1}), (\text{elevated\_CK, 0.7}), (\text{tachycardia, 0.8}), \ldots \text{ etc. } \ldots\}.$$

These examples demonstrate that the so-called diseases, reconstructed as fuzzy human conditions, are too different from one another to share common-to-all features that could provide *necessary and sufficient conditions* of their diseasehood. For this reason, the nosological class that comprises such fuzzy human conditions as 'diseases', cannot be based on, and represented by, a classical, reductively definable concept of disease. Despite the long history of medicine, it has not yet been possible to arrive at such a concept. The lack of common-to-all features of diseasehood raises the question, how is the irreducible category of diseases constituted so as to house completely different individual diseases as its members nonetheless?

On the one hand, there is no doubt that a number of so-called diseases are myths and conceptual illusions, e.g., drapetomania and hysteria. On the other hand, there are human conditions such as heart attack, breast cancer, epilepsy, and many others that have been known throughout the history of medicine and are encountered in all human societies today. What is usually meant by "diseases" are *'such real-world phenomena and similar things'* even though the belief in their existence depends on perspectives, e.g., the conceptual and epistemic systems that one holds (see Part VI). Although all of these human conditions are different from one another and lack any common-to-all features, they are placed, within the large class of human conditions, in the same category labeled "diseases". Our question above asks how this categorization may be understood and justified. The answer to this question we suggest is the following *prototype resemblance theory of disease*.

We assume that there are a few human conditions such as, for example, heart attack, breast cancer, stroke, epilepsy, pneumonia, measles, smallpox, schizophrenia, and the like which have existed for a long time, probably since the dawn of mankind. For reasons that we shall discuss shortly, each of these few human conditions is christened a disease by the society and is handled

---

[35] For detailed examples of fuzzy representation of individual diseases, see (Barro and Marin, 2002; Mordeson et al., 2000; Steimann, 2001b; Szczepaniak et al., 2000) and the journal *Artificial Intelligence in Medicine*.

as a prototype disease. This act of naming is an ostensive definition of the term "disease". Any other human condition that bears sufficient similarity to such a prototype disease, is also considered a disease. Thus, the category of diseases in a society emerges from two factors: (1) the existence of a few human conditions each of which is ostensively *named* a disease by the society and viewed as a prototype disease; (2) sufficient *similarity* of some other human conditions to a prototype disease. Viewed from a formal perspective, this emergence of the category of diseases may be understood as a recursive definition in the following way. (For the methods of ostensive and recursive definition, see pages 101 and 96.)

Let there be a few human conditions $H_1, \ldots, H_n$ such as heart attack, breast cancer, stroke, epilepsy, etc. The following two steps recursively define the term "disease":

Basis step: Any element of the base set $\{H_1, \ldots, H_n\}$ is a disease;
Recursion step: A human condition that is similar to a disease $H_i \in$
                           $\{H_1, \ldots, H_n\}$ is a disease.

A definition of this form is able to generate, through recursion, a potentially infinite set of diseases. But the definition is not yet good enough. We will now expand upon its recursive procedure to show how the concept of disease may be conceived.

Definition 37 (A crisp concept of disease). *Let $\mathcal{F} = \{F_1, F_2, \ldots, F_m\}$ be an agreed-upon feature space with $m \geq 1$ features. And let $\mathcal{H}$ be the set of all fuzzy human conditions over $\mathcal{F}$, i.e., the fuzzy powerset $F(2^{\mathcal{F}})$. If $\mathfrak{s}$ is a human society and $\{H_1, \ldots, H_n\}$ is a small subset of $\mathcal{H}$ with $n \geq 1$ members such as $\{$heart attack, breast cancer, stroke, epilepsy, pneumonia, measles, smallpox, $\ldots$, schizophrenia$\}$ each of which is named a disease by the society $\mathfrak{s}$, then in this society:*

1. *Any element of the set $\{H_1, \ldots, H_n\}$ is a disease, referred to as a pro-totype or core disease,*
2. *A fuzzy human condition $X \in \mathcal{H}$ is a disease if there is a disease H_i in $\{H_1, \ldots, H_n\}$ and an $\varepsilon > 0$ chosen by the society $\mathfrak{s}$ such that $simil(X, H_i) \geq \varepsilon$.*

Note that the concept of disease suggested in Definition 37 is non-classical because it does not reduce diseasehood to a set of common-to-all features. It only requires that there be at least one prototype human condition *named* "disease" by the society and that any other human condition be similar to such a prototype disease to a particular extent in order to count as *a* disease, too. Suppose, for instance, that in a society the following simplified fuzzy human condition is a prototype disease:

heart_attack $= \{(F_1, 1), (F_2, 0.4), (F_3, 0.9)\}$

The minimum degree of similarity to this prototype disease that a human condition is required to bear in order to be categorized as a disease, may be $\varepsilon = 0.5$. The degree of similarity between the following human condition:

$$\text{gastric\_ulcer} = \{(F_1, 0.8), (F_2, 0.6), (F_3, 0.3)\}$$

and heart attack above is 0.6. This is easily computed in the following way by using the Similarity Theorem above:

$$simil(\text{gastric\_ulcer, heart\_attack}) = \frac{c\,(\text{gastric\_ulcer} \cap \text{heart\_attack})}{c\,(\text{gastric\_ulcer} \cup \text{heart\_attack})}$$
$$= 0.8 + 0.4 + 0.3/1 + 0.6 + 0.9$$
$$= 1.5/2.5$$
$$= 0.6.$$

Since $0.6 > 0.5$, the human condition *gastric ulcer* above turns out a disease. By contrast, the human condition:

$$\text{pregnancy} = \{(F_1, 0.1), (F_2, 0.2), (F_3, 0.39)\}$$

cannot be considered a disease because it is similar to the prototype disease *heart attack* above only to the extent 0.3, i.e., $simil$(pregnancy, heart_attack) $= \frac{0.1+0.2+0.39}{1+0.4+0.9} = \frac{0.69}{2.3} = 0.3$. The required degree of similarity, $\varepsilon = 0.5$, partitions the set $\mathcal{H}$ of human conditions into two categories, diseases and non-diseases. The emerging category of diseases has sharp boundaries and is thus a crisp set with all-or-none membership. A human condition either is a disease or it is none. This crisp concept does not seem to reflect the real-world health care where the diseasehood of a human condition is considered to be something gradual, e.g., very severe, severe, moderate, mild or very mild. In real-world health care, a human condition does not constitute a subject of medical intervention because it is a disease, but because it is a disease to a particular extent that is no longer tolerable. This characteristic of clinical practice and nosology is taken into account by the following construct that yields a *fuzzy category of diseases* such that a human condition may be considered a disease to a particular extent. For example, it may turn out that according to such a concept, myocardial infarction is a disease to the extent 1, whereas alcoholism is a disease to the extent 0.5 and alopecia areata is a disease to the extent 0.1. A modified definition below will do justice to this alternative. To this end, we need first to generalize the binary functions $max(x, y)$ and $min(x, y)$ introduced in Definition 18 on page 94, to obtain the n-ary functions "maximum of more than two numbers" and "minimum of more than two numbers" with $n > 2$.

Definition 38 (Maximum and minimum of more than two numbers). *If* $(x_1, x_2, \ldots, x_n)$ *is an n-tuple of real numbers with $n > 2$, then:*

    a. $max(x_1, x_2, \ldots, x_n) = max\big(x_1, max(x_2, \ldots, x_n)\big).$

    b. $min(x_1, x_2, \ldots, x_n) = min\big(x_1, min(x_2, \ldots, x_n)\big).$

For example, $max(3, 5, 2) = max(3, max(5, 2)) = max(3, 5) = 5$. And $min(3, 5, 2, 1) = min(3, min(5, 2, 1)) = min(3, min(5, min(2, 1))) = min(3, min(5, 1)) = min(3, 1) = 1$.

Definition 39 (A fuzzy concept of disease). *Let* $\mathcal{F} = \{F_1, F_2, \ldots, F_m\}$ *be an agreed-upon feature space with* $m \geq 1$ *features. And let* $\mathcal{H}$ *be the set of all fuzzy human conditions over* $\mathcal{F}$*, i.e., the fuzzy powerset* $F(2^{\mathcal{F}})$*. If* s *is a human society and* $\{H_1, \ldots, H_n\}$ *is a small subset of* $\mathcal{H}$ *with* $n \geq 1$ *members such as* {*heart attack, breast cancer, stroke, epilepsy, pneumonia, measles, smallpox,* ..., *schizophrenia*} *each of which is named a disease by the society* s*, then in this society:*

1. *Any element of the set* $\{H_1, \ldots, H_n\}$ *is a* disease to the extent 1, *referred to as a* prototype *or* core disease,
2. *A fuzzy human condition* $X \in \mathcal{H}$ *is a* disease to the extent ε *if* $\varepsilon = max\big(simil(X, H_1), \ldots, simil(X, H_n)\big)$.

This fuzzy concept of disease differs from the first, crisp one given above in that the category of diseases created by this concept does not have sharp boundaries. A human condition may be a disease to an extent between 0 and 1. The degree of its maximum similarity with prototype diseases yields the degree of its diseasehood. For example, let the following human condition be, for simplicity's sake, the only prototype disease:

heart_attack $= \{(F_1, 1), (F_2, 0.4), (F_3, 0.9)\}$.

Then the human condition:

hemorrhoids $= \{(F_1, 0.6), (F_2, 0.1), (F_3, 0.22)\}$

turns out a disease to the extent 0.4 because $simil$(hemorrhoids, heart_attack) $= 0.4$. By contrast, the human condition:

homosexuality $= \{(F_1, 0), (F_2, 0), (F_3, 0)\}$

is a disease to the extent 0 because $simil$(homosexuality, heart_attack) $= 0$. The category of diseases established by a non-classical concept of disease of the type above is a fuzzy set. Any human condition is a member of the category, i.e., *a* disease, to a particular extent between 0 and 1. For instance, the above-mentioned human condition hemorrhoids $= \{(F_1, 0.6), (F_2, 0.1), (F_3, 0.22)\}$ is a member of the category to the extent 0.4. This peculiarity of fuzzy disease has far-reaching logical and metaphysical consequences that we shall discuss in Section 6.3.4 below. To prepare the discussion, we will now extensionally reformulate Definition 39 by the following equivalent that spotlights the fuzzy category of diseases, denoted $\mathbb{D}$.

Definition 40 (A concept of fuzzy disease: extensional). *Let* $\mathcal{F} = \{F_1, F_2, \ldots, F_m\}$ *be an agreed-upon feature space with* $m \geq 1$ *features. And let* $\mathcal{H}$ *be the set of all fuzzy human conditions over* $\mathcal{F}$*, i.e., the fuzzy powerset* $F(2^{\mathcal{F}})$.

*If ₅ is a human society and $\{H_1, \ldots, H_n\}$ is a small subset of $\mathcal{H}$ with $n \geq 1$
members such as {heart attack, breast cancer, stroke, epilepsy, pneumonia,
measles, smallpox, ..., schizophrenia} each of which is named a disease by
the society ₅, then in this society a fuzzy set $\mathbb{D}$ over $\mathcal{H}$ is the category of
diseases iff there is a function $\mu_\mathbb{D}$ with:*

$$\mu_\mathbb{D} : \mathcal{H} \mapsto [0, 1]$$

such that:

1. $\mu_\mathbb{D}(X) = \begin{cases} 1 & \text{if } X \in \{H_1, \ldots, H_n\}, \text{ called a prototype or core disease,} \\ \varepsilon & \text{if } \varepsilon = max\big(simil(X, H_1), \ldots, simil(X, H_n)\big). \end{cases}$

2. $\mathbb{D} = \big\{ \big(H_i, \mu_\mathbb{D}(H_i)\big) \mid H_i \in \mathcal{H} \big\}.$

The category of diseases, $\mathbb{D}$, is the fuzzy set $\{(H_i, \mu_\mathbb{D}(H_i)) \mid H_i \in \mathcal{H}\}$ consisting of all pairs of the form $\big(H_i, \mu_\mathbb{D}(H_i)\big)$ such that H_i is a human condition
in $\mathcal{H}$ and $\mu_\mathbb{D}(H_i)$ is the degree of its membership in $\mathbb{D}$, i.e., the degree of its
diseasehood. According to clause 1, the degree of diseasehood of a human
condition equals its maximum similarity to prototype diseases. Thus, the category of diseases is similarity-based and originates from its prototypes. It may
therefore be viewed as a *prototype resemblance category*.

A prototype resemblance category is irreducible because it is not defined
by a set of common-to-all features, but by similarity. Depending on the number n of the prototypes $\{H_1, \ldots, H_n\}$ in a prototype resemblance category,
we may distinguish between *monofocal* and *multifocal* categories. A category
is monofocal if $n = 1$, and multifocal if $n > 1$. Our example category above
with heart_attack $= \{(F_1, 1), (F_2, 0.4), (F_3, 0.9)\}$ as its only prototype disease was a monofocal one. However, the category of diseases in real-world
medicine is, like the categories of birds, fruits and vegetables, multifocal. It embraces many distinct prototype diseases giving rise to a number of nosological
subcategories such as *infectious diseases, cardiovascular diseases, metabolic
diseases, autoimmune diseases, genetic diseases, neoplasms, mental diseases,*
and so on. Since the category is irreducible, i.e., since individual diseases as its
members lack common-to-all features, an individual disease such as depression
that may sufficiently resemble a particular prototype disease, say schizophrenia, need not have anything in common with any other, remote, say 'somatic',
disease such as diabetes, glomerulonephritis, or cholelithiasis. No argument
by Thomas Szasz and others of like mind could then deny depression of diseasehood simply because its resemblance to schizophrenia as the supposed
prototype disease of the respective system is sufficient to categorize it as a
disease (see Section 19.3.3 on page 730).

The approach we have taken above is not the only possible way to demonstrate that the category of diseases is irreducible and is therefore best represented by a non-classical concept of disease. A clear and powerful philosophical

method to build the whole framework consists in analyzing the issue by constructing set-theoretical predicates. Such a set-theoretical predicate will now be briefly introduced to frame our theory and to apply it to our problem. Corresponding to Definitions 37 and 39 above, we will sketch a concept of *prototype resemblance frame* on the basis of which a concept of *prototype resemblance category* will be introduced. It is not a difficult task to interpret the real-world category of diseases as an instance of this latter concept, i.e., as a prototype resemblance category.[36]

Definition 41 (Prototype resemblance frame). ξ *is a prototype resemblance frame iff there are* Ω, A_1, ..., A_n, B, f, *and* $\mathfrak{s}$ *such that:*

1. $\xi = \langle \Omega, \{A_1, \ldots, A_n\}, B, f, \mathfrak{s} \rangle$;
2. Ω *is a non-empty set referred to as the universe of discourse;*
3. $\{A_1, \ldots, A_n\}$ *is a subset of* Ω *with* $n \geq 1$;
4. B *is a fuzzy set in* Ω;
5. f *is a similarity function like* simil *in Definition 35 on page 173 that maps pairs of* Ω *to* $[0, 1]$;
6. $\mathfrak{s}$ *is a human society;*
7. *Each member of* $\{A_1, \ldots, A_n\}$ *is a member of* B *to the extent* 1 *if it is considered a prototype in* B *by the society* $\mathfrak{s}$;
8. *A member* X *of* Ω *is a member of* B *to the extent* ε *iff* $\varepsilon = max\big(f(X, A_1),$ $\ldots, f(X, A_n)\big)$ *and* $\varepsilon > 0$.

To give a simple example, suppose that we have:

- Ω $\equiv$ the class of animals,
- $\{A_1, \ldots, A_n\}$ $\equiv$ {robin, sparrow, blackbird, crow} with $n = 4$,
- B $\equiv$ the class of birds, a fuzzy set in Ω,
- $\mathfrak{s}$ $\equiv$ the society of Western Europeans,
- f $\equiv$ *simil*, i.e., the similarity function introduced in Definition 35 on page 173

such that {*robin, sparrow, blackbird, crow*} are considered prototype birds by Western Europeans. So, according to axiom 7 of the definition above, each of these four animal species is to the extent 1 a member of the class of birds. In addition, according to axiom 8 any other species X in Ω, i.e., any other animal species, is to the extent $\varepsilon > 0$ a bird if $simil(X, A_i) = \varepsilon$ is the maximum degree of its similarity to the four above-mentioned prototypes in the class. Thus, the following structure satisfies all axioms of Definition 41 and is therefore a prototype resemblance frame: $\langle animals, \{robin,\ sparrow,$ *blackbird, crow*}, *birds, simil, Western Europeans* $\rangle$.

---

[36] In an earlier version of our theory, the notion of a "*fuzzy* prototype resemblance category" was used (Sadegh-Zadeh, 2008). The qualification "fuzzy" has now been dropped because it has proved to be gratuitous.

Definition 42 (Prototype resemblance category). *B is a* prototype resemblance category *iff there are* Ω, A_1, ..., A_n, f, *and* $\mathfrak{s}$ *such that* $\langle \Omega, \{A_1, ..., A_n\}, B, f, \mathfrak{s} \rangle$ *is a prototype resemblance frame.*

For instance, the class of birds in our above example is a prototype resemblance category because there are:

animals, {*robin, sparrow, blackbird, crow*}, *simil, and Western Europeans*

such that the supplemented 5-tuple:

$\langle$*animals,* {*robin, sparrow, blackbird, crow*}, **birds,** *simil,*

Western Europeans$\rangle$

is a prototype resemblance frame. Note that according to the concept presented in Definition 42, a class is a prototype resemblance category if it satisfies what is required by the preceding Definition 41. Specifically, membership in a *prototype resemblance category* is a matter of degree. The degree of category membership of an object equals 1 if the object is a prototype; otherwise, it equals the maximum degree of the object's similarity to prototypes. Thus, degrees of membership in the category smoothly decrease in the direction of non-membership such that the category has no sharp boundaries between full members and non-members. Most importantly, the category-generating, focal members of the category, i.e., its prototypes $\{A_1, ..., A_n\}$, are chosen by a human society to the effect that the society is in fact the inventor of the category. For example, it may be that what Australians view as the category of birds, vegetables, fruits, furniture, or cloths is not identical with what the Siberians do because the category-generating focal members of an Australian category differ from those of the Siberian category. An Australian category may partially overlap a Siberian one, though, they need not match completely. Thus, the question of whether a category "exists in the real world" becomes meaningless. Categories are cultural products. We are now in a position to state a hypothesis that is amenable to empirical examination:

Assertion 2. *The category of diseases in Western medicine, denoted* $\mathbb{D}$*, is a prototype resemblance category (as defined in Definition 42 above).*

To support this assertion, we will first assemble the required conceptual preconditions:

1. Let our universe of discourse be the class of all fuzzy human conditions, denoted $\mathcal{H}$, that we conceptualized on page 170 above;
2. Let $\{H_1, ..., H_n\}$ be a subset of $\mathcal{H}$, for example, fuzzy human conditions such as heart attack, breast cancer, stroke, epilepsy, pneumonia, measles, smallpox, and schizophrenia, as reconstructed above. We suppose that a couple of human conditions like these examples are considered *prototype diseases* in Western societies. This supposition will be discussed in Section 14.4 on page 572;

3. We have seen above that individual diseases are representable as fuzzy human conditions, i.e., as elements of $\mathcal{H}$. Thus, the category of diseases, $\mathbb{D}$, is a subset of $\mathcal{H}$;

4. The society $\mathfrak{s}$ may be Western Europeans;

5. Let the similarity function *simil*, introduced in Definition 35 on page 173, act as an instance of the similarity function f required in Definition 41;

6. Note that there are different degrees of similarity between fuzzy human conditions contained in $\mathcal{H}$ and the prototype diseases $\{H_1, \ldots, H_n\}$. For example, if in accord with the time-honored Hippocratic tradition, epilepsy is in fact considered a prototype disease $H_i \in \{H_1, \ldots, H_n\}$ by Western Europeans, then there is a considerable similarity between many neurological disorders, on the one hand, and epilepsy, on the other;

7. According to Definitions 40 and 41, set $\mathbb{D}$ emerges from 1–2 and 4–6. It is the category *disease* in Western European medicine.

These premises in conjunction with Definitions 40 and 41 imply the following statement:

Assertion 3. *The five-tuple* $\langle \mathcal{H}, \{H_1, \ldots, H_n\}, \mathbb{D}, simil, \text{ Western Europeans} \rangle$ *is a prototype resemblance frame.*

The following is a corollary of Definition 42 (after the rule "$\leftrightarrow$-Elimination" mentioned in Table 36 on page 895):

Corollary 1. *For every* $\mathbb{D}$, *if there are* $\mathcal{H}$, $\{H_1, \ldots, H_n\}$, *simil, and Western Europeans such that* $\langle \mathcal{H}, \{H_1, \ldots, H_n\}, \mathbb{D}, simil, \text{ Western Europeans} \rangle$ *is a prototype resemblance frame, then* $\mathbb{D}$ *is a prototype resemblance category.*

Assertion 2 follows from Assertion 3 and Corollary 1. That something is a prototype resemblance category implies that it is not a reducible category, but an irreducible one. It has already been outlined in Section 6.3.1 on page 162 why an irreducible category cannot be represented by a classical concept.

Our considerations above imply that the vast majority of the 50,000 individual diseases in current Western medicine are derived diseases in that their diseasehood is grounded on their similarity to some prototype diseases. Thus, the fundamental question of medicine "what is disease?" reduces to "what is a prototype disease?" or "where does a prototype disease come from?" This question will be discussed in the context of the moral construction of medical reality in Section 14.4 on page 572.

It is worth noting that a prototype disease may be *set-based* or *exemplar-based*. That is, it may refer to human conditions of a group of human beings such as, for example, recurring incidences of what has come to be termed "heart attack"; or to the human condition of a single individual such as, for instance, "the Kaspar Hauser Syndrome" (Money, 1992).[37]

In closing this section, two important remarks are in order. Until now, we have distinguished between classical and non-classical concepts to argue that *the concept of disease* belongs to the latter type. However, it must be emphasized that:

a. First, the notion of "non-classical concept" is not confined to concepts like the concept of disease that denote prototype resemblance categories. This subtype of non-classical concepts whose referents are prototype resemblance categories, may therefore be called *prototype resemblance predicates*. The concept of disease-in-general is such a prototype resemblance predicate. Do not try to explicate this predicate by enumerating a finite number of features that all diseases would have in common! This popular, traditional approach will forever remain a futile task. Other examples are the concepts of bird, fruit, and vegetable. As was suggested on page 147, the concept of a person may also be conceived as a prototype resemblance predicate.

b. Second, a classical, reducible category X with $m \geq 1$ necessary and sufficient features $\{F_1, \ldots, F_m\}$ such as "leucocytosis", "pulmonary tuberculosis", or "square figure" is representable as a fuzzy set of the form $X = \{(F_1, 1), \ldots, (F_m, 1)\}$ such that the membership degree of each feature F_i equals 1. For instance, the concept of a *square figure* that was classically defined in (15) on page 160, may be non-classically defined in the following way that is equivalent to (15):

$$\text{square figure} = \{(is\_a\_closed\_figure, 1),$$
$$(has\_four\_straight\_sides, 1),$$
$$(sides\_equal\_in\_length, 1),$$
$$(has\_equal\_angles, 1)\}.$$

Thus, a *classical concept* turns out the limiting case of non-classical concepts such that we may conclude:

The generality of non-classical concepts: The category of non-classical concepts is general enough to also include the classical concepts. In a nutshell, *every* concept is representable as a fuzzy structure such that its features are weighted in the unit interval [0, 1], the weights being the membership degrees of the features in the fuzzy structure.

---

[37] Kaspar Hauser (1812–1833) was a physically stunted 16-year-old boy with the mind of a child. He was found on May 26, 1828, in the streets of the city Nürnberg, South Germany, after sixteen years of neglect and isolation in a dungeon. See (Kitchen, 2001; Schiener, 2010).

6.3.2 Health

In this section and the next, a novel framework will be constructed, analogous to that of disease, that conceptualizes health and its fuzzy character. To aid us, we shall introduce a few new terms, and abandon others that are well-established, but inadequate. To begin with, we need not dwell on the World Health Organization's concept of health, as it is useless. In contrast to the customary practice in medicine and its philosophy, we shall also not consider the terms "health" and "disease" as mutual antonyms. We therefore abandon the view that "health is the absence of disease and vice versa". In our framework, the two terms are semantically independent of each other. As was emphasized previously, the antonym of "health" is "malady", denoting a much broader category than disease, that besides disease also contains injury, wound, lesion, defect, deformity, disorder, disability, impairment, and the like. See Figure 26 on page 154.

Suppose that someone consults her family physician because of a bee sting. Though she feels some pain in her right thumb where she has been stung, she doesn't feel ill in any sense of this term. Nor does she have a disease. She is simply *suffering*, a Homo patiens, i.e., a *patient*. This example demonstrates that there are patients who have no illness or disease. Our point of departure is thus the more general term "patient", defined as follows:

Definition 43 (Patient). *An individual is a patient if and only if the degree of her patienthood exceeds 0.*

The neologism "patienthood" in the definiens is our basic term. It serves as a handy substitute for "being afflicted by a malady" and will be defined in the next paragraph, followed by the concept of health as its antonym. To prepare its definition, let Ω be the set of all human beings at a particular instant of time, for example, right now. Suppose there is a fuzzy subset, $\mathbb{PAT}$, of Ω such that each member of the set $\mathbb{PAT}$ is characterized by a particular degree of each of the following features: *discomfort, pain, endogenously threatened life, loss of autonomy, loss of vitality,* and *loss of pleasure*. Thus, each member of $\mathbb{PAT}$ presents with a fuzzy human condition. An example is the human condition $\{(\text{discomfort}, 0.6), (\text{pain}, 0.5), (\text{endogenously\_threatened\_life}, 0.3), (\text{loss\_of\_autonomy}, 0.1), (\text{loss\_of\_vitality}, 0.3), (\text{loss\_of\_pleasure}, 1)\}$. The fuzziness of the set $\mathbb{PAT}$ means that a human being with such a human condition is its member to a particular extent between 0 and 1.

The extent to which an individual is a member of the fuzzy set $\mathbb{PAT}$, is called the degree of her *patienthood*. This degree of patienthood of an individual $x \in \Omega$ is indicated by the fuzzy set membership function $\mu_{\mathbb{PAT}}$, preferably written $\mu_{patienthood}$, such that $\mu_{patienthood}(x)$ is a real number in the unit interval $[0, 1]$. That means that we have the following mapping:

$$\mu_{patienthood} \colon \Omega \mapsto [0, 1]$$

that yields the above-mentioned fuzzy set $\mathbb{PAT}$ over Ω:

$$\mathbb{PAT} = \{(x,\, \mu_{patienthood}(x)) \mid x \in \Omega\}.$$

This set $\mathbb{PAT}$ contains every human being x from among Ω together with her $\mathbb{PAT}$ membership degree $\mu_{patienthood}(x)$. It may look like, for example, the following set:

$$\mathbb{PAT} = \{(Amy,\, 0),\, (Beth,\, 0.4),\, (Carla,\, 0),\, (Dirk,\, 0.7),\, (Elroy,\, 1),\, \dots\, \}.$$

Given any fuzzy set $A = \{(x_1, r_1),\, (x_2, r_2),\, (x_3, r_3),\, \dots\}$, its *support* is defined as the crisp set of those members whose membership degree exceeds 0. That is:

Definition 44 (Support of a fuzzy set). *If* $A = \{(x_1, r_1), (x_2, r_2), (x_3, r_3),\, \dots\}$ *is a fuzzy set, then* $support(A) = \{x_i \mid \mu_A(x_i) > 0\}$.

Thus, the support of fuzzy set $\mathbb{PAT}$ above is the crisp set of all human beings whose $\mu_{patienthood}$ degree exceeds 0. This is just the set of *patients* as this term was defined in Definition 43 above. *Patients* are the support of the fuzzy set $\mathbb{PAT}$, i.e., {Beth, Dirk, Elroy, ... } in the present example.

The fuzzy complement of patienthood, $\overline{\mathbb{PAT}}$, is referred to as *health*, i.e., 'the set of healthy people', and is written $\mathbb{H}$ instead of $\overline{\mathbb{PAT}}$. The degree of health of an individual $x \in \Omega$ is indicated by the membership function $\mu_{\mathbb{H}}$, preferably written μ_{health}. Thus, our terminology is:

$$\mu_{patienthood}(x) \quad \equiv\ \text{degree of patienthood of } x$$
$$\mu_{health}(x) \quad \equiv\ \text{degree of health of } x$$

where μ_{health} is defined as follows:

Definition 45 (Health membership function). $\mu_{health}(x) = 1 - \mu_{patienthood}(x)$.

It directly yields the health fuzzy set $\mathbb{H}$:

$$\mathbb{H} = \{(x,\, \mu_{health}(x)) \mid x \in \Omega\}.$$

For example, according to the arrangements above, an individual's degree of health is 0.6 if she has a patienthood of 0.4. Since that individual is to the extent 0.6 a member of set $\mathbb{H}$, and to the extent 0.4 a member of its complement, $\mathbb{PAT}$, she is to the extent $min(0.6,\, 0.4) = 0.4$ a member of the fuzzy intersection $\mathbb{H} \cap \mathbb{PAT}$. Hence, the intersection of *health* and *patienthood*, $\mathbb{H} \cap \mathbb{PAT}$, contains at least this member and is not empty. That means that health and patienthood, $\mathbb{H}$ and $\mathbb{PAT}$, are complementary in a fuzzy sense, but not disjoint and contradictory in a bivalent, Aristotelean sense. We shall come back to this issue in Section 6.3.4 below.

The term "patienthood" as an antonym of "health" could also be called "unhealth" to get the predicate "unhealthy" as an antonym of "healthy". However, to prevent a plethora of neologisms, we shall use the former throughout. Since the definition of degrees of patienthood is based on degrees of discomfort, pain, endogenously threatened life, loss of autonomy, loss of vitality, and loss of pleasure, it follows that its complement, fuzzy health $\mathbb{H}$, is also based on these dimensions. The weaker they are in an individual, the healthier she will be according to our terminology. Strictly speaking, this is a concept of 'negative health'. A concept of 'positive health' is obtained by directly characterizing health as something like feelings of physical and mental well-being, physical fitness, full functioning, experiencing pleasure, vitality, and autonomy (see the dimensions of patienthood).

Our considerations above show that, in contrast to bivalent views on health, there are indeed degrees of health. That means that health is measurable by simply introducing a quantitative concept of health and designing a scale (see Section 4.1.4). Note that our derived predicate "is healthy to the extent $\mu_{health}(x)$" is also holistic, having human individuals as its objects. In other words, it never applies to organs, tissues, cells, or other entities. Healthy or unhealthy are indivdiual human beings and not their organs, tissues, cells, or other body parts. It is meaningless in our framework to say, for example, that "Elroy Fox has a healthy heart" or that "he is healthy with respect to his heart". The term "is healthy" is a unary predicate. This will become apparent from Figure 28.

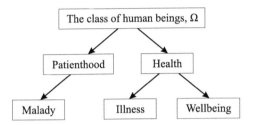

Fig. 28. The conceptual tree of our basic terminology about *health* and *illness* introduced in Sections 6.3.2 and 6.3.3. The root of the tree is the set of human beings at a particular instant of time. An edge from a node to another node means that the former defines the latter. Note that there is no reference to 'disease' in this graph. This is due to the fact that in our conceptual system, the terms "health" and "disease" are semantically independent of each other

6.3.3 Illness

An individual is usually said to be either *healthy* or *ill*, but not both at the same time. This crisp either-or terminology is inadequate, as health and illness are by no means mutual complements. They are not to be contrasted with each other. Rather, *ill* health, i.e. *illnes*, is in contrast to *well* health, i.e., wellness or *well-being*. As such, they are just two particular vague or fuzzy states of health among many others that create the multifarious granular structure of health. To unravel the granular, fuzzy structure of health, we shall in the first of the following two sections:

▶ Illness = *ill* STATE OF HEALTH
▶ Illness experience

introduce the phrase "state of health" as a linguistic variable and construct its syntax and semantics, and shall in the second section show that illness and illness experience are something different than disease. (For the theory of linguistic variables, see Section 30.4.1 on page 1018.)

Illness = *ill* State_Of_Health

What is usually nominalized and called *'illness'*, will be reconstructed as an *ill state of health*. To this end, the state of health of an individual is symbolized by the linguistic variable "*State_Of_Health*", written with capital initials, that assumes values such as *well, very well, ill, very ill* etc. Its term set, $T(State\_Of\_Health)$, may be conceived of as something like:

$$T(State\_Of\_Health) = \{\text{well, not well, very well, very very well, extremely well, ill, not ill, more or less ill, very ill, very very ill, extremely ill, not well and not ill, } \dots \text{ etc. } \dots\}. \quad (19)$$

The variable operates over the fuzzy set *health*, $\mathbb{H}$, introduced in the preceding section, and assigns to *degrees of health*, i.e., to μ_{health} values, elements of its term set (19). Each element τ of this term set is thus *the name of a particular fuzzy set* that is a fuzzy subset of *health*. It subsumes an entire spectrum of health values of the type $\mu_{health}(x)$ under a single fuzzy label τ such as "well", "ill", etc. (see Figure 29).

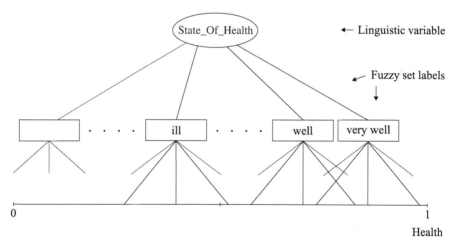

Fig. 29. See Figure 106 on page 1022. Analogous with that figure, possible values of the linguistic variable '*State_Of_Health*' may be {very well, well, not well, ill, not ill, … }. Each of these values is a label for an entire fuzzy set of degrees of health

For instance, let the term "well" designate one of those fuzzy sets. One can ask how compatible with this set, *well*, the health value of a particular individual such as $\mu_{health}(Pope) = 0.3$ may be. If the membership function of the fuzzy set *well* is denoted by μ_{well}, our question then reads: what is the value of $\mu_{well}(0.3)$, i.e., of $\mu_{well}\big(\mu_{health}(Pope)\big)$? Plots of two examples are displayed in Figure 30.

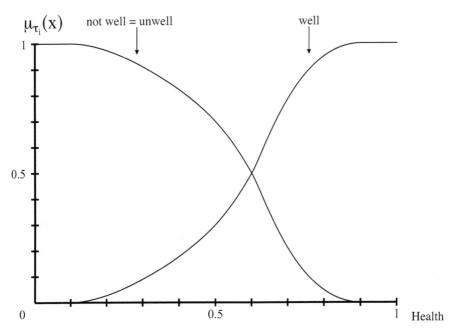

Fig. 30. A tentative illustration of the fuzzy set *well* and of its complement *not well* $\equiv$ unwell. The x-coordinate axis represents the fuzzy set *health* with its membership function μ_{health}. The y-axis demonstrates the compatibility degrees of values of μ_{health} with the fuzzy sets *well* and *unwell*, both represented by the membership function μ_{τ_i} where τ_i is a place-holder for the terms 'well' and 'unwell'. According to this tentative demonstration, we have $\mu_{well}(0.3) = \mu_{well}\big(\mu_{health}(Pope)\big) = 0.1$, and thus $\mu_{unwell}(0.3) = \mu_{unwell}\big(\mu_{health}(Pope)\big) = 0.9$. Note that complementation is a mirror image at point 0.5 of the y-axis

We are now in a position to understand what it means to say that illness is a *state of health* of an individual in the above sense and not something like a *disease* such as multiple sclerosis, diabetes, or myocardial infarction that is a state of the individual. "Illness" and "disease" are not synonyms.

As discussed in Section 30.4.1 on page 1018, the term set of a linguistic variable may be a more or less large set of linguistic terms based upon only a few primary terms. For example, the term set $T(State\_Of\_Health)$, as partly shown in (19) above, may have the term "well" as its only primary term. Its remaining terms such as "very well", "not well", "not well and not ill", and others are composed of primary terms by using semantic operators such as negation and linguistic hedges. A subset of $T(State\_Of\_Health)$, e.g., the minimum term set {well}, may therefore be used as a set of primary terms from which the remainder of $T(State\_Of\_Health)$ may be obtained by definition. Recall that if A is a fuzzy set, then according to (257) on page 1025:

very A	is a fuzzy set with	$\mu_{very(A)}(x) = \left(\mu_A(x)\right)^2$	$\equiv$ concentration
fairly A	is a fuzzy set with	$\mu_{fairly(A)}(x) = \sqrt{\mu_A(x)}$	$\equiv$ dilation.

According to these standard approximations, we obtain from the primary term set {well} by the calculations:

$$\mu_{very\_well}(x) = \left(\mu_{well}(x)\right)^2$$
$$\mu_{fairly\_well}(x) = \sqrt{\mu_{well}(x)}$$
$$\mu_{ill}(x) = \left(\sqrt{\mu_{ill}(x)}\right)^2 = \left(very\left(\mu_{unwell}(x)\right)\right)^2 = \left(\mu_{unwell}(x)\right)^4$$

a wide range of derived terms for $T(State\_Of\_Health)$ like the following:

$$very\ well = well^2$$
$$fairly\ well = \sqrt{well}$$
$$ill = very(fairly\ ill) = very\ very\ unwell = unwell^4.$$

See Figure 31. The figure demonstrates that according to the relationships above, being *ill*, i.e., *illness*, may be construed as a particular fuzzy set over *health*, specifically as the following state of health:

$$very\ very\ not\ well = very\Big(very\big(not(well)\big)\Big) = (unwell^2)^2 = unwell^4 = ill$$

which is a *concentration of the concentration of the complement* of the fuzzy set *well*. It should thus become clear what it means to say that illness is not the complement of health. In other words, the term "illness" is not the antonym of the term "health" and vice versa. Illness is a concentration of the concentrated complement of well-being. Due to additive-inverse relationships between health and patienthood:

$$\mu_{health}(x) = 1 - \mu_{patienthood}(x)$$
$$\mu_{patienthood}(x) = 1 - \mu_{health}(x)$$

according to Definition 45, the *State_Of_Health* fuzzy sets as illustrated in Figure 31 may also be founded on patienthood as the base variable. They will in this case reverse their positions to appear as mirror images of those in Figure 31. See Figure 32.

In closing this section, note that we have reconstructed the state of health by means of a many-valued linguistic variable referred to as "*State_Of_Health*" such that illness turns out to be only one of the many states of health. The linguistic variable we have proposed is of the following structure (see also Definition 253 on page 1023):

$$\langle v,\ T(v),\ \Omega,\ M \rangle$$

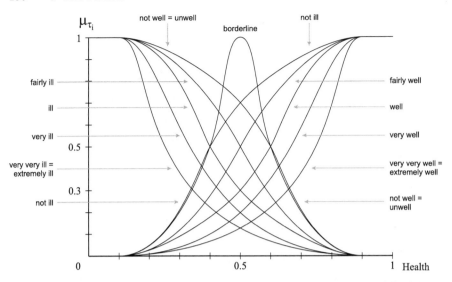

Fig. 31. A tentative illustration of some *State_Of_Health* fuzzy sets. All of them may be defined by complementation, dilation, and concentration of the primary fuzzy set *well*. Even *borderline* cases may be construed as some sort of 'not well and not ill'. Concentration by 'very' lowers membership degrees generating a deeper curve. Dilation by 'fairly' raises membership degrees generating a higher curve. Note that illness is $very\big(very(not(well))\big) = unwellness^4$. For instance, a health value of 0.4 corresponds to an illness of degree 0.5. An individual who is healthy to the extent 0.4, is ill to the extent 0.5, i.e., healthy and ill at the same time. Hence, health and illness are not disjoint. The same individual is also not ill to the extent 0.5. Hence, being ill and not being ill at the same time is possible, though a contradictory state. The logic of clinical language, and consequently the logic of medicine, is non-classical and admits of contradictions. This issue will be discussed in Part V

specifically:

⟨ *State_Of_Health*, {well, not well, very well, very very well, extremely well, ill, not ill, fairly ill, very ill, very very ill, extremely ill, not well and not ill, ... etc. ...}, [0, 1], M⟩

such that:

1. v is the name of the variable, i.e., *"State_Of_Health"*
2. $T(v)$ is its term set;
3. Ω is the universe of discourse, i.e., the unit interval [0, 1] comprising degrees of health upon which the terms of the term set $T(v)$ are interpreted as fuzzy sets such as *well, ill, very well*, etc.;
4. M is the method that associates with each linguistic value $\tau_i \in T(v)$ its meaning, i.e., a fuzzy set of the universe Ω denoted by τ_i. See Figures 31–32.

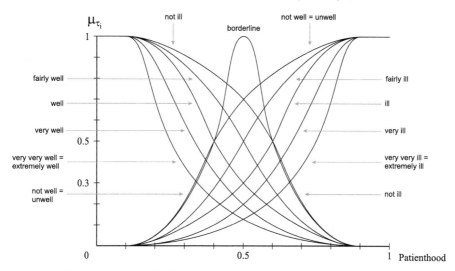

Fig. 32. The same *State_Of_Health* fuzzy sets as in Figure 31 based on patienthood

Illness experience

It was argued in previous sections that the conceptual network associated with the triad "health, illness, and disease" and related terms is a semantically underdeveloped and unkempt category with an abundancy of linguistic weeds. Pulling these weeds will help both medicine and the patients. Our recent service in this respect was to clarify the concept of illness; to show that illness and disease are in fact two different things; and to elucidate why there are no 'illnesses' like individual diseases. *Illness* means nothing more than "feeling ill", and as such, it is the *ill* state of health defined in the preceding section. A particular facet in this respect that nourishes controversies and sustains unfruitful criticisms of medicine by humanists and cultural anthropologists, is the so-called *illness experience* of the patient (Kleinman, 1981, 1988, 2006; Foucault, 1994).

What is commonly called *illness experience* is the mode of how, and the content of what, a patient experiences when she feels ill or believes that she feels ill, i.e., when she is or believes to be in an *ill state of health*. For instance, she may feel upper abdominal pain, suffer from stiffness and tenseness in her neck, be sleepless, anxious, and so on. She will try to interpret and explain this experience. Depending on group-specific, cultural, educational, linguistic, economic, and many other factors, some people will come to the conclusion that they are ill, or sick, and will consult experts, be they physicians, Ayurvedists, homeopaths, or others. Some other people will go to exorcists, psychologists, and the like. The decision whether a suffering individual seeks the advice of a physician or another authority, depends on whether she interprets her illness experience as something *medical*.

As a report by the patient's self-monitoring self-consciousness about *changes* in herself, her illness experience constitutes what we called a *self-diagnosis* of the organism on page 136. We encounter such self-diagnoses as *illness narratives* embedded in the so-called anamnesis or patient history that the physician elicits from the patients. In this sense, a patient's illness experience and illness narrative are episodes of her life history and are best understood in that context (see p. 11 f.).

In academic medicine, illness experience is viewed as an effect of a disease or pathological process behind it which causes those *changes* in the patient that constitute the subject of her illness experience. This is the reason why the diagnostic machinery is set in motion to diagnose that disease or pathological process. In some or most cases medicine succeeds in identifying 'the culprit'. But in some or many other cases no disease or pathological process is found. Patients of this type "suffering and complaining without having a disease" are often categorized as having some psychosomatic disorders, being psychopaths, malingerers, etc. There are many reasons for this failure of academic medicine. They include: (i) medical students are not trained in analyzing and understanding illness narratives that do not fit the language of medicine; (ii) thorough analyses of illness narratives are not paid for; (iii) it is not yet well known that the efficacy of psychosomatics is a myth. It will take some time to replace this myth with sociosomatics (see pp. 143 and 733).

6.3.4 Disease, Health, and Illness Violate Classical Logic

Our analysis has shown that health and disease are non-classical concepts denoting irreducible categories. This has far-reaching logical and metaphysical consequences, which will be briefly outlined below. The Aristotelean worldview that underlies classical logic and set theory and all traditional scientific disciplines, claims that the following two principles are universally valid:

$\alpha \lor \neg\alpha$ Principle of Excluded Middle $A \cup \overline{A} = \Omega$

$\neg(\alpha \land \neg\alpha)$ Principle of Non-Contradiction $A \cap \overline{A} = \varnothing$

See page 874 and Table 36 on page 895. Accordingly, it is assumed that like the crisp concept "even number", the concepts of health, illness, and disease are bivalent and therefore open to classical, bivalent reasoning of the Aristotelean type. It is said that:

- an individual is healthy or she is not healthy, but not both at the same time;
- an individual is ill or she is not ill, but not both at the same time;
- an individual has a disease or she does not have it, but not both at the same time.[38]

---

[38] Note that the predicates "healthy", "ill", and "diseased" used in clinical practice are *one-place* predicates. They apply to a person as a whole. A person x may be

However, imagine a world that violates the Aristotelean worldview and classical logic. In such a deviant world with no Law or Principle of Non-Contradiction, something may have a property P and its opposite not-P simultaneously. For instance, a rose may be red and not red; a fruit may be an apple and not an apple; a human being may be healthy and not healthy; and so on. Since such a world contains contradictory facts of the form 'is a P and is not a P', it is an inconsistent world in the classical-logical sense. We all have been taught to believe that an inconsistent world is impossible and does not exist. But our logical analysis of the concepts of health, illness, and disease demonstrates that we are living in exactly such an inconsistent, non-classical world. For example, we have seen above that an individual who is healthy to the extent 0.4, is not healthy to the extent 0.6. An individual who is ill to the extent 0.5, is not ill to the extent 0.5:

$$\mu_{health}(x) = 0.4$$
$$\mu_{patienthood}(x) = 1 - \mu_{health}(x) = 0.6$$

$$\mu_{ill}(x) = 0.5$$
$$\mu_{not\_ill}(x) = 1 - \mu_{ill}(x) = 0.5.$$

Thus, such an individual violates the Principles of Excluded Middle and Non-Contradiction because she both has a property and does not have it at once. The same holds for the concept of disease fuzzified in Definition 40 on page 178. An individual who has peptic ulcer disease to the extent 0.6, has a non-disease to the extent 0.4. The reason is this: A human condition that to the extent $\varepsilon = r > 0$ is a member of the fuzzy set $\mathbb{D}$ of diseases, i.e., is a disease to the extent ε, is a non-disease to the extent $1 - \varepsilon$ because to this extent it belongs to the complement fuzzy set $\overline{\mathbb{D}}$. Recall that $\overline{\mathbb{D}}$, as the complement of the fuzzy category $\mathbb{D}$ of diseases, can be represented as follows. If the category of diseases is:

$$\mathbb{D} = \left\{ \big(H_1, \mu_{\mathbb{D}}(H_1)\big), \ldots, \big(H_q, \mu_{\mathbb{D}}(H_q)\big) \right\},$$

characterized as healthy, ill, or diseased by saying that "x is healthy", "x is ill", or "x is diseased". For example, "Amy Fox is healthy", "Elroy Fox is ill", and the like. We should distinguish from such one-place predicates, *two-place* predicates such as "x is healthy with respect to y", e.g., "Elroy Fox is healthy with respect to his stomach", while "he is not healthy with respect to his liver". But these binary health predicates are semantically strange and should be avoided. In the same respect, consider the two-place, degenerate, comparative predicates of everyday language like "more healthy in one respect and less healthy in another". Such expressions are too artificial to deserve our attention and analysis here. A theory using the one-place predicate "is healthy" and another theory using the many-place ones, have nothing to do with each other simply on the grounds that the two predicate types have distinct objects. In our theory, the bearers of health, illness, and disease are only individual human beings and nothing else. Thus, objections like the following one miss the point: "An individual may arguably be healthy with respect to her stomach and not healthy with respect to her liver".

then the category of non-diseases is:

$$\overline{\mathbb{D}} = \{(H_1, 1 - \mu_{\mathbb{D}}(H_1)), \ldots, (H_q, 1 - \mu_{\mathbb{D}}(H_q))\}.$$

An individual's having a particular disease to the extent $\varepsilon = r > 0$ therefore means that to the extent $1 - r$ she does not have that disease. Thus, fuzzy disease is a non-classical, i.e., non-Aristotelean, attribute. You both have it *and* don't have it at once. It is perhaps more convincing to demonstrate the violation of classical-logical laws by set-theoretical means. Suppose there is a family $\Omega = \{\text{Amy, Beth, Carla, Dirk}\}$, conveniently symbolized by $\{a, b, c, d\}$. Two family members may be ill to a particular extent:

$$\Omega = \{a, b, c, d\},$$
$$ill = \{(a, 0), (b, 0.4), (c, 0), (d, 0.7)\}.$$

As a result, we have the set of those family members who are not ill:

$$\overline{ill} = \{(a, 1), (b, 0.6), (c, 1), (d, 0.3)\}.$$

and thus:

$$ill \cup \overline{ill} = \{(a, 1), (b, 0.6), (c, 1), (d, 0.7)\} \neq \Omega \quad \text{(maxima of both sets)}$$
$$ill \cap \overline{ill} = \{(a, 0), (b, 0.4), (c, 0), (d, 0.3)\} \neq \Omega \quad \text{(minima of both sets)}.$$

These two findings violate the two basic laws of classical logic mentioned on page 192: Principle of Excluded Middle and Principle of Non-Contradiction. We may thus draw the general conclusion that non-classical concepts do not obey classical logic. Since medical language and knowledge are replete with such concepts of the non-classical type and medical decisions are based thereon, classical logic cannot be the logic of medicine. We shall expand on this intriguing issue in Parts V–VI.

6.3.5 Summary

We have explicated the notions of health, illness, and disease and have provided a fuzzy-logical framework that demonstrates their fuzzy character. In this framework, health, illness, and disease turn out to be three completely different categories. Health is not a complement of illness. Varieties of illness characterized as ill, very ill, and so on are different *states of health*. Nor is health a complement of disease. It is the complement of *malady*, which contains disease as one of its subcategories. The concept of disease denoting this subcategory has been explicated by our *prototype resemblance theory of disease* according to which the category emerges from a few socially constructed prototype diseases and a similarity relation between other human conditions and these prototypes (see also Section 14.4 on page 572).

As a result of fuzzifying all three concepts, classical logic loses its capacity to be an appropriate logic of medicine. Particularly, the concept of fuzzy disease has consequences for clinical practice. Since individual diseases are fuzzified human conditions, diagnostic-therapeutic reasoning requires fuzzy logic. We shall come back to this issue in Part V.

6.4 Systems of Disease

6.4.0 Introduction

If you have a great many things to manage, use taxonomy to arrange them in classes. That is, *classify* them by introducing classificatory concepts. This advice reflects the experience that classification facilitates work. Because medicine deals with a lot of individual diseases, it has followed this principle since antiquity. Distinct diseases with some similarities between them are placed in the same group or class. Examples are classes such as 'infectious diseases', 'heart diseases', and others each containing, respectively, a number of infectious diseases, heart diseases, and so on. The emerging web of such disease classes with their subclasses, overclasses, over-overclasses, and inter-class relationships is called a *nosological system*. In this section, some important features of nosological systems are analyzed and a novel, abstract geometry of diseases is introduced. Our analysis divides into the following four parts:

  6.4.1 Symptomatology
  6.4.2 Nosological Systems
  6.4.3 Pathology *vs.* Nosology
  6.4.4 Nosological Spaces.

6.4.1 Symptomatology

The disease features used in constructing a nosological system include, among others, symptoms, signs, and findings. Usually, diseases are characterized by enumerating and describing their features, an activity traditionally referred to as *symptomatology*. The Greek term σύμπτωμα (symptoma) means "to occur together with", i.e., an event A that occurs together with another event B. In medicine, it refers to an event that 'occurs together with' a disease. For example, cough is a symptom of bronchitis because 'cough occurs together with bronchitis'. But due to the ambiguity of togetherness, the phrase "to occur together with" is much too ambiguous. We shall therefore have to clarify the term "symptom" in the next section.

As stated above, symptomatology is the art of characterizing diseases with reference to their symptoms, that is, the art of describing how symptoms and diseases are associated with one another. The symptomatological description of a particular disease such as myocardial infarction contains, among other things, *two* types of central statements. The first type indicates what features are present in a patient *if* she has the disease. In this case, the disease is the clue (disease → features). Conversely, the second type indicates what disease the patient has *if* she shows particular features. In this case, the features are the clues (features → disease). Regarding acute myocardial infarction, for example, we may have these two simplified statements:

1. If someone has myocardial infarction, then she may have an elevated creatine kinase enzyme of the type MB, denoted CK-MB;[39]
2. If someone has an elevated CK-MB enzyme, then she may have a myocardial infarction.

These statements are absolutely different from one another. The first one says: *If* disease D is present, *then* possibly symptom S is present. By contrast, the second statement means: If symptom S is present, *then* possibly disease D is present. We are thus faced with two distinct *if-then* relationships, symbolized by "$\rightarrow$", having different antecedents and consequents:

$$D \rightarrow \Diamond S$$
$$S \rightarrow \Diamond D.$$

Here the shorthands "S" and "D" mean, respectively, "symptom S is present" and "disease D is present". Thus "$\Diamond S$" and "$\Diamond D$" stand for "it is possible that symptom S is present" and "it is possible that disease D is present", respectively. (For the possibility operator $\Diamond$, see alethic modal logic in Section 27.1 on page 913.)

The disease-symptom associations sketched above will be thoroughly analyzed in Chapter 8. In the present section, we will focus on clarifying the concept of symptom itself. Accordingly, some characteristics of symptoms will be outlined and the medical-philosophically important distinction between the *description* and the *definition* of a disease will be explained. Our discussion thus divides into the following three parts:

▶ The concept of symptom
▶ Properties of symptoms
▶ Nosogram *vs.* nosological predicate.

The concept of symptom

The class of symptoms has been diversified over the centuries. Two classes that have been added are *signs* and *findings*. The term "symptom" is itself ambiguous and is used in a narrow and in a wider sense. In its narrow sense, a symptom is what the patient reports about her suffering, for example, her subjective chest pain. A sign is what the doctor perceives in the patient, for instance, her irregular pulse. A finding is what a laboratory examination reveals, for example, an elevated concentration in the blood of the CK-MB

---

[39] Creatine kinase, CK, is an intracellular enzyme present in the skeletal muscle fibers, myocardium, and brain. It is released into the bloodstream when muscle fibers are damaged or destroyed. Elevation of CK in the blood is therefore not specific for myocardial infarction. But CK has three different types, CK-MM, CK-BB, and CK-MB (MB = muscle-brain type). A significant concentration of CK-MB is found almost exclusively in the myocardium. So, elevation of CK-MB concentration in the blood is highly specific for acute myocardial infarction.

enzyme. All of these three features, i.e., symptoms, signs, and findings, are also called *symptoms* in a wider sense of the term. Symptomatology is concerned with symptoms in the latter sense. In this wider sense, everything associated with a particular disease is viewed as a symptom of this disease.

Thus, the ordinary notion of "symptom" is a binary predicate with the syntax "S is a symptom of D" and expresses a binary relation between S and D. It may be semiformally represented as follows: $Is\_a\_symptom\_of(S, D)$. That means that S is a symptom of disaese D, or $Symptom(S, D)$ for short. For example, the statement "chest pain is a symptom of myocardial infarction" is written "$Symptom(chest\_pain, myocardial\_infarction)$".

A feature may of course be a symptom of two or more diseases. For example, chest pain is a symptom of about 60 diseases. Such a symptom may be more indicative of a disease D_1 than another disease D_2. That means that if we encounter this symptom in a patient, it points to disease D_1 stronger than to disease D_2. For instance, acute chest pain in a 65-year-old male is more indicative of myocardial infarction than of gastritis. Thus, there are several characteristics of a symptom. To help us clarify these characteristics, we will first define what we understand by the term "symptom". The best way to define it is to consider it an event which, with a probability of greater than 0, is indicative of another event (for the probability terminology, see Chapter 29 on page 969):

Definition 46 (*S is a symptom of X*). *If S and X are events, then Symptom(S, X) iff $p(X \mid S) > p(X)$.*

That means that S is a symptom of X if and only if the probability of X conditional on S exceeds the absolute probability of X, i.e., the probability of X without considering S. In other words, if S is present or occurs, then the probability that X is also present or will occur, is greater than the probability of X without considering symptom S.

The event X may of course be a disease, D. Thus, we may conclude from the above definition that $Symptom(S, D)$ iff $p(D \mid S) > p(D)$. That is, S is a symptom of a disease D if and only if the probability of disease D conditional on S exceeds the absolute probability $p(D)$. For example, the probability of myocardial infarction, *MI*, in the German population may be 0.0001. That is, $p(MI) = 0.0001$. And the probability that someone in Germany has myocardial infarction on the condition that she has an elevated CK-MB enzyme, may be 0.93. That is, $p(MI \mid elevated\_CK\text{-}MB) = 0.93$. In this case, elevation of CK-MB enzyme in the blood is a symptom of myocardial infarction because $p(MI \mid elevated\_CK\text{-}MB) > p(MI)$.

The concept of symptom introduced above is a binary predicate. However, it is not good enough and formally sophisticated. Objections may be raised for the following reason. It is conceivable that according to Definition 46 above a particular feature, S, turns out a symptom of a disease X in a particular population, while it is not a symptom of the same disease in another population. We should therefore relativize the symptomaticity of an event to the population – background context or field – PO within which the relationship between it and a disease is considered. In this case, the above definition could be restated thus:

Definition 47 (S is a symptom of X in the population PO). *If S and X are events in the population PO, then $Symptom(S, X, PO)$ iff $p(X \mid PO \cap S) > p(X \mid PO)$.*

This concept of symptom is a ternary predicate. It means that S is a symptom of X in the population PO if and only if the probability of X conditional on S in the population PO exceeds the probability of X in PO without considering S. It may of course be that regarding some symptom S we have $Symptom(S, X, PO)$, while $\neg Symptom(S, X, PO')$ when $PO \neq PO'$. The term "population" is a general notion and covers all contexts in which the relationship between S and X is considered. For example, PO may be another disease X' or a particular genetic disposition whose presence in a patient influences the symptomaticity of S with respect to X.

Having said that, in order to simplify our discussion, we shall omit this aspect of relativization for the terminology introduced below. However, keep in mind that it is an implicit feature of our concepts. See our theory of probabilistic etiology in Section 6.5.3 where, because of its eminent importance, the relativity of causes is explicitly included in the concepts introduced.

Properties of symptoms

The association of a symptom with a disease has some properties that may be used to assess its diagnostic and differential-diagnostic value in clinical decision-making. Sketched below are four such properties: prognostic or predictive value, sensitivity, specificity, and pathognomonicity of a symptom.

We will conveniently symbolize the expression "symptom S is not present" by $\neg S$, and the expression "disease D is not present" by $\neg D$. We distinguish between positive predictive value and negative predictive value of a symptom S for a particular disease D, symbolized by $pv^+(S, D)$ and $pv^-(S, D)$, respectively. They are defined as follows:

Definition 48 (Positive predictive value, Negative predictive value).

    a) $pv^+(S, D) = p(D \mid S)$
    b) $pv^-(S, D) = p(\neg D \mid \neg S)$.

That is, the *positive predictive value* of a symptom S for a disease D, written $pv^+(S, D)$, equals the probability that a patient has disease D on the condition that she has symptom S, while the *negative predictive value* of a symptom S for a disease D, written $pv^-(S, D)$, is the probability that a patient does not have disease D on the condition that she does not have symptom S. Predictive value, either positive or negative, is obviously a binary function.

A simple example may explain. In a sample of 200 patients suspected of having acute myocardial infarction, the concentration of the enzyme CK-MB in their blood is determined. Some patients show the symptom "CK-MB is elevated". The remainder does not have this symptom. The patients are thoroughly examined and diagnosed. The 2×2 contingency table in Table 2 displays the results:

Table 2. A 2×2 contingency table for the association of elevated CK-MB enzyme with myocardial infarction. A plus or minus sign means that the feature is present or absent, respectively. TP = true positive, FP = false positive, TN = true negative, FN = false negative. These qualifications refer to the presence or absence of the symptom (CK-MB elevated). For CK-MB enzyme, see footnote 39 on page 196

	CK-MB elevated		
Myocardial infarction	Yes (+)	No (−)	Totals
present	90 (TP)	10 (FN)	100
not present	6 (FP)	94 (TN)	100

Positive and negative predictive values of the elevated CK-MB enzyme for myocardial infarction can be calculated directly from Table 2 in the following way. Here an acronym of the form XY means "the number of XY" (see caption of Table 2):

$$pv^+(S, D) = \frac{TP}{TP + FP} = \frac{90}{96} = 0.93$$

$$pv^-(S, D) = \frac{TN}{TN + FN} = \frac{94}{104} = 0.9.$$

As can be seen, the blood concentration of CK-MB has very high positive and negative predictive values for myocardial infarction.

There are two additional properties of symptoms which are of equal importance: the *sensitivity* and the *specificity* of a symptom for a disease. Both of them are binary functions. In what follows, the term "*sensitivity(S, D)*" reads "the degree of sensitivity of symptom S for disease D"; and the term "*specificity(S, D)*" means "the degree of specificity of symptom S for disease D". They are defined thus:

Definition 49 (Sensitivity and specificity of symptoms).

a) *sensitivity*$(S, D) = p(S \mid D)$
b) *specificity*$(S, D) = p(\neg S \mid \neg D)$.

For instance, by calculating the required conditional probabilities on the basis of the 2×2 contingency Table 2 above, we can determine to what extent the elevation of CK-MB enzyme is sensitive to, and specific for, myocardial infarction:

$$sensitivity(S, D) = p(S \mid D) = \frac{TP}{TP + FN} = \frac{90}{100} = 0.9$$

$$specificity(S, D) = p(\neg S \mid \neg D) = \frac{TN}{TN + FP} = \frac{94}{100} = 0.94.$$

The higher the predictive values, sensitivity, and specificity of a symptom for a disease, the more useful it is in clinical decision-making and vice versa. These values scarcely reach the maximum extent 1. A symptom with the maximum positive predictive value 1 is called a *pathognomonic* symptom:

Definition 50 (Pathognomonicity of a symptom). *S is pathognomonic of D iff* $pv^+(S, D) = 1$.

Definitions 48 and 50 jointly imply: S is pathognomonic of D iff $p(D \mid S) = 1$. Such a symptom S is pathognomonic of disease D because due to $p(D \mid S) = 1$ we have $p(\neg D \mid S) = 0$. And that means that the symptom is not associated with any other disease than D. Thus, a pathognomonic symptom is a diagnostically certain pointer to a given disease. For instance, Koplik's spots are pathognomonic of measles because $p(measles \mid Koplik's\_spots) = 1$. Pathognomonic symptoms are highly valuable, but very rare.

The term "symptom", as it has been defined above, is a general term that signifies everything that points to a particular event, for example, to the onset or presence of a disease. Therefore, a symptom need not be an 'elementary' feature of an individual like cough, chest pain, or the elevation of CK-MB enzyme. Two additional, important interpretations may be outlined:

1. What has been called a 'symptom' above, may also be a *disease* that points to another disease. For instance, pneumocystosis and Kaposi's sarcoma are diseases though, they are symptoms of AIDS because they point to AIDS. That is, the probability that someone has AIDS on the condition that she has pneumocystosis or Kaposi's sarcoma, exceeds the absolute probability that she has AIDS (without considering pneumocystosis and Kaposi's sarcoma).
2. Also test results, be they potitive or negative, may be interpreted as symptoms that are present or absent and thereby point to diseases to different extents, respectively. Examples are the results of radiography, blood counts, glucose tolerance test, etc. In this case, we obtain the following analogs of the above concepts: Positive predictive value of a test result; negative predictive value of a test result; test sensitivity; test specificity; and pathognomonicity of a test result. For example, the carbon 13 test, labeled urea breath test, has both high sensitivity and high specificity for peptic ulcer disease by Helicobacter infection (97.6% specific; 100% sensitive, and thus, pathognomonic).

Nosogram *vs.* nosological predicate

What the symptomatology of a disease D provides, is an empirical description of the disease, i.e., the representation of the associations between a number of symptoms $S_1, S_2, \ldots$, and the disease D. Such a description consists of statements informing us about which symptoms $S_1, S_2, \ldots$ occur when the disease occurs, and vice versa. For example, it is said that a patient with myocardial infarction *may* show angina pectoris, arrhythmia, sweating, elevation of CK-MB in the blood, depression of ST segment in ECG, and so on. It is not said that all these symptoms are necessarily present in all patients with myocardial infarction. There is no regular association between the disease and those symptoms. Some patients may have one subset of the symptoms, and other patients may have another. That is, the symptoms $S_1, S_2, \ldots$ encountered in the *description* of a disease are neither sufficient nor necessary for the presence of the disease. The description of the disease presented in textbooks is only a *nosogram* (Sadegh-Zadeh, 1977a).

There is a fundamental distinction between a nosogram and the *definition* of a disease, i.e., of the *nosological predicate* that denotes it. For example, different textbooks present different nosograms about myocardial infarction or schizophrenia. But *what* is the "myocardial infarction" and "schizophrenia" differently *described* by those nosograms? We can answer this question only by providing a *definition* of the respective nosological predicate. A nosogram will not do. The definition of a nosological predicate is absolutely necessary in order for the disease it denotes to be portrayed by a nosogram. If nosologists, clinicians, and medical researchers do not share a common definition of a nosological predicate such as "myocardial infarction", their research and communication will have the semantic chaos that results from each having her own private understanding of that nosological predicate. The best method of defining nosological predicates is the operational definition (see page 91).

6.4.2 Nosological Systems

To facilitate diagnostics, therapy, and clinical research and education, the plethora of diseases is arranged in more or less homogeneous classes such as "infectious diseases", "gastro-intestinal diseases", "degenerative diseases", and so on, and relationships are established between them. This system of interrelated classes and subclasses is usually referred to as a *nosological system*.

To put a number of distinct things, such as diseases, in the same class requires that they share some features to some extent. The features used in classifying diseases may be symptoms, signs, findings, causes of diseases, sites of the body they share, or something else. Their choice is deliberate. For instance, diseases bearing a particular symptom A may be put in the class of A-diseases. Diseases caused by a particular condition B may be accommodated in the class of B-diseases. Diseases originating from or affecting a particular site C of the body may be classified as C-diseases, and so on. Examples are:

- Lipid abnormalities   (symptomatologic classification)
- Viral diseases   (etiologic classification),
- Liver diseases   (topographic classification).

In building such classes, there are no binding rules governing the choice of the nosologist. This brings with it that all nosological systems are artificial. None is a natural system representing 'the true system of diseases'. That is, in contrast to a widespread opinion (Dragulinescu, 2010), diseases are not natural kinds. And there exists no natural order of diseases 'in the world out there' to be discovered and described. Both the contents as well as the structure of nosological *systems* in medicine change over time and from place to place. This is why the nosological systems built in different epochs of the history of medicine, and even in different schools of medical research and practice, are different from each other. For example, current medicine is not based on the Hippocratic nosological system. Nor do we employ a nosological system that was used fifty years ago. Even a nosological system established by a professional community or by the author of a clinical textbook does not remain constant over their lifetime. It is the author herself who builds and rebuilds the nosological system of her book according to her liking. New diseases such as AIDS, bulimia, borreliosis, and alcoholism enter the system when they are 'discovered'; another one is moved from a class X to another class Y; and still another one is completely removed. For example, we are currently witnessing the relocation of peptic ulcer disease from being a 'psychosomatic' disease to being an 'infectious' disease caused by Helicobacter pylori. Other diseases are eliminated from the nosological system. They simply sink into oblivion and disappear. For instance, homosexuality was a disease classified as a psychiatric entity until the 1950s. Today, it is none.

The observations above raise the following questions. How does something come to be considered or denied a disease and how does it come to enter or leave a nosological class of a nosological system? Also related to this issue is the intense discussion on whether a disease is a 'fact' that is discovered, or is it something 'value-laden' that is established by human beings (Boorse, 1997; Caplan et al., 1981; Engelhardt, 1975, 1976, 1986; Humber and Almeder, 1997; Margolis, 1969, 1976). Although this ongoing debate concerns a fundamental aspect of the genesis and development of a nosological system, it does not cover the whole problem. We shall tackle this issue in Chapter 14.

6.4.3 Pathology *vs.* Nosology

Like "nosos", the Greek term πάθος (pathos) means "suffering, illness, disease". Different from nosology, however, which has existed since antiquity, pathology is a recent, natural science-based discipline. Its practitioners investigate the biomedical, non-clinical manifestations of suffering, illness, and disease in body parts such as organs, tissues, cells, and molecules. The term "non-clinical manifestations" in this context means that pathology is concerned with only those symptoms, signs, and findings, say features, phenomena, and processes in the organism, which are not reported by the patient about herself, i.e., by making subjective, first-person statements about her suffering. Thus, pathology is not a science of the subjective sphere.

The Greek terms "nosos" ($\nu\acute{o}\sigma o\varsigma$) and "nosology" stem from the Hippocratic era. They reflect how medicine dealt with disease before *pathology* emerged in the eighteenth century. Prior to this innovation, suffering, illness, and diseases were studied and classified in living patients only. The microscope as a medical tool did not yet exist, and as a result, no autopsy and histopathological examinations were conducted. In describing and explaining a disease, the patients' subjective sphere, i.e., their *first-person reports* on their suffering and health condition such as "I feel a pain in my stomach", played a central role. Cadavers, tissues, and cells did not belong to the realm of nosology.

With the advent of *pathology* in the first half of the eighteenth century, the situation changed. Like nosology, this new branch was also studying the phenomenon of disease, including its causes, but this time from another perspective and with the aid of the microscope, chemicals, and additional tools of natural sciences. Disease was dealt with as a natural phenomenon; and the patient as a living and suffering individual with her *first-person reports* was no longer the subject of concern. Rather, cadavers, tissues, and cells of the diseased individuals had entered the field and attracted the interest of pathologists. Therefore, the systems of disease that pathologists were building, calling them 'nosological systems' once again, differed from those of the traditional, clinical nosology proper. We may therefore distinguish between two types of nosological systems today. The first type, i.e., clinical-nosological systems that are built and used in clinical medicine, refer to *Homo patiens*, whereas the nosological systems of pathology refer to cadavers. *Disease* (in the singular) and *diseases* (in the plural) as understood in clinical medicine, on the one hand, and in pathology, on the other, are two different things and are conceptualized differently. The two disciplines look at the world from two different perspectives, use distinct conceptual systems, and speak two different languages. An example will be given below.

As was outlined in previous sections, to place a disease X in a particular nosological class C constitutes a taxonomic task and means that disease X 'is_a' C (see Section 4.1.2 on page 59). For example, the inclusion of epilepsy and encephalitis in the nosological class of *brain diseases* is to indicate that both diseases are brain diseases. The feature used in this example to classify the diseases is a topographic one and concerns the anatomical localization of the disorders. However, in classifying a disease, non-anatomical features may be used as well. For instance, the now defunct, but huge, class of so-called 'fevers' of the well-known, eighteenth century nosological system of Francois Boissier de Sauvages (1706–1767) comprised diseases that displayed fever as a *symptom*. Depending on the features used in building such nosological classes, the classes and the nosological system itself will be different from other, competing ones.

Concerned with the living patient, a nosological system in clinical medicine includes diseases affecting a *person* with a subjective sphere. Thus, nosology in the clinical sense is an anthropological science. By contrast, pathology is a biological science concerned with cadavers, tissues, and cells lacking a subjective sphere. In a nutshell, clinical nosology is anthropology, while pathology is biology.

The obvious difference between nosology and pathology and between their viewpoints entails that they produce and advance conceptual systems which are different from, and partially incompatible with, one another. For example, a disease such as *carcinoma of the stomach* in clinical nosology is not the same entity as *carcinoma of the stomach* in pathology, although they are expressed by the same word. We must therefore conclude that many, or even most, disease names are ambiguous. This ambiguity has far-reaching epistemological and practical consequences, one of which may be briefly demonstrated here. We will use a very simple example to avoid further complicating an already complicated issue. Our example is the term "acute gastritis", used both in clinical medicine and pathology.

When one and the same term, e.g., "acute gastritis" or any other phrase, is defined and used in two scientific fields *differently,* then the two definitions jointly imply certain sentences because they share the definiendum. The consequences that they imply, are not empirically empty sentences any more, but statements with empirical content that may be true or false. The epistemological dilemma that is generated by this circumstance will be briefly outlined below.

We have seen in Sections 4.2 and 5.3.3 on pages 76 and 91 that disease names such as "acute gastritis" may be treated as dispositional terms. The best method of defining dispositional terms is operational definition. The current definition of the term "acute gastritis" as a clinical-nosological predicate was reconstructed by an operational definition on page 92, i.e. Definition 16. For the purpose of our analyses we now rewrite here that definition:

Definition 51 (Acute gastritis: clinical, 1). *If an individual is gastroscopically examined, then she has* acute gastritis *iff her gastric mucosa shows subepithelial hemorrhages, petechiae, and erosions.*

The currently used definition of the same term in pathology we may reconstruct, like above, by another operational definition thus:[40]

Definition 52 (Acute gastritis: in pathology, 1). *If a biopsy from gastroscopy of an individual is light-microscopically examined, then she has* acute gastritis *iff neutrophilic infiltration is present in her gastric epithelium and gastric lamina propria.*

These two definitions used in two different fields imply a host of statements as corollaries. We exemplify here three such corollaries. For their proof, see below.

---

[40] I would like to thank Dr. Harris G. Yfantis, VA Department of Pathology, Baltimore, for providing the basic information used in the histologic Definition 52.

Corollary 2. *If an individual is gastroscopically examined and her gastric mucosa shows subepithelial hemorrhages, petechiae, and erosions,* **then,** *if a biopsy from gastroscopy of the individual is light-microscopically examined,* **then** *neutrophilic infiltration is present in her gastric epitelium and lamina propria.*

Corollary 3. *If an individual is gastroscopically examined and her gastric mucosa shows subepithelial hemorrhages, petechiae, and erosions,* **then,** *if a biopsy from gastroscopy of the individual is light-microscopically examined,* **then** *neutrophilic infiltration is present in her gastric epitelium.*

Corollary 4. *If an individual is gastroscopically examined and her gastric mucosa shows subepithelial hemorrhages, petechiae, and erosions,* **then,** *if a biopsy from gastroscopy of the individual is light-microscopically examined,* **then** *neutrophilic infiltration is present in her gastric lamina propria.*

All these corollaries assert deterministic correlations of the following form between gastroscopic and histologic features:

$$\alpha \to (\beta \to \gamma). \tag{20}$$

The statement is not a definition. It has empirical content and may therefore be falsified *if* there is a patient who does not show the postulated association between clinical and histologic features, i.e., if $\neg(\beta \to \gamma)$. For example, it may be that clinically her gastric mucosa shows subepithelial hemorrhages, petechiae, and erosions (β), whereas histologically there is no neutrophilic infiltration in her gastric epithelium or lamina propria ($\neg\gamma$), and thus, $\beta \wedge \neg\gamma$ or equivalently $\neg(\beta \to \gamma)$. This evidence would falsify the assertion (20). Since the premises from which it follows, i.e., the two Definitions 51 and 52 above, are *definitions* used in two distinct areas and therefore cannot be false statements, we would have to conclude in such a case that they are logically incompatible. One or both of them should therefore be changed or abandoned.

As experience shows, however, in situations of the kind above a clinician who is informed by her pathology colleague about the negative histologic finding, almost always abandons her own *clinical diagnosis* which states that the patient has acute gastritis. She accepts the negative, histologic diagnosis instead. And both *definitions* are retained. This decision is neither logically nor epistemologically justifiable because the negative histologic finding has shown that the two definitions are logically incompatible. Nevertheless, it is pragmatically forced. Obviously, neither clinical definitions nor those in pathology can be changed or discarded every other day. Such a change would amount to conceptual change, and that would require that all knowledge, hypotheses, and theories containing, or based upon, those concepts be rewritten and republished every other day. This is clearly practically unfeasible. Thus, the two medical subdisciplines *clinical nosology and practice,* on the one hand, and *pathology,* on the other, will continue to operate on the basis of mutually incompatible conceptual systems.

To demonstrate how the three corollaries above are implied by the two different Definitions 51 and 52 of the term "acute gastritis", we will first provide some abbreviations. Some readers may want to skip this logical proof.

GEx	stands for:	x is gastroscopically examined
AGx		x has acute gastritits
$GMyx$		y is the gastric mucosa of x
SHy		y shows subepithelial hemorrhages
PEy		y shows petechiae
ERy		y shows erosions.

Using these symbols, the clinical definition of "acute gastritis" given in Definition 51 above may be rewritten as follows:

Definition 53 (Acute gastritis: clinical, 2)**.**

$$\forall x \forall y \big(GEx \wedge GMyx \rightarrow (AGx \leftrightarrow SHy \wedge PEy \wedge ERy) \big).$$

Analogously, the predicates contained in the histologic definition of "acute gastritis" given in Definition 52 may be briefly symbolized thus:

BGx	stands for:	biopsy from gastroscopy of the individual x is light-microscopically examined
$EPyx$		y is the gastric epithelium of x
$LPzx$		z is the gastric lamina propria of x
NIy		neutrophilic infililtration is present in y
NIz		neutrophilic infililtration is present in z.

By means of these abbreviations, we obtain the following formalization of the histologic Definition 52:

Definition 54 (Acute gastritis: in pathology, 2)**.**

$$\forall x \forall y \forall z \big(BGx \wedge EPyx \wedge LPzx \rightarrow (AGx \leftrightarrow NIy \wedge NIz) \big).$$

We will prove Corollary 2 only. The other corollaries can be proved similarly.

Assertion 4. *Definitions 53 $\wedge$ 54* $\vdash$ *Corollary 2.*

Proof 4:

1. $\forall x \forall y \big(GEx \wedge GMyx \rightarrow (AGx \leftrightarrow SHy \wedge PEy \wedge ERy) \big)$ Definition 53
2. $\forall x \forall y \forall z \big(BGx \wedge EPyx \wedge LPzx \rightarrow (AGx \leftrightarrow NIy \wedge NIz) \big)$ Definition 54
3. $GEx \wedge GMyx \rightarrow (AGx \leftrightarrow SHy \wedge PEy \wedge ERy)$ Iterated $\forall$-Elimination: 1
4. $GEx \wedge GMyx \rightarrow (SHy \wedge PEy \wedge ERy \rightarrow AGx)$ $\leftrightarrow$-Elimination: 3
5. $GEx \wedge GMyx \wedge SHy \wedge PEy \wedge ERy \rightarrow AGx$ Importation Rule: 4
6. $BGx \wedge EPyx \wedge LPzx \rightarrow (AGx \leftrightarrow NIy \wedge NIz)$ Iterated $\forall$-Elimination: 2
7. $BGx \wedge EPyx \wedge LPzx \rightarrow (AGx \rightarrow NIy \wedge NIz)$ $\leftrightarrow$-Elimination: 6
8. $AGx \rightarrow (BGx \wedge EPyx \wedge LPzx \rightarrow NIy \wedge NIz)$ Permutation of antecedents: 7
9. $GEx \wedge GMyx \wedge SHy \wedge PEy \wedge ERy \rightarrow$
            $(BGx \wedge EPyx \wedge LPzx \rightarrow NIy \wedge NIz)$ Chain Rule: 5, 8
10. $\forall x \forall y \forall z \big(GEx \wedge GMyx \wedge SHy \wedge PEy \wedge ERy \rightarrow$
            $(BGx \wedge EPyx \wedge LPzx \rightarrow NIy \wedge NIz) \big)$ Iterated $\forall$-Introduction: 9
11. $10 \equiv$ Corollary 2   QED

6.4.4 Nosological Spaces

A concept spans a semantic and ontological space that includes all of the instances of that concept. Every instance occupies a particular spatial region in that space. For the concept of disease introduced in Section 6.3.1, this opens up a unique facet of inquiry. Our steps thus far have led us to a novel area that might be termed the semantic geometry, or geometric semantics, of disease. It enables us to explore, using geometric and topological methods, the abstract space that *a* concept of disease spans. Our approach may be instrumental both in nosology and diagnostics as well as metanosology and metadiagnostics.

In what follows, we shall demonstrate that an individual disease, as a human condition, *is a point* in the semantic space of the concept of disease relative to which it is *a* disease. Within this space, we are able to determine *a* disease's location as well as the distance between any pair of diseases. To prepare our analysis, we shall first sketch a multidimensional space called "the fuzzy hypercube". The idea is due to Lotfi Zadeh who as early as 1971 suggested a geometric interpretation of fuzzy sets as points in unit hypercubes (Zadeh, 1971, 486). Many years later, his suggestion was taken up by Bart Kosko as the basis of a promising fuzzy-logical framework and geometry. Our abstract geometry of diseases discussed below is based on this geometry of fuzzy sets developed by Bart Kosko (1992, 1997). Our analyses divide into the following five sections:

▶   The fuzzy hypercube
▶   Diseases as points in the fuzzy hypercube
▶   The geometry of diseases
▶   Clarity *vs.* entropy of a disease
▶   The relativity and historicity of nosological spaces.

The fuzzy hypercube

The fuzzy hypercube is an abstract, multidimensional space that enables us to geometrically explore the irreducible category of diseases and its characteristics. To familiarize ourselves with the hypercube, we need some additional terminology. We will start by considering a simple example. The positive real line is the line of *positive real numbers,* denoted $\mathbb{R}^+$, beginning with 0 and extending to infinity $+\infty$ (Figure 33).

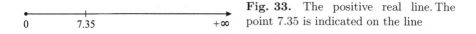

0   7.35 $+\infty$

Fig. 33. The positive real line. The point 7.35 is indicated on the line

A real number $a \geq 0$ such as 7.35 is a single point on the positive real line $\mathbb{R}^+$. The line is continuous in that it extends to infinity with no hole between each two points. Between any two adjacent points such as 7.35 and 7.36 there are still infinitely many other points. The line may be considered *one-dimensional* space, representable by a single coordinate axis extending from 0 to $+\infty$.

Two rectangular real lines as two coordinate axes x and y generate or span a plane, i.e., a *two-dimensional* space (Figure 34). In this space, a pair (a, b) of numbers a and b, each belonging to one of the coordinate axes, generates a point of the space. Put another way, a single point of a two-dimensional space is describable by a pair (a, b) of numbers on its coordinates.

We obtain a *three-dimensional* space if we use three real lines as three rectangular coordinate axes x, y, and z extending from 0 to $+\infty$ (Figure 34). A point in this space is generated by a triple (a, b, c) of numbers a, b, and c, each belonging to one of the three coordinate axes. That is, a single point of the three-dimensional space is describable by a triple (a, b, c) of numbers on three coordinates.

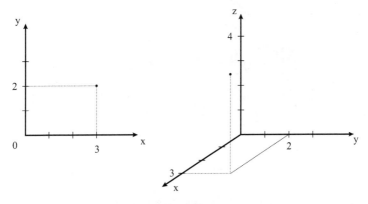

Fig. 34. A two-dimensional space (left) and a three-dimensional space (right). In the first space, a number pair (a, b) such as $(3, 2)$ yields a point in the space, whereas a point in the second space represents a number triple (a, b, c) such as $(3, 2, 4)$ each belonging to one of the three coordinate axes

One may introduce an additional, fourth coordinate axis to obtain a *four-dimensional* space. But a higher than three-dimensional space cannot be graphically illustrated, and hence, it cannot be visualized. It is an abstract space. Generalizing what we have already seen in the three concrete spaces above, a point in this abstract, four-dimensional space is represented by a quadruple (a, b, c, d) of four numbers such as $(15, 3, 8, 263)$ each of which belongs to a corresponding coordinate axis.

By introducing additional, fifth, sixth, $\ldots$, n-th coordinate axes in the same way, one obtains abstract spaces of five, six, $\ldots$, n dimensions, or in other words, *n-dimensional* spaces with $n \geq 1$. A point in such an n-dimensional space is described by an n-tuple $(a_1, a_2, \ldots, a_n)$ of numbers on its coordinate axes. In our analyses below, we shall be interested in an n-dimensional *cubic* space only referred to as an n-dimensional cube, or *hyper-*

cube for short. An hypercube is simply an n-dimensional space whose coordinate axes are of equal length. We are interested only in the *unit hypercube* the length of whose coordinate axes is 1. This notion will be introduced below. Since we shall need the notion of 'unit interval' throughout, it may be defined in a footnote.[41]

Given any closed interval $[p, q]$ such as $[5, 8]$, the difference $q - p$ is referred to as the *length* of the interval. The closed interval $[0, 1]$ is thus a line of length 1 called the unit interval or the *unit line*. A two-dimensional space consisting of two coordinate axes x and y, both of which are unit intervals $[0, 1]$, is a unit *square*, written $[0, 1] \times [0, 1]$, or $[0, 1]^2$ for short. A three-dimensional space consisting of three coordinate axes x, y, and z, all of which are unit intervals $[0, 1]$, is a unit *cube*, written $[0, 1] \times [0, 1] \times [0, 1]$, or $[0, 1]^3$ for short. In general, an n-dimensional space consisting of n coordinate axes $x_1, \ldots, x_n$, all of which are unit intervals $[0, 1]$, is an n-dimensional unit cube, called a *unit hypercube* and written $[0, 1] \times \cdots \times [0, 1]$, or $[0, 1]^n$ for short. Thus, an n-dimensional unit cube or hypercube is:

the unit line between 0 and 1 inclusive	if $n = 1$	$\equiv$	$[0, 1]$
the unit square	if $n = 2$	$\equiv$	$[0, 1]^2$
the ordinary unit cube	if $n = 3$	$\equiv$	$[0, 1]^3$
the unit hypercube	if $n \geq 1$	$\equiv$	$[0, 1]^n$.

For our discussion below, it is worth mentioning that a hypercube $[0, 1]^n$ has 2^n corners. For example, the unit line has $2^1 = 2$ corners. The unit square has $2^2 = 4$ corners. The unit cube has $2^3 = 8$ corners, and so on.

Diseases can be represented as points in an n-dimensional unit hypercube and can thus be geometrically analyzed and diagnosed in this abstract space. To understand this, we must convince ourselves that a fuzzy set is in fact a *point* in an n-dimensional unit hypercube. This may be illustrated as follows.

An ordered n-tuple $(a_1, a_2, \ldots, a_n)$ of numbers is referred to as a *vector*. The index n indicates its dimensionality; and for any $i \geq 1$ its i-th element a_i is called its i-th component. For example, the quadruple $(3, 1, 8, 2)$ is a four-dimensional vector of natural numbers with 8 being its third component. So, an n-dimensional vector $(a_1, a_2, \ldots, a_n)$ is a point in an n-dimensional

---

[41] The real line is the ordered set of singleton real numbers extending from 0 to positive infinity and negative infinity. A segment of this *real line* with the endpoints a and b, i.e., a set of real numbers lying between two real numbers a and b, is referred to as an *interval*. If both endpoints a and b are included, the interval is called *closed* and is written $[a, b]$. For example, the real interval '$[5, 11]$' is the closed interval between 5 and 11 containing all real numbers from 5 to 11 inclusive. If neither a nor b is included, the interval is called *open* and denoted (a, b). For instance, '$(5, 11)$' is the interval above excluding 5 and 11. If only one of a or b is included, the interval is written $(a, b]$ or $[a, b)$ and is called a left half-open interval or a right half-open interval, respectively. For example, the closed unit interval is $[0, 1]$. The open unit interval is $(0, 1)$, while the left half-open unit interval is $(0, 1]$ and the right half-open unit interval is $[0, 1)$.

space. For example, the vector (3, 2, 4) is a point in the three-dimensional space of natural numbers (Fig. 34 on page 208).

If $\{(x_1, a_1), \ldots, (x_n, a_n)\}$ is a fuzzy set with $n \geq 1$ members, the ordered n-tuple $(a_1, \ldots, a_n)$ of its membership degrees is referred to as its *membership vector*. For any $i \geq 1$, the component a_i of the membership vector $(a_1, a_2, \ldots, a_n)$ is the degree of membership of the object x_i in the set. For example, the membership vector of the fuzzy set $\{(chest\_pain, 1), (elevated\_CK, 0.4), (tachycardia, 0.8)\}$ is the triple $(1, 0.4, 0.8)$. Thus, it is three-dimensional, and its second component is 0.4.

Recall that the classical powerset, i.e., the set of all crisp subsets, of a *classical* set Ω with $n \geq 1$ members has 2^n members. It is therefore denoted by 2^Ω. For example, if our set is $\Omega = \{x, y\}$, then its powerset is $2^\Omega = \{\{x\}, \{y\}, \{x, y\}, \varnothing\}$ with $\varnothing$ being the empty set. Also recall that the set of all *fuzzy* subsets of a classical base set Ω is referred to as its fuzzy powerset and is denoted by $F(2^\Omega)$. This set has, in contrast to 2^Ω, infinitely many members (see Section 30.2.3 on page 1007).

Given a classical base set Ω with $n \geq 1$ members, its fuzzy powerset $F(2^\Omega)$ forms an n-dimensional unit hypercube such that each of its members, a fuzzy set, is a point in the cube. This is the central idea underlying our analysis.

Consider a simple example. Let $\Omega = \{x_1, \ldots, x_n\}$ be any base set. We will hold Ω in a constant order of n columns $x_1, x_2, \ldots, x_n$. We can thus use for any fuzzy set $\{(x_1, a_1), \ldots, (x_n, a_n)\} = A \in F(2^\Omega)$ the vector notation and represent it by its n-dimensional membership vector $(a_1, a_2, \ldots, a_n)$ with components in $[0, 1]$. For instance, if our base set Ω is $\{x_1, x_2, x_3\}$, we write:

(a_1, a_2, a_3) for fuzzy set: $\{(x_1, a_1), (x_2, a_2), (x_3, a_3)\}$

such as, for example:

$(1, 1, 1)$ for fuzzy set: $\{(x_1, 1), (x_2, 1), (x_3, 1)\}$
$(0.2, 0.8, 0.6)$ $\{(x_1, 0.2), (x_2, 0.8), (x_3, 0.6)\}$
$(1, 0, 1))$ $\{(x_1, 1), (x_2, 0), (x_3, 1)\}$.

The ith component a_i in a column $i \geq 1$ of such a fuzzy set vector $(a_1, \ldots, a_n)$ represents the membership degree $\mu_A(x_i) = a_i$ of the corresponding object x_i in set A. Our three example sets above are three-dimensional vectors. A membership function μ_A thus establishes a fuzzy set A as an n-dimensional vector $A = (\mu_A(x_1), \ldots, \mu_A(x_n))$ with $\mu_A(x_i) \in [0, 1]$.

If $\{(x_1, a_1), \ldots, (x_n, a_n)\}$ is a fuzzy set with $n \geq 1$ members, then allocate each of its objects $x_1, \ldots, x_n$ to one of the coordinate axes of an n-dimensional unit hypercube, and take into account that geometrically an n-dimensional vector $(a_1, a_2, \ldots, a_n)$ of real numbers with components in $[0, 1]$ defines:

a point on the unit line $[0, 1]$ if $n = 1$
a point in the unit square $[0, 1]^2$ if $n = 2$
a point in the cube $[0, 1]^3$ if $n = 3$
a point in the unit hypercube $[0, 1]^n$ if $n \geq 1$.

Thus, a fuzzy set $\{(x_1, a_1), \ldots, (x_n, a_n)\}$ as an n-dimensional vector of the form $(a_1, a_2, \ldots, a_n)$ with components in $[0, 1]$ is a *point* in an n-dimensional unit hypercube $[0, 1]^n$. Hence, given any base set Ω with $n \geq 1$ members, its fuzzy powerset $F(2^\Omega)$ forms an n-dimensional unit hypercube. The 2^n members of its ordinary powerset 2^Ω inhabit the 2^n corners of the cube with the empty set $\varnothing$ residing at the cube origin, and the n singletons x_i residing at the corners of the coordinate axes. The rest of the infinite fuzzy powerset $F(2^\Omega)$ fills in the lattice to produce the solid cube. The cube $[0, 1]^n$ may therefore be termed a *fuzzy hypercube*. See Figures 35 and 36.

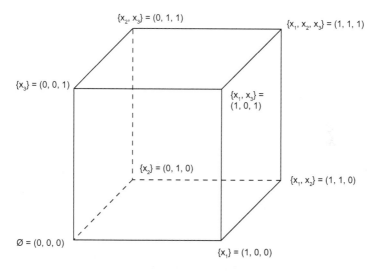

Fig. 35. Since more than three dimensions are not graphically representable, this illustration may be viewed as a proxy for all n-dimensional unit hypercubes $[0, 1]^n$. We have a three-element base set $\Omega = \{x_1, x_2, x_3\}$. The $2^n = 8$ vertices of the cube represent the eight fuzzified elements of the ordinary powerset 2^Ω with the three singletons $\{x_1\}$, $\{x_2\}$, and $\{x_3\}$ located at the corners of the coordinate axes. The entire fuzzy powerset $F(2^\Omega)$ forms the unit cube. The fuzzy set $A = \{(x_1, 0.5), (x_2, 0.4), (x_3, 0.7)\}$ is exemplified as a point within the cube in Figure 36

Diseases as points in the fuzzy hypercube

Let $\mathcal{F} = \{F_1, \ldots, F_n\}$ be the feature space of nosology referred to on page 168. And let $\mathcal{H}$ be the set of all fuzzy human conditions over $\mathcal{F}$, i.e., the fuzzy powerset $F(2^\mathcal{F})$. By interpreting each dimension, i.e., each coordinate axis $i \geq 1$, of the n-dimensional unit hypercube $[0, 1]^n$ as a feature F_i from the feature space $\mathcal{F}$, any human condition of the form:

$$\{(F_1, a_1), \ldots, (F_n, a_n)\} \tag{21}$$

presents itself as a single point in the hypercube such that its membership vector $(a_1, a_2, \ldots, a_n)$ describes that point on the dimensions $(F_1, \ldots, F_n)$, respectively. As a result, the uncountably infinite set of all fuzzy human conditions, $\mathcal{H}$, yields an n-dimensional fuzzy hypercube $[0,1]^n$. This fuzzy hypercube also represents the category of fuzzy diseases, $\mathbb{D}$, because according to Definitions 37 and 39, $\mathbb{D}$ is a fuzzy subset of $\mathcal{H}$. Thus, every fuzzy disease of the form (21) with the membership vector $(a_1, a_2, \ldots, a_n)$ is a point in the fuzzy hypercube $[0,1]^n$. For mnemonic reasons, this n-dimensional fuzzy hypercube with diseases as its points will be symbolized by $[\mathbb{D}]^n$ and referred to as the *nosological hypercube*.

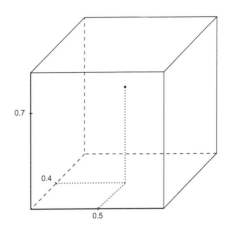

Fig. 36. The same hypercube as in Figure 35. The dot within the cube is the fuzzy set $A = \{(x_1, 0.5), (x_2, 0.4), (x_3, 0.7)\}$ with its fuzzy vector $(0.5, 0.4, 0.7)$

In our construct, diseases turn out to be spatial objects in the nosological hypercube. An example is $heart\_attack = \{(chest\_pain, 1), (elevated\_CK, 0.7), \ldots, (tachycardia, 0.8)\}$ with its membership vector $(1, 0.7, \ldots, 0.8)$. It characterizes, on the n dimensions $(chest\_pain, elevated\_CK, \ldots, tachycardia)$ of the cube $[\mathbb{D}]^n$, a single point in the cube. As spatial objects in the cube, diseases become amenable to a multitude of geometric analyses, as we shall see in the next section.

The geometry of diseases

According to the prototype resemblance theory of disease discussed on pages 174–183, a human condition is considered a disease by virtue of its similarity with a prototype disease. In this section, we will advance the geometric idea that the *similarity* between two diseases, A and B, equals their spatial *proximity* to each other in the nosological hypercube $[\mathbb{D}]^n$. Hence, the closer to a prototype disease A a human condition B is in the cube, the greater its diseasehood. To demonstrate these relationships, we need a notion of closeness or *proximity*, and a notion of *metric space* that enables the measurement of distances. To this end, a concept of metric space will be introduced first.

Definition 55 (Metric space: intuitive version). *Let Ω be a non-empty set of any objects. The structure $\langle \Omega, dist \rangle$ is called a metric space iff (i) dist is a binary function on $\Omega \times \Omega$ and assigns to each pair of elements, x and y, of set Ω a real number r such that $dist(x, y) = r$, to be read as "the distance between* *x and y is r"; and (ii) all elements x, y, and z of Ω satisfy the following axioms:*

1. $dist(x, y) \geq 0$ *non-negativity*
2. $dist(x, y) = 0$ *iff* $x = y$ *the identification property*
3. $dist(x, y) = dist(y, x)$ *symmetry*
4. $dist(x, y) + dist(y, z) \geq dist(x, z)$ *the triangle property.*

A function *dist* with these properties is called a *distance measure* in Ω or a *metric* on Ω. The elements of set Ω are referred to as the *points* of the metric space $\langle \Omega, dist \rangle$. For example, let d be a measure of physical distance between ordinary physical objects according to a scale such as meter, then the tuple $\langle Physical\_objects, d \rangle$ is a metric space consisting of the set of physical objects and the measure d. In this metric space, the distance between the centers of your eyes is, say, six centimeters, i.e., $d(\text{right\_eye, left\_eye}) = 6$. Note that we could have introduced the concept above more exactly by a set-theoretical definition. We will do so below for Definition 56, and thereafter use less formal, intuitive definitions as above to keep them more readable.

Definition 56 (Metric space: set-theoretical version). *ξ is a metric space iff there are Ω and* dist *such that:*

1. $\xi = \langle \Omega, dist \rangle$,
2. *Ω is a non-empty set of any objects,*
3. *dist: $\Omega \times \Omega \mapsto \mathbb{R}$, i.e., dist is a binary function from Ω to real numbers, referred to as a* distance measure, *such that for all $x, y, z \in \Omega$:*

    3.1. $dist(x, y) \geq 0$
    3.2. $dist(x, y) = 0$ *iff* $x = y$
    3.3. $dist(x, y) = dist(y, x)$
    3.4. $dist(x, y) + dist(y, z) \geq dist(x, z)$.

According to this definition, the structure $\langle [\mathbb{D}]^n, diff \rangle$ is a metric space with $[\mathbb{D}]^n$ being the nosological hypercube and *diff* being the function *diff* for fuzzy set difference introduced in Definition 34 on page 172. Also according to this definition, *diff* is a binary distance measure and maps $[\mathbb{D}]^n \times [\mathbb{D}]^n$ to $[0, 1]$. It satisfies all requirements of the definition to enable geometric analyses of diseases in the nosological hypercube $[\mathbb{D}]^n$. We shall come back to this issue below. First consider the following example.

Let Ω be the set of all n-dimensional vectors $(r_1, \ldots, r_n)$ of real numbers with $n \geq 1$. And let $(a_1, \ldots, a_n) = x$ and $(b_1, \ldots, b_n) = y$ be two such vectors defining the two points x and y in a metric space. An infinite class of distance measures, the so-called Minkowski class, is defined by the following sentence in which the variable "$dist^p$" signifies the p-th distance measure with $p \geq 1$:

$$dist^p(x, y) = \sqrt[p]{(|a_1 - b_1|^p + \cdots + |a_n - b_n|^p)} \qquad \text{for } n, p \geq 1.$$

Each $dist^p$ renders the structure $\langle \Omega, dist \rangle$ a metric space. (Recall that $|a - b|$ is the absolute value of the subtraction $a - b$. See Definition 33 on page

172.) The first two measures in the infinite series may be exemplified. The first and simplest one, named after the U.S.-American mathematician Richard Hamming (1915–1998), is the *Hamming distance* that is written $dist^1$ and defined thus:

$$dist^1(x,y) = |a_1 - b_1| + \cdots + |a_n - b_n| \qquad \text{(Hamming distance)}$$

And the second one, written $dist^2$, is the so-called *Euclidean distance:*

$$dist^2(x,y) = \sqrt[2]{|a_1 - b_1|^2 + \cdots + |a_n - b_n|^2} \qquad \text{(Euclidean distance)}$$

To demonstrate, we will use two overly simplified example diseases, and for simplicity's sake suppose that they consist of three features only, as if our disease hypercube were three-dimensional. Our example diseases are:

disease $A = \{(F_1, 1), (F_2, 0.7), (F_3, 0.8)\}$
disease $B = \{(F_1, 1), (F_2, 0.3), (F_3, 0.5)\}$

with their membership vectors:

$A = (1, 0.7, 0.8)$
$B = (1, 0.3, 0.5).$

They are two points in the 3-dimensional unit hypercube (Figure 37).

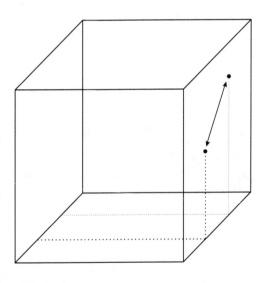

Fig. 37. The fuzzy sets $A = \{(F_1, 1), (F_2, 0.7), (F_3, 0.8)\}$ and $B = \{(F_1, 1), (F_2, 0.3), (F_3, 0.5)\}$ with their membership vectors (1, 0.7, 0.8) and (1, 0.3, 0.5), respectively, are two points in a 3-dimensional unit hypercube with the features F_1, F_2, and F_3 as their coordinate axes. The double arrow between the two points symbolizes their geometric distance in the cube. This distance may be measured by different Minkowski metrics, e.g., Hamming distance, Euclidean distance, etc. See body text

The Hamming distance between them is:

$$dist^1(A, B) = |1 - 1| + |0.7 - 0.3| + |0.8 - 0.5|$$
$$= 0 + 0.4 + 0.3$$
$$= 0.7$$

whereas their Euclidean distance is:

$$dist^2(A, B) = \sqrt[2]{|1 - 1|^2 + |0.7 - 0.3|^2 + |0.8 - 0.5|^2}$$
$$= \sqrt[2]{(0 + 0.16 + 0.09)}$$
$$= 0.5.$$

For a unit hypercube $[0, 1]^n$ with a metric $dist$ of this or another type, the resulting structure $\langle[0, 1]^n, dist\rangle$ is a *metric space*, and the distance $dist(x, y)$ between any two points x and y of the cube becomes measurable, as in the examples above. We will use the Hamming distance, $dist^1$, for two reasons. First, it is the simplest one. Second, it can be proved that all Minkowski distances are formally equivalent.

As stated above, our familiar function $diff$ is a distance measure for fuzzy sets and provides a metric on the unit hypercube. According to following theorem, which cannot be proved here, the difference between two fuzzy sets A and B, i.e. $diff(A, B)$, is proportional to their Hamming distance (Kosko, 1992):

Theorem 2. (Function $diff$ is a distance function):

$$diff(A, B) = \frac{dist^1(A, B)}{dist^1(A \cup B, \varnothing)}.$$

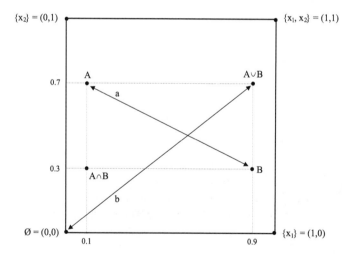

Fig. 38. A simple illustration of the *difference* relationship in a 2-dimensional hypercube. Set $A = (0.1, 0.7)$, set $B = (0.9, 0.3)$. According to Theorem 2 above, their difference is the Hamming distance a divided by the Hamming distance b, i.e., $diff(A, B) = \frac{a}{b} = 0.75$. We have thus $simil(A, B) = 1 - \frac{a}{b} = 0.25$

An example is depicted in Figure 38. What was told above about fuzzy sets, and human conditions as fuzzy sets, also holds true for diseases because we reconstructed them as fuzzy human conditions and single points of the nosological hypercube $[\mathbb{D}]^n$. For instance, our two example diseases A and B:

$$A = (1, 0.7, 0.8)$$
$$B = (1, 0.3, 0.5).$$

illustrated in Figure 37 have the following distance between them:

$$dist(A, B) = diff(A, B) = 0.28.$$

We can now further our notion of the nosological hypercube $[\mathbb{D}]^n$ by taking into account the distance measure $diff$ to obtain a metric space $\langle [\mathbb{D}]^n, diff \rangle$, referred to as a *nosological space*. A variety of metric analyses are feasible in this metric space. For instance, the proximity of a point A to a point B in the space is the inverse of their distance:

Definition 57 (Proximity). $prox(A, B) = 1 - diff(A, B)$.

As an example, consider the proximity of disease $A = (1, 0.7, 0.8)$ to disease $B = (1, 0.3, 0.5)$:

$$prox(A, B) = 1 - diff(A, B) = 1 - 0.28 = 0.72.$$

In Definition 35 on page 173, we defined similarity as follows: $simil(A, B) = 1 - diff(A, B)$. From this and Definition 57 above, we can infer that for any two diseases A and B:

$$simil(A, B) = prox(A, B).$$

Thus, the degree of similarity between any two points in the nosological space $\langle [\mathbb{D}]^n, diff \rangle$ equals their proximity to one another. For our two example diseases above, we obtain:

$$simil(A, B) = prox(A, B) = 0.72.$$

The closer to each other in the unit hypercube two diseases are, the more similar they are and vice versa (Figure 39). This is instrumental in similaristic reasoning in medicine and case-based diagnostic-therapeutic decision-making, discussed on page 639. It also implies our initial thesis: The closer to a prototype disease A a human condition B is in the unit hypercube, the greater its diseasehood.

Clarity *vs.* entropy of a disease

The more vague a disease is conceptualized, the more difficult is to differentiate it from its complement, i.e., to distinguish between its presence and absence in a patient, or in other words, to diagnose it. The degree of vagueness of a disease, referred to as its *entropy*, is measurable. There is an interesting method to do so that is discussed in Section 30.2.4 on page 1007.

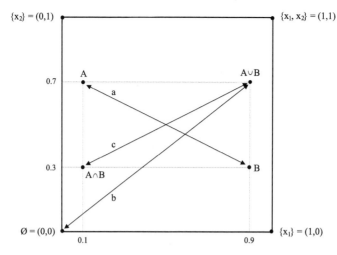

Fig. 39. An amendment to Figure 38 in which it was demonstrated that for fuzzy sets $A = (0.1, 0.7)$ and $B = (0.9, 0.3)$ we have $diff(A, B) = \frac{a}{b} = 0.75$. Since diagonal c equals diagonal a, $diff(A, B) = \frac{c}{b}$. And since $simil(A, B) = 1 - diff(A, B)$, we obtain $simil(A, B) = 1 - \frac{c}{b} = \frac{(b-c)}{b}$. Similarity between diseases is thus a geometric relationship in the unit hypercube of diseases

At this juncture, we prefer to use a simpler technique. Consider a disease of the form $A = \{(F_1, 0.5), (F_2, 0.5), (F_3, 0.5)\}$. Obviously, its complemet is $\overline{A} = \{(F_1, 0.5), (F_2, 0.5), (F_3, 0.5)\}$. Thus, it is undistinguishable from its complement because $A = \overline{A}$. As a result, it is absolutely unclear and undiagnosable. The entropy of a fuzzy set is a measure of its unclarity. It increases, the more the membership degrees of its features approach 0.5. The place of maximum entropy is thus the midpoint of the hypercube where a fuzzy set A as well as its complement $\overline{A}$ reside because they are identical as above and occupy the same point. The antonym of entropy is *clarity*. To increase its clarity, a fuzzy set must diverge from the hypercube midpoint. That is, the membership degrees of its features must increase their distance from 0.5. The term *"entropy of fuzzy set A"*, written $ent(A)$, is a unary function that maps the points of the unit hypercube to $[0, 1]$:

$$ent: [0, 1]^n \mapsto [0, 1].$$

To measure the entropy and clarity of a disease, we shall use the following Fuzzy Entorpy Theorem discussed as Thoerem 10 on page 1010:

$$ent(X) = \frac{c(X \cap \overline{X})}{c(X \cup \overline{X})}$$

(Kosko, 1992, 277). For instance, let there be three diseases:

disease $A = \{(F_1, 0.5), (F_2, 0.5), (F_3, 0.5)\}$

disease $B = \{(F_1, 1), (F_2, 0.4), (F_3, 0.8)\}$
disease $C = \{(F_1, 1), (F_2, 1), (F_3, 1)\}$,

then we have:

$$ent(A) = \frac{0.5 + 0.5 + 0.5}{0.5 + 0.5 + 0.5} = 1$$

$$ent(B) = \frac{0 + 0.4 + 0.2}{1 + 0.6 + 0.8} = 0.25$$

$$ent(C) = \frac{0 + 0 + 0}{1 + 1 + 1} = 0.$$

The clarity of a fuzzy set X, writen $clar(X)$, is defined as the antonym of its entropy (see Definition 250 on page 1009):

$$clar(X) = 1 - ent(X).$$

Thus, the above three example diseases have the following degrees of clarity:

$$clar(A) = 1 - ent(A) = 1 - 1 = 0$$
$$clar(B) = 1 - ent(B) = 1 - 0.25 = 0.75$$
$$clar(C) = 1 - ent(C) = 1 - 0 = 1.$$

The relativity and historicity of nosological spaces

In an n-dimensional nosological space $\langle [\mathbb{D}]^n, \mathit{diff} \rangle$, prototype diseases are the focal points relative to which other human conditions turn out individual diseases to particular extents. The choice of prototype diseases is therefore quite significant. Two different nosological spaces whose prototype diseases are not identical, will also have different derived diseases. Since the contents of a nosological space and the proximity relations between its disease points depend on its prototypes, there is no absolute nosological space $\langle [\mathbb{D}]^n, \mathit{diff} \rangle$. A nosological space is relative to its prototype diseases. In essence, any concept of disease generates a specific nosological space because it spans a specific semantic and ontological space that houses all of the instances of that concept. That is, any health care system depends on its underlying concept of disease. See Section 6.4.4 on page 207 above.

Prototype diseases have a long lifespan, and thus, determine the concept of disease for a long time. They are historical entities. For example, the prototype diseases of our Western concept of disease come from antiquity. Their historicity renders the concept of disease a historical construct.

6.4.5 Summary

The notions of symptomatology, nosology, pathology, and nosological system were analyzed and the concepts of symptom, predictive value, sensitivity, specificity, and pathognomonicity of symptoms were explained. We argued that all nosological systems are artifacts. In addition, we introduced a geometry of diseases. To this end, the concept of the unit hypercube was used to construct an abstract nosological hypercube $[\mathbb{D}]^n$ that houses all diseases as its points. With the distance measure *diff*, introduced in Definition 34 on page 172, the nosological hypercube yields a metric space $\langle [\mathbb{D}]^n, diff \rangle$ dubbed the *nosological space*. The space represents a highly ordered proximity structure of the diseases and allows analyses of distance, neighborhood, similarity, and dissimilarity between them. It demonstrates that the degree of diseasehood of a human condition depends on its proximity to a prototype disease.

The metric space $\langle [\mathbb{D}]^n, diff \rangle$ may also be used in diagnostics. For example, let $A = \{(F_1, a_1), (F_2, a_2), \ldots, (F_n, a_n)\}$ be a fuzzy set of any symptoms in a patient. In the metric space $\langle [\mathbb{D}]^n, diff \rangle$, one can easily find the disease, say $B = \{(F_1, b_1), (F_2, b_2), \ldots, (F_n, b_n)\}$, that is the nearest neighbor of A, by conducting a *nearest neighbor search:*

The *n*earest *n*eighbor of an object x in a region R is another object y, written $NN(x, R) = y$, if and only if among all elements of R it has the minimum distance, or the maximum proximity, to x. A *nearest neighbor search* is the query $NN(x, R) = ?$ with the aim of finding an object in the region R that can replace the question mark. It is conducted in the following way. Let $\langle \Omega, dist \rangle$ be a metric space with the region R being a subset of Ω. If $x \in R$ is any spatial object in the region R, one can always ask: Which spatial object in R is the nearest neighbor of x, i.e., $NN(x, R) = ?$, where NN is defined as follows:

Definition 58 (Nearest neighbor). *If $\langle \Omega, dist \rangle$ is a metric space and $R \subseteq \Omega$, then $NN(x, R) = y$ iff $dist(x, y) = min(\{dist(x, z) \mid z \in R \wedge z \neq x\})$ for all $x, y, z \in R$.*

Regarding our metric nosological space $\langle [\mathbb{D}]^n, diff \rangle$, let $A = \{(F_1, a_1), (F_2, a_2), \ldots, (F_n, a_n)\}$ be any set of symptoms whose membership vector $(a_1, \ldots, a_n)$ describes the point A in the region R of the cube $[\mathbb{D}]^n$. Find a disease $B = \{(F_1, b_1), (F_2, b_2), \ldots, (F_n, b_n)\}$ with the membership vector $(b_1, \ldots, b_n)$ in that region R such that $NN(A, R) = B$. This can easily be determined by an NN search, which minimizes the value $diff(A, X)$ for all elements X of the region R.

6.5 Etiology

In this section, the traditional language of causality used in medical etiology is carefully analyzed with the aim of improving it as it is not satisfactory. Specifically, it will be demonstrated that the received concept of cause as a *sufficient condition* for its effect is not tenable. In its place, we shall propose a concept of cause as a *probabilistic condition* for its effect.

6.5.0 Introduction

To begin, consider the following patient history. The patient Elroy Fox had been complaining of angina pectoris for some time and had to be hospitalized recently. The physicians in the cardiac intensive care unit diagnosed acute myocardial infarction and told him that this disease event was due to an occlusive coronary thrombosis in one of his main coronary arteries as a result of the atherosclerosis in their walls. Therefore, they immediately administered thrombolytic treatment to dissolve the blood clot in Elroy Fox's occluded coronary artery. The patient soon recovered and could be discharged from the hospital.

The onset of Mr. Elroy Fox's illness and his recovery are connected by the following two processes: (A) the genesis of his myocardial infarction and (B) the thrombolysis in his coronary arteries. They are viewed as two causal processes each of which starts with an event 1 that *causes* another event 2:

PROCESS A
event 1: thrombotic occlusion of a coronary artery
event 2: myocardial infarction

PROCESS B
event 1: thrombolytic treatment by the physician
event 2: recovery.

The first event is referred to as a *cause*. The second event is its *effect*. Why do we say, or what do we mean by saying, that event 1 *causes* event 2? What is this relation of causing or *causation?* What does it look like? And why do we believe that the two processes above are *causal* processes? Why is it necessary for both physicians and philosophers of medicine alike to concern themselves with such questions? The present section deals with these fundamental problems of etiology and may therefore be termed *metaetiology*.

Etiology, from the Greek term $\alpha \iota \tau \iota \alpha$ (aitia) meaning "the culprit" and "cause", is the inquiry into clinical *causation* or causality including the causes of pathological processes and maladies. For instance, when we assert that "the cause of AIDS is HIV" or "myocardial infarction is caused by occlusive coronary thrombosis", then we make etiologic statements. Etiology is not an individual medical specialty such as pediatrics or psychiatry. Etiologic knowledge originates from almost all medical disciplines, especially those concerned with nosology, pathology, epidemiology, and microbiology.

As emphasized in the Preface, medicine is a science and practice of intervention, manipulation, and control. The subject of medical intervention, manipulation, and control is primarily the suffering human being and her health and disease states. The physician intervenes in a disease process in an individual patient by some therapeutic acts to cure the patient or to relieve her suffering. As mentioned in Section 6.1 on page 111, it is customarily assumed that in order for such interventions and control to be successful, we must have knowledge about causes of diseases and pathological processes. This is a *protoetiologic,* metaphysical postulate that will be discussed in Section 21.5.[42] At this point, we will presume that it is true in order to ask what the notion of *knowledge about causes of diseases and pathological processes* means. To this end, we shall analyze the conceptual foundations of etiology and argue that we may sensibly distinguish between deterministic, probabilistic, and fuzzy etiology. We shall look at different types of conceptual structures for the relation of causation in order to reconstruct the notion of cause on four distinct levels and with two shapes, positive and negative:

A is a positive cause of B in class X	(qualitative)
A is a stronger positive cause of B in class X than is C	(comparative)
A is to the extent 0.8 a positive cause of B in class X	(quantitative)
A is a highly positive cause of B in class X	(fuzzy)
A is a negative cause of B in class X	(qualitative)
A is a stronger negative cause of B in class X than is C	(comparative)
A is to the extent -0.3 a negative cause of B in class X	(quantitative)
A is a weakly negative cause of B in class X	(fuzzy)

Examples of the qualitative level, which only indicates whether the relation is positive or negative, are given by the following two conjectures taken from current literature: (1) Chlamydophila pneumoniae infection is a positive cause of coronary heart disease in the population of non-diabetics; (2) aspirin is a negative cause of myocardial infarction in men with elevated C-reactive protein concentrations. The framework developed below may help deal with some of the methodological difficulties emerging in etiology and epidemiology, in systematizing nosology, and in causal diagnostics. It may also help with similar issues emerging in the engineering of causal knowledge in medical expert systems. Our analysis of etiology in this section precedes our discussion on diagnostics in Section 8.2, as the cause-effect terminology is also needed for the latter. Our discussion divides into the following four parts:

6.5.1   Cause and Causation
6.5.2   Deterministic Etiology
6.5.3   Probabilistic Etiology
6.5.4   Fuzzy Etiology.

6.5.1 Cause and Causation

As mentioned above, etiology is the inquiry into clinical causation. It deals with the question of how a particular *clinical event* such as:

---

[42] The term "protoetiologic" means that the postulate precedes and underlies etiology. For the notions of protoscience and protomedicine, see page 686.

a symptom or a set of symptoms,
a sign or a set of signs,
a finding or a set of findings,
a pathological state or a set of pathological states, and
a malady, e.g. a disease, or a set of maladies (diseases)

is generated at class lavel, not in an individual patient. For example, "what is the cause of myocardial infarction in human beings?" is an etiologic question. The goal is to identify the causes of human suffering insofar as this suffering presents itself as illness. Behind etiology lies the belief that causal knowledge is necessary for efficient clinical practice. Since this belief strongly governs both medical actions and public trust in medicine, the knowledge etiology produces should be well-grounded. However, a prerequisite for its being well-grounded is clarity about the foundational question: What is a cause? Let us consider this question along the lines of a recent etiologic hypothesis:

Is myocardial infarction an infectious disease? In the mainstream of the psychoanaly.ic movement in the first half of the 20th century, many diseases with empty or speculative etiology became 'psychosomatic' diseases. Among the prominent examples was peptic ulcer disease of the stomach and duodenum. Countless patients underwent gastrectomy or vagotomy because psychosomatic and other modes of treatment failed to cure their ulcer disease. In the 1980s, however, we began to see the dramatic move of this health disorder to another etiologic camp, i.e., to the theory of infectious diseases. *Helicobacter pylori* infection is now viewed as the main cause of peptic ulcer disease and is successfully treated by antibiotics.[43]

Another, even more dramatic move of a second disease group to the same etiologic camp seems to be underway: Atherosclerotic cardiovascular disease, well-known as ischemic heart disease, coronary artery disease, or *coronary heart disease*, is a major health problem in industrialized countries causing nearly half of the deaths through myocardial infarction and related clinical events. We were told that hypercholesterolemia, hypertension, stress, cigarette smoking, and lack of physical exercise were the main risk factors for coronary heart disease, and thus, for myocardial infarction. And we were advised accordingly: don't smoke, don't eat too much fat! There is a different, more recent version of the story, however. It seems that coronary heart disease is in the process of losing its venerable causes and assuming a new, major cause:

Chlamydophila pneumoniae is a Gram negative, intracellular bacterium, discovered in 1989 (Grayston et al., 1989), that causes acute respiratory infec-

---

[43] The term "Helicobacter pylori" derives from the Greek terms $\varepsilon\lambda\iota\xi$ (elix, helix) and $\pi\nu\lambda\omega\rho\acute{o}\varsigma$ (pyloros) meaning, respectively, (i) something wound in a continuous series of loops and (ii) "gatekeeper" that denotes the circular opening from the stomach into the duodenum, i.e, section of intestine below stomach. *Helicobacter pylori* is a spiral shaped bacterium that lives in the stomach and duodenum. It is so called because it was first found in the pyloric mucous membrane (see Section 11.2.4 on page 490).

tions in humans, horses, and koalas. Initially, it was named *Chlamydia pneumoniae* and was renamed recently.[44] We are now told that *Chlamydophila pneumoniae* is an important cause of coronary heart disease and may in the near future displace the classical risk factors mentioned above (Mendall et al., 1995; Miettinen et al., 1996; Saikku et al., 1988, 1992; Thom et al., 1992; Ouellette and Byrne, 2004). Should this etiologic hypothesis gain ground in the years ahead, myocardial infarction is likely to become an infectious disease. And we shall be advised anew: take antibiotics! "[...] the rise and fall of the incidence of coronary artery disease in the United States from the 1940s through the 1970s appears to emulate that of an infectious epidemic" (Muhlestein et al., 1996, 1555).

The medical community, more or less surprised by a new bacterium taking reign in a well-established clinical domain, is currently asking the question: Is it true that Chlamydophila pneumoniae infection is a major cause of coronary heart disease? "The simple demonstration of a prevalent microbe in atherosclerotic lesions does not prove a causal role for the agent" (Buja, 1996, 872). "Evidence includes elevated serologic titers as well as the presence of C. pneumoniae within atherosclerotic lesions. [...] However, these are preliminary and uncontrolled findings that do not yet prove an etiologic link. Whether C. pneumoniae exists as an 'innocent bystander' or has a direct causative role in the development of coronary artery disease remains to be seen" (Muhlestein et al., 1996, 1555).

That is true. But it remains to be seen when? The etiologic and clinical community will first need answers to following proto- and metaetiologic questions: What is an etiologic link? What is causation? What is a causative role? What is a cause at all, and what is a major or a minor cause? How do we prove whether or not a particular factor plays a causal role in the development of a clinical event? Without addressing these basic questions, it will only be a strange historical fact that clinical events from time to time change their etiologic camp. But we don't know why. Perhaps the reason is historical fluctuations in the quality of our therapies? Perhaps it is because of the publication policy of medical journals? In order to make headway, let us turn our attention to the questions above. Since we don't yet know what "cause" and "causation" mean, we have been using them colloquially. They will be clarified step by step. In the process, we shall look at the theories of causality that have played prominent roles in the history of this issue (Hume, 1748; Mill, 1843; Reichenbach, 1956; Lewis, 1973a; Mackie, 1974; Salmon, 1971; Suppes, 1970a).

---

[44] Grayston isolated Chlamydophila pneumoniae initially from a child's conjunctiva during a trachoma vaccine trial in Taiwan in 1965 and called the isolate TW-183 (Grayston, 1965). It was soon realized that TW-183 causes respiratory rather than ocular infections. Later, it was identified as belonging to chlamydial species and was renamed *Chlamydia pneumoniae* (Grayston et al., 1989). Its new name, *Chlamydophila,* means "similar to Chlamydia".

Usually, two main types of causation are distinguished. *Event causation* is the causation of an event by another event. A series of causally connected events is called a causal chain. By contrast, *agent causation* holds that in human action, e.g., "I open the window", the acting person is a cause that cannot be reduced to events. In our view the term "event" is a general term that covers both cases in that an agent produces a cause event by acting. So, we shall confine ourselves to event causation. Event causation is conceived of as a relation between two events one of which, the *cause*, causes the other one called its *effect*. The term "event" is also general enough to cover processes such as chains of time-sequential events, networks of simultaneous events, temporal dynamics of such networks as complex processes and histories, etc.

In natural languages, causal relationships between events are expressed by words and phrases like the following: because, due to, for, therefore, leads to, contributes to, develops, brings about, generates, engenders, affects, is effected by, etc. 'Due to' the laxity of these terms, in causal claims a clear distinction must be made between talks about (i) *singular* or token-level causes like "your hypercholesterolemia caused you to suffer coronary heart disease"; and about (ii) *generic* or type-level causes such as "hypercholesterolemia is a cause of coronary heart disease". Token-level causation is the concern of diagnostic reasoning, whereas etiology is concerned with type-level causation at the class or population level.

The typical use in conversation of the notions of cause and causation is a primary source of misconception. We often refer to an event as *the* cause of some other event as if there were or could exist no other causes of the same event. It is asked, for example, "what is *the* cause of myocardial infarction?". Granting that there may be, and in the vast majority of cases there is in fact, more than one cause of a given event, we abandon the doctrine of monocausationism and will follow John Stuart Mill in supposing a *multiplicity* of distinct causes instead. An event such as myocardial infarction may have a hundred or more different types of independent causes such as $Cause_1, Cause_2, Cause_3, \ldots$, and so on. Chlamydophila pneumoniae infection may be one of them. Cytomegalovirus infection a second one. Occlusive coronary thrombosis a third one, and so on (Figure 40).

A second step in our differentiation of causes is this: Each or some of the distinct causes $Cause_1, Cause_2, Cause_3, \ldots$ of an event may be a compound one comprising a *plurality* of partial causes $C_1, C_2, \ldots, C_n$, also called factors, co-factors, or conditions such that, for example, $Cause_i = C_{i_1} \& C_{i_2} \& \cdots \& C_{i_n}$ with $n > 1$ co-factors and $i \geq 1$. For instance, it may be that one of the causes of myocardial

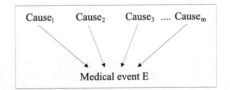

Fig. 40. Multiple causes of an event

infarction is the following complex event consisting of six co-factors: 'diabetes & hypercholesterolemia & hypertension & stress & cigarette smoking & lack of physical exercise'. The differentiation between multiplicity and plurality of causes shows that the usual term "multifactorial genesis" is unclear. Does it mean the multiplicity or does it mean the plurality of causes of an event? We shall come back to this issue in Section 6.5.3 on page 233 below.

Human knowledge rapidly changes and fades away. The search for causes, therefore, is useless if the causal knowledge it promises is void of practical value such as in cosmology and big bang research. In areas like medicine, knowledge of causes is meaningful only to the extent that it contributes to the advancement and efficacy of our actions against human and animal suffering. An action, generated and guided by a particular causal belief, is itself a cause, i.e., an intentional cause implemented by someone to produce an effect (Sadegh-Zadeh, 1979). Thus, alleged knowledge of *event causation* in medicine generates new causes in terms of *agent causation* in diagnostic, therapeutic, preventive, social, economic, and political domains. Due to this worldmaking impact of causal claims, it is morally imperative that causal knowledge be well-grounded.

Some quantum theorists claim that there is also 'backward causation'. That is, an effect may precede its cause in time. However, it is ontologically and action-theoretically problematic to presume that in the human sphere one could by doing something today produce an effect yesterday. In such a world, both orderly human cognition and human social life would be impossible. In the human sphere, including medicine, the arrow of causation is not directed backwards, so to speak. Moreover, in order for cause and effect to be distinguishable from one another, they must not be supposed to be simultaneous entities. Given two such events, we could never discern which one of them caused the other; they would always appear and vanish simultaneously. Hence, in etiology retrograde and simultaneous causation is excluded. The arrow of causation is directed forwards. The first axiom of an etiologic calculus therefore would run as follows: A cause precedes its effect in time. This temporal asymmetry of causation, recognized by David Hume, we call the *temporal priority* of causes or the *temporal succession* of effects. This criterion brings with it that causation is an asymmetric relation. If A causes B, then B does not cause A (see Definition 2 on page 68).

However, temporal succession is not sufficient for an event to be the effect of a preceding one. A frequent mistake made both in everyday life and in the sciences is the erroneous causal belief 'after this, therefore because of this'. An illustrative example of this *post hoc ergo propter hoc* fallacy is the assumption that the storm is caused by the rapid falling of barometric reading because it always occurs after the latter. A fallacious etiology of this type will be referred to as *the-barometer-causes-storm* fallacy. That both events have a common cause and that the falling of the barometric reading is only a spurious cause, or a symptom, of the storm is a warning sign to avoid doubtful etiologic studies which on a closer look exhibit a similar pattern of fallacious reasoning. Regarding the correlation between elevated Chlamydophila pneumoniae antibodies and the incidence of myocardial infarction reported above, the question arises whether this antibody increase is the barometer and myocardial infarction is the storm? We shall come back to this question below.

6.5.2 Deterministic Etiology

In the philosophical analysis of the problems sketched above, many attempts have been made during the last three centuries to find criteria that adequately characterize causation and causality. By and large, the harvest has been disappointing. That is, until recently. Earlier approaches were based on the philosopher David Hume's famous idea of the *constant conjunction* of cause and effect. It says that the association of cause and effect exhibits a general regularity in that whenever the cause event occurs, then the effect event occurs. "We may define a cause to be an object, followed by another, and where all the objects similar to the first, are followed by objects similar to the second" (Hume, 1748, section VII, part II). That is, the skeleton of a causal relationship is supposed to be a conditional of the form "If A occurs, then B occurs". For example:

> *If* a child is exposed to the measles virus and is not inoculated, *then* she will contract measles.   (22)

This Humean idea of causality known as 'the regularity theory of causality' is *deterministic* because the occurrence of the antecedent, i.e., the child's exposure to the measles virus in the present example (22), strictly determines the occurrence of the consequent, i.e., the contraction of measles. His deterministic conception dominated the philosophy on causality until 1970. In this section, we will show why it must be thrown into doubt, and consequently, cannot be used in medical etiology. Three well-known fruits of determinism will also be briefly mentioned and then dismissed: Robert Koch's postulates, John Mackie's acclaimed INUS theory, and David Lewis' counterfactuals. Our discussion thus consists of the following four sections:

▶ Determinism
▶ Koch's postulates
▶ INUS conditions
▶ Counterfactuals.

Determinism

In an etiologically simple, ideal world we would have clear-cut and logically well-treatable if-then relationships of the form (22) above between causes and their effects: If cause C_i occurs, then effect E_j occurs. Supposing that cause C_i consists of a plurality of $n \geq 1$ components $C_{i_1}, \ldots, C_{i_n}$, the general structure of such deterministic cause-effect relations would be:

If condition C_{i_1} & $\cdots$ & C_{i_n} occurs, then effect E_j occurs.

However, there are scarcely deterministic-etiologic relationships of this type. Most etiologic relationships are imperfect regularities such that a cause event is *not always* associated with an effect event. As we shall study in Section 6.5.3 below, the irregular association can be captured only *probabilistically* such as, for instance, "the exposure of a non-inoculated child to measles virus increases the probability of contracting the disease". That means that the world we presently live in, is etiologically complicated and not ideal. We will nevertheless clarify the logical structure of deterministic-etiologic relationships to convince ourselves that even if they did exist, they could be embedded in the more general, probabilistic etiology discussed below. To this end, we will first introduce the notion of a deterministic-causal law.

Let $\mathcal{L}$ be an interpreted language of the first order, for example, English or German. $P, Q, R, \ldots$ may be n-ary predicates of $\mathcal{L}$ with $n \geq 1$. Individual variables are symbolized by $x, y, z, \ldots, t, t_1, t_2, \ldots$, the latter ones being time variables denoting points in time. If P is an n-ary predicate, $Px_1 \ldots x_{n-1}t$ is an atomic sentence. It says that P at time t applies to $x_1, \ldots, x_{n-1}$. For instance, "Mr. Elroy Fox is suffering from myocardial infarction today", i.e., Pxt, where $P \equiv$ is suffering from myocardial infarction; $x \equiv$ Mr. Elroy Fox; and $t \equiv$ today.

An atomic sentence and the negation of an atomic sentence will be referred to as a *state description* in $\mathcal{L}$ and will be represented by Greek letters $\alpha, \beta, \gamma, \ldots$ If α and β are state descriptions in $\mathcal{L}$, their conjunction $\alpha \wedge \beta$ is also a state description in $\mathcal{L}$. Thus, state descriptions in $\mathcal{L}$ are temporalized simple statements or conjunctions of any length. They represent simple or complex events occurring at particular instants or periods of time.

If α is the positive, atomic state description $Px_1 \ldots x_{n-1}t$ or its negation $\neg Px_1 \ldots x_{n-1}t$, the set $\{t\}$ is called the time set of α and is written $time(\alpha)$. The set $\{P\}$ is referred to as its predicate set and written $predicate(\alpha)$. If $\alpha \wedge \beta$ is a state description, then $time(\alpha \wedge \beta) = time(\alpha) \cup time(\beta)$, and $predicate(\alpha \wedge \beta) = perdicate(\alpha) \cup predicate(\beta)$. For example,

- $time(\text{'Elroy Fox has a cough today and he had a fever yesterday'}) = \{today, yesterday\}$;
- $predicate(\text{'Elroy Fox has a cough today and he had a fever yesterday'}) = \{has\ a\ cough, has\ a\ fever\}$;
- $time(Pxt_1 \wedge Qxt_2 \wedge \neg Pxt_3) = \{t_1, t_2, t_3\}$;
- $predicate(Pxt_1 \wedge Qxt_2 \wedge \neg Pxt_3) = \{P, Q\}$.

Definition 59 (Deterministic law of succession). *Let $\mathcal{L}L$ be the extended language $\mathcal{L} \cup L$ with L being any system of the first-order predicate logic added to $\mathcal{L}$. If α and β are state descriptions in $\mathcal{L}L$ with the free individual variables $x_1, \ldots, x_m, t_1, \ldots, t_n$, then γ is a deterministic law of succession in $\mathcal{L}L$ iff:*

1. γ is the universal closure of $\alpha \rightarrow \beta$, i.e., the closed generalization $\forall x_1 \ldots \forall x_m \forall t_1 \ldots \forall t_n (\alpha \rightarrow \beta)$;

2. γ *is a contingent sentence; that means that it is consistent, not logically valid, and not undecidable in* $\mathcal{L}L$*;*

3. *every* $t_i \in time(\alpha)$ *is earlier than every* $t_j \in time(\beta)$*;*

4. *every predicate* $P \in predicate(\alpha)$ *is extensionally different from every predicate* $Q \in predicate(\beta)$*.*

For instance, the following statement is a deterministic law of succession: "If an acute occlusion occurs in a main coronary artery of someone now, she will suffer myocardial infarction within the next ten minutes".

For the sake of convenience, the quantifier prefix $\forall x_1 \ldots \forall x_m \forall t_1 \ldots \forall t_n$ of a deterministic law of succession is written $\mathcal{Q}$. If γ is a deterministic law of the form $\mathcal{Q}(\alpha \to \beta)$, the statements α and β are respectively referred to as its antecedent and consequent, symbolized by antecedent(γ) and consequent(γ). For example, if γ is $\mathcal{Q}(Pxt_1 \wedge \neg Qxt_2 \to Ryt_3)$, then we have: antecedent(γ) $= Pxt_1 \wedge \neg Qxt_2$; and consequent($\gamma$) $= Ryt_3$.

The conjunction $(\alpha_1 \wedge \ldots \wedge \alpha_n)$ minus its i-th link α_i, where $1 \leq i \leq n$, yields the pruned, or reduced, sentence $(\alpha_1 \wedge \ldots \wedge \alpha_n) - \alpha_i$. For instance, $(Pxt_1 \wedge \neg Qxt_2 \wedge Ryt_3) - Pxt_1$ is the reduced sentence $\neg Qxt_2 \wedge Ryt_3$.

Definition 60 (Deterministic relevance). *If* $\mathcal{Q}(\alpha_1 \wedge \ldots \wedge \alpha_n \to \beta)$ *is a deterministic law of succession in the extended language* $\mathcal{L}L$*, then the component* a_i *in the antecedent is, with respect to the reduced antecedent* $(\alpha_1 \wedge \ldots \wedge \alpha_n) - \alpha_i$*, deterministically relevant to the consequent* β *iff* $\neg \mathcal{Q}\Big(\big((\alpha_1 \wedge \ldots \wedge \alpha_n) - \alpha_i \big) \to \beta \Big)$ *is true in* $\mathcal{L}L$*.*

That means that the removal of the component a_i from the whole $(\alpha_1 \wedge \ldots \wedge \alpha_n)$ of the antecedent falsifies the law by verifying its pruned negation $\neg \mathcal{Q}\Big(\big((\alpha_1 \wedge \ldots \wedge \alpha_n) - \alpha_i \big) \to \beta \Big)$. For example, let our deterministic law of succession be the statement:

For all x :
IF x is a human being $\wedge$
            x is a male $\wedge$
            an acute occlusion occurs in a main coronary artery of x now,
THEN x will suffer myocardial infarction within the next ten minutes.

The second component "x is a male" in the antecedent of this statement is, with respect to being a human and having an acute occlusion in a coronary artery, *deterministically irrelevant* to myocardial infarction. It can therefore be discarded from the law. The reason is that by its removal the law is not damaged since the following negation *does not* become true:

Not for all x :
IF x is a human being $\wedge$
            an acute occlusion occurs in a main coronary artery of x now,
THEN x will suffer myocardial infarction within the next ten minutes.

That is, there exists someone in one of whose main coronary arteries an acute occlusion occurs, whereas she does not suffer myocardial infarction within the next ten minutes. But this assertion is not true.

Obviously, being a male is a redundant condition in the antecedent of the deterministic law of succession above. By contrast, consider the following law. "If a child is exposed to the measles virus and is not inoculated, she will contract measles within a few weeks". The component "is not inoculated" in its antecedent cannot be removed. It is, with respect to exposure to the measles virus, deterministically relevant to contracting measles. For an inoculated child will escape the disease. Deterministic relevance, to the effect, of all conditions included in the antecedent is an essential feature of a deterministic causal law:

Definition 61 (Deterministic-causal law). *A statement γ of the extended language $\mathcal{LL}$ is a deterministic-causal law in $\mathcal{LL}$ iff:*

1. *γ is a deterministic law of succession in $\mathcal{LL}$;*
2. *every $\alpha_i \in antecedent(\gamma)$ is, with respect to the reduced antecedent$(\gamma) - \alpha_i$, deterministically relevant to consequent(γ). That is, if its antecedent doesn't contain any redundant part.*

It is of course possible that for a particular clinical event such as myocardial infarction, there are $q > 1$ different deterministic causal laws:

$$\mathcal{Q}_1(\alpha_{1_1} \wedge \ldots \wedge \alpha_{1_m} \to \beta)$$
$$\vdots$$
$$\mathcal{Q}_q(\alpha_{q_1} \wedge \ldots \wedge \alpha_{q_n} \to \beta).$$

Each of them in its antecedent $\alpha_{i_1} \wedge \ldots \wedge \alpha_{i_k}$ refers to a particular $Cause_i = C_{i_1} \& C_{i_2} \& \ldots \& C_{i_k}$ with $k \geq 1$ factors. This is an example of what we have called *multiple causation* in the last section, contrasting monocausation.

Koch's postulates

After having discovered some important infectious germs such as Bacillus anthracis in 1876, Mycobacterium tuberculosis in 1882, and Vibrio cholerae in 1883, the German physician Robert Koch (1843–1910) in his speech at the 10th International Medical Congress in Berlin in 1890, put forward a few requirements that a micro-organism must satisfy to count as "the cause" of a disease. His requirements were codified by his colleague Friedrich Loeffler (1852–1915) and baptized *Koch's postulates*. They have been used as principles of medical causality ever since by bacteriologists, pathologists, nosologists, and other physicians concerned with etiology. In essence, the postulates say (Brock, 1988, 180):

1. The parasitic organism must be shown to be constantly present in characteristic form and arrangement in the diseased tissue;

2. The organism, which from its behavior appears to be responsible for the disease, must be isolated and grown in pure culture;
3. The pure culture must be shown to induce the disease experimentally.

A closer look reveals that these postulates are even much stronger than the causal determinism sketched above. For example, regarding the tuberculosis of the lung ("lung TB") and Mycobacterium tuberculosis ("Myco-TB"), the first and third postulates say, respectively, that "if an individual x has lung TB, then Myco-TB is present in x" and "if an individual x is infected with Myco-TB, then x develops lung TB". These two conditionals jointly imply the biconditional "lung TB develops in an individual x if and only if x is infected with Myco-TB". That is, lung TB is in every instance associated only with one causal factor, i.e., with Myco-TB, but with nothing else. There is no other causally relevant factor of lung TB. However, experience falsifies this assertion, as there are individuals infected with Mycobacterium tuberculosis who don't contract tuberculosis of the lung.

Koch's Postulates are obviously committed to monocausal and monofactorial determinism. They cannot serve as etiologic principles for two reasons. First, they are confined to infectious diseases only. Second, the history of medicine convincingly demonstrates that monocausal and monofactorial determinism is a simplistic myth. For multifactorial genesis, see page 259.

INUS conditions

In the light of Hume's regularity conception of causality sketched on page 226, the Australian philosopher John Leslie Mackie (1917–1981) suggested a concept of cause that has become popular in the last few decades. Nevertheless, it needs to be carefully evaluated. It is based on the notions of sufficient and necessary condition briefly discussed on page 161. We have seen that in a conditional of the form:

$$\text{If condition } C_{i_1} \& \ldots \& C_{i_n} \text{ occurs, then event } E_j \text{ occurs} \qquad (23)$$

the antecedent $C_{i_1} \& \ldots \& C_{i_n}$ is called a *sufficient condition* of event E_j occurring. On the other hand, condition $C_{i_1} \& \ldots \& C_{i_n}$ is called a *necessary condition* of event E_j occurring if it is true that whenever $C_{i_1} \& \ldots \& C_{i_n}$ does not occur, E_j does not occur. That is:

$$\text{If condition } \neg(C_{i_1} \& \ldots \& C_{i_n}) \text{ occurs, then event } \neg(E_j) \text{ occurs.}$$

Let us consider an example to explain Mackie's acclaimed concept of causality and to demonstrate its failure:

A middle-aged, male patient who recently had to undergo a minor abdominal surgery, died during the operation. The autopsy revealed that he had developed a sepsis, i.e., a systemic inflammatory response syndrome. It was induced by a tainted injection that he had received preoperatively. However, sepsis usually does not cause immediate death ('it is not a sufficient condition of immediate death'). In addition, the autopsy showed that the patient had died of an acute myocardial infarction that was due to an intraoperative, occlusive coronary thrombosis. Although he had a moderate coronary atherosclerosis, anginal symptoms were not known. His coronary atherosclerosis was not sufficient to cause occlusive thrombosis ('it was not a sufficient condition of occlusive thrombosis'). Moreover, the patient had a slightly pathologic clotting of blood, called hypercoagulopathy in medicine. This finding also could not provide a sufficient condition of the intraoperative accident.

The forensic pathologist argued that sepsis was *the cause* of death because it leads to disseminated intravascular coagulation. Since the patient suffered already from slight hypercoagulopathy, when intravascular coagulation occurred in an atherosclerotic plaque in one of his coronary arteries, it led to a thrombotic coronary occlusion, which in turn led to myocardial infarction.

To summarize, we have a couple of potential partial causes none of which is individually a sufficient condition of the patient's death, that is, slight coronary atherosclerosis, slight hypercoagulopathy, and sepsis. However, in the *context of these circumstances,* sepsis had increased the intravascular coagulability of the blood and had caused a local thrombosis in an atherosclerotic lesion of a coronary artery. All three partial, singly insufficient conditions had interactively reinforced each other to cause coronary thrombosis. The rationale behind this reasoning is the following deterministic-causal law:

Coronary atherosclerosis & hypercoagulopathy & sepsis → coronary thrombosis.

Now, according to John Mackie, "What is typically called a cause is an INUS condition" (Mackie 1974, 64). The acronym "INUS" he coined means "an *i*nsufficient but *n*on-redundant part of an *u*nnecessary but *s*ufficient condition" (ibid, 62). The forensic pathologist above who viewed *sepsis* as 'the cause' of the patient's death, had obviously identified a Mackie INUS condition. Such a Mackie cause is just a particular part C_{i_k} of the compound antecedent of a conditional such as (23) above.[45]

---

[45] The favorite example used in philosophical literature, also by Mackie himself, is a fire that burns a barn down. Many possible causes are conceivable for such an accident ('multiple causation'), for instance, a deliberate arson, a lightning strike, a lighted cigarette dropped by a smoker, and so on. Due to the multiplicity of these possible causes, none of them is a necessary condition. In the absence of one of them, another one will work as well. Suppose now that the fire department has identified the actual cause to be the dropping of a lighted cigarette. However, a careless action of this type cannot be viewed as a sufficient condition of a fire in a barn. Other inflammable material such as dry straw and wooden walls of the barn must also be present, i.e., a complex condition $C_{i_1} \& \ldots \& C_{i_n}$ comprising many components like in the body text above. In this inflammable context, the dropping of a lighted cigarette is an efficacious factor. It is an INUS condition. As it was emphasized in the body text, however, the selection of a particular INUS

The preceding considerations demonstrate that Mackie's concept of cause requires deterministic-causal laws to identify INUS conditions. For this reason, medical etiology cannot be recommended to search for INUS conditions simply because the set of deterministic-causal laws is nearly empty. There is another reason why Mackie's deterministic theory is gratuitous (see page 259).

Counterfactuals

David K. Lewis' (1941–2001) counterfactual approach suggests another understanding of causality based on a particular type of conditionals that have come to be termed contrary-to-fact or subjunctive conditionals, also known as counterfactuals. Lewis even reduces causality to counterfactuals (Lewis, 1973a, 1973b, 2000; Collins, 2007).

Counterfactuals are conditionals of the form "if A were to occur, B would occur" or "if it had been the case that A, it would have been the case that B". In this approach, causation is defined as follows: C is a cause of E iff (i) if C were to occur, then E would occur; and (ii) if C were not to occur, then E would not occur. An example is: "If sepsis had occurred, the patient would have died" and "if no sepsis had occurred, the patient would not have died". We need not go into the details of this widely acclaimed theory because its very basis is too speculative and beyond any accessible reality. Counterfactuals are interpreted by the possible-worlds semantics that is discussed in Section 27.1.2 on page 917. It is absolutely impossible to ground them in the experiential world and test them empirically. Accordingly, an advocate of a counterfactual will fail to reasonably answer the basic epistemological question "how do you know that?". Notwithstanding their intriguing metaphysical aura, counterfactuals cannot be relied upon and fruitfully used in empirical-practical domains such as medicine. Diagnostic-therapeutic decision-making ought not to rest on untestable etiologic speculation if more reliable knowledge is available. In addition, it has been convincingly demonstrated that counterfactuals lead to inferential absurdities in deductions and should therefore be avoided in argumentation (Stegmüller, 1970, 443).

Interestingly, the counterfactual conception of causality that is very different from Hume's regularity conception quoted on page 226, goes back to Hume himself who in the same breath expounded both ideas: "We may define a cause to be an object, followed by another, and where all the objects similar to the first, are followed by objects similar to the second. Or, in other words where, if the first object had not been, the second never had existed" (Hume, 1748, section VII, part II). But he never concerned himself with the alternative view expressed in this paraphrase. Two centuries later, it was taken up

---

condition rather than another one as *the cause* of the accident depends on the context. Here, the term "context" means what is usual and what is unusual in a barn. While dry straw and wooden walls belong to usual circumstances in a barn, dropping a lighted cigarette doesn't do so. We shall come back to this issue later on when discussing the contextuality of causes on page 245.

by others to give detailed counterfactual accounts of causality (Lyon, 1967; Mackie, 1974, ch. 2).

6.5.3 Probabilistic Etiology

We saw in the last section that deterministic etiology is an illusion. Indeterministic etiology is the only alternative. However, this does not imply the widespread belief that indeterminism would allow for 'uncaused', mysterious events. Such is not the case. Indeterminism merely permits the possibility of occurrences that lack sufficient causes, i.e., sufficient conditions in terms of antecedents of conditionals as in (23) above. What we are looking for, is a method of conceptualizing this indeterminism. Fortunately, probability theory has proven to be a promising methodology for this purpose. Thus, it seems reasonable to believe that the patient Elroy Fox's angina pectoris is *caused* by his coronary atherosclerosis and to act accordingly, although not all individuals having coronary atherosclerosis suffer from angina pectoris: ¬(every coronary atherosclerosis → angina pectoris). To justify our causal belief, we can point to the statistical finding that the probability of angina pectoris conditional on coronary atherosclerosis, is greater than when coronary atherosclerosis is not present. This simple idea is the basis of indeterministic, *probabilistic etiology* that we shall study in what follows. Our analysis is based on Patrick Suppes's theory of probabilistic causality (Suppes, 1970a), which superseded the Humean, deterministic causality philosophy. However, the conceptual framework we shall develop has a different structure and entails a new causal terminology and apparatus. We shall first introduce a concept of the probabilistic relevance of events to build upon that construct our probabilistic etiology. Our discussion comprises the following eight sections:[46]

- ▶ Dependence analysis
- ▶ Probabilistic relevance and irrelevance of events
- ▶ Spurious etiologic correlations
- ▶ Causal structures
- ▶ Quantitative causal structures
- ▶ Comparative causal structures
- ▶ Conjectural causal structures
- ▶ Subjective causal structures.

Dependence analysis

We now turn to our initial example. Does Chlamydophila pneumoniae infection play a *genuine* causative role in the development of coronary heart

---

[46] The history of the probabilistic-causal approach goes back to Hans Reichenbach (1956, section 23). Additional pioneering work was done by Wesley Salmon (1971). Patrick Suppes's theory, however, was the first comprehensive and well-founded work on the subject that opened a new direction in the philosophy of causality.

disease, or is it merely a *spurious* cause of the disease? In etiology, questions of this type are usually asked with regard to any factor suspected of playing a causative role in the pathogenesis of a particular clinical event. Thus, the main task of etiology is to discriminate genuine causal factors from spurious ones.

The sort of etiologically useless association between events we shall neglect, is the *spurious correlation*. And the sort of etiologically useful association between events we are interested in, is the *causal interaction*. What is a spurious correlation and what is a causal interaction? In our theory of etiology, we shall base these concepts upon the notion of the *probabilistic relevance of events*. To this end, we shall in the following two sections introduce some basic notions and the concepts of *probabilistic independence* and *conditional probabilistic independence* of events:

> ▷ Token events, type events, and conditional events
> ▷ Probabilistic independence and dependence.

Token events, type events, and conditional events

We distinguish between singular or token events, on the one hand; and generic or type events, on the other. A token event is an occurrence localized in space and time such as, for example, a particular patient's myocardial infarction occurring on a particular day. The class of token events of the same type is referred to as a type event, e.g., *the* myocardial infarction occurring in all patients who suffer this disease.

We shall tackle causation as a relation between type events and not between token events. Accordingly, we shall not be interested in the *causal explanation* of token events and in singular causal assertions such as "your smoking caused you suffer myocardial infarction". We shall be concerned with type events only, simply called *events*. They are symbolized by Roman capitals $A, B, C, \ldots$, and are treated as sets so that we may use methods of set theories and logics.

The notion of conditional probability, $p(B \mid A)$, will be extensively used that is introduced on page 978. The phrase $p(B \mid A)$ is the conventional notation of the two-place probability function $p(B, A)$ and reads "the probability of event B given event A", "the probability of event B on the condition that event A has already occurred", or simply "the probability of B conditional on A". For example, the statement "the probability that an individual x over 60 years of age suffers myocardial infarction on the condition that she has coronary heart disease, is 0.15" is written "$p($an individual x over 60 years of age suffers myocardial infarction $\mid$ the individual x has coronary heart disease$)$ $= 0.15$".

The construct "$B \mid A$" in a conditional probability $p(B \mid A)$ may be conceived as a conditional event. It is the event B on the condition that event A

has already occurred. An example is the event that someone suffers myocardial infarction on the condition that she has coronary heart disease. Maybe a conditional event $B \mid A$ will certainly occur or will never occur. The latter is the case if the event B never occurs. We may therefore speculate upon the probability of a conditional event in advance and ask how likely $B \mid A$ is. We do so by using the conditional probability function $p(B \mid A) = r$ to assert that "the probability of B given A is r" where r is a real number ranging from 0 to 1. We call $p(B \mid A)$ the probability of the conditional event $B \mid A$, or the *conditional* probability of event B given A. Note that $p(B)$ is the unconditional, *absolute* probability of event B. For the semantics of the term "probability", see page 982.

The syntactic convention in using the conditional event sign "$\mid$", i.e., "given", is this: intersection and union dominate "$\mid$". That is, $Y \cap Z \mid X$ is $(Y \cap Z) \mid X$, but not $Y \cap (Z \mid X)$; and $Y \cup Z \mid X$ is $(Y \cap Z) \cap X$, but not $Y \cap (Z \mid X)$.

Probabilistic independence and dependence

Recall first that the notion of conditional probability is *defined* in terms of absolute probability as follows (see page 979):

$$p(B \mid A) = \frac{p(B \cap A)}{p(A)} \qquad (24)$$

Definition 62 (Probabilistic independence). *As defined on page 978 in Part VIII, in the general theory of probability two events B and A are said to be stochastically or* probabilistically independent *of one another iff:*

$$p(B \cap A) = p(B) \cdot p(A) \qquad (25)$$

That is, if the probability of their joint occurrence equals the product of the probabilities of their individual occurrence. If we divide through both sides of the latter equation by $p(A)$, we obtain from Definition 62 the following conclusion.

Corollary 5. *Two events B and A are probabilistically independent of one another iff:*

$$\frac{p(B \cap A)}{p(A)} = p(B). \qquad (26)$$

This corollary and Equation (24) above imply a second corollary:

Corollary 6. *An event B is probabilistically independent of another event A iff:*

$$p(B \mid A) = p(B) \qquad (27)$$

that is, if and only if its probability conditional on A equals its unconditional probability. Its probability is not changed by A occurring. Otherwise put, event A has no influence on the occurrence of B. The two events are *uncorrelated*. Another consequence of the Corollary 6 and Definition 62 is:

Corollary 7. *An event B is probabilistically dependent on another event A iff:*

$$p(B \mid A) \neq p(B) \tag{28}$$

that is, if and only if event A changes the probability of event B. Obviously, "dependent" does not mean that there is any interaction between A and B. The relation of probabilistic dependence is, prima facie, merely a phenomenological feature we observe, usually referred to as *correlation*. It may in a particular case exhibit any of the following two directions of the inequality "$\neq$" mentioned:

$$p(B \mid A) > p(B) \qquad \text{(positive correlation)} \tag{29}$$
$$p(B \mid A) < p(B) \qquad \text{(negative correlation)} \tag{30}$$

The probabilistic dependence of B on A may be positive, as in case (29), or negative as in the latter case, (30). Thus, positive dependence or correlation turns out to be a *probability increase*. An event B is positively probabilistically dependent on an event A if the occurrence of A raises the probability of B. Conversely, negative dependence or correlation is a *probability decrease*. An event B is negatively probabilistically dependent on an event A if the occurrence of A lowers the probability of B.

Definition 63 (Probabilistic dependence). *An event B is:*

1. positively probabilistically dependent *on an event A iff $p(B \mid A) > p(B)$,*
2. negatively probabilistically dependent *on an event A iff $p(B \mid A) < p(B)$.*

For example, it may be that for a member of the German population the probability of suffering coronary heart disease is in general 0.00001, whereas the probability of the same event given Chlamydophila pneumoniae infection is 0.0001. By using the following shorthand notation:

chd   for: coronary *h*eart *d*isease is present
chlamydo   Chlamydophila pneumoniae infection is present,

we would then have the positive correlation:

$$p(chd \mid chlamydo) > p(chd) \qquad \text{(positive correlation)} \tag{31}$$

This example says that coronary heart disease is positively probabilistically dependent on Chlamydophila pneumoniae infection. Do we have reason to presume that, according to such a positive dependence, Chlamydophila pneumoniae infection is a *cause* of coronary heart disease, that it has a causal influence on this disease? Is an 'etiologic link' simply a *probability increase?* To answer this question, we will go a step further and introduce a second concept of dependence, i.e., the notion of *conditional dependence*.

Definition 64 (Conditional probabilistic independence). *Analogous to our terminology above, two events B and A are said to be* probabilistically independent *of one another* conditional on *a third event X iff::*

$$p(B \cap A \mid X) = p(B \mid X) \cdot p(A \mid X), \tag{32}$$

probabilistically dependent on one another conditional on *X, otherwise, i.e., iff:*

$$p(B \cap A \mid X) \neq p(B \mid X) \cdot p(A \mid X). \tag{33}$$

That means that two events B and A are probabilistically dependent on one another given a third event X if, according to (33), the probability of the conditional event $B \cap A \mid X$ differs from the product of the individual probabilities of the pruned conditional events $B \mid X$ and $A \mid X$. Otherwise put, two events B and A given a third event X are probabilistically dependent on one another if the probability of their joint occurrence $B \cap A$ conditional on X differs from the product of their individual probabilities conditional on X. They may be positively or negatively dependent on one another:

$$p(B \cap A \mid X) > p(B \mid X) \cdot p(A \mid X) \quad \text{(positive conditional dependence)} \tag{34}$$
$$p(B \cap A \mid X) < p(B \mid X) \cdot p(A \mid X) \quad \text{(negative conditional dependence)} \tag{35}$$

In what follows, this relation of *conditional dependence,* also called conditional correlation, will be of central importance. It will enable us to understand what it means to say that two events B and A are interactive, i.e., one of them exerts some kind of causal influence on the other. For instance, with reference to the recent epidemiologic study quoted below, let us conditionalize our two clinical example events (coronary heart disease, Chlamydophila pneumoniae infection) on the events of being a diabetic patient or a non-diabetic patient, respectively. Based on the study, we can postulate in advance that:

$$p(\textit{chd} \cap \textit{chlamydo} \mid \textit{diabetics}) =$$
$$p(\textit{chd} \mid \textit{diabetics}) \cdot p(\textit{chlamydo} \mid \textit{diabetics}) \tag{36}$$
$$p(\textit{chd} \cap \textit{chlamydo} \mid \textit{non-diabetics}) >$$
$$p(\textit{chd} \mid \textit{non-diabetics}) \cdot p(\textit{chlamydo} \mid \textit{non-diabetics}) \tag{37}$$

In this case, we would obviously have reason to assert that according to (36), coronary heart disease and Chlamydophila pneumoniae infection are, in the population of diabetics, probabilistically independent of one another. By contrast, in the population of non-diabetics they are, according to (37), probabilistically dependent on one another. Now, the following questions arise: Why are they independent in diabetics and dependent in non-diabetics? And what kind of dependence is it? Is it merely a spurious correlation like the one between the growth of a stork population in a particular area and the higher human birthrate in that area, or is it a causal interaction between the two clinical events? Which one of them may play the causative role? Does Chlamydophila pneumoniae cause atherosclerotic lesions in heart arteries and thus coronary heart disease, or is the atherosclerotic plaque a fertile ground for Chlamydophila to be deposited and grow? Or is there a third possibility, a common cause of both events? To account for etiologic questions of this type, we shall use the conceptual tools discussed above to construct and understand a concept of *probabilistic relevance* upon which we shall in turn build our concepts of causal relevance and causal irrelevance below.

Probabilistic relevance and irrelevance of events

The following two inequalities are, respectively, equivalent to the inequalities (34–35) above by which the conditional dependence of event B on event A was defined:

$$p(B \mid X \cap A) > p(B \mid X) \qquad \text{(positive conditional correlation)} \qquad (38)$$
$$p(B \mid X \cap A) < p(B \mid X) \qquad \text{(negative conditional correlation)} \qquad (39)$$

The first sentence says that the probability of event B conditional on $X \cap A$ is greater than conditional on X alone. The second sentence states that the probability of event B conditional on $X \cap A$ is less than conditional on X alone.

As the yield of our preceding discussion, these two interesting relationships will serve as the conceptual base of our probabilistic theory of causality below. Like the events B and A, the reference event X is always a more or less complex class in which something occurs, e.g., the class of diabetics, of warm summer days, of leucocytes, of cigarette smokers, etc. For both methodological and mnemonic reasons, we shall fix our reference event linguistically and shall call it a *population*. A population is sometimes referred to as a:

reference class,
context, background context,
causal field,
propensity field

and the like, and will be symbolized by the variable X throughout. Such a notion of background context is of great importance when analyzing issues of causality. As we shall see below, the causal impact of events is always relative to the background context ('contextuality of causes'). The background context will therefore constitute an essential element of our concept of causality.[47]

Definition 65 (Probabilistic relevance and irrelevance). *An event A is in a population X:*

1. positively probabilistically relevant *to an event B iff* $p(B \mid X \cap A) > p(B \mid X)$,
2. negatively probabilistically relevant *to an event B iff* $p(B \mid X \cap A) < p(B \mid X)$,
3. probabilistically irrelevant *to an event B iff* $p(B \mid X \cap A) = p(B \mid X)$.[48]

In part 1 of this triple definition, the addition of event A to event X raises the probability of event B. In part 2, the addition of event A to event X lowers the probability of event B. In part 3 nothing happens by adding A to X. The probabilistic relevance of an event A to an event B in a background context X is thus a change of the probability of B through A in the context X. In cases such as part 3 where factor A in presence of event X does not exert any probabilistic influence on event B, it is said, after terminology introduced by Hans Reichenbach (1956, section 23), that X *screens A off from B.* That is:

Definition 66 (Screening off). *X screens A off from B iff* $p(B \mid X \cap A) = p(B \mid X)$, *i.e., iff A is, in X, probabilistically irrelevant to B.*

We shall continue using this terminology below. Note that the notions of probabilistic relevance introduced above are three-place predicates with the following syntax:

    is_positively_probabilistically_relevant(A, B, X),
    is_negatively_probabilistically_relevant(A, B, X),
    is_probabilistically_irrelevant(A, B, X).

For instance, from the epidemiologic information given in the inequality (37) above we can infer, using the equivalence between (34) and (38), the following probabilistic relevance information about the relationship between Chlamydophila pneumoniae and coronary heart disease in the population of non-diabetics:

---

[47] The history of the concepts of probabilistic relevance and irrelevance introduced here goes back to Hans Reichenbach, Rudolf Carnap, and Wesley C. Salmon (Reichenbach, 1956, chh. III-IV; Carnap, 1962, ch. VI; Salmon, 1971, 1980).

[48] An alternative approach to probabilistic causality emerged in the 1990s which uses the inequalities $p(B \mid X \cap A) > p(B \mid X \cap \overline{A})$ and $p(B \mid X \cap A) < p(B \mid X \cap \overline{A})$ instead of those given in our Definition 65. See (Eells, 2008). Both approaches are equivalent, however. The advantage of our Suppes-based approach is that it is directly based on the well-established probability theory, and in addition, easier to manage. It is in fact a formal-mathematical extension of probability theory. This will be shown in Section "Causal structures" on page 243.

$$p(\mathit{chd} \mid \mathit{non\text{-}diabetics} \cap \mathit{chlamydo}) > p(\mathit{chd} \mid \mathit{non\text{-}diabetics}) \tag{40}$$

i.e., $p(B \mid X \cap A) > p(B \mid X)$, where:

$B \equiv$ chd
$X \equiv$ non-diabetics
$A \equiv$ chlamydo.

It says that in the population of non-diabetics, Chlamydophila pneumoniae infection is positively probabilistically relevant to coronary heart disease. There is no doubt that a probabilistic relevance information of this kind is *predictively* valuable in that it allows us to view the Chlamydophila pneumoniae infection as a prognostically unfavorable factor in non-diabetics, customarily called a *risk factor*. However, that does not yet mean that probabilistic relevance information is also *causally significant*. The rapid falling of a barometric reading on a warm summer day is positively probabilistically relevant to the subsequent storm, and thus predictively informative. But it does not cause the storm. Although we can reasonably view the falling of a barometric reading as a symptom of the storm in the offing, we should not attempt to prevent or to produce a storm by manipulating the barometric reading. The falling barometer is prognostically relevant and causally irrelevant, and it is rather a third factor that is causally operative behind both the barometer *and* the storm. Similarly, it is also possible that there is another, 'common cause' operating behind the joint occurrence of Chlamydophila pneumoniae infection and coronary heart disease. We shall try to find a solution to this problem in what follows.

Spurious etiologic correlations

Like the causal influence of the growth of the stork population on human birthrate, many alleged causes are spurious ones. To conceptualize this spuriousness, let there be a positive probabilistic relevance relationship between two events A and B in a particular population X as in (40) above, i.e.,

$$p(B \mid X \cap A) > p(B \mid X). \tag{41}$$

It is possible that this probabilistic relevance of A to B will vanish if an additional event C is introduced into the context, i.e.,

$$p(B \mid X \cap A \cap C) = p(B \mid X \cap C). \tag{42}$$

The previously positive correlation between A and B no longer exists in the presence of the new factor C that is equally able to bring about B in the absence of A (the right-hand side in Equation 42). Therefore, the question arises whether the positive correlation between A and B in (41) was only a spurious one. We will use as an example the well-known view that in the population of non-diabetics, smoking is a risk factor for coronary heart disease. In other words, it raises the probability of this disease:

$$p(chd \mid non\text{-}diabetics \cap smoking) > p(chd \mid non\text{-}diabetics). \tag{43}$$

However, on the basis of findings reported in an epidemiologic study on the association of Chlamydophila pneumoniae infection and acute coronary heart disease events, the following probabilistic relevance relationships must be supposed (Miettinen et al. 1996):[49]

$$p(chd \mid non\text{-}diabetics \cap smoking \cap chlamydo) =$$
$$p(chd \mid non\text{-}diabetics \cap chlamydo) \tag{44}$$

$$p(chd \mid non\text{-}diabetics \cap chlamydo) > p(chd \mid non\text{-}diabetics) \tag{45}$$

$$p(chd \mid diabetics \cap chlamydo) = p(chd \mid diabetics) \tag{46}$$

The statements (43) and (44) show that the positive probabilistic relevance of smoking to coronary heart disease in the population of non-diabetics, present in (43), disappears when Chlamydophila enters the scene in (44). Thus, the new factor Chlamydophila seems to degrade smoking to a spurious factor. Moreover, according to (45), Chlamydophila is with respect to non-diabetics positively probabilistically relevant to coronary heart disease. But once again, finding (44) demonstrates that Chlamydophila's relevance to heart disease is not changed by taking smoking into account. That is, Chlamydophila screens smoking off from coronary heart disease. We may therefore assert that in the presence of Chlamydophila, smoking loses its potential etiologic role. On the other hand, according to finding (46), in the population of diabetics Chlamydophila is probabilistically irrelevant to coronary heart disease. Otherwise put, diabetes mellitus screens Chlamydophila off from coronary heart disease.

---

[49] See, for example, (Miettinen, 1996): "It was found that the prevalence of elevated chlamydial antibodies at baseline was higher in non-diabetic subjects who had serious coronary heart disease events during the follow-up than subjects without coronary heart disease events (32 vs 15%, relative risk 2.56, p = 0.013) in East Finland. In non-diabetic subjects in West Finland we did not find this association. The association between C. pneumoniae antibodies and coronary heart disease events did not markedly change after controlling for other risk factors for coronary heart disease (OR 2.44, p = 0.055) in non-diabetic subjects living in eastern Finland" (ibid., 682).

"[...] The association between elevated chlamydial antibodies and incident coronary heart disease events before controlling for other risk factors for coronary heart disease was statistically significant [...]. This association remained similar after controlling for age, gender, and smoking" (ibid., 685).

"[...] We did not find any association between chlamydial antibodies and coronary heart disease events in diabetic patients from either East or West Finland. A possible explanation for the difference between diabetic and non-diabetic subjects could be that diabetes increases the risk for coronary heart disease events so much that it masks the effects of other, weak risk factors from coronary heart disease" (ibid., 686).

The first lesson we learn from these examples is that probabilistic relevance *is always relative to a particular population* (reference class, background context, propensity field, etc.). That means that if we change the background context against which we measure the relevance of Chlamydophila to coronary heart disease, the positive correlation might vanish. In the example above, we saw this happen first to smoking and then to Chlamydophila itself.

Let there exist an etiologic relationship of the type $p(B \mid X \cap A) \circledast p(B \mid X)$ where the variable "$\circledast$" stands for increase, decrease, or equality. It is not difficult to change the background context X of such etiologic research in order to see what will happen to $\circledast$. Just divide the reference population X into $n > 1$ disjoint subpopulations $X_1, X_2, \ldots, X_n$. Then inquire into the probabilistic relevance that factor A in each subpopulation $X_i \in \{X_1, X_2, \ldots, X_n\}$ has to factor B, i.e., ask the question:

$$p(B \mid X_i \cap A) \ ? \ p(B \mid X_i) \qquad \text{with } 1 \leq i \leq n \qquad (47)$$

where the question mark aks which one of the relations $>, <$, or $=$ obtains. What can happen now, is a collapse of the initial probabilistic relevance that A had to B in the undivided population X. Positive relevance may become negative relevance or irrelevance; irrelevance can become positive or negative; and negative relevance can become positive, etc. See findings (45) and (46) above where we divided the Chlamydophila infected population into diabetics and non-diabetics to the effect that the correlation varied. This dynamics of correlations by changing the reference population, known as Simpson's paradox, is due to the circumstance that in any of the subpopulations X_i, factor A may be associated with a particular, X_i-local factor C_i which modifies the effect, B, in a particular manner (Figure 41).

Fig. 41. Event A occurring in different contexts X_i where in each context a particular local, A-associated factor C_i may be present modifying effect B in a specific manner

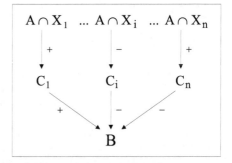

Figure 41 illustrates that the more intermediary associations between A and C_is enter the field, the more opaque and hopeless the etiologic situation between A and B may become. Something that is a risk factor in subclass $X_i \in X$, may surprisingly appear as a preventive factor in another subclass $X_j \in X$. But below, we shall see that Simpson's paradox, so named after its discoverer Edward H. Simpson (1951), is only apparently paradoxical.[50] For instance, it is well known that a particular drug used as a remedy in a certain diseased group, may have adverse effects in the presence of a specific, additional factor, called a 'contra-indication', such as a penicillin allergy. This example shows that *in an inhomogeneous reference class X almost anything is possible.* An event A may in a particular subpopulation of an inhomogeneous class X raise the probability of an event B while lowering it in another sub-population. Some philosophers have thus come to the erroneous conclusion that a cause need not be something that raises the probability of its effect. It may lower the probability of its effect as well, they say. This strange view followed an example provided by the Swedish philosopher Germund Hesslow on the thrombogenic effect of oral contraceptives (Hesslow, 1976).

Hesslow's argument runs as follows: "It has been claimed, e.g., that con-traceptive pills (C) can cause thrombosis (T), [...] But pregnancy can also cause thrombosis, and C lowers the probability of pregnancy. I do not know the value of $p(T)$ and $p(T \mid C)$ but it seems possible that $p(T \mid C) < p(T)$, and in a population which lacked other contraceptives this would appear a likely situation. Be that as it may, the point remains: *it is entirely possible that a cause should lower the probability of its effect*" (ibid., 291).

It will be shown in the next section that the conceptual base of Hess-low's reasoning is not sound and his conclusion has to be rejected. We must be able to rely upon the unambiguous, probability-increasing *or* probability-decreasing, modality of causes in order to be able to manipulate them thera-peutically and preventively. What is considered a cause of an effect, therefore, has to be definitely a positive or a negative one of that effect. Tertium non datur. An equivocal, 'mixed cause' which occasionally raises the probability of its effect and at other times lowers it, is not a cause at all and should be renamed. For example, we cannot allow for Chlamydophila pneumoniae to be a cause of coronary heart disease, on the one hand; and a protective factor for the same disease in the same group, on the other. The action-theoretic clarity we need for diagnostic and therapeutic decisions in clinical practice and preventive medicine requires that *causal structures* be unanimous. This characteristic is not an ontic one 'in the world out there'. The etiologist must construct it. To this end, we need clear concepts and adequate methods to be able to causally structure the world. (For the term "ontic", see Section 'ontic vagueness' on page 44.)

Causal structures

Since etiology is concerned with the question of how clinical events are causally associated with other events, we shall need to identify and precisely delimit

---

[50] Simpson (1951, pp. 240 f.) gives an interesting and amusing example that cannot be discussed here. Note that due to the changing background context, the so-called Simpson paradox is in fact a pseudo-paradox.

the class of causally associated events in order to understand what the term "causal association" means at all. To this end, a concept of causal structure will be introduced. A causal structure is characterized by causal association of its events. It will be conceived as a special extension of a probability space. We shall therefore need the latter concept and its concomitants, specifically the notions of sample space, event algebra, and event, introduced in Section 29.1.1 on page 973.

The goal of an etiologic inquiry into the causes of a particular clinical type event E such as myocardial infarction or schizophrenia consists in identifying those causal structures in which E is the effect. Before the investigation starts, the class of type events among which causal associations are being sought, must be known and designed. In a research setting, for instance, an etiologist inquiring into whether cigarette smoking has any causal relevance to coronary heart disease, is not allowed to tell us afterwards that she discovered Chlamydophila pneumoniae infection having a causal relevance to coronary heart disease. This infection didn't belong to the sample space she was considering. Therefore, in our discussion below we shall need the explicit characterization of the sample space and event algebra that are involved in a research setting. We shall frequently refer back to the following example:

We want to know whether our patient Mr. Elroy Fox is suffering from any of the two diseases 'Chlamydophila pneumoniae infection' and 'coronary heart disease'. In this case, we have the following sample space and event algebra, denoted Ω and $\mathcal{E}$, respectively. Because the latter is too large, only a minor part of it will be presented:

$\Omega = \{$Chlamydophila pneumoniae infection is present, Chlamydophila pneumoniae infection is not present, coronary heart disease occurs, coronary heart disease does not occur$\}$.

$\mathcal{E} = \{\{$Chlamydophila pneumoniae infection is present$\}, \{$Chlamydophila pneumoniae infection is not present$\}, \ldots, \{$Chlamydophila pneumoniae infection is present$\} \cup \{$coronary heart disease occurs$\}, \ldots, \{$Chlamydophila pneumoniae infection is present$\} \cap \{$coronary heart disease does not occur$\}, \ldots, \Omega, \varnothing\}$,

or equivalently:

$\mathcal{E} = \{\{$chlamydo$\}, \{\overline{\text{chlamydo}}\}, \{chd\}, \{\overline{\text{chd}}\}, \{$chlamydo$\} \cup \{chd\}, \{$chlamydo$\} \cup \{\overline{\text{chd}}\}, \{\overline{\text{chlamydo}}\} \cup \{chd\}, \{$chlamydo$\} \cap \{chd\}, \{$chlamydo$\} \cap \{\overline{\text{chd}}\}, \{\overline{\text{chlamydo}}\} \cap \{chd\}, \ldots, \Omega, \varnothing\}$

An *event* is conceived as an element of the event algebra. The events our inquiry is concerned with, are therefore the elements of set $\mathcal{E}$. They will be symbolized by Roman capitals A, B, C, etc.

Thus far we have the 2-tuple $\langle \Omega, \mathcal{E} \rangle$ that includes the sample space and the event algebra of our inquiry. By adding a probability function p that assigns to each element of $\mathcal{E}$, i.e., to each event, a real number in the unit interval

[0, 1], we obtain the triple $\langle \Omega, \mathcal{E}, p \rangle$. This triplet structure constitutes a finite *probability space* if it satisfies the Kolmogorov Axioms from Definition 237 on page 975. We may now demonstrate how a probability space $\langle \Omega, \mathcal{E}, p \rangle$ may be extended to a *probabilistic-causal structure*. Such a structure is usable in etiology as a methodological tool in searching for causes of clinical events and in etiologic and epidemiologic reasoning. An important syntactic innovation will be introduced first.

Traditionally, causation is conceived as, and represented by, a *two-place* relation of the form "*A* causes *B*", e.g., "HIV infection causes AIDS", or "trisomy 21 causes Down syndrome". However, the fruitless debates on causality since Aristotle demonstrate that this understanding and practice is logically defective. We should notice first of all that whatever else causation may be, it ensues from the interaction of causes with background contexts where they are operative. What is a cause in a particular context, e.g., HIV in humans, need not be a cause in another context, e.g., HIV in ants. Therefore, one cannot expect to find causes absolutely independent of the context in which they occur. The contextual dependence of their causal role and significance, their context sensitivity so to speak, ought to be taken into account by constructing an appropriate syntax for causal language, a syntax that makes a reasonable causal semantics possible in that it *contextualizes* causes. For it may be, for example, that the measles virus causes measles in a human population which is not inoculated against measles, whereas it doesn't do so in an inoculated population. To capture this *contextuality of causes*, we have decided to abandon the traditional, binary predicate "*causes(A, B)*" and to conceive the new verb "causes" as a *three-place* predicate with the syntax "*A* causes *B* in *X*" instead:

$$causes(A, B, X)$$

where *A* is the cause event, *B* is the effect event, and *X* is the population, context, or background context in which the relation between *A* and *B* is being considered. Examples of how this ternary predicate works, are: In a non-inoculated population the measles virus causes measles; in an inoculated population the measles virus does not cause measles; the measles virus does not cause measles in ants, although it causes measles in human beings. In a semi-formalized fashion we have predications and negations of the following form:

causes(measles-virus, measles, non-inoculated),
not causes(measles-virus, measles, inoculated),
causes(measles-virus, measles, humans),
not causes(measles-virus, measles, ants).

These examples demonstrate the fundamental, syntactic reason why it doesn't make any sense to ask questions of the form "does *A* cause *B*?", for instance, "does the measles virus cause measles?". We should always refer to a particular reference class *X* as above and put our question accordingly: "Does the measles virus cause measles in ants?". "Does Chlamydophila pneumoniae infection cause coronary heart disease in the reference class X?", e.g.:

causes(chlamydo, chd, humans)   ???
causes(chlamydo, chd, non-diabetics)   ???
causes(smoking, lung_cancer, teenangers)   ???
causes(smoking, lung_cancer, elderly)   ???
causes(helicobacter_pylori, peptic_ulcers, females)   ???
causes(oedipus_complex, peptic_ulcers, psychoanalysts)   ???
causes(anopheles, malaria, infants)   ???
causes(anopheles, malaria, sickle_cell_carriers)   ???

Thus, we may construe causation as a *three-place relation* of the structure "*causes*(A, B, X)" to be read in one of the following ways:

A causes B in the population X,
A causes B in the background context X,
A causes B in X,
A causes B with respect to X,
B is caused by A conditional on X,
B is caused by A relative to X,
B is caused by A with respect to X,

and the like. With little exaggeration, we may say that by so doing we have resolved *the stubborn, basic problem* of causality and etiology! And with help from the supplemental concepts below, we may say it without any exaggeration at all.

In what follows, we shall consider causes and effects as type events whose individual instances occur, as token events, at particular instants or periods of time. For this purpose, we shall use a discrete time interval $[t, t']$, denoted T, whose elements are points in time and linearly ordered as a *time line* according to the binary relation $<$ of precedence. The shorthand "$t_i < t_j$" means that the time point t_i is *earlier than t_j*; and "$t_i \leq t_j$" says that t_i is *earlier than or simultaneous* with t_j. These points in time will serve as the times of occurrence of our events. We will not complicate the temporal aspect of our analysis, although a detailed consideration of terms such as "occurrence", "duration", "overlapping occurrence", and "partial simultaneity" would be beneficial. An event A that occurs at time t_i is written A_{t_i} to indicate by the subscript t_i the time of its occurrence. In the following sections, we shall introduce in turn:

▷ Potential causal structures
▷ Spurious causal structures
▷ Genuine causal structures
▷ Multifactorial genesis.

Potential causal structures

Definition 67 below introduces the fundamental concept that everything else will be based on. A basic understanding of the concept is this: Let there be a particular probability space concerned with a random experiment, such as tossing a dice, whose events successively occur during a particular period of time. Thanks to mathematical laws of probability theory, we can calculate the probabilities of these events in advance presupposing they are independent of one another. Our observation may show, however, that among the actual occurrences in this experiment there are some events which prove probabilistically relevant to some later events, and thus, change their pre-calculated probabilities disproving our previous independence assumption. For instance, it may be that every time the dice falls with "1", the subsequent three events are "4", "5", and "6". When our actual experience so deviates from the mathematical calculations made before hand, we are forced to view the whole contraption as something in which the earlier events may be causally related to later events, i.e., as something that *possibly is a causal structure*. To capture such etiologically instructive situations, a concept of *potential causal structure* is introduced below. It will be presented in two versions, an elementary version and a general version. The elementary version, which we shall use throughout, represents a simplified adaptation of the general version. Therefore, the qualifying affix "elementary" is deliberately omitted. However, be aware of the affix "general" whenever we use it in the label "general potential causal structure".[51]

Definition 67 (Potential causal structure). *ξ is a potential causal structure iff there are $\Omega, \mathcal{E}, p, T, A_{t_1}, B_{t_2}$, and X such that:*

1. *$\xi = \langle \Omega, \mathcal{E}, p, T, A_{t_1}, B_{t_2}, X \rangle$,*
2. *$\langle \Omega, \mathcal{E}, p \rangle$ is a probability space,*
3. *T is a discrete, linearly ordered time interval,*
4. *A_{t_1} and B_{t_2} are elements of the event algebra $\mathcal{E}$ such that $t_1, t_2 \in T$ with $t_1 < t_2$. (That is, event A_{t_1} precedes event B_{t_2}.)*
5. *X is an element of the event algebra $\mathcal{E}$ referred to as the population, context, background context, or reference event X,*
6. *$p(B_{t_2} \mid X \cap A_{t_1}) \neq p(B_{t_2} \mid X)$.*

A probability space $\langle \Omega, \mathcal{E}, p \rangle$ thus qualifies as a potential causal structure if its event algebra $\mathcal{E}$ contains an event A_{t_1} that according to axiom 6 and relative to the reference event X is *probabilistically relevant* to a later event, B_{t_2}, of the event algebra. Thanks to the inequality relation in axiom 6, the probabilistic relevance of A_{t_1} to B_{t_2} may be positive or negative:

---

[51] In what follows, we shall make extensive use of definition by introducing a set-theoretical predicate. This method of concept formation was discussed on page 100 and will also be used for its epistemological advantages in Section 9.4.2.

$$p(B_{t_2} \mid X \cap A_{t_1}) > p(B_{t_2} \mid X) \quad \text{or}$$
$$p(B_{t_2} \mid X \cap A_{t_1}) < p(B_{t_2} \mid X).$$

In either case, the event A_{t_1} gives the prima facie impression to be causally relevant to B_{t_2} in X because it changes the probability of B_{t_2} occurring. Such an example is provided by the relationship between Chlamydophila pneumoniae infection and coronary heart disease in the population of non-diabetics. To demonstrate, let X be the population of non-diabetics and define:

$$\begin{aligned}
chlamydo_{t_1} &\equiv \text{Chlamydophila pneumoniae infection occurs at time } t_1 \\
chd_{t_2} &\equiv \text{coronary heart disease occurs at time } t_2.
\end{aligned}$$

According to inequality (45) on page 241, which we now restate as (48):

$$p(chd_{t_2} \mid non\text{-}diabetics \cap chlamydo_{t_1}) > p(chd_{t_2} \mid non\text{-}diabetics) \qquad (48)$$

we have this potential causal structure:

$$\langle \Omega, \mathcal{E}, p, T, chlamydo_{t_1}, chd_{t_2}, non\text{-}diabetics \rangle \qquad (49)$$

when $\langle \Omega, \mathcal{E}, p \rangle$ is its probability space and Chlamydophila pneumoniae infection, i.e. $chlamydo_{t_1}$, precedes coronary heart disease, chd_{t_2}, as required in Definition 67. The concept of potential causal structure is a convenient tool and will be used throughout. It is a simplified, elementary variant of the following, more general concept. We have seen that in an elementary potential causal structure of the form:

$$\langle \Omega, \mathcal{E}, p, T, A_{t_1}, B_{t_2}, X \rangle \qquad (50)$$

the potential cause-effect events A_{t_1} and B_{t_2} as well as the reference event X are *single elements* of the event algebra $\mathcal{E}$, i.e., elementary type events such as 'Chlamydophila pneumoniae infection occurs', 'coronary heart disease occurs', and 'diabetes occurs', or any combinations of them. But a *general* potential causal structure is of the form:

$$\langle \Omega, \mathcal{E}, p, T, \mathcal{A}, \mathcal{B}, \mathcal{X} \rangle, \qquad (51)$$

where the potential cause-effect components, $\mathcal{A}$ and $\mathcal{B}$, are more complex with $\mathcal{A} = \{A_1, \ldots, A_m\}$ and $\mathcal{B} = \{B_1, \ldots, B_n\}$ being *subsets* of the event algebra $\mathcal{E}$, and thus sets of events with $m, n \geq 1$; and $\mathcal{X} = \{X_1, \ldots, X_q\}$ being another subset of the event algebra $\mathcal{E}$ comprising $q \geq 1$ populations such that in a population X_k an event $A_{t_i} \in \mathcal{A}$ may have distinct probabilistic relevances to different events in $\mathcal{B}$. This general concept is an appropriate device to introduce a powerful theory of probabilistic causality. We will here merely illustrate the concept to demonstrate that it would be inconvenient to use it throughout. For simplicity's sake, we shall prefer elementary structures of the type (50) and shall seldom use the general type of causal structure. Both structures are easily distinguishable from each other by their format.

Definition 68 (General potential causal structure). ξ *is a general potential causal structure iff there are* $\Omega, \mathcal{E}, p, T, \mathcal{A}, \mathcal{B}$, *and* $\mathcal{X}$ *such that:*

1. $\xi = \langle \Omega, \mathcal{E}, p, T, \mathcal{A}, \mathcal{B}, \mathcal{X} \rangle$,
2. $\langle \Omega, \mathcal{E}, p \rangle$ *is a probability space,*
3. T *is a discrete, linearly ordered time interval,*
4. $\mathcal{A}$ *and* $\mathcal{B}$ *are subsets of the event algebra* $\mathcal{E}$ *such that if* $A_{t_i} \in \mathcal{A}$ *and* $B_{t_j} \in \mathcal{B}$, *then* $t_i, t_j \in T$ *with* $t_i < t_j$. (*That is, all events in* $\mathcal{A}$ *precede all events in* $\mathcal{B}$),
5. $\mathcal{X} = \{X_1, \ldots, X_q\}$ *with* $q \geq 1$ *is a subset of the event algebra* $\mathcal{E}$ *with each* X_k *referred to as a population, context, background context, or reference event* X_k, *where* $k \geq 1$,
6. *For every* $A_{t_i} \in \mathcal{A}$ *there is a* $B_{t_j} \in \mathcal{B}$ *and an* $X \in \mathcal{X}$ *such that* $p(B_{t_j} \mid X \cap A_{t_i}) \neq p(B_{t_j} \mid X)$.

In terms of this general concept, the elementary potential causal structure above:

$$\langle \Omega, \mathcal{E}, p, T, chlamydo_{t_1}, chd_{t_2}, non\text{-}diabetics \rangle.$$

turns out to be the general potential causal structure:

$$\langle \Omega, \mathcal{E}, p, T, \{chlamydo_{t_1}\}, \{chd_{t_2}\}, \{non\text{-}diabetics\} \rangle.$$

The advantage of the latter, general concept is that the cause-effect event sets $\mathcal{A}$ and $\mathcal{B}$ as well as the reference event set $\mathcal{X}$ are not confined to singletons. Rather, they may consist of an arbitrary number of events such that an event $A_{t_1} \in \mathcal{A}$ may be causally associated with different effects in $\mathcal{B}$, positively or negatively, and in different background contexts. For example, in the general potential causal structure:

$$\langle \Omega, \mathcal{E}, p, T, \{chlamydo_{t_1}\}, \{chd_{t_2}, longevity_{t_3}\}, \{non\text{-}diabetics, \ elderly\} \rangle$$

Chlamydophila pneumoniae infection may be probabilistically positively associated with coronary heart disease and probabilistically negatively associated with longevity in non-diabetics, while being probabilistically positively associated with coronary heart disease in the elderly. That is:

$$p(chd_{t_2} \mid non\text{-}diabetics \cap chlamydo_{t_1}) > p(chd_{t_2} \mid non\text{-}diabetics)$$
$$p(longevity_{t_3} \mid non\text{-}diabetics \cap chlamydo_{t_1}) < p(longevity_{t_3} \mid non\text{-}diabetics)$$
$$p(chd_{t_2} \mid elderly \cap chlamydo_{t_1}) > p(chd_{t_2} \mid elderly).$$

A general potential causal structure is obviously a whole system of $n \geq 1$ elementary potential causal structures. Otherwise put, an elementary potential causal structure is a general potential causal structure composed of only one elementary potential causal structure. This is the only difference between them. There is no conceptual difference. An elementary potential causal structure enables us to consider the association between two events only, whereas a general potential causal structure encompasses an arbitrary number of events whose associations may be simultaneously analyzed. Notwithstanding the immense instrumentality of general potential causal structures, we shall use elementary structures because they are easier to manage.

On the basis of the elementary Definition 67, the following conditional definition introduces two concepts of potential cause, a positive one and a negative one. Our definition says that an earlier event in a particular population is a *potential* positive or negative cause of a later event if it is, respectively, positively or negatively probabilistically relevant to that later event.

Definition 69 (Potential cause). *If* $\langle \Omega, \mathcal{E}, p, T, A_{t_1}, B_{t_2}, X \rangle$ *is a potential causal structure, then:*

1. A_{t_1} *is a* potential positive cause *of* B_{t_2} *in* X *iff* $p(B_{t_2} \mid X \cap A_{t_1}) > p(B_{t_2} \mid X)$,
2. A_{t_1} *is a* potential negative cause *of* B_{t_2} *in* X *iff* $p(B_{t_2} \mid X \cap A_{t_1}) < p(B_{t_2} \mid X)$.

A *potential cause* is simply a potential positive or a potential negative cause. In the potential causal structure $\langle \Omega, \mathcal{E}, p, T, chlamydo_{t_1}, chd_{t_2}, non\text{-}diabetics \rangle$ quoted in (49) above, Chlamydophila pneumoniae infection is due to (48) a potential positive cause of coronary heart disease in non-diabetics if it precedes the heart disease. On the other hand, because of the statement:

$$p(chd \mid diabetics \cap chlamydo) = p(chd \mid diabetics)$$

quoted in (46) on page 241, we are not allowed to suppose that Chlamydophila pneumoniae infection *also* plays a potentially positive causal role in the population of *diabetics*. As our statement shows, it clearly doesn't do so. In this population or context it is a probabilistically, and hence causally, irrelevant event, "an innocent bystander" as Muhlestein et al. would say (Muhlestein et al., 1996, 1555). In other words, diabetes mellitus screens Chlamydophila pneumoniae infection off from coronary heart disease. This may be the result of the high probabilistic relevance of diabetes itself to coronary heart disease, such that it cannot be additionally raised by Chlamydophila pneumoniae infection.

Another interesting example, showing both positive and negative potential causes, can be drawn from a study on the association of C-reactive protein, myocardial infarction, and the reduction of the latter by aspirin (Ridker et al., 1997). In this long-term study, known as *The Physicians' Health Study*, in a period of over 13 years (1982–1995) a total of 22.071 U.S.-American male physicians aged 40–84 years with no history of myocardial infarction, stroke, or cancer were assigned to different groups of a randomized, placebo-controlled trial of aspirin and beta carotene in the primary prevention of cardiovascular disease and cancer.[52] The authors report that an elevated plasma C-reactive

---

[52] Inflammation processes in heart and brain arteries are currently viewed as important etiologic factors in the pathogenesis of coronary heart disease, stroke, and

protein concentration, which indicates systemic inflammation, was statistically significantly correlated with myocardial infarction and stroke. These risks were stable over long periods and were not modified by smoking and lipid-related or non-lipid related risk factors. The use of aspirin was significantly associated with reductions in the risk of myocardial infarction (ibid, pp. 973, 977). "The aspirin component of the study was terminated early, on January 25, 1988, primarily because of a statistically extreme 44 percent reduction in the risk of a first infarction in the aspirin group" (ibid., 974). These findings have led to the widespread use of aspirin as a preventive agent in cardiovascular risk patients. To use them in our framework, let us first introduce the following shorthand notations:

infarction	for:	myocardial infarction occurs
C-reactive		C-reactive protein level is elevated
smoking		the patient is a smoker
cholesterol		hypercholesterolemia is present
aspirin		aspirin is used
men		the underlying population or context X.

We can now conclude from the study quoted above that:

$$p(\textit{infarction} \mid \textit{men} \cap \textit{C-reactive}) > p(\textit{infarction} \mid \textit{men}), \qquad (52)$$

$$p(\textit{infarction} \mid \textit{men} \cap \textit{C-reactive} \cap \textit{aspirin}) <$$
$$p(\textit{infarction} \mid \textit{men} \cap \textit{C-reactive}), \qquad (53)$$

$$p(\textit{infarction} \mid \textit{men} \cap \textit{C-reactive} \cap \textit{smoking}) =$$
$$p(\textit{infarction} \mid \textit{men} \cap \textit{C-reactive}), \qquad (54)$$

$$p(\textit{infarction} \mid \textit{men} \cap \textit{C-reactive} \cap \textit{cholesterol}) =$$
$$p(\textit{infarction} \mid \textit{men} \cap \textit{C-reactive}). \qquad (55)$$

Each of the findings (52) and (53) yields a potential causal structure when properly supplemented according to Definition 67 above. In all of them, the male population constitutes the background context. In the first one of these potential causal structures, based on finding (52), C-reactive protein seems to have a positive causal impact on the occurrence of myocardial infarction. In the second potential causal structure, based on finding (53), that impact is reversed by aspirin. One may thus suppose that in the reference population

---

related health catastrophes. As was pointed out previously, micro-organisms such as Chlamydophila pneumoniae, Helicobacter pylori, and others are therefore being studied as potential agents of the inflammation. C-reactive protein is a marker for systemic inflammation. Elevated plasma concentrations of C-reactive protein are known to be associated with acute myocardial ischemia and infarction. The major study referred to in the body text has analyzed, among many other things, the association of C-reactive protein and the diseases mentioned, on the one hand; and the effect of the antiinflammatory agent *aspirin* in this background context of pathogenesis, on the other (Ridker et al., 1997).

of *men*, elevated C-reactive protein is a potential positive cause of myocardial infarction (finding 52) and that in the population of *men having elevated C-reactive protein* (left-hand side of 53), aspirin is a potential negative cause of myocardial infarction. By contrast, neither smoking nor cholesterol is able to change the potential causal impact of C-reactive protein on myocardial infarction in men (findings 54–55).

In the next section, we shall examine whether the possibly causative roles given above remain the case when we delve a little bit deeper. Before doing so, it is worth noting that the so-called controlled clinical trials designed to test the efficacy of therapeutic and preventive interventions, e.g., the application of a particular new drug against multiple sclerosis or the use of aspirin to prevent myocardial infarction, are actually attempts to establish potential causal structures in which *human agency* is a potential cause of the recovery and prevention. The goal of such a trial is to examine whether:

$$p(B_{t_2} \mid X \cap A_{t_1}) > p(B_{t_2} \mid X)$$

is the case, where event X is, for example, any malady; $X \cap A_{t_1}$ is the treatment group whose members receive the therapy A_{t_1}; and B_{t_2} is recovery from malady X. The trial is considered controlled if the treatment group $X \cap A_{t_1}$ is compared against a control group X whose members do not receive the therapy A_{t_1}. We shall come back to this issue in Section 8.4.5 on page 359.

Spurious causal structures

Definition 69 above shows explicitly that a potential causal structure does not provide genuine causes yet, but merely *potential* causes. Genuine causes require us to ensure that the events appearing as potential causes are not spurious ones. To this end, a notion of spuriousness will be proposed with the following rationale behind it: A potential cause A_{t_1} cannot be reasonably said to have a causal impact if it is rendered ineffective by a preceding event, that is, if the potential cause A_{t_1} (e.g., the falling of barometric reading) of an event B_{t_2} is *preceded* by an event C_t with $t < t_1$ (e.g., decreasing air pressure) that generates the effect B_{t_2} (storm) to the same extent as A_{t_1} does. This rationale is given in the following provisional Definition 70 and will be made precise in a subsequent definition.

Definition 70 (Spurious cause). *In a population X, an event A_{t_1} is a spurious cause of an event B_{t_2} iff:*

1. *A_{t_1} is a potential cause of B_{t_2} in X,*
2. *There is an event C_t that precedes A_{t_1}, i.e., $t < t_1$,*
3. *C_t screens A_{t_1} off from B_{t_2}.*

A spurious cause like A_{t_1} in this definition does not represent a genuine cause of the effect B_{t_2} and must therefore be removed from the list of A_{t_1}'s causes.

Otherwise, we would be accused of the-barometer-causes-storm fallacy discussed on page 225. Here is a simple example. Suppose that, for whatever reasons, all newborns who are diagnosed with Down syndrome suffer perinatal meningitis caused by maternal bacteria infecting them during birth. The assertion that their Down syndrome was due to this perinatal meningitis refers to a spurious cause because *there is an earlier event*, trisomy 21, that screens any later event off from Down syndrome. However, the simplified definition above is not yet robust enough to cover more complex situations. To achieve this goal, recall the notion of a *partition* introduced on page 63. A partition of a set X is a collection $\pi = \{C_1, \ldots, C_n\}$ of $n > 1$ non-empty, pairwise disjoint subsets of X such that their union is X, i.e., $C_1 \cup \ldots \cup C_n = X$, or equivalently, $(X \cap C_1) \cup \ldots \cup (X \cap C_n) = X$. For example, a partition of the population of *men* examined in the aspirin trial above is provided by the set of those men who were administered aspirin and the set of those who were not, i.e., {{aspirin was administered}, {aspirin was not administered}}.

Definition 71 (Spurious causal structure). *If* $\langle \Omega, \mathcal{E}, p, T, A_{t_1}, B_{t_2}, X \rangle$ *is a potential causal structure, then it is a* spurious causal structure *iff there is a* $t \in T$ *and a partition* $\pi_t \subseteq \mathcal{E}$ *of* X *such that for all events* $C_t \in \pi_t$:

1. $t < t_1$,
2. $p(B_{t_2} \mid X \cap A_{t_1} \cap C_t) = p(B_{t_2} \mid X \cap C_t)$.

As clause 2 of this definition demonstrates, each of the earlier events C_t in the partition π_t is, without the later event A_{t_1}, equally effective in causing B_{t_2}, and thus disqualifies the later event A_{t_1} from being a genuine cause of B_{t_2}. It screens A_{t_1} off from B_{t_2}.

If a structure $\langle \Omega, \mathcal{E}, p, T, A_{t_1}, B_{t_2}, X \rangle$ is a spurious causal structure, then A_{t_1} is called a *spurious cause* of B_{t_2} in X. It may be a spurious positive cause or a spurious negative cause. With that in mind, let us turn back to our Chlamydophila example in non-diabetics: Should etiologic research be able to show in the near future that there is a partition of the reference class, e.g., {{coronary wall lesion occurs}, {coronary wall lesion does not occur}}, such that each of its events satisfies clause 2 of Definition 71 if it *precedes* the Chlamydophila pneumoniae infection (A_{t_1}):

$$p(chd_{t_2} \mid non\text{-}diabetics \cap wall\_lesion_t \cap chlamydo_{t_1}) >$$
$$p(chd_{t_2} \mid non\text{-}diabetics \cap wall\_lesion_t)$$
$$p(chd_{t_2} \mid non\text{-}diabetics \cap no\_wall\_lesion_t \cap chlamydo_{t_1}) =$$
$$p(chd_{t_2} \mid non\text{-}diabetics \cap no\_wall\_lesion_t)$$

then we shall have reason to view Chlamydophila pneumoniae as a spurious cause of coronary heart disease in non-diabetics (event X). Meanwhile we shall continue to believe the current epidemiologic hypothesis until we have proof to the contrary. Note, however, that we have not given any reason to believe that smoking and other classic risk factors have become spurious causes of coronary heart disease. Although we may have gotten this prima facie impression from the epidemiologic findings quoted above:

$$p(chd \mid non\text{-}diabetics \cap smoking \cap chlamydo) =$$
$$p(chd \mid non\text{-}diabetics \cap chlamydo)$$
$$p(infarction \mid men \cap smoking \cap C\text{-}reactive) =$$
$$p(infarction \mid men \cap C\text{-}reactive)$$
$$p(infarction \mid men \cap cholesterol \cap C\text{-}reactive) =$$
$$p(infarction \mid men \cap C\text{-}reactive).$$

these findings don't provide us with a partition of the respective reference class, which is required to judge the spuriousness of those risk factors. This research gap is especially awkward regarding the potential causal relevance of C-reactive protein to myocardial infarction (finding 52). Our current knowledge about the nature and role of C-reactive protein in the organism provides convincing evidence that it must be a spurious cause of myocardial infarction, i.e., a mere symptom like the falling of barometric reading, fever, pain, and erythrocyte sedimentation rate. As a non-specific, systemic reaction to infection, tissue injury, and necrosis, C-reactive protein has a multitude of factors behind it each of which may prove to be a preceding, *common cause* of both its increase and myocardial infarction. The life-saving merit of aspirin is not due to a conceivable lowering of C-reactive protein levels per se, but due to its anticoagulatory and presumably antiinflammatory effects, an idea which indirectly corroborates the Chlamydophila pneumoniae and other infection hypotheses. (For the notion of a *common cause*, see page 258.)

Genuine causal structures

From our discussion above it is obvious that a causal structure in etiology must not be a spurious one. That is, a potential causal structure is a *causal structure* if and only if it is not a spurious causal structure. Thus, we obtain directly the following definition:

Definition 72 (Causal structure). *If* $\langle \Omega, \mathcal{E}, p, T, A_{t_1}, B_{t_2}, X \rangle$ *is a potential causal structure, then it is a* causal structure *iff there is no* $t \in T$ *and no partition* $\pi_t \in \mathcal{E}$ *of* X *such that for every event* $C_t \in \pi_t$:

1. $t < t_1$,
2. $p(B_{t_2} \mid X \cap A_{t_1} \cap C_t) = p(B_{t_2} \mid X \cap C_t)$.

Likewise, a general potential causal structure yields a *general causal structure* of the form $\langle \Omega, \mathcal{E}, p, T, \mathcal{A}, \mathcal{B}, \mathcal{X} \rangle$ if it is void of any spurious elementary causal structures as above. But this general concept will not be defined separately. Rather, on the basis of Definition 72 two concepts of cause will be introduced that may be useful in etiology, clinical practice, preventive medicine, and treatment research:

Definition 73 (Genuine causes). *If* $\langle \Omega, \mathcal{E}, p, T, A_{t_1}, B_{t_2}, X \rangle$ *is a causal structure, then:*

1. A_{t_1} *is a* positive cause *of* B_{t_2} *in* X *iff* $p(B_{t_2} \mid X \cap A_{t_1}) > p(B_{t_2} \mid X)$,
2. A_{t_1} *is a* negative cause *of* B_{t_2} *in* X *iff* $p(B_{t_2} \mid X \cap A_{t_1}) < p(B_{t_2} \mid X)$.

Both concepts of cause are three-place predicates. An event A is a positive or a negative cause of another event B always with respect to a reference event, background context, or population X. Thus, we have the syntax:

is_a_positive_cause(A, B, X)
is_a_negative_cause(A, B, X).

This ternary predicate of causation reflects our causal contextualism outlined on page 245, and makes many traditional problems of causality in general, and of etiology in particular, disappear. Assuming that our preceding examples have not yielded spurious causal structures, one may presume that: (1) Chlamydophila pneumoniae infection is a positive cause of coronary heart disease in non-diabetics; and (2) aspirin is a negative cause of myocardial infarction in men with raised C-reactive protein levels.

As the exposition above indicates, it is our plan to distinguish *positive* and *negative* causes of different types. In what follows, we shall concentrate on the positive types only and shall not introduce separate definitions and concepts of negative causality, as they are more or less formal analogues of positive ones.

Definition 74 (Positive and negative causal structures). *If* $\langle \Omega, \mathcal{E}, p, T, A_{t_1}, B_{t_2}, X \rangle$ *is a causal structure, it is called a* positive *or a* negative *one, respectively, iff* A_{t_1} *is a positive or a negative cause of* B_{t_2} *in* X. *In a positive causal structure, we say "A_{t_1}* causes *B_{t_2} in X". In a negative causal structure we say "A_{t_1}* discauses *B_{t_2} in X".*

Causation and discausation are event relationships in causal structures. For example, in the positive causal structure $\langle \Omega, \mathcal{E}, p, T, chlamydo_{t_1}, chd_{t_2}, non\text{-}diabetics \rangle$ encountered above, Chlamydophila pneumoniae infection causes coronary heart disease in non-diabetics. And in the negative causal structure $\langle \Omega, \mathcal{E}, p, T, aspirin_{t_1}, infarction_{t_2}, men \cap C\text{-}reactive \rangle$, aspirin discauses myocardial infarction in men with increased C-reactive protein.

The phrase "to discause" is a new verb that we have coined for negative causation. Here is an additional example: All efficacious *preventive* measures discause the diseases they prevent. Thus, prevention is negative causation. This issue will be discussed in Section 8.5 on page 371. The following definition is meant to prepare that discussion.

Definition 75 (Prevention as discausation). *In a population X, an event A_{t_1} prevents a later event B_{t_2} iff it discauses the latter in X, i.e., iff it is a negative cause of B_{t_2} in X.*

Suppose an event A is a positive cause of an event B, and there is an *earlier* event C that is also a positive cause of B. Since A is not a spurious cause of B, event C obviously does not screen it off from B. This implies, by Definition 70 on page 252, that (i) the causal impact of A on B will not vanish when A and C jointly occur; and (ii) the causal impacts of both causes will interact; that is, one of them will either strengthen or weaken the other. The human organism and pathology are replete with such interactive causes. A more general concept of interactive causes is provided by the following definition:

Definition 76 (Interactive causes). *If $\langle \Omega, \mathcal{E}, p, T, \{A_{t_1}, C_t\}, \{B_{t_2}\}, \{X\}\rangle$ is a general causal structure, then A_{t_1} and C_t are interactive causes of B_{t_2} in X iff:*

1. $p(B_{t_2} \mid X \cap A_{t_1} \cap C_t) \neq p(B_{t_2} \mid X \cap A_{t_1})$,
2. $p(B_{t_2} \mid X \cap A_{t_1} \cap C_t) \neq p(B_{t_2} \mid X \cap C_t)$.

That means that two different causes A_{t_1} and C_t of an effect B_{t_2} are interactive if their joint occurrence in X has a different probabilistic relevance to the effect than their separate occurrence. The term "joint occurrence" does not mean that they must occur simultaneously, but merely that both of them, $A_{t_1} \cap C_t$, occur. In Definition 76, therefore, the occurrence times t and t_1 have been left indefinite. They may or may not be distinct. For instance, suppose that in addition to the previously-mentioned finding (45) on page 241:

$$p(chd \mid non\text{-}diabetics \cap chlamydo) > p(chd \mid non\text{-}diabetics)$$

we also have the following plausible probabilistic relevances extrapolated from the aspirin trial:

$$p(chd_{t_2} \mid non\text{-}diabetics \cap aspirin_t) < p(chd_{t_2} \mid non\text{-}diabetics), \tag{56}$$

$$p(chd_{t_2} \mid non\text{-}diabetics \cap chlamydo_{t_1} \cap aspirin_t >$$
$$p(chd_{t_2} \mid non\text{-}diabetics \cap aspirin_t), \tag{57}$$

$$p(chd_{t_2} \mid non\text{-}diabetics \cap chlamydo_{t_1} \cap aspirin_t <$$
$$p(chd_{t_2} \mid non\text{-}diabetics \cap chlamydo_{t_1}). \tag{58}$$

We may then conclude from this information that Chlamydophila pneumoniae infection and aspirin are interactive causes of coronary heart disease in non-diabetics. Depending on whether the joint occurrence of two interactive causes increases or decreases their separate probabilistic relevance to the effect, as in (57) and (58), positive and negative interaction may be distinguished. Our hypothetical example (58) above demonstrates a negative interaction: aspirin lowers, and even reverses, Chlamydophila's causal impact on coronary heart disease in non-diabetics. Positively interacting causes may be called *synergistic* causes or factors. Negatively interacting causes may be termed *antagonistic* causes or factors.

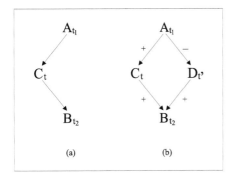

Fig. 42. Intermediaries between A_{t_1} and B_{t_2}. Part b displays two seemingly conflicting paths between A_{t_1} and B_{t_2}

If A_{t_1} and C_t are two interactive causes of an effect B_{t_2} such that A_{t_1} precedes C_t and causes or discauses it, then obviously C_t is an intermediate cause of B_{t_2}, or an intermediary for short (Figure 42a). Between a cause A_{t_1} and its effect B_{t_2} there may exist many intermediaries. A pseudoproblem arises whenever the earlier cause A_{t_1} has conflicting causal tendencies for intermediaries following it, such as, for example, causing C_t and discausing $D_{t'}$ (Figure 42b). In this case there are two seemingly incompatible paths between A_{t_1} and B_{t_2}, a contributory and an inhibitory one. Hesslow's example using contraceptive pills, given on page 243 above, may be viewed as such a pseudoproblem. Hesslow thinks his contraceptive pills may raise and lower the probability of thrombosis at the same time. However, the situation is quite different. As Figure 42b demonstrates, oral contraceptives (A_{t_1}) on the population level, not in an individual female, cause thrombosis (B_{t_2}) by triggering some thrombogenic intermediaries (C_t) over the left path, and discause thrombosis by preventing pregnancy ($D_{t'}$) over the right path. The overall statistical outcome in each emerging class yields a particular probability value for the thrombogenic relevance of Hesslow's contraceptive pills in an entirely distinct causal structure. This value may be different than their thrombogenic relevance in other background contexts such as, for example:

$p(\textit{thrombosis} \,|\, \textit{female}) = r_1$

$p(\textit{thrombosis} \,|\, \textit{female} \cap \textit{pill}) = r_2$

$p(\textit{thrombosis} \,|\, \textit{female} \cap \textit{pregnant}) = r_3$

$p(\textit{thrombosis} \,|\, \textit{female} \cap \overline{\textit{pregnant}}) = r_4$

$p(\textit{thrombosis} \,|\, \textit{female} \cap \textit{pregnant} \cap \textit{pill}) = r_5$

$p(\textit{thrombosis} \,|\, \textit{female} \cap \overline{\textit{pregnant}} \cap \textit{pill}) = r_6$

$p(\textit{thrombosis} \,|\, \textit{female} \cap \overline{\textit{pregnant}} \cap \overline{\textit{pill}}) = r_7$

$p(\textit{thrombosis} \,|\, \textit{female} \cap \textit{diabetics} \cap \textit{pill}) = r_8$

$p(\textit{thrombosis} \,|\, \textit{female} \cap \textit{aspirin} \cap \textit{pill}) = r_9$

and so on. None of these values will equal another one. The positive or negative causal impact and the strength of causal relevance that one factor has to another factor is relative to the causal structure and background context in which it operates, or equivalently, in which it is being considered. There is no such thing as *the* absolute, positive or negative, causal relevance of something to something else. This is the essence of our relativistic theory of causality that may also be referred to as causal contextualism (see page 245).

Definition 77 (Dominant causes). *If $\langle \Omega, \mathcal{E}, p, T, A_{t_1}, B_{t_2}, X \rangle$ is a causal struc-ture, then A_{t_1} is a dominant cause of B_{t_2} in X iff there is no partition $\pi_t \in \mathcal{E}$ of X and no $t \in T$ such that for all events $C_t \in \pi_t$:*

1. $t_1 \leq t < t_2$,
2. $p(B_{t_2} \mid X \cap A_{t_1} \cap C_t) = p(B_{t_2} \mid X \cap C_t)$.

This definition says that a cause is dominant if no simultaneous or later event is able to screen it off from the effect. It makes its mark on the effect. For instance, genetic or chromosomal abnormalities such as trisomy 21 may be viewed as dominant causes. They cannot be hindered from being effective. A cause A_{t_1} of an event B_{t_2} in X is said to be a *recessive cause* of B_{t_2} if and only if it is not dominant.

Theorem 3 (Dominant causes). *Dominant causes are interactive.*

To state the theorem precisely, let $\langle \Omega, \mathcal{E}, p, T, \{A_{t_1}, C_t\}, \{B_{t_2}\}, \{X\} \rangle$ be a gen-eral causal structure such that A_{t_1} and C_t are dominant causes of B_{t_2} in X. Theorem 3 says that A_{t_1} and C_t are interactive causes of B_{t_2} in X.[53]

The concept of common cause that was postponed on page 254, can now be introduced. Intuitively, if in a background context X two events B_1 and B_2 are approximately simultaneous and correlated, i.e., probabilistically positively or negatively dependent on each other, e.g., elevated C-reactive protein and myocardial infarction; then they have a common cause A if (i) event A precedes them, and (ii) both A as well as $\overline{A}$ renders them conditionally independent of each other. When the correlation between B_1 and B_2 is positive, one may also want to require that A be a cause of B_1 and of B_2. Concisely, we have (Reichenbach, 1956, 158–159; Suppes, 1984, 68):

Definition 78 (Common cause). *If in a population X two events B_{1_t} and $B_{2_{t'}}$ are correlated, i.e., $p(B_{1_t} \cap B_{2_{t'}} \mid X) \neq p(B_{1_t} \mid X) \cdot p(B_{2_{t'}} \mid X)$, then event A_{t_1} is a common cause of B_{1_t} and $B_{2_{t'}}$ in X iff:*

---

[53] Proof of Theorem 3. Two disjoint cases are to be distinguished: (1) Either $t_1 \leq t$, or (2) $t < t_1$. In case 1, A_{t_1} and C_t are simultaneous events or C_t is later than A_{t_1}. In this case, the theorem follows directly from Definitions 76–77. Clause 1 of Definition 76 is fulfilled because A_{t_1} is a dominant cause of B_{t_2}. Clause 2 of Definition 76 is also fulfilled because C_t is a dominant cause of B_{t_2}. In case 2 which says that a dominant cause interacts with an earlier dominant cause of its effect, the theorem follows from Definition 71 of the notion of spuriousness and Definition 76 of causal interaction. Clause 1 of the latter is fulfilled because otherwise A_{t_1} would be a spurious cause of B_{t_2}. But by hypothesis this is not the case. Clause 2 of Definition 76 is also satisfied. Otherwise, C_t would be a recessive cause of B_{t_2}. But by hypothesis this is not the case. QED

1. $t \cong t'$,
2. $t_1 < t, t'$; that is, event A_{t_1} precedes B_{1_t} as well as $B_{2_{t'}}$,
3. $p(B_{1_t} \cap B_{2_{t'}} \mid X \cap A_{t_1}) = p(B_{1_t} \mid X \cap A_{t_1}) \cdot p(B_{2_{t'}} \mid X \cap A_{t_1})$,
4. $p(B_{1_t} \cap B_{2_{t'}} \mid X \cap \overline{A}_{t_1}) = p(B_{1_t} \mid X \cap \overline{A}_{t_1}) \cdot p(B_{2_{t'}} \mid X \cap \overline{A}_{t_1})$.

Obviously, a common cause of two events screens off their correlation. Additional types of cause cannot be discussed here. However, a particular type of cause, i.e., the notion of a *sufficient cause* discussed in the context of deterministic causation in Section 6.5.2 on page 226, must be mentioned to show that deterministic causation is also covered by the probabilistic approach we are here presenting. A sufficient cause is simply the limiting case where the probability of its effect reaches 1:

Definition 79 (Sufficient causes). *If* $\langle \Omega, \mathcal{E}, p, T, A_{t_1}, B_{t_2}, X \rangle$ *is a causal structure, then* A_{t_1} *is a sufficient cause of* B_{t_2} *in* X *iff* $p(B_{t_2} \mid X \cap A_{t_1}) = 1$.

A deterministic-causal law, as explicated on page 229, may now be rewritten as a causal structure with the limiting probability 1:

$$p(B_{t_2} \mid X \cap C_{t_1} \cap C_{t_2} \cap \ldots \cap C_{t_n}) = 1 \tag{59}$$

such that $n \geq 1$ and all partial causes in a composite cause $C_{t_1} \cap \ldots \cap C_{t_n}$ are interactive. A Mackie INUS condition discussed on page 230 turns out to be just a C_{t_i} factor of such a composite cause in a causal structure with limiting probability 1 such as (59). Thus, John Mackie's deterministic, INUS theory of causality is gratuitous because its message is included in our more general theory of probabilistic causality.

Multifactorial genesis

In our theory of probabilistic etiology, the multifactorial genesis of an event B_{t_2} may be understood as a general causal structure $\langle \Omega, \mathcal{E}, p, T, \mathcal{A}, \{B_{t_2}\}, X \rangle$ whose cause events, $\mathcal{A}$, consist of $n > 1$ partial causes or factors $A_{t_1}, \ldots, A_{t_n}$ such that their joint occurrence $A_{t_1} \cap A_{t_2} \cap \ldots \cap A_{t_n}$ may, or may not, yield a determinsistic causation of the form (59). An example is the pathogenesis of coronary heart disease in the population of alcoholics ($= X$) who have diabetes and hypertension and hypercholesterolemia and smoke and do not physically exercise. The *multifactorial cause* in this case is the following compound cause: Diabetes mellitus $\cap$ hypertension $\cap$ hypercholesterolemia $\cap$ smoking $\cap$ lack of physical exercise (Sadegh-Zadeh, 1981e).

Quantitative causal structures

Among its numerous methodological advantages, the framework sketched above also possesses the virtue of enabling us in different ways to view and treat the causal impact of causes as a measurable quantity. We shall choose

the most obvious and simple measurement: The measurement of the causal
relevance of causes. As we shall see, this is a useful methdological tool that allows us to answer etiologically important questions such as: What is the degree
of causal relevance of smoking to coronary heart disease in men? Is Chlamydophila pneumoniae infection causally more relevant to coronary heart disease
in men than smoking is?

To measure the causal strength of causes, we shall need an appropriate
terminology and syntax. For our purposes, we shall consider all of the following expressions as synonyms: causal strength, causal impact, causal relevance,
causal influence, causal support, causal significance, causal propensity, causal
contribution, degree of causation. We prefer the term "degree of causal relevance" or simply "causal relevance" and use it in the following way: "The
causal relevance of A to B in X is r" symbolized by $cr(A, B, X) = r$ and
defined as follows:

Definition 80 (Degree of causal relevance). *If $\langle \Omega, \mathcal{E}, p, T, A_{t_1}, B_{t_2}, X \rangle$ is a
causal structure, then $cr(A_{t_1}, B_{t_2}, X) = r$ iff $r = p(B_{t_2} \mid X \cap A_{t_1}) - p(B_{t_2} \mid X)$.*

That means that in a causal structure as introduced in Definition 72 on page
254, the causal relevance of an event A_{t_1} to the effect event B_{t_2} in a population X is just the extent to which it raises or lowers the probability of the
occurrence of the effect event in that population. For example, we have:

$$cr(chlamydo, chd, non\text{-}diabetics) =$$
$$p(chd \mid non\text{-}diabetics \cap chlamydo) - p(chd \mid non\text{-}diabetics).$$

Causal relevance, cr, is thus a three-place, numerical function. Depending
on the magnitudes of the two involved probabilities whose difference yields
$cr(A, B, X)$, the causal relevance function cr assumes values in the real interval $[-1, +1]$. For instance:

$$cr(chlamydo, chd, non\text{-}diabetics) = 0.25$$
$$cr(chlamydo, chd, diabetics) = 0$$
$$cr(smoking, chd, non\text{-}diabetics \cap chlamydo) = 0$$
$$cr(aspirin, infarction, men \cap C\text{-}reactive) = -0.44.$$

The first and the last one of these quantities are fictitious as it was not possible
to extract accurate base probabilities from the literature sources referred to
previously (Miettinen et al., 1996; Ridker et al., 1997). The definitions and
examples above demonstrate that:

causal irrelevance amounts to	$cr(A, B, X) \approx 0$	(null-causing)
positive causal relevance is	$cr(A, B, X) > 0$	(causing)
negative causal relevance is	$cr(A, B, X) < 0$	(discausing, preventing)
maximum positive causal relevance	$cr(A, B, X) = 1$	(maximum efficiency)
maximum negative causal relevance	$cr(A, B, X) = -1$	(maximum prevention)

It goes without saying that at least due to its range [-1, +1], the causal relevance function cr is not a probability, possibility, necessity, belief, or plausibility. It is simply a conditional measure over the event algebra. This is evident from the following definition, which in its axiom 4 also includes Definition 80. We shall not use Definition 81, which displays a genuine *space* in the mathematical sense, for our purposes. But it demonstrates how our theory of causation may be extended stepwise. The intuitive idea behind it is that if a *general* causal structure $\langle \Omega, \mathcal{E}, p, T, \mathcal{A}, \mathcal{B}, \mathcal{X} \rangle$ is supplemented by a causal relevance measure cr, it yields a measurable space $\langle \Omega, \mathcal{E}, p, T, \mathcal{A}, \mathcal{B}, \mathcal{X}, cr \rangle$.

Definition 81 (Causal space). ξ *is a* causal space *iff there are* $\Omega, \mathcal{E}, p, T, \mathcal{A}, \mathcal{B},$ $\mathcal{X}$, *and* cr *such that:*

1. $\xi = \langle \Omega, \mathcal{E}, p, T, \mathcal{A}, \mathcal{B}, \mathcal{X}, cr \rangle$,
2. $\langle \Omega, \mathcal{E}, p, T, \mathcal{A}, \mathcal{B}, \mathcal{X} \rangle$ *is a general causal structure,*
3. $cr \colon \mathcal{A} \times \mathcal{B} \times \mathcal{X} \mapsto [-1, +1]$,
4. *If* $\langle \Omega, \mathcal{E}, p, T, A_{t_1}, B_{t_2}, X \rangle$ *is a causal structure, then* $cr(A_{t_1}, B_{t_2}, X) = r$
   iff $r = p(B_{t_2} \mid X \cap A_{t_1}) - p(B_{t_2} \mid X)$,
5. *For all non-empty* $Y, X \in \mathcal{E}$: $cr(Y, \varnothing, X) = cr(Y, \Omega, X) = 0$,
6. *For all non-empty* $Y, Z_1, Z_2, X \in \mathcal{E}$: *If* $Z_1 \subseteq Z_2$, *then*

   6.1. $cr(Y, Z_1, X) \leq cr(Y, Z_2, X)$ *if* $cr(Y, Z_2, X) \geq 0$,
   6.2. $cr(Y, Z_1, X) \geq cr(Y, Z_2, X)$ *if* $cr(Y, Z_2, X) < 0$.

Obviously a causal space is an extension of a causal structure by adding the quantitative function cr that measures the context-relative causal impact of events. Axiom 5 says that no event is causally relevant to the impossible event $\varnothing$ and the sure event Ω.

Comparative causal structures

A causal space as just introduced, provides a strong ordering for causes in the real interval [-1, +1] rendering metric causal and metacausal studies feasible. For example, in analogy to random functions, one may construct causal functions to analyze causal relevance distributions and their temporal changes ('causal kinematics') over the event algebra. The space also enables us to lend a comparative order to associations between causes and effects by comparing their quantitative causal relevances $cr(A, B, X)$. We may thus introduce a wide-ranging comparative causal terminology such as "A is a *stronger* positive cause of B in class X than is C"; "A is causally *more relevant* to B in X than is C in Y"; "A is causally *less relevant* to B in X than is C", and so on. For example, the statement:

$$cr(chlamydo, chd, non\text{-}diabetics) > cr(smoking, chd, non\text{-}diabetics)$$

says that Chlamydophila pneumoniae infection is a stronger cause of coronary heart disease in non-diabetics than is smoking. Similar examples are:

$$cr(chlamydo, chd, diabetics) =$$
$$cr(chlamydo \cap smoking, chd, non\text{-}diabetics),$$
$$cr(chlamydo, chd, diabetics) < cr(chlamydo, chd, non\text{-}diabetics),$$
$$cr(helicobacter, peptic\_ulcers, men) > cr(oedipus, peptic\_ulcers, men),$$
$$cr(contraceptives, thrombosis, pregnant) >$$
$$cr(contraceptives, thrombosis, non\text{-}pregnant).$$

Conjectural causal structures

The numerical probabilities needed for calculating the causal relevance $cr(A, B, X)$ that an event A has to another event B, are unfortunately not always available in medicine. For this reason, we have to guess in most cases whether an event like depression exerts any causal influence on something else, e.g., stomach cancer. How do we do that? Is it even possible to advance our etiologic conjecturing when such quantitative knowledge is lacking? Based on our discussion above, we are in fact able to do so. Below, we shall sketch methods that can be used to this end.

Next to actually having numerical probabilities, the best situation would be if one could say which of the events whose cause-effect associations are being judged, is *more likely than* another. Fortunately, in most cases comparative probabilities should be available. They are obtainable by, for example, frequency analyses and comparisons. The comparative probabilities we need are conditional ones between pairs of conditional events of the form $(B \mid A)$ and $(D \mid C)$. The two-place relation "ist at least as likely as" or any of its synonyms may serve as the basic predicate. We symbolize it by "$\succcurlyeq$" to use the shorthand notation:

$$(B \mid A) \succcurlyeq (D \mid C) \tag{60}$$

that reads "B given A is *at least as likely as* D given C". For example, "myocardial infarction given coronary heart disease is at least as likely as stroke given cerebral atherosclerosis". By standard definitions, on the basis of (60) we may introduce the relations:

$(B \mid A) \succ (D \mid C)$	more likely than	(61)
$(B \mid A) \approx (D \mid C)$	as likely as	(62)
$(B \mid A) \not\approx (D \mid C)$	not as likely as	(63)
$(B \mid A) \prec (D \mid C)$	less likely than	(64)

The first one says "B given A is *more likely than* D given C"; the second one reads "B given A is *as likely as* D given C"; the thid one means "B given A is *not as likely as* D given C"; and the last one stands for "B given A is *less likely than* D given C". Overly simplified, the standard definitions referred to are of the following structure:

$$(B \mid A) \succ (D \mid C) \quad \textit{iff} \quad (B \mid A) \succcurlyeq (D \mid C) \ \textit{and not} \ (D \mid C) \succcurlyeq (B \mid A) \tag{65}$$

$$(B \mid A) \approx (D \mid C) \quad \textit{iff} \quad (B \mid A) \succcurlyeq (D \mid C) \ \textit{and} \ (D \mid C) \succcurlyeq (B \mid A) \tag{66}$$

$$(B \mid A) \not\approx (D \mid C) \quad \textit{iff} \quad \textit{not} \ ((B \mid A) \approx (D \mid C)) \tag{67}$$

$$(B \mid A) \prec (D \mid C) \quad \textit{iff} \quad (D \mid C) \succ (B \mid A). \tag{68}$$

We shall not deal with a calculus for handling these comparative probability relations here. For details, see, e.g., (Krantz et al., 2007; Suppes, 1970a). Based on such a calculus, we define: A triple $\langle \Omega, \mathcal{E}, \succcurlyeq \rangle$ is a *comparative probability space* iff Ω is a sample space, $\mathcal{E}$ is an event algebra on Ω, and $\succcurlyeq$ is a comparative probability relation on $\mathcal{E}$ such that the axioms of that calculus are satisfied.

Definition 82 (Conjectural potential causal structure). *ξ is a conjectural potential causal structure iff there are $\Omega, \mathcal{E}, \succcurlyeq, T, A_{t_1}, B_{t_2}$, and X such that:*

1. *$\xi = \langle \Omega, \mathcal{E}, \succcurlyeq, T, A_{t_1}, B_{t_2}, X \rangle$,*
2. *$\langle \Omega, \mathcal{E}, \succcurlyeq \rangle$ is a comparative probability space,*
3. *T is a discrete, linearly ordered time interval,*
4. *A_{t_1} and B_{t_2} are elements of the event algebra $\mathcal{E}$ such that $t_1, t_2 \in T$ with $t_1 < t_2$. That is, event A_{t_1} precedes event B_{t_2},*
5. *X is an element of the event algebra $\mathcal{E}$ referred to as the population, context, background context, or reference event X,*
6. *$(B_{t_2} \mid X \cap A_{t_1}) \not\approx (B_{t_2} \mid X)$.*

There are obvious analogies with Definition 67 on page 247 where elementary potential causal structures were constructed on quantitative probability spaces. The only difference is that now the comparative probability relation $\succcurlyeq$ replaces the quantitative probability function p. For example, supposing that myocardial infarction given both diabetes and obesity is more likely than given diabetes only,

$$(infarction_{t_2} \mid diabetes \cap obesity_{t_1}) \succ (infarction_{t_2} \mid diabetes),$$

then, supplemented by remaining components, we have the following conjectural potential causal structure: $\langle \Omega, \mathcal{E}, \succ, T, obesity_{t_1}, infarction_{t_2}, diabetes \rangle$. Note that no statistical knowledge on quantitative probabilities is required.[54]

Also analogous to the quantitative case, we may introduce additional formal causal terminology. However, we will not parallel that procedure here. Only the following two will be demonstrated:

Definition 83 (Conjectural causes). *If $\langle \Omega, \mathcal{E}, \succcurlyeq, T, A_{t_1}, B_{t_2}, X \rangle$ is a conjectural potential causal structure and is not a spurious one, then:*

---

[54] There is a second difference between potential causal structures of the first type based upon quantitative probabilities and conjectural potential causal structures. It is a philosophical one. The latter are beyond any doubt subjective structures because comparative probabilities are subjective probabilities.

1. A_{t_1} is a conjectural positive cause *of B_{t_2} in X iff* $(B_{t_2} \mid X \cap A_{t_1}) \succ (B_{t_2} \mid X)$,
2. A_{t_1} is a conjectural negative cause *of B_{t_2} in X iff* $(B_{t_2} \mid X \cap A_{t_1}) \prec (B_{t_2} \mid X)$.

Definition 84 (Conjectural causal structure). *If $\langle \Omega, \mathcal{E}, \succcurlyeq, T, A_{t_1}, B_{t_2}, X \rangle$ is a conjectural potential causal structure, then it is a* conjectural causal structure *iff A_{t_1} is a conjectural positive or a conjectural negative cause of B_{t_2} in X.*

Subjective causal structures

If in addition to quantitative probabilities we are also without comparative ones, we shall depend on qualitative probabilities. They are usually communicated by expressions like "probable", "likely", "unlikely", "improbable", and similar ones representing fuzzy probabilities (see page 1032). For instance, "lung cancer in men given smoking is likely". Major parts of personal knowledge and belief used in everyday life and medical practice belong to this type of qualitative-probabilistic knowledge and belief. The question arises whether it is possible to elicit etiologic knowledge and belief from this subjective part of one's epistemic sphere. To this end, a qualitative probability space was constructed and extended to a *subjective causal structure* in (Sadegh-Zadeh, 1998, 256–259).

6.5.4 Fuzzy Etiology

When dealing with the conjectural and subjective causal structures above, we already entered the realm of fuzzy etiology. The comparative and qualitative probabilities those structures are based on, are fuzzy probabilities. This is evinced by terms such as "is at least as likely as", "improbable", "likely", and so on that we used as our basic probability notions. All of them are fuzzy predicates denoting fuzzy sets. If we take into account that even a quantitative probability may be a fuzzy number such as $p(B \mid A) =$ approximately 0.7, we shall recognize how serviceable in medical etiology fuzzy logic may be. This service is not confined to the fuzzy probability component of causation, however. Causal speech in which causal relevance itself is used as a relation among events, may also benefit from fuzzy logic. To illustrate this possibility, we shall in the following two sections briefly introduce:

▶ Fuzzy causal structures
▶ Fuzzy causal spaces.

Fuzzy causal structures

To begin with, it appears quite sensible to use fuzzy predicates in etiology and to state that:

> *A* causes *B* in *X* to a *low* extent,
> *A strongly* causes *B* in *Y*,
> *A moderately* discauses *B* in *Z*,

when an appropriate semantics is available. To this end, let us fix a uniform syntax that will represent all fuzzy statements of the type above. We write:

$$CR(A, B, X) = \tau$$

to say that:

> *The causal relevance of A to B in X is τ.*

In this sentence, τ is a linguistic term and denotes a fuzzy strength of causation such as "low" in the following statement:

$$CR(smoking, \; lung\_cancer, \; students) = low.$$

This new notion of *causal relevance* is written in capitals, *CR*, so as to distinguish it from the numerical function or variable of causal relevance, *cr*. *CR* is a ternary *linguistic variable* with the following example term set, $T(CR)$:

$$T(CR) = \{low, \; very \; low, \; not \; low, \; medium, \; high, \; fairly \; high,$$
$$very \; high, \; not \; high, \; very \; very \; high, \; extremely \; high,$$
$$more \; or \; less \; high, \; neutral, \; null, \; negative, \; weakly$$
$$negative, \; very \; negative, \; \ldots, \; etc. \ldots \}.$$

Elements of this term set may be symbolized by τ_1, τ_2, τ_3, and so on. As a three-place linguistic variable, *CR* will assign to a triple such as $\langle A_{t_1}, B_{t_2}, X \rangle$ a linguistic value $\tau_i \in T(CR)$. Using this method, we are able to understand what it means to say, for example, that in non-diabetics the causal relevance of Chlamydophila pneumoniae infection to coronary heart disease is fairly high:

$$CR(chlamydo, \; chd, \; non\text{-}diabetics) = fairly \; high.$$

We have seen already that due to the contextuality of causes it is of course possible that in different reference classes, Chlamydophila pneumoniae infection is differently causally relevant to the same disease. For instance, we may face the following situation:

$$CR(chlamydo, chd, diabetics) = null,$$
$$CR(chlamydo, chd, diabetics \cap rheumatism) = low,$$
$$CR(chlamydo, chd, non\text{-}diabetics \cap rheumatism) = very \; high.$$

And it is also conceivable that by causal intervention the very high causal relevance may be reversed, e.g., by using antibiotics, aspirin, etc.:

$$CR(chlamydo \cap antibiotics, chd, non\text{-}diabetics \cap rheumatism) =$$
$$moderately\ negative,$$
$$CR(chlamydo \cap antibiotics \cap aspirin, chd, non\text{-}diabetics \cap rheumatism)$$
$$= highly\ negative.$$

These examples demonstrate how causal relevances may be expressed and dealt with linguistically rather than numerically, provided they are available. But in order for them to be available, we need an appropriate framework of fuzzy etiology. We will not go into details for that here. We will only introduce elementary and general fuzzy causal structures to illustrate fuzzy-causal inquiries.

Definition 85 (Fuzzy causal structure). ξ *is a fuzzy causal structure* **iff** *there are* $\Omega, \mathcal{E}, p, T, A_{t_1}, B_{t_2}, X, CR,$ *and* τ *such that:*

1. $\xi = \langle \Omega, \mathcal{E}, p, T, A_{t_1}, B_{t_2}, X, CR, \tau \rangle$,
2. $\langle \Omega, \mathcal{E}, p, T, A_{t_1}, B_{t_2}, X \rangle$ *is a causal structure,*
3. *CR is a linguistic variable with* $T(CR) = \{low,\ very\ low,\ not\ low,\ medium,\ high,\ fairly\ high,\ \dots etc.\ \dots\}$,
4. $\tau \in T(CR)$,
5. $CR(A_{t_1}, B_{t_2}, X) = \tau.$

Suppose, for instance, that we have the following statistical information:

a)   The probability that a non-diabetic over 70 years old will suffer myocardial infarction or stroke, is 0.1;
b)   The probability that a non-diabetic over 70 years old who has coronary heart disease, will suffer myocardial infarction or stroke, is 0.7.

That is:

a′) $p(infarction_{t_2} \cup stroke_{t_2} \mid non\text{-}diabetics\_over\_70_{t_1}) = 0.1$
b′) $p(infarction_{t_2} \cup stroke_{t_2} \mid non\text{-}diabetics\_over\_70_{t_1} \cap chd_{t_1}) = 0.7.$

By Definition 67 on page 247, we can infer from the statistical information above that the following septuple, supplemented by the components of its probability space, is a potential causal structure:

$$\langle \Omega, \mathcal{E}, p, T, chd_{t_1}, infarction_{t_2} \cup stroke_{t_2}, non\text{-}diabetics\_over\_70_{t_1} \rangle.$$

After Definition 72 on page 254, it is in addition a *causal structure* if it is not a spurious one. If according to an agreed-upon definition of the linguistic variable *CR* we have the statement:

$$CR(infarction_{t_2} \cup stroke_{t_2}, non\text{-}diabetics\_over\_70_{t_1} \cap chd_{t_1}) = high$$

then the following nonuple is a *fuzzy causal structure:*

$$\langle \Omega, \mathcal{E}, p, T, chd_{t_1}, infarction_{t_2} \cup stroke_{t_2}, non\text{-}diabetics\_over\_70_{t_1},$$
$$CR, high \rangle.$$

Fuzzy causal structures of the type above are elementary ones. Introduced below is the concept of a general fuzzy causal structure, which we shall need in the next section:

Definition 86 (General fuzzy causal structure). ξ *is a* general fuzzy causal structure *iff there are* Ω, $\mathcal{E}$, p, T, $\mathcal{A}$, $\mathcal{B}$, $\mathcal{X}$, CR, *and* $T(CR)$ *such that:*

1. $\xi = \langle \Omega, \mathcal{E}, p, T, \mathcal{A}, \mathcal{B}, \mathcal{X}, CR, T(CR) \rangle$,
2. $\langle \Omega, \mathcal{E}, p, T, \mathcal{A}, \mathcal{B}, \mathcal{X} \rangle$ *is a general causal structure,*
3. CR *is a linguistic variable with* $T(CR) = \{low, \; very \; low, \; not \; low,$ *medium, high, fairly high, ... etc. ...*$\}$,
4. *For every* $A_{t_1} \in \mathcal{A}$ *there is a* $B_{t_2} \in \mathcal{B}$, *an* $X \in \mathcal{X}$, *and a term* $\tau \in T(CR)$ *such that* $CR(A_{t_1}, B_{t_2}, X) = \tau$.

An example is provided by a couple of diseases and their supposed causes, i.e., event sets $\mathcal{A}$ and $\mathcal{B}$, which in a probability space $\langle \Omega, \mathcal{E}, p \rangle$ yield a general fuzzy causal structure when to each cause-effect association is assigned a linguistic value from the term set $T(CR)$ such as:

$$CR(chd_{t_1}, stroke_{t_2}, non\text{-}diabetics\_over\_70_{t_1}) = low$$
$$CR(chd_{t_1}, infarction_{t_2}, non\text{-}diabetics\_over\_70_{t_1}) = not \; high$$
$$CR(chd_{t_1} \cap hypertension_{t_1}, infarction_{t_2}, non\text{-}diabetics\_over\_70_{t_1}) =$$
$$medium$$
$$CR(chd_{t_1} \cap smoking, infarction_{t_2} \cup stroke_{t_2}, non\text{-}diabetics\_over\_70_{t_1}) =$$
$$high$$
$$CR(HIV\_infection_{t_1}, AIDS_{t_2}, adults_{t_1}) = very \; high.$$

But how do we obtain a fuzzy causal relevance value τ such as "medium" for use in our fuzzy causal structure? Clause 2 of Definitions 85 and 86 shows that an underlying probabilistic-causal structure is required, which means two things. First, without probability there is no fuzzy causality. Causal structures rest on (quantitative, comparative, or qualitative) probability spaces. Second, the fuzzy, linguistic value τ must be derived from them. To this end, a concept of fuzzy causal *space* is constructed below that will allow us to fuzzify causality.

Fuzzy causal spaces

The idea behind, and the intuitive understanding of, the concept of a fuzzy causal space we are aiming at is this: We may be faced with a particular type of system displaying a more or less complex causal behavior, e.g., with the pathology and epidemiology of all or some infectious diseases in a human population. We need not describe this causal system crisply-numerically. Rather, we may describe it fuzzily-linguistically by stating that, for instance, "event A is *strongly* causally associated with event B, but only *moderately* causally associated with event C, and *highly negatively* causally associated with event D", etc. The totality of such fuzzy causal statements about the system under discussion represent a fuzzy causal space where the set of italicized, fuzzy CR values used such as:

strongly causally associated,
moderately causally associated,
highly negatively causally associated,

may be $\{\tau_a, \tau_b, \ldots, \tau_m\} \subseteq T(CR)$. It appears quite promising to view this set $\{\tau_a, \tau_b, \ldots, \tau_m\}$, in analogy to probability distribution, as a fuzzy causal relevance *distribution* over the event algebra $\mathcal{E}$ and to assume that (i) the distribution is controlled by a socially, biologically, or meteorologically induced fuzzy causal function; and (ii) may exhibit a fuzzy causal kinematics over time depending on factors that need to be traced by etiologists.

Definition 87 below extends general fuzzy causal structures, introduced by Definition 86 above, to fuzzy causal *spaces* by standardizing the linguistic variable *CR*. To this end, the term set $T(CR)$ must be rank-ordered in some appropriate fashion. We will order our ranking according to whether a term $\tau_j \in T(CR)$ expresses a stronger causal association between two events than another term $\tau_i \in T(CR)$ does. Such is the case, for example, regarding the two terms "strongly associated" and "moderately associated". Let us string the elements of $T(CR)$ in the order of their increasing strength, as just described, to obtain an ordinal or rank-ordered scale such that $\tau_1 \in T(CR)$ denotes the most negative association, τ_{i+1} denotes a stronger association than τ_i, while $\tau_n \in T(CR)$ represents the most positive association:

$$T(CR) = \langle \text{highly negative}, \tau_2, \ldots, \text{null}, \ldots, \tau_{n-1}, \text{highly positive} \rangle$$

Definition 87 (Fuzzy causal space). *ξ is a fuzzy causal space iff there are $\Omega, \mathcal{E}, p, T, \mathcal{A}, \mathcal{B}, \mathcal{X}, CR,$ and $T(CR)$ such that:*

1. *$\xi = \langle \Omega, \mathcal{E}, p, T, \mathcal{A}, \mathcal{B}, \mathcal{X}, CR, T(CR) \rangle$,*
2. *$\langle \Omega, \mathcal{E}, p, T, \mathcal{A}, \mathcal{B}, \mathcal{X}, CR, T(CR) \rangle$ is a general fuzzy causal structure,*
3. *CR is a linguistic variable with $T(CR) = \langle \tau_1, \ldots, \text{neutral}, \ldots, \tau_n \rangle$ being its rank-ordered term set,*
4. *For all non-empty $Y, X \in \mathcal{E}$: $CR(Y, \varnothing, X) = CR(Y, \Omega, X) = \text{null}$,*
5. *For all non-empty $Y, Z_1, Z_2, X \in \mathcal{E}$: If $Z_1 \subseteq Z_2$, then*

    5.1. $CR(Y, Z_1, X) \leq CR(Y, Z_2, X)$ if $CR(Y, Z_2, X) \geq \text{null}$,
    5.2. $CR(Y, Z_1, X) \geq CR(Y, Z_2, X)$ if $CR(Y, Z_2, X) < \text{null}$.

The linguistic causal relevance function *CR* has been standardized by axioms 3–5. It remains undefined, however.

Thus far we have two types of causal space at our disposal, the crisp ones produced by the numerical causal relevance measure *cr*, on the one hand (Definition 81); and the fuzzy ones supplied by the linguistic causal relevance measure *CR*, on the other. Both spaces may be interrelated with one another in the following way: A crisp causal space can be transformed into a fuzzy causal space. That is, it can be fuzzified such that given any numerical causal relevance value such as:

$$cr(A, B, X) = r$$

we can find out whether r is low, medium, high, very high, not very low and not very high, and so on by determining the fuzzy value:

$$CR(A, B, X) = \tau_i$$

where $\tau_i \in T(CR)$. That means, according to the theory of linguistic variables discussed on pages 78 and 1019, that every linguistic value of the measure CR, e.g., "high", may be defined as a name of a fuzzy subset of the range $[-1, +1]$ of the measure cr such that any point in $[-1, +1]$ can be linguistically classified in the term set $T(CR)$. That is, we may semantically interpret CR values in the following way (for details, see Sections 30.4.1 and 6.3.3):

The term set $T(CR) = \langle \tau_1, \ldots, neutral, \ldots, \tau_n \rangle$ may be a more or less large set of linguistic terms. It may rest on only a few undefined primitives such as "low", "medium", and "high". They may therefore be called the *primary terms* of CR, represented by the set "*primary-$T(CR)$*". The remaining elements of $T(CR)$, such as "very high", "not low", "not very high and not very low", and others are defined by applying to primary terms semantic operators of different type, e.g., connectives like "not"; linguistic hedges like "very"; etc. Thus, the semantic interpretation of primary terms will suffice to obtain an entirely interpreted $T(CR)$ because semantic operators obey specified rules. This basic semantic interpretation and definition of primary terms is provided by a *compatibility function* μ.

Let μ be a binary function which maps the Cartesian product of the range of the function cr and the primary terms of CR to the unit interval:

$$\mu: [-1, +1] \times primary\text{-}T(CR) \rightarrow [0, 1].$$

It evaluates, in $[0, 1]$, the compatibility of a cr value $x \in [-1, +1]$ with a linguistic term $\tau_i \in primary\text{-}T(CR)$. For example, it determines the extent to which a causal relevance 0.6 is to be called *high*. Thus, it assigns to a pair $\langle x, \tau_i \rangle$ the grade of membership of x in τ_i. That means that μ is a binary, fuzzifying membership function. For instance, we may carry out the definition of our function μ above in such a way as to obtain:

$$\begin{aligned}
\mu(1, high) &= \mu(-1, high) &= 1 \\
\mu(0.8, high) &= \mu(-0.8, high) &= 1 \\
\mu(0.6, high) &= \mu(-0.6, high) &= 0.8 \\
\mu(0.5, high) &= \mu(-0.5, high) &= 0.3 \\
\mu(0.2, high) &= \mu(-0.2, high) &= 0.
\end{aligned}$$

For the sake of convenience, we abbreviate $\mu(x, \tau_i) = y$ to a pseudo-unary membership function $\mu_{\tau_i}(x) = y$. The above examples then read:

$$\begin{aligned}
\mu_{high}(1) &= \mu_{high}(-1) &= 1 \\
\mu_{high}(0.8) &= \mu_{high}(-0.8) &= 1 \\
\mu_{high}(0.6) &= \mu_{high}(-0.6) &= 0.8 \\
\mu_{high}(0.5) &= \mu_{high}(-0.5) &= 0.3 \\
\mu_{high}(0.2) &= \mu_{high}(-0.2) &= 0.
\end{aligned}$$

And we obtain a large number of local membership functions such as μ_{high}, μ_{medium}, μ_{low}, μ_{very_high}, etc. Each of them may be interpreted as a particular restriction of μ on the range $[-1, +1]$ of the numerical causality function cr as a base variable. Plots of some of these restrictions are displayed in Figures 43–46. The figures illustrate what it means to say that linguistic CR values such as "high", "very high", "not low", and others have now become interpreted labels for fuzzy subsets of the values of the numerical function cr.

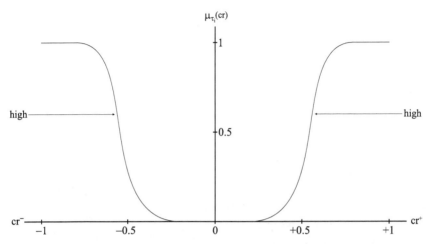

Fig. 43. A tentative compatibility function for *highly causally relevant* on both banks of the numerical causal relevance function cr, that is, *highly positively causally relevant* and *highly negatively causally relevant*, both abbreviated to "high"

We may understand the fuzzy-logical interpretation and definition of linguistic causal relevance in the following way. With reference to the definition of a fuzzy set as a set of ordered pairs $\langle x, f(x) \rangle$ such that x is an element of a crisp base set Ω and f is a function that maps Ω to unit interval $[0, 1]$, we can use any of the functions μ_{high}, μ_{medium}, μ_{low}, ... as a particular fuzzifying function on the range $[-1, +1]$ of the numerical causal relevance function cr. For instance:

$$\mu_{high} : [-1, +1] \mapsto [0, 1].$$

We shall thus obtain "high, positive causal relevance" and "high, negative causal relevance" as fuzzy sets, e.g., *highly positively causally relevant* = $\{(1, 1), (0.8, 1), (0.6, 0.8), (0.5, 0.3), (0.2, 0)\}$.

The same kind of fuzzification applies to key notions of etiology, epidemiology, and clinical medicine such as *indicator, risk factor, preventive factor,* and *protective factor*. Each of them may be fuzzily partitioned into different grades of strength ("weak risk factor", "medium risk factor", etc.), and these grades may be interpreted as linguistic labels of degrees of causal impact. See Section 16.5 on page 603.

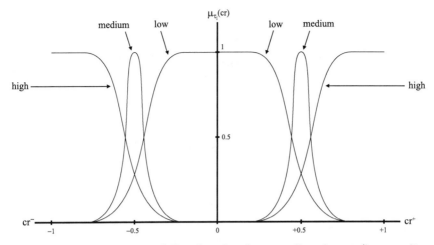

Fig. 44. A tentative compatibility function for *causally relevant* (low, medium, high) on both banks of the causal relevance function *cr*, positive and negative

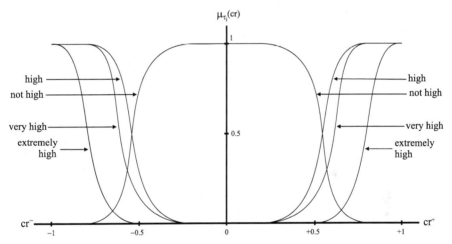

Fig. 45. A tentative compatibility function for *causally relevant* (not high, high, very high, extremely high) on both banks of the causal relevance function *cr*

6.5.5 Summary

As additional information about a patient's suffering, knowledge about its causes may enhance diagnostic, therapeutic, and preventive decision-making. In the preceding sections, we tried to explicate the notions of cause and causation needed for this purpose. To this end, we distinguished between deterministic and probabilistic etiology and added a new, third type called fuzzy etiology. We paid particular attention to probabilistic etiology, as the concept of cause is best conceived as a particular probabilistic relation between

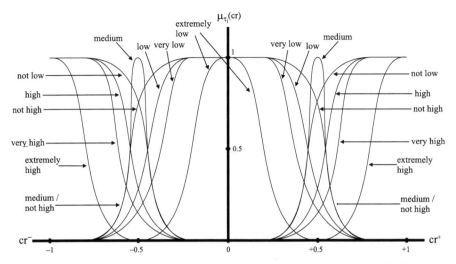

Fig. 46. A summary visualization of positive and negative fuzzy causal relevances *low, high, not low, not high, very low, very high,* etc. One may of course also consider additional values such as *not very high and not very low,* and the like. But we have tried to keep the present figure readable

events. Specifically, we chose the familiar, well-defined concept of stochastic or *probabilistic independence* as our point of departure and interpreted causation as a ternary relation of probabilistic dependence between an event A and an event B in a background context X consisting of $n \geq 1$ partial events $X_1, \ldots, X_n$, provided there is no other event C that renders this dependency relation between A and B spurious. Our ternary concept of causation also explicitly articulates the contextuality of causes in terms of the relationships between the cause event A and the context X.

A complex system involving a number of events and a relationship of causation between them we called a *causal structure*. A causal structure is simply an extension of a probability space by including a period of time, a couple of events, and the information that there is a non-spurious, probabilistic dependency between these events. Because it is an *extended probability space*, the entire theory of probability is directly applicable to our theory of etiology.

We distinguished positive and negative causation depending on whether an event A increases or decreases the probability of a later event B in a background context X. This ternary relation of causation resolves many age-old, stubborn philosophical problems of causality. Moreover, it allows for a quantitative concept of causality that measures the *degree of causal relevance* of an event to its effect. With the aid of this numerical function, denoted cr, causes may be compared with each other regarding their causal impact. It also enables us to fuzzify causality using a linguistic variable of causal relevance, CR.

7

The Physician

In Western culture, human medicine has evolved as a healing profession, and as such, it is oriented toward curing sick people, caring for sick people, preventing maladies, and promoting health. This orientation is primarily centered around the *healing relationship,* a relationship that is usually thought of as a dyadic structure, comprising the physician and the patient. Venerable terms such as "the physician-patient relationship" and "the doctor-patient interaction" reflect this view.

The healing relationship is also referred to as "the clinical encounter". The latter term, however, is a meaning-laden word that gives rise to unrealistic expectations, e.g., in (Pellegrino, 2008; Pellegrino and Thomasma, 1981). The increasing mistrust of the population toward the health care system demonstrates that these expectations are not satisfied in clinical practice. Yet, trust in the doctor and in the medical sciences and professions is a prerequisite for a *genuine encounter* in Martin Buber's sense (Buber, 1958). That is, there must be trust between the patient and the doctor in order that the healing relationship be successful. We must therefore ask the question, what qualities of a doctor tend to elicit trust from her patients and potential patients? Among the conceivable qualities, the following ones are commonly viewed as necessary conditions: (i) The doctor should be an expert of her specialty and should not have a bad reputation; (ii) she must possess a sound knowledge of the medical sciences; (iii) she must be interested in the patient's health and be capable of communicating with her; (iv) she must preserve confidentiality of knowledge about the patient; and (v) she must be committed to continuing education to update her diagnostic-therapeutic knowledge and skill.

A closer look at the structure of a healing relationship reveals, however, that it is more complex than a dyadic structure. For the doctor is not the only determinant of the healing relationship. There are additional components that shape it and its success or failure. Among these components are, for example, the physician's assistants and the patient's family members. This complex, polyadic healing structure with its function, effects, and defects will be the subject of our concern in the next chapter. It embraces the physician as one of

K. Sadegh-Zadeh, *Handbook of Analytic Philosophy of Medicine,*
Philosophy and Medicine 113, DOI 10.1007/978-94-007-2260-6_7,
© Springer Science+Business Media B.V. 2012

its most important components. In contrast to what is typically assumed, in this polyadic structure she is not the sole agent responsible for the patient's trust. As a human being, she plays multiple roles and is at the same time a member of numerous groups that obey different, and possibly conflicting, norms. Such groups are, for example, her family, the hospital workers, the personnel of a laboratory, a doctors' association, scientific communities, a religious denomination, the larger society, the state, and others. Her healing role and skill, and her moral as well as legal responsibilities in the healing structure are shaped by these groups and their rules and norms, and thus, by external factors and traditions. That means that the physician as an acting component of the healing relationship is embedded in a surrounding system as one of its components. It would therefore be interesting to empirically investigate physician performance depending on the surrounding system within which it takes place. Research of this type could best be named "iatrology", from the Greek term ιατρός" (iatros) meaning "the physician". The term "iatrology" with a more general meaning was introduced by Karl Eduard Rothschuh (1978).

The healing relationship between the doctor and the patient emerges and develops in a process that is traditionally called *clinical practice,* from the Greek terms "κλινη" (kline) for *bed, sick-bed;* and "πραξις" (praxis) for *doing, acting, action.* Like the physician, it is embedded in a surrounding system with a variety of components and relations between them such as science, professional communities, economics, technology, politics, religion, and others. In Western societies, its most important characteristic is its embeddedness in the world of science and scientific knowledge and methodology. The following Chapter 8 is an inquiry into clinical practice to analyze the clinical encounter, its foundations, and outcomes.

8

Clinical Practice

8.0 Introduction

Clinical practice is where the clinical encounter occurs. It constitutes the focus of medicine. Since the time of Hippocrates, it has been composed of five activities. They are fundamental features of the healing relationship and have come to be known as *anamnesis,* i.e., history taking or clinical interview, *diagnosis, prognosis, therapy,* and *prevention.* The present chapter is devoted to the analysis and discussion of the logical, methodological, and philosophical problems of these activities.

As was pointed out above, the patient expects the physician to be an expert of her specialty devoid of a bad reputation. This constitutes what may be called a *good doctor,* i.e., one whose clinical decisions are *right and good* in most cases, at least in as many cases as another expert in the same area also achieves. In what follows, we shall analyze the characteristics and presuppositions of such right and good clinical decisions. To this end, we shall undertake a conceptual analysis of the clinical encounter and its outcomes, in order to develop a theory of clinical practice. Our analysis consists of the following five parts:

    8.1   The Clinical Encounter
    8.2   Anamnesis and Diagnosis
    8.3   Prognosis
    8.4   Therapy
    8.5   Prevention.

8.1 The Clinical Encounter

8.1.0 Introduction

This section lays the foundations for a relativistic theory of clinical practice that will follow in the next sections. The theory implies that there is no

K. Sadegh-Zadeh, *Handbook of Analytic Philosophy of Medicine,*
Philosophy and Medicine 113, DOI 10.1007/978-94-007-2260-6_8,
© Springer Science+Business Media B.V. 2012

true state of the patient to be discovered by anamnesis and diagnosis, and to be used in making a prognosis and a therapeutic decision. What is usually considered to be the patient's true state, is a construct of medical knowledge and methods of reasoning applied to the patient in clinical decision-making. This view has far-reaching philosophical and practical consequences. It will enable us to prove that in contrast to its mystification in medicine and philosophy of medicine, clinical decision-making is a computable task and does not necessarily require human intelligence, mind, and intuition.

The traditional view of the clinical encounter goes as follows: A patient seeks the advice of a physician and reports to him her complaints and symptoms. By interviewing and examining the patient, the doctor elicits additional information about her health condition. On the basis of all collected *patient data,* she eventually:

- makes a diagnosis to account for patient data, and
- administers the appropriate treatment suggested by the diagnosis.

The only interesting characteristic of this widespread view is that it is wrong. An individual seeks medical care and advice either as a reaction to her own interpretation of her current health condition, or she is committed to medical care because her health condition is interpreted by someone else to be serious. The latter is the case when the patient is too ill or incompetent, for example, when she is unconscious and was found in the ditch, or is an infant that is brought to the doctor by her mother. In any event, the search for medical advice and assistance follows the interpretation of a *problem,* which may be real or merely imaginary, by the patient or others. On the basis of that antecedent interpretation and some particular values, it is decided to resolve the pre-shaped problem by a doctor. The decision not to consult someone else, for example, a bricklayer, an attorney, or the employment exchange, demonstrates that the problem has already been pre-classified as a *medical* one. Maybe this critical pre-classification was a misclassification. Be that as it may, the choice of a physician will determine the outcome. It is predictable that the outcome will be a medical diagnosis and treatment, although the problem is *perhaps* non-medical or might better be resolved by non-medical interventions. The same applies to the choice of a particular medical specialist rather than another. It does indeed make a difference whether an internist, a urologist, an orthopedist, or another specialist is chosen since a specialist will automatically try to shape the initial problem of the patient into the subject of her own specialty. When analyzing the clinical encounter, all of these aspects have to be taken into account.

The clinical encounter serves many purposes. Among the most important of them is the task of establishing a relationship of mutual trust between the physician and her patient, and inquiring into *what should be done for this patient.* The clinical interview of the patient, usually called history taking or anamnesis, constitutes the verbal component of the inquiry. Its non-verbal expression is the examination of the patient, including laboratory tests as well as analyses of other types. By the interview and examination of the patient, the physician elicits information that she needs in deciding *what should be done for this patient*. To this end, she generates and tests diagnostic hypotheses from the very beginning of the clinical encounter. Based on only a few facets such as the patient's initial problem, gender, age, voice, and appearance, she automatically forms an *initial idea* of 'what the patient might have'. Let us have a quick look at an example interview in Table 3:

Table 3: Patient interview: An example

1. DOCTOR:	How may I help you?	
2. PATIENT:	I have been having sporadic chest pain and also an increasing physical weakness for some time.	
3. DOCTOR:	(thinks: "a 49-year-old man complaining of chest pain and weakness. Maybe he has a heart problem? She asks:) Please tell me more about your chest pain.	
4. PATIENT:	Well, it is pressure-like, Doctor.	
5. DOCTOR:	(thinks: "Does he suffer perhaps from angina pectoris due to myocardial ischemia?" She asks:) When does your chest pain occur and how long does it last?[55]	
6. PATIENT:	Often it occurs after meals and lasts for hours.	
7. DOCTOR:	(thinks: "No heart problem, it seems". To test this hypothesis, she asks:) Does the pain radiate to your left arm?	
8. PATIENT:	No.	

To get more clear about her initial idea of 'what the patient might have', the doctor continues asking specific questions. In so doing, she is guided by the following three types of queries:

a. *Why* did this event (symptom, complaint, problem, or finding) occur?
b. *How* did it come about?
c. *What if* the patient has *X?*

Why- and how-questions require the physician to reason by the backward-chaining of her hypotheses, while what-if-questions induce forward-chaining. The entire interview and the examination of the patient following it, constitute a hypothesis-driven and hypothesis-testing, cyclic process (Figure 47).

Clinical reasoning in the cyclic process of generating and testing diagnostic hypotheses is traditionally referred to as *differential diagnostics*. The qualifying adjective "differential" reflects the common belief that in clinical reasoning, the physician (i) considers *all* diseases that may account for the current problem the patient presents; (ii) *"differentiates"* between them according to their probability, plausibility, or potential causal relevance; and

---

[55] "Myocardial ischemia" means "reduced blood supply to the heart muscle".

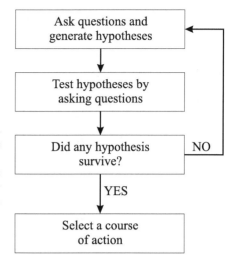

Fig. 47. The hypothesis-driven and hypothesis-testing, cyclic process of the clinical interview. The doctor's intellectual acts to get through this process is called 'clinical reasoning'. She may or may not explicitly apply logic in this reasoning process. The term "reasoning" is not synonymous with "logical reasoning". See Part V

(iii) *"differentiates"* between the true and false diagnoses by testing them. This belief cannot be true simply because no method of clinical reasoning and differential diagnostics is taught to medical students. As a result, physicians usually lack differential-diagnostic skill. They lack expert methodological knowledge about how to generate meaningful diagnostic hypotheses, how to test them according to a specific theory of testing hypotheses, and how to use patient data correctly in this process. Rather, it is claimed that "In spite of the recent perfusion of high-technology diagnostic procedures and tests, the majority of patient problems can still be solved during the first two minutes of the patient interview" (Cutler, 1998, vii). It is therefore no surprise that there are still about 30–38% misdiagnoses in medicine (Gross and Löffler, 1997; Sadegh-Zadeh, 1981c).

Since misdiagnoses entail misconceptions about the patient's health condition, they give rise to inappropriate treatments and malpractices. For this reason, the quality of physician performance cannot be enhanced without reducing misdiagnoses. This goal, however, requires a theory of clinical reasoning that transforms clinical practice from being conducted as an 'art' into a scientific endeavor. In what follows, we will demonstrate how such a transformation may be conceived. Our discussion divides into these four parts:

8.1.1   The Patient Elroy Fox
8.1.2   Dynamic, Branching Clinical Questionnaires
8.1.3   Clinical Paths
8.1.4   The Clinical Process.

We start by considering a clinical case report on an anonymous patient whom we shall call Dr. Elroy Fox. This case report is a short excerpt from a real patient history. We shall use it in developing our theories and frameworks.

8.1.1 The Patient Elroy Fox

Dr. Elroy Fox was a 49-year-old physiologist when he got ill for the first time. One day he found evidence to suspect that he had fatty stool. Upon this suspicion, he had a lightning explanation of the continuing loss of his physical energy that he had been experiencing for some time. As a physiologist, he correctly concluded that he certainly had exocrine pancreatic insufficiency. The next day he consulted an internist to ask him to evaluate his suspicion. The internist took some blood and stool tests. A few days later he informed Dr. Elroy Fox of the outcome. "My diagnosis is", he said:

DIAGNOSIS 1: You don't have exocrine pancreatic insufficiency.[56]

Elroy Fox was happy to hear this good news. Over time, however, he developed some additional symptoms. Therefore, he consulted the same internist and complained of:

  a. increasing adynamia,
  b. night sweat,
  c. feeling of pressure in the left chest,
  d. pain in the same region,
  e. paroxysmal tachycardia.[57]

Before going into details, the outcome may be reported right now to understand in what follows why things in clinical practice often go wrong. After finishing the diagnostic process, the doctor said:

DIAGNOSIS 2: You have a psychosomatic syndrome that manifests
             itself in cardiac symptoms.

Elroy Fox was a well-informed physiologist. He found this diagnosis to be not only wrong, but simply absurd, and for this reason he never returned to this doctor. He consulted another physician and received the diagnosis:

DIAGNOSIS 3: a. Angina pectoris due to stress,
              b. Nicotine abuse,
              c. mild hypercholesterolemia.

He was advised to stop smoking, to do physical exercise, and to reduce fat intake. But in spite of compliance, he didn't get rid of his symptoms in the next two years. Due to his distrust in the doctors he had consulted, Elroy Fox changed his doctors one after another and successively received the following diagnoses. "Elroy Fox has", they said:

---

[56] The term "exocrine" refers to pancreatic secretion of digestive enzymes.

[57] Paroxysmal tachycardia is the acceleration of heart rate having sudden onset and cessation. The adjective "paroxysmal" means "sudden, violent". It derives from the Greek terms παρά (para) for "by, beside"; οξυς (oxys) for "acute". The phrase "tachycardia" is composed of the Greek terms ταχυς (tachys) for "rapid", and καρδιά for "heart".

DIAGNOSIS 4: Ulcerative gastritis.

DIAGNOSIS 5: a. Latent diabetes,
              b. polyneuropathy.

DIAGNOSIS 6: Ectopic atrial tachycardia.

DIAGNOSIS 7: a. Exocrine pancreatic insufficiency,
              b. endocrine pancreatic insufficiency (type 2 diabetes),
              c. peptic esophagitis,
              d. Helicobacter pylori gastritis,
              e. sorbitol intolerance,
              f. no hepatitis.

It was only with the last, seventh diagnosis that the patient's initial, correct suspicion was confirmed. After six years had passed, Elroy Fox was finally provided with the basis of appropriate therapy and advice. We must therefore ask ourselves how it could take six years to confirm the patient's own, initial interpretation, after so many misdiagnoses. Is it conceivable that other patients are victims of similar misfortunes? How could such misfortunes be prevented? To answer these questions, we are pursuing a theory of clinical reasoning suitable to the clinical encounter. We shall be guided by Elroy Fox's case, further described below.

Usually it is said that the physician 'interprets' the patient's symptoms, or that she tries 'to explain' and to 'understand' why the patient presents them, in order to choose an appropriate treatment. This widespread view sheds no light on the reasons for the diagnostic failures above. Independently of whether or not it is true, to identify a more efficient method of reasoning we will look at the interview with the patient Elroy Fox, continued from Table 3 on page 277. See Table 4.

Table 4: Patient interview: Continued from Table 3

9. DOCTOR:	Did you have any diseases in your childhood?
10. PATIENT:	Yes, I have had measles.
11. DOCTOR:	Did you have any other diseases thereafter?
12. PATIENT:	No.
13. DOCTOR:	Are there any serious diseases in your family, hereditary or non-hereditary ones?
14. PATIENT:	Yes. My cousin suffers from hemophilia A.
15. DOCTOR:	(thinks: "Hm, hemophilia A. There is no relationship between the patient's state and that". She asks:) What is your job?
16. PATIENT:	I am a physiologist working at a university institute.
17. DOCTOR:	Please tell me something about your work atmosphere.
18. PATIENT:	Well, I am head of the neurophysiology department and have fifteen colleagues. We have a very good atmosphere in the department. I think everything is OK.

Table 4: Patient interview: Continued from Table 3

19.	DOCTOR:	When did you feel pressure in your thorax for the first time?
20.	PATIENT:	About six years ago.
21.	DOCTOR:	When did you feel chest pain for the first time?
22.	PATIENT:	Approximately at the same time.
23.	DOCTOR:	Is your chest pain brought on by exertion?
24.	PATIENT:	No.
25.	DOCTOR:	Is it brought on by breathing or cough?
26.	PATIENT:	No.
27.	DOCTOR:	Do you become short of breath when climbing stairs?
28.	PATIENT:	No.
29.	DOCTOR:	Are you a smoker?
30.	PATIENT:	Not any more.
31.	DOCTOR:	(thinks: "His chest pain is independent of exertion, breathing and cough, and it does not radiate. It is dependent on meals and lasts for hours. So, it does not seem to be a heart problem. Peptic ulcer disease and pancreatic or esophageal affection are more likely". She asks:) Please tell me something more about your night sweat and adynamia.
32.	PATIENT:	Well ...

The doctor-patient interaction almost always starts and continues like the dialogue above. Throughout the interaction, the physician forms diagnostic hypotheses about the patient's health condition. Usually they are of the following structure:

a. The patient might have A, B, C, but not X, Y, Z;
b. She possibly has A, B, C, but not X, Y, Z;
c. It is likely that she has A, B, C, but not X, Y, Z;
d. She has perhaps A, B, C, but not X, Y, Z.

One of them may be, for example, this assumption:

- Elroy Fox has perhaps myocardial ischemia, but not pancreatic insufficiency.

Modal expressions – such as "might", "possibly", "likely", "perhaps" – in the sentences above indicate that the doctor is only hypothesizing and doesn't know yet if her hypotheses are true. In order to examine the believability, plausibility, and certainty of such a hypothesis, she adapts the dialogue accordingly, asking the patient questions she considers suitable for the task. For example, in question No. 27 above our physician asked Elroy Fox:

- Do you become short of breath when climbing stairs?

She was testing the hypothesis that the patient's complaints might be due to myocardial ischemia. Since such an ischemia hinders the heart from functioning sufficiently during exertion, thereby causing shortness of breath, the physician asked just that question and not, for example, "do you sleep well?". We simplified the dialogue above to prevent confusion. However, we could have made these generate-hypotheses-and-test-them relationships more apparent, by including the steps of the physician's reasoning taking place in the background. After she successively formed and confirmed or disconfirmed a number of diagnostic assumptions by, and during, the dialogue, there eventually remains a certain set of $n \geq 1$ diagnostic hypotheses whose testing requires additional, non-verbal data. These data she will try to collect by a physical examination of the patient and by laboratory tests such as blood analyses, ECG, etc. The final diagnostic hypotheses that will eventually yield the *final diagnosis* may be, for example:

Elroy Fox might have:
a. Insufficient functioning of the adrenal cortex (Morbus Addison),
b. peptic esophagitis,
c. exocrine pancreatic insufficiency,
d. endocrine pancreatic insufficiency.

What additional data does the doctor need in order to decide "what is wrong with this patient?", i.e., to decide which one of the presumptive diagnoses above should be accepted and which one should be rejected? This type of inquiry would aim at selecting from among *all* possible alternatives the final diagnosis by differentiating between 'right' and 'wrong' ones. It has therefore come to be termed *differential diagnostics*. As mentioned on page 277 above, it is commonly assumed that the physician is conducting differential diagnostics during the entire interview and examination of the patient. However, from a wider, action-theoretic perspective we shall argue that from the very beginning of the clinical encounter the physician's problem is not the question "what is wrong with this patient?", but rather another one, namely *"should anything be done for this patient?* And if so, what among the many things that can be done, ought to be done?". That means that clinical reasoning may be reconstructed not as an inquiry into differential diagnosis, but more appropriately as differential indication. For the concept of differential diagnosis, see Section 8.2.8 on page 332.

Roughly, *differential indication* in a given situation is the task of selecting from among a set of alternative *actions* an action A that is indicated in that situation. This view, which favors action selection by differential indication over truth selection by differential diagnostics, will be discussed in detail in Section 8.2.4 below (Sadegh-Zadeh, 1981d, 194).

8.1.2 Dynamic, Branching Clinical Questionnaires

Based on the considerations above, in this section we will prepare the framework for our action-theoretic view on clinical decision-making, presented in Section 8.2 below. It says that clinical reasoning is concerned with *differential indication* rather than with differential diagnostics. Throughout our discussion, we shall understand by the general term "patient data" the problems, complaints, symptoms, and signs a patient presents. That is,

Patient data ≡ the patient's problems, complaints, symptoms, and signs.

In the last section, the case history of the patient Elroy Fox showed that he had consulted six doctors to obtain seven different diagnoses. Only the treatment and advice based on the seventh one ameliorated his health condition. Thus, the question is, why had the previous five doctors arrived at six useless diagnoses, although Elroy Fox reported the same patient data to each doctor? There is a simple answer to this question which will guide us in our analysis below. It says that in their clinical decision-making those five physicians:

a. asked the patient the wrong questions,
b. failed to ask him the right questions,
c. drew wrong conclusions from the available patient data,
d. so, the diagnostic hypotheses that they generated and tested, were inappropriate and useless.

This is the general, causal pattern of clinical misdiagnoses. Given this alarming observation, we plan to reconstruct clinical reasoning as a method of *information-seeking by questioning* based on a *dynamic branching clinical questionnaire*, or branching questionnaire for short. Only a doctor who follows the best dynamic, branching clinical questionnaire will arrive at the best diagnostic-therapeutic decisions. Roughly, a questionnaire of this type is a questionnaire whose questions have no fixed, static order. They are asked in an order determined by the answers to the preceding questions. That is, the order in which the questions are asked is dynamic, and depends on the patient's answers. To clearly define the concept, we shall proceed in three steps. First, the patient will be conceived as a black box with an unknown 'content' that has to be uncovered by the doctor, i.e., by 'diagnostics'. Second, an approach will be developed to exploring the black box by closed, structured questions. Third, on the basis of these two steps, the concept of a dynamic, branching questionnaire will be introduced. Our discussion thus divides into the following four sections:

▶ Initial data and initial action
▶ The patient as a black box
▶ Examination of the black box
▶ Dynamic, branching questionnaires.

Initial data and initial action

In the clinical encounter the physician collects patient data upon which to base her clinical reasoning. By this reasoning, she aims at a judgment about *"should anything be done for this patient?* If so, what among the many things that can be done, ought to be done?"*. We want to understand what kind of reasoning is best suited to answer these two questions. To this end, let us reconstruct how the clinical encounter starts. When consulting a doctor, a patient presents at the beginning of the dialogue a particular:

- non-empty set of patient data,

i.e., a set of problems, complaints, symptoms, and signs that we refer to as initial patient data, *initial data,* or patient data for short. Since the initial data set is never empty, the patient at the very beginning of the encounter is never a tabula rasa. Even an unconscious patient found in a ditch unable to provide any information on herself presents the initial data "the patient is unconscious". For example, we had the following initial data about the patient Elroy Fox:

a. Feeling of pressure in the left chest,
b. sporadic pain in the same region,
c. night sweat,
d. paroxysmal tachycardia,
e. increasing adynamia.

Provided with the initial data, the physician has to decide what action to take. Should the data be taken seriously and the clinical encounter be continued, or should the encounter be terminated because the patient data is harmless and needs no medical intervention? To answer this initial question, the physician must make a decision and perform an action, referred to here as an *initial action.* This initial action may simply be a question asked of the patient or her companions and relatives, which may lead to taking the patient history. It is also possible that the initial action is an emergency measure, e.g., an injection, an X-ray, a more or less extended physical examination of the patient, a surgical operation, or some other action. In any event, the initial action yields particular information about the patient. The physician follows this new data with a new action, and so on. The process ends at some later time with the physician's final action, e.g., giving the patient a drug or advice, referring the patient to a colleague or hospital, and the like.

Thus, the entire process of the clinical encounter, which started with the patient's initial data and the physician's initial action, consists of a series of *data gathering and acting* by the physician. This series includes, of course, the questions she asks the patient. We will now analyze and structure this process.

The patient as a black box

The patient in her entirety, including her body, mind, environment, biography, future life, etc., will be considered a black box about which nothing else is known at the beginning of the interview besides the initial data (Figure 48).

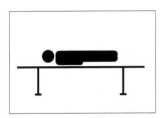

Fig. 48. The patient as a black box. The only knowledge we have about the box at the beginning of the clinical encounter is the initial patient data

The whole life of the patient lies as a riddle in the black box. It is not known whether or not it is a 'healthy life' or harbors pathological processes or diseases emitting the initial data from within the black box. To solve the riddle, the physician is allowed to ask the box any possible question whatever. In addition, she also has the option of drawing from the answers that the box emits, any conclusion she likes. From her knowledge and conjectures on what goes in (= input) and what goes out (= output), she must conclude what is in the box.

Examination of the black box

Almost always the initial patient data are not sufficient to form a clinical judgment about the patient's health condition. This task requires additional data about her. The best way to acquire such data is to examine the black box by addressing questions to it. This interrogative examination we refer to as *information-seeking by questioning*. A question that the physician addresses to the black box may either be a verbal question in the usual sense such as "do you become short of breath when climbing stairs?", or a non-verbal question in the form of a specific inquiry she undertakes to find out the value of a variable, for instance, by scratching the box to learn how it reacts; looking at the tongue of the box to judge its color; taking an X-ray photograph of the thorax; recording an ECG; conducting a glucose tolerance test; and the like. The goal is to draw conclusions about the contents of the black box from how it reacts to the interrogation. Thus, any *question* that is addressed to the patient or to her companions and relatives in the clinical encounter, represents a *test,* and vice versa, any test the patient is subjected to is a more or less complex question. For this reason, we shall consider these two terms as synonyms in what follows: question ≡ test.[58]

---

[58] By considering the patient as a black box and the questions asked by the physician as tests, clinical judgment becomes amenable to the *theory of testing* that is a significant methodological tool in psychology and social sciences.

The clinical encounter as an inquiry may also be characterized as an interrogative two-person game, referred to as a *question-answering game*, with the
following proviso. On the one hand, the interrogator need not be an individual
physician, but can also be a team or even a scientific community. On the other
hand, the black box as the answerer need not be an individual patient. It may
also be a couple, a family, or a larger group. For simplicity's sake, we shall
use the singular terms "the doctor" and "the patient" nonetheless.

A question, or a test, is in general an investigation to find out to which
one of the categories A, B, C, ... an object belongs or what numerical value
on a particular scale it has. For example, when looking at the tongue of her
patient, Mr. Elroy Fox, to examine what color it is, the doctor aims to answer
the question "what is the color of Elroy Fox's tongue?". In so doing, she is
exploring whether Elroy Fox is a member of the class 'has a red tongue', or
of the class 'has a blue tongue', or of any other tongue-color class. Likewise,
the question "what is the patient Elroy Fox's current heart rate?" is searching
for a quantitative value, for example, whether Elroy Fox's current heart rate
is 60, or 61, or 62, etc. By and large, we may conceive a question either as a
linguistic variable v or a *numerical variable f* applied to a tuple $(x_1, \ldots, x_n)$
with $n \geq 1$ to search for the missing value "?" in an interrogative sentence of
the following form:

$$v(x_1, \ldots, x_n) = ?$$
$$f(x_1, \ldots, x_n) = ?$$

For instance, our above-mentioned examples read:

$$\text{Tongue\_Color(Elroy Fox)} = ? \tag{69}$$
$$\text{heart\_rate(Elroy Fox)} = ?$$

The first example asks after the value of the linguistic variable *Tongue_Color*
as applied to Elroy Fox. In the second example, the value of the numerical
variable *heart_rate* as applied to Elroy Fox is sought. Perhaps we receive from
the black box the following answers: "Elroy Fox has a red tongue" and "Elroy
Fox has a heart rate of 76". That is:

$$\text{Tongue\_Color(Elroy Fox)} = \text{red}$$
$$\text{heart\_rate(Elroy Fox)} = 76.$$

In what follows, we shall show that clinical reasoning is best understood and
managed if the questions, such as (69) above, that are posed to the black
box are constructed as a *dynamic, branching questionnaire*. To introduce this
concept, we need the following three notions: *closed* questions, *open* questions,
and the *answer set* of a question. They may be defined first.[59]

---

[59] The inspiration for the concept of a branching questionnaire and its application
comes from Lotfi Zadeh (1976b).

Let Q be a verbal or non-verbal question as conceived above. The set of all admissible answers to Q is referred to as the answer set of Q, denoted $ans(Q)$ where "ans" is a set-valued function that identifies the set of all admissible answers to Q. For example, if our question is $Q = \text{“}Tongue\_Color(x) = ?\text{”}$, then its answer set may be $ans(Q) = \{red, white, green\}$. That means that the answer to an instance of this question, such as " Tongue_Color(Elroy Fox) $= ?$ ", is an element of the answer set $\{red, white, green\}$. Other answers are not considered or allowed.

An *atomic question* is a pair $\langle Q, ans(Q)\rangle$ such that Q is a question and $ans(Q)$ is its answer set. Q is referred to as the body of the atomic question. An example is provided by the tuple $\langle Tongue\_Color(Elroy\ Fox) = ?, \{red, white, green\}\rangle$. The body of this atomic question is the question "what is Elroy Fox's tongue color?".

Consider the questionnaire one must fill out when applying for a document, say a passport. It contains questions like the following ones: What is your name? What is the date of your birth? What is your birth place? Are you male or female? What is your marital status: unmarried, married, divorced, or widowed? And so on. It is obvious that each of these questions is, in principle, answerable. Likewise, questions that are directed to the patient as a black box, should be in principle answerable. First of all, they ought to be closed questions. We shall see that open questions should be avoided since they are a main source of physician idiosyncrasies and reasoning errors.

Definition 88 (Closed question). *An atomic question $\langle Q, ans(Q)\rangle$ is a* closed question *iff:*

1. *its answer set $ans(Q)$ consists of a determinate number of answers;*
2. *the answers in $ans(Q)$ are known and may in principle be made available to the client in order for her to choose the right one (e.g., 'multiple choice');*
3. *the client is allowed to choose from $ans(Q)$ an element that she considers to be the right answer.*

Definition 89 (Open question). *An atomic question $\langle Q, ans(Q)\rangle$ is an* open question *iff it is not a closed one.*

For instance, a question that can only be answered Yes or No is closed. The same is true of the following one: "Is the color of your tongue red, white, green, or none?". By contrast, the following is an open question: "What is the color of your tongue?". It is open because it leaves to the client the choice to give any answer she likes, for example, "fantastic". In this case, the nature, the content, and the range of admissible answers is left *open*. Answers to open questions may lead the physician astray and out of her medical knowledge into speculations about the patient's suffering.

Definition 90 (Questionnaire: closed and open). *A questionnaire is a set of $n \geq 1$ questions. It is said to be a* closed questionnaire *iff it comprises only closed questions; an* open questionnaire, *otherwise.*

The following example illustrates a closed questionnaire in which the right answers are to be ticked:

1.	Gender:	female	male	
2.	Marital status:	unmarried	married	divorced	widowed
3.	Do you have headaches?	no	weakly	moderately	severely
4.	Childhood diseases:	none	scarlet	smallpox	measles
	etc. ...	...	...	...	...

By contrast, an open questionnaire contains at least one open question, which has no available set of predetermined, admissible answers. For instance, if the above questionnaire is continued by adding the following questions, we obtain an open questionnaire consisting of 4 closed and 4 open questions:

5. When did your chest pain occur for the first time?
6. What do you feel when I now press on your abdomen?
7. A blood count is taken. The result is ...
8. An ECG is recorded. The result is ...
etc. ...

As was stated above, ordinary clinical reasoning may be viewed as a question-answering game between the physician or other health care personnel involved, on the one hand; and the patient as a black box, on the other. The course of the game may be conceived of as a path through a complex questionnaire, where clinical reasoning constitutes a pathfinding endeavor. This perspective comes from interpreting the set of all questions the physician addresses to the patient, as a questionnaire. The physician's knowledge serves as the source of her questionnaire; and her reasoning methodology, if she has any, guides her through the jungle of its questions. This view brings with it several philosophical and methodological consequences which we will study in what follows.

Dynamic, branching questionnaires

Clinical reasoning will be conceived as the implementation of a dynamic, branching clinical questionnaire. This new concept will be introduced in the following two sections:

▷ branching questionnaires
▷ dynamic, branching clinical questionnaires.

Branching questionnaires

A branching questionnaire is not a fixed questionnaire in the usual sense of this term and does not consist of explicit, verbal, or written questions that would require explicit, verbal, or written answers. Rather, it is the physician's *procedural knowledge,* i.e., her more or less ordered expert knowledge on how to proceed with her patient. Our aim is to inquire into the methodology and philosophy of applying this know-how. To this end, we distinguish between *unstructured* and *structured* questionnaires. A branching questionnaire is a particular type of structured questionnaire explained below.

In a clinical encounter, the number of questions posed to the patient is usually greater than 1. In the light of the theory of testing, the set of all questions posed to the patient may be viewed as a macro-test such that the outcome of the test depends on the order in which the constituent micro-questions are asked. For example, if we have a suspicion that a patient such as Mr. Elroy Fox might have a problem with the functioning of his heart, it makes a difference in what order we ask him the following:

1. Do you become short of breath when climbing stairs?
2. An exercise ECG is recorded,
3. Coronary angiography is performed.

If question 3 is posed before question 1, it will be useless and even ridiculous to ask the patient, after this costly and highly informative examination, whether he becomes short of breath when climbing stairs. The reason is that the goal of question 1 is to acquire evidence for or against the hypothesis that the patient might have a narrowing of his coronary arteries. But when asked after step 3, its result will not change the value of the pictorial information obtained by coronary angiography. Thus, question 3 asked before question 1 renders the latter completely uninformative and irrelevant. It would therefore be useful if the set of questions to be asked could be arranged in a particular *sequence*, i.e., could be conceived as an ordered set of the type $\langle Q_1, Q_2, Q_3, \ldots \rangle$ such that each Q_i is a question, and the subscripts 1, 2, 3, ... indicate the order of their use. Our goal is to find a suitable concept to do so.

An *unstructured questionnaire* is a questionnaire whose questions may be asked or answered in an arbitrary order. The answer to a particular question does not have any influence on the order in which subsequent questions are posed. Any question of the questionnaire may succeed any other without increasing or decreasing the information the entire questionnaire would yield. For example, when applying to a city authority for a passport, it is all the same to the authority whether their questionnaire asks about the date of your birth first and then asks about your name and the color of your eyes, or vice versa. A questionnaire of this type is obviously amorphous.

In a clinical encounter, a question is not an end in itself. It serves as a decision aid. The information a patient provides by answering a doctor's questions, has an impact on the doctor's response by way of a decision, as the expected outcome of that decision is valued conditional on the information provided by the patient. Put another way, the *expected value* of a decision to be made on the basis of a question, depends on the actual answer to the question. For example, when a blind fellow asks a pedestrian the question "is the traffic light for pedestrians green?", each of the two possible answers {yes, no} will influence his decision to cross the street or to stop because in each case his decision to act assumes a particular expected value. The *informational yield* of a question in a questionnaire is the impact that the answer to it will exert on the decision planned on the basis of *preceding* questions. When our above-mentioned blind fellow learns the current state of the traffic light by touching the traffic light post, the verbal question "is the traffic light for pedestrians green?" that he might ask a pedestrian, becomes informationally irrelevant because it is now void of any informational yield. In an amorphus, unstructured questionnaire the order of its questions does not influence their informational yield and may be changed without any loss or gain.

By contrast, in a *structured questionnaire* the questions are ordered as they are interactive such that their order is relevant to their informational yield. If we change their order, some of them may lose their informational yield and become informationally empty. For instance, we have already pointed out above that in a patient such as Elroy Fox it would be unreasonable if his coronary angiography preceded the recording of an exercise ECG or the question of whether he becomes short of breath when climbing stairs. That is, regarding the following three questions:

a   perform a coronary angiography,
b. record an exercise ECG
c   do you become short of breath when climbing stairs?

the performance order $\langle c, b, a \rangle$ should be preferred to $\langle a, b, c \rangle$, for test a is much more costly and risky than the cheap and harmless tests b and c, whereas the latter two may render test a unnecessary if they do not uncover any abnormalities. This example demonstrates what it means to say that in an ordered questionnaire a test result is relevant to the significance and performance order of the remainder. The constituent questions of such a questionnaire are asked in an order that is determined by the answers given to the preceding questions. For these reasons, it is advisable to array the questions that will be directed to the black box, i.e., the patient, and to fix in advance how the outcome of a test will influence the subsequent course of action. The act of ordering will lend a structure to the questionnaire.

To better understand what specific structure an ordered clinical questionnaire should have, we will consider an example. First we must be aware that if Q is any question, its answer set $ans(Q)$ always has $n > 1$ elements because the smallest answer set has two elements, i.e., {yes, no}. The individual answers in an answer set may be symbolized by $a_1, a_2, \ldots, a_n$ such that the answer set is, in general, of the form $ans(Q) = \{a_1, a_2, \ldots, a_n\}$ with $n \geq 2$. For instance, the question "Do you become short of breath when climbing stairs?" may be answered in at least four different ways:

a_1 = No
a_2 = weakly
a_3 = moderately
a_4 = severely.

Thus, we have $ans($"Do you become short of breath when climbing stairs?"$)$ = {No, weakly, moderately, severely} = {a_1, a_2, a_3, a_4}. Let $\langle Q, ans(Q)\rangle$ be an atomic question as above. The question Q is representable as a node from which the elements of its answer set $ans(Q)$ originate pointing in different directions (Figures 49–50).

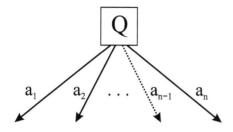

Fig. 49. An atomic question $\langle Q, ans(Q)\rangle$ with Q being its body and $ans(Q) = \{a_1, a_2, \ldots, a_n\}$ the set of its possible, admissible answers. The answers point in different directions like the branches of a tree. Figure 50 illustrates a concrete example

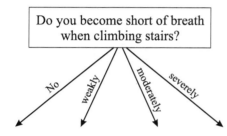

Fig. 50. An atomic question $\langle Q, ans(Q)\rangle$ with $ans(Q) = \{$No, weakly, moderately, severely$\}$

After having asked 'the black box' a question Q and having received an answer $a_i \in ans(Q)$, the doctor never remains passive. She always reacts to the answer in some way. Depending on its informational yield, her reaction will be a particular new question, that is, a new test, because she still aims at solving 'the riddle' in the black box. Her situation is comparable to that of someone who in a strange city asks a pedestrian directions to the train station, and is told:

a. Go straight on until the next traffic light for pedestrians;
b. if it is red, stop. If it is yellow, press the button;
c. if it is green, cross the street;
d. etc.

Depending on the conditions at the next traffic light for pedestrians, the visitor will stop, press the button, or cross the street. In a clinical encounter, the physician acts likewise. She receives from the black box a particular answer to her question. Depending on the information the answer conveys, i.e., the information on 'whether the traffic light is red, yellow, or green', she acts accordingly. This new action consists in asking the next question. Recall, for example, that in the dialogue with the patient Elroy Fox above in Table 4 on page 281, she asked the patient question No. 27:

Question 27: Do you become short of breath when climbing stairs?

and received the answer "No". If the patient had responded Yes, the doctor's reaction would have been something like the question "weakly, moderately, or severely?" instead of the question "are you a smoker?" that she actually has posed (Figure 51).

Our examples demonstrate that the clinical encounter (interaction, decision-making) may be construed as a question-answering game between the physician and the patient in a growing question-answering network. The game takes its course through the Q nodes of the network. Depending on what answer a_{i_j} to a question Q_i the doctor actually receives from the black box when passing through that node, she uses the corresponding edge a_{i_j} as an access path to arrive at the next accessible node Q_k, and so on. This idea may be elaborated on in the following way to make clinical reasoning amenable to graph-theoretical tools (see page 114).

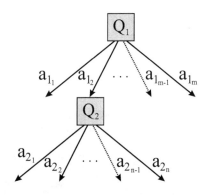

Fig. 51. The answer a_{1_2} that the black box has emitted evokes a new question, Q_2. Another answer, e.g., a_{1_m}, would have evoked another question than Q_2. See below

In the doctor-patient interaction, there are a number of different ways $a_1, a_2, \ldots, a_n \in ans(Q_i)$ to answer a question Q_i the physician asks. Each possible answer $a_{i_j} \in ans(Q_i)$ points to a particular question Q_{i+1} that may follow if this answer is emitted by the black box. The two questions, Q_i and Q_{i+1}, are interpreted as two adjacent nodes of a graph connected by the answer $a_{i_j} \in ans(Q_i)$ as a directed edge between them. The answer that is actually given by the patient, evokes a new question to which it leads as an edge. Since in this way the question-answering game assumes the structure of a branching tree, it will be referred to as a *branching questionnaire* (Figure 52).

A number of $n > 1$ questions $Q_1, \ldots, Q_n$ asked successively is referred to as a sequence of questions and written $\langle Q_1, \ldots, Q_n \rangle$ with Q_1 being the initial, and Q_n being the terminal question that concludes the dialogue. In order for the dialogue to really come to an end, the terminal question must remain unanswered. Otherwise, a new question would be evoked and the sequence would steadily grow. Below it will be interpreted as the final action of the physician terminating the clinical encounter.

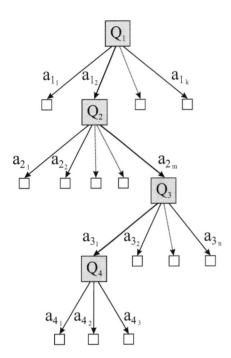

Fig. 52. A branching questionnaire is a collection of closed, atomic questions such that each actual answer to a question evokes a particular, unique question. It may therefore be represented as a directed graph. Its nodes are bodies of atomic questions (tests), and its edges are possible answers to those questions consisting of the patient's reactions (test results, findings, signs, etc.). In the present figure, the root node Q_1 represents the initial question. Each of the subsequent questions Q_2–Q_4 is a test evoked by the answer the black box actually emits. The initial question, $Q_1 =$ "How may I help you?", posed by the doctor has an answer set, $ans(Q_1)$, that may contain several millions of admissible answers. The answer that the patient actually gives, is $a_{1_2} =$ "I have been having sporadic chest pain and also an increasing physical weakness for some time". It terminates on the question node $Q_2 =$ "Please tell me more about your chest pain". The patient's answer to this new question is $a_{2_m} =$ "Well, it is pressure-like, Doctor", and so on. See the doctor-patient dialogue in Table 3 on page 277 and its continuation in Table 4 on page 281

Definition 91 (Composite question). ξ *is a composite question iff there are* $Q_1, \ldots, Q_n$ *such that:*

    1. $\xi = \langle Q_1, \ldots, Q_n \rangle$ with $n > 1$,

    2. Each Q_i in $\langle Q_1, \ldots, Q_n \rangle$ is a closed atomic question of the form $\langle Q_i, ans(Q_i) \rangle$,

    3. Each question Q_{i-1} with $1 \leq i \leq n$ has in its answer set an answer that terminates on the subsequent question Q_i.

Figure 52 above provides an example which represents the tetradic composite question $\langle Q_1, \ldots, Q_4 \rangle$. More generally, a sequence $\langle Q_1, \ldots, Q_n \rangle$ is called an *n-adic composite question,* or an *n*-adic question for short, if there are $n > 1$ closed atomic questions $\langle Q_1, ans(Q_1) \rangle, \ldots, \langle Q_n, ans(Q_n) \rangle$ such that for each question Q_{i-1} there is an answer a_{i-1_k} that terminates on question Q_i. Note that a composite question is *a* question, even though a complex one. We are now in a position to define a branching questionnaire as a directed, acyclic graph consisting of a network of n-adic composite questions in the following way:

Definition 92 (Branching questionnaire). *ξ is a branching questionnaire iff there are $\boldsymbol{Q}$ and $ANS(\boldsymbol{Q})$ such that:*

1. *$\xi = \langle \boldsymbol{Q}, ANS(\boldsymbol{Q}) \rangle$,*
2. *$\langle \boldsymbol{Q}, ANS(\boldsymbol{Q}) \rangle$ is a directed, acyclic graph,*
3. *There is a set of n-adic composite questions of the form $\langle \langle Q_1, ans(Q_1) \rangle,$ ..., $\langle Q_n, ans(Q_n) \rangle \rangle$ such that $\boldsymbol{Q}$, the set of nodes of the graph, is the set of their bodies, i.e., $\boldsymbol{Q} = \{Q_1, Q_2, \ldots, Q_n\}$,*
4. *$ANS(\boldsymbol{Q})$, the set of edges, is the union of the answer sets of those bodies.*

The question-answering game played by the physician and the patient in the clinical encounter may be conceived of as a dialogue conducted in a branching clinical questionnaire of the form above. However, if such a questionnaire is to be useful, it must be a *dynamic* one.

Dynamic, branching clinical questionnaires

As emphasized above, in a structured questionnaire the answers given to the preceding questions are relevant to the significance and performance order of the remaining tests. This characteristic brings with it that the order of questions in a braching questionnaire to ask after time t is a dynamic one and depends on the data available at time t about 'the patient in the black box'. A dynamic questionnaire of this type concerned with clinical affairs will be referred to as a *dynamic, branching clinical questionnaire*.

Due to both the vast number of clinical questions that can be asked and the huge number of the admissible answers to them terminating on other questions, there are innumerable composite questions in a dynamic, branching clinical questionnaire. By considering the large set of all possible *initial questions* which may initiate the doctor-patient dialogue, the complexity of the dynamic, branching clinical questionnaire will become apparent. It is impossible to represent it on a two-dimensional book page. As a graph, it includes all possible *clinical paths* one of which the clinical reasoning will actually take in an individual clinical encounter.

8.1.3 Clinical Paths

The dynamic, branching clinical questionnaire will be referred to simply as the *clinical questionnaire*. By the term "clinical path" we understand the route that clinical decision-making *actually takes* in the clinical questionnaire. Since the way that leads from the initial patient data to a final diagnostic-therapeutic decision, may be considered such a *clinical path*, this concept will be constructed in what follows. It will be instrumental in developing our theory of clinical practice.

As was noted above, the clinical questionnaire is representable as a directed, acyclic graph. To this end, we need only to interpret a node Q of the graph as a question (test) that the physician asks the patient, whereas the edges originating from the node are the admissible answers to that question, i.e., the answer set $ans(Q)$. Figures 49–53 illustrate this idea.

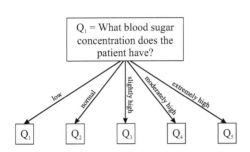

Fig. 53. A small question-answering game as a directed acyclic graph representing the inquiry into the blood sugar level of the patient. Admissible answers are: $ans(Q_1) = \{$low, normal, slightly high, moderately high, extremely high$\}$. For the interpretation of these linguistic values, see Figure 67 on page 613. Each answer leads to a subsequent, specific question Q_i

Figures 49–53 demonstrate that the admissible answers to a question Q evoke new questions and tests, one of which the physician will conduct depending on the answer she actually receives from the patient. This reconstruction is by no means artificial. As we shall see below, each question in the clinical questionnaire the doctor asks the black box, is a clinical *action* she performs in the diagnostic-therapeutic process. Thus, each node of the graph is a clinical action that generates some information about the patient as a black box. From a proximal to distal route in the graph the information *is connected* with subsequent actions and information, and so on. Each stretch of the route starts at a node and terminates at another node. The latter may also be a terminal node consisting of the physician's farewell "See you again!". By compiling all of the partial graphs of which the clinical questionnaire consists, we obtain a huge, complex, directed, acyclic graph a segment of which is depicted in Figure 54.

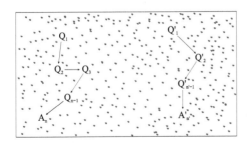

Fig. 54. The directed graph of the entire clinical questionnaire. Two paths are exemplified therein. Each of them leads from the initial action of the doctor to a corresponding final node, i.e., the final actions A_n and $A'_{n'}$, respectively

At this point in our discussion, we may now introduce the notion of a *clinical path*. In the graph-theoretical terminology sketched on page 114, a clinical path is simply a path in a clinical questionnaire. Apparently there exist a large number of clinical paths from one action node to another, distal action node (Figure 55).

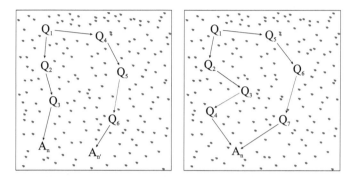

Fig. 55. In the first graph on the left-hand side, two different paths lead from the same initial question Q_1 to two different final actions. The second graph on the right-hand side shows two different paths that in two different patients lead from the same initial question Q_1 to the same action

For example, let the node 23 be the doctor's action consisting of the question No. 23 in Table 4 on page 281: "Is your chest pain brought on by exertion?". This action node in the directed graph is connected with a number of possible actions as its consequences. Depending on the answer that the doctor receives from the patient, one of these consequent actions will be taken, and so on. Thus, a node induces an actual path from among the huge number of potential paths that originate from that node. Now several problems arise. For instance, what is the length of a clinical path? Is it the number of the edges that constitute the path? Is it the time required to go along this path? Or does it consist of the benefits, damages, and financial costs it causes? Do we have to always use the shortest path that in the diagnostic-therapeutic process would lead us from the initial patient data to a final decision? How do we have to search for and to find in the tangle of the branching, clinical questionnaire the best clinical path from initial patient data to diagnosis, and from diagnosis to therapy? Is it possible to build a methodology of clinical pathfinding? This is the problem we shall be dealing with in what follows to explore whether and how the doctor can avoid such wrong routes as occurred in Mr. Elroy Fox's case report in Section 8.1.1 on page 279.

8.1.4 The Clinical Process

The doctor-patient interaction in clinical practice starts with the patient's initial problem that we have termed "initial patient data", or *initial data* for short. For example, in the case report on the patient Elroy Fox we had the following initial data:

a. increasing adynamia,
b. night sweat,
c. feeling of pressure in the left chest,
d. pain in the same region,
e. paroxysmal tachycardia.

An ideal doctor-patient interaction that aims at resolving such an initial problem, will search for *the best clinical path* in the dynamic, branching clinical questionnaire. The search will be referred to by the following terms that may be used interchangeably:

- Clinical judgment
- clinical reasoning
- diagnostic-therapeutic reasoning
- clinical decision-making
- diagnostic-therapeutic decision-making
- the clinical process.

These terms are synonymous and designate one and the same process in which the physician tries to resolve the patient's initial problem by answering the question: "What is the case and what shall I do?". The process will be referred to as *the clinical process*. Traditionally, it is partitioned into anamnesis, diagnosis, prognosis, therapy, and prevention.

The clinical process represents the emergence of a concrete clinical path that winds through the jungle of the branching clinical questionnaire, i.e., a path used by the doctor and her patient in moving toward the yet unknown goal of their encounter. We shall unfold this process in order to uncover some fundamental issues in the philosophy of clinical practice. Our requirement that the graph of the clinical questionnaire be a closed and structured one, is of course an ideal that serves to reduce diagnostic-therapeutic idiosyncrasies and errors.

The closedness of the clinical questionnaire means (see Definition 90 on page 287), first, that it contains only closed questions according to our Definition 88 on page 287. It prevents those answers, i.e., 'reactions of the black box', that would be differently understood and interpreted by different doctors. For example, when the patient is asked an open question such as the following one:

- What additional symptoms do you, or did you, have?

more often than not she will leave out some particular symptoms because the language she uses to describe them is insufficient. For the same reason, she may also end up exaggerating or obscuring her symptoms. Therefore, a closed question of the following type should be preferred to an open one:

- Which one of the symptoms *A, B, C, D* do you, or did you, have in addition?

In this way, the risk of bias by both the patient and the doctor is minimized. The closedness of the clinical questionnaire means, second, the following: In the clinical process, each step that leads from a reaction X of the patient to an action Z of the doctor, i.e., the association of a particular, directed edge X with a particular node Z of the clinical graph, is based on an *imperative* of the form:

- If the patient's condition is X and you want to know whether Y is the case, then do Z.

Or more generally:

- If the patient's condition is $X_1, X_2, \ldots, X_m$ and you want to know whether $Y_1, \ldots, Y_n$ is the case, then do $Z_1, Z_2, \ldots, Z_q$.

For example,

- If the patient has fever, cough, and dyspnea,
- and you want to know whether she has community acquired pneumonia,
- then examine her chest and search for altered breath sounds and rales and perform chest radiography and search for opaque areas in both lungs.

The clinical process consists of a multitude of such single steps based on imperative *action rules*. It aims at finding the best clinical path to manage the health affairs of an individual patient. It may therefore be viewed as *clinical pathfinding*. The analysis and reconstruction of this clinical pathfinding is the subject of our discussion after the following summary.

8.1.5 Summary

The clinical encounter starts with the patient's initial problem A and eventually enables a solution or final decision B. The attempt to arrive at this final decision we have termed the clinical process of pathfinding such that the path leads from A to B. The space where the pathfinding occurs, is the dynamic, branching clinical questionnaire. This questionnaire has been conceived as a directed, acyclic graph that represents the procedural medical knowledge of the physician. An edge of the graph is constituted by the information that the physician obtains about the patient's health condition as an answer to a question (examination, test). It connects the question (examination, test) with the next one that is necessitated thereby. This process of knowledge-based action selection will be analyzed and discussed in the remainder of the present Chapter 8.

8.2 Anamnesis and Diagnosis

8.2.0 Introduction

As noted above, the clinical process of pathfinding is traditionally partitioned into anamnesis, diagnosis, prognosis, therapy, and prevention. We consider the taking of the patient history, i.e., *anamnesis,* as part of the diagnostic process referred to as *diagnostics.* It will therefore be integrated into our analyses and discussions on diagnostics. Diagnostics starts with the clinical interview considered in preceding sections. We shall continue and detail our considerations in this section, which consists of the following parts:

8.2.1   The Clinical Goal
8.2.2   The Logical Structure of Medical Statements
8.2.3   Action Indication and Contra-Indication
8.2.4   Differential Indication
8.2.5   The Computability of Differential Indication
8.2.6   The Logical Structure of Diagnosis
8.2.7   The Syntax of Diagnosis
8.2.8   The Semantics of Diagnosis
8.2.9   The Pragmatics of Diagnosis
8.2.10   The Methodology of Diagnostics
8.2.11   The Logic of Diagnostics
8.2.12   The Epistemology of Diagnostics
8.2.13   The Relativity of Diagnosis.

This plan indicates that we shall study diagnosis and diagnostics from multiple perspectives to present our theory of the relativity of clinical diagnosis. We start by considering the goal of the clinical practice.

8.2.1 The Clinical Goal

Medical information technology, which goes under such different labels as "medical informatics", "medical computer science", and "artificial intelligence in medicine", includes as a subdiscipline a new field concerned with the logic, methodology, and technology of clinical judgment. Since the 1970s, this new science has led to the production of computer programs sophisticated enough to compete with the clinical reasoning competence of expert physicians. These computer programs are used to support doctors' clinical decision-making. They have therefore come to be known as 'computer-aided medical decision support systems', 'medical knowledge-based systems', or 'medical expert systems' and the like. Under the umbrella name 'medical artificial intelligence' they are continually invading clinical practice, including hospitals. We shall come back to this issue on page 784.[60]

---

[60] An expert system ('knowledge-based system', 'computer-aided decision-support system') is a computer program that is capable of providing solutions to specific

Although most physicians are aware of the 60% reliability limit of their clinical judgment, they don't believe that medical expert systems will increase their chances of a correct clinical decision. Their doubts are reinforced by the practical shortcomings of current expert-system techniques. Like the source of many doctors' diagnostic failures, these shortcomings are mainly due to the lack of a theory and methodology of clinical reasoning. A direct consequence of this is that most medical expert-system researchers hold an inadequate view of clinical reasoning. Two notions that are crucial to an adequate understanding of clinical reasoning, are *indication* and *differential indication*. Their central role is widely overlooked both by doctors and clinical expert-system researchers. However, in order to develop a successful theory of clinical practice and of knowledge-based clinical expert systems, we must first have a logic and methodology of indication and differential indication. The present section suggests a framework for discussing the basic problems of this task.

To begin with, we may recall that the subjects the physician is dealing with, are sick persons and not symptoms, findings, diseases, or treatments. Since sick persons, different than physical devices, are moral agents governed by internal and external moral values and norms, clinical judgment is not comparable to trouble-shooting in physical devices. Therefore, the theories on trouble-shooting in physical devices that have been proposed by artificial intelligence researchers and that are also spreading in medicine, cannot provide the foundations needed for our task. Raymond Reiter's acclaimed "theory of diagnosis from first principles" as a theory of trouble-shooting is no exception (Reiter 1987; de Kleer et al., 1992).

The starting-point of clinical judgment is a particular person, denoted "p", who is ill or believes herself to be ill, and thus presents a non-empty set of initial data consisting of some problems, complaints, symptoms, and signs. Let us call this initial data, patient data set D_1 such that $D_1 = \{\delta_1, \ldots, \delta_m\}$ with $m \geq 1$ and each δ_i being a sentence that provides any information on the patient p. For instance, D_1 may be one of the following sets of sentences:

- {p is a male of about 49, p is complaining of sporadic chest pain};
- {p is a 12-year-old boy, p is bleeding from the nose};
- {p has just been involved in a car accident, p is unconscious, p's heart rate is 124 per minute, p's blood pressure is 80/60 mm Hg};
- {p has undergone gastrectomy last year, p is complaining of acute pain in the upper left abdomen}.

---

problems in a given domain, such as cardiology, at a level of performance comparable to that of domain experts. It consists of (i) a knowledge component referred to as its *knowledge base,* and (ii) a problem-solving component. The latter is called an *inference engine* because it uses some logic to reason and to draw conclusions from the knowledge base and available information about a current problem. The construction of expert systems has come to be known as *knowledge engineering.* For details, see, e.g., (Buchanan and Shortliffe, 1984; Giarratano and Riley, 2004; Kendal and Creen, 2007).

It is commonly assumed that clinical judgment primarily aims at finding a *diagnosis* which will explain why D_1 occurred. For various reasons, however, this widespread opinion must be considered a metapractical misconception about the nature and purpose of clinical practice (Sadegh-Zadeh, 1979). A more realistic and fruitful view is provided by treating D_1 as a clinical problem that provokes a problem-solving process, where the solution aimed at is *not* a diagnosis, but rather a remedial action, including advice and a *wait and watch* recommendation, which is meant to ameliorate the patient's present suffering and make her problem disappear. This clinical goal may be termed *praxiognosis*, i.e., recognizing *what should be done* for this patient, in contradistinction to diagnosis that says "what is wrong" with this patient. That the search for and the optimization of the remedial action often requires additional information about the patient, part of which may be termed diagnosis, is an accidental feature of the praxiognostic process due to the particular course the history of medicine has taken since about 1750. It could have been otherwise (see Section 8.3.1 on page 349).

The term "praxiognosis", from the Greek $\pi\rho\alpha\xi\iota\varsigma$ (praxis) and $\gamma\nu\tilde{\omega}\sigma\iota\varsigma$ (gnosis) for *cognition* and *recognition*, means the same as the Latin term "differential indication" briefly introduced on page 310. Our postulate of praxiognosis above, i.e., differential indication, becomes plausible by considering the truism that if there were only one unique remedial action for all kinds of patients, no problem-solving and thus no diagnosis would be necessary. Every patient could enjoy that unique remedial action without regard to the nature and causes of her problem. But unfortunately, the therapeutic inventory of medicine offers a variety of therapeutic measures, say $T_1, \ldots, T_n$ with $n > 1$, including the empty action 'doing nothing'. And each of these numerous therapies may be viewed as a potential remedy for every patient with the initial data set D_1. The problem-solving task is to select from among the large therapeutic inventory $\{T_1, \ldots, T_n\}$ a minimum subset $\{T'_1, \ldots, T'_m\}$ that is considered the best solution to the problem D_1 (Figure 56).

The initial patient data set D_1 provides us with a root problem, and the appropriate, minimum remedial set $\{T'_1, \ldots, T'_m\} \subseteq \{T_1, \ldots, T_n\}$ we are searching for, is the solution goal of the problem-solving process provoked by D_1. The entirety of all possible paths from the root problem to the unknown solution goal $\{T'_1, \ldots, T'_m\}$ may be conceived of as a structured, closed, branching clinical questionnaire discussed previously. The patient is the black box containing her organism, illness experience, personality, pathogenetically relevant factors, environment, and history. We have the opportunity of asking the box any closed question, e.g., any anamnestic question we may ask, any physical examination and laboratory test we are allowed to perform, etc. Through its responses to our closed questions the object in the black box guides us through the labyrinth of the candidate clinical paths to the desired solution goal.

Clinical judgment thus presents itself as a path-searching, or pathfinding, endeavor based on a question-answering and information-producing process, and controlled by the physician and her clinical questionnaire. The process is

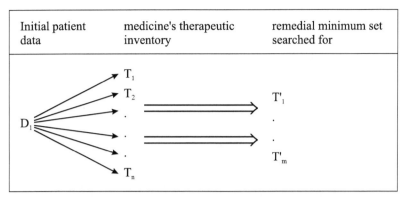

Initial patient data	medicine's therapeutic inventory	remedial minimum set searched for

Fig. 56. The initial patient data set D_1 points to a large subset of the total set $\{T_1, \ldots, T_n\}$ of available treatments ("symptomatic therapy"). Each element of set $\{T_1, \ldots, T_n\}$ is a potential remedy for the patient. The non-trivial problem to be solved is to find out which one of the trivial paths $\longrightarrow$ is a solution path $\Longrightarrow$ leading to the appropriate, minimum, remedial action set $\{T'_1, \ldots, T'_m\} \subseteq \{T_1, \ldots, T_n\}$. The diagnosis is only part of the solution path

initiated by the initial patient data set D_1 which provokes the first question and test, i.e., the initial clinical action A_1 the physician takes, and is terminated by her final action A_n. To formulate the problem, the microstructure of this clinical process will first be reconstructed (Sadegh-Zadeh, 1977b, 1994):

Any particular instance of clinical judgment is initiated at a particular instant of time, t_1, and is terminated at a later instant of time, t_n. A doctor d at t_1 starts inquiring into whether or not the patient p presenting the data set D_1, suffers from any disorder and needs any treatment. The total period of this inquiry, $[t_1, t_n]$, can be partitioned into a finite sequence of discrete sub-periods $t_1, t_2, t_3, \ldots, t_n$. Proceeding from the root data set D_1 at t_1, the physician chooses from among *all possible actions* she might consider, a particular set of actions, A_1, and performs it. This action set A_1 may be any verbal questions she asks the patient, a diagnostic inference she makes, a particular physical examination, laboratory test, treatment or the like. For instance, A_1 may be one of the following action sets:

- {how long has this problem been going on?};
- {is there any genetic disease in your family?};
- {measure p's body temperature, determine her heart rate};
- {an ECG should be recorded first, followed by postero-anterior chest radiography and Coomb's test};
- {I believe that p suffers from systemic lupus erythematosus};
- {give the patient a nitroglycerin tablet of 0.3 mg}.

The outcome of the action set A_1 the physician performs, is some information about the patient she obtains. This new information changes the original data set D_1 to data set D_2 at t_2, e.g., to the set $\{p$ is a male of about 49, p is complaining of sporadic chest pain, p's body temperature is 38 °C, p's heart rate is 102 per minute$\}$.

Proceeding from D_2 at t_2, a second set of actions, A_2, is chosen and performed whose result changes the preceding data set D_2 to data set D_3 at t_3, and so forth until a final action set A_n is performed at time t_n terminating the clinical process.

We have thus partitioned the whole period $[t_1, t_n]$ of clinical decision-making into the discrete sub-periods $t_1, t_2, t_3, \ldots, t_n$ such that the sequence of patient data sets available in these temporal granules is $D_1, D_2, \ldots, D_n$, and the corresponding action sets performed are $A_1, A_2, \ldots, A_n$, respectively. Clinical judgment may now be viewed as a linear clinical path of the form depicted in Figure 57.

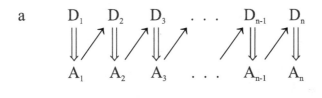

$$ \text{b} \qquad D_1 \Rightarrow A_1 \rightarrow D_2 \Rightarrow A_2 \rightarrow \ldots \rightarrow D_n \Rightarrow A_n $$

Fig. 57. The clinical path (the solution path). Figure a shows how each data set D_i provokes a corresponding action set A_i to be performed. Figure b demonstrates the linearity of the process

The path consists of a finite sequence of data-based selection of the actions $A_1, A_2, \ldots, A_n$, on the one hand; and successively building the patient data sets $D_1, D_2, \ldots, D_n$, on the other, which are then used in identifying and selecting the corresponding actions. A double arrow in Figure 57 says that the data set D_i leads the clinical decision-maker to the action set A_i, whereas a simple arrow represents the A_i-mediated acquisition of the data set D_{i+1}. By reconstructing this sequence of data-based action selection in the language of our *branching clinical questionnaire* concept presented in Section 8.1.2, we shall recognize that the action sets $A_1, A_2, \ldots, A_n$ the physician performs at $t_1, t_2, t_3, \ldots, t_n$ are the questions she asks the patient, and the data sets $D_1, D_2, \ldots, D_n$ are the respective answers she receives. This question-answering game creates a *clinical path* that represents the route the clinical process in an individual case has actually taken through the jungle of the branching clinical questionnaire (Figure 58).

The basic idea above may be formalized in the following way. It is advantageous in clinical decision-making to represent patient data with the aid of *linguistic variables* and *numerical variables*. For example, *gender* may

Fig. 58. The same clinical path as in Figure 57 represented within the clinical questionnaire. This figure demonstrates that the clinical process takes its path through the clinical questionnaire by an *n*-adic composite question $\langle A_1, A_2, \ldots, A_n \rangle$. Otherwise put, clinical judgment as *praxiognostics* proceeds by asking an *n*-adic question to recognize "what shall I do?". The action sequence $A_1, A_2, \ldots, A_n$ consists of the bodies of the composite question $\langle A_1, A_2, \ldots, A_n \rangle$ directed to the black box. The data sequence $D_1, D_2, \ldots, D_n$ represents the corresponding answers each of which terminates on a particular action $A_i \in \langle A_1, A_2, \ldots, A_n \rangle$. The terminal question, A_n, of the composite question remains unanswered. It is simply the closing word that the doctor says to the patient, e.g., "see you next week!"

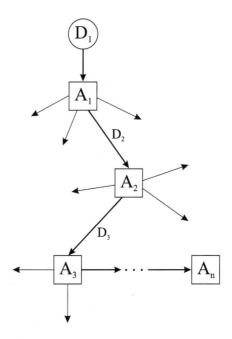

be conceived of as a linguistic variable that takes values such as *male, female,* and *hermaphroditic,* i.e., with the term set $T(\text{gender}) = \{\text{male, female, hermaphroditic}\}$. Likewise, *heart rate* is a numerical variable that takes numerical values between 0 and 300 and more. Using such variables, a statement about the patient such as "the patient is about 49 years old" can be formulated as an ordered pair $\langle \text{age, about 49 years} \rangle$. Thus, patient data may be represented as ordered pairs of attribute-value type of the form $\langle A, B \rangle$ where A is a linguistic or numerical variable (representing an 'attribute'), and B is the value it takes in the patient. Here is an example:

$\langle$gender, male$\rangle$	$\equiv$ statement δ_1
$\langle$age, about 49 years$\rangle$	$\equiv$ statement δ_2
$\langle$sporadic chest pain, moderate$\rangle$	$\equiv$ statement δ_3
$\langle$night sweat, intensive$\rangle$	$\equiv$ statement δ_4
$\langle$heart rate, 102 per minute$\rangle$	$\equiv$ statement δ_5

In special analyses, the core data structure above may be supplemented by a variety of additional dimensions, e.g., by adding patient name and time period to yield temporal quadruples of object-time-attribute-value type such as, for example, $\langle$Elroy Fox, February 20; night sweat, intensive$\rangle$. We will symbolize:

- statements describing singular data by $\delta, \delta_1, \delta_2, \ldots$ to connote data;
- sets of such data statements by $D_1, D_2, \ldots$ to connote *data set;*
- statements describing single actions by $\alpha, \alpha_1, \alpha_2, \ldots$ to connote *action;*
- sets of such action statements by $A_1, A_2, \ldots$ to connote *action set.*

The set of all data patients may present in the course of clinical decision-making, the *data space*, will be denoted by $\mathfrak{D}$. The physician's *action space* comprising all clinically relevant and possible actions she may consider, will be termed $\mathfrak{A}$. 'Clinically relevant actions' means methods of clinical inquiry in history taking, diagnosis, prognosis, therapy, and prevention. Note that the omission of an action that is described by a statement α is also an action, i.e., the negation $\neg\alpha$, and is thus included in the action space $\mathfrak{A}$. The powerset of a set X is written $powerset(X)$. Thus we have:

$$\mathfrak{D} = \{\delta \mid \delta \text{ is an attribute-value statement about the patient}\}$$
$$\mathfrak{A} = \{\alpha \mid \alpha \text{ is a sentence describing an action the physician may consider}\}$$
$$powerset(\mathfrak{D}) = \{D \mid D \subseteq \mathfrak{D}\}$$
$$powerset(\mathfrak{A}) = \{A \mid A \subseteq \mathfrak{A}\}.$$

Succinctly stated, the basic problem in the methodology of clinical reasoning is the following question (Sadegh-Zadeh, 1977b, 77):

Basic Query: Supposing that the temporal sequence of the decision-making process is $t_1, t_2, t_3, \ldots, t_n$ with $n \geq 1$, is it possible to construct an effective procedure, e.g., an algorithm, which can be initiated at time t_1 such that when the patient data set at time t_i is $D_i \subseteq \mathfrak{D}$ with $1 \leq i \leq n$, the optimal action set $A_i \subseteq \mathfrak{A}$ can be selected unambiguously from among the action space $\mathfrak{A}$, the next data set $D_{i+1} \subseteq \mathfrak{D}$ can be built as objectively as possible, and the particular doctor d is in principle exchangeable by any doctor x? Put another way, is there a mapping:

$$f : \mathfrak{D} \mapsto \mathfrak{A}$$
$$f : \mathfrak{A} \mapsto \mathfrak{D}$$

such that f is a computable function so as to render the process of clinical judgment sketched in Figures 56–58 above a computable path-searching with:

$$f(D_i) = A_i$$
$$f(A_i) = D_{i+1}$$

and to unambiguously provide the physician in all possible clinical situations with an optimal guide for her decisions? A computable function of this type will be referred to as a computable clinical decision function, *ccdf* for short.

The good news is that the answer to the Basic Query above is Yes. This is a philosophically remarkable claim, which will be proven in what follows. To this end, the conceptual framework needed for constructing a *ccdf* will be introduced first. Note, however, that the ordered sequence of patient data sets $D_1, D_2, \ldots, D_n$ above reflects only a chronological order. They are not supposed to possess a monotonic, material relationship of the type $D_1 \subseteq D_2 \subseteq D_3 \subseteq \ldots \subseteq D_n$. Such monotonicity is never found in clinical practice. Otherwise, neither healing nor recovery could exist. Patient data change over time by changing their size as well as the truth values of their individual statements. For example, the patient has a fever right now, but she has a normal body temperature after two hours. Note, secondly, that no material distinction has been made between patient data and diagnosis. What is usually called diagnosis, may be part of any of the patient data sets $D_1, D_2, \ldots, D_n$. Thus, we shall avoid both the impracticable partition of clinical decision-making into anamnestic, diagnostic, and therapeutic phases, and the old-fashioned differentiation between anamnestic, diagnostic, and therapeutic actions.

8.2.2 The Logical Structure of Medical Statements

One of our goals is to demonstrate that the institution of clinical practice may be conceived of as *practiced morality*, and clinical research may be conceived of as *normative ethics*. We begin by considering two fundamental concepts of clinical decision-making, i.e., "indication" and "contra-indication". In studying these concepts, we will first look at the logical structure of statements used in medical reasoning. The important ones are, first:

- Singular statements such as "Elroy Fox coughs",
  i.e., coughs(Elroy Fox),
  $\equiv Pa$
- simple universal statements such as "if someone has bronchitis, then she coughs",
  i.e., for all $x, has\_bronchitis\,(x) \rightarrow coughs(x)$
  $\equiv \forall x(Px \rightarrow Qx)$
- compound universal statements such as "if a human being has bronchitis and hepatitis, then she coughs and is icteric",
  i.e., for all $x, is\_a\_human\_being\,(x) \wedge has\_bronchitis\,(x) \wedge$
  $\qquad\qquad\qquad has\_hepatitis\,(x) \rightarrow coughs(x) \wedge is\_icteric(x)$
  $\equiv \forall x(Hx \wedge Px \wedge Qx \rightarrow Rx \wedge Sx)$
- existential statements such as "some human beings have bronchitis and cough",
  i.e., there are human beings who are P and Q
  $\equiv \exists x(Hx \wedge Px \wedge Qx)$
- probability statements of all types, e.g., "the probability that someone has fever given that she has pneumonia, is 0.9",
  $\equiv p(B \,|\, A) = 0.9$

and their combinations by employing ubiquitous extensional operators such as the usual propositional connectives "not", "or", "and", etc. In dealing with statements of this type, the classical predicate logic and probability calculus are of course sufficient tools. But medical knowledge also includes, second:

- Fuzzy statements of all types, e.g., "many patients with pneumonia have fever" which cannot be handled by classical logic or probability calculus because they contain vague notions such as the fuzzy quantifier "many" in the present example. They require fuzzy logic, introduced in Chapter 30. A third type of statements are non-extensional (= intensional, *modal*) ones containing modal operators. They are studied in Chapter 27. Modal operators are ingredients of all natural languages, and thus, of medical language and knowledge too. Of particular importance in the current context are the following three *deontic operators:*

Natural language usage:	**logical names:**	**symbol:**
• may, is allowed	permission operator ("it is permitted that")	*PE*
• must, should, ought, is required	obligation operator ("it is obligatory that")	*OB*
• omit, don't do, avoid, must not	prohibition operator ("it is forbidden that")	*FO*

The acquaintance with the syntax and logic of these three operators, i.e., with deontic logic, will be presupposed in what follows (see Section 27.2 on page 927). They will be used below to explicate the notions of *"indication"*, *"contra-indication"*, and *"differential indication"*. Our analysis will demonstrate why the logic of clinical reasoning must be something beyond predicate logic, probability calculus, and fuzzy logic. To recall their use, let α be any first-order sentence. By prefixing deontic operators, we shall write $OB\alpha$, $FO\alpha$, and $PE\alpha$ to express, respectively, it is obligatory that α, it is forbidden that α, it is permitted that α. For instance, if α is the atomic sentence "the doctor records an ECG", then:

- $OB\alpha$ means: it is obligatory that the doctor records an ECG,
- $FO\alpha$ it is forbidden that the doctor records an ECG,
- $PE\alpha$ it is permitted that the doctor records an ECG.

As is obvious from their syntax, these three deontic operators refer to actions that are morally or legally obligatory, forbidden, or permitted, respectively. Using these notions, it will be shown below that not only are the two fundamental concepts of clinical practice, *indication* and *contra-indication*, essentially deontic concepts, but that all clinical actions performed by the physician are deontic actions, and further, that disease as a fundamental subject of medicine is a deontic entity. To this end, we need some formal notions and tools.

Let ∇ be a variable representing any of the three deontic operators OB, FO or PE. We write $\nabla\alpha$ to express any of the propositions $OB\alpha$, $FO\alpha$, and $PE\alpha$. If $x_1, \ldots, x_m$ are the free individual variables of a sentence β, the universal closure $\forall x_1 \forall x_2 \ldots \forall x_m \beta$ says that for all objects $x_1, \ldots, x_m$, the statement β obtains. For the sake of convenience, however, a universal statement of the form $\forall x_1 \forall x_2 \ldots \forall x_m \beta$ will be abbreviated to β omitting the cumbersome quantifier prefix $\forall x_1 \forall x_2 \ldots \forall x_m$.

8.2.3 Action Indication and Contra-Indication

In this section and the next, it will be shown that the concepts of indication and contra-indication as two fundamental tools of clinical practice are deontic concepts. From the outset, we should be aware that clinical reasoning is a knowledge-based task. It does not take place in an epistemic vacuum. More specifically, it is based on knowledge of different types and sources. Examples are anatomical, biochemical, physiological, pathophysiological, and nosological knowledge. Clinical decisions are also made on the basis of clinical-practical knowledge, which we shall briefly sketch below in order to introduce our deontic concepts of indication and contra-indication. A detailed analysis of clinical-practical knowledge will be undertaken in Sections 10.7, 15.1, and 21.5.3.

Biomedical knowledge originating from anatomy, biochemistry, physiology and similar, non-clinical sources is merely declarative and may be viewed as belonging to zoology in the widest sense. Such knowledge can be formalized and represented at the level of logic beneath that of modal logics. Pathophysiological and nosological knowledge deals with processes in human beings and will require at least temporal logic, probability theory, and fuzzy set theory. But what kind of logic does the appropriate understanding, representation, and management of *clinical* knowledge require?

Clinical knowledge deals with suffering human beings, with maladies, say diseases, and with the question of how to act in particular circumstances. It is thus anthropological knowledge with its core being diagnostic-therapeutic knowledge. In clinical textbooks, diagnostic-therapeutic knowledge concerned with a particular disease, e.g., myocardial infarction, is disseminated over different sections of a chapter. In a section entitled "symptoms and signs", the disease is described, while in another section entitled "diagnosis" the use of particular techniques such as ECG, blood tests, and the like is recommended to diagnose the disease; and still in another section on "therapy", therapeutic recommendations are put forward. A thorough, logical analysis reveals that these building blocks of diagnostic-therapeutic knowledge implicitly express complex *commitments* stating that:

$$\begin{aligned} \text{under circumstances } \delta &\equiv X \\ \text{action } \alpha \text{ should be performed or omitted} &\equiv Y. \end{aligned}$$

The implicit commitments, of which clinical knowledge in fact consists, are made explicit in Sections 10.6 and 10.7 on pages 450–457. The X component of such a commitment as above is the description of the disease or disease state δ presented in the section on 'symptoms and sings'; and the Y component is recommended either in the section on 'diagnosis' if action α is a diagnostic technique, or in the section on 'therapy' if action α is a therapeutic measure. Note that the general scheme of clinical knowledge sketched above is a conditional of the form $X \rightarrow Y$ that associates circumstances with actions.

The artificially separated presentation of its components X and Y in different sections of a textbook chapter hides the fact that by such a conditional a commitment with the following structure is being extended: Circumstance δ commits you to α. Thus, the commitment is reconstructible as a universal deontic conditional of the form:

$$\forall x_1 \forall x_2 \ldots \forall x_m \text{ If } \delta, \text{ then } \nabla \alpha$$

which, simply stated, says that if the circumstance is δ, then do, or omit, α. For instance, "if the patient complains of angina pectoris and her ECG is unknown, then record an ECG". For simplicity's sake, we will briefly formalize it as:

$$\delta \to \nabla \alpha \qquad (70)$$

omitting the quantifier prefix. The antecedent δ is an atomic or compound sentence describing symptoms, signs, findings, pathological states, any boundary conditions such as patient gender, age, her social environment, the physician's goal, etc. An example is the statement "the patient complains of angina pectoris and her ECG is unknown". The consequent, $\nabla \alpha$, is a deontic statement in which the deontic operator, ∇, is expressed by deontic phrases such as "should be performed", "is required", "must be applied", "is recommended", "do!", "omit!", "may be used", and the like. Simple examples are the following diagnostic-therapeutic commands, recommendations, or rules:

1. If the patient complains of angina pectoris and her ECG is unknown, then an ECG should be recorded.
2. When someone has acute myocardial infarction, taking an exercise ECG is forbidden.
3. In acute myocardial infarction, one may administer oxygen to the patient.

These examples demonstrate that depending on the nature of the operator ∇ in the consequent of the formula (70), we have to distinguish between sentences of the type:

- conditional obligation: $\delta \to OB\alpha$
- conditional prohibition: $\delta \to FO\alpha$
- conditional permission: $\delta \to PE\alpha$

referred to as *deontic conditionals*. For details about the notion of a deontic conditional, see Section 27.2.4 on page 935. Example 1 above is a conditional obligation; example 2 is a conditional prohibition; and example 3 is a conditional permission. A clinical indication rule is, in general, a more or less complex sentence of this type prescribing what actions are permitted, forbidden, or obligatory provided that the patient data is δ. More specifically, what is usually called a *clinical indication* rule prescribing some particular diagnostic or therapeutic measures, may be construed as a conditional obligation, $\delta \rightarrow OB\alpha$. And a *contra-indication* rule, on the other hand, may be construed as a conditional prohibition, $\delta \rightarrow FO\alpha$. The sentences δ and α in the antecedents and consequents of these rules may be of arbitrary complexity designating a set of data or actions, respectively. A profound logical and philosophical analysis of this issue has been conducted by the psychiatrist Markus Schwarz (Schwarz, 1993).[61]

Suppose a particular item of clinical knowledge contains, among other things, the following indication and contra-indication rules:

$$\delta_1 \rightarrow OB\alpha_1$$
$$\delta_2 \rightarrow OB\alpha_2$$
$$\vdots$$
$$\delta_m \rightarrow FO\alpha_m.$$

If x is a patient with the data set $\{\delta_1, \ldots, \delta_m\}$, a deontic-logical inference will yield the conclusion $\{OB\alpha_1, OB\alpha_2, \ldots, FO\alpha_m\}$ that says, action α_1 is indicated and ... and action α_m is contra-indicated. Thus, from the considerations above we may see why clinical-practical knowledge cannot be appropriately formalized and handled below the level of deontic predicate logic (see Section 27.2).

8.2.4 Differential Indication

In this section, clinical judgment will be reconstructed as a *deontic-logical* process of pathfinding for indications in the dynamic, branching clinical questionnaire discussed in Section 8.1.2 above. To enhance the expressive power of the framework, however, we shall not confine ourselves to individual deontic conditionals. Suppose there is a patient with the data set D such that:

$$D = \{\delta_1, \ldots, \delta_m\} \qquad \text{with } m \geq 1 \text{ data.}$$

Given a particular clinical knowledge base, a set-valued function f will identify from among this knowledge base a bundle of deontic rules whose antecedents match D:

$$\delta_1 \rightarrow \nabla\alpha_1$$
$$\delta_2 \rightarrow \nabla\alpha_2$$
$$\vdots$$
$$\delta_m \rightarrow \nabla\alpha_m$$

---

[61] There are considerable disagreements in the literature as to how conditional obligations, prohibitions, and permissions are to be formalized. We have conceived them as conditional sentences as above. For details, see Sections 10.6 and 27.2.4.

and will infer their consequents, $\{\nabla\alpha_1, \ldots, \nabla\alpha_m\}$. This deontic conclusion informs us about the actions $\alpha_1, \ldots, \alpha_m$ each of which, depending on the pre-fixed operator ∇, is obligatory, forbidden, or permitted in this situation. Thus, the whole procedure can be simply formalized as a set-functional relationship between the black box's, i.e., the patient's, reactions to the questions asked and the actions that are to be taken accordingly:

$$f(D) = \{\nabla\alpha_1, \ldots, \nabla\alpha_m\}. \tag{71}$$

On the basis of the available patient data D and the given clinical knowledge base, the set-valued function f selects a set of actions that are permitted, oblig-atory, or forbidden in this situation. If the operator ∇ in $\{\nabla\alpha_1, \ldots, \nabla\alpha_m\}$ is exclusively one of the three operators OB, FO, or PE, one may also conven-iently write $OB\{\alpha_1, \ldots, \alpha_m\}$, $FO\{\alpha_1, \ldots, \alpha_m\}$, or $PE\{\alpha_1, \ldots, \alpha_m\}$ to ex-press that the whole action set $\{\alpha_1, \ldots, \alpha_m\}$ is obligatory, forbidden, or per-mitted, respectively. That means:

Definition 93. *If $A = \{\alpha_1, \ldots, \alpha_m\}$ is a set of sentences, we write:*

- *$OB(A)$ instead of: $\{OB\alpha_1, \ldots, OB\alpha_m\}$*
- *$FO(A)$ instead of: $\{FO\alpha_1, \ldots, FO\alpha_m\}$*
- *$PE(A)$ instead of: $\{PE\alpha_1, \ldots, PE\alpha_m\}$.*

In the following frameworks, the set function f used in (71) above that selects the action set A, will be of particular importance. For the sake of simplicity and convenience, we may suppose that our set function is a triple of the type (72):

$$f = \left\{ \begin{array}{c} \text{a set G of goals,} \\ \text{a knowledge base KB,} \\ \text{a methodology M of applying KB} \end{array} \right\} \tag{72}$$

consisting of:

- $G \equiv$ the goals that the decision-maker, e.g., a doctor, pursues in the process of decision-making. These goals play a basic role in determining the course of decision-making;
- $KB \equiv$ a particular system of knowledge that she applies in decision-making, e.g., a cardiologic knowledge base;
- $M \equiv$ a set of methods of how to apply the knowledge base KB in decision-making to achieve the goals G, e.g., Bayes's Theorem, hypothetico-deductive approach, probabilistic-causal analysis, case-based reasoning, etc. (The term "method" derives from the Greek word $\mu\acute{\epsilon}\theta o\delta o\varsigma$ (metho-dos) meaning "way, access, pursuit".)

The methods component M may also explicitly or implicitly include, or be based upon, any particular system of classical or non-classical logic. We shall come back to this issue in Sections 8.2.10 and 8.2.13 below when analyzing the methodology and relativity of diagnosis, respectively.

Definition 94 (Decision-making frame). *ξ is a decision-making frame iff there are c, d, t, 𝔇, 𝔄, D, A, f, and ∇ such that:*

    1. $\xi = \langle c, d, t, \mathfrak{D}, \mathfrak{A}, D, A, f, \nabla \rangle$,

    2. c is a non-empty set of clients, i.e., $c = \{c_1, \ldots, c_m\}$ with $m \geq 1$,

    3. d is a non-empty set of decision-makers ('doctors'), i.e., $d = \{d_1, \ldots, d_n\}$ with $n \geq 1$, not necessarily distinct from c,

    4. t is a time period,

    5. 𝔇 is the data space, i.e., a set of statements about c's possible states,

    6. 𝔄 is d's action space at t, i.e., the set of all possible actions d may take,

    7. $\langle \mathfrak{D}, \mathfrak{A} \rangle$ is a branching questionnaire (see Definition 92),

    8. D is a subset of 𝔇 accepted by d at t,

    9. A is a subset of 𝔄,

    10. There are goals G, a knowledge base KB, and a methodology M such that $f \equiv \{G, KB, M\}$ and $f: powerset(\mathfrak{D} \cup \mathfrak{A}) \mapsto powerset(\mathfrak{D} \cup \mathfrak{A})$,

    11. ∇ is a deontic operator, provided by knowledge base KB or methods M.

For example, the client set *c* may consist of an individual patient or a group of patients such as {Amy, Elroy Fox}, whereas *d* represents one or more decision-makers, e.g., an individual doctor, a team of doctors, or other health care providers. It is not required that *c* is different from *d*, for sometimes a decision-maker is a client at the same time when, for example, a doctor examines and treats herself. The time period of decision-making is indicated by *t*.

The definition above axiomatizes only the frame of a decision-making situation. The function *f* maps the set of all possible data and actions to this set itself. Thus, it will enable us to choose the appropriate action, given a particular data set *D* at time *t*. For this reason, it will be referred to as the *decision function* of the frame. In the following definitions, this decision function is characterized and specialized yielding indication, contra-indication, and differential indication structures.

Definition 95 (Permissive structure). *ξ is a permissive structure iff there are c, d, t, 𝔇, 𝔄, D, A, f, and PE such that:*

    1. $\xi = \langle c, d, t, \mathfrak{D}, \mathfrak{A}, D, A, f, PE \rangle$,

    2. ξ is a decision-making frame,

    3. $f(D) = A$,

    4. PE(A).

Suppose, for example, *D* is any of the patient data sets $D_1, D_2, \ldots, D_n$ presented to the physician, respectively, over the time periods $t_1, t_2, \ldots, t_n$ during the decision-making process. According to axioms 3–4, the decision function *f* will identify the action set $A \subseteq \mathfrak{A}$ which is permitted in this situation. A permissive structure may also be termed a weak indication structure. The following definitions determine indication, contra-indication, and differential indication structures as deontic-logical ones.

Definition 96 (Indication structure). *ξ is an* indication structure *iff there are c, d, t, $\mathfrak{D}$, $\mathfrak{A}$, D, A, f, and OB such that:*

1. $\xi = \langle c, d, t, \mathfrak{D}, \mathfrak{A}, D, A, f, OB \rangle$,
2. ξ *is a decision-making frame,*
3. $f(D) = A$,
4. $OB(A)$.

Definition 97 (Contra-indication structure). *ξ is a* contra-indication structure *iff there are c, d, t, $\mathfrak{D}$, $\mathfrak{A}$, D, A, f, and FO such that:*

1. $\xi = \langle c, d, t, \mathfrak{D}, \mathfrak{A}, D, A, f, FO \rangle$,
2. ξ *is a decision-making frame,*
3. $f(D) = A$,
4. $FO(A)$.

By interpreting the set D as patient data at time t, and the action set A as a set of diagnostic or therapeutic measures, in Definition 96 the decision function f assigns to D the diagnostic or therapeutic action set A that is obligatory in this situation, i.e., *indicated*. By contrast, in Definition 97 the selected action set A is forbidden, i.e., *contra-indicated*. In this way, diagnostic and therapeutic reasoning will become a model for the axiom systems introduced by Definitions 94–97. We may therefore term the decision function f a *clinical decision function*. (For the general notion of a model, see Section 26.2.2 on page 886.)

What is particularly important in understanding the deontic nature, and in representing the methodology, of clinical reasoning is the clinical decision function f used in the axiomatizations above. It assigns to a given patient data set a particular set of actions that are permitted, obligatory, or forbidden in this situation. Informally, the physician's goals, knowledge, experience, logic, and morality act as a function of this type, though not as a perfect one. In Section 8.1.2, we tried to enhance this imperfect conduct by constructing our concept of branching clinical questionnaire referred to in axiom 7 of Definition 94. In fact, the clinical decision function f is a tool for clinical pathfinding in this questionnaire. An action set A that the decision function f selects and suggests to perform, is a particular *node* in that questionnaire as a network.

It is shown in Definition 232 on page 929 that the obligation operator OB may be used as the basic deontic operator by which the other deontic operators are definable. We thus obtain the following inverse relationships between obligation, prohibition, and permission where α is any sentence and $\neg\alpha$ is its negation to be read 'not α':

1. $FO\alpha$ *iff* $OB\neg\alpha$ (73)
2. $PE\alpha$ *iff* $\neg FO\alpha$
3. $PE\alpha$ *iff* $\neg OB\neg\alpha$.

The first one of these relationships says that a particular action, represented by sentence α, is forbidden if and only if it is obligatory to omit this action.

The second relationship says that an action is permitted if and only if it is not forbidden. These two sentences imply the third one which shows that an action is permitted if its omission is not obligatory. Thanks to these relationships, every contra-indication turns out to be the indication of the *omission* of the contra-indicated action as expressed by:

Theorem 4. $\delta \to OB\neg\alpha$ *is equivalent to* $\delta \to FO\alpha$

that follows from (73) above. It means that the omission ('$\neg\alpha$' on the left-hand side) of a contra-indicated action ('α' on the right-hand side) is indicated. In this way, a contra-indication structure:

$$\langle c, d, t, \mathfrak{D}, \mathfrak{A}, D, \{\alpha_1, \ldots, \alpha_m\}, f, FO \rangle \tag{74}$$

as defined in Definition 97 above, becomes equivalent to an indication structure of the form:

$$\langle c, d, t, \mathfrak{D}, \mathfrak{A}, D, \{\neg\alpha_1, \ldots, \neg\alpha_m\}, f, OB \rangle. \tag{75}$$

The action set $\{\neg\alpha_1, \ldots, \neg\alpha_m\}$ is the omission of the actions $\{\alpha_1, \ldots, \alpha_m\}$. The relationship between 74 and 75 is based on the following theorem that is implied by Definitions 96–97 and Theorem 4 above.

Theorem 5. $\langle c, d, t, \mathfrak{D}, \mathfrak{A}, D, \{\neg\alpha_1, \ldots, \neg\alpha_m\}, f, OB \rangle$ *is an indication struc-ture if* $\langle c, d, t, \mathfrak{D}, \mathfrak{A}, D, \{\alpha_1, \ldots, \alpha_m\}, f, FO \rangle$ *is a contra-indication structure.*

For this reason, we may integrate contra-indications as *obligatory omissions* into our theory of indication structures and thus omit the additional term "contra-indication".

When a particular set $A = \{\alpha_1, \ldots, \alpha_m\}$ of clinical actions is indicated, it is natural to assume that there is a clinical priority ordering $\succ$ that determines the temporal sequence of performing the elements or subsets of A, say in the order $\alpha'_1 \succ \ldots \succ \alpha'_m$. A performance order of this type defined over an action set A will be written $\langle A, \succ \rangle$. It renders an indication structure a well-ordered one.

Definition 98 (Well-ordered indication structure). ξ *is a* well-ordered indi-cation structure *iff there are* c, d, t, $\mathfrak{D}$, $\mathfrak{A}$, D, A, f, OB, *and* $\succ$ *such that:*

1. $\xi = \langle c, d, t, \mathfrak{D}, \mathfrak{A}, D, A, f, OB, \succ \rangle$,
2. $\langle c, d, t, \mathfrak{D}, \mathfrak{A}, D, A, f, OB \rangle$ *is an indication structure,*
3. $\succ$ *is a linear ordering on powerset(A),*
4. $\langle A, \succ \rangle$ *is the performance order induced by f over A.*

Since in clinical settings individual clinical actions may be differently urgent, invasive, risky, productive of information, valuable, and expensive, there are distinct advantages to a performance ordering $\succ$ of the type above. Depending on the degree of its sophistication, such an ordering may contribute to a well-ordered indication structure. And the search for an adequate and acceptable performance ordering $\succ$ is among the central ethical problems of medicine. "What action A_i must be preferred to what action A_j?". An ordering relation of the type $\succ$ will be proposed on page 662.

Well-ordered indication structures are necessary even though they are not sufficient for optimal patient management. There are clinical situations where a patient presents, as a partition of her data set D, various data sets $D_1, \ldots, D_m$ at the same time such that D is their union, e.g., multiple disorders to be treated or multiple groups of coherent symptoms and signs to be interpreted. Each of these partial data sets, considered separately, necessitates a particular diagnostic or therapeutic indication set A_i such that an array $A_1, \ldots, A_m$ of action sets appears to be indicated corresponding to the data sets $D_1, \ldots, D_m$. For instance, after a kidney operation, a patient must be given several drugs, while her postoperative pneumonia requires in addition antibiotics that may increase her current renal insufficiency. In such a case, the physician is faced with the problem of whether or not there is any conflict of action among the indication set $\{A_1, \ldots, A_m\}$ and of how to resolve this conflict and minimize the action union $A_1 \cup \ldots \cup A_m$. The solution aimed at is a minimum, proper subset $B \subseteq A_1 \cup \ldots \cup A_m$ such that B is indicated due to the present data set $D_1 \cup \ldots \cup D_m$. Conflict analysis, optimization, and resolution of this type is referred to as making a *differential indication* decision that differentiates between *what ought to be done for this patient* and what should be omitted or postponed.

Note that every patient data set D is the union $D_1 \cup \ldots \cup D_m$ of its covering subsets $D_1, \ldots, D_m \subseteq D$. Since these subsets may necessitate a large indication set $A_1 \cup \ldots \cup A_m$ as above that requires differentiation and reduction, it appears reasonable to view every diagnostic-therapeutic setting as one that is best managed by a differential indication decision.

Definition 99 (Differential indication structure). *ξ is a differential indication structure iff there are c, d, t, $\mathfrak{D}$, $\mathfrak{A}$, $D_1, \ldots, D_m, A_1, \ldots, A_m$, B, f, and OB such that:*

1. *$\xi = \langle c, d, t, \mathfrak{D}, \mathfrak{A}, \{D_1, \ldots, D_m\}, \{A_1, \ldots, A_m\}, B, f, OB \rangle$,*
2. *For each pair $\{D_i, A_i\}$, the tuple $\langle c, d, t, \mathfrak{D}, \mathfrak{A}, D_i, A_i, f, OB \rangle$ is an indication structure,*
3. *$B \subset A_1 \cup \ldots \cup A_m$,*
4. *$\langle c, d, t, \mathfrak{D}, \mathfrak{A}, D_1 \cup \ldots \cup D_m, B, f, OB \rangle$ is an indication structure.*

Definition 100 (Well-ordered differential indication structure). *ξ is a well-ordered differential indication structure iff there are c, d, t, $\mathfrak{D}$, $\mathfrak{A}$, $D_1, \ldots, D_m$, $A_1, \ldots, A_m$, B, f, OB, and $\succ$ such that:*

1. *$\xi = \langle c, d, t, \mathfrak{D}, \mathfrak{A}, \{D_1, \ldots, D_m\}, \{A_1, \ldots, A_m\}, B, f, OB, \succ \rangle$,*
2. *$\langle c, d, t, \mathfrak{D}, \mathfrak{A}, \{D_1, \ldots, D_m\}, \{A_1, \ldots, A_m\}, B, f, OB \rangle$ is a differential indication structure,*
3. *$\succ$ is a linear ordering on powerset(B),*
4. *$\langle B, \succ \rangle$ is the performance order induced by f over B.*

The last three definitions imply that every differential indication structure is an indication structure.

A re-examination of the clinical solution path in Figure 57 on page 303 above will demonstrate that each of the proposed action steps $D_i \Rightarrow A_i$ in clinical decision-making may be construed as the outcome of a differential indication structure where a clinical decision function f selects, from among the physician's action space $\mathfrak{A}$, the action set A_i as the indicated one in this situation. The entirety of the concatenated action steps in that figure may thus be viewed as a trajectory or clinical path:

$$D_1 \Rightarrow A_1 \to D_2 \Rightarrow A_2 \to \cdots \to D_n \Rightarrow A_n \tag{76}$$

of data-based action planning in a dynamical system of differential indication structures consisting of the following sequence of well-ordered indication structures:

$$\langle c, d, t_1, \mathfrak{D}, \mathfrak{A}, D_1, A_1, f, OB, \succ \rangle \qquad \text{with} \quad \langle D_1, A_1 \rangle \ \text{ at } \ t_1 \tag{77}$$
$$\langle c, d, t_2, \mathfrak{D}, \mathfrak{A}, D_2, A_2, f, OB, \succ \rangle \qquad \text{with} \quad \langle D_2, A_2 \rangle \ \text{ at } \ t_2$$

$$\vdots$$

$$\langle c, d, t_n, \mathfrak{D}, \mathfrak{A}, D_n, A_n, f, OB, \succ \rangle \qquad \text{with} \quad \langle D_n, A_n \rangle \ \text{ at } \ t_n$$

The Basic Query that we formulated on page 305 above ["... is it possible to construct an effective procedure, e.g., an algorithm, which can be initiated at time t_1 such that when the patient data set at time t_i is $D_i \subseteq \mathfrak{D}$ with $1 \le i \le n$, the optimal action set $A_i \subseteq \mathfrak{A}$ can be selected unambiguously from among the action space $\mathfrak{A}$, the next data set $D_{i+1} \subseteq \mathfrak{D}$ can be built as objectively as possible, and the particular doctor d is in principle exchangeable by any doctor x?"] may now be restated as follows: Is it possible to render the data-action path (76) computable? To show that the answer to this question is Yes, one needs only to demonstrate that the clinical decision function f is a computable function.[62]

8.2.5 The Computability of Differential Indication

There has been much discussion in the philosophy of medicine during the last decades on whether computers are, or will one day become, able to 'diagnose' diseases or make the appropriate clinical 'decision' like a doctor does or is able to. The standard position on this question has been, and still seems to remain, No. A famous argument goes as follows: Clinical judgment has an essential component of the same cognitive sensibility or style that is required in catching

---

[62] For our purposes, we may understand by a "computable function" a function that can be computed by an algorithm. Well-known examples are the arithmetical operations of addition, subtraction, multiplication, and division. For details, see (Cooper SB, 2003; Hermes, 1971; Rogers, 1987).

on to a joke. Therefore, a theory of jokes may shed some light on the logic of diagnosis. But computers and computer programs cannot catch on to a joke; therefore, computers and computer programs cannot diagnose (Wartofsky, 1986, 82). However, this position itself has been turned into a joke by recent medical expert-systems research and practice. As part of artificial intelligence, this research is based on the fundamental concept of computability introduced in the 1930s by Alan Turing (1936, 1937). In line with this concept, it is briefly shown below that our clinical decision function f above is computable. Therefore, it may be replaced with a computer program. The computability of the decision function f will be demonstrated by constructing two series of computable sub-functions,

$f_1, f_2, \ldots, f_n$ whose arguments are the patient data sets $D_1, \ldots, D_n$
$g_1, g_2, \ldots, g_n$ whose arguments are the action sets $A_1, \ldots, A_n$

of which f will be composed. Given the above series (77) of differential indication structures with the initial patient data $D_1 = \{\delta_1, \ldots, \delta_m\}$ at time t_1, it is not hard to design a computable function f_1 such that:

$f_1(D_1) = A_1$,

$OB(A_1)$,

$\langle A_1, \succ \rangle$ is the performance order of the action set A_1.

To this end, one may take a branching clinical questionnaire $\langle \mathfrak{A}, \mathfrak{D} \rangle$ and from it write a definite computer program, say $Progr_1$, that returns the output $A_1 \subseteq \mathfrak{A}$ as an answer to the input D_1 and says "action set A_1 is obligatory with the performance order $\langle A_1, \succ \rangle$". Thus, $Progr_1$ computes a function, f_1, with $f_1(D_1) = A_1$. Hence, f_1 is a computable function.

Now, write a second definite program, say $Progr_2$, that proceeds as follows. It asks the doctor (i) to perform action set A_1 in a particular manner; (ii) to answer a list of specific questions concerning the outcome of the performed action set A_1; and (iii) to answer another list of specific questions – regarding the black box 'the patient' – so as to update the preceding data set D_1. Based on (i) through (iii), the program then composes the patient data set $D_2 = \{\text{outcome of step (ii)}\} \cup \{\text{outcome of step (iii)}\}$. Thus, $Progr_2$ computes a function, g_1, such that $g_1(A_1) = D_2$. Hence, g_1 is a computable function.

Now, write a third definite program, $Progr_3$, that provides the output "action set A_2 is obligatory with the performance order $\langle A_2, \succ \rangle$" as an answer to the input D_2. Thus, $Progr_3$ computes a function, f_2, with $f_2(D_2) = A_2$. Hence, f_2 is a computable function.

And so forth ... until the final action set A_n is recommended by the final program, i.e., $Progr_n$ at time t_n. We shall in this way have available two series of computable functions:

$f_1, f_2, \ldots, f_n$

$g_1, g_2, \ldots, g_n$

such that:

$$f_1(D_1) = A_1$$
$$f_2(D_2) = A_2$$

$$\vdots$$

$$f_n(D_n) = A_n = \{\textit{terminate decision-making!}\},$$

and:

$$g_1(A_1) = D_2$$
$$g_2(A_2) = D_3$$

$$\vdots$$

$$g_n(A_n) = \{\textit{decision-making terminated}\}.$$

The concatenation of the partial programs $Progr_1, Progr_2, \ldots, Progr_n$ will yield a composite program that interleaves the two function series above in the following order:

$$\langle f_1, g_1, f_2, g_2, \ldots, f_n, g_n \rangle.$$

Thus, it executes a computable function $f \equiv \langle f_1, g_1, f_2, g_2, \ldots, f_n, g_n \rangle$ as a composition:

$$f \equiv \langle g_n \circ f_n \circ g_{n-1} \circ f_{n-1} \circ \cdots \circ g_1 \circ f_1 \rangle$$

which, successively executed as above, provides the mapping:

$$f: powerset(\mathfrak{D}) \mapsto powerset(\mathfrak{A})$$
$$f: powerset(\mathfrak{A}) \mapsto powerset(\mathfrak{D}),$$

that is:

$$f: powerset(\mathfrak{D} \cup \mathfrak{A}) \mapsto powerset(\mathfrak{D} \cup \mathfrak{A})$$

for the management of clinical judgment, and acts as required regarding the computability question posed in Basic Query on page 305. Hence, *there is a ccdf*, a computable clinical decision function *f*, that may be defined by cases as follows:

$$f(X) = \begin{cases} f_1(D_1) & \text{if } X = D_1 \\ g_1(A_1) & \text{if } X = A_1 \\ \vdots \\ f_n(D_n) & \text{if } X = D_n \\ g_n(A_n) & \text{if } X = A_n \end{cases} \tag{78}$$

Sufficient empirical evidence is available in favor of the existence claim given in the last sentence. Every clinical expert system designed to provide advice in a particular clinical domain, is a restriction of the ccdf f to that domain. Analogously, a comprehensive clinical expert system covering all of clinical medicine would represent an instance of the total function f, i.e., a particular global *ccdf*.

This, of course, suggests that one may conceive of a variety of different, competing ccdfs each of which will render clinical judgment computable in a particular manner. The question of how to decide which one of them may be preferred to the rest, is among the core problems of the experimental science of clinical practice that is emerging from current medical knowledge engineering research.

As is obvious from the design of the sub-function series $g_1, g_2, \ldots, g_n$ above for performing the indicated actions, the argument of any such function g_i is a set of actions, A_i, having the data set D_{i+1} as its value, i.e., $g_i(A_i) = D_{i+1}$. The physician is currently involved in each g_i of the series in that the computation of $g_i(A_i)$ requires her to perform the recommended action set A_i and to assist g_i in collecting data for building the next data set D_{i+1}. Thus, the physician is physically involved in the computation of the whole function f. For this reason, one may raise the objection that none of the sub-functions $g_1, g_2, \ldots, g_n$ is a computable one in the proper sense of this term, and may conclude that there is no ccdf as maintained above.

This objection is based on the assumption that the doctor's physical involvement in the execution of the sub-functions $g_1, g_2, \ldots, g_n \in f$ is necessary to this execution. However, this necessity is a mere physical necessity for the time being, but not a logical necessity. To prove this claim, replace the doctor with a robot that acts as a mobile peripheral of the machine that computes f. This seeming 'science fiction' era has already begun in university health centers where a huge *hospital information system* in collaboration with Intranets and the Internet acts as a *clinical process control system* using the doctors and other health personnel themselves as mere mobile peripherals. The circumstance that robots are not yet able to match the sensorimotor proficiency of doctors as machine peripherals, does not concern the computational aspect of our problem. So, we need not enter into a philosophical discussion on robotics. See also Section "Clinical decision-engineering" on page 784.

8.2.6 The Logical Structure of Diagnosis

As was pointed out on page 300, an applicable theory of medical diagnosis and diagnostics will necessarily differ from proposals originating in computer sciences, such as Reiter and de Kleer's theory on trouble-shooting in physical devices (Reiter 1987; de Kleer et al., 1992). To arrive at a satisfactory one, however, we first need some conceptual and logical clarifications. For example, what is to be understood by "medical diagnosis"? How does diagnosis emerge? What role does it play in patient management? Is there a logic of diagnostics?

These and related issues will be dealt with in what follows to further develop our theory. See also (Sadegh-Zadeh, 1977b, 1981d, 1982b).

From the perspective of, and within, the framework presented above, the concept of indication structure will be further specialized to anchor our meta-diagnostic inquiries. A *diagnostic structure* will be laid out first. Based upon that, we shall reconstruct and analyze the concept of clinical *diagnosis*. The analysis will reveal that clinical diagnostics is a deontic endeavor because the diagnostic actions (questions, tests, examinations) performed are deontically required in the given circumstances. Our aim in formalizing these subjects is to bring clarity to some unduly simplified and distorted issues of clinical philosophy.

The intuitive idea in medicine of diagnosis is that some condition causally accounts for patient data, and that the diagnosis is just the description of that condition. The appropriate understanding and refinement of this vague idea must be based on the awareness that (i) patient data must be something pathological in a medical sense to require a diagnosis at all; (ii) a clear concept of causality will be needed; and (iii) the diagnosis should be based upon specific diagnostic information to avoid as much as possible diagnostic methods and deliberations that depend upon chance similar to tossing a coin. All of these criteria are met by Definition 101 below.

Let the phrase 'normality value', written nv, be a binary linguistic variable whose term set, $T(nv)$, may be a set of fuzzy evaluation predicates like {normal, pathological, fairly pathological, very pathological, extremely pathological, not pathological, ... }:

$$T(nv) = \{\text{normal, pathological, fairly pathological, very pathological,}$$
$$\text{extremely pathological, not pathological, ... etc. ...}\}.$$

Within a particular population, denoted 'PO', to which the patient belongs, any term of $T(nv)$ can be used to categorize a given patient data δ as normal, pathological, very pathological, etc. The term set $T(nv)$ will therefore be referred to as *normality* values. In this way, the *normality value*, nv, of a patient data δ with respect to the population PO may be symbolized by a statement of the form:

$$nv(\delta, PO) = y \qquad \text{where } y \in T(nv).$$

It says that the normality value of δ in PO is y. For example, severe chest pain in the population of men_over_40 is pathological, that is:

$$nv(\langle chest\_pain, severe \rangle, men\_over\_40) = pathological.$$

Finally, let the following functional statement:

$$cr(X, Y, PO) = z$$

express that the causal relevance, cr, of event X to event Y in the population PO equals z. For instance, it may be that cr(smoking, angina_pectoris, diabetics) $= 0.1$, whereas cr(smoking, angina_pectoris, non-diabetics) $= 0.03$. This numerical causality function cr was introduced in Definition 80 on page 260. Roughly, the causal relevance of an event X to an event Y in a population PO is the extent to which in this population the occurrence of X raises or lowers the probability of the occurrence of Y, given that some additional requirements are satisfied (for details, see pp. 259–261).

A diagnosis does not fall from the heavens. It does not originate in the physician's mind either. It emerges from a more or less complex social-historical context that includes the medical machinery in a practice or hospital, the diagnostician(s), the assistants, the patient, her family, the medical community, health authorities, and many other factors. As will be shown below, all of them contribute to the diagnosis given to an individual patient.

The following definition axiomatizes the complex structure of the *diagnostic context* that generates a diagnosis, *dg*, for a patient p who presents with the data set D, and is a member of the population PO. See axiom 14. The other 13 axioms are preparatory ones. They say, in essence, that in the specified context a set of statements, Δ, is identified as *diagnosis* for a patient's data set D in a particular population PO, i.e., $dg(D, PO) = \Delta$, if Δ in that population is causally-positively relevant to D (axiom 13) and some additional conditions are satisfied.

Definition 101 (Diagnostic structure). ξ *is a* diagnostic structure *iff there are* $p, d, t_1, \mathfrak{D}, \mathfrak{A}, D_1, A_1, f, OB, t_2, D_2, D, \Delta, PO, nv, T(nv), cr,$ *and* dg *such that:*

1. $\xi = \langle p, d, t_1, \mathfrak{D}, \mathfrak{A}, D_1, A_1, f, OB, t_2, D_2, D, \Delta, PO, nv, T(nv), cr, dg \rangle$
2. $\langle p, d, t_1, \mathfrak{D}, \mathfrak{A}, D_1, A_1, f, OB \rangle$ *is an indication structure*
3. $t_2 \geq t_1 (i.e., t_2$ *is the same time as or later than* t_1
4. $f(A_1) = D_2$
5. D_2 *is a subset of* $\mathfrak{D}$ *accepted by d at* t_2
6. $D \subseteq D_1 \cup D_2$
7. *Also* $\Delta \subseteq D_1 \cup D_2$
8. PO *is a population to which the patient(s) belong(s), i.e.,* $p \subseteq PO$
9. nv *is a linguistic variable such that its term set* $T(nv) = \{normal, pathological, very pathological, \ldots etc. \ldots\}$
10. $cr: powerset(\mathfrak{D}) \times powerset(\mathfrak{D}) \times \{PO\} \mapsto [-1, +1]$
11. $dg: powerset(\mathfrak{D}) \times PO \mapsto powerset(\mathfrak{D})$
12. $nv(\delta, PO) = y \in T(nv)$ *and* $\neq normal,$ *for all* $\delta \in D$
13. $cr(\Delta, D, PO) > 0$
14. $dg(D, PO) = \Delta.$

The definition requires, first of all, that the base of the structure be an indication structure. This property of being an indication structure, stated in axiom 2, implies that there is an initial patient data set D_1 and an initial action set A_1 (question, test, examination) that is indicated due to that data. Axioms 3–5 say that a diagnostic inquiry by performing the indicated action set A_1 has updated the information on the patient, i.e., the data set D_2. Axioms 6–11 characterize the respective ingredients of the diagnostic structure. Axiom 12 says that some part, D, of total patient data is pathological in the reference population PO. Axiom 13 states that to some extent, another subset Δ of patient data is positively causally relevant, in the population PO, to the pathological part D of patient data. In Axiom 14, the function dg ('diagnosis') assigns to the pathological part D of patient data in the reference population PO the set Δ as *diagnosis*. Note that due to the time points or periods, t_1 and t_2, the structure is a temporally dynamic one, i.e., a process usually referred to as "the diagnostic process". Now, on the basis of the structure above, Definition 102 below introduces a concept of diagnosis as a ternary set function. The functional relation:

$$diagnosis(p, D, KB \cup M) = \Delta$$

in its definiendum reads:

> the diagnosis for patient p with data set D and relative to the knowledge base KB and its application methods M is Δ.

Set Δ has been defined in Definition 101 above as a set of sentences, being a subset of $D_1 \cup D_2$. The knowledge base and the methods of its application, $KB \cup M$, have already been included in our basic Definition 94 on page 312 (see axiom 10 of that definition).

Definition 102 (Diagnosis). $diagnosis(p, D, KB \cup M) = \Delta$ *iff there are d, t_1, $\mathfrak{D}, \mathfrak{A}, D_1, A_1, f, OB, t_2, D_2, PO, nv, T(nv), cr$, and dg such that:*

1. *$\langle p, d, t_1, \mathfrak{D}, \mathfrak{A}, D_1, A_1, f, OB, t_2, D_2, D, \Delta, PO, nv, T(nv), cr, dg \rangle$ is a diagnostic structure,*
2. *KB is the knowledge base and M is the methodology of the functions f and dg.*

One may of course rewrite the concept of diagnosis above, introduced as a ternary function, as a quaternary predicate in the following way:

Definition 103 (Diagnosis*). $diagnosis^*(\Delta, p, D, KB \cup M)$ *iff there are d, t_1, $\mathfrak{D}, \mathfrak{A}, D_1, A_1, f, OB, t_2, D_2, PO, nv, T(nv), cr$, and dg such that:*

1. *$\langle p, d, t_1, \mathfrak{D}, \mathfrak{A}, D_1, A_1, f, OB, t_2, D_2, D, \Delta, PO, nv, T(nv), cr, dg \rangle$ is a diagnostic structure,*
2. *KB is the knowledge base and M is the methodology of the functions f and dg.*

We shall use Definition 102. We call the knowledge base and the methods of its application, $KB \cup M$, the *frame of reference* of the respective diagnosis. Below we shall see that one and the same patient may receive different diagnoses from distinct frames of reference. For instance, it may be that a diagnostic examination of our patient Elroy Fox above undertaken within a particular frame of reference, say gastroenterological knowledge and methodology, suggests (see diagnosis No. 7 on page 280):

diagnosis ({Elroy Fox}, {⟨pressure in the left chest, mild⟩, ⟨sporadic chest pain, moderate⟩, ⟨night sweat, intensive⟩, ⟨heart rate, 102⟩, ⟨adynamia, increasing⟩}, KB ∪ M) = {⟨exocrine pancreatic insufficiency, moderate⟩, ⟨peptic esophagitis, severe⟩, ⟨gastritis by Helicobacter pylori, severe⟩, ⟨sorbitol intolerance, moderate⟩, ⟨type 2 diabetes, mild⟩, ⟨hepatitis, none⟩}.

Overly simplified, that means that "Elroy Fox has moderate exocrine pancreatic insufficiency, severe peptic esophagitis, severe Helicobacter gastritis, moderate sorbitol intolerance, mild type 2 diabetes, and no hepatitis". The theory of diagnosis that we are developing will make it apparent that it is most realistic to assume that another frame of reference may, and would, generate another diagnosis (Sadegh-Zadeh, 1977b, 1981d). In addition, Definition 101 implies that every diagnostic structure is also an indication structure, i.e., a context where individual diagnostic actions are deontically required by clinical knowledge. It goes without saying that the computability proof demonstrated in Section 8.2.5 above can be extended to the diagnostic function dg sketched in Definition 101, and to the ternary function 'diagnosis' defined in Definition 102.

As alluded to on page 313, the physician's goals, knowledge, experience, logic, and morals act as her *frame of reference* in the sense given above. In the current era of clinical knowledge-based or so-called expert systems research and practice, the frame of reference is included in the expert system, i.e., in the computer program used in a hospital or in a doctor's practice. The entirety of such an expert system may be conceived of as a computable clinical decision function *ccdf*, as outlined in (78) on page 318, that controls diagnostic and differential indication structures, and replaces physicians' confined and biased clinical judgment. Due to the experimental and technological nature of clinical knowledge-based systems research, it seems realistic to view this emerging discipline as an *experimental engineering science of clinical practice* that continually produces different species of computable clinical decision functions: $ccdf_1, ccdf_2, ccdf_3$, and so on (Sadegh-Zadeh, 1990).

The clinical implementation of any such function will be referred to as a 'clinical operator', *cop* for short. For example, cop_1 may be a MYCIN machine that executes the expert system MYCIN; cop_2 may be a CADUCEUS machine that executes the expert system CADUCEUS; cop_3 may be a QMR machine; cop_4 may be a CADIAG-2 machine, and so on. Let cop_i be a particular type $i \geq 1$ of clinical operator with its domain-specific knowledge base KB_i and its underlying methodology M_i as its frame of reference. Let p be a patient with the data set D; and let d be her doctor using the clinical operator cop_i to obtain a diagnosis or advice X. Upon receiving this output X, we have that:

$$cop_i(p, d, D, KB_i \cup M_i) = X \qquad \text{for } i \geq 1. \tag{79}$$

That is, the machine cop_i operates as a mathematical operator on the quadruple $\langle p, d, D, KB_i \cup M_i \rangle$ as its argument and produces the value X that may be the recommendation of an indicated action, a diagnosis, or something else. The objectivity of an indication or diagnostic structure governed by the operator cop_i is provided by the fact that for all patients p with the same data set D and for all doctors d, the output X in (79) remains the same guaranteeing the exchangeability of doctors. We can therefore remove the doctor variable d and agree upon the pruned syntax:

$$cop_i(p, D, KB_i \cup M_i) = X \qquad \text{for } i \geq 1 \qquad (80)$$

replacing formula (79). The three-place function cop_i in formula (80) may be construed as a composite operator consisting of at least two parts, a diagnostic operator written $diag_i$, and an indication operator termed $indic_i$, such that:

$$diag_i(p, D, KB_i \cup M_i) = \Delta$$
$$indic_i(p, D, KB_i \cup M_i) = OB(A_i).$$

This syntax may be based upon, and interpreted by, our familiar conceptual apparatus as follows:

Definition 104 (Indication operator). $indic(p, D, KB \cup M) = OB(A)$ iff there are d, t, $\mathfrak{D}$, $\mathfrak{A}$, and f such that:

1. $\langle p, d, t, \mathfrak{D}, \mathfrak{A}, D, A, f, OB \rangle$ is an indication structure,
2. $KB \cup M$ is the knowledge base and methodology ("the frame of reference") of the function f.

Definition 105 (Diagnostic operator). $diag(p, D, KB \cup M) = \Delta$ iff there are d, t_1, $\mathfrak{D}$, $\mathfrak{A}$, D_1, A_1, f, OB, t_2, D_2, PO, nv, $T(nv)$, cr, and dg such that:

1. $\langle p, d, t_1, \mathfrak{D}, \mathfrak{A}, D_1, A_1, f, OB, t_2, D_2, D, \Delta, PO, nv, T(nv), cr, dg \rangle$ is a diagnostic structure,
2. $KB \cup M$ is the knowledge base and methodology ("the frame of reference") of the functions f and dg.

Apparently, the diagnostic component of a clinical operator, the function $diag$, is formally identical with our ternary concept of diagnosis, i.e., $diagnosis(p, D, KB \cup M) = \Delta$, constructed in Definition 102 above. The only difference is that $diag$, executed by a machine, is unbiased, whereas fallible human doctors execute $diagnosis(p, D, KB \cup M) = \Delta$.

A clinical knowledge-based or expert system, reconstructed in this fashion as a composite operator, maps patient data to diagnoses and therapies. And it does so always relative to its frame of reference, i.e., its underlying knowledge base and methodology, $KB \cup M$. Any change in the variable $KB \cup M$ will engender changes in diagnoses and action recommendations. That means, explicitly, that if a patient p is subjected to two clinical operators such that for p with the data set D we have:

$$diag_i(p, D, KB_i \cup M_i) = \Delta_i$$
$$indic_i(p, D, KB_i \cup M_i) = OB(A_i).$$

and:

$$diag_j(p, D, KB_j \cup M_j) = \Delta_j$$
$$indic_j(p, D, KB_j \cup M_j) = OB(A_j).$$

then:

it is almost certain that $\Delta_i \neq \Delta_j$ and $A_i \neq A_j$ if $i \neq j$.

Diagnoses and therapies are thus context dependent in that they are epistemically and methodologically relative. There are no such things as *the patient's true state* such as *the patient's disease* or *the patient's health* independently of the respective frame of reference, i.e., theories, methodologies, and epistemologies applied. This fact diminishes the value of quality research endeavors exploring the reliability and validity of diagnoses and treatment decisions, or exploring treatment efficacy (Sadegh-Zadeh, 1977b, 1981c–d, 1982b, 1983).

Moreover, due to the inevitable vagueness of medical language, most parts of patient data and clinical knowledge are based on inherently vague concepts and are therefore vague statements, independently of how they are internally represented. For these reasons, it will be of vital relevance to medical expert systems technology to produce fuzzy *cops* rather than unrealistic, crisp constructs incapable of competing with the cerebral fuzzy machines of physicians.

8.2.7 The Syntax of Diagnosis

In clinical textbooks and education, individual diseases such as hepatitis A, B, C, diabetes mellitus, and myocardial infarction are given descriptions followed by instructions about how to diagnose each disease described. However, in spite of the long and honorable history of medicine, there is as yet no general *science of diagnostics* taught to medical students and young doctors instructing them how to diagnose in general. That is, there is no science which shows them how to learn and implement a dynamic, branching clinical questionnaire as introduced in Section 8.1.2, and to seek and find in this questionnaire the best clinical path from the patient's initial data, D_1, to a diagnosis by forming and testing diagnostic hypotheses. Every individual doctor develops her own, idiosyncratic mode of diagnostic reasoning and decision-making. The bitter fruit of this methodological vacuum was demonstrated in the case report on the patient Elroy Fox in Section 8.1.1 on page 279. In this report, we saw that the patient had consulted six doctors, getting seven different diagnoses for the same data $D = \{$feeling of pressure in the left chest, sporadic pain in the same region, night sweat, paroxysmal tachycardia, increasing adynamia$\}$. What is even worse is that only a few physicians are aware of how they achieve their diagnoses at all. Usually, a diagnosis seems to happen to a physician much as a dream or headache does. Therefore, it is not surprising that there are about 30–38% misdiagnoses. It is to be expected that these diagnostic errors bring with them at least as many wrong treatments. For this reason, medicine in the 21st century will urgently need to develop a *methodology of clinical practice* to guide the physician's clinical reasoning (Sadegh-Zadeh, 1977c). The emerging disciplines of clinical knowledge-based systems research and medical decision-making may be viewed as the advent of such a methodology, called 'experimental science of clinical practice' on page 319. It is very likely that this new science of clinical methodology will produce competing theories of medical diagnostics because it continually produces new and competing diagnostic operators. We symbolized such operators by the ternary function $diag_i$ in Definition 105 above. Recall that this function operates on a triple $\langle p, D, KB \cup M \rangle$:

$$diag_i(p, D, KB_i \cup M_i) = \Delta_i$$

consisting of a patient p such as Elroy Fox, his data set D, and a frame of reference comprising the knowledge base KB_i together with the methods of reasoning applied, M_i, to yield a particular diagnosis Δ_i. As we have already seen, the diagnosis Δ_i is a set of $n \geq 1$ singular statements about the patient such as {Elroy Fox has mild type 2 diabetes; he does not have hepatitis; he has moderate exocrine pancreatic insufficiency; he has severe peptic esophagitis; he has severe Helicobacter gastritis; he has moderate sorbitol intolerance}. In this section, the syntax of such diagnoses is analyzed. To this end, we shall use a very simple example to fix some terminology, which we shall use throughout.

A particular patient, say Mr. Elroy Fox, consults his doctor and five additional ones complaining of pressure in the left chest, sporadic pain in the same region, night sweat, tachycardia, and increasing adynamia. After performing a routine examination and some non-routine tests, the sixth doctor concludes that Elroy Fox has diabetes and some additional disorders (see above).

The patient data Elroy Fox presents with at any instant t in the diagnostic process, i.e., his problems, complaints, symptoms, and signs, is described by a set of singular statements $\{\delta_1, \ldots, \delta_n\} = D$ where each δ_i is a statement describing a problem, a complaint, a symptom, or a sign. The set of judgments that the doctor holds about what might be wrong with Elroy Fox at that instant t of the diagnostic process, will be referred to as the *diagnosis*, symbolized by $\{\alpha_1, \ldots, \alpha_n\} = \Delta$ where each α_i is a statement about the patient.

Not every statement about a patient is a diagnosis, however. Both the structure and the content of the statement, i.e., its syntax and semantics, must be taken into account. To this end, we distinguish between two types of diagnosis that are discussed in the following two sections:

- ▶ Categorical diagnoses
- ▶ Conjectural diagnoses.

Categorical diagnoses

A *categorical diagnosis* is a statement about the patient that the diagnostician considers true, and for this reason, it is an *idiogram* about the patient. This is explained in two steps below.

Recall that an atomic sentence is of the structure $P(t_1, \ldots, t_n)$ or $t_1 = t_2$ where P is an n-place predicate, and $t_1, t_2, \ldots, t_n$ are $n \geq 1$ terms in logical sense. See Definition 205 on page 862. Examples are simple atomic sentences such as $P(x_1, \ldots, x_n)$ and $f(x_1, \ldots, x_m) = y$ where P is an n-ary predicate; f is an m-ary function symbol; and $x_1, \ldots, x_m, x_n, y$ are $m, n \geq 1$ individual variables or constants.

A statement in a language $\mathcal{L}$ is referred to as a *literal* in $\mathcal{L}$ if it is an atomic sentence or the negation of an atomic sentence in $\mathcal{L}$. For instance, both "Elroy Fox has diabetes" and "Elroy Fox does not have diabetes" are literals in English, i.e. $P(a)$ and $\neg P(a)$.

An *idiogram*, in a language $\mathcal{L}$, about an individual a is a conjunction $\alpha_1 \wedge \ldots \wedge \alpha_n$ of $n \geq 1$ literals α_i about this individual a such that all literals are variable-free and contain the proper name of the individual, i.e., "a". For instance, each of the following statements is, in English, an idiogram about Elroy Fox: "Elroy Fox has diabetes", "Elroy Fox does not have hepatitis", "Elroy Fox has diabetes and Elroy Fox does not have hepatitis". To give some general examples, let P, Q, and R be unary predicates of a language $\mathcal{L}$ such as English or German; let f be a unary function symbol; and let a and b be individual constants of $\mathcal{L}$. The following statements are literals:

$$P(a), \quad \neg Q(a), \quad f(a) = b$$

and the following ones are *idiograms* in this language about the individual a:

$$P(a), \quad P(a) \wedge \neg Q(a), \quad P(a) \wedge \neg Q(a) \wedge R(a), \quad P(a) \wedge f(a) = b.$$

Natural language examples are:

Elroy Fox has diabetes	$\equiv P(a)$
Elroy Fox has diabetes and he does not have hepatitis	$\equiv P(a) \wedge \neg Q(a)$
Elroy Fox's blood sugar is 215 mg%	$\equiv f(a) = b$
Elroy Fox has diabetes and his blood sugar is 215 mg%	$\equiv P(a) \wedge f(a) = b.$

Since a fuzzy-set membership function such as μ_A is a function f as above, fuzzy statements such as $\mu_{diabetes}(\text{Elroy Fox}) = 0.9$ and their occurrence in conjunctions are also covered by the concept of categorical diagnosis above.

Conjectural diagnoses

Not all diagnoses in clinical practice are categorical ones, however. A considerable part of them may be called conjectural diagnoses.

A *conjectural diagnosis* is a conjecture about a patient. That means that the diagnostician does not yet consider it true, but only a hypothesis. For this reason, it may have a variety of syntactic structures. For example, it may be a *disjunction* such as "Elroy Fox has diabetes or he has hepatitis"; or it may be a *modal* statement such as "it is possible that Elroy Fox has gastritis". A probabilistic diagnosis is also a conjectural diagnosis. It may be either a qualitative-probabilistic diagnosis such as "it is likely that Elroy Fox has diabetes", or a quantitative-probabilistic diagnosis such as "the probability that Elroy Fox has diabetes, is 0.7". We may succinctly express this notion in the following way.

Let ∇ be the qualitative-probability operator "it is probable that ...";
or a modal operator, e.g., an alethic-modal operator such as "it is possible that ..."; or an epistemic-modal operator such as "I consider it possible that ..."; or "I believe that ...". A statement β about a patient is a conjectural diagnosis if there is a statement α about her such that (i) either β is $\nabla\alpha$, for example:

- *It is probable that* Elroy Fox has diabetes, $\equiv$ it is probable that α_1
- *it is possible that* Elroy Fox has appendicitis $\equiv$ it is possible that α_2
- *I believe that* Elroy Fox has cystitis $\equiv$ I believe that α_3

or (ii) α is a disjunction and β is α, as for instance:

- Elroy Fox has diabetes, or Elroy Fox has appendicitis, or Elroy Fox has cystitis.

The diagnosis $p(\alpha) = r$ is also a conjectural diagnosis where p is the probability function with $0 < r < 1$. For example, $p(\text{Elroy Fox has diabetes}) = 0.7$, i.e., the probability that Elroy Fox has diabetes, is 0.7. For details, see (Sadegh-Zadeh, 1982b).

The diagnosis set Δ

In our analyses above a patient's diagnosis, made at any instant during the diagnostic process, was considered to be a set of $n \geq 1$ statements about her, referred to as the diagnosis set $\Delta = \{\alpha_1, \ldots, \alpha_n\}$. Each of these statements may be a categorical or a conjectural diagnosis.

8.2.8 The Semantics of Diagnosis

Not every categorical or conjectural statement about a patient is a medical diagnosis. Examples are the statements "Elroy Fox has a fever" and "Elroy Fox is blonde". Obviously, then, the content of the statement is also a critical factor. We must therefore ask *what* it is that a physician is diagnosing? To answer this question we distinguish between several types of diagnosis that we shall consider in the following sections:

▶ Nosological diagnosis
▶ Abnormality diagnosis
▶ Causal diagnosis
▶ Fuzzy diagnosis
▶ Differential diagnosis.

Nosological diagnosis

It is commonly assumed that a diagnosis identifies the disease or diseases from which the patient suffers, e.g., "Elroy Fox has diabetes". This traditional notion of diagnosis may be called a *nosological diagnosis*.

A nosological diagnosis would require that every predicate and function symbol occurring in a diagnosis, e.g., in the idiogram $P(a) \land \ldots \land f(a) = b$, be a nosological term that signifies a disease ("nosos" ≡ disease). However, the actual usage of the term in medicine deviates from this view. Many physician judgments in clinical practice are handled as diagnoses which are by no means nosological ones. For instance, statements of the type "the patient has hypercholesterolemia of 280 mg%", which identify an abnormality, are also used as diagnoses. But abnormalities are not always diseases. For this reason, a second notion of diagnosis may be useful, i.e., the notion of *abnormality diagnosis*.

Abnormality diagnosis

An abnormality diagnosis is a statement that identifies any abnormality in the patient. According to this notion, any predicate or function symbol contained in a diagnosis would have to be the name of an abnormality, i.e., a malady, be it a disease, disorder, injury, wound, lesion, defect, deformity, disability, and the like. A nosological diagnosis is an abnormality diagnosis, but not vice versa.

Causal diagnosis

For a statement to be a diagnosis it is not enough to be the identification of a disease or an abnormality. There needs to be some relationship between the diagnosis and what it is a diagnosis for, i.e., the patient data. We have already required in our basic Definition 101 on page 321 above that this relationship be a *causal* one. That means that if $\Delta = \{\alpha_1, \ldots, \alpha_n\}$ is a diagnosis for patient data $D = \{\delta_1, \ldots, \delta_n\}$, there should be a link ⊛ between them of the form $\Delta \circledast D$ with ⊛ being a causal relation which says that elements of Δ causally account for elements of D. What does this causal relation ⊛ look like?

It is usually required that the diagnosis *causally explain* the patient data. According to this requirement, the doctor would have to causally explain, for example, why Elroy Fox has pressure in the left side of his chest, and has sporadic chest pain and other symptoms and signs. As will be shown on page 343, this apparently reasonable pursuit that is also referred to as the "hypothetico-deductive approach", is unrealistic because it is not always satisfiable. For this reason, we envisage a weaker causal relationship than causal explanation that requires a deterministic world. It suffices if the diagnostic process undertakes a *probabilistic-causal analysis* of the patient's health state to provide a diagnosis describing an event that to some extent is *causally positively relevant* to patient data (see Section 16.4.2 on page 598). The concept of causal relevance was developed on pages 259 ff. Roughly, the degree of causal relevance, *cr*, of an event A to an event B in a population PO is a number in the interval [-1, 1]:

$$cr(A, B, PO) = r \in [-1, 1]. \tag{81}$$

It indicates the extent $r \in [-1, 1]$ to which the occurrence of event A changes the probability of the occurrence of event B in the population PO provided that some additional requirements, discussed in Section 6.5.3, are satisfied. The relationship may be a positive, negative, or neutral one:

$$cr(A, B, PO) = r > 0,$$
$$cr(A, B, PO) = r < 0,$$
$$cr(A, B, PO) = 0.$$

For example, we may have these positive causal relevance relationships:

$$cr(influenza, cough, smoker) = 0.7 \tag{82}$$
$$cr(influenza, cough, non\text{-}smoker) = 0.2.$$

The former one says that in the population of smokers, influenza is causally positively relevant to cough to the extent 0.7. According to the latter, influenza in the population of non-smokers is causally positively relevant to cough to the extent 0.2.

Let $\Delta = \{\alpha_1, \ldots, \alpha_n\}$ be a diagnosis for patient data $D = \{\delta_1, \ldots, \delta_n\}$. By interpreting the diagnosis as a set of statements that describe the cause event A, and patient data as another set of statements that describe the effect event B in a respective population PO, it becomes apparent how through this interpretation:

$$cr(\Delta, D, PO) = r > 0$$

our concept of *positive* causal relevance, $cr(A, B, PO) = r > 0$, enters the theory of diagnostics. For instance, with reference to relationships (82) above we may suggest the following diagnosis about the patient Elroy Fox who is a smoker:

$$cr(\{Elroy\ Fox\ has\ influenza\}, \{Elroy\ Fox\ coughs\}, smoker) = 0.7.$$

As stated above, there are also negative causal relevances such as, for example:

$$cr(aspirin,\ myocardial\_infarction,\ men) = -0.44 \tag{83}$$

where 'men' is a shorthand for the population of 'men with elevated C-reactive protein concentration'. A negative causal relevance such as (83) amounts to prevention. Thus, (83) says that to the extent 0.44, aspirin prevents myocardial infarction in the population mentioned. In this way, preventive and protective factors are cause events with negative causal relevance to the effect events they prevent or protect from. By contrast, the generating of an effect event is a positive causal relevance such as in (82) above. Examples are diseases, risk factors, and other abnormalities that generate patient data, i.e., problems, complaints, symptoms, and signs. We shall come back to these issues in Section 8.5 on page 371.

Fuzzy diagnosis

It seems reasonable to define diagnosis as a set $\Delta = \{\alpha_1, \dots, \alpha_n\}$ of statements that signify the cause event being causally positively relevant to patient data D in a population PO:

$$cr(\Delta, D, PO) = r > 0.$$

Now the following problem arises. In the wake of this concept, the diagnosis for patient data D will seldom be unique. Almost always there will exist a large number of such diagnoses $\Delta_1, \dots, \Delta_n$ since a lot of different, positive causal relevance relationships of the following type will be available:

$$cr(\Delta_1, D, PO) = r_1$$

$$\vdots$$

$$cr(\Delta_n, D, PO) = r_n$$

such that each Δ_i to a particular extent r_i causally accounts for the same patient data D. For example, even at the end of the diagnostic inquiry it may turn out that as many as twenty different diseases appear to be causally responsible for Elroy Fox's ill health. Since not all of them can be regarded as being of equal weight, it may be useful to search for how to assess their *diagnostic relevance*. We may do this using the notion of fuzzy diagnosis, which is introduced below.

It is commonly assumed that a statement is either a diagnosis or is not a diagnosis about a patient. We have tacitly subscribed to this traditional, bivalent view until now. For example, the true statement "Elroy Fox has diabetes" is classified as such a diagnosis for his adynamia, whereas the equally true statement "Elroy Fox is blonde" is viewed as a non-diagnosis for the same problem. Thus, the category of diagnoses is handled as a crisp set with clear-cut boundaries such that diagnoses definitely reside within the boundaries and non-diagnoses definitely stand outside. The fuzzifying of these clear-cut boundaries will yield a fuzzy set, denoted by *Diag*, such that a collection of statements, $\Delta = \{\alpha_1, \ldots, \alpha_n\}$ with $n \geq 1$, is a member of this fuzzy set only to a particular extent $r \in [0, 1]$, and thus, a diagnosis to that extent. Let μ_{Diag} be the membership function of the fuzzy set *Diag* we are constructing. We shall in this way obtain a notion of fuzzy diagnosis which says that the degree of membership of a statement set Δ in the emerging fuzzy set *Diag* of diagnoses for patient data D in the population PO is $\mu_{Diag}(\Delta, D, PO) = r \in [0, 1]$. For example, if D is Elroy Fox's patient data set, it may be that we have:

$$\mu_{Diag}(\{Elroy \ Fox \ has \ diabetes\}, D, PO) = 0.9 \tag{84}$$

$$\mu_{Diag}(\{Elroy \ Fox \ has \ hepatitis\}, D, PO) = 0.3$$

$$\mu_{Diag}(\{Elroy \ Fox \ has \ diabetes \ or \ hepatitis\}, D, PO) = 1$$

$$\mu_{Diag}(\{Elroy \ Fox \ is \ blonde\}, D, PO) = 0.$$

The degree of membership of a statement set Δ in the fuzzy set *Diag*, denoted μ_{Diag}, will be referred to as the *degree of its diagnostic relevance,* or the *degree of its diagnosticity,* or simply, as its *diagnosticity*. We define the diagnosticity of a statement set Δ to be the degree of its causal relevance, that is:

Definition 106 (Diagnosticity). $\mu_{Diag}(\Delta, D, PO) = cr(\Delta, D, PO)$.

For instance, we have $\mu_{Diag}(\{Elroy \ Fox \ has \ diabetes\}, D, PO) = cr(\{Elroy \ Fox \ has \ diabetes\}, D, PO) = 0.9$. Thus, the diagnosticity of Elroy Fox's diabetes for his data is 0.9. The higher a statement set is causally relevant to patient data, the greater its diagnosticity. On the basis of this terminology, we may also observe that our concept of causality presented in Section 6.5.3 induces a *diagnosticity distribution* such as (84) over the universe of statements describing a patient.

Note that the diagnosticity of a statement set Δ for patient data derives from its causal relevance, but not from its probability, truth, or plausibility. Hence, diagnosticity is not a measure of probability, truth, plausibility, or any other epistemic quality of a statement. It is an ontological measure indicating the extent to which a statement is a diagnosis for something. In this way, the totality of all possible diagnoses $\Delta_1, \ldots, \Delta_n$ for a particular patient data set D may be arranged in the order of their increasing diagnosticity to suggest an idea of how to plan therapeutic steps. Thus, *diagnosticity* constitutes a quantitative concept of diagnosis. We shall return to this aspect below.

Differential diagnosis

The present context is an appropriate place to briefly explicate the notion of differential diagnosis, a term which is used throughout clinical medicine without a clear meaning. Consider as a simple example a particular patient with $m \geq 1$ patient data $\{\delta_1, \ldots, \delta_m\} = D$ such as:

$D = \{$Elroy Fox has an acute fever, Elroy Fox has a severe cough$\}$.

The set of 'all diseases' that, relative to the knowledge base used, potentially-causally account for patient data D is commonly referred to as 'differential diagnoses'. In the present example, it may comprise the diseases:

$\{$bronchitis, pneumonia, pleurisy$\}$.   (85)

However, the received view is mistaken because diseases are *diseases,* not diagnoses. The issue is much more complicated than it seems prima facie, and calls for a sophisticated concept. In what follows, we shall suggest such a concept, which may also be used in clinical decision support systems. For details, see (Westmeyer, 1975; Sadegh-Zadeh, 1978a).

Two possibilities are to be distinguished: (i) On the one hand, 'all diseases' that come into consideration in a patient as being potentially-causally relevant to her data D, may not be mutually exclusive to the effect that some or all of them may be present simultaneously. This is the case in the above example where Mr. Elroy Fox may have all three diseases (85), or two of them, at the same time. Thus, the hypothesis "Elroy Fox has bronchitis, pneumonia, and pleurisy" is an admissible differential diagnosis. (ii) On the other hand, the presence of some diseases in a patient may exclude the presence of others to the effect that not 'all diseases' that are hypothesized, can be present at the same time. For example, it is not sensible to assume that a 60-year-old patient, *b,* with acute chest pain might have myocardial infarction, diaphragmatic rupture, *and* intrapleural bleeding. The presence of each of these three diseases excludes, empirically and not logically, the presence of the other two.

To account for the differences above and to formulate differential diagnoses more adequately, we recommend putting them into one *grand disjunctive sentence* of the form "the patient has A, or B, or C, ..., or Z". To this end, recall the difference between inclusive Or and exclusive OR outlined on page 884. Since exclusive OR, i.e., either-or-but-not-both, is defined by means of the inclusive Or, i.e. $\vee$, as follows:

$$\alpha \text{ OR } \beta \ \textit{iff} \ (\alpha \vee \beta) \wedge \neg(\alpha \wedge \beta),$$

differential diagnoses should be articulated by means of the inclusive Or, $\vee$, taking the exclusive OR into account whenever necessary. For instance, let us call the patient Elroy Fox in the first example above simply "a". Then it is reasonable to suppose that:

a has bronchitis $\vee$ a has pneumonia $\vee$ a has pleurisy.

In the same fashion, the differential diagnoses in the second example above, i.e. patient b, where mutually exclusive diseases are being considered, may be represented by the conjecture:

$(b$ has $P \lor b$ has $Q \lor b$ has $R)$
$\land \neg(b$ has $P \land b$ has $Q)$
$\land \neg(b$ has $P \land b$ has $R)$
$\land \neg(b$ has $Q \land b$ has $R)$

where $P \equiv$ myocardial infarction; $Q \equiv$ diaphragmatic rupture; $R \equiv$ intrapleural beeding. Independent of whether we obtain a uniform disjunctive statement as in the first example, or a logically mixed statement as in the second example, there is a method that unifies both of them in terms of the so-called *disjunctive normal form* that we shall propose as a means of representing differential diagnoses. We will first explain the new term "disjunctive normal form" with the aid of the phrase "elementary formulas of a formula", discussed on page 876. Instead of "elementary formula" we shall here say "elementary sentence". This may be exemplified by the statement "Elroy Fox has bronchitis and there are no leprous people in London" whose elementary sentences are {Elroy Fox has bronchitis, there are leprous people in London}.

For any sentence α, there are two sentences each of which is equivalent to α, while one of them is a disjunction and the other one is a conjunction. They are referred to, respectively, as a *disjunctive normal form* for α and as a *conjunctive normal form* for α. Here, we need only the former one.

Definition 107 (Disjunctive normal form). *Let α be any sentence with $m \geq 1$ elementary sentences $\{\alpha_1, \ldots, \alpha_m\}$. A sentence β is a* disjunctive normal form *for α iff:*

1. *β is a sentence of the form $\beta_1 \lor \ldots \lor \beta_n$ with $n \geq 1$,*
2. *Each β_i is a conjunction of the form $\alpha'_1 \land \ldots \land \alpha'_m$ with $m \geq 1$,*
3. *Each α'_i is an elementary sentence $\alpha_i \in \{\alpha_1, \ldots, \alpha_m\}$ or its negation $\neg\alpha_i$,*
4. *β is equivalent to α, i.e. $\vdash \beta \leftrightarrow \alpha$.*

For instance, let our sentence α be the statement "either patient b has myocardial infarction or diaphragmatic rupture, but not both", i.e.:

$$(Pb \lor Qb) \land \neg(Pb \land Qb). \tag{86}$$

The disjunctive normal form for this sentence is:

$$(Pb \land \neg Qb) \lor (\neg Pb \land Qb). \tag{87}$$

In accord with Definition 107, the components of this disjunction are conjunctions such that each component of a conjunction is either an elementary formula of (86) or its negation; and (87) is equivalent to (86). Thus, all clauses of Definition 107 are satisfied. There are algorithms that produce for any sentence its disjunctive normal form.[63]

---

[63] As mentioned above, there is also for every sentence α a *conjunctive normal form* of the structure $(\gamma_1 \lor \ldots \lor \gamma_m) \land \ldots \land (\phi_1 \lor \ldots \lor \phi_m)$ as a dual to disjunctive normal forms and with analogous characteristics such that each component of a disjunction is either an elementary sentence of α or its negation.

We are now in a position to introduce a concept of differential diagnosis that is superior to the one traditionally used. We shall need the terms "literal" and "idiogram", introduced on page 327, as auxiliaries.

Let $D = \{\delta_1, \ldots, \delta_k\}$ be the data set of a patient a, and let there be $m \geq 1$ maladies that relative to the knowledge base and reasoning method $KB \cup M$ are considered potentially-causally relevant to D, and are therefore presumptively ascribed or denied to the patient by the literals $\{\alpha_1^*, \ldots, \alpha_m^*\}$ such as "Elroy Fox has myocardial infarction", "Elroy Fox has diaphragmatic rupture", "Elroy Fox has intrapleural bleeding", "Elroy Fox does not have carcinoma of the lung", etc. Depending on the peculiarities of the setting in the clinical encounter, the physician formulates a *grand hypothesis* by means of inclusive Or, or exclusive OR, or in any other way, to hypothesize what might be wrong with the patient. In any event, there is a disjunctive normal form for her grand hypothesis that we suggest taking as the *grand differential diagnosis*.

Definition 108 (Grand differential diagnosis). *Let a be a patient and D be the set of her patient data. If α is a hypothesis, referred to as a grand hypothesis, that by means of the knowledge base and reasoning method $KB \cup M$ ascribes or denies $n \geq 1$ maladies to the patient and has $\{\alpha_1, \ldots, \alpha_n\}$ as its elementary sentences, then GDD is a grand differential diagnosis about the patient with respect to $\langle D, KB \cup M \rangle$ iff:*

1. *GDD is a disjunctive normal form for α, i.e., a sentence of the form $(\gamma_1 \wedge \ldots \wedge \gamma_m) \vee \ldots \vee (\phi_1 \wedge \ldots \wedge \phi_m)$,*
2. *Each component of the disjunction, i.e., each of the conjunctions, is an idiogram about the patient, i.e., each component of the conjunction is a literal.*

Definition 109 (Differential diagnosis). *If in a particular setting the sentence $(\gamma_1 \wedge \ldots \wedge \gamma_m) \vee \ldots \vee (\phi_1 \wedge \ldots \wedge \phi_m)$ is a grand differential diagnosis about a patient, then the set of its conjunctive components, i.e., $\{(\gamma_1 \wedge \ldots \wedge \gamma_m), \ldots, (\phi_1 \wedge \ldots \wedge \phi_m)\}$, is the set of all differential diagnoses about the patient in this setting. Each member of the set is a differential diagnosis with respect to the rest.*

In the example (87) above, the sentence $(Pb \wedge \neg Qb) \vee (\neg Pb \wedge Qb)$ is a grand differential diagnosis about the patient b; the set $\{(Pb \wedge \neg Qb), (\neg Pb \wedge Qb)\}$ is the set of all differential diagnoses; and each of its elements is a differential diagnosis with respect to the other element. It is interesting to observe that a grand differential diagnosis is, as a disjunction, a *conjectural diagnosis* as defined on page 327.

8.2.9 The Pragmatics of Diagnosis

Independently of its syntax and semantics, a diagnosis has additional characteristics that are usually overlooked, but are at least as important as those considered. This is the case because the diagnosis establishes social realities and roles for the patient, the physician, and their communities. These central *pragmatic* features of diagnosis are discussed in the following two sections:

▶ Diagnosis is a speech act
▶ Diagnosis is a social act.

Diagnosis is a speech act

On pages 22 and 54, we divided declarative sentences into constatives and performatives. The latter we called speech acts. In addition, we differentiated between three aspects or dimensions of a speech act: locution, illocution, perlocution. We will now demonstrate that clinical diagnoses are *speech acts* with these three dimensions. In this capacity, they establish social realities and roles independently of whether they are true or not, and state or communicate any facts. What does that mean?

Syntactically and semantically, a diagnosis such as "Elroy Fox has diabetes" or "to the extent 0.9 Elroy Fox has diabetes" seemingly resembles a constative statement such as "it is raining" or "to the extent 0.4 it is raining". Since constative statements are usually viewed as truth-evaluable assertions of facts, a physician considers her diagnoses as constatives which she believes report facts. Because of its far-reaching consequences, however, this view merits critical examination (Sadegh-Zadeh, 1976, 1983).

The *diagnostic context* discussed on page 321 includes the patient, the doctor, her practice, the hospital, the patient's family, medical knowledge, and other factors, and produces the diagnosis as one of its outputs. It may metaphorically be characterized as a *machinery* that like a Turing machine consists of a tape and a control unit. An individual tape containing everything we know and learn about the patient, is assigned to each individual patient throughout the clinical encounter. The tape is a potentially infinite sequence of cells, with each cell containing a particular sentence about the patient. The control unit of the *machinery* has a tape head that moves over the tape and successively reads the contents of its cells. Sometimes the tape head stops for a second and attaches the label "diagnosis" to a sentence after reading it in the cell. Thus, the machinery selects from among the set of all possible sentences about the patient, say set $\mathcal{S}$, a finite subset that it calls "diagnosis". So the question arises how this machinery generates and justifies its diagnoses. *Why* does it label sentence $\alpha \in \mathcal{S}$ a diagnosis, e.g., the sentence "Elroy Fox has diabetes", but not another sentence $\beta \in \mathcal{S}$, e.g., "Elroy Fox is blonde"?

The real-world context or 'machinery' of diagnostics is highly complex with regard to the genesis of diagnoses. For example, a diagnosis such as "Elroy Fox has AIDS" emerging from a molecular-biological context of the 21st century would never emerge from a context of the Hippocratic humoral pathology that produced diagnoses such as "Elroy Fox has black fever". If we consider this aspect, i.e., the context of genesis of a diagnosis, as a base variable on which the diagnosis depends, it will become apparent that the diagnosticity of a sentence is a construct of the context of its genesis in the 'machinery'. The sentence "Elroy Fox has black fever" gets the label "diagnosis" attached in a Hippocratic context, but not in a molecular-biological one. This contextual dependence of the diagnosis may be called its context sensitivity or *contextuality*. The contextuality of diagnosis may of course be viewed and analyzed from different perspectives, e.g., from a technological, social, scientific, economic, or historical one.

The ontological import of diagnosis as an alleged *constative* that purportedly reveals truth or some truth about the patient, is called into question by its contextuality. The adherents of the Hippocratic school considered their diagnoses true. In our view today they are not false, but simply meaningless. In a future system of health care, our current diagnoses may earn a comparable judgment.

Notwithstanding the quarrel about whether or not a diagnosis narrates truths and facts, it *generates* truths and facts in that it triggers individual, group, and organizational behavior. Specifically, the patient assumes the role her doctor's diagnosis suggests; her family members, relatives, and the hospital personnel do what the diagnosis implies; the health insurance pays for what the diagnosis costs; and so on. The doctor's utterance "you have diabetes" or "you have myocardial infarction" makes it appear so in the real-world context. The patient is treated and behaves as if she had diabetes or she had myocardial infarction even though the doctor's diagnosis may in fact be a misdiagnosis. That means that a diagnosis belongs to the second type of declarative sentences. Rather than being a constative, it is a *performative*.

On page 55 we distinguished between implicit and explicit performatives depending on whether they explicitly contain a performative verb or not. The diagnosis in its usual form, such as "Elroy Fox has diabetes" or "you have diabetes", is an implicit performative. It can be transformed into an explicit performative by inserting the missing performative verb, e.g., "*I assert* that you have diabetes". For the notion of a performative verb, see page 55.

The verb "to diagnose" is also a performative verb. This will become apparent by reconstructing the context of communicating the diagnosis in a clinical encounter. Let $\Delta = \{\alpha_1, \ldots, \alpha_n\}$ be the diagnosis set the physician has arrived at. The diagnosis she communicates to the patient has the structure of an *explicit performative:*

I diagnose you as having Δ. (88)

Examples are "I diagnose you as having type 2 diabetes" or "I diagnose you as having type 2 diabetes, exocrine and endocrine pancreatic insufficiency, peptic esophagitis, Helicobacter gastritis, sorbitol intolerance, and no hepatitis".

The diagnosis proper, e.g., the supposed 'fact' that the patient has type 2 diabetes, is the *illocutionary* act of the diagnostician. And its impact on the patient, her family, the hospital, and community is her perlocutionary act (see Section 3.3 on page 53). A clinical diagnosis as a speech act thus belongs to the following, particular category of speech acts.[64] Like a judicial verdict, it is a *verdictive*. As a verdictive, it imposes a social status on the patient, a status that is created by the physician or a group of decision-makers on behalf of the society, and is regulated by:

- *the state:* health care laws, patient rights, physician duties,
- *professional communities:* oaths, taxonomies, terminologies, recommendations,
- *medical sciences:* medical language, medical knowledge, diagnostic criteria.

The physician's status-establishing decision says "you have the malady X and must therefore do Y". We have added to the diagnosis (88) in the narrow sense the supplement *"and must therefore do Y"* because the diagnostic judgment of the physician in a wider sense also includes her recommendation as to *what must be done* in this situation, i.e., treatment and advice. We shall continue our discussion on this issue in Section 8.4 on page 353.

Diagnosis is a social act

It is well-known that a judicial verdict has significant social effects. It not only affects the life of the accused when, for example, she is to be imprisoned, but also the lives of a more or less large group directly or indirectly related with her. This perlocutionary dimension of the speech act is unquestionably a *social act*. We should be aware that a clinical diagnosis as a verdictive also develops similar, socially efficacious perlocutionary effects in that it imposes a social status on the patient, the well-known *sick role,* including particular rights and obligations (Parsons, 1951, 436). It affects her family, colleagues, employer, the hospital personnel caring for her, the health insurance, and even the state. She becomes the client of a care group that looks after her: medically, psychologically, socially, financially, spiritually, etc. Thus, diagnosis as a speech act alters social reality, and the diagnostician turns out a social agent who creates *social facts.* "Appropriate diagnoses can exempt individuals from military service, provide special financial compensations, and render persons accused of a crime non-culpable by reason of insanity. On the other hand,

---

[64] John Austin, the founder of speech act theory, has distinguished the following five types of speech acts (Austin, 1962, lecture 12). 1. *Verdictives* are speech acts giving a verdict, e.g., court decisions; 2. *Exercitives* are speech acts exercising power, rights, and influence, e.g., orders and requests; 3. *Commissives* are speech acts that commit the speaker to a course of action, e.g., promises and guarantees; 4. *Behabitives* are speech acts concerning social behavior and interaction, e.g., apologies and congratulations; and 5. *Expositives* are an heterogeneous group of speech acts expounding views on how utterances fit into a present discourse, e.g., arguing, replying, and conceding.

diagnoses can brand individuals as deviant, as lepers, as appropriate for hospitalization against their will as insane. That is to say, the act of diagnosis renders individuals subject to various sick-roles, each endowed with its own sanctions and privileges" (Engelhardt, 1980, 43).

Although diagnosis as a verdictive is usually enacted by the doctor, it is brought about by a collective action of the group that participates in the diagnostic process. This collective action, i.e., diagnostics, is a recurrent one that takes place daily in numerous practices and hospitals. On page 514, we shall term this type of recurrent collective actions a *social practice*. Medical diagnostics represents a social practice par excellence. As we shall observe in the above-mentioned context, social practices are generative of social facts. Such facts are referred to as *institutional facts* because they emerge, through social practices, from and within *social institutions*. The sick role imposed by diagnosis is an institutional fact that is generated, through the social practice of diagnostics, by the institution of medicine and supporting state authorities. It is not a natural fact, such as rain and earthquakes, beyond human will and control. Since a social institution consists of a number of ought-to-do rules or norms that are constitutive of a social practice, the sick role as a social fact is an institutional fact brought about by the social institution of diagnostic ought-to-do rules. It is completely a human construct (see Section 15.1 on page 578).

8.2.10 The Methodology of Diagnostics

Methodology of diagnostics is that part of the metadiagnostic inquiry which is concerned with the methods of diagnostic reasoning, i.e., the component M in our concept of diagnosis:

$$diagnosis(p, D, KB \cup M) = \Delta \tag{89}$$

introduced in Definition 102 on page 322. As was mentioned in preceding sections, medical students are not taught any general diagnostic method that would enable them to find the right clinical path through the jungle of the branching clinical questionnaire, a deficiency that is partially responsible for physician fallibility. Explicit methods to guide the diagnostic process were something that medicine had to wait for until 1959 when a seminal paper by the engineer Robert Steven Ledley and the physician Lee B. Lusted appeared. This publication on the foundations of reasoning in medical diagnosis gave rise to the field of medical decision-making which also contributed to the emergence of medical artificial intelligence in the 1970s (Ledley and Lusted, 1959; Lusted, 1968; Buchanan and Shortliffe, 1984). Thanks to these research efforts, a true methodology of diagnostics is emerging. We have already stated on page 323 that the advent of this methodology may be viewed as the beginning of an engineering science of clinical practice, including diagnostic reasoning. The so-called diagnostic decision support systems, clinical knowledge-based systems, or expert systems are in fact the products of this clinical engineering science.

The responsibilities of the methodology of diagnostics will also include the analysis of the conceptual and logical structure of the clinical knowledge used in diagnostics, i.e., the component *KB* in the concept (89) above, the construction of new methods and tools of diagnostic reasoning, and comparative diagnostic methodology. A comparative diagnostic methodology may examine, compare, and evaluate:

- the diagnostic goodness of different knowledge bases KB_1, KB_2, and so on;
- different diagnostic operators dg_1, dg_2, and so on (see Section 8.2.6 on page 319);
- competing methods $M_1, M_2, \ldots$ of diagnostic reasoning to compare their diagnostic accuracy, moral impacts, economic, and other social aspects.

For example, to compare two diagnostic methods M_1 and M_2, one may define, on the basis of the conceptual apparatus provided in preceding sections, simplified notions of diagnosis such as "the diagnosis for patient p with data set D relative to knowledge base KB and method M is Δ", symbolized by $diagnosis(p, D, KB \cup M) = \Delta$. The application of two distinct methods, M_1 and M_2, will enable us to evaluate them by comparing their diagnostic outcomes, Δ_1 and Δ_2, if the other components are held constant:

$$diagnosis(p, D, KB \cup M_1) = \Delta_1$$
$$diagnosis(p, D, KB \cup M_2) = \Delta_2.$$

If in a clinical setting both diagnostic methods yield the same diagnoses, $\Delta_1 = \Delta_2$, then no epistemological problems will arise. However, if the two diagnoses differ from one another, $\Delta_1 \neq \Delta_2$, questions of the following type will ensue: Which one of the two diagnoses is true? Which one of them is more reliable? Which one of them is preferable to the other? Is the diagnostic difference $\Delta_1 \neq \Delta_2$ due to a difference between M_1 and M_2, to any vagueness of the knowledge base KB used, or to any inter-diagnostician differences? Of course, a method M_i is more accurate if in the same sample of patients it yields more accurate diagnoses than another method M_j. But there are two cases and two questions regarding this hypothesized accuracy:

First, assuming that both diagnostic methods operate on the same knowledge base KB, it must be asked relative to what background frame of reference their diagnostic outcomes are being evaluated. For example, when in comparing two diagnoses about the same patient the frame of reference consists of an alternative diagnosis provided by histopathology, the question will arise whether this alternative diagnosis is acceptable. What guarantees its acceptability? Furthermore, if we were to continue with this necessary epistemological question, we would unavoidably get into an infinite regress (see Section 20.3 on page 759).

Second, assuming that the two diagnostic methods operate on two distinct knowledge bases KB_i and KB_j, it must be ensured that their diagnostic yields are comparable at all. For instance, diagnoses emerging from a system of psychoanalysis or traditional Chinese medicine can never be compared with those generated by the theory of autoimmune pathology. Therefore, the underlying knowledge bases, KB_i and KB_j, need to be commensurable. That is, they must have a comparable ontology that is referred to by a comparable terminology and language. Otherwise, we would face the problem that no diagnosis generated by the knowledge base KB_i has a greater diagnosticity than 0 with respect to the second knowledge base KB_j, and vice versa. An example is a psychoanalytic diagnosis such as "Elroy Fox has a regression to anal phase" that in a system of autoimmune pathology has a diagnosticity of 0 indeed (see Section 20.3).

To further illustrate the issue of commensurability of knowledge bases, suppose that KB_1, KB_2, KB_3, and KB_4 are four different cardiology knowledge bases of current medicine. They are used, respectively, with the aid of the following four reasoning methods M_1–M_4 to obtain a diagnosis for the same patient p with the data set D:

$M_1 \equiv$ hypothetico-deductive approach (see page 343);
$M_2 \equiv$ Bayes's Theorem (see pages 980 and 988);
$M_3 \equiv$ case-based reasoning (see page 639);
$M_4 \equiv$ possibilistic reasoning (see page 628).

Four different diagnoses will emerge because the contents and the logical structure of the four knowledge bases KB_1–KB_4 as well as the inference strategies of the reasoning methods M_1–M_4 are different from one another. This example demonstrates once again that diagnoses are dependent on a variable frame of reference, i.e., the theories, methodologies, and epistemologies applied (see Section 8.2.6 on page 319).

Comparative diagnostic methodology may contribute to the enhancement of diagnostic certainty, accuracy and efficiency, and may thereby help reduce the vast amount of misdiagnoses. However, as the brief discussion above demonstrates, diagnostic methodology is inextricably intertwined with epistemological and logical issues.

8.2.11 The Logic of Diagnostics

Is diagnostics a logical process? Is it governed by a particular logic? These questions, of course, ask whether there is a logic of diagnostics. This problem will be analyzed in Chapter 17 on "The Logic of Medicine" (see page 675).

8.2.12 The Epistemology of Diagnostics

We have seen in preceding sections that clinical knowledge is an indispensable basis of medical diagnostics. For this reason, the reliability of diagnosis depends on the reliability of the underlying knowledge. We shall have a number of occasions in later chapters to address this issue. But among the epistemological issues concerning the diagnostic process are also the following ones: Does diagnostics generate knowledge? Does it lead to discoveries? What relationships exist between diagnosis and patient data? In addition, we asked on page 329 whether the diagnostics provides a causal explanation of patient data as is generally claimed. These questions constitute the subject of the following four sections:

- ▶ The epistemic status of diagnosis
- ▶ Is diagnosis a discovery?
- ▶ The hypothetico-deductive approach
- ▶ The truth status of diagnosis.

The epistemic status of diagnosis

Usually, a diagnosis is viewed as some item of knowledge about the patient's health condition. This view is based on the assumption that the diagnosis belongs to the class of declarative sentences such as 'it is raining', 'Elroy Fox has diabetes' or, in the fuzzy case, 'to the extent 0.4 it is raining', and 'to the extent 0.9 Elroy Fox has diabetes'. However, knowledge and opinion are to be distinguished from one another. We shall argue in Section 8.2.13 below that due to its context relativity, a diagnosis conveys an opinion rather than knowledge.

Is diagnosis a discovery?

A diagnosis is usually considered to be a discovery. But a discovery of what? First, a physician who diagnoses some diseases or abnormalities in a patient, does not discover any new category. She only allocates the patient to categories that are already known, or rather, are ones the physician has learned in the past. Second, supposing that she encounters something novel in a patient that was previously unknown, the discovery of such a new feature in only one patient, comparable to the discovery of a unique object such as a mountain on the backside of Mars, can never be a diagnosis. The causal rule that could justify the diagnosticity of that feature for patient data D does not even exist yet. The rule needs to be empirically established first. This rule-finding requires the examination of a large number of patients. Once the rule has eventually been 'found' and formulated, then it is a general rule, but not a diagnosis. It is a rule such as "most, or all, human beings infected with HIV develop AIDS". Even if we were prepared to call such a rule-finding process a 'discovery', i.e., a discovery of a relationship, it would be a mere slip of the tongue to refer to it as a diagnosis because a diagnosis as an idiogram has to bear the name of an individual patient, whereas a rule lacks any patient name. For these reasons, no diagnosis is a discovery.

The hypothetico-deductive approach

It is a rather widely held view that the aim of science is to explain natural phenomena and to predict future events. In accord with this deeply-rooted traditional dogma, clinical diagnostics is also supposed to provide explanations of the patient's suffering. To examine whether this claim is an appropriate account of medical diagnostics, we must first ask ourselves what an explanation is.

The most influential theory of scientific explanation today, first proposed by Carl Gustav Hempel and Paul Oppenheim in 1948 (Hempel and Oppenheim; 1948; Hempel, 1965), has come to be known as the *covering-law model*. To understand this proposal, we need a few auxiliary terms. An event that is to be explained, is called the *explanandum*, e.g., a patient's fever and cough. The statement that describes it, is referred to as the *explanandum statement*, e.g., "Elroy Fox has fever and coughs". An explanandum is explained by a set of other statements. They are called the *explanans*.

Roughly, the covering-law model says that a scientific explanation is a logical argument whose conclusion is the explanandum statement and whose premises comprise the explanans consisting of (i) one or more scientific laws, and (ii) some additional statements describing those particular circumstances, called *antecedent conditions,* which made the occurrence of the explanandum possible. The authors distinguish several subtypes the main representative of which is the so-called *deductive-nomological explanation,* or D-N explanation for short. A D-N explanation is a deductive argument such that the explanandum statement deductively follows from the explanans. The explanans consists of $m \geq 1$ universal generalizations, referred to as laws, and $n \geq 1$ statements of antecedent conditions. The explanandum statement describes a singular event such as, for example, the event that the patient Elroy Fox has suffered myocardial infarction. A D-N argument may be schematically represented in the following way:

Explanans:	$L_1, \ldots, L_m$
	$A_1, \ldots, A_n$
Explanandum statement:	E

This is the so-called Hempel-Oppenheim scheme, or H-O scheme, of D-N explanation. $L_1, \ldots, L_m$ are $m \geq 1$ universal generalizations, i.e., laws; $A_1, \ldots, A_n$ are $n \geq 1$ singular statements of antecedent conditions; and the conclusion E is the explanandum statement implied by the explanans. A *causal explanation* is a D-N explanation whose explanans contains at least one deterministic-causal law defined in Definition 61 on page 229. A simple example may demonstrate. Our explanandum is the event that the patient Elroy Fox has suffered myocardial infarction. *Why* did this event occur? The following D-N argument causally explains why:

L :   If one of the main coronary arteries of the heart of a human being occludes at time t_1, then she suffers myocardial infarction shortly after t_1;

A_1 :   Elroy Fox is a human being;

A_2 :   A main coronary artery of Elroy Fox's heart occluded at time t_1 (e.g., ten minutes ago);

A_3 :   time t_2 is shortly after time t_1;

E :   Elroy Fox suffers myocardial infarction at time t_2.

The explanandum statement E deductively follows from the causal explanans $L \wedge A_1 \wedge A_2 \wedge A_3$. The law statement L in the explanans is a causal law of the form $\forall x \forall t_1 \forall t_2 (Px \wedge Qxt_1 \wedge t_2$ *is shortly after* $t_1 \rightarrow Rxt_2)$ where $Px \equiv$ "x is a human being"; $Qxt_1 \equiv$ "one of the main coronary arteries of x's heart occludes at time t_1"; and $Rxt_2 \equiv$ "x suffers myocardial infarction at time t_2". In the example above, the explanandum is the patient's suffering; and the antecedent statement $A_1 \wedge A_2 \wedge A_3$ suggests a cause of this event and is therefore a *causal diagnosis*.

We will not go into the details of the D-N theory here. It provides an explication of the so-called hypothetico-deductive approach where the laws in the explanans represent the 'hypothetico' component. The idea behind it is that a D-N argument explains an event by demonstrating that this event was nomically expectable ("nomos" $\equiv$ *law*). An extensive analysis, evaluation, and criticism of the theory may be found in (Stegmüller, 1983).

The D-N theory of explanation was suggested and extensively analyzed as a reasoning method in psychological diagnostics by Hans Westmeyer (1972). We must emphasize, however, that for the following reason it has only limited value in medical diagnostics: As was discussed on page 227, the universal generalizations required by the explanans, i.e., the deterministic-causal laws as above, are scarcely available in medicine. Most statements in empirical-medical knowledge are probabilistic statements that describe non-deterministic associations between events, and therefore do not enable the deduction of the explanandum statement from the explanans. That is, only a limited number of "causal diagnoses" can be obtained using the method of D-N explanation.

Hempel and Oppenheim's theory also includes as a subtype a method of 'inductive-statistical explanation'. An explanation of this type, it is said, is an argument whose explanans contains at least one statistical law and inductively implies the explanandum statement (Hempel, 1965, 381 ff.). We need not speculate about whether or not the method of inductive-statistical explanation might be used as a device of diagnostic reasoning in medicine because it has been shown that Hempel and Oppenheim's proposal is objectionable. There are no such things as inductive-statistical explanations (Stegmüller, 1973b, 1983). We shall show in Section 16.4.2 on page 598, that there is a more workable method instead, called statistical or *probabilistic-causal analysis* that may be used as a diagnostic procedure in all cases with lack of deterministic-causal laws (Westmeyer, 1975; Sadegh-Zadeh, 1978a, 1979).

The truth status of diagnosis

As was pointed out previously, the traditional conception of diagnostics rests upon the assumption that a patient is suffering from something definite and factual, and that the task of diagnostics is to uncover what it is. Correspondingly, it is usually assumed that the diagnosis is a constative describing the uncovered fact, e.g., "Elroy Fox has diabetes". Our considerations above will now be extended to explain why this naïve-realistic view is a misconception.

A major part of the diagnostic process consists of communication and interaction between persons and groups involved, e.g., the patient, members of her family, doctors, nurses, laboratory personnel, and others. The diagnostic process must therefore be viewed as a complex *communal action*. The diagnostician who eventually makes the diagnostic decision and says "Elroy Fox has diabetes", is only seldom in the position to know whether the information about the patient, e.g., test results, that she has received from the co-agents participating in that communal action, consists of true statements. As will be outlined in Sections 20.2–20.3, she must trust them. However, the communal action which occurs in the foreground, is shaped by a second one that occurs in the background. Through long-term analyses and negotiations, medical-professional and medical-scientific communities determine both the class of abnormalities and the ways they are to be diagnosed. For example, cardiological communities fix the class of cardiovascular disorders and the modes of cardiological diagnostics. Other communities such as medical taxonomy and terminology committees, e.g., on ICD and SNOMED, prescribe the conceptual substructures that are used in diagnostic categorization. For these reasons, diagnostics may be considered a spatio-temporally distributed network of collective action that is influenced by particular social processes occurring in medical communities. A diagnosis as the outcome of this collective action turns out a *social construct* generated by a complex social-historical process (Sadegh-Zadeh, 1983).

The diagnostic process is also shaped by available technological facilities, i.e., the action space that a diagnostician has at her disposal. For instance, if no microscope, no electrocardiograph, no PET and no immune cytology were available today, one could not obtain patient data that only these techniques are able to elicit. But patient data play an eminent role in the production of a diagnosis. A patient who fifty years ago would have been diagnosed as having several unrelated diseases such as Kaposi's sarcoma, intermittent pneumonia, pneumocystis carinii, and non-Hodgkin's lymphoma, is said today to have a retro-viral infectious disease, i.e., AIDS, a categorization that would not have occurred without the technology behind retro-virology and immunology. Hence, a diagnosis is also a *technological construct*.

We have repeatedly demonstrated that the context of diagnostics contains, among other things, two variables on which the diagnosis essentially depends, i.e., the method of diagnostic reasoning, M, and the knowledge base, KB. The instances of both variables that are used in diagnostics come from scientific and professional communities. The authority of such a community or group that recommends one method of diagnostic reasoning, M_i, over another method M_j is the only justification in clinical practice for preferring the former over the latter. The same applies to the choice of knowledge bases. A particular medical knowledge, e.g., evidence on the causal role of blood cholesterol level or of Chlamydophila pneumoniae infection in the pathogenesis of cardiovascular diseases, is never used on the grounds that it is true or that one knows it is true. The reason is simply that the concept of truth does not apply to scientific knowledge. Support for this is given in Section 9.3, where we shall see that no scientific knowledge is true. A particular medical knowledge is employed only because it appears more useful than a competing one. But 'appearing more useful than something else' is a pragmatic feature whose recognition and appreciation by the knowledge user is not independent of the propaganda campaign undertaken by the knowledge seller. Even the production of scientific knowledge does not rest on methods that could equip their products with a grain of truth or truth-likeness. The production of knowledge is itself a social, economic, and technological process occurring in epistemic factories (see Chapter 12).

Given that diagnosis depends on a number of generating factors, it appears more convincing than not to assume that diagnosis as a context-dependent sentence does not report facts. This holds true especially for conjectural diagnoses because their truth values, as mentioned on page 327, are unknown. Nevertheless, as speech acts diagnoses themselves generate facts, and thus, truths if they are enacted as successful speech acts. A diagnosis that as a speech act proves unsuccessful, has come to be termed a *misdiagnosis*. This issue will be discussed in Section 20.3 on page 759.

8.2.13 The Relativity of Diagnosis

As a verdictive, medical diagnosis is a product of the diagnostic process. That means, in contrast to identifying diagnostics with trouble-shooting in inanimate physical devices (Reiter 1987; de Kleer et al., 1992)(see page 300), that clinical diagnostics produces verdictives. Clinical diagnostics is a spatio-temporal network of collective actions a node of which accommodates an individual patient or a group of patients, e.g., a married couple, for whom a diagnosis is sought. The context dependence of diagnosis suggests that this diagnostic network is embedded in a social-historical context where a number of variables are operative to bring about the diagnosis as a construct of the whole context. We have already identified the frame of this context in Definition 94 on page 312, which is key to our discussion and has served as the basis of the host of concepts we have constructed thus far. As we have thoroughly studied, the main variables of the context are:

- The patient or a group of patients: Distinct patients have distinct diagnoses.
- Patient data $D = \{\delta_1, \ldots, \delta_m\}$ for which a diagnosis is sought: A data set D usually evokes another diagnosis than a data set D' does if $D \neq D'$.
- The diagnostician or a group of diagnosticians who are searching for the diagnosis: Since different diagnosticians usually have different knowledge backgrounds and reasoning strategies, they may arrive at different diagnoses for the same patient data D.
- The goals that the diagnostician is pursuing: For example, does she want to 'explain' the data? Does she want to collect additional patient data? Or does she pursue something else?
- The action space that the diagnostician has at her disposal to achieve the aforementioned goals: The collecting of data, for instance, is dependent on the available facilities.
- The frame of reference consisting of the knowledge base, *KB,* and the methods of inquiry and reasoning, *M,* which the diagnostician employs.

Obviously, a number of variables are at work in a diagnostic context. If they vary in distinct contexts, different diagnoses for one and the same patient will result when she is subjected to them. Let C_1 be such a diagnostic context. A diagnosis $\Delta_1 = \{\alpha_1, \ldots, \alpha_n\}$ produced in this context C_1 for a particular patient with her data $D = \{\delta_1, \ldots, \delta_m\}$ need not be equivalent to another diagnosis $\Delta_2 = \{\beta_1, \ldots, \beta_q\}$ for the same patient if it emerges from another context C_2. Given our familiar patient Elroy Fox with his data set $D = \{$Elroy Fox complains of pressure in the left chest, pain in the same region, paroxysmal tachycardia, night sweat, increasing adynamia$\}$, we saw in Section 8.1.1 that from six different doctors in different practices and hospitals he received seven different diagnoses: see pages 279–280. Each of these diagnoses must be evaluated relative to a corresponding context C_i with $i \geq 1$. By changing any of the above-mentioned variables in the diagnostic context, the diagnostic outcome, i.e. *the diagnosis,* will vary. Thus, diagnosis is relative to the context of its production. The relativity sketched thus far we term the *relativity of diagnosis* (Sadegh-Zadeh, 1977b, 1981d).

Among the whole context of relativity, the most important subcontext comprises the *knowledge base* and the *methods* of its application used, $KB \cup M$, that serves as the frame of reference of the diagnostician and diagnosis. Relative to this partial context, we introduced in Definition 102 on page 322 our three-place concept of diagnosis:

$$diagnosis(p, D, KB \cup M) = \Delta.$$

We have sufficient evidence to assert that a diagnosis, Δ, heavily depends on the structure and content of the knowledge base used, *KB,* and the reasoning methods M. The reasoning methods M may or may not include particular diagnostic algorithms, expert systems, and any kind of logic, e.g., a classical-logical system or a non-classical one. Since a doctor is never certain whether KB consists of true and reliable knowledge, whether the entire patient data set D is reliable, and also doesn't have the guarantee that her reasoning methods M are the best available ones, a diagnosis she arrives at for a patient will never be knowledge, but a mere opinion built in the respective diagnostic context. In another context, she may arrive at another opinion for the same patient data D. See Section 8.2.10.

8.2.14 Summary

The conceptual and logical foundations and structure of clinical reasoning were analyzed. A concept of dynamic, branching clinical questionnaire was introduced that serves as a tool to graph-theoretically reconstruct clinical reasoning as a process of pathfinding on the basis of patient data and medical knowledge. The concepts of differential diagnosis, indication, contra-indication, and differential indication were explicated to show that clinical pathfinding is a computable, deontic process of differential action indication. A concept of diagnosis was introduced and its syntax, semantics, and pragmatics were analyzed. On the basis of the whole framework, a relativistic theory of diagnostics and diagnosis was suggested in the light of which medical diagnosis turns out a context-dependent speech act.

8.3 Prognosis

8.3.0 Introduction

To make a prognosis about a system means to predict how the system will behave in a specified future time. For example, "Elroy Fox's hyperglycemia will decrease this afternoon" is a prognosis about the patient Elroy Fox's sugar metabolism. Like a diagnosis, a prognosis is made through a process. This process or act of making is called *prognostics*. To parallel the verb "to diagnose", we coin the verb "to prognose" that means "to prognosticate", "to predict", and "to make a prognosis". In prognostics, you prognose to obtain a prognosis just like in diagnostics you diagnose to obtain a diagnosis. In the present section, we will inquire into the concept, logic, and pragmatics of clinical prognostics. Our study has four parts:

8.3.1   The Clinical Role of Prognosis
8.3.2   The Structure of Prognosis
8.3.3   The Uncertainty of Prognosis
8.3.4   Prognosis is a Social Act.

8.3.1 The Clinical Role of Prognosis

There is a frequently cited adage in the German medical literature, which is erroneously attributed to the famous internist and pioneer of nephrology Franz Volhard (1872–1950), and says "The gods have placed diagnosis before therapy". This popular dictum is used in German medicine to emphasize the fundamental importance of diagnosis.[65] However, before medicine began in the eighteenth century to profit from the then emerging natural sciences and to gradually assume their methodology, prognostics was the central intellectual and practical concern of physicians in clinical practice. With the advent of natural-scientific, diagnostic techniques and devices such as the stethoscope, thermometer, microscope, and clinical chemistry, diagnostics displaced prognostics between approximately 1750 and 1850 (Hartmann, 1977).

Clinical medicine is an institution of intervention in the lives of patients in particular, and of human beings in general. Its responsibility is *to intervene in order to prevent* harm and fatal development. At first glance, its actions seem to be guided by diagnosis. This first glance is deceptive, however. The diagnosis-orientedness of clinical practice notwithstanding, prognosis remains the basis of the practice on the grounds that no reasonable physician will perform a particular diagnostic or therapeutic action A without considering its benefits and costs. For example, suppose that action A is the use of a particular drug. When a physician knows or supposes that this drug will harm the patient more than it will benefit her, she will not use it. Only few physicians are aware that this basic principle of clinical decision-making, i.e., the principle of non-maleficence mentioned on page 680, is prognosis-oriented. It requires two prognoses about the patient, one about the natural course of her health condition in the event that action A is omitted, and another one in the event that action A is performed. That is:

    a. What state will develop in the patient if I do not do A, i.e., if I do $\neg A$?

    b. And what state will develop if I do A?

---

[65] The wrong attribution to Franz Volhard of the adage is due to the title of the book "The gods placed diagnosis before therapy" that was posthumously published as an homage to him by the pharmaceutical company Hoffmann-La Roche two years after his death (Volhard, 1952). However, with reference to a famous textbook on differential diagnosis by the Swiss internist and hematologist Otto Naegeli (1871–1938), Volhard has borrowed the dictum from Naegeli in 1939 (Volhard, 1942). It had been created by Naegeli in the following epigraph on the title page of his above-mentioned textbook: "The immortal gods placed diagnosis before therapy (in analogy to the well-known verse by Hesiod)" (Naegeli, 1937). The ancient Greek poet Hesiod (approx. 740–670 BC), to whom Naegeli alludes, wrote in his *Works and Days:* "But between us and Goodness the gods have placed the sweat of our brows" (Hesiod, 2007, § 286–292). The information given in this footnote was compiled on the basis of an illuminating brief note by a grand-child of Volhard, Fritz S. Keck (2007, 388).

Note that both prognoses are action-dependent ('... if I do ...'), and thus, possible consequences of actions. The rationale behind requiring these two prognoses is to compare the consequences of doing action A with those of doing action $\neg A$ in order to decide which one of these alternative actions is preferrable. That means that the question of whether or not such an action will be performed or omitted, be it a diagnostic or a therapeutic action, takes prognostic considerations into account. This circumstance is reflected in our basic concept of the decision-making frame in Definition 94 on page 312. The goals of decision-making in a clinical setting permanently change depending on the prognosis suggested by the health condition of the patient. We shall expand on this idea in Section 8.4.2.

8.3.2 The Structure of Prognosis

A clinical prognosis at a particular time about a patient's health condition says that in this patient something will occur at some later time. Thus, it is a singular statement at some time t_1 about an event at some other time t_2 such that $t_1 < t_2$. After t_2, it belongs to history and is no longer a prognosis. That is, a clinical prognosis is a temporally confined, singular statement about the future behavior of a system, called "the patient". It may have different sources. However, in order to be taken seriously, the prognostics producing it must be distinguishable from fortune-telling. To this end, it must obey explicit methods and criteria accessible to critical analysis and discussion.

For instance, the diabetic patient Elroy Fox may have hyperglycemia. Let the sentence "Elroy Fox's hyperglycemia will decrease this afternoon" be a prognosis suggested by her doctor. The first prerequisite is that such a prognosis be based on an explicit knowledge base and a particular method of inference such that both of them, the knowledge base and the method, are accepted in the professional community. To illustrate, let our knowledge about the physiology and pathology of the organism be represented in the form of general sentences each of which says what happens in the organism the next time if it is in the states $s_1, \ldots, s_k$ in a particular prior time. An example is provided by the general, deterministic law that the level of its blood sugar will decrease if it is injected with insulin. This general law together with a singular statement about the patient Elroy Fox yields the following prognostic argument:

- If someone is injected with insulin, then her blood   (90)
  sugar level decreases;
- Elroy Fox is injected with insulin;

- Elroy Fox's blood sugar level will decrease.

It is usually required that the knowledge used in prognostics be scientific knowledge and the prognosis be its logical consequence as in (90) above. Both requirements are problematic, however. First, it is by no means clear what "scientific knowledge" is. Second, there are a variety of logics. Which one of them are we to apply in prognostics?

It has been claimed that prognosis is structurally identical with causal explanation. We have already sketched the concept of deductive-nomological or hypothetico-deductive, causal explanation on page 343. According to the first part of the claim, which says that "explanation is structurally identical with prognosis", a D-N argument of the form:

$$L_1, \ldots, L_m$$
$$A_1, \ldots, A_n$$
$$\overline{}$$
$$E$$

that at a particular time explains the explanandum event described by E, could have been used as a prognostic argument at an earlier time to yield E as a prognosis before the explanandum event occurred. This part of the thesis is undisputed (Hempel, 1965, 364 ff.). However, its second part – "prognosis is structurally identical with explanation" – does not hold in general. The example (90) above demonstrates such exceptions. A prognostic argument of D-N structure as (90) cannot in general be used as an explanation after the predicted event has occurred. For details, see (Stegmüller, 1983, 153 ff.).

The concept of prognosis sketched above may be termed a *deterministic* one because it is based on deterministic laws in the premises of the prognostic argument. But we know that deterministic knowledge is scarcely available. Most prognoses are made using *probabilistic* knowledge about the probability of events, or using *possibilistic* knowledge about their possibility (see next section).

Unlike an explanation, a prognostic argument need not contain general sentences (laws) in its premises. Its premises may also consist of mere singular statements. General statements about an individual herself who is the subject of prognosis are admissible as well, be it a patient in the hospital or a rat in the laboratory. By employing a particular method M, whenever a set π of prognostic statements about a patient p follows from patient data D and knowledge base KB, then π is a prognosis about p relative to D, KB, and M. That is, $prognosis(p, D, KB \cup M) = \pi$.

The formal analogy between this concept and our concept of diagnosis is obvious. By and large, our philosophy of diagnostics also applies to this concept. We will therefore not define and further analyze it.

8.3.3 The Uncertainty of Prognosis

Depending on the syntax of the knowledge base KB and on the reasoning method M used in prognostic argumentation, a prognostic statement will have a different structure. It may be categorical such as "Elroy Fox's blood sugar level will decrease" as in the deductive argument (90) above. However, due to the lack of deterministic knowledge in medicine, most prognoses will not be categorical ones. They are usually qualitative-probabilistic statements such as "it is unlikely that without chemotherapy the patient's leukemia will improve", and express only the physician's subjective belief. Whenever statistical knowledge is available, one may attain quantitative-probabilistic prognoses such as "the probability that without chemotherapy the patient's leukemia will improve, is 0.1". In expected value therapeutic decision-making, one tries to obtain such prognoses from statistical data. See Section 8.4.2 on page 355. For formal analogies with diagnosis, see Section 8.2.7 on page 325. Another option is the formation of quantitative-possibilistic prognoses such as "the possibility that without chemotherapy the patient's leukemia will improve, is 0.5". See Section 16.5.2 on page 616.

8.3.4 Prognosis is a Social Act

We saw in Section 8.3.1 above that clinical decisions are based on prognoses. In this way the prognosis impacts the behavior of the physician, the lives of the patient and her family, what the hospital personnel does for the patient, health insurance, and so on. We will try to understand this phenomenon.

The new verb "to prognose", coined on page 348 above, is a performative verb. For instance, when a physician says to her patient "I prognose that without chemotherapy your leukemia will not improve", this statement is a speech act having *the prognosis* as its illocution. As an explicit performative, it also brings about a perlocutionary act to the effect that, for example, the patient's chemotherapy is indirectly justified, the patient is moved to accept it, the health insurance has to pay for it, etc. Like diagnosis, the prognosis obviously influences the decisions and lives of a group of individuals that includes the patient and other persons and institutions. It may therefore be considered a verdictive with social consequences, and thus, a social act. As a prognostician, the physician turns out a social agent. (For the notion of a verdictive, see footnote 64 on page 338.)

8.3.5 Summary

Diagnostics displaced prognostics between approximately 1750 and 1850. Nevertheless, prognosis remains a critical component in clinical decision-making and patient management today. Deductive prognoses can scarcely be formed because the deterministic knowledge needed for this purpose is rare. Most prognoses are made on the basis of probabilistic or fuzzy knowledge and data. Therefore, they are uncertain. Like diagnosis, prognosis may be interpreted as a speech as well as social act. Thanks to its perlocutionary social effects, the prognostician plays the role of a social agent.

8.4 Therapy

8.4.0 Introduction

The issue of therapy does not seem to arouse much interest in the philosophy of medicine, as there are few published analyses of its philosophical problems. What we often encounter is the common belief that diagnosis is a prerequisite of therapy. However, this belief is disproved not only by the important role that prognosis plays, as we saw in Section 8.3.1, but also by emergency measures where the physician has no available diagnosis and must intervene nonetheless. This and the practice of therapeutic intervening even in the absence of diagnostic certainty demonstrate that therapeutic decisions do not depend primarily or merely on diagnosis. At least as important as diagnosis is the assessment of the probability that the omission of immediate remedial action would increase discomfort, be harmful, or even life-threatening. This follows from our theory of praxiognosis, or differential indication, developed in Section 8.2.4.

There is enough reason to suppose that therapeutic intervention is based on prognosis and risk assessment rather than on diagnosis. In this section, we shall briefly examine this issue to inquire into the logic and pragmatics of therapeutic decision-making and to provide a basis for further investigations. We shall also include in our considerations the concepts and problems of therapeutic knowledge and efficacy. Our discussion divides into the following five sections:

8.4.1   Therapeutic Decisions
8.4.2   Expected Value Therapeutic Decision-Making
8.4.3   Treatment Threshold Probability
8.4.4   Treatments are Social Acts
8.4.5   Therapeutic Efficacy.

8.4.1 Therapeutic Decisions

When trying to understand and analyze the clinical goal in Section 8.2.1, we introduced on page 301 the concept of *praxiognosis*, or differential indication, which said that clinical reasoning is an inquiry into 'what should be done for this patient?' rather than into 'what is wrong with this patient?'. We showed that the dynamic, branching clinical questionnaire provides an appropriate praxiognostic tool. After evaluating all available patient data, the physician arrives at a decision node of the questionnaire where she receives an imperative of the form "perform action *A!*". The recommended action *A* is one of the following options:

- Do nothing,
- Terminate decision-making,

- Ask question Q to obtain additional information on the patient, e.g., record an exercise ECG,
- Intervention of the type X is indicated, e.g., laparotomy, immunization against tetanus, etc.,
- Therapeutic action T_i is indicated, e.g., appendectomy.

Options of the latter category are treatment indications proper referred to as therapies, therapeutic decisions, or therapeutic actions. According to our concepts of indication and differential indication discussed in Sections 8.2.3–8.2.4, the physician is obliged to choose a particular treatment of the recommended type T_i. This *type* may be appendectomy, antihypertensive therapy, chemotherapy, physiotherapy, or something else. For example, the treatment indication in a particular patient with acute appendicitis may be this: "perform an appendectomy!". Note that in terms of an *indication structure*, a therapeutic imperative of this form is an obligation in the deontic sense: "It is obligatory that you perform an appendectomy in this patient", i.e., "OB(appendectomy is performed)". See Definition 96 on page 313.

A therapeutic imperative to treat a particular patient, e.g., Elroy Fox, by performing a particular remedial action A is a deontic obligation of the form $OB(A)$ because it is the consequence of a deontic, therapeutic argument. The obligation follows from the therapeutic rule:

$$\text{If patient data is } D \text{ and your goal is } G, \text{then } OB(A) \tag{91}$$

and the information that the patient, Elroy Fox, presents with the data set D und you want to save his life (see Section 8.2.4). For instance, the premises:

- If a patient has acute appendicitis and you want to save her life, then it is obligatory that you perform an appendectomy on her,
- Elroy Fox has acute appendicitis and you want to save his life,

deontic-logically imply that:

- It is obligatory that you perform an appendectomy on Elroy Fox.

The fact that a therapeutic recommendation like the one above is a deontic obligation, is usually obscured by the inadequate presentation of clinical knowledge in medical textbooks. We pointed out on page 308 that diagnostic and therapeutic knowledge about a given disease is artificially spread over different sections of a textbook chapter. It is presented as if it were descriptive knowledge informing us about the symptoms of the disease and how it is actually diagnosed and treated by individual physicians. But how individual physicians 'actually' deal with diseases is certainly uninteresting as well as unimportant to talk about in the context of a canonical textbook. We shall explicitly demonstrate later on in Sections 10.6, 15.1, and 21.5.3 that clinical knowledge is of deontic character.

8.4.2 Expected Value Therapeutic Decision-Making

The therapeutic rule (91) used above gives the impression that all therapeutic decision-making is easy and unproblematic. However, the imperative "it is obligatory that you perform an appendectomy on the patient" instituted by the rule hides two important aspects:

First, in almost every patient there are alternative courses of therapeutic action, i.e., $n > 1$ competing therapies $T_1, T_2, \ldots, T_n$. They are called possible actions, treatments, or alternatives. At the very least, the set of possible alternatives comprises a single treatment T and its omission, $\neg T$, in terms of "doing nothing". For example, in the above patient with acute appendicitis, one can perform an appendectomy and one can refrain from performing an appendectomy (2 alternatives). A cancer patient can be treated with drugs, surgery, chemotherapy, radiotherapy, or left untreated (5 alternatives).

Second, it is not certain that a recommended treatment will have the desired therapeutic effect. Most treatments also have unfavorable side-effects, including death. That is, the causal association between a treatment and its desired therapeutic effect is not deterministic, but indeterministic, traditionally measured in degrees of probability. An example is "the probability that the appendectomy will cure the patient, is 0.98".

Thus, the question arises whether a categorical therapeutic rule such as "if a patient has acute appendicitis, then it is obligatory to perform an appendectomy on her" is plausible. It appears more reasonable to give the physician and patient the opportunity to compare the positive and negative effects of the alternatives and to choose the best one from among them. Below, we shall look at how such a decision can be made.

The sum of the benefits and costs of an action constitutes its utility or *value*. Decision theory provides a methodology of selecting therapeutic actions on the basis of their therapeutic values. There are two main types of decision theory, the classical probability-based theory, on the one hand; and the recently developed, fuzzy logic-based theory, on the other. We will not enter into a detailed discussion here. Rather, we shall discuss the fuzzy logic-based theory in a later chapter. For details of the classical decision theory, see (Jeffrey, 1990; Luce and Raiffa, 1989; Lusted, 1968; Sox et al., 2006).

To prepare the way for our later discussion, we will briefly mention several types of decision-making. *Individual decision-making* involves a single decision maker, while *multiperson decision-making* involves more than one decision maker. Therapeutic decisions are usually of the latter type. They involve at least the physician and the patient as decision makers. Furthermore, a therapeutic decision is either made in one stage, referred to as *single-stage decision-making;* or it derives from *multistage decision-making*. Finally, it may involve a *simple optimization* of the decision; an *optimization under constraints,* e.g., "the treatment should not incapacitate the patient"; or an *optimization under multiple criteria*. Although most therapeutic decisions are of the latter two types, for the sake of simplicity we shall consider only the simplest type, i.e., individual, single-stage therapeutic decision-making with simple optimization. To this end, we must take into account that decision situations may be of three different types:

▶ Decisions under certainty
▶ Decisions under risk
▶ Decisions under uncertainty.

Therapeutic decisions under certainty

A therapeutic decision is a *decision under certainty* if each of the treatments that could be administered is associated with a unique outcome. That is, the causal relationship between a treatment T and its effect E is described by a deterministic sentence of the form "if T occurs, then E occurs". The decision strategy in such cases is simple: choose the action leading to the outcome with the greatest therapeutic value. But what is the therapeutic value of an outcome?

The therapeutic value of an outcome must in principle be assessed by the patient or her proxy, but not by the physician or someone else. For example, she may evaluate the possible outcomes of the treatment alternatives, i.e., the prognoses, on a scale from -100 to $+100$ so as to render them comparable with one another. Costs get attached negative values. Positive values are assigned to benefits. For instance, our above patient Elroy Fox with acute appendicitis may attach to the traditional appendectomy the value 80 on the grounds that although it is therapeutically effective, it also causes pain and discomfort, and costs money. Endoscopic appendectomy gets the value 100 attached because it causes less pain and discomfort than the competing treatment does. Thus, in this case, due to $100 > 80$, endoscopic appendectomy has the greatest therapeutic value and will therefore be preferred by the patient.

Therapeutic decisions under risk

A therapeutic *decision under risk* is made when (i) each treatment alternative is associated with more than one consequence, e.g., with positive therapeutic effects and negative effects such as incapacitation, coma, or death; and (ii) the probability of occurrence of each consequence is known. Here the usual decision strategy is the *Bayesian decision rule* that says: Maximize the *expected value!* That is, choose the action with the greatest expected value. To explain this concept and strategy, suppose for simplicity's sake that in a patient with acute appendicitis we consider only two treatment alternatives, {appendectomy, palliative therapy}, and know that:

- the probability of a cure is 0.98 if she receives an appendectomy,
- the probability of death is 0.02 if she receives an appendectomy,
- the probability of a cure is 0.7 if she is treated palliatively,

- the probability of death is 0.3 if she is treated palliatively.

Thus, we have for the two treatment alternatives the following four matrices:

1. A *consequence matrix* of all possible outcomes of treatment alternatives (Table 5).
2. A *probability matrix* that shows the probability of each outcome (Table 6).
3. A utility or *value matrix* that results from the evaluation of treatment effects, listed in the consequence matrix, by the patient or her proxy (Table 7).
4. Now, multiply the value of each action consequence, given in the value matrix, by the probability of its occurrence given in the probability matrix. The product is the *expected value* of that consequence. We thus obtain the *expected value matrix* (Table 8).

Table 5. The *consequence matrix* of the treatment alternatives 'appendectomy' and 'palliative therapy' in a patient with acute appendicitis

Therapy	Outcome	
	1	2
Appendectomy	cure	death
Palliative therapy	cure	death

Table 6. The consequence *probability matrix*, i.e. probabilities of the treatment results, in the same patient as in Table 5

Therapy	Outcome	
	1	2
Appendectomy	0.98	0.02
Palliative therapy	0.7	0.3

Table 7. The *value matrix* in a patient with acute appendicitis. The consequences listed in the matrix in Table 5 are evaluated by the patient on a scale from -100 to $+100$

Therapy	Outcome	
	1	2
Appendectomy	80	-100
Palliative therapy	80	-100

Table 8. The *expected value matrix* of the consequences in the same patient. The expected value ev of a consequence c is the product of its value with its probability: $ev(c) = v(c) \cdot p(c)$

Therapy	Outcome	
	1	2
Appendectomy	78,4	-2
Palliative therapy	56	-30

The *expected value of an action,* i.e., of a treatment in the present context, is the sum of the expected values of its single consequences. For instance, according to Table 8 the expected value of an appendectomy is $78.4 + (-2) = 76.4$, whereas the expected value of palliative therapy is $56 + (-30) = 26$.

Thus, an appendectomy has the greatest expected therapeutic value for our patient. If she and her physician follow the Bayesian decision rule ('maximize the expected value of your decision!'), they will prefer an appendectomy to palliative therapy. A 90-year-old patient with the same disease might have evaluated both treatment alternatives differently than our younger patient Elroy Fox did. Note that there are also other decision rules such as 'minimize costs of your decision'. They would favor other decisions. We will not enter into details here, however (see Luce and Raiffa, 1989).

Our aim here was to show that therapeutic decision-making, as multi-person decision-making, is based on value considerations. As a clinical expert, the physician provides the patient or her proxy with the consequence and probability matrixes, and the patient or her proxy creates the value matrix to attain the expected value matrix. With reference to the role of prognosis discussed in Section 8.3, we can now state why in clinical decision-making prognosis is at least as important as diagnosis: It determines the expected value of diagnostic tests as well as treatments. The treatment consequences evaluated by the patient are *prognoses,* and eventually the physician acts on the basis of such evaluated prognoses. That is, her actions are goal-driven and not diagnosis-driven. This also remains true in those cases where treatment decisions are made on behalf of incapacitated patients or are imposed upon those who avoid health care even though they have a dangerous contagious disease.

Therapeutic decisions under uncertainty

A therapeutic *decision under uncertainty* is made when each treatment alternative is associated with more than one possible outcome, while their probabilities are not known. We will not discuss this decision situation because it can be replaced with a decision under risk by using the subjective probabilities given by the physician, i.e., her *degrees of belief.* We shall come back to this issue later on page 635.

8.4.3 Treatment Threshold Probability

Because making a therapeutic decision depends on prognosis, the severity of the predicted course of a disease state influences the degree of diagnostic certainty needed by the doctor making it. The higher the imminent risk of damage by a supposed disease, the more uncertain the diagnosis is allowed to be when administering an urgent therapy or emergency measure. This treatment threshold certainty is measured by the probability of the disease state and referred to as the *treatment threshold probability.* It is the probability of the disease state at which therapeutic intervention becomes mandatory. Furthermore, as it is of more practical importance than diagnostic certainty, it is also influenced by the relevance of additional testing, i.e., the extent to which additional diagnostic tests will or will not change the probability of diagnosis. There are decision-analytical methods of calculating the treatment threshold probability (Pauker and Kassirer, 1980).

8.4.4 Treatments are Social Acts

It is commonly assumed that after having made a treatment decision, the physician acts accordingly, for example, by intervening in biological functions of the patient's body. However, like diagnostics and prognostics, therapeutics is also a performance that takes place in, and shapes, a larger context that we usually call a community or society. To substantiate this claim, note that when the physician decides to treat the patient with a particular treatment *T,* her explicit or implicit decision may be expressed by the following statement directed to the patient: "I recommend that you undergo treatment *T*", for instance, "I recommend that you undergo an appendectomy". Obviously, the statement is a speech act performed using the performative verb "to recommend". Its illocution is *the recommendation* itself. The doctor's treatment decision proper may be identified with this illocutionary act.

Once the patient or her proxy has given her consent to the physician's decision, the effects of the physician's perlocutionary acts maneuver the patient into a therapy role. There is sufficient evidence that even the patient's or her proxy's consent is one of those perlocutions. This implies that like diagnosis and prognosis the doctor's treatment decision, via her recommendation, is *also a verdictive* in that it has the effect of a verdict when spoken.

As a verdictive, the treatment decision sets a huge social machinery in motion, including the physician's and her collaborators' intervention in the patient's life and death affairs, the hospital departments' and workers' actions, the involvement of health authorities, of the patient's family, employer, colleagues, and health insurance. That is to say, the doctor's treatment is operating not only at the level of the patient's cells, organs or psyche, but also in the larger context of society. It alters, and creates, social realities and processes. Thus, it is a *social act.*

8.4.5 Therapeutic Efficacy

In order for the doctor and patient to determine the expected values of treatment alternatives and to make a therapeutic decision, they must know what the *therapeutic efficacy* of those treatments are. Probabilistic statements of the form "in a patient with acute appendicitis, the probability of a cure on the condition that she receives an appendectomy, is 0.98" are simple examples of the knowledge required. Therapeutic efficacy is tested in so-called *randomized, controlled clinical trials,* or RCCTs for short. An RCCT is a genuine, scientific experiment in the proper sense of this term. It is a well-designed investigation consisting of specified intervention in, and manipulation of, some condition to determine the effect of the intervention and manipulation. More specifically, it constitutes a systematic, prospective study of the efficacy of an intervention in human affairs designed to prevent, cure, or ameliorate a malady. The intervention consists in the application of pharmaceutical substances, surgical procedures, technological devices, balneological techniques, or other measures to examine their causal contribution to recovery, referred to as their therapeutic efficacy. The notion of *therapeutic efficacy,* however, has been fairly mystified since the advent of RCCTs. Advocates of the so-called "alternative, complementary, unconventional, unorthodox, or innovative" health care theories and practices such as homeopathy, anthroposophical medicine, bioharmonics, and others are primarily responsible for this mystification. They are of the opinion that therapeutic efficacy is something unmeasurable and transcends scientific methodology. So, they abandon RCCTs and do not subject their therapeutic techniques to such examinations. Viewed from a psychological perspective, their control phobia reflects their fear that their therapeutic approaches might turn out inefficacious. However, the orthodox adherents of RCCTs who oppose such 'alternative' health care, especially the traditional pharmacologists and pharmacists, display an equally sloppy semantics, since they overlook the distinction between *therapeuticum* and *therapy,* say drug and treatment. In this section, we shall shed some light on this difference in order to better understand the nature of therapeutic efficacy claims, on the one hand; and of therapies as complex bio-psycho-social processes, on the other. Our discussion consists of the following four parts:

▶   Randomized and controlled clinical trials
▶   The placebo effect
▶   Therapeuticum *vs.* therapy
▶   The myth of evidence-based medicine.

Randomized and controlled clinical trials

As mentioned above, a randomized and controlled clinical trial (RCCT) is an experimental, prospective study of the effect and effectiveness of a systematic, human, clinical intervention. We shall here concern ourselves with RCCTs insofar as their subject is the effectiveness, or efficacy, of therapeutic interventions. The instruments used in such interventions, include chemical-pharmacological substances such as acetylsalicylic acid (= aspirin), or procedures and devices such as a particular type of surgical operation, balneological technique, dietary measure, technical apparatus, and the like. Since not all therapeutic means are drugs, we shall use the term "therapeuticum" as a general label to denote the class of all agents, procedures, devices, and regimens of the type above used to attain a therapeutic goal. Below we shall see that a therapeuticum is not identical with therapy. It constitutes only a single component of a complex *treatment structure* intended to develop a therapeutic effect on the patient. Therefore, therapeuticum and therapy should not be confused.

Designed as a therapeutic experiment, an RCCT examines the efficacy and safety of a *therapy* – not of a therapeuticum – in human subjects, usually patients, with a specified malady such as a disease, disorder, syndrome, injury, lesion, defect, wound, deformity, disability, impairment, and the like. We shall use the common term "disease" to refer to any kind of such malady. For instance, the subject of a particular efficacy research may be the question whether the consumption of citrus fruits has any therapeutic effect in patients with scurvy.[66]

An RCCT has four phases. But we will not go into details here. For details, see (Friedman et al., 1998; Gallin and Ognibene, 2007; Hackshaw, 2009; Matthews, 2006; Piantadosi, 2005). As its name indicates, it has two characteristic features. It is both *randomized* and *controlled* to prevent possible biases such as selection bias, allocation bias, observer bias, assessment bias, etc.

The term "randomized" means that by applying special methods of random allocation, like 'tossing a coin', the sample space of the patients used in the trial is randomly divided into two groups: (i) the intervention or *treatment group*, and (ii) the *control group* against which the former is compared. That is, a patient is allocated at random to one of these two groups.

The second characteristic feature of the experiment is that it is controlled in such a way as to determine whether the intervention is a causal structure, which we discussed on pages 247 ff. That is, the experiment is a pursuit for action types that may be conducted in clinical practice as *causes* to prevent, cure, or ameliorate a malady. To this end, the treatment and control groups must be sufficiently similar with respect to relevant features, say malady X, in order that the outcome of the experiment may justifiably be attributed to the intervention. Only patients in the treatment group receive the new therapeuticum, A, that is being tested. To enable a comparison of the experimental results between the treatment group and the control group, patients in the latter group do not receive A, they receive *non-A*. Non-A is either nothing or something else, say B, that is either a standard therapeuticum or a placebo that does not contain any therapeutically active agent.

In order to further exclude extraneous influences on the outcome and to increase control of the experiment as far as possible, it may be blinded whenever applicable. It is a double-blind experiment when neither the doctor nor the patient knows whether she, the patient, is a member of the treatment or control group, i.e., when neither the doctor knows whether the therapeuticum

---

[66] The evolution of efficacy research dates from the eighteenth century. The English naval physician James Lind (1716–1794) discovered in 1747 that citrus fruits were an effective therapeutic and preventive measure against scurvy. "On the 20th May, 1747, I took twelve patients in the scurvy on board of the *Salisbury* at sea. Their cases were as similar as I could have them. They all in general had putrid gums, ..." (Lind, 1753). The first controlled clinical trial in the strict sense of this term, however, was conducted by the Danish physician Johannes Andreas Grib Fibiger (1867–1928) in 1896–97. He studied the effect of serum treatment on the mortality of patients suffering from diphtheria. He clearly introduced the principles of control and randomization (Fibiger, 1898).

that she gives a patient is an *A* or *B,* nor a patient knows whether she receives *A* or *B.* Thus, we obtain a *randomized, double-blind, controlled clinical trial.* When the therapeutically active component of a therapeuticum cannot be hidden like in drugs, as occurs, for example, when the intervention is a surgical operation, blinding is not possible. In such cases, efficacy experiments are *open* trials. In either case, the main feature of the trial is its comparative nature. It enables us to compare therapeuticum *A* with therapeuticum *B.* We shall show below that it is due to this feature that controlled clinical trials fit our theory of probabilistic causality, discussed in Section 6.5.3 on page 233.

However, even with the use of an RCCT in testing a given treatment, an intractable problem remains. Suppose patients in the treatment group receiving the therapeuticum *A* show a number of symptoms, signs, and findings. What effect of *A* in these patients is to be considered its 'therapeutic effect' so as to be compared with the 'therapeutic effect' of the competing therapeuticum *B* used in the control group? The total spectrum of *A*'s effect will range from death to complete recovery, including every conceivable occurrence between these two extremes ranging from the normalization of an elevated enzyme level to pathological elevation of another enzyme level. Usually, the most favorable effect is chosen by the experimenters and referred to as a *cure.* The question of who decides in a controlled clinical trial what the term "cure" means or should mean, is a fundamental one in the philosophy of therapy. The only criteria that are unquestioned are mortality and the duration of survival. Of course, at first glance a therapeuticum seems to be superior to another one if it saves more lives and prolongs life. Let us consider a simple example:

A set of 500 patients suffering from disease *X,* say peptic ulcer disease, was randomly partitioned into two groups of equal size. The members of the first group received the new therapeuticum, say *A,* whereas the members of the second, control group didn't receive any therapeuticum. The experiment lasted two months. The comparison of the figures and a careful follow-up showed that in the treatment group 230 patients were 'cured' as compared with 30 patients 'cured' in the control group (see Table 9). According to this table, the proportion of the cured in the treatment group is $\frac{230}{250} = 0.92$, and in the

Table 9. This 2×2 contingency table demonstrates the results of an RCCT in 250 patients with peptic ulcer disease. Patients in the treatment group received antibiotics (metronidazole, amoxycillin, and clarithromycin), while patients in the control group didn't receive any therapy

	Cured	Not cured	All
Treatment A	230	20	250
No treatment	30	220	250

control group is $\frac{30}{250} = 0.12$. If we consider these numbers as estimates of probabilities in the long run, we obtain the following conditional probabilities, where *X* is the population of patients with disease $X \equiv$ peptic ulcer disease; *A* is the application of the therapeuticum *A;* and *C* means 'cured':

$$p(C \mid X \cap A) = 0.92 \qquad\qquad (92)$$
$$p(C \mid X) = 0.12.$$

Obviously, it is more likely for a patient to be cured by treatment A than without it. Here we shall not be concerned with the mathematics of statistical significance tests. Such a test shows, however, that the results are statistically significant, i.e., that the difference of 80% between the cure rates in the treatment group and control group is not a random effect. If the therapeuticum A has no serious negative side-effects, it may be preferred to non-treatment.

According to our theory of probabilistic etiology, the above result (92) of the experiment demonstrates that in the population of patients suffering from disease X, the therapeutic intervention A is positively probabilistically relevant to C because $p(C \mid X \cap A) > p(C \mid X)$. The intervention A may therefore be viewed as a potential positive cause of the cure. However, in order for it to be viewed as a genuine positive cause of the cure, there must not be another, earlier intervention, Y, in the treatment group that would screen A off from C, i.e., it must not be the case that $p(C \mid X \cap A \cap Y) = p(C \mid X \cap Y)$. Usually, it is tacitly supposed that this requirement is fulfilled. But the supposition is never explicitly analyzed. (For the notion of "screening off", see Definition 66 on page 239.)

Our experiment above was not blinded because patients in the control group didn't receive a therapeuticum and could thus recognize that they were in the control group. To prevent this extraneous influence, and for moral reasons, they may be given an alternative therapeuticum, B, to enable a comparison between its effect, $p(C \mid X \cap B)$, and the effect of A by examining whether $p(C \mid X \cap A) > p(C \mid X \cap B)$ or not. Here the notion of placebo effect enters the scene because the alternative therapeuticum B may be either a standard therapeuticum or a placebo. We shall study in the next section whether a specific therapeutic effect can be distinguished from the famous placebo effect or not.

The placebo effect

The well-known Latin term "placebo" is derived from the verb "placere", *to please*, and means "I shall please". It has been used in medicine since the last quarter of the 18th century and is borrowed from the Latin version of Psalm 116, verse 9, which reads "Placebo domino in regione vivorum" (Brody, 1980, 9).[67]

---

[67] "I shall please the Lord in the land of the living". It is said that the Latin translation of this verse 9 from the Hebrew (– et'halekh liphnay adonai b'artzot hakhayim –) is not correct. As in our current Bibles, the correct wording is "I shall walk before the Lord in the land of the living". In the 12th century, the Latin verse was sung in the Vespers of the Office of the Dead. Its initial word, "Placebo", soon became the name of those Vespers. Since about the 14th century,

In order to please or to appease a patient rather than to cure her inexistent disease, physicians sometimes administer pharmacologically inert medications in the form of dummy tablets, e.g., sugar pills, starch pills, or even 'fake surgery'. The experience shows that about 30% of the patients indeed feel improvement in their health nonetheless. The term "placebo" is used to denote this kind of empty treatment, and its effect is called the *placebo effect.* Although no therapeuticum with a specific effect is employed, there is an observable and measurable therapeutic effect, the placebo effect. How does this effect arise?

The placebo effect is of course not the effect of the fake, dummy tablet, e.g., a sugar pill, called the *placebo,* since it is void of any chemically effective substance. It is the therapeutic effect of the treatment setting as a whole including the doctor-patient relationship, the physician's positive attitude, the information about the patient's health condition and the instructions she gives her, the confidence in the treatment she expresses, and the therapeutic environment. All of these factors influence the patient's attitudes, behavior and life, her sick role and self-perception. A sugar pill would not develop such an effect if it were given to a diseased animal or if the patient unwittingly received it in her breakfast.

Therefore, one must conclude that a particular amount of the specific, therapeutic effect of a genuine therapeuticum such as aspirin or penicillin is placebo effect because the therapeutic setting is *efficacious* in the same manner and to the same extent as in the case of placebo treatment. This brings with it the idea that the efficacy, E, of a therapeuticum is composed of its specific therapeutic effect S and the placebo effect P, i.e., $E = S + P$. This implies that $S = E - P$. That means

Table 10. Results of an RCCT in 250 patients with peptic ulcer disease, where A = treatment, and B = placebo. For a comparable study, see (Lam et al., 1997)

	Cured	Not cured	All
Treatment A	230	20	250
Treatment B	80	170	250

that the specific therapeutic effect equals gross effect minus placebo effect. As an illustration, consider in Table 10 the extension of the RCCT reported in Table 9 on page 362. A second control group, also consisting of 250 patients with peptic ulcer disease, were given an alternative treatment, B, that was a

often the chorus didn't consist of genuine mourners only. Strangers also attended, sang the Placebo, and were paid by the dead's relatives. In this way, the word acquired connotations such as "fake", "substitute", "Ersatz", and "sycophant". In exactly this sense, disaggregated from its ecclesiastical role, it entered medical-therapeutic terminology by the end of the 18th century. It first appeared in 1785 in the second edition of George Motherby's New Medical Dictionary. With an improved meaning close to the current usage of the term, we find it somewhat later in Hooper's Medical Dictionary (1811): "Any medicine adapted more to please than benefit the patient" (Aronson, 1999).

placebo. According to Table 10, the proportion of the cured in the treatment group is $\frac{230}{250} = 0.92$ and in the placebo group is $\frac{80}{250} = 0.32$. As estimates of probabilities in the long run, these numbers yield the following conditional probabilities. Again, X is the population of patients with disease $X \equiv$ peptic ulcer disease, while A is the application of the therapeuticum A in the treatment group; B is the application of a placebo in the control group, and C means 'cured':

$$p(C \mid X \cap A) = 0.92 \tag{93}$$
$$p(C \mid X \cap B) = 0.32.$$

Thus, the specific therapeutic effect of the therapeuticum A now amounts to $0.92 - 0.32 = 0.60$. For moral reasons, however, genuine placebos are not used in all clinical trials in order not to harm the patients in control groups by withholding another, specific treatment, e.g., a standard treatment. Supposing that in an experimental trial such as (93) a new therapeuticum A is being tested against another, established therapeuticum B used in the control group, we are allowed to assess the efficacy of A by comparing it with the efficacy of B as in the example above. In such comparisons not only the arcane 'cure effect', but also the lethality and other negative and positive side-effects of both therapeutica must be taken into account and evaluated. As yet there is no acceptable methodology of doing such multi-criteria efficacy analyses.

Analogous to the positive placebo effect above, there is also a negative placebo effect called *nocebo* effect. The term "nocebo", i.e., "I shall harm", is derived from the Latin verb "nocere" meaning "to harm". The effect consists in the increase of existing, and creation of additional, adverse symptoms, signs, and findings such as pain, anxiety, nausea, fatigue, weakness, stomachaches, headaches, etc. Like a self-fulfilling prophecy or Pygmalion effect, the nocebo effect is the phenomenon that a patient who is told the treatment will cause harm actually experiences negative effects. For moral reasons, nocebos are taboos in clinical practice and research. Therefore, the nocebo phenomenon is not well-established in medical literature. However, it is well-known that particular types of physician behavior and therapeutic styles cause nocebo effects.

Due to their origin, placebo as well as nocebo effects unavoidably contaminate the therapeutic efficacy of a therapeuticum because they are effects of the therapeutic setting as a whole. The essential component of this setting is the therapeutic action of human agents participating in the setting. It cannot be *eliminated* from the therapeutic setting, be it in the treatment group, in the control group, or in the day-to-day practice. Therapy or treatment is the control of the patient's health condition by human therapeutic action that uses the therapeuticum as an *amplifier*. The amplifier is eliminable from the therapeutic setting in that a placebo is used. But its elimination will considerably reduce the efficacy of the therapeutic action. For instance, nobody will be able to cure breast cancer, AIDS, or myocardial infarction by employing any kind of placebo. Thus, some understanding of causality is necessary to understand therapeutic efficacy. It is a sheer exaggeration to maintain that all therapy is placebo effect (Lindahl and Lindwall, 1982).

Therapeuticum *vs.* therapy

On the basis of the foregoing considerations we distinguish between treatment *with* and treatment *without* a specific therapeuticum as a genuine amplifier. The predicate "is a genuine amplifier" means, first, that a specific therapeuticum such as a betablocker or anticoagulant is a causally relevant agent even without the therapist, for example, when the patient unwittingly receives it in her breakfast; and second, that it increases the placebo effect of the therapeutic setting. That is, the therapeutic setting and the amplifier are *interactive causes* according to the definition of this notion in Definition 76 on page 256. By contrast, a sugar or starch pill is not a genuine amplifier because without the therapeutic setting it is causally irrelevant and does not influence the patient's disease in any sense if, for example, it is hidden in her breakfast. Thus, we have arrived at a clear definition of placebo and therapeuticum: (i) A *therapeuticum* is something that without a therapeutic setting is causally positively relevant to a cure; (ii) a *placebo* is something that without a therapeutic setting is causally irrelevant to a cure.

What is conducted in controlled clinical trials in particular, and in therapeutic settings in general, is the *therapeutic action*. On the one hand, the efficacy of this action is increased by therapeutica, but not by placebos. On the other hand, the increments caused by distinct therapeutica, called their specific therapeutic efficacy, are different. For example, in infectious diseases penicillin is more efficacious than betablockers.

To conceptualize the views put forward above, we must distinguish between therapeuticum and therapy. A therapeuticum τ, e.g., a drug, is not a therapy. It is merely one single component of a complex *treatment structure* that we have referred to above as the therapeutic setting. A treatment structure includes, among other things, living subjects, situations and actions, and consists of at least the following eight components (Sadegh-Zadeh, 1982c):

a. therapeuticum τ,
b. the species of the treated patient, e.g., human, dog, cat, male, female, adult, child, newborn, etc.,
c. her specific disease state, e.g., endocarditis,
d. her boundary health conditions, e.g., penicillin allergy,
e. her specific social environment, e.g., single, married, wealthy, prisoner, homeless person, unemployed,
f. the treatment goal, e.g., cure, pain relief,
g. the image and psychological type of the therapist,
h. her modus therapeuticus placed somewhere between the two extremes 'prescribing without further ado' and 'being the ideal physician every patient dreams of'.

Thus, we have the 8-tuple $\langle a, b, c, d, e, f, g, h \rangle$ as our treatment structure or 'therapeutic setting'. Although the extent of therapeutic efficacy considerably depends on the component h that is also responsible for placebo as well as nocebo effects, all other components are equally important because all of them contribute to the efficacy. For example, a particular therapeuticum may be efficacious in the species cat, whereas it is inefficacious in the species *human*. Even in the human species females, males, and infants show different reactions to therapeutica. For instance, aspirin does not have the same preventive efficacy against cardiovascular diseases in females as in males. Thus, efficacy is relative to the species of the treated subject. Generalizing to the remaining components of the therapeutic setting $\langle a, b, c, d, e, f, g, h \rangle$, therapeutic efficacy must be viewed as something relative to the entire setting. Phrases such as "the drug x is efficacious" and "the substance y is inefficacious" are outdated and inappropriate. A complex structure of the form $\langle x_1, \ldots, x_n \rangle$ cannot be handled by using a one-place predicate such as 'is efficacious' or 'is inefficacious'. A corresponding n-place predicate or function is needed to yield a formally suitable and correct concept of efficacy. We will now sketch the formal structure of such a concept. To this end, let each of the variables $\langle \tau, S, D, C, E, G, T, M \rangle$ respectively represent a generic element of the:

1. space of therapeutica, $\{\tau_1, \tau_2, \tau_3, \ldots\}$,
2. species space, $\{S_1, S_2, S_3, \ldots\}$,
3. disease space, $\{D_1, D_2, D_3, \ldots\}$,
4. space of boundary conditions, $\{C_1, C_2, C_3, \ldots\}$,
5. space of social environments, $\{E_1, E_2, E_3, \ldots\}$,
6. space of therapy goals, $\{G_1, G_2, G_3, \ldots\}$,
7. space of therapist types, $\{T_1, T_2, T_3, \ldots\}$,
8. space of modi therapeutici, $\{M_1, M_2, M_3, \ldots\}$.

Thus, any treatment structure is of the form $\langle \tau, S, D, C, E, G, T, M \rangle$. The following 8-tuple represents an example: $\langle$bisoprolol, man, tachycardia, penicillin _allergy, prisoner, normal_heart_rate, friendly, excellent$\rangle$. Of course, it may be that in this structure bisoprolol will turn out efficacious, whereas by changing any of the parameters it will develop no effect at all. For instance, it will not work when the disease is 'leukemia' instead of 'tachycardia', and the treatment goal is 'cure'. Thus, efficacy as well as inefficacy is an attribute not of a substance or tangible object, say drug, but of the whole of a treatment structure. Otherwise put, the bearer of therapeutic efficacy is *the therapy* and not the therapeuticum. This can be conceptualized by introducing classificatory, comparative, and quantitative concepts of efficacy in the following way:

a. Syntax of an 8-place classificatory concept: $EF(\tau, S, D, C, E, G, T, M)$, to be read as "$\tau$ is efficacious with respect to S, D, C, E, G, T, M".
b. Syntax of a 16-place comparative concept: $EFF(\tau, S, D, C, E, G, T, M, \tau', S', D', C', E', G', T', M')$, to be read as "$\tau$ is, with respect to S, D, C, E, G, T, M, at least as efficacious as is τ' with respect to

$S', D', C', E', G', T', M'''$. This syntax can be simplified as follows: $(\tau, S, D, C, E, G, T, M) \succcurlyeq (\tau', S', D', C', E', G', T', M')$ where "$\succcurlyeq$" represents the 16-place predicate "... is at least as efficacious as ...". From this basic predicate, the following three comparative efficacy predicates (*more efficacious than, less efficacious than, as efficacious as*) may be obtained in the usual way (see definition schemes 65–68 on page 263):

- $(\tau, S, D, C, E, G, T, M) \succ (\tau', S', D', C', E', G', T', M')$
- $(\tau, S, D, C, E, G, T, M) \prec (\tau', S', D', C', E', G', T', M')$
- $(\tau, S, D, C, E, G, T, M) \approx (\tau', S', D', C', E', G', T', M')$.

c. Syntax of an 8-place quantitative concept: $ef(\tau, S, D, C, E, G, T, M) = r$, to be read as "the efficacy of τ with respect to S, D, C, E, G, T, M equals r", where r is a real number.

EF is an 8-place predicate; *EFF* is a 16-place predicate; and *ef* is an 8-place numerical function. We shall not try to suggest definitions of these concepts because this would require a whole theory of efficacy and a separate book volume. However, from our intuitive understanding of "therapeutic efficacy", which depends so strongly on moral values and worldview, we can presume that a consensus on its definition may be very difficult or even impossible to reach. Nevertheless, the use of a sophisticated language such as above may help reduce fruitless debates in therapy research and efficacy analysis. For example, it may be that regarding a particular drug τ we have $EF(\tau, S, D, C, E, G, T, M)$, whereas $\neg EF(\tau, S', D, C, E, G, T, M)$ if $S \neq S'$, and $\neg EF(t, S, D, C, E, G, T, M')$ if $M \neq M'$. Efficacy is something relative to treatment structures.

The myth of evidence-based medicine

The results of RCCTs have been subjected to critical review and evaluation in recent years from which the so-called *evidence-based medicine*, EBM for short, has emerged. This is not the right place for detailed expositon and criticism of EBM. A few words will suffice to show why it is nothing more than a dubious myth.

Several new research approaches gave rise to EBM. The main representatives of them were *systematic reviews* and *metaanalyses*. They will be briefly sketched first.

Systematic reviews

Literature reviews have existed for several centuries under the umbrella names "overview articles" or "review articles". They are *narrative reviews* insofar as they are conducted unsystematically, adressing any clinical or non-clinical questions dealt with in the antecedent literature.

What has come to be called a *systematic review*, is in essence a literature review to find out how a particular issue, e.g., the therapy of Alzheimer's disease, is dealt with in a collection of different research works; what results or solutions have been put forward; and how to compare and evaluate these results and suggestions. Most systematic reviews address issues of the effect and efficacy of therapeutic interventions, RCCTs so to speak. But they may also focus on other clinical and non-clinical research topics such as diagnosis, diagnostic tests and devices, prevention, etc. Although there are attempts to establish a roadmap for systematic reviews, e.g. (Guyatt et al., 2008a–b), there are as yet no specific methods underlying them. Approaches range from qualitative ('narrative') to statistical analyses. In the latter case, no sharp borderlines exist between a systematic review and a so-called metaanalysis.

Metaanalyses in medicine

Metaanalysis evolved in psychology and education as a method of statistical integration of the findings of independent studies of the same subject (Glass, 1976). Today, the term "metaanalysis in medicine" is understood to mean a systematic and structured analysis, synthesis, and evaluation of a problem as investigated by a number of different, independent studies of that problem, be it a treatment efficacy, the efficiency of a diagnostic procedure, an etiological problem, or something else (Jenicek, 1995; Petitti, 2000).

Such problems are, for example: Has antibiotic treatment of peptic ulcer disease been able in recent decades to decrease the incidence of gastric cancer? Is a carbon 13 test more sensitive for diagnosing gastric Helicobacter infection than a biopsy? Does Chlamydophila pneumoniae infection play a causative role in the genesis of coronary heart disease? A problem of this type is investigated not by new observations, experiments, or field research, but by analyzing the available, published results of a collection of studies of that problem. The aim is to examine whether the results and conclusions can be endorsed, and to search for additional results or ideas. In any event, a metaanalysis is itself *new research* to the effect that its results do not necessarily mirror the underlying findings. It is virtually a statistical, systematic review as discussed in the preceding section, and as such, it is meta-research that is subject to critical evaluation like any other scientific study.

The so-called evidence-based medicine: EBM

Impressed by the usefulness of results of systematic reviews and metaanalyses, a Canadian research group suggested in the early 1990s the popular doctrine of EBM (Guyatt et al., 1992). They started with the slogan:

A new paradigm for medical practice is emerging. Evidence-based medicine de-emphasizes intuition, unsystematic clinical experience, and pathophysiologic ratio-nale as sufficient grounds for clinical decision-making and stresses the examination of evidence from clinical research. Evidence-based medicine requires new skills of the physician, including efficient literature searching and the application of formal rules of evidence evaluating the clinical literature (Guyatt et al., 1992, 2420).

The proponents recommend to use in clinical practice *the best evidence* obtained through personal observations, systematic reviews, metaanalyses, experimental research, etc. According to its well-known, official definition, "Evidence based medicine is the conscientious, explicit, and judicious use of current best evidence in making decisions about the care of individual patients. The practice of evidence based medicine means integrating individual clinical expertise with the best available external clinical evidence from systematic research" (Sackett et al., 1996, 71).

The doctrine spread like wildfire by the end of the twentieth century as if it were something original, a "new paradigm" as they say, and more importantly, as if it were a novel medicine competing with the existing, academic medicine-based clinical practice and health care. However, the whole undertaking is based on a misnomer. A more appropriate label for what is called "evidence-based" medicine would have been "research-based" or "scientific" medicine. The misnomer is due to the meaning-laden term "evidence" that is uncritically used in the English language.

If "evidence" means results of scientific research, then the proclamation of "evidence-based medicine as a new paradigm" has been much ado about nothing, and our suggestion above to equate it with scientific medicine is justified to the effect that the new label is gratuitous. Otherwise, two possible interpretations of the term are:

a. Evidence is experience-based and research-based personal belief, or
b. any data that increase the strength of one's belief in a particular hypothesis.

In either case, EBM is in fact an old hat that has constantly been proclaimed since the emergence of modern, natural science-based medicine in the eight-eenth century (see, e.g., Tröhler, 2001; Naunyn, 1909), and every physician who is committed to continuing education already is doing it. Thus, the new term "evidence-based medicine" turns out a mere label for a mishmash of platitudes to draw a line of demarcation between academic medicine-based clinical practice, on the one hand; and esoteric services such as alternative, complementary, or unconventional health-care approaches, on the other, e.g., homeopathy, anthroposophical medicine, and bioharmonics. However, should proponents of these alternative approaches insist that "their clinical decision-making and practice is also evidence-based", what would you say? To answer such foundational questions, it is necessary first to define what is to be under-stood by the basic term "evidence". After all, what is evidence? Everything else being equal, it is not reasonable to define "evidence" such that scientific knowledge, hypotheses, and theories would count as evidence, for their epistemological status is uncertain and permanently under debate. But EBM explicitly categorizes them as evidence. For a more detailed analysis of this issue, see page 482.

8.4.6 Summary

Therapeutic decisions are usually multiperson and multistage decisions and are often made under risk or uncertainty. Although diagnostic-therapeutic knowledge is of deontic, imperative character, it leaves enough room to the physician to choose among therapeutic alternatives. Her decision is based on prognosis rather than diagnosis. Diagnosis constitutes only one part of the information she uses in therapeutic decision-making. Therapeutic decisions are value decisions because they depend on the value that the expected outcome of the therapeutic interventions has for the patient. This requires substantiated information on the therapeutic efficacy of therapeutic actions. Randomized controlled clinical trials provide the best method to obtain this information. In contrast to the customary view, such a trial is not a natural-scientific experiment to inquire into the efficacy of a therapeuticum, e.g., a chemical substance, physical procedure, or device. It is an *interventional-causal* investigation of the efficacy of a therapeutic setting a single part of which is the therapeuticum. What is being analyzed are in fact social acts in a complex context. For the term "interventional-causal", see sections 10.3 and 21.5.2.

There is a long-standing debate on whether therapeutic efficacy and placebo effect are distinguishable properties. We have answered this question in the affirmative by defining both notions. Taking into account that any substance can be furtively administered to the patient "in her breakfast", a substance can be defined to be a placebo against a malady if its furtive administration to the patient is causally irrelevant to curing this malady, while a substance can be defined to be a therapeuticum against a malady if its furtive administration to the patient is causally relevant to curing the malady.

8.5 Prevention

8.5.0 Introduction

Prevention in medicine means *intervening in the natural order of things* when there is a risk for the occurrence of harm such as suffering, disease, or death in an individual or population. For example, a physician may administer to a schoolboy a particular vaccine so that measles will not spread from his classmates to him. As a science and practice of prevention in medicine, *preventive medicine* is systematically concerned with the investigation, planning, and conduct of such preventive actions. The discipline that provides the data and their interpretation, is *epidemiology*. (The term "epidemiology" is composed of the Greek terms $\varepsilon\pi\iota$ (epi) for "upon, among"; $\delta\tilde{\eta}\mu\circ\varsigma$ (demos) for "people"; and $\lambda\acute{o}\gamma\circ\varsigma$ (logos) for "stuty". It means "the study of the social dimension of maladies", i.e., *what is upon the people.*)

The terms "prevention" and "protection" are related and interdefinable. To prevent an occurrence A in an individual or population B is synonymous with protecting B from A. We shall not be concerned with all of the philosophical and metaphysical problems of prevention, preventive medicine, and epidemiology. We shall reconstruct the concept of prevention only in order to show later on in Section 21.5 that thanks to its subdisciplines like preventive medicine, medicine is not a natural science, but a *science of praxis* par excellence, i.e., a pursuit of rules of efficacious doing and acting. In our discussion we shall confine ourselves to prevention in individuals and shall not include populations. We shall also not consider the differentiation between primary, secondary, and tertiary prevention. For a definition of the verb "to prevent", see Definition 75 on page 255.

The fundamental concept of preventive medicine is the notion of a "risk factor". For example, many features and habits such as the breast cancer gene, hypercholesterolemia, obesity, and smoking are considered risk factors for disease and death. A risk factor usually gives rise to actions to eliminate it. But the term "risk factor" is far from being clear. In addition, it is often overlooked that a risk factor is relative with respect to a population. We saw in Section 6.5.3 that a feature or habit may lose its property of being a risk factor from one population to another. Concisely, given a feature or event E that is *disvalued* in a particular population *PO,* then a risk factor for event E in that population *PO* is a *positive cause* of the event in that population. This idea will be expanded upon in what follows in order to reconstruct the concept of prevention. Our analyses divide into the following two sections:

8.5.1   What is a Risk Factor?
8.5.2   Prevention is Goal-Driven Practice.

8.5.1 What is a Risk Factor?

Whether or not a preventive action against an event is to be taken depends on whether there is a risk for the occurrence of that event. For example, prevention of coronary heart disease and stroke by anticholesterol therapy in a 50-year-old male is necessary only when he has hypercholesterolemia because hypercholesterolemia in men of this or older age is a risk factor for atherosclerosis, and consequently, for coronary heart disease and stroke.

A risk may be permanently or temporarily present. Correspondingly, there are, on the one hand, preventive actions that are regularly and systematically taken to protect people from a group of maladies because the risk for their occurrence is permanently present. Examples are pest control, sewage systems, clean water supply, and state-supervised hygiene in general to prevent infectious diseases. On the other hand, some other preventive actions need to be taken only when a particular person or a group of persons are at risk of being harmed or afflicted, e.g., a yellow fever vaccination for a visitor to Nigeria or the collective vaccination of German people against the imminent Mexican swine influenza epidemic in 2009. In any event, prevention is undertaken depending on whether there is a risk present. Thus, the concept of prevention requires a concept of risk. There are different types and concepts of risk such as the individual risk, the risk ratio, the risk difference, the attributable risk, the odds ratio, and the hazard rate ratio. We will explicate only the first two risks for developing a disease. In the following three sections, the currently used concepts are explicated in a probability-based and in a possibility-based version, followed by a criticism and improvement:

▶ Individual risk and risk ratio: Probability-based
▶ Individual risk and risk ratio: Possibility-based
▶ Individual risk and risk ratio: Criticism and improvement.

Individual risk and risk ratio: Probability-based

Customarily, individual risk is defined in the following fashion: "The probability of an individual developing a disease (or dying) in a defined time, given the characteristics of the individual and his community, represents an individual risk" (Jenicek, 2003, 87). This standard definition used in epidemiology, however, is both imprecise and inadequate and needs to be improved. To demonstrate, we will first make the definition precise. To this end, let there be a particular population PO with its members characterized by a condition C, e.g., "is a schoolchild", "is not inoculated", or "has hypercholesterolemia". Syntactically purified, the above definition says that the *individual risk* of a person $x \in PO$ for developing a disease D in the population PO with condition C in a defined time is the probability of developing the disease D conditional on C in that population. That is:

$$individual\_risk(x, D, PO, C) = p(D \mid PO \cap C) \qquad (94)$$

Obviously, "individual_risk" is a four-place function. As we know from our considerations on etiology on page 239, however, condition C in a statement of the type $p(D \mid PO \cap C) = r$ in the formula (94) above may be probabilistically irrelevant to D in the population PO simply because of the following relationship that may hold in that population:

$$p(D \mid PO \cap C) = p(D \mid PO).$$

For instance, it may be that for developing coronary heart disease, *chd,* we have:

$$p(chd \mid diabetics \cap obese) = p(chd \mid diabetics).$$

That means that in diabetics, obesity is probabilistically irrelevant to coronary heart disease. In such a case, it would not be justified to view obesity as a risk factor for developing coronary heart disease because its addition to the base attribute *diabetic* does not change the base probability $p(chd \mid diabetics)$. This consideration suggests to include in the definition of "individual risk" the feature that the supposed risk factor is, with respect to the base population *PO*, probabilistically relevant to developing the disease. The mere conditional probability of developing the disease as required in the standard definition (94) does not suffice. An example may demonstrate the significance of the probabilistic relevance. Suppose we had the following data on the incidence of measles in the population of German schoolchildren in 2009 (Table 11):

Table 11. A 2×2 contingency table on the incidence of measles in German school-children of the year 2009 (dressed up)

	Contracted	Not contracted	All
Inoculated	9	8 999 991	9 000 000
Non-inoculated	89	355 911	356 000
All	98	9 335 902	9 356 000

From the contingency table given in Table 11 we can calculate the following conditional probabilities. The mean probability of contracting measles in the base population of German schoolchildren is $\frac{98}{9356000} = 0.0000104$, whereas the conditional probability of contracting measles in the subpopulation of non-inoculated is 24 times higher, i.e., $\frac{89}{356000} = 0.00025$, and in the subpopulation of inoculated 10 times lower:

$p(measles \mid German\_schoolchild) = 0.0000104$

$p(measles \mid German\_schoolchild \cap inoculated) = 0.000001$

$p(measles \mid German\_schoolchild \cap non\text{-}inoculated) = 0.00025.$

These data demonstrate that not being inoculated is probabilistically positively relevant to contracting measles in the population of German schoolchildren, whereas inoculation is probabilistically negatively relevant on the grounds that:

$p(measles \mid German\_schoolchild \cap non\text{-}inoculated) >$
$$p(measles \mid German\_schoolchild)$$

$p(measles \mid German\_schoolchild \cap inoculated) <$
$$p(measles \mid German\_schoolchild).$$

According to this information we can say that in the population of German schoolchildren, inoculation is a preventive factor, whereas not being inoculated is a risk factor for measles. Inoculation lowers, while its absence raises the probability of contracting the disease. The notion of prevention was introduced in Definition 75 on page 255 as a relation of negative causation or *discausation*. With reference to that definition, we may provisionally define the notions of risk and preventive (= protective) factor in the following way.

Definition 110 (Risk factor). *A condition C is a* risk factor *for an event D in a population PO iff:*

  1. *D is disvalued in the population PO,*
  2. *$p(D \mid PO \cap C) > p(D \mid PO)$.*

Definition 111 (Preventive factor). *A condition C is a* preventive (= protective) *factor for an event D in a population PO iff:*

  1. *D is disvalued in the population PO,*
  2. *$p(D \mid PO \cap C) < p(D \mid PO)$.*

Obviously, risk assessment in the traditional sense is not based on any explicit or recognizable causal relation between the risk factor and the disease. It is only an assessment of the factor's probabilistic relevance, and thus, of its *potential-causal* impact. A traditional risk factor is a positive potential cause, while a protective factor is a negative potential cause. A risk factor or a protective factor may of course be actually a negative or positive cause, respectively. (For the notions of potential cause, positive cause, and negative cause, see pages 250–255.)

Based on the preliminaries above, we may now introduce a concept of individual risk. As our preceding discussions suggest, the degree of *individual risk* of an inoculated schoolchild x for contracting measles equals *the probability of* contracting the disease conditional on inoculation. And the degree of *individual risk* of a non-inoculated schoolchild x for contracting measles equals *the probability of* contracting the disease conditional on not being inoculated:

$$individual\_risk(x, measles, German\_schoolchild, inoculated) =$$
$$p(measles \mid German\_schoolchild \cap inoculated)$$
$$individual\_risk(x, measles, German\_schoolchild, non\text{-}inoculated) =$$
$$p(measles \mid German\_schoolchild \cap non\text{-}inoculated).$$

In the following definition, the expression "individual_risk(x, D, PO, C)" reads "the individual risk of a person x for developing an attribute D in the population PO with condition C".

Definition 112 (Individual risk). *If in a population PO a condition C is a risk factor for an attribute or event D, then for every member x of that population:*

$$individual\_risk(x, D, PO, C) = p(D \mid PO \cap C).$$

In this definition, the term "individual risk" is introduced as a function defined by the probability of a risk factor in a population. A stronger concept of risk is the *risk ratio,* which is more useful in making preventive decisions because it also considers those people in the population who contract the disease without having condition C. On the basis of the conceptual framework introduced above, we may explicate it as the ratio of two conditional probabilities where the term "risk_ratio(x, D, PO, C)" reads the "risk ratio of an individual x for developing an attribute D in the population PO with the risk factor C":

Definition 113 (Risk ratio). *If in a population PO a condition C is a risk factor for an attribute or event D, then for every member x of that population:*

$$risk\_ratio(x, D, PO, C) = \frac{p(D \mid PO \cap C)}{p(D \mid PO \cap \textit{non-}C)}.$$

This is a conditional definition, and written in its complete form, means that:

IF 　　　 1. $p(D \mid PO \cap C) > p(D \mid PO)$

　　　　　 2. D is disvalued in the population PO

THEN 　　 3. $risk\_ratio(x, D, PO, C) = r$ iff $r = \dfrac{p(D \mid PO \cap C)}{p(D \mid PO \cap \textit{non-}C)}.$

The more the risk ratio of an individual exceeds 1, the greater is her risk. Whatever concept of risk is used in a given case for preventive decision-making, a practically and philosophically significant question concerns the *intervention threshold risk* above which preventive action becomes necessary and mandatory. For example, what risk ratio should a 50-year-old patient with hypercholesterolemia have for coronary heart disease to receive preventive anticholesterol therapy? There is as yet no satisfactory solution to this problem, although the intervention threshold decreases with increasing harmfulness of the event to be prevented. Professional communities today try to fill this knowledge gap by recommending so-called *clinical practice guidelines.* See page 581. This example further demonstrates that the practice of health care more and more depends on communal decisions rather than on explicit-empirical knowledge

Individual risk and risk ratio: Possibility-based

We have frequently pointed out in preceding chapters that in real-world medicine, the probabilistic knowledge one needs in order to make a decision, is often not available. This also holds true in preventive medicine where conditional probabilities of the type required in the definitions above are often lacking. Additionally, the events that are to be prevented, e.g., diseases, are fuzzy events, processes, or states. To prevent a fuzzy event such as "contracting pneumonia", however, crisp probabilities will not work because a fuzzy event cannot be assigned a crisp probability such as 0.7. Therefore, a complementary approach is needed that does not use probabilities. Such an approach may use, instead of degrees of probability, *degrees of possibility*, a notion that has emerged from fuzzy set theory and logic in the last decades. Degrees of possibility will be introduced on page 618. For now we will use this term in an intuitive sense.

The expression "the possibility of X is r" is written $poss(X) = r$. Analogous to conditional probability, *conditional possibility* is symbolized thus: $poss(D \mid PO \cap C) = r$. That is, the possibility that disease D occurs conditional on $PO \cap C$, is r. For instance, the statement "the possibility that a non-inoculated German schoolchild contracts measles, is 0.5" may be written: $poss(measles \mid German\_schoolchild \cap non\text{-}inoculated) = 0.5$. Using this terminology, a possibilistic concept of risk ratio may be introduced, as an analog of the probabilistic one above, in the following way. The possibilistic risk ratio of an individual x for developing an attribute D in a population PO with condition C is:

$$risk\_ratio(x, D, PO, C) = \frac{poss(D \mid PO \cap C)}{poss(D \mid PO \cap non\text{-}C)}.$$

An example is:

$$risk\_ratio\,(x, measles, German\_schoolchild, inoculated) =$$
$$\frac{poss(measles \mid German\_schoolchild \cap inoculated)}{poss(measles \mid German\_schoolchild \cap non\text{-}inoculated)}.$$

We will not go into further details of this approach here. Profound analyses of how useful such fuzzy-logical considerations are in the theory and practice of preventive medicine and beyond, may be found in (Massad et al., 2008).

Individual risk and risk ratio: Criticism and improvement

As was emphasized on page 373, the customary concepts of individual risk and risk ratio that we have made precise above, are inadequate and need to be improved. The reason is that they are conceived as the probabilistic relevance of a condition C for developing a disease D in a population PO. See Definitions 110–113 in the preceding sections. But this may lead to the categorization of useless features as risk factors because mere probabilistic relevance reflects potential causal relevance only, but not genuine causal relevance, as was discussed on page 252. For example, consider our improved version given in Definition 110:

$$p(D \mid PO \cap C) > p(D \mid PO)$$

of the commonly used notion of a risk factor. According to our theory of probabilistic etiology, a condition C with such a characteristic may well be a mere symptom of D like the rapid falling of barometric reading is a symptom of the imminent storm. In spite of its positive probabilistic relevance to storm, it is not reasonable to view the rapid falling of barometric reading as a risk factor for storm and to manipulate the barometer in order to prevent storm because no feature of the barometer is *causally relevant* to storm. To avoid the-barometer-causes-storm falacies of this type in preventive medicine, discussed on pages 225 and 253, a condition C that is supposed to be a risk factor for a disease D in a population PO, must be guaranteed not to be a spurious causal factor, but a genuine causal factor for that disease. That is, there must not be an earlier condition C' that screens C off from D. Put another way, it must not be true that there is a C' preceding C such that:

$$p(D \mid PO \cap C \cap C') = p(D \mid PO \cap C').$$

See Definitions 70–71 on page 252. Accordingly, the definitions given in the preceding two sections need to be amended. We will do so with respect to the general concepts of risk factor and preventive factor only. The remaining definitions should be adapted analogously.

Definition 114 (Risk factor: improved). *A condition C is a* risk factor *for an event D in a population PO iff:*

1. *D is disvalued in the population PO,*
2. *$p(D \mid PO \cap C) > p(D \mid PO)$,*
3. *There is no C' that precedes C such that $p(D \mid PO \cap C \cap C') = p(D \mid PO \cap C')$.*

Definition 115 (Preventive factor: improved). *A condition C is a* preventive (= protective) factor *for an event D in a population PO iff:*

1. *D is disvalued in the population PO,*
2. *$p(D \mid PO \cap C) < p(D \mid PO)$,*
3. *There is no C' that precedes C such that $p(D \mid PO \cap C \cap C') = p(D \mid PO \cap C')$.*

The essence of our suggestion above is that risk and preventive factors should be conceived as positive causes and negative causes, respectively. Mere probabilistic relevance is not sufficient. An example was given in Formula (52) on page 251:

$$p(infarction \mid men \cap C\text{-}reactive) > p(infarction \mid men)$$

which, according to the customary concept of risk, implies that an elevated plasma C-reactive protein concentration in the population of men is a risk factor for myocardial infarction. Such categorizations are semantically absurd and should be avoided because the production of C-reactive protein is itself the effect of an underlying process X that causes myocardial infarction. The process X is a common cause of both, the production of C-reactive protein *and* myocardial infarction.

8.5.2 Prevention is Goal-Driven Practice

An essential part of medical knowledge is *practical knowledge*. This concept will be introduced and thoroughly discussed in Sections 10.6 and 21.5.3. In the present context, we can anticipate that concept only to the extent that is necessary to understand the goal-driven, practical character of the preventive-medical knowledge that regulates preventive interventions.

In contrast to descriptive, non-practical knowledge types such as number theory or cytology, *action rules* are needed in preventive medicine to guide the physician in situations where she has to decide whether and how a preventive action is to be taken, for example, whether a schoolchild ought to receive vaccination against measles, a 50-year-old male ought to receive anticholesterol therapy, and so on. Declarative knowledge of the type "in such circumstances one does such and such" is not helpful because it describes the actual behavior of physicians that may be a bad habit, and does not take the goal of the action into account. The action rules that underlie the preventive practice in medicine, are imperative action rules of the following type to be found in Section 10.6 on page 450:

If condition C obtains and goal G is pursued, then *do* action $A!$

This conditional may semi-formally be represented by the sentence:

$$C \ \& \ G \rightarrow \ \text{do } A! \tag{95}$$

A simple example is: If a schoolchild is not sufficiently immune against measles (condition C) and you want to protect her from contracting the disease (goal G), then inoculate her against measles. The rule is obviously a goal-driven imperative. Medicine, including preventive medicine, rests upon such imperatives. We shall discuss their origin, logic, and metaphysics in Sections 10.6 and 21.5.

To implement a prevention rule of the form (95) in preventive practice, the preventive efficacy of the action type A needs to be experimentally, or at least empirically, examined and compared with the efficacy of alternative preventive intervention types. The optimum method is *randomized, controlled clinical trials,* discussed as RCCTs for therapeutic studies in Section 8.4.5 above.

8.5.3 Summary

In these sections, we explicated the customary notions of risk factor, individual risk, and risk ratio, and suggested an improvement. We showed that a risk, as a condition C for an event in a population, is associated with the disvaluedness of the event in that population and may be identified with the positive causal contribution of C to the occurrence of the event. Conversely, prevention of an event that is disvalued in a population is identified with an action that is negatively causally relevant to the occurrence of the event. Thus, both risk and prevention are value-laden concepts. Due to the lack of probabilistic knowledge, they may also be based on possibilistic knowledge to make preventive medicine amenable to fuzzy logic. In general, prevention in medicine rests upon goal-driven, conditional imperatives, which we shall discuss in later chapters.

Part III

Medical Epistemology

9

The Architecture of Medical Knowledge

9.0 Introduction

Fragmentary medical-epistemological thoughts are put forward in medical journals and books every day. But there is as yet no medical epistemology as an established area of inquiry. As a result, no methodology is available to instruct us about how to conduct medical epistemology. To establish a field of medical epistemology with well-identified problems, issues, and a specific methodology, requires an answer to the question: What is medical epistemology and what is it needed for?

Epistemology, also called *the theory of knowledge,* initially emerged as a branch of philosophy dealing with questions concerning knowledge, such as "what is knowledge?", "what can we know?", "how can we know?", etc. It is a multidisciplinary branch today, also including psychology, sociology, and the history of knowledge, inquiring into the nature, source, scope, and limits of human knowledge, whether it be scientific or everyday knowledge. In line with this general understanding, *medical epistemology* may be conceived as an epistemology of medicine, i.e., the theory of medical knowledge.

Medical-epistemological questions are of the following type: What is medical knowledge? What can we know in medicine? How can we acquire medical knowledge? How can we justify, support, confirm, or disconfirm a particular knowledge claim? How can we differentiate between theoretical-medical knowledge and practical-medical knowledge? What is the best way of acquiring medical knowledge? What is a medical theory? Are medical theories true? What does the theory of, say, immune pathology look like? Is everything that we call 'knowledge' in medicine really knowledge or maybe something else? The analysis of these and related issues may contribute to a better understanding of the nature of medical knowledge, its significance and role, the process of its acquisition, and the way it may be successfully acquired and applied. The present Part III undertakes such an analysis and is divided into the following four chapters:

K. Sadegh-Zadeh, *Handbook of Analytic Philosophy of Medicine,*
Philosophy and Medicine 113, DOI 10.1007/978-94-007-2260-6_9,
© Springer Science+Business Media B.V. 2012

We should be aware at the outset that almost all epistemological inquiries into a particular item of knowledge require familiarity with its structure because epistemological properties such as truth, justifiability, falsifiability, and reliability of scientific knowledge are dependent on its syntax. Therefore, before praising any theory, e.g., the theory of evolution (Coyne, 2009), a scientist ought to know that due to its logical structure, a *theory* cannot be true. For these reasons, we shall first of all analyze the structure of medical knowledge. Our analysis will deal with these issues:

9.1 Detachment of Medical Knowledge from the Knower

What is medical knowledge? This question is basic to medical epistemology. To answer it by stating that medical knowledge is knowledge about medical subjects, does not solve the problem. It only transfers the problem to the more general question "what is knowledge?". We therefore have to concern ourselves with this general issue before proceeding to specific medical-epistemological topics. In the present context, we will familiarize ourselves with the received, *classical* concept of knowledge that Western science and culture have inherited from the Greek antiquity. Alternative views will be discussed in later chapters.

The subject of our discussion is the so-called propositional knowledge, *know-that,* that was distinguished from the procedural knowledge, *know-how,* in Sections 1.1–1.2. There we saw that propositional knowledge is traditionally considered a mental state of the knower. The mental state consists in an individual x's epistemic propositional attitude described by a sentence of the form "x knows that α" where "α" is the statement representing the known proposition. For example, "you know that *AIDS is an infectious disease*". Given such a statement "α", e.g., "AIDS is an infectious disease", a person x knows that α whenever she is in the mental state of knowing that α. We called this type of knowledge propositional knowledge. We shall be concerned with propositional medical knowledge only. To inquire into the properties of propositional medical knowledge, we need an idea of what it means to say that someone knows that α, i.e., a definition of the two-place epistemic predicate "... knows that ..." (for this predicate, see Section 27.3.1 on page 938).

Since Plato (428–347 BC), there has existed in the tradition of Western philosophy a popular concept of knowledge that considers knoweldge to be a particular type of belief. But what is it that makes a belief into knowledge? This *knowledge-conducive* force or factor is, according to Plato, the truth and justifiedness of a belief. That is, *knowledge is justified true belief* (Plato, 1973, 201c–d: "Knowledge is true belief with an account"). Thus, knowledge is defined by the features *belief, justifiedness,* and *truth.* Surprisingly, this objectionable, classical concept of knowledge attracts philosophers, epistemologists, and scientists still today. It has three characteristics: belief condition, justifiedness condition, and truth condition:

Definition 116 (The classical concept of knowledge). *A person x knows that α, i.e., $K(x, \alpha)$, iff:*

1. *x believes that α,*
2. *x is justified in believing that α,*
3. *"α" is true.*

Condition 1 is unproblematic since every competent person has privileged, direct access to her beliefs. She knows when she *believes that* something is the case. As we shall see in Section 11.1, however, conditions 2 and 3 are problematic because there is as yet no agreement on the concepts of justification and truth. At least for this reason, the classical concept of knowledge remains problematic. See, for example (Lehrer, 2000; Audi, 2003).

In addition, the classical concept of knowledge is seriously challenged by the so-called *Gettier problem.* According to a highly influential paper of merely three pages by Edmund Gettier, Jr., the classical concept of knowledge as *justified true belief* leads to the awkward consequence that someone may be justified in believing a true statement, which she cannot be said to know because the justification for her belief is based on assumptions that are false (Gettier, 1963). The example used by Gettier himself is difficult to understand. We will look at another, simpler one:

A 65-year-old female patient of Dr. Smith has died. Dr. Smith certifies her death by diagnosing that she has died of cardiac arrest. He justifies his belief in the diagnosis by adding the information that the patient had consumed plentiful amounts of deadly nightshade that her granddaughter had harvested in the adjacent forest mistaking them for bilberries. Deadly nightshade, also called atropa belladonna, contains toxic substances such as scopolamine and hyoscyamine which are responsible for the well-known belladonna intoxication. They cause, among other things, cardiac arrest. We have thus these data:

(a) Dr. Smith's belief: The patient has died of cardiac arrest;
(b) His justification of his belief: The patient had eaten atropa belladonna. The consumption of atropa belladonna causes cardiac arrest by belladonna intoxication;
(c) Dr. Smith's belief stated in (a) is true.

The authorities consider Dr. Smith's death certificate as an acceptable diagnosis and approve the funeral. Dr. Smith's epistemic attitude is, according to Definition 116, *knowledge* because it is a justified true belief. Surprisingly and in contrast to Definition 116, however, for the following reason Dr. Smith cannot *know* what he asserts:

Two weeks after the funeral, the criminal police has some reason to doubt that the death of the patient can have been caused by the consumption of deadly nightshade because the sort of blueberries harvested by her granddaughter turn out the fruit of a harmless mutant that is void of toxic substances. An autopsy of the exhumed body reveals that the patient has died of cardiac arrest nonetheless. This, however, was not due to belladonna intoxication. Rather, it was caused by a pacing system malfunction of the patient's pacemaker that consisted in a pulse generator failure.

Thus, Dr. Smith's justification of his belief was wrong. How can one *know* what one believes when one wrongly justifies the belief? This is an awkward question because it indicates that the time-honored classical concept of knowledge reconstructed in Definition 116 above is indeed problematic.[68]

In a nutshell, Gettier's argument is that one cannot be said to *know* that something is true without also *knowing why* it can be said to be true. This brings with it the pitfall of infinite regress of knowing-that. The lessons we learn from this sobering observation are two-fold. First, all empirical knowledge is in principle Gettierizable because every justification can be shown to be imperfect. Second, knowledge cannot be reduced to (i) other *epistemic* notions such as "belief" and (ii) the semantic notion of *truth*. It must have anchors of another, non-epistemic and non-semantic, type. We shall come back to this basic issue later on in Section 11.5 on page 498 when discussing the *pragmatic* anchors of what is called knowledge.

It is worth noting that conditions 1 and 3 of the above-mentioned, classical concept of knowledge recur as axioms of the epistemic logic discussed in Section 27.3. See Axiom T in Table 43 on page 942, and Axiom KB 1 in Table 45 on page 943:

$$K(x, \alpha) \rightarrow \alpha \qquad \text{(what one knows is the case)}$$
$$K(x, \alpha) \rightarrow B(x, \alpha) \qquad \text{(one believes what one knows).}$$

A sentence of the form "*x* knows that *α*" that ascribes propositional knowledge to a person *x*, obviously *describes* a particular property of a knower by the predicate "*x* knows that ...". Thus, propositional knowledge, or simply knowledge, is a part, or an attribute, of a knower, and as we have supposed previously, does not exist as a subject-independent, objective entity. Taken at face value, that means that epistemology as an inquiry into knowledge would have to examine the subjective, mental states of knowers. Such an epistemology would be a branch of psychology, however, to concern itself with cognitive

---

[68] In the present author's opinion, the Gettier problem is a secondary one caused by the extremely vague notion of *justification* that allows everybody to qualify a belief state as "justified" or "unjustified" according to her liking. A generally agreed-upon concept of justification does not yet exist. See Section 11.1.2 on page 467.

capacities of the human mind. As a subdiscipine of the philosophy of science, the epistemology of scientific knowledge has chosen another way. It has artificially detached from the knower her knowledge as a subjective state so as to analyze it as an intersubjective, say 'objective', entity. This detachment may be construed as a simple process of defining a notion of intersubjective knowledge, say knowledge*, in the following way:

Definition 117 (Knowledge). *A statement "α" is knowledge* iff there is an individual x such that x knows that α.*

The statement "α" that is labeled *knowledge** describes the proposition that a knower knows. For example, consider an AIDS researcher who knows that AIDS is an infectious disease. The statement "AIDS is an infectious disease" describing the proposition that our AIDS researcher privately knows, is, according to Definition 117, knowledge* and may now be dealt with as a public entity. In what follows, we shall be concerned with such detached, public knowledge* after the definition above. Therefore, we shall henceforth use simply the term "knowledge" instead of the asterisked one.

Definition 117 has two important features. First, it shows that the existence of knowledge presupposes the existence of knowers expressed in its definiens "there is an individual x such that ...". All books and all other reservoirs of statements and information will cease to contain knowledge if human beings cease to exist. Knowledge known by nobody cannot and does not exist.

Second, it has an epistemologically important effect. It transforms knowledge as a known proposition, i.e., state of affairs, into a *statement* in that the object-linguistic sentence, "α", representing the proposition, is metaliguistically tagged by inverted commas. Knowledge thus becomes a public, linguistic entity. Such knowledge is available in the form of single, declarative sentences or collections of such sentences in medical books, journals, or whatever. We are speaking of sentences because they represent statements. But from here onward we shall not differentiate between sentences and statements.

What is usually referred to as knowledge, is detached knowledge of the type above. It is important to add that viewed from a formal perspective, this type of knowledge is denoted by a one-place predicate, "... is knowledge", extracted from the two-place basic predicate "... knows that ..." presented in Definition 116.

9.2 The Syntax of Medical Knowledge

Suppose you are a proponent of the molecular-genetic hypothesis of carcinogenesis which amounts to the assertion that cancer is, ultimately, caused by defective genes. In order for you to collect supporting evidence in favor of your hypothesis and to defend it, or to re-evaluate it in the face of unfavorable evidence, you need to explicitly present your hypothesis and its ancillaries: What do they really look like and what do they claim? The analysis of the syntax of an item of medical knowledge requires acquaintance with all of the syntactic structures that we encounter in medicine. There is a large variety of them. In this section, the following five main types are identified.

9.2.1   Problematic Sentences
9.2.2   First-Order Sentences
9.2.3   Modal Sentences
9.2.4   Probabilistic Sentences
9.2.5   Fuzzy Sentences.

9.2.1 Problematic Sentences

Unfortunately, only seldom is medical knowledge formulated clearly enough to betray its logical structure. For instance, nobody knows what the theory of autoimmune diseases or the psychoanalytic theory of neurosis exactly looks like, and whether a particular sentence does or does not belong to such a theory. The reason is that medical language, as the medium of medical knowledge, is merely an extension of the vague, natural language that lacks a specific and clear syntax and semantics. As a result, the analysis of the logical structure of medical statements may sometimes require extensive reconstruction. To demonstrate, consider the following simple example. We are told that:

> Angina pectoris is usually due to atherosclerotic heart disease (Tierney et al., 2004, 329).

What does this statement mean? Specifically, which one of the following sentences is a suitable reconstruction of its hidden syntax?

a. Usually angina pectoris occurs if atherosclerotic heart disease is present,
b. usually atherosclerotic heart disease is present if angina pectoris occurs,
c. if atherosclerotic heart disease is present, then usually angina pectoris occurs,
d. if angina pectoris occurs, then usually atherosclerotic heart disease is present.

Obviously, these are different assertions. This may be demonstrated by the following formalization where $\alpha \equiv$ "atherosclerotic heart disease is present"; $\beta \equiv$ "angina pectoris occurs"; and ∇ is the fuzzy operator "usually":

- $\nabla(\alpha \to \beta)$
- $\nabla(\beta \to \alpha)$
- $\alpha \to \nabla\beta$
- $\beta \to \nabla\alpha$.

We encounter a similar difficulty in other, modal and fuzzy, sentences which use particles such as "possibly", "necessarily", "probably", "typically", and

the like. It is often not noticed that syntactic ambiguities have serious semantic consequences because syntax directly affects the semantics. We shall
demonstrate this in our discussion about medical hypotheses in Section 9.3
below.

9.2.2 First-Order Sentences

In the simplest cases we have sentences whose structure may be reconstructed
by means of the first-order predicate-logic. Examples are statements such as
the following ones:

    a. Every patient with acute pneumonia has a fever and cough,
    b. Some diabetics do not suffer stroke,
    c. The heart of a human being has four chambers.

The first statement says:

$$\forall x \big(is\_a\_patient(x) \land has\_acute\_pneumonia(x) \rightarrow$$
$$has\_a\_fever(x) \land has\_a\_cough(x)\big).$$

Thus it has the following structure:

$$\forall x (Px \land Qx \rightarrow Rx \land Sx).$$

The second sentence means:

$$\exists x \big(is\_a\_diabetic(x) \land \neg\, suffers\_stroke(x)\big).$$

That is:

$$\exists x (Px \land \neg Qx).$$

The third sentence says:

$$\forall x \forall y \big(is\_a\_human\_being(x) \land is\_the\_heart\_of(y, x) \rightarrow$$
$$number\_of\_chambers\_of(y) = 4\big).$$

That is:

$$\forall x \forall y \big(Px \land Qyx \rightarrow f(y) = 4\big).$$

By employing the *numerically definite existential quantifier* "there are exactly
n xs such that", with $n \geq 1$, the consequent of the latter sentence may also
be formulated thus: "There are exactly 4 zs such that each z is a chamber
and y possesses z". But we cannot use this option here because we have
not introduced a numerically definite existential quantifier in Part VIII. See
(Quine, 1966, 231).

9.2.3 Modal Sentences

The examples above are formulated in a language of the first order. But medical language goes far beyond that limited language. It is in addition a modal language whose vocabulary contains a wide variety of modal operators which will be discussed in Chapter 27, e.g., alethic modal operators such as "possible" and "necessary"; deontic operators such as "obligatory" and "forbidden", etc. Consider as an example the following two simple alethic-modal sentences:

a. If a patient has hyperglycemia, she possibly has diabetes.
b. There are patients with hyperglycemia who need not necessarily have diabetes.

The first sentence says:

$$\forall x \Big(has\_hyperglycemia(x) \rightarrow it\_is\_possible\_that\big(has\_diabetes(x)\big)\Big).$$

That is:

$$\forall x (Px \rightarrow \Diamond Qx).$$

The second example means:

$$\exists x \Big(has\_hyperglycemia(x) \wedge \neg\, it\_is\_necessary\_that\big(has\_diabetes(x)\big)\Big).$$

That is:

$$\exists x (Px \wedge \neg \Box Qx).$$

The latter sentence turns out equivalent to:

$$\exists x (Px \wedge \Diamond \neg Qx).$$

because $\Diamond \alpha$ is $\neg \Box \neg \alpha$ and $\neg\neg\alpha$ is α. See Definition 229 on page 914 and the equivalence rule $\vdash \alpha \leftrightarrow \neg\neg\alpha$ in Table 37 on page 898. In addition to alethic modalities above, medical language also uses a host of other modalities the most important ones being the deontic modalities of obligation, permission, and prohibition. We have already touched this aspect when reconstructing the concetps of indication and contra-indication in Section 8.2.3, and shall thoroughly analyze it in later chapters to demonstrate the deontic character of medicine (see Sections 10.7, 14.4, and 21.5.3).

9.2.4 Probabilistic Sentences

We have seen in Section 6.5.2 that the medical world is not a deterministic one where regularities of the type "if A then B" guarantee certainty about what will happen when we know that A is the case. Most occurrences are *random* and can only be characterized as *subjectively uncertain*. Random as well as subjectively uncertain events are said to be likely or *probable*. Therefore, the notion of probability is used to talk about both random and subjectively uncertain events and states. For a clear distinction between randomness and uncertainty, see Section 16.4.1 on page 596. According to our taxonomy of concepts in an earlier section, we distinguish between qualitative, comparative, and quantitative probability. Simple examples are:

a. It is *probable* that Elroy Fox has diabetes (qualitative),
b. that he has diabetes is *more probable than* that he has hepatitis (comparative),
c. the *probability* that he has diabetes, is 0.7 (quantitative).

We encounter in medicine all of these three types of probabilistic utterances with the last, quantitative type being the most important. Such a quantitative sentence says "the degree of probability that Elroy Fox has diabetes, is 0.7". The probability theory sketched in Chapter 29 provides a calculus for dealing with this quantitative notion of probability, which is represented by the numerical function "p" for the term "probability of". Thus, sentence c above reads:

$$p(\textit{Elroy Fox has diabetes}) = 0.7. \tag{96}$$

If we symbolize events by Roman capitals $A, B, C, \ldots$, a sentence of the form (96) may be rewritten:

$$p(A) = 0.7 \qquad \text{where } A \equiv \textit{Elroy Fox has diabetes.} \tag{97}$$

This is an *absolute* probability because the probability of A is not conditional on any other event. But almost all probability statements in medicine are conditional probabilities of the form:

$$p(A \mid B) = r \tag{98}$$

which says that the probability of event A conditional on event B is r. An example is the statement "the probability that a patient has coronary heart disease on the condition that she has angina pectoris, is 0.4". That is, $p(chd \mid angina\_pectoris) = 0.4$. From this we can conclude that $p(\overline{chd} \mid angina\_pectoris) = 0.6$. Additional examples may be found in Sections 29.1.5 and 6.5.3.

9.2.5 Fuzzy Sentences

In preceding chapters we pointed out in several places that medical knowledge is vague due to the vagueness both of medical language and medically relevant entities such as cells, metabolic processes, laboratory results, symptoms, and diseases. An example presented on page 37 demonstrates that medical knowledge is formulated using a variety of vague terms such as fuzzy predicates, fuzzy quantifiers, fuzzy temporal notions, and fuzzy frequency notions listed in Table 1 on page 37. Additional fuzzy terms used in medical language and knowledge are:

- fuzzy numbers such as *about 8, approximately 12, close to 67,*
- fuzzy intervals such as *approximately in the range of 1 to 5,*
- fuzzy probabilities such as *probable, improbable, likely, very likely,*

and others. Although the use of such fuzzy terms in medicine is unavoidable as well as highly valuable, one should be aware that they are the source of many epistemological and practical difficulties for at least two reasons:

1. Their denotations are vague entities to the effect that the determination of the truth value of a fuzzy statement containing a fuzzy term confronts unsolvable problems. For example, in the descriptions of diseases in our textbooks we are accustomed to finding statements such as "cough often occurs in bronchitis", which we learn and use in clinical decision-making and patient management. Let us ask, however, whether it is true that cough *often* occurs in bronchitis. How would you, in principle, determine the truth value of the claim that cough *often* occurs in bronchitis? Where would you draw the demarcation line between *often* and *not often?* Should you come to the conclusion that, in principle, you cannot, the second question that would arise then is this: Do we have any reason to rely on medical knowledge that mainly consists of fuzzy statements?
2. Due to their vagueness, everyone interprets them in a different way.

Attempts are therefore being made to fuzzy-logically reconstruct the syntax of vague medical knowledge so as to render it efficiently usable, e.g., in computer-aided knowledge processing in clinical decision-making. One of the most interesting and powerful approaches is the representation of medical knowledge with the aid of *fuzzy relations* and *linguistic variables* discussed in Chapter 30. Since we shall make use of these techniques in later chapters, a sketch may be given here using a nosological example that deals with relationships between symptoms and maladies and vice versa. Because of its complexity, we will not elaborate on this example here, but only present it briefly in order to show that even vague medical knowledge can be employed with precision. To this end, consider the above-mentioned vague sentence once again:

1. Cough *often* occurs in bronchitis.

It contains the vague frequency indicator "often" that specifies the strength of association between the symptom *cough* and the disease *bronchitis*. Clinical knowledge is replete with such statements. To appropriately understand and apply such statements, however, we must ask ourselves what a fuzzy term such as "often" means. In how many cases of a disease does a symptom occur which *often* occurs? In 10, 20, 50, 80 or more percent of cases? And what can we do with a symptom that *often* occurs? Analogously, there may be other symptoms which *seldom* occur or *very often* occur in the same disease such as, for example:

2. Headache *seldom* occurs in bronchitis,
3. fever *very often* occurs in bronchitis.

On the other hand, fever may *fairly seldom* occur in acute gastritis, while abdominal pain *almost always* occurs:

4. Fever *fairly seldom* occurs in acute gastritis,
5. abdominal pain *almost always* occurs in acute gastritis.

The vague frequency notions "fairly seldom", "seldom", "often", "very often", and "almost always" used in the statements above indicate the frequency of joint occurrence of some symptoms and maladies. If we represent the joint occurrence of two events A and B by the binary linguistic variable *Joint_Occurrence* of A and B (Adlassnig, 1980, 145):

$Joint\_Occurrence(A, B)$

written with capital initials, such as:

$Joint\_Occurrence(cough, bronchitis)$,

then the statements 1–5 above say that:

$Joint\_Occurrence(cough, bronchitis) = often$
$Joint\_Occurrence(headache, bronchitis) = seldom$
$Joint\_Occurrence(fever, bronchitis) = very\ often$
$Joint\_Occurrence(fever, acute\_gastritis) = fairly\ seldom$
$Joint\_Occurrence(abdominal\_pain, acute\_gastritis) = almost\ always.$

According to the theory of linguistic variables discussed in Sections 4.3 and 30.4.1, the term set of the linguistic variable Joint_Occurrence, written $T(\text{Joint\_Occurrence})$, may be conceived of as something like the following:

$$T(Joint\_Occurrence) = \{\text{never, almost never, seldom, fairly seldom, very seldom, very very seldom, often, fairly often, very often, very very often, not seldom, not often, not seldom and not often, almost always, always, } \ldots \text{ etc. } \ldots \}. \qquad (99)$$

The vague terms of this term set may be used as values of the linguistic variable *Joint_Occurrence* to characterize the association between symptoms and diseases. To come closer to their precise meaning, we will now introduce a binary *numerical variable*, denoted "joint_occurrence" and written with lower-case initials and with the following syntax:

$joint\_occurrence(A, B)$

where A and B are any events. It measures the percentage of joint occurrence of two events A and B, and may get assigned a range of 0 to 100% such that we have:

$$range(joint\_occurrence) = \{0, 1, 2, \ldots, 100\}$$

and a number $n \in \{0, 1, 2, \ldots, 100\}$ means the percentage of joint occurrence of two given events A and B, i.e., joint_occurrence$(A, B) = n$. For example, a statistical analysis may reveal that the symptom cough is present in 65% of patients with bronchitis. We would in this case have $joint\_occurrence(cough, bronchitis) = 65$. The theory of linguistic variables enables us to relate both statements:

$$Joint\_Occurrence(cough, bronchitis) = often,$$
$$joint\_occurrence(cough, bronchitis) = 65$$

with one another as shown in Figure 59. The figure demonstrates that the linguistic variable *Joint_Occurrence* with its terms set T(Joint_Occurrence) operates on the numerical variable *joint_occurrence* and transforms subsets of its range $\{0, 1, 2, \ldots, 100\}$ into fuzzy sets that have come to be called *never, almost never, seldom, fairly seldom, often, very often*, etc. For example, a particular numerical value on the x-axis such as 65% representing the value "joint_occurrence(cough, bronchitis)" is a member of the fuzzy set *often* to the extent 0.7. That is: $\mu_{often}(65\%) = \mu_{often}$ (joint_occurrence(cough, bronchitis)) $= 0.7$. The Z- and S-shaped graphs in Figure 59 illustrate the membership functions of some elements of T(Joint_Occurrence) as fuzzy sets, or granules, of numerical joint_occurrences.

We may take the linguistic values "often" and "always" to be the primary terms of the term set T(Joint_Occurrence) from which all other terms such as "never", "almost never", "almost always", "seldom", "very seldom", and "fairly seldom" may be obtained on the basis of the definition of the linguistic modifiers "very", "fairly", and "almost" discussed in Section 30.4.1 on page 1024. A prerequisite is the definition of the membership functions of the primary terms themselves. Because of its complexity, however, we will avoid this task here (see Adlassnig 1980, 143–145). Figure 59 depicts all membership functions and demonstrates, in terms of intervals of its x-axis, the corresponding subsets of the numerical joint_occurrences which constitute the fuzzy sets *never, almost never, seldom, often*, and others (Table 12 on page 396).

The above construction may be expanded upon in order to create a persuasive framework for use in clinical decision-making that would facilitate the application of vague frequency indicators. See, for instance, (Adlassnig, 1980). For our present discussion, we need not do so. But a similar example will be demonstrated in Section *Possibilistic diagnostics* on page 628.

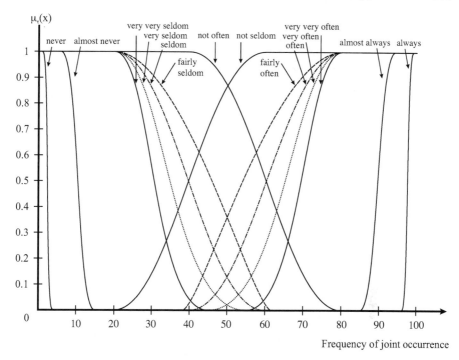

Fig. 59. S- and Z-shaped graphs of membership functions of the fuzzy sets *never, seldom, often, always,* etc. (Modified after Adlassnig, 1980, 145.) They are fuzzy sets over the universe of discourse $\Omega = \{0, 1, 2, \ldots, 100\}$ representing the values of the numerical variable *joint_occurrence* of two events, such as cough and bronchitis, on the x-axis. The value $\mu_{\tau_i}(x)$ on the y-axis is the membership value of $x \in \{0, 1, 2, \ldots, 100\}$ in a fuzzy set denoted by the term $\tau_i \in T(\text{Joint\_Occurrence})$ such as "seldom", "often", etc.

9.3 Medical Hypotheses

The problematic character of the classical concept of knowledge sketched in Definition 116 on page 385 notwithstanding, its truth condition stated in clause 3 is generally deemed necessary. That means that according to the conceptual apparatus of the traditional, classical epistemology, only what is true can constitute knowledge. What is not true cannot be the content of *knowledge*. For example, nobody can reasonably claim to know that AIDS is caused by high blood pressure simply because this causal assertion is definitely not true. Analogously, the statement that multiple sclerosis is an autoimmune disease cannot be viewed as knowledge because we do not know yet whether it is true, although there is some evidence that it might be so. These remarks demonstrate why in traditional epistemology one should carefully distinguish between *episteme* and *doxa,* i.e., knowledge and opinion such as conviction, belief, and conjecture (see page 911).

Table 12. The linguistic variable *Joint_Occurrence* on the left-hand side of the table transforms intervals of the range of the numerical variable *joint_occurrence* on the right-hand side into fuzzy sets such as *never, almost never, very very seldom,* etc. The graphs of these fuzzy sets are depicted in Figure 59 on page 395

Joint_Occurrence	Range of joint_occurrence
never	[0, 3]
almost never	[0, 15]
very very seldom	[0, 45]
very seldom	[0, 55]
seldom	[0, 60]
fairly seldom	[0, 60]
not seldom and not often	[20, 80]
fairly often	[40, 100]
often	[40, 100]
very often	[45, 100]
very very often	[55, 100]
almost always	[85, 100]
always	[97, 100]

It is worth noting that whether or not a statement qualifies as knowledge in the traditional sense above depends, among other things, on its syntactic structure. There are statements which can never constitute knowledge because, due to their structure alone, they are not verifiable and thus cannot turn out, or be considered, true. For instance, the famous statement that "all human beings are mortal" cannot be verified.[69] Its domain of reference, i.e., the set of *all human beings,* is potentially infinite. So, nobody will be able to examine it exhaustively, and we can and shall never know whether every human being is mortal. That is, a general sentence of the structure $\forall x(Px \rightarrow Qx)$ is not verifiable if the universal quantifier $\forall x$ ranges over an actually or potentially infinite domain. It should preferably be viewed as an opinion, *doxa,* i.e., a hypothesis, but not as knowledge.

For our purposes, we may define the term "hypothesis" as follows: A statement is said to be a *hypothesis* if it is a meaningful assertion whose truth value is not yet known. Meaningless assertions are thus excluded. To demonstrate that most of what is usually considered 'knowledge' in fact consists of hypotheses, we will briefly mention a few main types of sentences which are hypotheses simply due to their syntactic structure. They may be of non-probabilistic (1.1–1.5), probabilistic (2.1–2.2) or fuzzy character (3.1.–3.2), or negations (4.1–4.2):

---

[69] The Latin term "veritas" means *truth.* To *verify* a statement means to demonstrate that it is true. Conversely, to *falsify* a statement means to show that it is false. Verification and falsification are the acts or processes of verifying and falsifying, respectively.

1. **Non-probabilistic hypotheses:**
   1.1. Indefinite existential hypotheses: $\exists x \alpha$. A hypothesis of this form asserts that there is something with a particular property, e.g., "there are diabetics" or "some diabetics have Marfan syndrome". Since such a hypothesis does not specify any time or place where the object it speaks about is to be found, it is not falsifiable. 'The world is large, the time is long'. However, it is verifiable because as soon as at least one object of the required type is found, the stipulation is verified.
   1.2. Definite existential hypotheses: $\exists x \alpha$, when α specifies time or place or both such as, for example, "there are diabetics in London" or "some diabetics in London have Marfan syndrome". Hypotheses of this type are both verifiable and falsifiable.
   1.3. Unbounded universal hypotheses: $\forall x \alpha$. The quantifier $\forall x$ ranges over an actually or potentially infinite domain. For instance, "the heart of a human being has four chambers". Such hypotheses are not verifiable because the set of human beings is potentially infinite, whereas they are falsified by a single counterexample.
   1.4. Bounded universal hypotheses, e.g., "the heart of any current inhabitant of London has four chambers". Like hypotheses of type 1.2, they are both verifiable and falsifiable.
   1.5. Mixed, universal-existential hypotheses: $\forall x \exists y \alpha$. A statement of this form is, according to 1.3 above, unverifiable if its $\forall x$ component is unbounded, and according to 1.1 above unfalsifiable if its $\exists y$ component is indefinite. Examples are the famous biological postulate put forward by the German pathologist Rudolf Virchow (1821–1902) in his theory of cellular pathology which says "omnis cellula e cellula", i.e., every cell stems from another cell (Virchow, 1855, 23), as well as everyday truisms such as "every human being has a father". That is, for every cell x there is another cell y such that x stems from y; and for every human being x there is another human being y such that y is the father of x. We shall never be able *to know* whether such a hypothesis of the structure $\forall x \exists y (Px \wedge Py \rightarrow Qxy)$ is true or false.

2. **Probabilistic hypotheses:**
   2.1. Unbounded probabilistic hypotheses, also called statistical hypotheses, e.g., the probability that an individual with hypercholesterolemia will suffer coronary heart disease, is 0.3. That is, $p(\text{chd} \mid \text{hypercholesterolemia}) = 0.3$. Hypotheses of this type are neither verifiable nor falsifiable.
   2.2. Bounded probabilistic hypotheses are both verifiable and falsifiable. For instance, 30% of the current inhabitants of London with hypercholesterolemia will suffer coronary heart disease.

3. **Fuzzy hypotheses:**
   3.1. Unbounded, fuzzily quantified hypotheses are neither verifiable nor falsifiable, e.g., *most* diabetics have glucosuria.

3.2. Fuzzy temporal conditionals are neither verifiable nor falsifiable, e.g., if the body temperature of a patient is high, then she often has tachycardia.

4. **Negative hypotheses:**

4.1. A negative indefinite existential hypothesis of the form $\neg \exists x \alpha$ is not verifiable because it is equivalent to the unverifiable universal hypothesis $\forall x \neg \alpha$ as in 1.3 above;

4.2. A negative unbounded universal hypothesis of the form $\neg \forall x \alpha$ is not falsifiable because it is equivalent to the indefinite existential hypothesis $\exists x \neg \alpha$ as in 1.1 above (see Table 13).

Table 13. A tabular illustration of the verifiability and falsifiability of the 11 hypotheses types listed in the body text. Regarding fuzzy hypotheses, see also Section 16.5 on page 603

Hypotheses of the type	Verifiable	Falsifiable
1.1	+	−
1.2	+	+
1.3	−	+
1.4	+	+
1.5	−	−
2.1	−	−
2.2	−	−
3.1	−	−
3.2	−	−
4.1	−	+
4.2	+	−

The unverifiability or unfalsifiability of a hypothesis does not suggest that the hypothesis is meaningless or unacceptable. These are semantic and pragmatic issues and will be discussed below. Our aim in the present section was only to demonstrate that the syntax of a sentence affects its qualification as *knowledge* because it may stand in the way of the truth condition required by clause 3 of Definition 116 on page 385. Thus, there are reasons why the notion of "knowledge" should be used with caution. What is usually called medical knowledge, is unavoidably replete with *hypotheses*. This may be demonstrated by the following passage from a clinical textbook:

The most common symptom of cardiac failure is shortness of breath, chiefly exertional dyspnea at first and then progressing to orthopnea, paroxysmal nocturnal dyspnea, and rest dyspnea. A more subtle and often overlooked symptom of heart failure is a chronic nonproductive cough, which is often worse in the recumbent position. Nocturia due to excretion of fluid retained during the day and increased renal perfusion in the recumbent position is a common nonspecific symptom of heart failure ... (Tierney et al., 2004, 374).

A fundamentally important notion usually confused with "hypothesis" is "theory". Most people erroneously believe that a theory is a hypothesis, i.e., something hypothetical and uncertain that is 'merely probable', or 'probably true', or whose truth is not yet known. Even a prominent philosopher of science, Karl Popper, says that "All scientific theories are conjectures, even those that have successfully passed many and varied tests" (Popper, 1978). Such sloppy uses of the term "theory" are inappropriate and ought to be avoided in medicine. A theory is not a hypothesis. A hypothesis is not a theory either. The terms "hypothesis" and "theory" denote two distinct entities. Since medical knowledge also necessarily contains *theories,* we will take a closer look at this notion to understand what medical theories are and for what purpose they are made and used.

9.4 Theories in Medicine

To understand what a scientific theory in general and a medical theory in particular is, at the outset we must distinguish between theories in formal sciences, e.g., mathematical theories, and theories in empirical fields such as chemistry, biology, and medicine. Theories in medicine are empirical in the sense that the domain of their application is the experiential world and not artificial-formal objects such as numbers in mathematics. Since we shall not be concerned with formal-scientific theories such as mathematical theories, the qualifying adjective "empirical" will be omitted in what follows.

Theories in medicine, whether they be biomedical or clinical, are either not explicitly represented or misrepresented in medical literature because there exists in medicine no clear idea of what a medical theory in fact is and what it looks like. Even nonsensical word salads are not uncommon such as, for example, "By the term theory we mean a tentative explanation of a portion of reality, derived from principles independent of the phenomena to be explained" (Rosse and Mejino, 2008, 64). This careless use of language has led to some stubborn and harmful misunderstandings in medicine, among them being the beliefs that (i) a theory, e.g., Hodgkin and Huxley's biomedical theory of excitable membranes, consists of any statements and hypotheses about objects or phenomena in the world; (ii) constitutes knowledge or even an explanation of those phenomena; and (iii) can therefore be true, false, or probably true to some extent. All three assumptions are wrong. A theory neither comprises statements or hypotheses nor represents any true or false knowledge or explanation. Rather, it is a *conceptual structure* like a machine is a mechanical structure, and is used to *produce knowledge* like a machine is used to produce something else. Theories are the most complex entities ever created by scientific endeavor. For this reason, their analysis and understanding requires suitable methods and methodologies.

The view of theories as highly complex conceptual structures has significant consequences in constructing, applying, and analyzing medical theories and the relationships between them, on the one hand; and in utilizing formal sciences such as fuzzy logic to enhance them, on the other. In what follows, we shall explain and illustrate these consequences by reconstructing the theory of active immunity and creating ex nihilo a theory of toxic hyperpyrexia. Our inquiry will start with some introductory remarks on the genesis of the view and consists of the following six parts:

The statement view will be briefly described first. Somewhat more extensively, the non-statement view will be introduced to show how it may be applied in medical epistemology to reconstruct and analyze medical theories. A meager clone of the latter which has come to be known as *the semantic view of theories* will also be briefly mentioned.

9.4.1 The Statement View of Theories

A scientific theory in the empirical sciences is not commonly equated with myth or astrology. The essential difference is identified with the notion of a theory's *empirical testability*. Whereas the fantastic nature of myths and astrology put them beyond the limits of our experience, it is said that scientific theories are carriers of scientific knowledge and may be tested by exposing them to the tribunal of empirical 'facts' in the so-called real or experiential world. We are told that 'facts' confirm a theory if they accord with what the theory says or implies. Otherwise, the theory is disconfirmed or falsified. This is the widespread, *received view* of scientific theories. For example, it is said that Hodgkin and Huxley's theory of excitable membranes may be empirically tested by examining whether it is true that the action potential of a nerve membrane has something to do with the flux of sodium and potassium ions through the membrane channels as the theory asserts.

On the one hand, empirical 'facts' are observable states of affairs. They may be either (i) directly observable such as the fact that *the Eiffel Tower is in Paris;* the fact that *Elroy Fox coughs;* and the fact that *this apple is red;* or (ii) indirectly observable by means of devices such as microscopes and telescopes. Examples are the fact that *Elroy Fox has hyperglycemia,* or *this apple consists of cells.* On the other hand, however, theories deal with objects and processes which are neither directly nor indirectly observable, e.g., electrons, cell membrane channels, neurosis, risk ratio, and protective factors. Thus, the obvious gap between theories and supposed facts, which confirm or disconfirm them, gives rise to the following serious problem:

A basic problem of epistemology: How can a scientific theory talking about unobservables be tested by observables? The unobservable is not observable. And the observable is not unobservable. There is an unbridgeable gap between the two categories.

If there is no viable answer to this basic question of the empirical sciences, one may advance any theory at all, including astrological theories, and explain everything by occult processes, forces, particles, fields, attractors, 'energies', and the like. The philosophy of science, therefore, has struggled with this problem since the early twentieth century. Eventually a solution emerged in the latter part of the century. In Section 9.4.2 below, we shall sketch that solution with a view to making use of it in our medical epistemology.

As was mentioned previously, both in everyday language as well as in empirical sciences the terms "hypothesis" and "theory" are dealt with as if they were synonymous. We should avoid this mistake, however. There is no doubt that a hypothesis is a statement or a network of statements. For instance, a system such as a cell, or a disease such as AIDS may be described by a collection of such hypotheses consisting of statements that say something about the experiential world and are therefore empirically testable. A *theory*, e.g., Hodgkin and Huxley's theory of membrane excitation, is erroneously identified with such a collection of hypotheses, and is thus considered to be something that consists of statements. This traditional, received view is therefore called the *statement view* of theories. In contrast to this view is a recent, *non-statement view* of theories which says that a theory does not consist of statements and, for this reason, is not empirically testable.

According to the statement view, the statements of which a theory is composed contain, like other statements, besides logical signs the following two types of descriptive terms:

- observational terms,
- theoretical terms.

Observational terms denote observable objects or processes, e.g., apples, cells, kidneys, myocardial infarctions, heart transplantations, cities, unemployment, countries, etc. *Theoretical terms* denote unobservable, 'hidden' objects or processes such as electrons, cell membrane channels, neurosis, big bangs, etc. The basic epistemological problem mentioned above is, in essence, this: How are theoretical terms interpreted by observable entities in 'the world out there'? How can statements be empirically tested which contain theoretical terms? For example, consider the following cardiological statements:

Ventricular tachycardia is most frequently observed after a heart attack, in otherwise diseased hearts, and occasionally in apparently normal and healthy individuals. In most cases, it is due to a short-circuiting of electrical activity within the myocardium of ventricles of the heart, thus giving rise to a circular movement of the electrical waves. This mechanism, referred to as *re-entry,* continuously re-excites the heart, causing it to beat at rapid rates. It shows a typical pattern in ECG.[70]

These statements contain the theoretical term "re-entry". Defined by the phrase "circular movement of the electrical waves in the myocardium", it refers to something unobservable. The question arises how the supposition of such an unobservable phenomenon, i.e., re-entry, as a cause of ventricular tachycardia can be empirically tested so as to be distinguishable from astrology and mythology. The response of the statement view of theories is that theoretical terms in a theory are interpreted by observable phenomena in the following way:

"A scientific theory might be likened to a complex spatial network: Its terms are represented by the knots, while the threads connecting the latter correspond, in part, to the definitions and, in part, to the fundamental and derivative hypotheses included in the theory. The whole system floats, as it were, above the plane of observation and is anchored to it by rules of interpretation. These might be viewed as strings which are not part of the network but link certain points to the latter with specific places in the plane of observation. By virtue of these interpretive connections, the network can function as a scientific theory: From certain observational data, we may ascend, via an interpretive string, to some point in the theoretical network, thence proceed, via definitions and hypotheses, to other points, from which another interpretive string permits a descent to the plane of observation" (Hempel, 1952, 36).

The statement view of theories sketched above has two serious shortcomings that render it unacceptable. First, it is a mere metaphor. No real scientific theory has ever been reconstructed in this fashion to show that it contains knots, threads, strings, and so on, and to demonstrate that the metaphor works. Second, the metaphor presupposes that the descriptive language of a scientific field such as medicine consists of two disjoint parts, one containing observational terms and the other comprising theoretical terms. This two-level conception of scientific languages is a dogma. There is no clear-cut distinction between the so-called observational terms and theoretical terms. Neutral observational terms such as "red" and "water" independent of background theoretical knowledge of the observer are only trivial phrases and very rare. For instance, a lay-patient is unable to observe in her ECG what the cardiologist *observes,* e.g., ventricular tachycardia. Thus, in contrast to what is usually assumed, the term "observable" does not have the structure of the unary predicate "x is observable". It should be conceived as an at least three-place predicate of the form "x is observable by y relative to the background knowledge K". When speaking of the observability of an object or phenomenon, one must always ask the question "observable by whom and relative to which background knowledge?", e.g., is it observable by the patient relative to her everyday knowledge, or by the cardiologist relative to her expert knowledge?

---

[70] Modified after http://www.mmrl.edu/ExcitableHeart.asp. Last access 15 October, 2010.

An elderly observes more and other things than a child does, and an erudite person observes more and other things than a simple-minded individual is able to, for observation is heavily infused with past learning experiences and pre-observational, conceptual systems used by the observer. That is, what counts as *observational* is often produced and construed on the basis of the *theoretical*. Otherwise put, observation is a theory-laden performance (Hanson, 1958; Feyerabend, 1960). The theory-ladenness of observations makes it impossible to empirically test a theory independently of other theories. A scientist who tests a theory is thus subject to an obvious circularity.

It is worth noting that the theory-ladenness of observation was recognized by the French physicist Pierre Duhem as early as 1906. We will here quote a famous passage from his work to refer to it later on:

Go into this laboratory; draw near this table crowded with so much apparatus: an electric battery, copper wire wrapped in silk, vessels filled with mercury, coils, a small iron bar carrying a mirror. An observer plunges the metallic stem of a rod, mounted with rubber, into small holes; the iron oscillates and, by means of the mirror tied to it, sends a beam of light over to a celluloid ruler, and the observer follows the movement of the light beam on it. There, no doubt, you have an experiment; by means of the vibration of this spot of light, this physicist minutely observes the oscillation of the piece of iron. Ask him now what he is doing. Is he going to answer: "I am studying the oscillations of the piece of iron carrying this mirror"? No, he will tell you that he is measuring the electrical resistance of a coil. If you are astonished and ask him what meanings these words have, and what relation they have to these phenomena he has perceived and which you have at the same time perceived, he will reply that your question would require some very long explanations, and he will recommend that you take a course in electricity (Duhem, 1954, 145).[71]

9.4.2 The Non-Statement View of Theories

The theory-ladenness of observations pointed out above shows that the dichotomy 'observational versus theoretical terms' does not work. To attain a solution to the basic problem of epistemology mentioned on page 401, we need to introduce the correct dichotomy 'observational versus non-observational terms' on the one hand; and 'theoretical versus non-theoretical terms', on the

---

[71] Pierre Maurice Marie Duhem (1861–1916) was a French physicist and a historian and philosopher of science. Thanks to his extension and application of thermodynamics to chemistry, he is viewed as one of the founders of physical chemistry. He was of the opinion that the failure of a theory to pass an empirical test is a failure of the theory as *a systematic whole,* not of a particular part of it. This view was later adopted by the U.S.-American philosopher and logician Willard Van Orman Quine (1908–2000) who held that no particular experiences are linked with any particular statements of a theory. Recalcitrant experience affects the whole system of knowledge used (Quine, 1951, 43). "Our statements about external reality face the tribunal of sense experience not individually but as a corporate body" (Quine, 1966, xii). This *holistic* view, which we shall refer to in later chapters, has come to be known as the *Duhem–Quine Thesis.*

other. While the first one of these two dichotomies is of semantic, and maybe pragmatic, character, the second one is an epistemological dichotomy giving rise to the question "what is a theoretical term?".

We saw in the previous section that a theoretical term cannot be characterized negatively by supposing that "what is not observational is theoretical". We should be able to identify a term such as "Oedipus complex", "membrane depolarization", or "antibody" as a theoretical one by positively indicating *the theory from which it originates*. We cannot reasonably say, for example, that "schizophrenia" or "HIV immunity resistance" is a theoretical term if we are unable to clearly demonstrate the *theory* the term comes from. "A theoretical term, properly so called, is one which comes from a scientific theory" (Putnam, 1962, 243).

The considerations above transfer the problem "what is a theoretical term?" to the higher-level question of *what is a theory?* This question requires that scientific theories be explicitly presented in order for us to be able to explore what they are, and in specific cases to identify a particular theory. However, theories are unambiguously presented only in mathematics and mathematical physics, e.g., probability theory in mathematics and quantum theory in mathematical physics. In the literature of these sciences, one can exactly identify where a theory begins, where it ends, on which concepts it is based, what it looks like, what it implies, and so on. In all other branches, theories are put forward more or less implicitly, loosely, vaguely, and often chaotically. In medicine, for example, Rudolf Virchow's theory of cellular pathology and the theories of infectious diseases and immune pathology have been discussed for a long time. Nevertheless, it is astonishing that nobody knows what any of these theories qua a theory proper explicitly looks like, of what principles, axioms, or postulates it consists, and whether a particular sentence does or does not belong to it.

Patrick Suppes, a Stanford philosopher of science, and his collaborators took up these epistemological issues in the 1950s and developed valuable tools for reconstructing scientific theories (Suppes, 1951, 1957, 1959, 1967; Adams, 1955; Jamison, 1956; McKinsey et al., 1953; McKinsey and Suppes, 1955). Their pioneering work led Joseph D. Sneed, a Ph.D. student of Suppes in the 1960s, to the lucid concept of a theory that we shall study below. It has a far-reaching consequence which says that a scientific theory does not assert anything about 'the world out there'. In other words, it does not consist of statements. Rather, it is a *conceptual structure*. This view is therefore called the non-statement or *structuralistic* view of theories (Sneed, 1971; Suppes, 1970b, 2002).[72]

We will try to outline this novel, structuralistic approach to scientific theories in the present section, and shall utilize it in subsequent sections by in-

---

[72] The present terms "structuralism" and "structuralistic" that are used in analytic philosophy of scientific theories should be carefully distinguished from the French structuralism that is something different and began in linguistics with the work of the Swiss linguist Ferdinand de Saussure (1857–1913) (Saussure, 1916). It was

quiring into the structure of some real-world theories and of an ad hoc theory that we shall construct. For this purpose, the following notions will be needed: set-theoretical predicate, models for a theory, constraints of a theory, core of a theory, intended applications of a theory, the structure of a theory. These notions will be introduced and discussed in the following thirteen sections in turn:

- ▶ Representing a theory by a set-theoretical predicate
- ▶ Models for a theory
- ▶ Theoretical terms
- ▶ Potential and partial potential models for a theory
- ▶ The frame of a theory
- ▶ The constraints of a theory
- ▶ The core of a theory
- ▶ The intended applications of a theory
- ▶ What a theory is
- ▶ A first example: The theory of active immunity
- ▶ Empirical claims made using a theory
- ▶ A second example: Diagnosis and diagnostics
- ▶ The empirical content of a theory.

Our discussion is based on the original works by Suppes, Sneed, and Stegmüller (Suppes, 1957, 1970b, 2002; Sneed, 1971; Stegmüller, 1976].[73]

Representing a theory by a set-theoretical predicate

As a critic of the statement view of theories, Patrick Suppes developed an alternative methodology well-elaborated as early as 1957 (Suppes, 1957, 246–

---

adopted and developed into a movement by Claude Lévi-Strauss, Michel Foucault, Jacques Lacan, and Jacques Derrida. See (Hawkes, 2003; Sturrock, 2003).

[73] Patrick Suppes (born in 1922 in Tulsa, Oklahoma) is a mathematically and logically oriented philosopher of science. He worked at the Stanford University from 1950 until his retirement in 1992. His broad area of research includes mathematical physics, foundations of physics, theory of measurement, decision theory, foundations of probability and causality, mathematical psychology, foundations of psychology, philosophy of language, education and computers, and philosophy of science. The basic idea and method of the structuralistic view of theories is originally due to him (Suppes, 1957, 1970b, 2002). His Ph.D. student Ernest W. Adams conducted the first improvement (Adams, 1955). The structuralism proper is an achievement of another Ph.D. student of his, Joseph D. Sneed, who made significant improvements (Sneed, 1971). His innovative metatheory was adopted and further developed by the Austrian-born German philosopher of science Wolfgang Stegmüller (1923–1991) and his students (Stegmüller, 1973a, 1976; Moulines, 1975; Balzer, 1978; Balzer and Moulines, 1996). Additional structuralistic analyses of theories in psychology may be found in (Westmeyer, 1989, 1992), and of theories in medicine in (Müller and Pilatus, 1982; Müller, 1985; Pilatus, 1985; Sadegh-Zadeh, 1982a).

305). According to him, a theory is difficult or impossible to reconstruct and analyze by means of weak linguistic tools such as first-order logic, which are used by the advocates of the statement view, because the entities that the theory refers to almost always go beyond the expressive power of such weak tools. Its models, i.e., the structures 'in the world out there' in which the theory is satisfied, are non-linguistic entities that can best be handled by set theory (Suppes, 1960, 290). Our understanding of theories can be enhanced by concentrating on their models. Thus, the best way of inquiring into a theory is to reconstruct or even to construct it by means of set theory rather than of logic.

Suppes's discovery underlying this idea is expressed in his well-known slogan: "to axiomatize a theory is to define a predicate in terms of notions of set theory. A predicate so defined is called a *set-theoretical predicate*" (Suppes, 1957, 249). To adequately understand this ingenious idea, one may replace the word "to axiomatize" with any of the following terms: to construct, to clearly formulate, to reconstruct, to analyze, to inquire into, or to identify the structure of.[74]

A set-theoretical predicate is simply a predicate that is defined by means of set theory in a formal way. Thus, it is introduced by a *set-theoretical definition*. This method of concept formation was presented on page 100 and extensively used in previous chapters. To Suppes-reconstruct and analyze a theory by defining a set-theoretical predicate, is to introduce a predicate of the form "is a *P*" by a definition of the form:

- x is a P iff there are $A_1, \ldots, A_n$ such that $x = \langle A_1, \ldots, A_n \rangle$ and A_1 is such and such ... and A_n is such and such.

The definiens following the iff-particle reflects the structure of the theory that is being explicated by introducing the predicate "x is a P". $A_1, \ldots, A_n$ are its conceptual constituents that are characterized by the specifications "A_1 is such and such ... and A_n is such and such". We will now illustrate the procedure using an elementary example, since the structuralist metatheory is itself relatively complex. Also, for the sake of simplicity and understanding, we shall in

---

[74] Axiomatization is a usual method of theory formation in mathematical sciences. See, e.g., arithmetic or the Euclidean geometry. "Axiomatization" means to formulate the theory by explicitly providing its sentences. However, empirical sciences have not made use of this excellent technique until now. Suppes's suggestion to axiomatize a theory by introducing a set-theoretical predicate is an amended application to empirical sciences of the formal *Bourbaki* method. The name "Nicolas Bourbaki" is a collective pseudonym under which a group of mostly French, twentieth century mathematicians have written some fifty volumes on pure mathematics. The group has jokingly adopted the pseudonym from General Charles Bourbaki because of his disastrous defeat in the Franco-Prussian war (1870–1871). Their aim was to provide a solid foundation for the whole body of mathematical knowledge. The method they used for the first time was axiomatization by employing set theory (see Bourbaki, 1950, 1968).

this introductory context avoid medical examples, as they would gratuitously complicate our discussion. See, for instance, the structuralistic reconstruction of Hodgkin and Huxley's complicated theory of excitable membranes (Müller und Pilatus 1982; Müller 1985).

The example we shall use in presenting the metatheory, is the theory of mechanical equilibrium which dates back to the ancient Greek mathematician Archimedes, and is therefore known as the Archimedean equilibrium theory, or *Archimedean static* for short. In its original version, it says that a beam balance with two arms of length a and length b from which two weights x and y are suspended, respectively, is in equilibrium if the product of weight x and arm a equals the product of weight y and arm b (Figure 60).

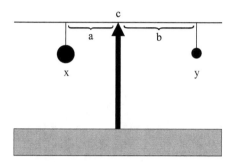

Fig. 60. A beam pivots at a center of gravitation, c, and has two arms of length a and length b, respectively. A weight x is suspended from a, and a weight y is suspended from b. The beam is in equilibrium if $x \cdot a = y \cdot b$

A generalization of this theory to more than two weights will be presented below. To simplify the presentation, we will suppose that the beam has a fulcrum, i.e., a center of gravitation or rotation, c, and a right and a left arm. Objects suspended from the left arm are denoted x_1, x_2, etc.; and objects suspended from the right arm are denoted y_1, y_2, etc. Let d be a distance function that measures the distance of a point z on the beam from its fulcrum c such that "$d(z,c) = r$" means that the distance of z from c is r. We now axiomatize *the theory of Archimedean static*, conveniently referred to as *AS*, by introducing the set-theoretical predicate "x is an Archimedean static".

Definition 118 (AS). ξ *is an* Archimedean static ($\equiv \xi$ *is an AS*) *iff there are* Ω, b, d, *and* w *such that:*

1. $\xi = \langle \Omega, b, d, w \rangle$,
2. Ω *is a finite set of* $n \geq 1$ *objects*,
3. b *is a beam that pivots on a fulcrum* c,
4. d *is a function from* Ω *to* $\mathbb{R}^+$, *(called the distance function),*
5. w *is a function from* Ω *to* $\mathbb{R}^+ - \{0\}$, *(called the weight function),*
6. *if every element of* Ω *is suspended from* b, *then* b *is in equilibrium,*
7. $\sum w(x_i) \cdot d(x_i, c) = \sum w(y_j) \cdot d(y_j, c)$ *for* $\forall x_i, y_j \in \Omega$ *with* $1 \leq i, j \leq n$.

The sentences of such a set-theoretical definition are called *axioms* because they are stipulations, but not assertions. As part of the definiens, they delimit the structure, i.e. the structure $\langle \Omega, b, d, w \rangle$ in the present example, that is being introduced by the definition of the set-theoretical predicate "ξ is an Archimedean static".[75]

When introducing the technique of set-theoretical definition on page 100, we distinguished two types of axioms of a set-theoretical predicate, structural and substantial ones. The first five axioms of our miniature theory above are structural axioms. They merely characterize the constituents of the structure. The structure under discussion is what is baptized an *Archimedean static, AS*. Our theory has in addition two substantial axioms, i.e., axioms 6–7. Axiom 6 requires that the beam be in equilibrium. Axiom 7, the main substantial axiom, requires that the arithmetical product of weights and their respective distances from the fulcrum on the right-hand and left-hand sides of the beam, be equal. Whenever an entity of the structure $\langle \Omega, b, d, w \rangle$ satisfies all axioms of the predicate "ξ is an Archimedean static", it may be called an *Archimedean static*.

Models for a theory

According to the general notion of a *model* introduced on page 886, a structure $\langle \Omega_1, \ldots, \Omega_m; R_1, \ldots, R_n; a_1, \ldots, a_p \rangle$ with $m, n \geq 1$ and $p \geq 0$ is a model for, or of, a sentence if the sentence is satisfiable in that structure, i.e., if there exists an interpretation that renders the sentence true in the structure. The set of *all* models for a sentence α will be denoted by "$\mathcal{M}(\alpha)$". If S is a set of sentences, a structure $\langle \Omega_1, \ldots, \Omega_m; R_1, \ldots, R_n; a_1, \ldots, a_p \rangle$ is a model for S if it is a model for each sentence in S. The set of *all* models for S is written $\mathcal{M}(S)$. $\mathcal{M}$ is a set-valued function that assigns to a single sentence α, or a set of sentences, S, the set of its models, respectively. In summary, a crisp sentence, and a set of crisp sentences as well, divides the world into two families of structures such that one of them comprises its models, the other one none.

In line with the considerations above, we can meaningfully talk of the models for a theory. If a theory is axiomatized by introducing a set-theoretical predicate "x is a P" like in Definition 118 above, a structure in which all axioms defining this predicate are satisfiable, constitutes a model for the theory. It is clear that a sentence, and likewise a theory, may have many and even an infinite number of models depending on the number of structures in which it is satisfiable.[76]

---

[75] Archimedes (287–212 BC) is reported to have said, in the spirit of his theory, "Give me a place to stand, and with a lever I will move the whole world". See axiom 7.

[76] Note that the basic concept of mathematical *model theory* sketched above is something different from what is colloquially understood by the term "model" in empirical sciences and everyday life. As outlined on page 886, in empirical sciences theories and hypotheses are considered as *models for* some aspects of reality. In everyday life, a certain artifact, e.g., a toy car, is said to be a *model*

Let x and y be two objects of the weight 5 and 2 kg, respectively, and b' be a beam balanced on a fulcrum c. Objects x and y may be suspended from the beam at a distance of 20 cm and 50 cm from the fulcrum, respectively. We have thus a concrete structure $\langle \{x, y\}, b', d', w' \rangle$ such that:

- $d'(x, c) = 20, \quad d'(y, c) = 50$
- $w'(x) = 5, \quad w'(y) = 2.$

The beam may be in equilibrium. Thus, axioms 1–6 of the set-theoretical predicate "ξ is an AS" defined in Definition 118 above are satisfied. Since its axiom 7 is also satisfied:

- $5 \cdot 20 = 2 \cdot 50$

the structure $\langle \{x, y\}, b', d', w' \rangle$ is an Archimedean static. That is, the structure $\langle \{x, y\}, b', d', w' \rangle$ is a model for our miniature theory axiomatized by the set-theoretical predicate "ξ is an Archimedan static". This predicate provides a general concept of mechanical equilibrium. It is applicable to a great many cases such as levers, beam balances, and seesaws.

The first obvious achievement of axiomatizing a theory by way of a set-theoretical predicate is this: The predicate delimits the class of all structures that are models for the theory. Let AS be our theory of Archimedean static above and let $\mathcal{M}(AS)$ be the class of all of its models. Then the set-theoretical predicate "ξ is an Archimedan static" delimits the class $\mathcal{M}(AS)$. Thus, the class $\mathcal{M}(AS)$ consists of only those structures that satisfy the predicate. It turns out that an object x is an Archimedean static if and only if $x \in \mathcal{M}(AS)$. Below we shall further analyze this class in order to reveal the details of our theory. To this end, we need the structuralistic notion of a "theoretical term".

Theoretical terms

As was emphasized in Section 9.4.1 above, the dichotomy between observational terms and theoretical terms conceived prior to the emergence of the structuralistic view of theories is problematic. For instance, I am incapable of observing what *Hodgkin and Huxley* 'observe' when examining the membrane potential of a neuron, although I too look at their multiamplifier and oscilloscope and have no visual defects. What Sigmund Freud allegedly 'observes' in a patient, e.g., an Oedipus complex, when analyzing the patient's free associations, is not seen by behaviorists. The arbitrariness of the dichotomy is due to the circumstance that what someone 'observes', depends on the background knowledge, say the theory, that she employs while observing. The structuralistic approach stops this arbitrariness by characterizing a theoretical term positively as one "which comes from a theory". This idea is the main

---

for something. In the present context, however, a particular sector or aspect of the world is considered to be a *model for* some sentence.

motive of Joseph D. Sneed's decision to introduce his own criterion of term *theoreticity,* pointed to above (Sneed, 1971, 31–33).

Syntactically, the old concept of term theoreticity was a unary predicate in that of a term t it was said "t is a theoretical term". By contrast, the new concept of term theoreticity is a binary predicate of the form "t is a theoretical term with respect to theory T". It enables a clear-cut partitioning of the terms of a theory into theoretical and non-theoretical terms, which has beneficial epistemological consequences. Since it is a relatively complex predicate, we will present it here in a simplified form.

We start with an elementary consideration. When we want to know whether something is a P, for example, whether Elroy Fox has pneumonia, we often need first to know whether it is a Q, for instance, whether Elroy Fox has a fever. In such a case, we say that the application of the predicate P is Q-dependent. In the present example, the application of the term "pneumonia" is "fever"-dependent. In an analogous fashion, a concept of *theory dependence* will be introduced below which says that a term is a theoretical term with respect to a particular theory T if its application is T-dependent. This theory dependence of the application of a term is the core feature of term theoreticity.

Let the variable t denote any term, e.g., the term "AIDS", "pneumonia", or "hypertension". A *method* that can be used to determine whether or not t applies to a particular case, will be called a method of t-determination. For example, an HIV test provides a method of AIDS-determination in that it enables us to diagnose whether someone has AIDS or not. The rules of postero-anterior chest radiography and film inspection provide a method of pneumonia-determination that enables us to judge whether someone has pneumonia or not. The standard method of blood pressure measurement is a method of hypertension-determination that enables us to make out whether someone has high blood pressure or not. Of course, for a term t there may exist numerous methods of t-determination.

For any term t, a *method M* of t-determination is said to be epistemically t-dependent if in determining by method M whether or not t applies to a particular case x, one needs to know that there is another case y to which t already applies. For example, the standard method of hypertension-determination by a sphygmomanometer is not epistemically hypertension-dependent. For when using this method to test whether or not a particular patient has high blood pressure, one does not need to know whether any other individual has, or had, high blood pressure or not. However, every method of perception-determination one may use or conceive, is epistemically perception-dependent. In determining whether or not some act of an ameba, animal, or human being is a perception, another $perception_1$ is needed; but to know whether or not $perception_1$ is a perception, another $perception_2$ is needed; but to know whether or not $perception_2$ is a perception, another $perception_3$ is needed; and so on. This is so because perception is an integral part of every method of perception-determination. In short, the term "perception" is epistemically perception-dependent, i.e., self-referential.

Overly simplified, the structuralistic criterion of term theoreticity introduced by Joseph D. Sneed amounts to this: A term t occurring in a theory T that is represented by a set-theoretical predicate S, "ξ is an S", is a theoretical term *with respect to this theory* T if every existing method of t-determination is epistemically T-dependent, that is, if the application of the term t to a particular case x presupposes that there be another case y such that T applies to y. In such a case, the term t *comes from* the theory T in question in that its meaning is the same as its T-dependent, i.e., theory dependent, use. Although Sneed's criterion gives the impression that it might lead to an infinite regress, it does not do so. An example will be demonstrated below.

After the intuitive remarks above, we will now present a simplified definition of term theoreticity. Note, however, that we must differentiate between theoretical functions and theoretical predicates. We shall consider them in turn.

Regarding theoretical functions, the structures dealt with will generally be of the form $\langle \Omega_1, \ldots, \Omega_k, f_1, \ldots, f_n \rangle$ where $\Omega_1, \ldots, \Omega_k$ with $k \geq 1$ are the universes of the structure; and $f_1, \ldots, f_n$ with $n \geq 1$ are functions on any, or any Cartesian product, of them. For the sake of convenience, the universes will be symbolized by the single variable Ω which in any special case may represent the entire domain of a function f_i in question, $1 \leq i \leq n$. Thus, $\langle \Omega, f_1, \ldots, f_n \rangle$ will be our simplified structure variable. The definition captures those structures in which $f_1, \ldots, f_n$ are functions. Such functions are ubiquitous in medicine. A function f_i may simply be a body parameter such as blood pressure, heart rate, blood sugar, or blood cholesterol concentration and the like (see Section 4.1.4).

Definition 119 (T-dependent functions). *Let T be any theory constructed or reconstructed by defining the set-theoretical predicate "ξ is an S" and whose models are of the form $\langle \Omega, f_1, \ldots, f_n \rangle$. Then:*

1. *If the structure $\langle \Omega', f_1', \ldots, f_n' \rangle$ is a new application of T to find out whether it is an S, then a concrete m-ary function f_i' occurring therein, with $m \geq 1$, is measured in a T-dependent way if and only if there is at least one $\langle x_1, \ldots, x_m \rangle \in \Omega'$ such that every existing method of $f_i'(x_1, \ldots, x_m)$-determination presupposes that there is another structure $\langle \Omega'', f_1'', \ldots, f_n'' \rangle$ which is an S.*
2. *The concrete function f_i' is measured in a T-independent way if and only if it is not measured in a T-dependent way.*

The term "concrete function f_i'" in an application of the theory T means an instance of the function variable f_i in theory T. Suppose, for example, that the theory T under discussion is the theory of the Archimedean static axiomatized in Definition 118 on page 407. When measuring the weight of the present copy of this book by a particular beam balance, the function "weight of" that we use, is an instance of the weight function w used in our theory of the Archimedean static. From the concept introduced in Definition 119 above, we easily obtain the concept of term theoreticity as follows.

Definition 120 (T-theoretical functions). *Let T be any theory constructed or reconstructed by defining the set-theoretical predicate "ξ is an S" and whose models are of the form $\langle \Omega, f_1, \ldots, f_n \rangle$. Then:*

1. *The term f_i occurring in the theory T is theoretical with respect to T, or T-theoretical for short, if and only if in every structure $\langle \Omega', f'_1, \ldots, f'_n \rangle$ which is an application of T, i.e., is an S, the concrete function f'_i is measured in a T-dependent way.*

2. *The term f_i is non-theoretical with respect to T, or T-non-theoretical for short, if it is not T-theoretical.*

This concept of T-theoreticity of terms may be illustrated using our miniature theory of the Archimedean static, *AS*, axiomatized in Definition 118 on page 407. To this end, first recall that in ancient Greece when Archimedes developed his theory, beam balance was the only method of weight measurement. Suppose beam balance had remained the only method of weight measurement.

Let b' be a beam on a fulcrum, and $\Omega' = \{child_1, child_2, \ldots, child_7\}$ be a group of seven children who play seesaw on b'. In addition, d' and w' may be a distance function and a weight function, respectively, to determine the distance of a child from the fulcrum of b' and her weight. Now, we want to know whether the contraption $\langle \Omega', b', d', w' \rangle$ *is an Archimedean static*, i.e., a model for the set-theoretical predicate "ξ is an Archimedean static". To this end, we must measure both the weight of each child and her distance from the fulcrum of the beam b' to examine whether the contraption $\langle \Omega', b', d', w' \rangle$ satisfies axioms 6–7 of Definition 118. A requirement of our theory is that we must know the weight of at least one child in advance, that is, we must have measured it previously using *another* beam balance structure $\langle \Omega'', b'', d'', w'' \rangle$ that we already know is an Archimedean static. In determining the weights of the other six children by the current seesaw we have to judge six times whether this beam balance $\langle \Omega', b', d', w' \rangle$ is in equilibrium, i.e., whether it is an Archimedean static. Thus, it turns out that in our present setting $\langle \Omega', b', d', w' \rangle$, the concrete weight function w' is measured *AS*-dependently because it presupposes the existence of another *AS* structure $\langle \Omega'', b'', d'', w'' \rangle$. Since beam balance is supposed to be the only available method of weight measurement, clause 1 of Definition 120 will be satisfied in every application of our miniature theory. Therefore, the weight function w occurring in this theory is an *AS*-theoretical term. By contrast, the distance function d of the theory is an *AS*-non-theoretical one because distance is measured *AS*-independently.

The definition of term theoreticity above dealt with numerical functions, i.e., quantitative terms. However, it can easily be reformulated for predicates to cover qualitatively formulated theories, which are more usual in medicine. In this case, the core concept of T-dependent measurement is to be replaced with a concept of T-dependent determination of truth values of statements. Suppose, for example, that there is a theory of *autoimmune diseases*, call it AutoID theory, containing the predicate "has an autoimmune disease". This predicate is *AutoID*-dependent provided that regarding an individual patient

x, whenever it is to be determined whether the sentence "x has an autoimmune disease" is true or false, the determination of this truth value presupposes that there be another case to which the theory AutoID has already been successfully applied, i.e., that there be at least one patient $y \neq x$ of whom it is definitely known that *she has an autoimmune disease*. Thus we may define our term (see also Stegmüller, 1976, 53):

Definition 121 (T-theoretical predicates). *Let T be any theory constructed or reconstructed by defining the set-theoretical predicate "ξ is an S" and whose models are of the form $\langle \Omega, R_1, \ldots, R_n \rangle$. Then:*

1. *In a new application $\langle \Omega', R_1', \ldots, R_n' \rangle$ of theory T the truth value of an R_i'-sentence is determined in a T-dependent way if and only if there are $x_1, \ldots, x_m \in \Omega'$ such that the determination of the truth value of the sentence $R_i'(x_1, \ldots, x_m)$ presupposes that there be another structure $\langle \Omega'', R_1'', \ldots, R_n'' \rangle$ which is a model for the theory.*
2. *The predicate R_i in theory T is T-theoretical if and only if in all applications of the theory the truth value of an R_i-sentence is determined in a T-dependent way; it is T-non-theoretical, otherwise.*

Below are three epistemologically most important aspects of term theoreticity as defined thus far:

- The T-dependence of a term shows that the meaning of a T-theoretical term is produced and controlled by the theory itself in that the theory prescribes how it is to be used.
- The phrase "T-theoretical", or "theoretical with respect to T", makes apparent that the theoreticity of a term is always relative to a particular theory T. A term t, such as "has an autoimmune disease", may be a theoretical one with respect to a theory T_i, e.g., theory of autoimmunity, while being a non-theoretical one with respect to another theory T_j, e.g., theory of genes. That is, T_i-theoreticity and T_j-theoreticity of a term are two different properties if $T_i \neq T_j$.
- The T-theoreticity of terms is historically relative in that a term t that is a T-theoretical one at a particular time, may lose this property later when new methods of t-determination emerge which are independent of T. An example is the weight function w that was an AS-theoretical term from the inception of Archimedes's theory AS until new methods of weight measurement were developed.

Potential and partial potential models for a theory

The class of models for a theory T, denoted $\mathcal{M}(T)$, was delineated on page 408. Before we can proceed to the question of what a theory is, two additional types of models for a theory will be characterized in what follows, i.e., potential models and partial, potential models.

We have seen in previous sections that a set-theoretically axiomatized theory such as the miniature theory of the Archimedean static, AS, has structural axioms as well as substantial axioms. The former characterize the constituents of the entities which are capable of becoming models for the theory if they also satisfy its substantial axioms. Substantial axioms in our example theory AS are axioms 6–7 in Definition 118 on page 407.

Now, consider any theory minus its substantial axioms, e.g., axioms 6–7 of our miniature theory AS in Definition 118. An entity that satisfies this pruned theory is called a *potential model* for the theory. It is so called because it is possible that it will also satisfy the substantial axioms if they are added. To illustrate, we will remove axioms 6–7 from our AS theory. A structure that satisfies the remaining mini theory we shall refer to as a *potential Archimedean static*, or AS_p for short:

Definition 122 (AS_p). ξ *is a potential Archimedean static* ($\equiv \xi$ *is an AS_p*) *iff there are Ω, b, d, and w such that:*

1. *$\xi = \langle \Omega, b, d, w \rangle$,*
2. *Ω is a finite set of $n \geq 1$ objects,*
3. *b is a beam that pivots on a fulcrum c,*
4. *d is a function from Ω to $\mathbb{R}^+$, (called the distance function),*
5. *w is a function from Ω to $\mathbb{R}^+ - \{0\}$, (called the weight function).*

As an example, let A be a group of seven children, b' a seesaw, and d' and w' measures for distance and weight, respectively. Then the structure $\langle A, b', d', w' \rangle$ is a potential Archimedean static, i.e., a *model* for AS_p. But it is a *potential model* for the predicate "ξ is an Archimedean static". Thus, the set-theoretical predicate defined in Definition 122 delineates the class of all potential models for an Archimedean static, denoted $\mathcal{M}_p(AS)$. $\mathcal{M}_p$ is a set-valued function that assigns to a single sentence, or a set of sentences, the set of its potential models. We have that $\mathcal{M}_p(AS) = \mathcal{M}(AS_p)$. As its name betrays, a potential Archimedean static will also *possibly* satisfy the following two substantial axioms of the structure AS that we removed:

6. if every child is riding on the seesaw, then the seesaw is in equilibrium,
7. the sum of the products of the weights of all children on the right-hand side of the seesaw with their respective distances from the fulcrum equals the sum of the products of the weights of all children on the left-hand side of the seesaw with their respective distances from the fulcrum.

Note that a potential model still contains T-theoretical components. For example, a potential Archimedean static, i.e., an AS_p of the structure $\langle \Omega, b, d, w \rangle$ above, contains a weight function w, which under our earlier supposition that beam balance is the only method of weight measurement, turned out an AS-theoretical term. Now, if we also remove all T-theoretical entities from potential models for a theory, we obtain elementary structures which are void of any

T-theoreticity. These interesting entities are called *partial, potential models* for the theory under consideration. Below is the definition of partial, potential models for our miniature theory of the Archimedean static, referred to as AS_{pp} :

Definition 123 (AS_{pp}). ξ *is a partial, potential Archimedean static* ($\equiv \xi$ is an AS_{pp}) *iff there are* Ω, *b, and d such that:*

1. $\xi = \langle \Omega, b, d \rangle$,
2. Ω *is a finite set of* $n \geq 1$ *objects,*
3. *b is a beam that pivots on a fulcrum c,*
4. *d is a function from* Ω *to* $\mathbb{R}^+$, *(called the distance function).*

A partial, potential Archimedean static of the structure $\langle \Omega, b, d \rangle$ contains no *T*-theoretical terms any more. It comprises completely *T*-non-theoretical entities as opposed to our theory of the Archimedean static, which has both *T*-theoretical and *T*-non-theoretical entities. It is something 'empirical' with respect to *T,* so to speak. For example, seven children $\{a_1, \dots, a_7\}$ *playing* on a seesaw and having a measuring tape with which to measure their individual distances from the fulcrum, constitute a partial, potential Archimedean static, an AS_{pp}, of the form $\langle \{a_1, \dots, a_7\}, seesaw, measuring\_tape \rangle$.

The set-theoretical predicate from Definition 123 above delineates the class of *all* partial, potential models for an Archimedean static, denoted $\mathcal{M}_{pp}(AS)$. $\mathcal{M}_{pp}$ is a set-valued function that assigns to a single sentence, or a set of sentences, the set of its partial, potential models. We have that $\mathcal{M}_{pp}(AS) = \mathcal{M}(AS_{pp}) = \mathcal{M}_p(AS_p)$. Regarding our above example with seven children $\{a_1, \dots, a_7\}$, it can be observed that:

$$\langle \{a_1, \dots, a_7\}, seesaw, measuring\_tape \rangle \in \mathcal{M}(AS_{pp})$$
$$\langle \{a_1, \dots, a_7\}, seesaw, measuring\_tape \rangle \in \mathcal{M}_p(AS_p)$$
$$\langle \{a_1, \dots, a_7\}, seesaw, measuring\_tape \rangle \in \mathcal{M}_{pp}(AS).$$

That a partial, potential model for a theory *T,* e.g., $\langle \Omega, b, d \rangle$, consists only of *T*-non-theoretical terms means that any such entity is completely independent of the theory *T* and can be hypothesized to become a model thereof when it is extended to a larger structure, say $\langle \Omega, b, d, w \rangle$. We shall return to this epistemologically important issue below.

It is worth noting that while a partial, potential model is void of any *T*-theoretical terms, it may contain terms which are theoretical with respect to *another* theory T'. For example, a partial, potential Archimedean static of the structure $\langle \Omega, b, d \rangle$ contains a distance function *d,* e.g., a measuring tape in the example above, that is non-theoretical with respect to an Archimedean static. But the measurement of distance requires a particular geometry. Therefore, *d* will turn out to be a theoretical term with respect to a particular geometric theory, which is of course something different than our miniature theory of the Archimedean static.

The frame of a theory

In the last sections, we have identified the following three types of models for a theory: models; potential models; and partial, potential models. Categories of these three model types may be denoted by:

$$\mathcal{M}(T) \quad \equiv \text{ set of all models for the theory } T,$$
$$\mathcal{M}_p(T) \quad \equiv \text{ set of all potential models for the theory } T,$$
$$\mathcal{M}_{pp}(T) \quad \equiv \text{ set of all partial, potential models for the theory } T.$$

Let T be a theory that has been axiomatized by defining the set-theoretical predicate "x is an S". Then we have:

$$\mathcal{M}(T) \quad = \{x \mid x \text{ is an } S\} \qquad \text{e.g., } \{x \mid x \text{ is an } S\} \text{ as above,}$$
$$\mathcal{M}_p(T) \quad = \{x \mid x \text{ is an } S_p\} \qquad \text{e.g., } \{x \mid x \text{ is an } S_p\} \text{ as above,}$$
$$\mathcal{M}_{pp}(T) \quad = \{x \mid x \text{ is an } S_{pp}\} \qquad \text{e.g., } \{x \mid x \text{ is an } S_{pp}\} \text{ as above.}$$

Note that $\mathcal{M}_{pp}(T)$ is the largest set, because the most tolerant one, such that $\mathcal{M}(T) \subseteq \mathcal{M}_p(T) \subseteq \mathcal{M}_{pp}(T)$. The ordered triple $\langle \mathcal{M}_{pp}(T), \mathcal{M}_p(T), \mathcal{M}(T) \rangle$ of these three sets is referred to as the *frame* of the theory. That is:

Definition 124 (The frame of a theory). *If S is a set-theoretical predicate that axiomatizes a theory T, then $\mathcal{FR}(T)$ is the frame of the theory T iff there are $\mathcal{M}_{pp}(T), \mathcal{M}_p(T),$ and $\mathcal{M}(T)$ such that:*

1. $\mathcal{FR}(T) = \langle \mathcal{M}_{pp}(T), \mathcal{M}_p(T), \mathcal{M}(T) \rangle$,
2. $\mathcal{M}(T) = \{x \mid x \text{ is an } S\}$,
3. $\mathcal{M}_p(T) = \{x \mid x \text{ is an } S_p\}$,
4. $\mathcal{M}_{pp}(T) = \{x \mid x \text{ is an } S_{pp}\}$.

With two additional components, we may enrich the frame $\langle \mathcal{M}_{pp}(T), \mathcal{M}_p(T), \mathcal{M}(T) \rangle$ in order to obtain the concept of a theory. The two components needed are the *constraints* and the *intended applications* of the theory discussed below.

The constraints of a theory

In order to prevent models for a theory from behaving deviantly, they must be constrained by certain requirements. For instance, it would be astounding if the same object exhibited two different weights in two different models for the theory of the Archimedean static, *AS*. An example is a child that plays seesaw on two different beams and exhibits two different weights. Anomalies of this type must be kept out of the theory by stipulating that "the same object has the same weight in two different models". Such a constraining condition, or *constraint* for short, is equivalent to the a priori requirement that the *AS*-theoretical function w, i.e., weight, should behave consistently in all applications of the theory. Thus, it is a non-empirical sentence that *declares* weight to be a constant property of objects. This constraint establishes internal cross-connections between different models for the theory in that it constrains the weight function w to select from among the set of *potential models* for the theory those exemplars as models which in the measurement process obey the requirement, and to rule out those that deviate from it.

A theory T may have a set of $n > 1$ constraints, denoted $\mathcal{C}(T)$. It constitutes the set of those potential models for a theory which are selected to yield models for the theory. Thus, it is a subset of the powerset of $\mathcal{M}(T)$, i.e., $\mathcal{C}(T) \subseteq powerset(\mathcal{M}(T))$. For details of the concept of constraint, see (Balzer and Moulines, 1996; Sneed, 1971; Stegmüller, 1976).

The core of a theory

The frame of a theory, $\langle \mathcal{M}_{pp}(T), \mathcal{M}_p(T), \mathcal{M}(T) \rangle$, supplemented by the constraint $\mathcal{C}(T)$ for $\mathcal{M}_p(T)$ yields the kernel or *core* of the theory, denoted by $\mathcal{K}(T)$. Thus, we have $\mathcal{K}(T) = \langle \mathcal{M}_{pp}(T), \mathcal{M}_p(T), \mathcal{M}(T), \mathcal{C}(T) \rangle$. That is:

Definition 125 (The core fo a theory). *If S is a set-theoretical predicate that axiomatizes a theory* T, *then* $\mathcal{K}(T)$ *is the core of the theory* T *iff there are* $\mathcal{M}_{pp}(T), \mathcal{M}_p(T), \mathcal{M}(T),$ *and* $\mathcal{C}(T)$ *such that:*

   1. $\mathcal{K}(T) = \langle \mathcal{M}_{pp}(T), \mathcal{M}_p(T), \mathcal{M}(T), \mathcal{C}(T) \rangle$,
   2. $\langle \mathcal{M}_{pp}(T), \mathcal{M}_p(T), \mathcal{M}(T) \rangle$ is the frame of the theory,
   3. $\mathcal{C}(T)$ is a set of constraints, i.e. $\mathcal{C}(T) \subseteq powerset(\mathcal{M}(T))$.

As we shall see below, the core is the main part of a theory and is applied to T-non-theoretical entities to produce *knowledge* about them. For details, see (Balzer and Sneed, 1977, 1978; Sneed, 1976; Stegmüller, 1979).

The intended applications of a theory

The class of all entities to which at a particular time it is claimed that a theory T applies, we call the set of intended applications of the theory, or its *intended applications* for short, denoted $\mathcal{I}(T)$.

What type of entities are the intended applications of a theory? An intended application of a theory T is a partial, potential model for T, i.e., something that is void of T-theoretical components, something 'empirical', so to speak. This feature is a prerequisite because the entity must be something *independent of the theory* in order to prevent the obscurantism that characterizes, for example, astrology, demonology, and exorcism. The aim of applying the theory to an entity is to find out whether it covers that entity, i.e., whether the entity can be supplemented by T-theoretical components to yield a potential model that, in addition, is able to satisfy the substantial axioms of the theory and to become a model thereof. For example, two children and a seesaw on a fulcrum c together with a distance function, i.e., an entity of the structure $\langle \Omega, b, d \rangle$ such that:

$$\Omega = \{child_1, child_2\} \tag{100}$$

b is a seesaw,

d is a distance function with, e.g.,

$$d(child_1, c) = 210 \ cm,$$

$$d(child_2, c) = 126 \ cm$$

constitute an *AS*-non-theoretical collection of objects. This collection is a partial, potential model for an Archimedean static, i.e., $(100) \in \mathcal{M}_{pp}(AS)$. Is it also possibly a model for an Archimedean static? That is, does the theory of Archimedean static cover that entity? We can answer this question by adding the *AS*-theoretical function *weight, w*, with e.g.:

$$w(child_1) = 15 \ kg \tag{101}$$

$$w(child_2) = 25 \ kg$$

to obtain the potential model $\langle \Omega, b, d, w \rangle$. If this *AS*-theoretically enriched entity $(100) \cup (101)$ also satisfies the substantial axioms 6–7 of Definition 118 on page 407, then we obtain a model for *AS* theory, i.e., an *application* of the theory of the Archimedean static to the *empirical entity* (100) in the experiential 'world out there'.

Consider now the powerset of partial, potential models for a theory, i.e., $powerset(\mathcal{M}_{pp}(T))$. This set contains sets of different size, i.e., singletons such as (100) above, 2-tuples, 3-tuples and, in general, n-tuples of partial, potential models. The set of intended applications, $\mathcal{I}(T)$, is a subset of $powerset(\mathcal{M}_{pp}(T))$, i.e., $\mathcal{I}(T) \subseteq powerset(\mathcal{M}_{pp}(T))$. For instance, the set of intended applications of our miniature theory of the Archimedean static, $\mathcal{I}(AS)$, contains the above application (100) and all of the other examples mentioned in previous sections, i.e., all seesaws, beam balances, and levers.

The set $\mathcal{I}(T)$ of intended applications of a theory is not closed and static. Instead, it is an open and dynamic collection that usually changes during the theory's life. These changes occur when new applications are added or previous ones are deleted. An application is deleted from the set of intended applications when it is discovered that it is a false application of the theory. For example, it may be that at a particular period in the history of psychosomatics, a disease such as peptic ulcer disease is considered psychosomatic, but at a later point in time this view is abandoned because peptic ulcer disease turns out to be an infectious disease caused by Helicobacter pylori. In such a case, the disease that was previously viewed as an intended application of psychosomatics, is deleted from $\mathcal{I}(\text{psychosomatics})$ and included in $\mathcal{I}(\text{infectiology})$. Most importantly, the set of intended applications $\mathcal{I}(T)$ includes the following two particular elements:

The entities to which a theory is successfully applied for the first time, constitute the initial set of intended applications, denoted by $\mathcal{I}_0(T)$. Sometimes this initial set with which a theory starts, is also referred to as *paradigmatic applications,* from the Greek term παράδειγμα (paradeigma) meaning "example, exemplar, sample". It is always presented as a list of examples to which the inventor of the theory has initially applied her theory, and is *never deleted* from set $\mathcal{I}(T)$. In medical theories, for example, such paradigmatic applications may be the first cells, tissues, animals, or patients to whom a new, emerging theory is successfully applied.

At every instant t of a theory T's life history, there is a set of *actual applications,* $\mathcal{I}_t(T)$, that contains all entities which are considered models for the theory. It is obvious that $\mathcal{I}_0(T) \subseteq \mathcal{I}_t(T) \subseteq \mathcal{I}(T)$. The scientific community holding the theory may delete any elements from $\mathcal{I}(T)$, including any elements of $\mathcal{I}_t(T)$, which are different from $\mathcal{I}_0(T)$. Peptic ulcer disease mentioned above was such an example.

It is interesting to observe how the set of intended applications of a theory, $\mathcal{I}(T)$, grows and changes over time. Given some paradigmatic applications with which a theory T starts, i.e. $\mathcal{I}_0(T)$, additional partial, potential models that *resemble* them are considered as new candidates that might turn out models for the theory when analyzed according to the theory's methodology. Thus, set $\mathcal{I}(T)$ grows on the basis of *similarity relationships* between its actual members and other entities. This is a similaristic process, like the process of nosological categorization that we studied in our prototype resemblance theory of disease on pages 174–183. Thus, the initial applications of a theory may be viewed as its prototype applications. Due to lack of space, this idea of a *prototype resemblance theory of knowledge* cannot be pursued here.

What a theory is

Following the steps above we are now in a position to understand what a theory is according to the structuralistic approach:

Definition 126 (Theory). *T is a theory iff there are $\mathcal{K}(T)$ and $\mathcal{I}(T)$ such that:*

> *1. $T = \langle \mathcal{K}(T), \mathcal{I}(T) \rangle$,*
> *2. $\mathcal{K}(T)$ is the core of the theory,*
> *3. $\mathcal{I}(T)$ is the set of its intended applications.*

A theory is thus an ordered pair consisting of the core of the theory and the set of its intended applications. Note that due to $\mathcal{K}(T) = \langle \mathcal{M}_{pp}(T), \mathcal{M}_p(T), \mathcal{M}(T), \mathcal{C}(T) \rangle$, the theory is the ordered set of its different model types, constraints, and intended applications:

$$T = \langle \langle \mathcal{M}_{pp}(T), \mathcal{M}_p(T), \mathcal{M}(T), \mathcal{C}(T), \mathcal{I}(T) \rangle \tag{102}$$
$$= \langle core, intended\ applications \rangle$$
$$= \langle frame, constraints, intended\ applications \rangle.$$

Suppose, for example, that $\mathcal{K}(AS)$ is the core of our miniature theory of the Archimedean static, i.e., the set of its partial, potential models; the set of its potential models; the set of its models; and the set of its constraints. And suppose further that $\mathcal{I}(AS)$ is a class comprising all levers, beam balances, and seesaws. Then, $\langle \mathcal{K}(AS), \mathcal{I}(AS) \rangle$ represents our miniature theory of Archimedean static.

It is now possible to be more explicit about what the non-statement, or structuralistic, view of theories amounts to. It says: We have the core $\mathcal{K}(T)$ of the theory, on the one hand; and the set of its intended applications, $\mathcal{I}(T)$, on the other. These two entities constitute a *structure*, $\langle \mathcal{K}(T), \mathcal{I}(T) \rangle$, called a *theory*. The structure obviously does not consist of statements. Rather, it consists of two more or less complex sets. Accordingly, it does not say anything about the world. In what follows, we shall see that only its core $\mathcal{K}(T)$ is *applied* to entities of that world to generate knowledge about them. As a structure, like a building or machine, the theory itself does not represent knowledge. In the next section, we shall evaluate this important epistemological consequence by analyzing a medical theory. For a further development of the Sneedean metatheory, see (da Costa and French, 2003).

A first example: The theory of active immunity

In this section, the familiar concept of active immunity is reconstructed by introducing the set-theoretical predicate "x is an active immunity structure" to show that it denotes a genuine *theory* of the type $\langle \mathcal{K}(T), \mathcal{I}(T) \rangle$ demonstrated above.

It is well known that medical theories are not formulated in such a way that easily reveals them as structures of the type $\langle \mathcal{K}(T), \mathcal{I}(T) \rangle$. They need first to be reconstructed by means of the methodology sketched in the preceding sections. Suppose that we explicitly reconstruct some medical theories in order to lay bare what they look like. The well-established theories of immunity, autoimmunity, and cellular pathology recommend themselves as candidates. Should any of these theories turn out to be a structure of the type $\langle \mathcal{K}(T), \mathcal{I}(T) \rangle$, then we shall have reason to abandon the view that the theory says something about the organisms or processes to which it is applied, and is testable by empirical analyses and observations. We shall then want to inquire into other virtues or shortcomings it may have instead. To provide an impetus for such inquiries, we will attempt our own reconstruction of the theory of active immunity.

The starting point is always the reconstruction of *the basis* of a theory, on which the whole edifice rests, as a set-theoretical predicate. The basis of the theory of immunity is as simple as this:

- **The basic idea of the theory of immunity:** An organism is immune if it is able to defend itself against invading agents.

Although this stipulation sounds like an empirical statement about abilities of organisms, it is in fact a pruned definition of the term "is immune" that to a first approximation may be rewritten as follows:

Definition 127 (Immune). *An organism is immune iff it is able to defend itself against invading agents.*

Unfortunately, this commonly held basic idea of the theory of immunity is defective for two reasons. First, it is an ill-formulated one and straightforwardly leads to inconsistencies in that an organism may turn out *immune* if it can defend itself against some particular agents, e.g., common influenza virus H1N1, and *not immune* at the same time because it cannot defend itself against some other agents, e.g., HIV. Second, it is unstructured and thus too undifferentiated to yield a solid theory. Both shortcomings may be avoided if we represent the idea by means of a set-theoretical predicate. This would in addition enable us to use, in the emerging theory and in dealing with it, all of the facilities of set theories, logics, and other formal sciences. Before we do so below, we must be clear about the constituents involved. These are:

a. one or more organisms, maybe a whole species, which constitute the universe of our discourse ("the immune entities"),
b. a bunch of harmful agents that invade or attack a host. They may be (i) living micro-organisms; (ii) viruses; or (iii) other objects such as prions, allergens, toxins, and irritating substances,
c. a collection of defenders in the host, e.g., phagocytes, antibodies, etc.

We will now axiomatize the basic idea of immunity quoted above by defining a set-theoretical predicate, baptized "is an immunity structure", to show that it is indeed the basic element of the whole network of the huge theory of immunity.

Definition 128 (Immunity structure: IS). *ξ is an immunity structure iff there are Ω and X such that:*

1. *$\xi = \langle \Omega, X \rangle$,*
2. *Ω is a non-empty set of living organisms,*
3. *X is a non-empty set of harmful organisms, viruses, or substances, referred to as agents,*
4. *If some elements of X invade or attack any members of Ω, then these members destroy or render them harmless.*

For example, the following pairs:

$\langle \{Elroy\ Fox\}, measles\_viruses \rangle$
$\langle Current\_students\_of\_MIT, smallpox\_viruses \rangle$

satisfy the structural axioms 1–3 of the set-theoretical predicate "ξ is an immunity structure" above. If they also satisfy the substantial axiom 4, then they are models for the predicate, i.e., immunity structures. However, the pairs:

$\langle \{Elroy\ Fox\}, HIV \rangle$
$\langle Current\_students\_of\_MIT, HIV \rangle$

are not immunity structures. That is, they don't constitute models for the same predicate because they violate axiom 4. No human organism is able to combat HIV.

It is worth noting that for the inquiry into whether a given entity $\langle A, B \rangle$ is an immunity structure or not, there need not exist another immunity structure $\langle A', B' \rangle$ on which our judgment depends. Thus, according to the criterion of T-theoreticity provided in Definitions 120–121 on pages 412–413, an immunity structure does not contain T-theoretical terms. As before, the affix "T" in the phrase "T-theoretical" refers to a theory under discussion. That means in the present context that the concept of *immunity structure*, suggested in Definition 128 above, does not include a term that is a theoretical term with respect to that concept itself, an immunity-structure-theoretical term, so to speak.

Note also that in Definition 128, the base domain Ω of an immunity structure has been conceived as a set such that it may be a singleton like {Elroy Fox} or comprise any group of organisms such as the set of current students of MIT, the human species, or any animal species. In virtue of its capacity to be applicable to groups, the concept also covers "military defense" and thus demonstrates that the idea of immunity is related with conflict, war, and defense. Tellingly, the immune system of the organism is called its "defense system" in German ("Abwehrsystem").

The set-theoretical predicate "ξ is an immunity structure" introduced above should not be mistaken for what is called the "immune system" of the organism. It is meant to delineate the class of those entities that exhibit immunity to specified infections and other types of violence. On this account, it may serve as the basic theory-element of the whole network of the received theory of immunity to enable the reconstruction of all of its partial theories such as the theories of active immunity, passive immunity, adaptive immunity, natural immunity, humoral immunity, cell-mediated immunity, autoimmunity, and others. One example may suffice here to illustrate. Stepwise, we shall show that the *theory of active immunity* is a specialization of the basic, set-theoretical predicate "ξ is an immunity structure" above by adding a third component, Y, that will be a T-theoretical term. To this end, we should note that by "active immunity" is usually understood the immunity of the organism through its production of specific antibodies against particular agents. Active immunity is acquired in two ways: naturally by contracting an infectious disease, or artificially by vaccination.

Definition 129 (Active immunity structure: AIS). ξ *is an* active immunity structure *iff there are* Ω, X, *and* Y *such that:*

1. $\xi = \langle \Omega, X, Y \rangle$,
2. Ω *is a non-empty set of living organisms,*
3. X *is a non-empty set of harmful organisms, viruses, or substances, referred to as agents,*
4. Y *is a non-empty set of objects called antibodies against agents X,*

5. *The production of Y is an acquired feature of members of Ω,*
6. *The organism of each member of Ω produces a subset Z of Y,*
7. *If some elements of X invade or attack any members of Ω, then these members destroy or render them harmless by using Z.*

An active immunity structure according to Definition 129 is also an immunity structure according to Definition 128 because the structure $\langle \Omega, X, Y \rangle$ includes the structure $\langle \Omega, X \rangle$. But a major epistemological difference emerges by adding the component Y to $\langle \Omega, X \rangle$. While an immunity structure $\langle \Omega, X \rangle$ according to Definition 128 is void of any *IS*-theoretical terms, an active immunity structure contains the binary *AIS*-theoretical relation Y that in the structural axiom 4 has been characterized by the binary predicate "*a is an antibody against b*". The *AIS*-theoreticity of this predicate and its epistemological impact will be demonstrated and analyzed below. To this end, consider first the following example:

$$\langle \{Elroy\ Fox\}, measles\_viruses, measles\_antibodies \rangle. \tag{103}$$

This triple satisfies the structural axioms of the set-theoretical predicate "ξ is an active immunity structure". If it also satisfies the remaining, substantial axioms 5–7, then it is an active immunity structure. That is, the triple (103) is a model for the set-theoretical predicate "ξ is an active immunity structure" on the condition that it satisfies axioms 5–7 in Definition 129. These axioms say that if Elroy Fox is exposed to measles viruses, then he will be able to destroy them or render them harmless by using specific antibodies against them that his own organism has produced. Now the following question arises:

How are we to determine whether or not the triple (103) satisfies axioms 5–7 to be considered an active immunity structure? The least is to show that (i) Elroy Fox's organism houses *antibodies against measles viruses* produced by itself, and (ii) they destroy or defuse invading measles viruses. This, however, requires that the following experiment be conducted: Expose Elroy Fox to measles viruses and show measles antibodies in action! Since such an experiment in vivo is morally and legally prohibited, the physician or the immunologist will argue instead: "We have taken a blood test that demonstrates that measles antibodies are present in Mr. Elroy Fox's organism. We cannot prove that they have been produced in his own organism and are able to destroy or defuse invading measles viruses. But on the basis of innumerable animal experiments conducted since the early work done by Emil Behring (1854–1917) and Paul Ehrlich (1854–1915), we are convinced that it is so". This reference to *another* setting, other than Elroy Fox's own case, amounts to the use of Sneedean criterion of T-theoreticity of predicates presented in Definition 121 on page 413. It says: To determine whether it is true that Elroy Fox in the triple (103) above possesses efficacious measles antibodies to yield an active immunity structure, requires that there be *another* entity of the same form $\langle \Omega', X', Y' \rangle$ which is an active immunity structure. Thus, the predicate "antibodies against agents X" occurring in Definition 129 is an *AIS*-theoretical term, the only one in the concept.

Thus far we have been concerned only with the set-theoretical "active immunity structure" itself and have shown that it contains the AIS-theoretical predicate "antibodies against agents X". We will now identify the remaining components to demonstrate the *theory of active immunity structure*, i.e., an entity of the form $\langle \mathcal{K}(AIS), \mathcal{I}(AIS) \rangle$ characterized in Definition 126 on page 419. To this end, the following notational symbols will be used:

$$\mathcal{M}(AIS) \quad = \quad \text{\textit{set of models for the theory of active immunity structure,}}$$
$$\mathcal{M}_p(AIS) \quad = \quad \text{\textit{set of potential models for the theory of active immunity structure,}}$$
$$\mathcal{M}_{pp}(AIS) \quad = \quad \text{\textit{set of partial, potential models for the theory of active immunity structure.}}$$

The set of models, $\mathcal{M}(AIS)$, is delimited by Definition 129. This set is obviously a huge collection containing all human beings, animals, and any of their groups and species characterized by active immunity against any agents. It is worth noting that if an entity x such as (103) is an active immunity structure, then that means that $x \in \mathcal{M}(AIS)$. Thus, the measles immunity of an individual such as Mr. Elroy Fox is representable by the statement $x \in \mathcal{M}(AIS)$ where $x = \langle \{\text{Elroy Fox}\}, \text{measles\_viruses}, \text{measles\_antibodies} \rangle$, while we know a priori that $y \notin \mathcal{M}(AIS)$ if $y = \langle \{\text{Elroy Fox}\}, \text{HIV}, \text{HIV\_antibodies} \rangle$.

To obtain $\mathcal{M}_p(AIS)$, remove the substantial axioms 5–7 from Definition 129. All structures of the form $\langle \Omega, X, Y \rangle$ consisting of a set of organisms, a set of agents, and a set of antibodies against such agents satisfy the remaining, structural axioms 1–4 and yield the set of potential models, $\mathcal{M}_p(AIS)$. That is:

Definition 130 (Potential, active immunity structure: AIS$_p$). ξ *is a potential, active immunity structure iff there are Ω, X, and Y such that:*

1. *$\xi = \langle \Omega, X, Y \rangle$,*
2. *Ω is a non-empty set of living organisms,*
3. *X is a non-empty set of harmful organisms, viruses, or substances, referred to as agents,*
4. *Y is a non-empty set of objects called antibodies against agents X.*

Given such an entity, e.g., $\langle \{\text{Elroy Fox}\}, \text{Swine\_influenza\_viruses}, \text{antibodies\_against\_SIV} \rangle$, which satisfies axioms 1–4, it will indeed make sense to ask whether the entity *possibly* satisfies the substantial axioms 5–7 as well. It is this open possibility that justifies the name "potential model for AIS". But the set-theoretical structure AIS_p still contains the AIS-theoretical component Y characterized by the structural axiom 4. By also removing this component we obtain the partial, potential models $\mathcal{M}_{pp}(AIS)$, i.e., those minimal structures which satisfy the following elementary set-theoretical predicate:

Definition 131 (Partial, potential, active immunity structure: AIS$_{pp}$). ξ *is a partial, potential, active immunity structure iff there are Ω and X such that:*

1. $\xi = \langle \Omega, X \rangle$,
2. Ω is a non-empty set of living organisms,
3. X is a non-empty set of harmful organisms, viruses, or substances, referred to as agents.

A closer look will reveal that a model for AIS_{pp} is just a potential model for the basic predicate "ξ is an immunity structure" introduced in Definition 128, i.e., a potential immunity structure.

The three types of models we now have at our disposal, constitute the *frame* of the theory of active immunity structure. That is:

$$\mathcal{FR}(AIS) = \langle \mathcal{M}_{pp}(AIS), \mathcal{M}_p(AIS), \mathcal{M}(AIS) \rangle.$$

By adding the constraint $\mathcal{C}(AIS)$ we obtain the core of the theory:

$$\mathcal{K}(AIS) = \langle \mathcal{M}_{pp}(AIS), \mathcal{M}_p(AIS), \mathcal{M}(AIS), \mathcal{C}(AIS) \rangle.$$

A first constraint of this type is provided by the following postulate of *antibody specificity*. It is well known in the theory of immunity and will be referred to as constraint $\mathcal{C}_1$: "Antibodies act with great specificity, i.e., distinct antibodies are directed against distinct types of agents". This will prevent an antibody from having different effects in different active immunity structures. It cannot be, for example, that measles antibodies destroy measles viruses in Elroy Fox's organism, whereas they target Koch's bacilli in another patient. Interestingly, another, converse constraint, $\mathcal{C}_2$, was put forward by the German pioneer of immunology Paul Ehrlich in 1891: "If two substances give rise to two different antibodies, then they themselves must be different" (Ehrlich, 1891, 1218–1219). The constraint $\mathcal{C}(AIS)$ above may be conceived as $\mathcal{C}_1 \& \mathcal{C}_2$. It selects from among the $powerset(\mathcal{M}_p(AIS))$ only those structures which behave as required to become models for AIS.

The last component we need to finalize the theory AIS is the set of its intended applications, $\mathcal{I}(AIS)$. Intended applications of the theory are elementary structures of the type $\langle \Omega, X \rangle$ consisting of organisms and agents without further characterization. They are partial, potential models of the AIS theory as introduced in Definition 131 above. That is, $\mathcal{I}(AIS) \subseteq powerset(\mathcal{M}_{pp}(AIS))$. Elements of this set may be conceived of as human beings or animals exposed to any infections and allergens. It makes sense to ask of such an entity $x \in \mathcal{I}(AIS)$ whether it will be possible to show that it is an active immunity structure, i.e., an application of the AIS theory. Researchers concerned with AIS ask just such questions. The initial patients and animals exposed to infections or antigens and examined by the two pioneers of immunology, Paul Ehrlich and Emil Behring, constitute the set of *initial applications*, $\mathcal{I}_0(AIS)$. All infectious diseases and allergies that in current medicine are viewed to give rise to acquired immunity in the hosts constitute, together with the hosts and the antibodies they induce, AIS structures of the type $\langle \Omega, X, Y \rangle$. They yield the set of *actual applications* of the theory, i.e.,

$\mathcal{I}_t(AIS)$ where t is the current date. As was mentioned on page 419, we have that $\mathcal{I}_0(AIS) \subseteq \mathcal{I}_t(AIS) \subseteq \mathcal{I}_0(AIS)$. The theory of active immunity we have explicated thus far, consists of the following core and intended applications:

$$AIS = \langle \mathcal{K}(AIS), \mathcal{I}(AIS) \rangle.$$

That is:

$$AIS = \langle \mathcal{M}_{pp}(AIS), \mathcal{M}_p(AIS), \mathcal{M}(AIS), \mathcal{C}(AIS), \mathcal{I}(AIS) \rangle.$$

Empirical claims made using a theory

In the preceding section, we saw that the basic theory of active immunity is the structure $\langle \mathcal{K}(AIS), \mathcal{I}(AIS) \rangle$. Obviously, it does not consist of any statements. That a theory as a structure of the type $\langle \mathcal{K}(T), \mathcal{I}(T) \rangle$ does not consist of statements, and therefore, does not say anything about 'the world out there', does not mean that it is something empirically sterile, neutral, and worthless. By contrast, it provides a most effective *tool that is used* to make empirical claims, and by examining these claims, to *produce* empirical hypotheses and knowledge. Also a hammer does not make statements about the world. It is a useful tool nonetheless.

What does an empirical claim made using a theory $\langle \mathcal{K}(T), \mathcal{I}(T) \rangle$ look like? And where does the meeting point of a theory as an abstract structure, on the one hand, and 'the world out there', on the other, lie? These central epistemological questions are briefly discussed in this section to show how a theory as an abstract structure is tied to reality. To begin with, let there be a tuple such as:

$$\langle \{Elroy\ Fox\}, Swine\_influenza\_viruses, SIV\_antibodies \rangle \tag{104}$$

consisting of our patient Elroy Fox who has been exposed to Swine influenza viruses and has produced antibodies against them in his organism. Suppose that Mr. Elroy Fox goes through the infection unmolested, not showing any symptoms of the disease. The tuple (104) thus turns out a model for the *AIS* theory axiomatized by the set-theoretical predicate "ξ is an active immunity structure" in Definition 129 on page 422. Now, an *empirical* claim that can be made on the basis of the *AIS* theory is *not* a statement of the form:

$$(104)\ is\ an\ active\ immunity\ structure. \tag{105}$$

For a model, i.e., (104) in the present example, is something *that has T-theoretical components and satisfies all axioms of the theory*. Thus, the statement (105) is a logical consequence of this information plus Definition 129 itself, and is therefore true of logical reasons. It cannot be something empirical. Rather, an empirical claim is provided by the statement that an *AIS-non-theoretical,* partial, potential model for the theory such as:

$$\langle \{Elroy\ Fox\}, Swine\_influenza\_viruses \rangle \qquad (106)$$

can be enriched to a model for the theory AIS. This may be explained in the following way:

A partial, potential model for our theory, i.e., a structure of the type $\langle \Omega, X \rangle$ such as (106), can be supplemented by a set Y of antibodies against X to yield the structure $\langle \Omega, X, Y \rangle$ that in principle may, or may not, *satisfy the substantial axioms of the theory AIS.* Provided that it does satisfy them, we obtain an entity that is a model for the theory, i.e., "$\langle \Omega, X, Y \rangle$ is an active immunity structure". Thus, it is an empirical claim to say that:

(106) can be enriched to a model for AIS. $\qquad (107)$

Empirical statements made using a theory are sentences of this latter type. Below, this idea will be briefly conceptualized in a very simplified fashion. For details, see (Sneed, 1971; Stegmüller, 1976).

Definition 132 (Enrichment). *If x_{pp} is a partial, potential model for a theory T, then y is an extension, or enrichment, of x_{pp} iff there are $n \geq 1$ functions (relations) $f_1, \ldots, f_n$ that can be added to x_{pp} to yield y such that y is a model for T.*

Regarding our example above, the tuple $\langle \{$Elroy Fox$\}$, Swine_influenza_viruses$\rangle$ with following characteristics:

- $\{$Elroy Fox$\}$ is a set of organisms,
- Swine influenza viruses are a set of harmful viruses,

is a partial, potential model for our *AIS* theory. It could be extended to $\langle \{$Elroy Fox$\}$, Swine_influenza_viruses, SIV_antibodies$\rangle$ with the characteristics:

- SIV antibodies are a set of antibodies against Swine influenza viruses,
- their production is an acquired feature of Elroy Fox,
- Elroy Fox's organism has produced some such antibodies,
- some Swine influenza viruses have invaded his organism and have been destroyed or rendered harmless by his SIV antibodies

to become a model for *AIS* because it satisfies all axioms of the theory *AIS*. Thus, an empirical claim made using our theory is an assertion of this form:

There is an extension, i.e., enrichment, $\langle \Omega, X, Y \rangle$ of $\langle \Omega, X \rangle$ such that $\langle \Omega, X, Y \rangle$ is a model for *AIS*. $\qquad (108)$

This has been exemplified above by the empirical claim (107) which says that:

There is an extension $\langle \{Elroy\ Fox\}, Swine\_influenza\_viruses,$ $SIV\_antibodies \rangle$ of $\langle \{Elroy\ Fox\}, Swine\_influenza\_viruses \rangle$ such that $\langle \{Elroy\ Fox\}, Swine\_influenza\_viruses, SIV\_antibodies \rangle$ is a model for *AIS*.

The result may now be generalized to cover all other cases:

Definition 133 (Empirical claim made using a theory). *A statement is an empirical claim made using a theory T iff it says that "The partial, potential model x_{pp} for T can be extended to the structure y such that y is a model for T".*

Otherwise put: ... iff it says that:

$$\text{There is an extension of } x_{pp} \text{ which is a model for theory } T, \tag{109}$$

or simply, "it can be shown that this *fact* is a model for the theory such and such".

A second example: Diagnosis and diagnostics

An interesting practical example is the diagnosis of non-trivial diseases which require extensive diagnostics, e.g., autoimmune diseases. Suppose we conceive or reconstruct the nosological predicate, *P,* that represents such a disease in medical knowledge, as a set-theoretically defined one with possibly *T*-theoretical components. A diagnostician who on the basis of some easily observable patient data hypothesizes that this patient might be a *P*, e.g., possibly "she has Hashimoto's thyroiditis", does indeed make an emprirical claim of the type above about a patient using a nosological *theory*. She claims that the persent patient data can be extended, by adding Hashimoto-theoretical functions or predicates such as measurement results, to render the patient's disease state a model for Hashimoto's thyroiditis. That means that the non-statement view is not only epistemology. It is also highly recommendable as a methodology, e.g., in medical diagnostics. A prerequisite in this case is that individual diseases be represented by set-theoreticaly defined nosological predicates. This is not difficult to realize in knowledge-based clinical decision-support systems. See Section 'A fourth example' on page 437 below and (Mueller-Kolck, 2010).

The empirical content of a theory

What we have achieved thus far can also be used to determine the *empirical content* of a theory. The empirical content of a theory $\langle \mathcal{K}(T), \mathcal{I}(T) \rangle$ is the class of all entities to which the core $\mathcal{K}(T) = \langle \mathcal{M}_{pp}(T), \mathcal{M}_p(T), \mathcal{M}(T), \mathcal{C}(T) \rangle$ applies. Therefore, it is also called the *application set* of $\mathcal{K}(T)$, denoted $\mathbb{A}(\mathcal{K}(T))$. It is defined as follows.

Definition 134 (Empirical content of a theory). *If $\mathcal{K}(T)$ is the core of a theory T, then a subset X of $\mathcal{M}_{pp}(T)$ is in the application set of $\mathcal{K}(T)$, written $X \in \mathbb{A}(\mathcal{K}(T))$, if and only if each of its members can be extended to a structure that turns out a subset of $\mathcal{M}(T)$ satisfying the constraint $\mathcal{C}(T)$.*

Concisely, the application set of a set-theoretically axiomatized theory T is the category of all entities which are (i) void of any T-theoretical components, and thus, completely independent of the theory; (ii) can be extended to models of the theory; and (iii) satisfy its constraints. For example, all patients who have a fever belong to the application set of the theory of infectious diseases if they satisfy the constraints of this theory.

It is worth noting that an empirical claim such as (109) made on the basis of a theory T is equivalent to $\mathcal{I}_i(T) \in \mathbb{A}(\mathcal{K}(T))$ where $\mathcal{I}_i(T)$ is any element of the intended applications $\mathcal{I}(T)$. The total, or *central*, empirical claim that can be made using the theory is the single, big statement $\mathcal{I}(T) \subseteq \mathbb{A}(\mathcal{K}(T))$. It says that the set of intended applications of the theory is included in the application set of its core, i.e., in those sets of T-non-theoretical, 'empirical' or 'observable', entities which pass through the filter of $\mathcal{K}(T)$. For details, see (Stegmüller, 1976, 1979, 1980).

In closing this section and on the basis of our preceding framework, we state a medical-ontologically significant thesis which will be referred to in a later chapter as the *nosological categorization postulate*. The postulate explains what it actually means when someone claims that a particular attribute, e.g., a specific human condition, belongs to a particular nosological class, for example, "schizophrenia is a mental disease", or "bipolar disorder is a mental disease".

Nosological categorization postulate: Let X be a category of patients with a number of features $F = \{F_1, \ldots, F_n\}$. If a claim of the form "the feature set F is a disease of the type D" is put forward (e.g., "schizophrenia is a genetic disease"), then it means: If T is a theory of disease D, then any structure $\langle \{x\}, F \rangle$ consisting of an individual patient x with the feature set F can be extended, by adding T-theoretical components of the nosological predicate D, to become a model for theory T. If all patients of the category X in addition also satisfy the constraints of the theory T, then this category of patients belongs to the application set $\mathbb{A}(\mathcal{K}(T))$ of the theory.

9.4.3 The Semantic View of Theories

There is an additional approach to understanding scientific theories that has come to be known as the semantic view or conception of theories (Suppe, 1977, 1989; van Fraassen, 1980). It is slightly related to the non-statement view because it has been inspired by the same Stanford source (Suppes, 1960, 1962, 1967). It considers a scientific theory to be a collection of models. But it is not well-developed and lacks precision to be transparently applicable to medical theories. It will therefore not be considered here.

9.4.4 Theory-Nets and Intertheoretic Relations

A theory may grow into a large unit consisting of a great number of sub-theories which are interconnected in a particular manner. For instance, the theories of inflammation, microbiology, infectious diseases, and immunology are interconnected in different ways. The yield of such intertheoretic relations is a more or less complex network whose single elements are called *theory-elements*. A theory-element of a theory network is simply what we have reconstructed above as a theory $\langle \mathcal{K}(T), \mathcal{I}(T) \rangle$. One may conceive a network of theory-elements as a graph whose nodes are the theory-elements and whose arcs are the intertheoretic relations between them. There is a variety of such intertheoretic relations. In the present section, we will briefly study a few important ones. To this end, we shall first construct an appropriate theory-element that will grow into a small network. Our study divides into the following four sections:

▶ A third example: The theory of toxic hyperpyrexia
▶ Theory specialization and expansion
▶ Theory reduction and equivalence
▶ A fourth example: Nosology and diagnostics.

A third example: The theory of toxic hyperpyrexia

For the following two reasons, we will present here an additional medical theory in the spirit of the non-statement view. *First,* the miniature theory of active immunity structure (*AIS*) discussed in preceding sections plays an important and interesting role within the network of the theory of immunity. Unfortunately, we could not unambiguously demonstrate on page 423 that it has an *AIS*-theoretical term, i.e., the binary predicate "a is an antibody against b". Term theoreticity, however, is the central feature of a genuine theory and ought to be ensured in order that the three types of models for the theory can be differentiated and identified. This is a prerequisite for the identification of the theory. *Second,* in the next section we shall inquire into the relationships that may exist between different theories, for example, whether one of them follows from the other or is a specialization thereof. For these purposes, we need appropriate example theories. We shall construct here an ad hoc theory that fulfills the requirements described above.

Dr. Timothy Smith, an internist, has delimited a class of patients with a new, previously unkown disease. This new disease is an acute and lethal disorder. It has a rapid onset and results in death within a few days. Its salient symptom is a sudden, high body temperature above 40 °C. Since a high fever of this magnitude may occasionally occur in other diseases which are not life-threatening, one will have to determine as early as possible whether a patient with a body temperature of above 40° has the new lethal disease or not. How may one do that?

The class of patients with a body temperature higher than 40° is heterogeneous because the temperature increase may have different causes. In the subclass of those patients who die within a few days, Dr. Smith found a novel molecule in their blood. Later, he discovered that in their stored blood specimens the molecule changed into another substance by oxidization within two weeks. He observed that by adding a few milliliters of a *new patient's* blood to 5 milliliters of the older blood of a patient who had died, the following reaction occurred if the older blood was at least two weeks old: The red color of the older blood turned into green. He said that the patients who die, had *toxic hyperpyrexia* (the term "pyrexia" means *fever*. From Greek πυρετός (pyretos) for "fever") to be distinguished from malignant hyperthermia caused by some drugs used for general anesthesia. And he considered the ratio:

$$5 \div \text{amount of milliliter of the new blood added} \qquad (110)$$

as a measure of that toxicity in the new patient. In this measure, 5 milliliter is the amount of the old blood used to cause *color conversion* described above. Dr. Smith called the ratio (110) above the degree of *hyperpyrexia toxicity* of the new patient x, symbolized by the quantitative function "*ht*":

$$ht(x) \qquad \equiv \text{ hyperpyrexia toxicity of the patient } x.$$

The less blood of the new patient is required to cause color conversion, the higher her hyperpyrexia toxicity. Finally, Dr. Smith baptized the measurement of the function ht "color conversion test", which he proposed to use as a diagnostic device, and defined a new patient x as having the disease if her hyperpyrexia toxicity equalled or exceeded 5, i.e., if $ht(x) \geq 5$. On the basis of what we have sketched thus far, we can now conceptualize the new disease by the following set-theoretical predicate that defines it extensionally:

Definition 135 (Toxic hyperpyrexia system: THS). *ξ is a toxic hyperpyrexia system iff there are Ω, f, and ht such that:*

1. *$\xi = \langle \Omega, f, ht \rangle$,*
2. *Ω is a non-empty set of human beings,*
3. *f, i.e. 'fever', is a function from Ω to $\mathbb{R}^+$,*
4. *ht, i.e. 'hyperpyrexia toxicity', is a function from Ω to $\mathbb{R}^+$,*
5. *$f(x) > 40\ °C$ for every member x of Ω,*
6. *$ht(x) \geq 5$ for every member x of Ω.*

Since the universe of discourse, Ω, is a set of human beings, a toxic hyperpyrexia system may include a single patient or a group of patients. Axioms 1–4 are structural. The substantial axiom 5 says that any individual in set Ω has an elevated body temperature of above 40 °C. The substantial axiom 6 says that the hyperpyrexia toxicity of an individual in Ω equals or exceeds 5. The theory that is being axiomatized by the set-theoretical predicate above, will be referred to as the theory of *THS*, or *THS* for short ('toxic hyperpyrexia system').

Let $\mathcal{M}(THS)$ denote the class of models for the set-theoretical predicate "ξ is a toxic hyperpyrexia". Each element of $\mathcal{M}(THS)$ is an entity of the structure $\langle \Omega, f, ht \rangle$ that satisfies all six axioms. For instance, the triple:

$\langle \{Elroy\ Fox\}, f', ht' \rangle$

with following characteristics:

> f' is fever function (= body temperature)
> ht' is the hyperpyrexia toxicity
> $f'(Elroy\ Fox) = 41\ °C$
> $ht'(Elroy\ Fox) = 10$

is such a model for *THS*. The interesting question to ask, is: Does the theory *THS* contain any *T*-theoretical terms? Let us analyze this question using the patient Elroy Fox above as an example. The theory contains two functions, f for the measurement of body temperature, and ht for the measurement of the degree of hyperpyrexia toxicity. Regarding f' as an instance of f, to determine whether Elroy Fox's body temperature exceeds 40 °C (axiom 5), we need not know whether there is another patient who ever had such a body temperature. Regarding ht' as an instance of ht, however, the measurement of Elroy Fox's hyperpyrexia toxicity (axiom 6) requires, according to *color conversion test* sketched above, that there be another patient who has suffered from toxic hyperpyrexia and has died, and whose stored blood specimen is needed for use in the color conversion test. Thus, for the determination of the $ht'(Elroy\ Fox)$ value in the entity $\langle \{Elroy\ Fox\}, f', ht' \rangle$, a prerequisite is that there be another entity of the structure $\langle \Omega'', f'', ht'' \rangle$ that *is already* a model for the theory. Since this requirement holds for all models of the theory, the function ht in the structure $\langle \Omega, f, ht \rangle$ is a *THS*-theoretical term according to the criterion of term theoreticity given in Definition 120 on page 412.

By removing its substantial axioms 5–6 we can identify the set of potential models for our theory, $\mathcal{M}_p(THS)$. This set comprises all entities which satisfy the following pruned set-theoretical predicate:

Definition 136 (Potential, toxic hyperpyrexia system: THS$_p$). *ξ is a potential, toxic hyperpyrexia system iff there are Ω, f, and ht such that:*

> *1. $\xi = \langle \Omega, f, ht \rangle$,*
> *2. Ω is a non-empty set of human beings,*
> *3. f, i.e. 'fever', is a function from Ω to $\mathbb{R}^+$,*
> *4. ht, i.e. 'hyperpyrexia toxicity', is a function from Ω to $\mathbb{R}^+$.*

If in addition we also remove the *THS*-theoretical function ht from the structure $\langle \Omega, f, ht \rangle$, what remains is a partial, potential model of the form $\langle \Omega, f \rangle$ void of any *THS*-theoreticity:

Definition 137 (Partial, potential, toxic hyperpyrexia system: THS$_{pp}$). *ξ is a partial, potential, toxic hyperpyrexia system iff there are Ω, f such that:*

> *1. $\xi = \langle \Omega, f \rangle$,*
> *2. Ω is a non-empty set of human beings,*
> *3. f, i.e. 'fever', is a function from Ω to $\mathbb{R}^+$.*

Recall that a partial, potential model is a *THS*-non-theoretical, 'empirical' entity. In the present example, any human individual and group whose body temperature is measurable, is such a partial, potential model for toxic hyperpyrexia. Let $\mathcal{M}_{pp}(THS)$ denote the set of all partial, potential models for our theory. An *intended application* of the theory is any subset of $\mathcal{M}_{pp}(THS)$.

As a *constraint* of the theory it seems reasonable to require that an individual x who at the same time is a member of the universe A in a potential model $\langle A, f', ht' \rangle$, and a member of the universe B in another potential model $\langle B, f'', ht'' \rangle$, should possess exactly or approximately the same hyperpyrexia toxicity values, i.e., the fuzzy relation $ht'(x) \approx ht''(x)$ should hold. The set of those potential models for the theory which satisfy this constraint, may be denoted by $\mathcal{C}(THS)$. Thus we obtain the following core of our theory:

$$\mathcal{K}(THS) = \langle \mathcal{M}_{pp}(THS), \mathcal{M}_p(THS), \mathcal{M}(THS), \mathcal{C}(THS) \rangle.$$

Together with the set of intended applications of the theory, $\mathcal{I}(THS)$, it yields the following theory of toxic hyperpyrexia:

$$THS = \langle \mathcal{K}(THS), \mathcal{I}(THS) \rangle.$$

For instance, the set of intended applications, $\mathcal{I}(THS)$, may include, among many others, the following three patients:

$$\langle \{Elroy\ Fox\}, f' \rangle, \quad \langle \{Amy\}, f'' \rangle, \quad \langle \{Beth\}, f''' \rangle.$$

Note that all of these entities are elements of $\mathcal{M}_{pp}(THS)$ satisfying Definition 137. Someone may claim that by adding an instance of the *THS*-theoretical function ht to any of these entities and measuring the hyperpyrexia toxicity of the respective patient thereby, the entity *can* be extended to a model for the theory if it also satisfies axiom 6 of the basic set-theoretical predicate "ξ is a toxic hyperpyrexia system" introduced in Definition 135 above. Such a claim is an *empirical claim* made using the theory *THS*. It says that a particular partial, potential model x_{pp}, e.g., $\langle \{Elroy\ Fox\}, f' \rangle$, is an element of the application set of $\mathcal{K}(THS)$, i.e., $x_{pp} \in \mathbb{A}(\mathcal{K}(THS))$. To confirm or disconfirm the claim, the hyperpyrexia toxicity of Elroy Fox needs to be determined. If the result $ht'(Elroy\ Fox)$ exceeds 5, then Elroy Fox has toxic hyperpyrexia and is thus a model for the theory *THS*.

We have chosen the example theory above for these four reasons: (i) it is simple and transparent enough to avoid laborious analyses; (ii) it has an easily recognizable T-theoretical term, i.e., the function ht, that allows for structuralistic inquiries, which we shall undertake below; (iii) as a nosological example, it demonstrates that diseases, at least in pathology, can best be represented by set-theoretical predicates. Accordingly, we may recognize that nosological concepts, the so-called individual diseases, are in fact theories; and (iv) diagnostics may be viewed as an examination of the question whether the patient is a model for the respective nosological concept.

On the basis of the theory constructed thus far, we will now sketch the following intertheoretic relations: specialization, expansion, reduction, and equivalence. For details, see (Balzer and Sneed, 1977, 1978; Sneed, 1976; Stegmüller, 1979).

Theory specialization and expansion

A theory is a specialization of another theory if it has additional axioms or constraints. Consider, for example, the following set-theoretical structure:

Definition 138 (Heterogeneous toxic hyperpyrexia system: HTHS). ξ *is an heterogeneous toxic hyperpyrexia system* iff *there are* Ω, f, *and* ht *such that:*

1. $\xi = \langle \Omega, f, ht \rangle$,
2. Ω *is a non-empty set of human beings,*
3. f, *i.e. 'fever', is a function from* Ω *to* $\mathbb{R}^+$,
4. ht, *i.e. 'hyperpyrexia toxicity', is a function from* Ω *to* $\mathbb{R}^+$,
5. $f(x) > 40\ {}^\circ C$ *for every member* x *of* Ω,
6. $ht(x) \geq 5$ *for every member* x *of* Ω,
7. *If* $x \neq y$, *then* $ht(x) \neq ht(y)$ *for all* x, $y \in \Omega$.

Let us compare it with the structure THS delineated in Definition 135 on page 431. The new structure emerges as a *specialization* of the latter by adding the substantial axiom 7 which says that in an heterogeneous toxic hyperpyrexia system, the extent of the hyperpyrexia toxicity of any two distinct patients is different. It is such additions that cause differences between models for theory-elements in a theory-net. If a theory $T' = \langle \mathcal{K}(T'), \mathcal{I}(T') \rangle$ is a specialization of another theory $T = \langle \mathcal{K}(T), \mathcal{I}(T) \rangle$, then we have $\mathcal{M}_{pp}(T') \subseteq \mathcal{M}_{pp}(T)$; $\mathcal{M}_p(T') \subseteq \mathcal{M}_p(T)$; $\mathcal{M}(T') \subseteq \mathcal{M}(T)$; $\mathcal{C}(T') \subseteq \mathcal{C}(T)$; and $\mathcal{I}(T') \subseteq \mathcal{I}(T)$. For example, an heterogeneous toxic hyperpyrexia system is automatically a toxic hyperpyrexia system, whereas the converse is not true.

An *expansion* T_j of a theory-element T_i emerges by adding new T-non-theoretical or T-theoretical components and corresponding axioms and/or constraints to T_i. Suppose, for instance, someone discovers that toxic hyperpyrexia is caused, like hepatitis, by different types of viruses, say virus A and virus B, and thus differentiates between two types of toxic hyperpyrexia, type A and type B, in the following manner:

Definition 139 (Toxic hyperpyrexia system of type A: THS-A). ξ *is a toxic hyperpyrexia system of type A* iff *there are* Ω, f, ht, *and* V_A *such that:*

1. $\xi = \langle \Omega, V_A, f, ht \rangle$,
2. Ω *is a non-empty set of human beings,*
3. V_A *is a bunch of virus A,*
4. f, *i.e. 'fever', is a function from* Ω *to* $\mathbb{R}^+$,
5. ht, *i.e. 'hyperpyrexia toxicity', is a function from* Ω *to* $\mathbb{R}^+$,
6. $f(x) > 40\ {}^\circ C$ *for every member* x *of* Ω,

7. $ht(x) \geq 5$ for every member x of Ω,

8. Elements of V_A are present in the blood of every member x of Ω.

Analogously, one may formulate a toxic hyperpyrexia system of type B. Each of these new concepts expands the basic theory-element *toxic hyperpyrexia system*. If any of the new components contained in the emerging theory-element is T-theoretical, the expansion is called theoretization. It is referred to as non-theoretical expansion, otherwise. While the new hyperpyrexia theories, *THS-A* and *THS-B*, are non-theoretical expansions of our initial theory-element *toxic hyperpyrexia system,* the latter itself may be viewed as a theoretization of the following structure (Figure 61):[77]

Definition 140 (Hyperpyrexia system: HS). ξ *is a hyperpyrexia system iff there are Ω and f such that:*

1. $\xi = \langle \Omega, f \rangle$,
2. Ω is a non-empty set of human beings,
3. f, i.e. 'fever', is a function from Ω to $\mathbb{R}^+$,
4. $f(x) > 40\,°C$ for every member x of Ω.

We saw some other interesting examples of specialization and expansion in Section 6.5.3 on probabilistic etiology on pages 233–264. The basic set-theoretical predicate "potential-causal structure" introduced in Definition 67 on page 247 is an expansion of the concept of probability space introduced in Definition 237 on page 975. It is further specialized to spurious causal structures, genuine causal structures, etc. Thus, the basic theory-element of our probabilistic etiology is in fact the mathematical concept of probability space. Otherwise put, medical-causal processes are specific probability spaces.

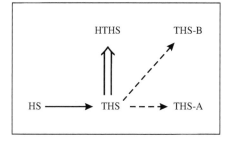

Fig. 61. A theory-net as a directed graph. The nodes are theory-elements. The edges represent intertheoretic relations between them, i.e.: "→" ≡ theoretization; "⇒" ≡ specialization; "-→" ≡ non-theoretical expansion. The theory-elements constituting the theory-net are: HS ≡ hyperpyrexia system; THS ≡ toxic HS; HTHS ≡ heterogeneous THS; THS-A ≡ THS of type A; THS-B ≡ THS of type B. Obviously, the basic theory-element is HS

---

[77] A real-world example of non-theoretical expansion is the group of diseases *hepatitis A, B, C, ..., G,* and *non-A-non-G* as an expansion of hepatitis.

Theory reduction and equivalence

Reductionism is the thesis that the results of research in one domain, e.g., principles, laws, or theories in biology, can be derived from or explained by the results of research of another, more fundamental domain, e.g., of chemistry. For example, it is said that chemistry is reducible to physics. In this sense, some scientists and philosophers of science are interested in the question of whether a particular branch of science is reducible to another, 'more fundamental' one, for instance, psychology, psychiatry, and psychosomatics to neuroscience; neuroscience to biology; biology to physics; and the like. This interest in *domain reductionism* is not new. Nevertheless, it remains as fruitless now as it has been in the past. A similarly unsuccessful attempt has been the famous doctrine of *semantic physicalism* held by some prominent logical empiricists in the early twentieth century according to which "the language of physics is the universal language of all science" (see footnote 138 on page 724). But there are also more specific reductionistic interests, beliefs, and claims such as "mind is reducible to neural mechanism"; "disease is reducible to genetics and pathobiochemistry"; and so on. The only remedy against such misguided exaggerations is to call the attention of the proponents to the art of argumentation. More important and promising than top-down reductionism is the modest metatheoretical question of whether a particular theory-net or theory-element is reducible to another one. For instance, it is said that thermodynamics is reducible to the kinetic theory.

A theory that is being reduced to another one is called the *reduced* theory. That theory to which it is reduced is referred to as the *reducing* one. The reduction of a theory T to another theory T' has to be conducted by introducing a reduction relation which demonstrates what the reduction looks like. Such a relation should satisfy at least the following criteria.

First, the relation should map each intended application of the reduced theory T to at least one intended application of the reducing theory T' to guarantee that the latter is 'anchored in the same world' and covers the same phenomena and facts, i.e., partial, potential models, as the reduced theory does. Second, if α is a sentence that is formed using T and describes something in the 'world out there', there must be a sentence α' that is formed using T' and is true whenever α is true. That means that the laws of the reduced theory T should logically follow from the laws of the reducing theory T'. These brief remarks on theory reduction may suffice in this context. The concept as a whole is too complex to be discussed here in detail. See (Sneed, 1971; Stegmüller, 1976).

Besides reduction, there is also a relation of equivalence between theories. In some disciplines, especially physics and chemistry, it is sometimes said that two different expositions of a particular theory are *equivalent,* for example, that Werner Heisenberg's formulation of quantum mechanics is equivalent to Erwin Schrödingers's. The main criterion of equivalence between two theory-elements, $\langle \mathcal{K}(T), \mathcal{I}(T) \rangle$ and $\langle \mathcal{K}(T'), \mathcal{I}(T') \rangle$, is that the application sets of their cores, i.e., $\mathbb{A}\big(\mathcal{K}(T)\big)$ and $\mathbb{A}\big(\mathcal{K}(T')\big)$, be equivalent. We will not concern ourselves with additional criteria because the concept of theory equivalence is also too complex and cannot be discussed here. For details, see (Sneed, 1971, ch. VII; Stegmüller, 1976, ch. 8).

A fourth example: Nosology and diagnostics

As was pointed out above, the non-statement view is not merely epistemology. It may also serve as a methodological device, e.g., in building nosological systems as well as in diagnostics in the following way.

On the one hand, nosological predicates are unfortunately seldom defined, or well-defined, in clinical medicine. We are usually provided with a vast amount of symptom-disease associations, i.e., disease descriptions. However, since the description of a disease, which we have previously referred to as a *nosogram* (p. 200), is commonly mistaken for the definition of the disease, the explicit delimitation of a disease by defining the corresponding nosological predicate is almost always omitted.

On the other hand, medical knowledge engineering that is gradually developing into an experimental science of clinical practice (see page 319), is methodologically sophisticated enough to implement the differentiation made above between partial potential models, potential models, and models for a theory. Within the confines of this framework, a nosological predicate such as "myocardial infarction" may be set-theoretically defined to represent the disease as a theory-element which in combination with other theory-elements may form a nosological theory-net when there are intertheoretic relations of expansion or specialization between them. This approach may be viewed as nosological theory construction. As far as diagnostics is concerned, a patient x to whom such a disease is ascribed, is a model for the theory. At a lower level prior to the making of the final diagnosis, she is a potential model for the theory because she does not yet satisfy all axioms of the theory. The information about the patient that would justify the diagnosis, is still lacking. At the lowest level, when initial patient data set D only is available, she is a partial potential model for the theory. And the entire diagnostic plan to examine which one of the numerous differential diagnoses is true of her, amounts to *empirical claims* of several theories $T_1, T_2, \ldots$ each of which says that the patient x together with her patient data D can be extended to a structure $y = \langle x, D' \rangle$ such that y is a model for the theory T_i, where T_i is any of the hypothesized differential diagnoses (see page 426).

For example, a patient complaining of acute angina pectoris, is a partial potential model for the above-mentioned theory of myocardial infarction. If the diagnostic examination reveals that the enzyme CK-MB is elevated in her blood, then she becomes a potential model for that theory. The question of whether or not she has in fact myocardial infarction, presupposes the concept, or theory, of myocardial infarction we are talking about. Every cardiologist making such diagnoses ought to know the answer to the question: What does it explicitly look like?

9.4.5 Untestability of Theories

It is usually assumed that by means of a theory we predict events. If a predicted event fails to occur, this is evidence against the theory and falsifies it. The scientist then abandons her theory and seeks a new one.

We are thus told that theories are empirically tested by means of their predictions. Einstein's general theory of relativity is the prime example used in such contexts. It is said, for example, that the observation of the redshift of the light of distant stars by the gravitational field of the sun confirms his theory because the gravitational deflection of the light is just a prediction made by that theory (Dyson et al., 1920).

Unfortunately, there is not a single grain of truth in this commonly held view. Otherwise, no theories would exist at all because, for whatever reasons, most of the events predicted using our theories do not occur. In the light of the non-statement, or structuralistic, metatheory sketched in preceding sections, a theory turns out something that cannot be subjected to empirical testing in order to verify, falsify, support, confirm, or disconfirm it. None of these and related semantic predicates is sensibly applicable to a theory because, as a structure of the type $\langle \mathcal{K}(T), \mathcal{I}(T) \rangle$, a theory does not assert anything that might be true, false, probable, improbable, confirmable, disconfirmable, etc. So, it is informationally empty and does not predict anything. Examples are our theories of the active immunity structure (AIS) and the toxic hyperpyrexia system (THS), presented on pages 422 and 431, respectively. They describe nothing, assert nothing, explain nothing, and predict nothing. They are syntactic networks based on set-theoretical definitions. Thus, they are neither true nor false, neither close to nor far from truth, neither probable nor improbable, and so on. Each of them can only be *used* as a structure to inquire into whether there are entities of this structure in the world. A theory is thus a *tool* for structuring the world, acquiring knowledge about it, and forming a worldview. For example, suppose that there is a partial, potential model x_{pp} of the theory of toxic hyperpyrexia such as the patient Elroy Fox who has a body temperature above 41 °C. We may try to extend this partial, potential model x_{pp} and examine whether Elroy Fox has a hyperpyrexia toxicity above 5 to become a model for the theory. If this attempt succeeds, then its success does not verify or confirm the theory because the theory does not assert that the extended entity is a model for it. Only our following *empirical claim*, which we made *using* the theory, is verified:

There is an extension, i.e., enrichment, of x_{pp} which is a model for *THS* theory,

specifically:

There is an extension of $\langle \{Elroy\ Fox\}, f \rangle$, where $f(Elroy\ Fox) >$ 41 °C, which is a model for *THS* theory.

The verification of this claim does not touch the theory itself. The same obtains when the empirical claim fails. The failure does not disconfirm or falsify the theory. The theory remains untouched. Predictions made on the basis of a theory are such *empirical claims made using the theory*, e.g., the prediction of the gravitational deflection of the starlight by the sun mentioned above. If a predicted event fails to occur, then this is by no means evidence against the theory. It only falsifies the empirical claim. So, the theory will be retained. In this way every theory is able to survive any recalcitrant circumstance. Only the *persistent failure* of empirical claims that are made using a particular theory will be a reason to modify or abandon the theory on the grounds that it seems, or turns out, to be void of models in 'the world out there', and is thus *an inapt tool* for structuring and systematizing the world to produce knowledge about it. That means that theories are *evaluated* with respect to their potential to be instruments of knowledge acquisition. They are judged with respect to their truth, falsehood, verisimilitude, probability, or plausibility just as little as a screwdriver, hammer, or microscope is so judged. A theory is never abandoned because it turns out false, but because it is considered the wrong and incompetent device, while there exists a *better* one to replace it. See also Thomas Kuhn's judgment on this issue on page 508. For a profound analysis of the issue, see (Stegmüller, 1976; Kuhn, 1996).[78]

9.4.6 Theories Fuzzified

The structuralistic metatheory is based on classical set theory to the effect that it is confined to the reconstruction, analysis, and construction of crisp theories. Although it was developed at Stanford University, its creators (Sneed, 1971; Suppes, 1957, 1970b, 2002) did not adapt it to fuzzy set theory, which was developed around the same time just across the San Fransisco Bay at the University of California, Berkeley.[79] For this reason, it requires an overhaul. This desideratum has also been overlooked by the epigones of its creators, e.g., (Stegmüller, 1973a, 1976; Moulines, 1975; Balzer, 1978; Balzer and Moulines,

---

[78] Verisimilitude or truthlikeness is a concept introduced by Karl Popper (1963, 47–52 and 329–335) to compare theories with one another according to the degree of their closeness to truth. It is a complex concept that we will not discuss here. It represents a useless speculation and has not survived the criticism. For example, see (Miller, 1974; Tichy, 1974).

[79] This is surprising because it cannot be supposed that the inventors of the structuralistic metatheory have been ignorant of fuzzy set theory. Although nowhere in their publications do they mention fuzzy set theory, Patrick Suppes as the father of the structuralistic metatheory has been and is acquainted with Lotfi Zadeh, the inventor of fuzzy set theory and fuzzy logic. As Zadeh admits, "Patrick Suppes is a good friend. Unlike many logicians, he has never been hostile to fuzzy logic" (Lotfi Zadeh, personal communication on 20 November, 2009).

1996; Westmeyer, 1989, 1992). To render the metatheory applicable to real-world scientific theories, it needs to be fuzzified because like everything else in science, scientific theories are vague entities and implicitly or explicitly fuzzy. According to Zadeh's Principle of Fuzzifiability mentioned on page 1041 ("Any crisp theory can be fuzzified by replacing the concept of a set in that theory by the concept of a fuzzy set"), their explicit fuzzification may be carried out in the following two ways:

▶ Fuzzy set-theoretical predicates: Type 1
▶ Fuzzy set-theoretical predicates: Type 2.

Fuzzy set-theoretical predicates: Type 1

The first option is the introduction of a set-theoretical predicate itself as a fuzzy predicate instead of a crisp one. It may be expressed, for instance, as "ξ is a fuzzy S" instead of "ξ is an S". This may be illustrated by replacing the crisp set-theoretical predicate "ξ is a hyperpyrexia system", introduced in Definition 140 on page 435, with the new, fuzzy set-theoretical predicate "ξ is a fuzzy hyperpyrexia system" by fuzzifying the set of those human beings who have hyperpyrexia:

Definition 141 (Fuzzy hyperpyrexia system: FHS). *ξ is a fuzzy hyper-pyrexia system iff there are Ω, f, and μ_{FHS} such that:*

1. *$\xi = \langle \Omega, f, \mu_{FHS} \rangle$,*
2. *Ω is a non-empty set of human beings,*
3. *f, i.e. 'fever', is a function from Ω to $\mathbb{R}^{+}$,*
4. *μ_{FHS} is a function from Ω to $[0, 1]$ referred to as degree of hyperpyrexia,*

$$
5. \ \mu_{FHS}(x) = \begin{cases} 0 & \text{if } f(x) \leq 39 \ °C & \text{for all } x \in \Omega, \\ f(x) - 39 & \text{if } 39 < f(x) < 40 \ °C & \text{for all } x \in \Omega, \\ 1 & \text{if } f(x) \geq 40 \ °C & \text{for all } x \in \Omega. \end{cases}
$$

Suppose, for example, that Amy, Beth, and Carla have contracted Mexican swine flu and have a very high body temperature. Then the structure $\langle \{Amy, Beth, Carla\}, g, \mu_{FHS} \rangle$ is a fuzzy hyperpyrexia system if $g(Amy) = 39.4 \ °C$, $g(Beth) = 39.9 \ °C$, and $g(Carla) = 42 \ °C$. Their membership degrees in the set of hyperpyrexia patients, i.e., the degrees of their hyperpyrexia, are $\mu_{FHS}(Amy) = 0.4$; $\mu_{FHS}(Beth) = 0.9$; and $\mu_{FHS}(Carla) = 1$. This example shows that the set of patients suffering from hyperpyrexia has been fuzzified by the new, fuzzy set-theoretical predicate to the effect that Amy, Beth, Carla, and other human beings are members thereof to different extents.

Fuzzy set-theoretical predicates: Type 2

The second option is this: In addition to fuzzifying the set-theoretical predicate itself as above, any other component of the theory appearing in the structure

$\langle \Omega, R_1, \ldots, R_n \rangle$ that defines the predicate, may also be fuzzified. For example, the fever function f in the structure $\langle \Omega, f, \mu_{FHS} \rangle$ above may be constructed as a fuzzy function by introducing it as an approximate fever degree, e.g., as a fuzzy number, fuzzy interval, or as a linguistic variable "Body_Temperature" with a linguistic term set such as {very low, low, normal, slightly high, fairly high, extremely high}. See page 1019.

Fuzzifications of both types will impact the application and applicability of theories as well as the nature of the knowledge produced by using them. This is true because fuzzification will change the conception of models; potential models; partial, potential models; and the core and intended applications of a theory, on the one hand; and the epistemological relationships between empirical claims of the theory and the 'real world', on the other, e.g., support, confirmation, falsification, etc. For instance, if our set-theoretical predicate is a fuzzy set-theoretical predicate as introduced in Definition 141 above, the set $\mathcal{M}(T)$ of models for the corresponding theory T will also be a fuzzy set. An entity will be a member of $\mathcal{M}(T)$, i.e., a model for the theory, only to a particular extent between 0 and 1. A fuzzy set-theoretically formulated theory is more tolerant and flexible than a crisp one because both the set of its intended applications and the set of its models are fuzzy to the effect that it is more compatible with the 'real world' than a crisp theory.

The above considerations suggest that the entities a theory is concerned with, be construed as vague entities. And that means in medicine that the intended applications of a medical theory, e.g., the theory of autoimmune diseases, are vague objects, vague sets, and vague relations. Since almost all physiologic and pathologic objects, states, and processes in medicine are vague, the reconstruction of medical theories as fuzzy theories seems to be more realistic than the crisp, non-statement view suggests. Such reconstructions are interesting desiderata for research in medical epistemology in the years ahead. For similar analyses and assessments, see (Seising, 2007b–c, 2009).

9.5 Summary

Knowledge is a subjective state of the knower. It may be artificially detached from the knower by means of transforming it into intersubjectively available sentences. In this way it becomes amenable to scientific and metascientific epistemological analyses. We examined the syntax of medical knowledge and distinguished between problematic sentences, first-order sentences, modal sentences, probabilistic sentences, and fuzzy sentences to show that, for the most part, medical knowledge is represented by fuzzy sentences. The impact of the syntax of medical knowledge on its semantics was demonstrated by analyzing the logical structure of medical hypotheses and their possible truth values. We pointed out that the term "theory" plays an important role in medicine and medical epistemology. To inquire into the nature of medical theories and their epistemology, we concerned ourselves with the concept of theory and discussed (i) the traditional view that has come to be termed the "statement view"; (ii) the so-called semantic view; and (iii) a recent view in the general philosophy of science referred to as the "non-statement view" of theories or "structuralism". We briefly introduced the latter, which is a well-elaborated metatheory. In light of this metatheory we provided some elementary steps in the direction of a structuralistic analysis of medical theories and theory-nets. The structuralism discussed here should not be confused with (a) the Swiss and French structuralism in linguistics and the humanities, and (b) structuralism in mathematics because the three structuralisms are different things.

Types of Medical Knowledge

10.0 Introduction

The axiomatization of theories by set-theoretical predicates in the preceding chapter demonstrated that a theory cannot be, and is not, knowledge. Like a building or machine, a scientific theory T is a relational structure. But unlike buildings and machines, it is a *conceptual structure* consisting of a core, $\mathcal{K}(T)$, and intended applications, $\mathcal{I}(T)$. Thus, it is a pair of the form $\langle \mathcal{K}(T), \mathcal{I}(T) \rangle$. As a structure, a theory $\langle \mathcal{K}(T), \mathcal{I}(T) \rangle$ does not consist of, and does not make, statements. It is created by some individuals or groups in a particular period of history, grows over time in that generations of scientists modify and develop its core and intended applications, and dies in a later period when it is displaced by other, or better, conceptual structures. It then languishes in obsolete books, stored in the cellars of libraries, and becomes a mere subject of historical studies like cosmologists study the graveyard of deceased stars and galaxies that they call 'the universe'.

During its lifetime, a theory is *used* as a conceptual tool to acquire knowledge. Suppose the theory used is the theory of the Archimedean static, the theory of toxic hyperpyrexia, or any other theory. The *products* of applying such a theory as a tool to acquire knowledge are statements of the form "Elroy Fox has toxic hyperpyrexia" or "this seesaw is an Archimedean static". A statement of this form is of course *knowledge*. As we have seen earlier, it says that a particular entity x is an element of the application set of the theory's core, i.e., $x \in \mathbb{A}\big(\mathcal{K}(T)\big)$.

Much medical knowledge – experimental and clinical knowledge, for instance – is acquired using medical theories. But not all medical knowledge is arrived at in this way. A considerable amount of it emerges from mere description of phenomena without using any background theory. First of all, experimental and clinical knowledge is produced by theories in medicine. To analyze these interesting issues in later chapters, a classification of medical knowledge types is undertaken in the current chapter. Our analysis divides into the following eight parts:

K. Sadegh-Zadeh, *Handbook of Analytic Philosophy of Medicine*,
Philosophy and Medicine 113, DOI 10.1007/978-94-007-2260-6_10,
© Springer Science+Business Media B.V. 2012

10.1 Shallow and Deep Medical Knowledge

Information technology in general and medical information technology in particular are extremely productive of novel epistemological terms. Not all of these terms are meaningful, however. For instance, in medical expert systems research it has become customary to distinguish between shallow and deep expert systems. A shallow expert system is defined as one which uses "shallow medical knowledge", and a deep expert system is defined as one which uses "deep medical knowledge". Deep systems are preferred to shallow systems because it is said that the latter ones do not allow for diagnostic and therapeutic reasoning (Chandrasekaran et al. 1989; Keravnou and Washbrook, 1989; Washbrook and Keravnou, 1992).

"Shallow knowledge" means simply non-causal knowledge, whereas "deep knowledge" refers to causal knowledge. Due to the evaluative connotations of the phrases "shallow" and "deep", these terms insinuate that non-causal knowledge is superficial and may not be good enough. That is by no means true. The terms "causal" and "non-causal" should, therefore, be preferred, and the new dichotomy *shallow* versus *deep* knowledge should be avoided.

In clinical medicine, many statements about the relationships between patient data such as symptoms, signs, and findings, on the one hand; and diseases, on the other, are not causal ones. An example is the statement "if a patient coughs and has a fever, then she has bronchitis". This conditional does not report any causal connection between the phenomena referred to in its antecedent and consequent. Nevertheless, it is diagnostically highly valuable. Although causal knowledge may in many cases enable more efficient decisions, diagnosis as well as therapy do not always require causal knowledge about the present state of the patient. Causal medical knowledge will be discussed in Section 10.3 below.

10.2 Classificatory Knowledge

A considerable amount of medical knowledge is classificatory knowledge and informs us either about the belonging of *individual* objects to any classes and relations such as "Elroy Fox is ill"; or about the taxonomy of classes, i.e., belonging of classes to other classes and relations such as, for example, melanoma is a skin disease; hyperglycemia is a symptom of diabetes mellitus; and so on (see page 60).

To adequately understand their meaning, we must clearly differentiate between class membership or elementhood, $\in$, on the one hand; and subsethood $\subseteq$ or $\subset$, on the other. Both are expressed by the ambiguous natural language predicate "is" or "is_a". While "Elroy Fox is ill" says that 'Elroy Fox $\in$ the class of ill people', "melanoma is a skin disease" means that the class of those people who have melonoma is a subcalss of those who have a skin disease, i.e., melanoma patients $\subset$ skin disease patients. Like the membership predicate "$\in$" used in the first example, a predicate such as "has" in a statement like "Elroy Fox has myocardial infarction" also represents the predicate "is_a", i.e., Elroy Fox *is_a* member of the class of those who are suffering from myocardial infarction: Elroy Fox $\in$ the class of people suffering from myocardial infarction (see also Section 5.4.2 on page 105).

The examples above may also be interpreted and formalized in another fashion. For instance, "melanoma is a skin disease" may be understood as a statement about the membership of melanoma as an *abstract individual*, M, in the larger class of skin diseases, $\{A, B, \ldots, M, \ldots\}$, that consists of many such abstract individuals such that $M \in \{A, B, \ldots, M, \ldots\}$, i.e., melanoma $\in$ the class of skin diseases. The interpretation depends both on the context and the goal. Depending on the ontological level one chooses, melanoma may appear as an individual object or as a class. This example shows that sometimes the decision whether an entity is an individual or a class is arbitrary (see also pages 58 and 696).

10.3 Causal Knowledge

What causality is and what causal statements look like, we studied in Section 6.5. But it is not only medical-etiologic knowledge about the genesis of maladies that consists of causal statements. Even simple statements in biomedical disciplines such as physiology and biochemistry about the functioning of organs, cells, or molecules often deal with causal relationships. For example, a chemical formula representing a chemical reaction such as $H_2 + O \rightarrow H_2O$ is a causal statement. It says that "the joining of two hydrogen atoms and one oxygen atom causes the emergence of one water molecule". We saw in Section 6.5 that causal statements may be deterministic or probabilistic. The latter predominate in medicine.

There are two types of causal statements, *non-interventional* and *interventional*. (i) Non-interventional causal statements report about causal relationships that are independent of interventions by the observer. In such a case, the researcher simply observes the processes which she studies. But she does not actively manipulate the events constituting them. For example, she examines whether babies born to mothers who drink excessively during pregnancy, or have diabetes mellitus, are at a high risk of developing any disorders. If the answer is Yes, then by employing our probabilistic theory of etiology discussed in Section 6.5, the causal assertion can be made that "excessive use of alcohol, or diabetes mellitus, during pregnancy is positively causally relevant to pathological disorders X, Y, Z". This causal statement is non-interventional because the allegedly causal factors, i.e., "excessive drinking during pregnancy" and "diabetes during pregnancy", have not been produced or manipulated by the researcher. By contrast, (ii) interventions are conducted in some other cases when a researcher is interested to know what effect a particular action has when it is performed in a particular situation, i.e., when *the action is used as a cause to bring about an effect*. A statement reporting about the effect of such interventions is an interventional-causal statement. An example is the statement "if a patient has angina pectoris and at least one of her coronary arteries is narrowed and *coronary artery by-pass surgery is performed,* then her suffering will be relieved". Formally generalized, that means the following:

If condition C obtains and action A is performed, then result R occurs.

That is:

$$C \,\&\, A \to R \tag{111}$$

such that:

- C is some elementary or compound condition $C_1 \cap \ldots \cap C_k$ with $k \geq 1$ like in the patient above who "has angina pectoris $\wedge$ at least one of her coronary arteries is narrowed";
- A is some elementary or compound action $A_1 \cap \ldots \cap A_m$ with $m \geq 1$. In the example above, coronary artery by-pass surgery is the single action A performed;
- R is some elementary or compound result $R_1 \cap \ldots \cap R_n$ with $n \geq 1$. In the example above, the patient's relief is the single result R.

The sentence (111) above is, according to Exportation and Importation Rules of deduction in Table 36 on page 895, equivalent to the following conditional:

$$C \to (A \to R)$$

which states: Given condition C, if action A is performed, then result R occurs. This simple example demonstrates that an interventional-causal statement is an assertion about *human agency*, i.e., about the causal consequence of a human action, A, performed in a particular situation C. Its subject is not an agent-independent, 'objective', process in a human-independent world. While the above statement is deterministic, the causal relationship between an action and its effect may also be probabilistic and assume the following form:

$$p(R \,|\, C \cap A) = r.$$

For instance, "the probability of relief on the condition that a patient has angina pectoris and takes sublingual nitroglycerin tablet, is 0.6". We shall consider additional examples in the next section.

10.4 Experimental Knowledge

Although medicine is not exclusively an empirical science, it belongs to empirical sciences in that it acquires knowledge through experience and making observations, and applies its theories and knowledge to the experiential world, e.g., patients, cells, micro-organisms, and other entities. This feature of being an experiential science includes, among other things, conducting genuine experiments. Today experimentation represents the main avenue to knowledge in all empirical disciplines. Therefore, no medical epistemology can be taken seriously if it does not pay attention to the nature and significance of medical experimentation. In the present section, we will concern ourselves only briefly with this issue. But we shall examine it thoroughly in Chapter 12 and Section 21.7.1.

Scientific experimentation emerged after the so-called Scientific Revolution in the sixteenth and seventeenth centuries to free science from the authority of tradition. A prominent example of this authoritative tradition is the intellectual dependence on, and reference to, Aristotle by way of Scholasticism and speculation. The following anecdote illustrates the point:

"During the thirteenth century, professors at the University of Paris decided to find out whether oil would congeal if left outdoors on a cold night. They launched a research project to investigate this question. To them, research meant searching through the works of Aristotle. After much effort, they found that nothing Aristotle had written answered their question, so they declared the question unanswerable" (Starbuck, 2006, 1).

One of the most original and influential leaders of the revolution was Francis Bacon (1561–1626). In his philosophical writings, he advocated *observation, experimentation,* and *induction* as the only acceptable methods of scientific inquiry. For the notion of induction, see Section 29.2 on page 984.[80]

The first disciplines to have followed Bacon's doctrine were physics and chemistry, which together would later constitute what would be termed natural sciences. Biology and medicine joined the ranks of the natural sciences in the late eighteenth and early nineteenth centuries. A fundamental misunderstanding about the nature of experimentation also emerged in that early period, and still persists today. An experiment is, it says, (i) a question that scientists put to the world to examine phenomena whose occurrence is inde-

---

[80] Lord Francis Bacon, born in London to a prominent and well-connected family and known as the Baron of Verulam, was a lawyer, statesman, historian, intellectual reformer, essayist, and philosopher. In his philosophical treatise *Novum Organum,* published in 1620 as part 2 of his major work *Instauratio Magna,* he championed a new direction of thought that would later be termed empiricism or British *empiricism.* In this work he introduced the method of induction to replace the Aristotelean deductive syllogisms and to guide us in acquiring scientific knowledge. According to him, we must in addition intervene in nature and manipulate it by means of experimental control (Verulam, 1893).

pendent of the experimenter, e.g., blood coagulation, neurotransmitter secretion in the brain, base sequences of DNA and RNA, seizures, etc. The aim is (ii) to obtain *true and objective knowledge* about them. Accordingly, experimentation has ascended to be the preeminent method of testing hypotheses and theories in order to differentiate between true and objective ones, on the one hand; and false and subjective ones, on the other. However, we shall have to examine this received view critically.

A medical experimenter does not test ready-made hypotheses or theories. She does not differentiate between true and false ones either. Rather, she only intervenes in experimental conditions and elicits experimental data to investigate the causal relevance that human intervention has to the genesis of these data. Roughly, a token experiment consists of a setup comprising:

- some elementary or compound initial condition $C \equiv C_1 \cap \ldots \cap C_k$ with $k \geq 1$, prepared by the experimenter. For instance, the experimenter uses a dog and makes sure that the animal is free of diabetes mellitus;
- some elementary or compound action $A \equiv A_1 \cap \ldots \cap A_m$ with $m \geq 1$, to which that condition C is subjected. For example, the experimenter removes the pancreas of the dog;
- some elementary or compound data $D \equiv D_1 \cap \ldots \cap D_n$ with $n \geq 1$, obtained as the supposed effect of action A. For instance, the experimenter measures the blood sugar concentration of the dog and observes hyperglycemia. She also measures the urine sugar concentration and observes glucosuria.

After conducting a series of such token experiments and on the basis of some available knowledge from disciplines such as anatomy, physiology, and others, the researcher interprets the experimental data as diabetes mellitus. Thus, an item of knowledge that a series of token experiments of the same type provides, may be described either (a) by a conditional statement of the form:

1. If condition C obtains and action A is performed, then D occurs,

that is $C \& A \rightarrow D$, when the relationship between the experimental setup $C \& A$ and data D is deterministic; or (b) by a probabilistic statement of the following type, otherwise:

2. $p(D \mid C \cap A) = r$

where $0 \leq r \leq 1$. Examples are:

- If a dog with no diabetes mellitus gets its pancreas removed, then it develops hyperglycemia and glucosuria (Frederick Banting und Charles Best, 1921; see Bliss, 2007);
- The probability that in a rat with epileptic convulsions the injection of Gamma Amino Butyric Acid (GABA) decreases the frequency of its convulsions, is 0.8.

The examples above are items of experimental knowledge. Since they report about the effects of human actions, they constitute *interventional-causal knowledge* as discussed in the preceding section. They demonstrate that, for the following two reasons and in contrast to the common doctrine, a medical experiment does not supply (i) true and objective knowledge about phenomena, which supposedly (ii) occur naturally and independently of the experimenter:

First, the first example is an unbounded universal hypothesis and thus not verifiable. It has no determinate truth value. The second example is an unbounded probabilistic hypothesis and thus neither verifiable nor falsifiable. It is incapable of possessing a truth value at all (see Section 9.3 on page 395).

Second, an experimenter is not a spectator passively observing the domain of her investigation, say *nature,* and then reporting what she has seen. Rather, she is a manipulator of the observed. By virtue of a more or less complex action $A = A_1 \cap \ldots \cap A_m$, she intervenes in the initial conditions $C = C_1 \cap \ldots \cap C_k$ of the experiment and produces a set $D = D_1 \cap \ldots \cap D_n$ of data such as blood sugar measurements, diagrams, and blood counts. In the light of antecedently available systems of knowledge originating from different disciplines, she then interprets these data to put forward assertions about causal relationships between events or processes in the artificial experimental arrangement. However, a central constituent of the experimental arrangement is the experimenter herself. She designs the experiment in a particular fashion and intervenes in its initial conditions according to a particular algorithm to study what will occur when particular actions are performed. Thus, an experiment is essentially based on, and includes, human intervention to the effect that its yield is interventional-causal knowledge about the causal consequences of that very intervention. Some philosophers of science have used this fact as a reason to consider science a *praxis* and to view scientific research as the study of *human agency* (Dingler, 1928; Holzkamp, 1968).

Most experimenters are not aware of their agency and overlook or hide the active role they play in the experimental knowledge that they attain. Having eliminated themselves from the scene, they present that knowledge "objectively" without mentioning their operational part. For example, the two experimental statements given above are presented in the literature thus:

- If in a dog with no diabetes mellitus the pancreas dies, then it develops hyperglycemia and glucosuria;
- The probability that in a rat with epileptic convulsions Gamma Amino Butyric Acid (GABA) decreases the frequency of its convulsions, is 0.8.

Apparently, then, experimental knowledge reported by the experimental scientists is not quite correct. The experimenters prune the outcome of their research and present something artificially reduced to pure, non-interventional knowledge, whereas it is in fact interventional knowledge concerned with the consequences of human action. We shall consider these issues further in Chapter 12 and Section 21.7.1.

10.5 Theoretical Knowledge

It has become customary to contrast *theoretical* knowledge with *practical* knowledge. However, this dichotomy is problematic because both italicized terms are highly ambiguous. We must therefore make them precise first.

To begin, "theoretical knowledge" does not necessarily refer to knowledge that is based on theories or contains theories and theoretical terms. And "practical knowledge" does not necessarily refer to knowledge that is not based on theories or that does not contain theories and theoretical terms. Rather, we define an item of knowledge to be (i) a *theoretical* one if and only if it asserts what was, is, or will be the case, and (ii) a *practical* one if and only if it says something about what to do. Theoretical knowledge is *declarative* knowledge; practical knowledge is *procedural* knowledge. Another criterion of distinction is that theoretical knowledge is justified by what is called *theoretical reasoning*, i.e., any type of logic, whereas practical knowledge is justified by what is called *practical reasoning*. These two types of reasoning or rationality will be discussed in Section 22.3 on page 799. For example, our knowledge about the nature and genesis of AIDS is theoretical knowledge, while our knowledge about how to diagnose AIDS and treat AIDS patients, is practical knowledge. See next section.

Theoretical knowledge is what we termed propositional knowledge, or *know-that*, on page 15. It describes some object or relation, for example,

- a. Elroy Fox has diabetes,
- b. AIDS is caused by HIV,
- c. Man is an offspring of the apes,
- d. Every Romance language is a daughter language of Latin,
- e. Streptomycin inhibits the growth of strains of tubercle bacilli.

As descriptive information about its subject, theoretical knowledge enables explanations and predictions, e.g., diagnoses and prognoses. Theoretical-medical knowledge begins first of all in the biomedical sciences, nosology, and pathology. For instance, anatomy, physiology, biochemistry, and medical physics provide theoretical knowledge about the body, its parts and their functions, their chemistry, and their physics.

Linguistically, theoretical knowledge consists of declarative sentences, or more accurately, *constatives*. It may therefore also be called descriptive, declarative, or constative knowledge. These synonymous characterizations of theoretical knowledge are highly significant epistemologically, and enable us to discriminate between types of sciences and to identify the logics they require in their management. See Sections 17.3 and 22.1.4.

10.6 Practical Knowledge

Practical knowledge abounds in medicine. As we shall observe later on in Section 21.5, this is why medicine must be viewed not as a natural or applied science, but as a practical science. This may easily be shown by inspecting the type of knowledge medicine produces, i.e., practical knowledge. We must therefore clarify what practical knowledge is. To begin with, recall that the term "practical" is an adjective of the term "practice". As pointed out on page 109, the term "practice" derives from the Greek word $\pi\rho\alpha\xi\iota\varsigma$ (praxis) for "doing", "acting", and "action". Hence, practical knowledge must be something concerned with doing, acting, and action. This will be explicated in what follows.

Practical knowledge is a subtype of know-how, specifically a subtype of what is called procedural knowledge in the information sciences. An item of procedural knowledge consists of $n \geq 1$ rules that prescribe *what to do under some particular circumstances in order to achieve a particular goal.* Suppose, for instance, that you want to go from your home to your office. There are five different routes, numbered ROUTE 1 through ROUTE 5, each of which you may take. The fastest one is ROUTE 5. It is a shortcut and consists of the concatenation of the streets A, B, and C. Sometimes, street C is blocked. In this case, you have to drive back and take ROUTE 1, which is much longer than ROUTE 5 and requires much more time. If you want to go to your office and are in a rush, then you may use the following prescriptive algorithm as your procedural knowledge:

a. If you want to go from home to your office and you are in a rush, then call the traffic information hotline and ask whether street C is open. Go to b.
b. If street C is open, then take ROUTE 5 and go to d. Otherwise, go to c.
c. If street C is blocked, then take ROUTE 1 and go to d.
d. End.

Like this example, practical knowledge comprises imperatives and commands: do! go! take!, and the like. Thus, it is always *normative* and never descriptive. It does not describe how people actually act. Rather, it prescribes *how to act in a particular situation to attain a particular goal,* for instance, to diagnose community acquired pneumonia in a patient with fever, cough, dyspnea, etc. In a nutshell, the subject and concern of practical knowledge is goal-directed or *goal-driven practice.*

The core of practical medicine consists of practical knowledge. To analyze this momentous feature of medicine, we must be aware that practical knowledge may be put forward in the following two different forms:

- implicit practical knowledge,
- explicit practical knowledge.

Implicit practical knowledge is syntactically degenerate, and therefore, it does not betray that it is in fact practical knowledge, i.e., something normative. Examples are ubiquitous statements of the type "in such a situation *one analyzes* the patient's blood to see whether she has antibodies against HIV". The descriptive phrase "one analyzes" is mistakable and confusing because it is not the aim of such knowledge to inform the student what people actually do in such a situation – maybe they do something wrong –, but rather to instruct her: In such a situation, *analyze* the patient's blood to see whether she has antibodies against HIV!

In what follows, we shall show that in medical literature *practical knowledge* is communicated primarily as implicit practical knowledge, and shall make it *explicit* to inquire into the epistemological, moral, metaphysical, and practical consequenes of the fact that *clinical knowledge is practical knowledge*. It is usually put forward in very complex textual structures and is therefore not easily discernible as such knowledge. These 'practical' texts may be reconstructed as nested sentences whose deep structure reveals that they are by no means constatives, but represent conditional imperatives, commands, and commitments of the form:

Circumstances of the type C commit you to do A when you want to attain goal G,

or equivalently:

Under circumstances C, if you want to attain goal G, then do A.

This may be convenietly formalized by the sentence:

$C \rightarrow (G \rightarrow do\ A)$

that according to Exportation and Importation Rules of deduction in Table 36 on page 895 is equivalent to:

$$C \wedge G \rightarrow do\ A. \tag{112}$$

Consider as a simple example the following incomplete clinical conditional:

If a patient has fever, cough, and dyspnea, and you want to know whether ...

This incomplete sentence can, after the phrase "whether", be continued in numerous different ways which point to completely different directions and lead to differnt goals such as, for instance:

... she has disease D_1, then do A_1
... she has disease D_2, then do A_2
... she has disease D_3, then do A_3

and so on. Here, $D_1, D_2, D_3, \ldots$ are different diseases that come into consideration in the present patient; and $A_1, A_2, A_3, \ldots$ are distinct, more or less complex diagnostic actions that can be performed to diagnose those diseases, respectively. We will exemplify only one of the above-mentioned possible clinical situations:

If a patient has fever, cough, and dyspnea, AND $\qquad(113)$

- you want to know whether she has community acquired pneumonia,
- then
    a. examine her chest and search for altered breath sounds and rales, and
    b. conduct chest radiography and search for opaque areas in both lungs.

Sentence (113) has the structure of sentence (112) above and is, according to Exportation and Importation Rules of deduction in Table 36 on page 895, equivalent to the following conditional:

If a patient has fever, cough, and dyspnea, THEN (114)

- if you want to know whether she has community acquired pneumonia,
- then
    a. examine her chest and search for altered breath sounds and rales, and
    b. conduct chest radiography and search for opaque areas in both lungs.

The nested sentence (114) will now be formalized to uncover its micro-logical structure. To this end, the following shorthands will be used:

α_1 ≡ the patient has fever,
α_2 ≡ the patient has cough,
α_3 ≡ the patient has dyspnea,
β ≡ you want to know whether the patient has community acquired pneumonia,
γ_1 ≡ the patient's chest is examined to search for altered breath sounds,
γ_2 ≡ the patient's chest is examined to search for rales,
γ_3 ≡ chest radiography is conducted to search for opaque areas in both lungs.

A closer look at the above nested sentence (114) shows that it is a *conditional imperative* of the following form:

$$\text{If } \alpha_1 \wedge \alpha_2 \wedge \alpha_3, \text{ then } \left(\text{if } \beta, \text{ then do } (\gamma_1 \wedge \gamma_2 \wedge \gamma_3)\right). \tag{115}$$

An imperative is a do-sentence of the form "do action such and such!". The term "conditional imperative" means that the imperative has a precondition, i.e., it has the structure of the conditional:

If X, then do A

with X being the precondition. This precondition is in the present example the antecedent $\alpha_1 \wedge \alpha_2 \wedge \alpha_3 \wedge \beta$ of the conditional:

$$\text{If } \alpha_1 \wedge \alpha_2 \wedge \alpha_3 \wedge \beta, \text{ then do } (\gamma_1 \wedge \gamma_2 \wedge \gamma_3)$$

that is equivalent to the conditional imperative (115) above. The precondition may of course consist of more than only 4 elements as in the present case. Likewise, the terminal imperative may include more than only 3 actions to be performed. Thus, a conditional imperative has in general the following structure:

$$\text{If } \alpha_1 \wedge \ldots \wedge \alpha_k \text{ then } \big(\text{if } \beta_1 \wedge \ldots \wedge \beta_m, \text{ then do } (\gamma_1 \wedge \ldots \wedge \gamma_n)\big)$$

with $k, m, n \geq 1$. Still more generally, the imperative in the terminal consequent may include many complex *alternative* actions of the form:

$$(\gamma_1 \wedge \ldots \wedge \gamma_n)_1 \vee \ldots \vee (\delta_1 \wedge \ldots \wedge \delta_p)_q$$

with $n, p, q \geq 1$ among which the physician is allowed to choose. An example is:

(a resting ECG is taken and echocardiography is performed) or
(an exercise ECG is taken and a 24 hour ECG is recorded) or
(a diagnostic electrophysiology study of the heart is performed).

Thus, we obtain the following, general, conditional imperative:

$$\text{If } \alpha_1 \wedge \ldots \wedge \alpha_k \text{ then } \Big(\text{if } \beta_1 \wedge \ldots \wedge \beta_m, \text{ then} \tag{116}$$
$$\text{do } \big((\gamma_1 \wedge \ldots \wedge \gamma_n)_1 \vee \ldots \vee (\delta_1 \wedge \ldots \wedge \delta_p)_q\big)\Big)$$

with $k, m, n, p, q \geq 1$. Sentence (116) represents the basic structure of sentences expressing *practical knowledge*. In medicine, the imperative is expressed, implicitly, in terms of a *conditional obligation* in which "do" is represented by the much stronger predicate "you should" (for the notion of "conditional obligation", see Section 27.2.4 on page 935):

$$\text{If } \alpha_1 \wedge \ldots \wedge \alpha_k \text{ then } \Big(\text{if } \beta_1 \wedge \ldots \wedge \beta_m, \text{ then} \tag{117}$$
$$\text{you\_should } \big((\gamma_1 \wedge \ldots \wedge \gamma_n)_1 \vee \ldots \vee (\delta_1 \wedge \ldots \wedge \delta_p)_q\big)\Big).$$

That is:

$$\alpha_1 \wedge \ldots \wedge \alpha_k \rightarrow \Big(\beta_1 \wedge \ldots \wedge \beta_m \rightarrow \tag{118}$$
$$OB\big((\gamma_1 \wedge \ldots \wedge \gamma_n)_1 \vee \ldots \vee (\delta_1 \wedge \ldots \wedge \delta_p)_q\big)\Big).$$

Here the predicate *"OB"* stands for "you_should" and represents the deontic obligation operator *it_is_obligatory_that* discussed in Section 27.2. It applies to the whole disjunction following the operator OB in sentence (118). The disjunction means that at least one of its members indicating a simple or complex action has to be performed. A simple example is:

> If a patient has episodes of severe tachycardia and the episodes have an abrupt onset and termination, then (119)
> - if you want to know whether she has a Wolff-Parkinson-White (WPW) syndrome,
> - then it_is_obligatory_that:
>   a. a resting ECG is taken and echocardiography is conducted or
>   b. an exercise ECG is taken and a 24 hour ECG is recorded or
>   c. a diagnostic electrophysiology study of the heart is conducted.

This *conditional clinical obligation* demonstrates a simplified item of highly complex diagnostic knowledge on how to diagnose a particular disease, i.e., WPW syndrome in the present example. Its terminal consequent, $OB\big((\gamma_1 \wedge \ldots \wedge \gamma_n)_1 \vee \ldots \vee (\delta_1 \wedge \ldots \wedge \delta_p)_q\big)$, is an obligation sentence, and thus a command that may also be represented by using a command term such as "do action such and such!". Obviously, then, medical-diagnostic knowledge does not tell us 'what is the case' or 'what physicians usually do', but how to act under certain circumstances. Therefore, it is not true or false. It enables us to *know how* to proceed and is thus normative, practical rather than theoretical, i.e., descriptive and declarative, knowledge. *Conditional obligations* as the units of this practical knowledge are exactly the clinical indication and contra-indication rules we were concerned with in Sections 8.2.3–8.2.4 (pp. 308–316).

Note that we have overly simplified the issue. In real-world medical knowledge, things are much more complicated. When introducing our framework for differential indication structures, we analyzed the question of how the application of practical knowledge may be tackled logically. We shall give further thought to issues of practical-medical knowledge in Chapters 15 and 21.

10.7 Clinical Knowledge

What is usually called *medical knowledge* may be unsharply partitioned into clinical and non-clinical knowledge. Non-clinical knowledge consists of pre-clinical , or biomedical, knowledge. It is not concerned with clinical subjects such as nosology, disease, diagnosis, treatment, and other clinical aspects and issues. It deals with 'normal' anatomy, physiology, physics, and chemistry of the human organism and some animal species such as mice, rats, cats, and dogs that serve as subjects of biomedical experimentation. The usual label for the production of this type of knowledge in medicine is "animal experimentation". Most of what is erroneously called "medical knowledge", stems from such animal experimentation. Therefore, it belongs in fact to *zoology* and not to medicine.

Medicine proper is clinical medicine comprising clinical research and clinical practice. It produces and uses clinical knowledge. Clinical knowledge may either be *non-practical,* i.e., theoretical knowledge, or *practical* knowledge. Non-practical clinical knowledge is concerned with theoretical aspects of human maladies, i.e., pathology and nosology. It consists of many subtypes, e.g., (i) pathophysiological knowledge on the pathological behavior of cells, tissues, organs, organ systems, and the organism; and (ii) phenomenological knowledge on subjective illness and on symptoms and signs of maladies, e.g., "symptoms of pneumonia are fever, cough, and dyspnea". The main type of clinical knowledge, however, is *practical-clinical knowledge.* It belongs to the category of practical knowledge that we analyzed in the preceding section.

In the preceding section we exemplified practical-clinical knowledge by way of a simple sentence. The practical knowledge conveyed by such a sentence is opaquely communicated in medical literature because it is typically divided into parts, which are then presented in different sections of more or less complex medical texts. And though, as we have seen, practical knowledge is not descriptive knowledge, it is presented as if it were. On page 451, we labeled this syntactically degenerate type of practical knowledge as implicit practical knowledge. Accordingly, it is difficult to recognize at first glance that the deep structure of practical-clinical knowledge consists of imperatives and commitments, which can in turn be reconstructed as conditional obligations. Consider, for example, a clinical textbook on internal medicine. There we shall find that a chapter on a particular disease or disease group, e.g., community acquired pneumonia, is composed of several sub-chapters each of which is devoted to a special aspect, for example, nosology, diagnosis, or treatment of the disease in the following fashion:

- Chapter on nosology: Symptoms of community acquired pneumonia are cough with or without sputum, acute or subacute onset of fever, dyspnea, ... etc.
- Chapter on diagnosis: Community acquired pneumonia is diagnosed by chest examination, chest radiography, thoracentesis with pleural fluid analysis, ... etc. In chest examination, altered breath sounds and rales are heared. Chest radiography shows that ... etc.
- Chapter on treatment: Antibiotic options for patients with community acquired pneumonia include the following: (1) clarithromycin, 500 mg orally twice a day, (2), ... etc.

The diagnosis chapter maintains that the disease "is diagnosed by chest examination, ... etc.". Pseudo-descriptive formulations of this type are usual in medical textbooks. However, they must not be mistaken for reports about how physicians actually diagnose the disease in their practice. Such reports would be irrelevant simply because the physicians' actual conduct might be a poor example to follow. Rather, they *recommend* that certain measures be taken in order to test a diagnostic hypothesis, e.g., the hypothesis that the patient may have community acquired pneumonia. That is, the artificially separated sections of a chapter in a textbook on the nosology and diagnosis of the disease in fact comprise disintegrated parts of a conditional command of the following form:

> If a patient has a cough with or without sputum, has acute or subacute fever, and has dyspnea, then
>
> - if you want to know whether she has community acquired pneumonia,
> - then *you should*:
>   a. examine her chest and search for altered breath sounds and rales, and
>   b. conduct chest radiography and search for opaque areas in both lungs.

Treatment of the disease is also based on a command sentence, which is similarly divided over different sections of a chapter on the disease. It may be of the following type:

> If a patient has a cough with or without sputum, has acute or subacute fever, and has dyspnea, then
>
> - if she has community acquired pneumonia, then
> - *you should* choose a treatment from among the following options:
>   a. clarithromycin, 500 mg orally twice a day,
>   b. etc.

In the philosophy of medicine, there is an enduring debate on the 'nature of medicine'. Specifically, it is asked whether medicine is a science or an art. We shall see in Chapters 15 and 21 that our analysis of the logical structure of clinical knowledge as practical knowledge may effectively contribute to a solution of this problem. Our foregoing studies have demonstrated that clinical knowledge mainly consists of rules for clinical action indication and contra-indication as explicated in Sections 8.2.3–8.2.4 (pp. 308–316).

10.8 Medical Metaknowledge

Metaknowledge is knowledge about knowledge, for instance, "it is not yet certain whether the hypothesis on the causative role of Chlamydophila pneumoniae in the genesis of myocardial infarction is acceptable". Medical meta-knowledge is explicitly available only in artificial knowledge-based systems, i.e., medical expert systems, characterizing their structure and logic. Medical metaknowledge in a field such as cardiology or psychiatry could provide valuable information about the syntax, semantics, and pragmatics of the knowledge and methods in that field, for example, about their structure, quality, and efficiency. It could serve as a guide for application, research, and methodological studies. Here we are doing medical epistemology in pursuit of just such metaknowledge.

10.9 Summary

We distinguished several types of medical knowledge – classificatory, causal, experimental, theoretical, practical, and clinical knowledge – and clearly explicated each type. We saw that the terms "shallow knowledge" and "deep knowledge" have misleading connotations and should therefore be avoided. All of the types of knowledge mentioned above will be of assistance in later chapters when we shall concern ourselves with the so-called nature of medicine.

11

The Semantics and Pragmatics of Medical Knowledge

11.0 Introduction

At least as important as a particular item of medical knowledge itself is to know something about the relationships of that knowledge to the experiential world it is talking about. The reason is that the patients the physician is concerned with are parts of that experiential world. So, when using any knowledge in her practice, e.g., some knowledge on infectious diseases, a morally conscientious doctor will be interested in whether, and in what way, this knowledge relates to the 'world out there'. Does the medical knowledge she employs bear any relevance to the bodies and souls of her patients? Does it enable her to understand the patient's suffering, illness experience, and illness narrative? Will it help her find useful diagnoses and treatments? Are there in fact any indicators of such qualities of medical knowledge? Why not use astrology, Ayurveda, or exorcism instead of the theory of infectious diseases?

A prerequisite for dealing with such questions is the awareness of the relationships between medical knowledge and its referent, i.e., of the semantics of medical knowledge, on the one hand; and of the pragmatic factors beyond this semantics, which influence the role medical knowledge plays in health care, on the other, e.g., social and economic processes. In the present chapter, we shall look at these issues with an eye toward understanding why some particular information is allowed to enter the medical world as knowledge, whereas other information is considered unacceptable or quackery. Is there a clear line of demarcation between medical knowledge and self-deception?

To begin with, we will discuss the issues of truth and justification because, as pointed out in Section 9.1 on page 384, knowledge is traditionally defined as *justified true belief*. These two defining features of knowledge, *truth* and *justifiedness*, are due to the classical conception of knowledge as the representation of some 'reality'. This ancient, representational postulate brings with it that the predominant view on the semantics of medical knowledge is *realism*, i.e., the view that medical knowledge is concerned with and represents 'the real world out there'. We shall therefore need to inquire into the philosophy

K. Sadegh-Zadeh, *Handbook of Analytic Philosophy of Medicine*,
Philosophy and Medicine 113, DOI 10.1007/978-94-007-2260-6_11,
© Springer Science+Business Media B.V. 2012

and medical relevance of this doctrine before we proceed to alternative views. Our discussion thus divides into the following five parts:

11.1 Justified True Belief

If knowledge is required to be *justified true belief,* the question arises how much of a physician's alleged medical knowledge is justified true belief. For instance, consider the patient Elroy Fox who is suffering from angina pectoris and has been diagnosed as having coronary heart disease. His family doctor is going to treat him with a recently developed remedy. She assures the patient that his angina pectoris will be relieved in a few days because this treatment will dissolve the atherosclerotic plaques in his coronary vessels and thereby normalize the supply of blood to the myocardium. "Do you really believe that?", the patient asks the doctor. "I not only believe that", she replies, "I even know that. It is well known in informed groups of angiologists that the novel drug I am prescribing you is capable of dissolving atherosclerotic plaques. This truth has been discovered by experimental research. And there is sufficient cardiologic evidence that justifies my belief. So, *I know that* this treatment is capable of relieving your suffering". Although the patient is skeptical, he complies nonetheless because he is in need of help. We will now inquire into whether his skepticism is reasonable and whether his doctor used the concepts of *truth* and *justification* properly to make a knowledge claim. To this end, we shall briefly discuss these two concepts in turn to examine whether there are justified true beliefs in medicine. Our discussion thus consists of the following three sections:

11.1.1 Truth

According to the traditional view of science, its goal is the pursuit and discovery of the truth about the world and its phenomena. Like their colleagues in other areas of inquiry, medical scientists also share this view. They believe that they uncover such truth when they apply their expert methods of research and analysis in order to acquire evidence through both their senses and artificial devices, and then are able to draw conclusions from what they have observed. The following brief discussion on the concept of truth shows why this traditional view is problematic and in need of revision.

The concept of truth is a constituent part of the foundations of our sciences and culture that we have inherited from Greek antiquity, especially from Aristotle. In this book, especially in Part VIII, we have frequently referred to this heritage as the Aristotelean worldview. For example, see page 874. We have seen that its characteristic feature is bivalence: the two-valued notion of truth consisting of the pair {true, false}, and the two-valuedness of the classical logic used in our sciences. Aristotle defined the bivalent truth thus:

Aristotle's concept of truth: To say that what is is not, or that what is not is, is false; but to say that what is is, and what is not is not, is true (Metaphysics, Book IV, 1011 b 25).

This Aristotelean concept that is still effective in the foundations of our sciences today, can be traced back to Plato. See, for example, his (Cratylus 385 b 2; Sophist 263 b). As usual, the above concept has found proponents as well as opponents in the course of history. Accordingly, there are currently many competing conceptions of truth called "theories of truth" each of which tries to explicate what it means to say that something is true or false. We shall briefly sketch the following main representatives to see whether any of them may be useful in medicine. For detailed analyses and discussions, see (Armour-Garb and Beall, 2005; Kirkham, 1995; Künne, 2003; Lynch MP, 2001; Pitcher, 1964):

- ▶ The correspondence theory of truth
- ▶ The coherence theory of truth
- ▶ The semantic theory of truth
- ▶ The consensus theory of truth
- ▶ The pragmatist theory of truth
- ▶ The deflationary theories of truth.

The correspondence theory of truth

In the Middle Ages, the Aristotelean concept of truth quoted above assumed the following shape, given to it by Thomas Aquinas (1225–1274): "A judgment is said to be true when it conforms to the external reality" (Aquinas, 1994, Q.1, A.1 & 3). The correspondence theory of truth conveys exactly this Thomist version of the Aristotelean conception. It defines truth as correspondence to facts. Truth-bearers are statements, sentences, ideas, judgments, or beliefs. The theory says that a statement, sentence, idea, judgment, or belief is true if and only if it corresponds to a state of affairs that obtains, and false, otherwise. It reflects what almost all scientists mean when they talk about truth, for example, when they say that the theory of AIDS is true. They mean, in the present example, that the theory of AIDS 'corresponds to facts'. Thus, correspondence theory defines truth as a binary relation, termed *correspondence,* between a truth-bearer and a fact: "statement α corresponds to fact X", i.e., corresponds(α, X). However, it does not make the relation explicit and does not betray what the correspondence between a truth-bearer α and a fact X looks like and how it could be demonstrated. Otherwise put, it does not define the predicate "corresponds". For this reason, it must be considered basically incomplete, and therefore, useless. Bertrand Russell and Ludwig Wittgenstein have tried to improve it by their 'logical atomism'. However, they have failed (Russell, 1918; Wittgenstein, 1922; Armstrong, 1997, 2004; O'Connor, 1975).

The coherence theory of truth

According to this theory, a statement is true if it *coheres* with a specified set of other statements. Contrary to correspondence theory, the truth conditions of a statement are not objective features of an independent reality, but other statements. And the truth relation is not correspondence, but coherence. For details, see (Blanshard, 1939; Rescher, 1973).

The coherence theory of truth is also faced with many problems. We will mention only two. First, there is no agreement on the nature of the relation of coherence. Often it is identified with consistency such that a statement is considered true if it is consistent with a specified set of other statements. However, we must take the plurality of logics into account and ask with respect to which system of logic the consistency is to be adjudicated. Second, there is no agreement on how to identify the specified set of statements with which our candidate statement is to cohere. A statement such as "peptic ulcer disease is an infectious disease" may cohere with the Helicobacter theory of peptic ulcer disease, whereas it will not cohere with the psychosomatic theory of this disease group. For example, see (Schüffel and von Uexküll, 1995, 825–838).

The semantic theory of truth

While other theories of truth lack a clear concept of truth, the most precise one is provided by the semantic theory. It originated with the Polish-American logician Alfred Tarski (1933, 1983) (see footnote 162 on page 874). On the one hand, it may be viewed as an exact reconstruction and formal elaboration of the above-mentioned, arcane correspondence theory. On the other hand, it represents a novel approach to truth and therefore contrasts with correspondence theory. The semantics of the classical, first-order predicate logic discussed in Section 26.2.2 on page 873, is based on this theory of truth. It will be presupposed in what follows.

In Tarski's view, truth-bearers are sentences. His primary aim was to define the notion of a "true sentence" in a way that could prevent logical and semantic paradoxes. Consider, for example, the well-known Liar paradox, LP, that is touched in footnote 183 on page 966:

This sentence is false.   (LP)

It is easily checked that the sentence LP above implies a contradiction and is, therefore, classical-logically inconsistent. For it is both true and false at the same time. If it is false, as it states, then it is true. And if it is true, then, as it states, it is false. This result yields a paradoxical biconditional of the form LP $\leftrightarrow \neg$ LP from which any contradiction follows. The presence of a sentence of this form in, or its derivability from, a scientific theory trivializes the theory. By means of the deduction rule *Ex Contradictione Quodlibet* mentioned in Table 36 on page 895, the theory implies, due to its inconsistency, everything, including its own negation.

Tarski observed that detrimental paradoxes of the type above emerge in so-called semantically closed languages, i.e., languages that are not able to distinguish between metalinguistic and object-linguistic levels such that a statement, like LP above, may metalinguistically refer to itself. To prevent paradoxes, such self-references ought to be blocked. That is, terms such as "true" and "false" should be handled as metalinguitsic notions that only by means of a meta-statement can be applied to an object statement, e.g., by the following meta-statement:

The sentence LP is false

to its object-statement LP. By contrast, sentence LP above has declared itself as false. It plays the role of an object statement and of a meta-statement about that object statement at the same time. This semantic self-reference, being the cause of the paradox, was only possible because LP is a natural language sentence, and natural languages are obviously semantically closed. This peculiarity renders them sources of paradoxes par excellence. For this reason, Tarski decided to define the notion of truth not for natural, but for formal languages. The latter ones are sufficiently precise and enable one to strictly differentiate between an object language and metalanguage. His definiendum "is true" was therefore of the binary form "is true in language $\mathcal{L}$" where $\mathcal{L}$ is a specified formal language, for example, the language of the first-order predicate logic studied in Section 26.2.1.

Note that Tarski's two-place notion of truth, 'sentence "α" is true in language $\mathcal{L}$', does not use the dictum 'sentence "α" is true' and thus breaks with the tradition of *absolute* truth. It *relativizes* truth to a particular language $\mathcal{L}$ and does not mean truth simpliciter. It means, for example, true-in-English, true-in-German, true-in-language-$\mathcal{L}_1$, etc. We could, for example, create two artificial languages and interpret the sentence "Blobelines snurgle dwiftly" differently such that it would mean "AIDS is an infectious disease" in one of them, and "AIDS is not an infectious disease" in the other. The sentence has different truth values in the two languages without being inconsistent because "sentence 'α' is true in language A" does not contradict "sentence 'α' is false in language B".

If we fix the language for which we want to define a truth predicate, we may for simplicity's sake use the one-place notion "is true". Tarski required that any truth definition in a fixed language to be materially adequate must fulfill the following condition, referred to here as "Convention T", where "α" is any arbitrary, declarative statement in that language:

$$\text{"}\alpha\text{" is true iff } \alpha. \tag{T}$$

That means that the statement "α" is true if and only if the state of affairs α described thereby obtains. For example:

- "Elroy Fox has diabetes" is true iff Elroy Fox has diabetes;   (120)
- "Belligerism is a disease" is true iff belligerism is a disease.   (121)

Convention T avoids self-reference. While ' "α" ' on the left-hand side enclosed in quotation marks is a metalinguistic *name* that denotes the statement, 'α' on the right-hand side without quotation marks is the statement *itself* denoting the state of affairs. This clear distinction between *mentioning* and *using* a linguistic string, i.e., between metalinguistic level and object-linguistic one, is demonstrated by the examples (120–121). Thus, Convention T is obviously the refined, correspondence-theoretic component of Tarski's truth theory. It says in effect that a true statement corresponds to a fact. For instance, our first example (120) above may be re-read as follows: the statement that Elroy Fox has diabetes is true due to the fact that Elroy Fox has diabetes. Tarski calls his approach 'a semantic conception of truth' because, according to him, the predicate "is true" is, as a metalinguistic term, a semantic term and deals with the relation – of correspondence – between a sentence and the state of affairs denoted thereby. The substantial contribution of his theory to the definition of a truth predicate is his semantics of the language of classical, first-order logic, $\mathcal{L}_1$, that is briefly introduced in Section 26.2.2 on page 873.

The consensus theory of truth

The U.S.-American philosopher and semioticist Charles Sanders Peirce (1839–1914) supplemented the concept of truth with a pragmatic dimension. He included in the meaning of the truth predicate the role that language users play, thereby creating a consensus theory of truth, which heavily influenced William James's pragmatist theory of truth (see below). The consensus theory says, in essence, that "the opinion which is fated to be ultimately agreed by all who investigate is what we mean by truth" (Peirce, 1931–1958, vol. 5, § 407). "Human opinion universally tends in the long run to ... the truth ... There is, then, to every question a true answer, a final conclusion, to which the opinion of every man is constantly gravitating" (ibid., vol. 8, § 12).

It is worth noting that an ancient criterion, or property, of truth has been the so-called consensus omnium or consensus gentium, i.e., agreement of the people, that goes back to Cicero. It says that what is accepted by all carries the weight of truth (Oehler, 1961). Peirce's consensus theory referred to above may be viewed as a revival of this old conception. The German philosopher Jürgen Habermas elaborated on this tradition, suggesting a discourse-theoretic version of consensus theory (Habermas, 1973). According to him, truth is a discursive property of constative speech acts, e.g., "Elroy Fox has diabetes". He distinguishes between the context of experience ('life-world'), on the one hand; and the context of argumentation ('discourse'), on the other. By asserting a constative we make a *validity claim,* i.e., a claim that our assertion obtains. The question of whether or not we are right, is dealt with in a discursive context to justify the acceptability of our validity claim. "True is a constative that we can justify ... A precondition for truth is the potential approval by all other people ... Truth means the promise to achieve a rational consensus" (ibid., 219).

The pragmatist theory of truth

The main proponent of this theory was the U.S.-American psychologist and philosopher William James (1842–1910) who advocated that *true* be equated with *expedient* or useful: "[..] what is *better for us* to believe is true unless the belief incidentally clashes with some other vital benefit" (James, 1907, 77). Sometimes James's theory is counted as an instance of instrumentalism. *Instrumentalism* is the view that scientific concepts and theories are instruments developed by human beings to solve problems. Their worth is measured not by whether they are true or false, but by how effective they are to achieve some specified goal. "You must bring out of each word its practical cash-value, set it at work within the stream of your experience. It appears less as a solution, then, than as a program for more work, and more particularly as an indication of the ways in which existing realities may be changed. *Theories thus become instruments, not answers to enigmas, in which we can rest.* We don't lie back upon them, we move forward, and on occasion, make nature over again by their aid" (ibid., 53) [emphasis by William James].

The deflationary theories of truth

Deflationism denotes a family of theories whose proponents hold the view that the word "is true" is a gratuitous phrase. It is not a predicate and does not involve the ascription of a property called 'truth' to sentences or anything else. We shall here mention the main representatives of deflationary theories, i.e., the redundancy theory, disquotationalism, the prosentential theory, and the performative theory of truth.

The redundancy theory of truth

This theory originated with Frank Plumpton Ramsey (1903–1930). Its core idea is that a statement such as "it is true that Caesar was murdered" means no more than that Caesar was murdered. So, the that-clause "it is true that" is redundant and is used only for emphasis. The same applies to the predicate phrase "is true" in a statement like "'Caesar was murdered' is true". For this sentence too is equivalent to "Caesar was murdered". The phrase "is true" is used as a convenient linguistic device and does not carry any additional information. Ramsey concludes that "there is really no separate problem of truth but merely a linguistic muddle" (Ramsey, 1927, 142 f.) An initial version of the redundancy theory, which Ramsey wrote in 1922 when he was only 19 years old (Ramsey, 1922), was posthumously published in 1990.

The disquotational theory of truth

A similar approach was put forward by the U.S.-American philosopher and logician Willard Van Orman Quine (1908–2000). His theory of truth tries to dethrone the concept of truth by what he calls *disquotation*. He argues that to ascribe truth to a sentence such as "snow is white" is to ascribe whiteness to snow. Using Tarski's Convention T, which we looked at on page 464, we could reformulate the example above as "'snow is white' is true if and only if snow is white". This would show that the use of the truth predicate "is true" on the left-hand side of the convention cancels the metalinguistic quotation marks to yield the object-linguistic fact description on the right-hand side of the convention. Thus, truth is merely disquotation and the truth predicate is redundant (Quine, 1995, 113 ff.; see also Quine, 1973, 21).

The prosentential theory of truth

An even more astounding idea than the preceding two deflationary views is the interpretation of the term "truth" as a *prosentence* (Grover et al., 1975; Grover, 1992). To understand this approach, consider the third-person pronouns "she", "he", and "it". A *pronoun* such as "he" in a sentence like "Elroy Fox has bronchitis, but *he* doesn't cough" acquires its meaning from a name preceding it, to which it anaphorically refers, i.e., "Elroy Fox". A *proverb* operates similarly. For example, "did" in the sentence "Elroy Fox went to the hospital, his wife did so too" is a proverb that refers to the verb "went" preceding it. By analogy, the prosentential theory of truth interprets the truth predicate as a *prosentence,* i.e., as a phrase with anaphoric reference to an antecedent sentence which it represents to prevent repetition. For example, when we are told "Dr. Smith says 'Elroy Fox has bronchitis'. And *that is true"*, the latter phrase "that is true" represents the sentence "Elroy Fox has bronchitis" that precedes it. An alternative would therefore be to repeat the sentence itself in the following fashion: "Dr. Smith says 'Elroy Fox has bronchitis'. And *Elroy Fox has bronchitis"*. The phrase "that is true" may thus be viewed as a prosentential expression. It is of course replaceable by another, equivalent prosentence such as, for example, "that is so". We thus obtain "Dr.

Smith says 'Elroy Fox has bronchitis'. And *that is so*". The truth predicate seems indeed to be a stylistic element and thus something dispensable. The seed of the prosentential theory can be found in Ramsey's early work on the redundancy of the truth predicate quoted above (Ramsey, 1922/1990, 10 ff.).

The performative theory of truth

This deflationary view was advanced by Peter Strawson (1949, 1950). It contends that the ascription of truth to a sentence is a performative utterance like "I promise ..." and "I do ...". To utter that "what Dr. Smith says is true" is not to *state* anything at all but *to do* something, i.e., to *agree* with him. The use of the phrase "is true" by someone indicates that she is *agreeing to* or *endorsing* the statement to which she ascribes truth. "What you have just said is true" means "I endorse what you have just said". To say that the diagnosis "Elroy Fox has bronchitis" is true is to say that one agrees to the diagnosis or with the diagnostician. Thus, truth ascription to a statement α, interpreted as agreement and endorsement, is a speech act of the form "I agree to the statement α" or "I endorse the statement α". It is the performance of an act of doing rather than a constative about a semantic or metaphysical property of a statement.

11.1.2 Justification

Despite the problematic character of truth sketched above, the second problematic feature that the classical concept of knowledge requires of a belief, in addition to its being true, is that it be justified. To understand the crucial role of this issue in medical practice and research, we need to be clear about what it means to say that a belief is justified, e.g., the belief of a physician in a diagnosis or prognosis, and the belief of an epidemiologist in the hypothesis that AIDS is caused by HIV.

We distinguish between *justification* as an act, and *justifiedness* as its result. Unfortunately, both terms are vague. We shall use them here only in an epistemic sense. That is, we are dealing with *epistemic justification* and not with moral, political, or other types of justification, and shall consider justifiedness as a property ascribed to doxastic-epistemic attitudes, i.e., conjectures, beliefs, convictions, and knowledge.

The justifiedness of a belief may be viewed as an indicator of its epistemic goodness. In our Western culture, justified beliefs are traditionally considered to be epistemically 'better than' unjustified ones. A belief counts as justified if it is based on some reason. It is this reason that justifies the belief. For instance, Elroy Fox has angina pectoris. For this reason, his doctor believes that he has coronary heart disease. Thus, provisionally we may conceive justification as a binary relation of the form "reason A justifies belief B", or $J(A, B)$ for short. By so doing, two questions arise:

1. What is it that qualifies something, A, to serve as a justifying reason for a belief B?
2. What does the justification relation J in "$J(A, B)$" look like?

As regards the second question, all *deductive logics* considered in Part VIII are methods of justification par excellence. The justification relation J in such deductive cases is an inferential relation, i.e., simply the relation of inference with respect to a particular logic. A justifies B when A implies B. However, justification cannot in general be confined to deduction because such a confinement would restrict the amount of justifiable beliefs to a negligible minimum, especially in the empirical sciences. We know, for example, that most of what is called empirical-scientific knowledge, is not deductively justifiable because such knowledge types, e.g., universal hypotheses, do not follow from a finite number of observations. Therefore, methods of non-deductive justification will be indispensable in science. A prominent example of such a method is *inductive logic* discussed in Section 29.2 on page 984.

Regarding the first question above, we must be aware of the following basic problem. The requirement that the reason A of a belief B ought to be justified itself, would lead to an infinite regress of reasons. Specifically, the justifying reason of a belief B may itself be a belief, say belief A_1. But this can only work if this justifying belief A_1 itself is justified. How did it become justified? There must be another belief A_2 that justifies A_1. How did belief A_2 become justified? There must be another belief A_3 that justifies A_2, and so on. To prevent such paralyzing regress, there are two main positions in epistemology, *foundationalism* and *coherentism*. We shall discuss them in turn to examine which one of them is appropriate for use in medicine. There are several important ramifications of foundationalism used in all sciences. As their main representatives, confirmation, reliabilism, and statistical inference will be analyzed below. So, our discussion divides into these six parts:[81]

▶ Foundationalism
▶ Coherentism
▶ Reliabilism
▶ Confirmation
▶ Statistical inference
▶ What is evidence in medicine?

---

[81] The age-old problem of skepticism will not be considered because it can be shown that skepticism is an utenable mythos. Whoever is interested in living, cannot be a genuine skeptic and *must take a position* because skepticism is self-defeating. For its basic postulate says, in essence, that none of our beliefs is more justified than its negation. A simple test may help recognize that this postulate is not acceptable: Ask the skeptic the question "do you believe that your postulate is itself more justified than its negation?". What can she reasonably reply? It makes no difference whether she replies Yes or No. In either case, her position will turn out awkward. While the answer Yes falsifies her postulate, the answer No disqualifies it from being something preferable to its negation.

The phrase "evidence" used in the latter item is one of the favorite, technical terms in the philosophy of epistemic justification. It is a vague and ill-defined term, however, that is usually employed carelessly. We shall define it at the end of our discussion on page 482. Up until then, we shall take it to mean *data* that affect the credibility of a statement, e.g., attacks of angina pectoris in a patient that make the hypothesis believable that she might have coronary heart disease. In this example, the patient's angina pectoris is evidence for the presence of coronary heart disease. (Data are *accepted or believed sentences* describing singular events of any complexity. It is obvious that we don't define "evidence" by recourse to "truth". "Evidence" is not a semantic, but a pragmatic notion. See page 482.)

Foundationalism

Foundationalism in epistemology is a view that takes into account the whole of a belief system. To prevent infinite regress, it considers such a system to contain some basic beliefs upon which the remainder depends. Foundationalism says that the reasons-based chain of justification cannot be infinitely long and should not contain circular, vacuous self-justification. Thus, it is not allowed that a belief B be justified by reason A_1 which is justified by reason A_2, and so on until we reach a reason A_n that is based on belief B itself. There must exist some beliefs that are basic, or foundational, and linearly justify a set of other beliefs. Foundational beliefs are not based on, and thus not justified by, other beliefs. They obtain initial warrant of their own. In order to avoid grounding beliefs on something arbitrary and dogmatic, however, empirically oriented branches of science such as physics, biology, and medicine require that the foundational beliefs be based upon some evidence that is anchored 'in the world out there' that we perceive, observe, analyze by experimentation, etc. We shall revert to this issue below.

Coherentism

Coherentism in epistemology denies that there are any foundational beliefs by allowing justification circles. A belief B may be justified by belief A_1 which is justified by belief A_2, and so on until we reach a belief A_n which directly or indirectly is based on belief B itself. According to the coherentist's view, the justifiedness of a belief depends on how well it coheres with a background system of beliefs rather than on any foundations. The holistic Duhem–Quine Thesis mentioned in footnote 71 on page 403 is a version of coherentism. There are different versions of coherentism and foundationalism. For details, see (Alston, 1989; Bender, 1989; DePaul, 2000; Pollock, 1986).

Reliabilism

Reliabilism is a class of theories in epistemology which say that the epistemic goodness of a belief depends on some kind of reliable linkage to what is believed. For example, when someone believes that there are white mice in front of her, her belief must be reliably linked to some existing objects in front of her that she calls "white mice". There are reliabilist theories of knowledge (Armstrong, 1993a) as well as those of justification (Goldman, 1979, 1986, 2004). We are here interested in the latter.

Among reliabilist theories of justification, the most viable one is the so-called *process reliabilism*. It says that a belief is justified if it is produced by cognitive processes that are generally reliable. The critical determinants are thus belief-forming and belief-preserving psychological processes such as, for example, perception, memory, conjecturing, introspection, reasoning, etc. Epistemically 'good' processes are those which in most cases produce true beliefs, i.e., whose belief outputs have a high ratio of true beliefs. A belief's justificational status thus depends on the truth-ratio of the type of processes that are causally responsible for it (Goldman, 2004, 433).

Obviously, process reliabilism is a mentalistic *theory* of justification with "justified belief" as its theoretical term. This is so because the act of determining whether a particular belief B_1 such as "I believe there are white mice in front of me" is justified, presupposes that there is another justified belief B_2 which adjudicates that question. The individual having the belief B_1 cannot make this decision herself, for the question would emerge anew whetehr her second belief that judges about B_1 is justified, and so on. This impending infinite regress shows that *belief justification* is a T-theoretical term of process reliabilism as discussed on pages 409–413.

Confirmation

We must distinguish two types of relation between sentences: (i) *inferential relation*, on the one hand, when according to a particular system of logic some sentences imply another sentence; and (ii) *evidential relation*, on the other, when there is no inferential relation between them, but any non-logical relation of justification and support by some data obtained through perception, observation, experiment, etc., usually referred to as "evidence".

Confirmation is primarily an evidential relation of justification between data, i.e. 'evidence', and belief. We shall elaborate on this notion to examine whether confirmation is useful for the acquisition and management of medical knowledge. To avoid the psychologism associated with much of the terminology of the theories above, we shall replace beliefs with their contents. The content of a belief attitude "x believes that α" is representable by the believed statement α. We shall therefore focus on the confirmation of such believed statements (sentences, assertions, hypotheses) instead of beliefs themselves as mental attitudes, states, and processes. For example, we shall not say:

1. The fact that Elroy Fox has acute fever and cough confirms the
   belief that he has a respiratory tract disease.

Rather, we shall say:

2. The fact that Elroy Fox has acute fever and cough confirms the *statement* that he has a respiratory tract disease.

A confirmation claim of this form may be represented as a binary relation between the confirming and confirmed statements it contains:

3. α confirms β

such that the statement α says that Elroy Fox has acute fever and cough, and the statement β says that he has a respiratory tract disease. The confirming statement, i.e., α in the present example, reports the result of some perception, observation, experience, or experiment referred to as data or *evidence*. This explains what it means to say that confirmation is an evidential relation between evidence and any statement it supports.

It may be that an evidential statement α such as "Elroy Fox has acute fever and cough" confirms another statement β which confirms another statement γ ... which confirms still another statement δ that finally confirms the statement ϕ, e.g., $\phi \equiv$ 'Elroy Fox has a primary immune deficiency syndrome'. We are thus usually faced with confirmation chains, or justification chains, of arbitrary length. Our example shows that the theoreticity of the confirmed statements increases as one ascends from evidence statements toward the final statement to be confirmed, ϕ. In evidential justification chains, evidence statements are the most basic ones with which a chain starts and which cannot be, or are not, justified themselves. For example, you cannot justify the observation that Elroy Fox's body temperature is increased. It is increased, period. Thus, any theory of confirmation belongs to the category of epistemic foundationalism, which we looked at above. All empirically oriented scientists, including medical researchers and professionals, implicitly or explicitly endorse this foundationalist type of epistemology. They suppose that knowledge in their disciplines is empirically grounded and has no other sources and dependencies, e.g., axioms and postulates, metaphysics, religion, magic, and the like. Later in our discussion, we shall examine whether and to what extent this supposition is true in medicine.

To begin with, we must distinguish between deductive and non-deductive confirmation. In a deductive confirmation, the confirming sentence implies the confirmed one. Thus it is a trivial inferential relationship of logical implication, $\models$, discussed in Part VIII. It does not play the role of evidential justification relation in medicine or other empirical disciplines because empirical-scientific knowledge never deductively follows from evidence. The subject of our discussion will therefore be non-deductive confirmation, which has come to be termed *inductive confirmation*. In an inductive confirmation, the confirming sentence does not imply the confirmed one. To analyze this relationship, it is helpful to note that the concept of confirmation may be formulated in three ways as listed in Table 14. In what follows, we shall consider the pros and cons of these three alternatives in order to examine whether they are useful in medicine.

Table 14. Three types of confirmation

Name:	Syntax:	Formalized:
qualitative	α confirms β	$C(\alpha, \beta)$
comparative	α_1 confirms β_1 at least as strongly as α_2 confirms β_2	$C_{\succcurlyeq}(\alpha_1, \beta_1, \alpha_2, \beta_2)$
quantitative	α confirms β to the extent r	$c(\alpha, \beta) = r$

Qualitative confirmation

A qualitative or classificatory concept of confirmation enables only an affirmative or negative judgment about whether some item of evidence supports a given statement. This may be explained by using the simple, standard example "All ravens are black". This example was introduced by Carl Gustav Hempel to demonstrate a paradox of confirmation, later called Hempel's Raven paradox. The paradox shows that the received, qualitative concept of confirmation is inadequate and alternate forms of confirmation are required. For more details, see (Hempel, 1943, 1945, 1965).

Formally, the universal generalization "All ravens are black" says that $\forall x(Rx \rightarrow Bx)$ where "R" is shorthand for "is a raven" and "B" stands for "is black". This hypothesis may therefore exemplify all universal hypotheses of the structure $\forall x_1 \ldots \forall x_k(\alpha_1 \wedge \ldots \wedge \alpha_m \rightarrow \beta_1 \wedge \ldots \wedge \beta_n)$ that we may encounter in medicine, for instance, "All patients who have acute fever and cough have a respiratory tract disease". A hypothesis of this type is formed by inductive generalization of a finite number of observations. For instance, a scientist encounters a raven and notes that it is black. Some time later she sees another raven and notes that it is also black. After making some additional observations of this type, she correctly states that "All of the ravens that I have seen so far have been black". From this finite number of observations, however, she generalizes about *all* ravens and asserts that "All ravens are black". This statement does not deductively follow from the finite number of observations referred to. According to the terminology we used in Section 9.3 on page 395, it represents an unbounded universal hypothesis about the class of *all* ravens. This is a potentially infinite class consisting of those ravens which currently exist on earth and elsewhere, those which no longer exist, and those which do not yet exist.[82]

The above inductive process of forming a hypothesis is usually viewed as a process of 'discovery'. It is generally supposed that thereafter comes the

---

[82] To obtain a medical example, replace ravenhood in $\forall x(Rx \rightarrow Bx)$ with patients who have some symptoms $A, B, C, \ldots$ And replace blackness with disease X. The generalization obtained will say that "All patients with symptoms $A, B, C, \ldots$ have disease X". We can thus see by analogy that our simple hypothesis "All ravens are black" indeed exemplifies all of the unbounded universal hypotheses that we may encounter in medicine.

process of 'justification'. That is, after acquiring some item of hypothetical knowledge of the type "All ravens are black", scientists try to confirm or disconfirm it by systematic observations, e.g., experimentation. They do so by examining as many ravens as possible to see if they are black, and thus confirm the hypothesis. Surely, each new observation of a black raven tends to confirm it. Only the sight of the first red, white, or otherwise non-black raven, say raven a, will disconfirm the hypothesis. The reason is that such an evidence says "a is a raven and a is not black", i.e., $Ra \wedge \neg Ba$. This sentence, however, is classical-logically incompatible with the hypothesis $\forall x(Rx \rightarrow Bx)$ and falsifies it. For $Ra \wedge \neg Ba$ implies $\exists x(Rx \wedge \neg Bx)$; and this is equivalent to the negation of our hypothesis, i.e., $\neg \forall x(Rx \rightarrow Bx)$. The proof goes as follows. For the derivation rules used in the proof, see Section 26.2.3:

Assertion 5 (Disconfirmation). $Ra \wedge \neg Ba \vdash \neg \forall x(Rx \rightarrow Bx)$

Proof 5:

1.	$Ra \wedge \neg Ba$	Premise (evidence)
2.	$(Rx \wedge \neg Bx) \rightarrow \exists x(Rx \wedge \neg Bx)$	$\exists$-Introduction Rule
3.	$(Ra \wedge \neg Ba) \rightarrow \exists x(Rx \wedge \neg Bx)$	Substitution Rule: 2
4.	$\exists x(Rx \wedge \neg Bx)$	Modus ponens: 1, 3
5.	$\neg \forall x \neg (Rx \wedge \neg Bx)$	Equivalence of $\exists$ and $\neg \forall \neg$: 4
6.	$\neg \forall x(\neg Rx \vee Bx)$	De Morgan's Law: 5
7.	$\neg \forall x(Rx \rightarrow Bx)$	Equivalence of $\neg \vee$ and $\rightarrow$: 6. QED

The conclusion of this proof in line 7 that follows from our evidence in line 1 says that not all ravens are black. Thus, it contradicts the hypothesis that all ravens are black, disconfirming it by falsification. What is surprising is that so long as no such falsification occurs, the observation of *every object* whatsoever will confirm our hypothesis, be it a black raven, the Eiffel Tower, or something else. For example, the evidence that this tomato in my hand is red or the grass in your garden is green are confirming instances of "All ravens are black". To see this, we need to be aware of the following fact F, which we will not prove here:

If α and β are two classical-logically equivalent statements and   (F)
there is a statement γ that confirms α, then it also confirms β.

This is so because in the assertion $C(\gamma, \alpha)$ the statement α is exchangeable by its equivalent β to yield the assertion $C(\gamma, \beta)$. That is, all equivalent statements are confirmed by the same evidence. The red tomato in my hand, say object b, is not black. It is also not a raven. So we have $\neg Bb \wedge \neg Rb$. This evidence confirms the hypothesis that "All non-black objects are non-ravens", i.e., $\forall x(\neg Bx \rightarrow \neg Rx)$. But this latter statement is equivalent to the statement $\forall x(Rx \rightarrow Bx)$ which says that all ravens are black. Thus, according to fact F above, the evidence that the red tomato b is not black and not a raven, confirms our hypothesis "All ravens are black". A still more strange finding is that every non-raven is a confirming instance of our hypothesis. To prove this claim, let the object c be a non-raven, e.g., the book that is currently in front of you. Then we have $\neg Rc$. This evidence implies, according to the rule $\vee$-Introduction in Table 36 on page 895, the following two sentences:

1. $Rc \vee \neg Rc$
2. $\neg Rc \vee Bc$

On the other hand, our hypothesis $\forall x(Rx \rightarrow Bx)$ is equivalent to $\forall x(\neg Rx \vee Bx)$, and this to:

3. $\forall x\big((Rx \vee \neg Rx) \rightarrow (\neg Rx \vee Bx)\big)$.

The latter sentence says "Anything which is or is not a raven is either no raven or black". It is obvious that our evidence in 1 and 2 above confirms the sentence 3. Thus, it also confirms our hypothesis $\forall x(Rx \rightarrow Bx)$ as its equivalent. That means that the book in front of you, as a non-raven, supports the claim that all ravens are black. Since any other object may also serve as a confirmation instance of the hypothesis "All ravens are black", this hypothesis is confirmed by everything. We can reason analogously with respect to any other unbounded universal statement.

Comparative confirmation

Hempel's Raven paradox sketched above shows that the received, qualitative concept of confirmation is unsuitable for use in medicine because medical hypotheses, which are unbounded universal statements such as "All patients who have acute fever and cough have a respiratory tract disease", may also be confirmed by everything. Although a comparative concept of confirmation would be superior to the qualitative one, such a concept is not yet available. At this time, we may only present its formal structure to perhaps stimulate inquiry into the subject. Like any comparative concept, its syntax may be conceived as follows:

> Evidence e_1 confirms hypothesis h_1 at least as strongly as evidence e_2 confirms hypothesis h_2. (122)

An example may illustrate:

> That Elroy Fox has acute fever and cough confirms the hypothesis that he has bronchitis, at least as strongly as his angina pectoris confirms the hypothesis that he has coronary heart disease.

Note that sentence (122) represents only the definiendum. No definition for it is available yet. To indicate a direction toward such a definition and to assess its value, we may according to the general method discussed in Section 4.1.3 on page 65, introduce on the basis of the four-place predicate in (122) three special, comparative predicates. To this end, the syntax of the four-place predicate is uncovered in the following way. Concisely, sentence (122) says:

e_1 confirms h_1 at least as strongly as e_2 confirms h_2.

That means, by infix notation:

(e_1, h_1) confirms at least as strongly as (e_2, h_2),

and by prefix notation:

confirms_at_least_as_strongly_as(e_1, h_1, e_2, h_2),

or simply:

$C_{\succcurlyeq}(e_1, h_1, e_2, h_2).$

This is a notational scheme that will be defined on page 480. On the basis of this scheme, we may now introduce the following three predicates of comparative confirmation:

1. e_1 confirms h_1 as strongly as e_2 confirms h_2 iff $C_{\succcurlyeq}(e_1, h_1, e_2, h_2)$ and $C_{\succcurlyeq}(e_2, h_2, e_1, h_1)$;
2. e_1 confirms h_1 more than e_2 confirms h_2 iff $C_{\succcurlyeq}(e_1, h_1, e_2, h_2)$ and not $C_{\succcurlyeq}(e_2, h_2, e_1, h_1)$;
3. e_1 confirms h_1 less than e_2 confirms h_2 iff e_2 confirms h_2 more than e_1 confirms h_1.

To render these notions transparent, one could also formalize them in the following way. For all e_1, h_1, e_2, h_2 :

1'. $C_{\approx}(e_1, h_1, e_2, h_2)$ *iff* $C_{\succcurlyeq}(e_1, h_1, e_2, h_2) \wedge C_{\succcurlyeq}(e_2, h_2, e_1, h_1)$;   (123)
2'. $C_{\succ}(e_1, h_1, e_2, h_2)$ *iff* $C_{\succcurlyeq}(e_1, h_1, e_2, h_2) \wedge \neg C_{\succcurlyeq}(e_2, h_2, e_1, h_1)$;
3'. $C_{\prec}(e_1, h_1, e_2, h_2)$ *iff* $C_{\succ}(e_2, h_2, e_1, h_1)$.

To lend meaning to these three comparative predicates, demands a definition of the basic, four-place predicate $C_{\succcurlyeq}(e_1, h_1, e_2, h_2)$. As mentioned above, there exists no such definition yet. But this is clearly feasible by means of the concept of *comparative support* introduced below. A proposal will be made in Definition 144 on page 480.

Quantitative confirmation

If we had a quantitative concept of confirmation at hand, it would also allow us to form a comparative concept by defining the quaternary predicate $C_{\succcurlyeq}(e_1, h_1, e_2, h_2)$. *Inductive logic,* considered in Section 29.2 on page 984, is such an attempt to introduce, on the basis of probability theory, a concept and theory of quantitative confirmation, $c(e, h) = r$. The attempt has failed, however. Viable, alternative approaches exist in the guise of statistical theories of empirical support. We shall concern ourselves with these approaches in what follows to examine whether they may be of any assistance in solving our problem of justification of medical hypotheses.

Statistical inference

The above discussion on confirmation covers only an exceedingly small category of scientific hypotheses. All of the hypotheses that we considered thus far are universal statements, e.g., "all patients with acute cough and high fever have a respiratory tract disease". They are *deterministic* sentences and mostly representable in a first-order language. A cursory glance at medical and other scientific publications shows, however, that a considerable part of empirical-scientific knowledge is of *statistical* nature and uses the vocabulary of statistics and probability theory. We may be told, for example, that:

> 30% of people with hypercholesterolemia suffer from coronary heart disease;

or equivalently:

> The probability that an individual with hypercholesterolemia will suffer coronary heart disease, is 0.3. That is, $p(CHD \mid HC) = 0.3$.

We have seen in Section 9.3 that unbounded statistical, or probabilistic, hypotheses of this type are neither verifiable nor falsifiable. The term "unbounded" means that the size of the universe of discourse they talk about, i.e., the set of human beings in the present example, is unlimited. It is therefore impossible to find sufficient data that prove the truth or falsehood of a statement like above. In this awkward situation, one would be interested at least to know which of the several, alternative statistical hypotheses on a particular subject is best *supported* by some given empirical evidence. For instance, suppose there are additional hypotheses put forward by other researchers on the association between hypercholesterolemia and coronary heart disease that compete with the above-mentioned hypothesis, e.g., the following one:

> The probability that an individual with hypercholesterolemia will suffer coronary heart disease, is 0.016. That is, $p(CHD \mid HC) = 0.016$.

Suppose in addition that we have the following empirical evidence at our disposal. In a sample of 100 patients with chronic hypercholesterolemia, it has been found that 16 patients are suffering from coronary heart disease. Which one of the two hypotheses above is better supported by this evidence and could be preferred to the other, and why? To answer questions of this type, a variety of statistical tests and theories have been constructed that may help differentiate between acceptable and unacceptable statistical hypotheses. We will here briefly sketch only two classes of tests, i.e., the *likelihood tests* and tests of *statistical significance*. They have been designed to determine whether, and to what extent, some empirical evidence *supports* a statistical hypothesis. In this capacity they can be viewed as devices for epistemological judgment and decision-making. Our following discussion of these issues is based on (Cox, 2006; Hacking, 1965, 2001; Stegmüller, 1973b).

Likelihood tests: Comparative support of type 1

Likelihood tests are interesting and useful methods of analyzing whether a particular medical hypothesis may or may not be accepted on the basis of some available evidence. The central term needed is the notion of "support". To understand this notion, we shall first introduce the auxiliary term "likelihood of a hypothesis". Suppose a particular event has occurred, e.g., the patient Elroy Fox who has hypercholesterolemia *has coronary heart disease*. Given an item of evidence of this type, say *e,* and two hypotheses like above, say h_1 and h_2, we will say that evidence *e* supports hypothesis h_1 better than hypothesis h_2 if it lends a greater likelihood to h_1 than to h_2. But what is *likelihood?*

Due to its connotations with 'probability', the term "likelihood" is very confusing in the context of assessing hypotheses. The term "plausibility" would have been a better choice. But the prominent British statistician Ronald Aylmer Fisher (1890–1962) was responsible for introducing it into the literature and thus it remains ineradicable. Note at the outset that likelihood is *not* probability. This will be demonstrated below. To this end, it is advisable to use simple examples because the concepts and theories we have to illustrate are themselves complicated enough. We shall therefore unduly simplify their presentation.

Suppose that a doctor who is practicing in a large city has just received from health authorities the current figures on the prevailing flu epidemic. They say that the prevalence of flu in the city is currently 80%. This yields our first statistical hypothesis, denoted "$hypo_1$":

$hypo_1$ $\equiv$ 80% of the population have the flu.

The doctor doubts the veracity of this hypothesis because according to her own statistic, the prevalence is much lower and amounts to 10%. Of all the patients treated by her in the last few days, only one out of every ten suffered from the flu. So, our second hypothesis is:

$hypo_2$ $\equiv$ 10% of the population have the flu.

We shall use empirical evidence to help us judge which of these two hypotheses is 'true'. According to $hypo_1$, the probability that a randomly selected inhabitant of the city under discussion has the flu, is 0.8, whereas according to $hypo_2$, the probability is 0.1. For simplicity's sake, we will assume that patients visiting the doctor's practice are randomly selected inhabitants of the city, and moreover, their disease states are independent of one another.

The first patient of the day enters the examination room. The doctor examines her. She does not have gastritis. She does not have rheumatism. She does not have diabetes. She has the flu. Intuitively it is clear that the finding "this patient has the flu" affects the two hypotheses above, $hypo_1$ and $hypo_2$, differently. To elucidate the issue, we will introduce the following two-place notion: "the likelihood of hypothesis *h* in the light of evidence *e*" symbolized by "$L(h, e)$". In this context, "evidence" means an event that has occurred.

Definition 142 (Likelihood). *The* likelihood of hypothesis h *in the light of evidence e equals the probability of evidence e conditional on hypothesis h. That is, $L(h, e) = p(e \mid h)$.*

In the expression $L(h, e)$, the symbol "L" is shorthand for "likelihood of" and signifies the binary likelihood function. To illustrate the definition, consider our example above. In the practice of the doctor in our example, evidence e was her first patient's case of the flu. Thus we have the following two likelihoods where the expression "patient_1_flu" means that the first patient has the flu:

$$L(hypo_1, patient\_1\_flu) = 0.8 \quad \text{because:} \quad p(patient\_1\_flu \mid hypo_1) = 0.8$$
$$L(hypo_2, patient\_1\_flu) = 0.1 \qquad\qquad\qquad p(patient\_1\_flu \mid hypo_2) = 0.1.$$

Obviously, an event that has actually occurred, lends the hypothesis that predicted it, as much likelihood as the probability that the hypothesis assigned to the event before it occurred. The likelihood of a hypothesis is something like its plausibility or credibility in light of the respective evidence. It is by no means a probability value because it does not obey the Kolmogorov Axioms of probability put forward in Definition 237 on page 975. We can easily see this from the following example. Suppose we have not only two, but an infinite number of mutually exclusive hypotheses about the prevalence of the flu in the city. Hence, after the first patient is diagnosed with the flu, we have infinitely many different likelihoods of our distinct hypotheses. Since the number of the hypotheses is infinite, the sum of their likelihoods exceeds 1. This violates the second Kolmogorov Axiom.

Definition 143 below introduces a four-place comparative concept of empirical support. We write "$supp(h_1, e_1, h_2, e_2)$" to say that "evidence e_1 supports hypothesis h_1 better than evidence e_2 supports hypothesis h_2". For clarity's sake, the following shorthand at the left-hand side will be used which at first glance appears pseudo-binary, but is in fact a quaternary predicate:

$$h_1 \mid e_1 > h_2 \mid e_2 \qquad \equiv \quad supp(h_1, e_1, h_2, e_2).$$

Definition 143 (Comparative support). *If evidence e is predicted by two hypotheses h_1 and h_2, then $h_1 \mid e > h_2 \mid e$ iff $L(h_1, e) > L(h_2, e)$.*

Otherwise put, the higher the likelihood of a hypothesis in the light of a particular evidence, the better that evidence *supports* the hypothesis. For example, in the practice mentioned above, the first patient's case of the flu supported the hypothesis of the health authorities, which said that "80% of the population have the flu", *better than* that of the doctor because:

$$L(hypo_1, patient\_1\_flu) = 0.8$$
$$L(hypo_2, patient\_1\_flu) = 0.1.$$

Hence:

$hypo_1 \mid patient\_1\_flu > hypo_2 \mid patient\_1\_flu.$

The interesting question that arises in comparing such hypotheses is this: How can we use the comparative concept of support above to judge which hypothesis is to be rejected and which one is to be accepted? It is clear that in the present context we shall not reject the doctor's hypothesis, $hypo_2$, on the basis of only the first patient's case of the flu. It could happen that none of the subsequent patients in that practice will present with the flu. This negative evidence will support $hypo_2$ much better than the alternative hypothesis $hypo_1$. The lesson we learn from this example is that the decision of whether a hypothesis is to be accepted or rejected, requires much more data, i.e., 'a sufficient, good statistic'. For instance, suppose the doctor examines an additional four patients and obtains, in total, the following series of five diagnoses:

FNNNF

where "F" means that the respective patient in the series has the flu, whereas "N" means that she does not have the flu. The complex event above, consisting of a series of five randomly chosen patients, has a probability of $0.8 \cdot 0.2 \cdot 0.2 \cdot 0.2 \cdot 0.8 = 0.00512$ according to the hypothesis $hypo_1$ of health authorities, and a probability of $0.1 \cdot 0.9 \cdot 0.9 \cdot 0.9 \cdot 0.1 = 0.00729$ according to the hypothesis $hypo_2$ of the doctor. Note that we have assumed the individual patients' disease states are probabilistically independent of one another. Thus, in the present stage of hypothesis testing, the hypothesis of the doctor ($hypo_2$) is better supported by the evidence than the health authorities' hypothesis ($hypo_1$) because $hypo_2 \mid \text{FNNNF} > hypo_1 \mid \text{FNNNF}$.

Definition 143 above implies that an evidence e supports a hypothesis h_1 better than an alternative hypothesis h_2 if their *likelihood ratio* exceeds 1, i.e., when $\frac{L(h_1,e)}{L(h_2,e)} > 1$. However, it is not reasonable to use this finding as a criterion of hypothesis acceptance without further qualification, even though a sufficient and good statistic in favor of h_1 may be available. The reason is that the likelihood ratio already exceeds 1 when the likelihood difference between both competing hypotheses is close to 0 and thus negligible, e.g., $\frac{0.3}{0.29} > 1$. A hypothesis should only be rejected if there is an alternative hypothesis that is much better supported than it is. We will here not go into details to explain what the requirement "much better supported" means. It is the task of *likelihood tests* to explicate this comparative predicate and to suggest stringent methods of support analysis. A critical ratio, say r, will be associated with each test. The greater the critical ratio r, the more stringent the test will be. A hypothesis will be rejected in favor of an alternative hypothesis just in case their likelihood ratio exceeds r. For further details, see (Hacking, 1965, 89 ff.).

A concept of comparative confirmation that was envisaged on page 475 may now be introduced by defining the notational scheme $C_{\succ}(e_1, h_1, e_2, h_2)$ in the following way:

Definition 144 (A comparative concept of confirmation). *Evidence e_1 confirms hypothesis h_1 at least as strongly as evidence e_2 confirms hypothesis h_2 iff e_1 supports h_1 at least as strongly as e_2 supports h_2. That is:*

$$C_{\succcurlyeq}(e_1, h_1, e_2, h_2) \leftrightarrow h_1 \,|\, e_1 \geq h_2 \,|\, e_2.$$

In anticipation of this concept three specific, comparative confirmation predicates have already been defined in (123) on page 475.

Significance tests: Comparative support of type 2

Although the well-known tests of statistical significance are widely used in empirical sciences, it is almost unknown that they are in fact based on the idea of comparative support discussed above. Their exposition is usually veiled in an inscrutable vocabulary and symbolism to the effect that in medicine they are poorly understood and often mystified. To easily explain their underlying philosophy, and their function and benefit, we must choose a simpler example than the one concerning the flu used in the preceding section.

Suppose a surgeon has found a high correlation between peptic ulcer disease caused by Helicobacter pylori, and the incidence of stomach cancer. A significance test is simply a test for determining *the probability that* a given result, such as the high correlation under discussion, could not have occurred by chance, but reports 'facts'. To explain this typical yet cryptic characterization, we will use the customary, transparent example of tossing a coin to simulate an empirical experiment. The aim of our coin-tossing experiment is to find out whether the coin is (i) fair, i.e., whether the probability of tossing heads or tails is 0.5; or (ii) biased toward one of its sides, and if so, to what extent. To this end, the coin must be tossed a sufficient number of times to explore its long run behavior by counting the proportion of heads and tails.

After a few playful tosses, we may have the prima facie impression that *the coin is biased.* To inquire into whether or not this hypothesis is true, we do not test it directly. Rather, we test it indirectly by testing whether its opposite is false. This procedure is an analog of the indirect proof in deductive logic that will be sketched on page 590. Thus, we negate our hypothesis by supposing that *the coin is fair.* This latter hypothesis is called the *null hypothesis*, written h_0. The null hypothesis is the position of the Advocatus diaboli who argues that "what you suppose is not true". Thus, significance tests are in fact tests of a null hypothesis (Hacking, 2001, 222).

That is, by a significance test a hypothesis h_0 is tested against its negation to find out which one is to be rejected. We have therefore to demonstrate in the present example that there are good reasons to reject the null hypothesis, h_0. If we succeed, then we shall have reason to accept its opposite called the *alternative hypothesis*, written h_A, which says that *the coin is biased.* We have thus the hypotheses:

$$\begin{aligned} h_0 \quad &\equiv \text{ the coin is fair} \\ h_A \quad &\equiv \text{ the coin is biased.} \end{aligned}$$

One should always try to show that the null hypothesis h_0 is unacceptable, thereby *justifying* that the alternative hypothesis h_A is acceptable. But this goal is not always attainable. Nevertheless, to achieve it we must design a suitable experiment that indicates in advance a reject class, say R, that comprises possible outcomes such that if the experimental results fall within this class, the null hypothesis must be rejected. We decide to toss the coin $10,000$ times and count the frequency of heads. We calculate in advance the behavior of the coin. If it is an absolutely *fair* coin, then the number of heads will be 5000. Otherwise, the probability that the number of heads in $10,000$ tosses lies:

- between 4950 and 5050   is about 0.66
- between 4900 and 5100   is about 0.95
- between 4850 and 5150   is about 0.99.

And that means, conversely, that the reject class R comprises a frequency of heads:

- outside of the interval $[4950, 5050]$ with $p = 0.33$
- outside of the interval $[4900, 5100]$ with $p = 0.05$
- outside of the interval $[4850, 5150]$ with $p = 0.01$.

We start tossing the coin. After $10,000$ tosses we stop. To our surprise, we observed 5386 heads and 4614 tails. We think this surplus of $5386 - 5000 = 386$ heads speaks for itself. The event, i.e., the surplus of heads, is *significant* in that it represents a marked deviation from the behavior of a fair coin specified above. If the null hypothesis, h_0, is true and the coin is fair with $p(head) = p(tail) = 0.5$, then the probability of an event like "5386 heads" is about 0.01. It is a highly improbable event and falls into the reject class, R. *Either* the null hypothesis is true, in which case we have just observed something practically improbable, *or* the null hypothesis is false. This *either-or* is the philosophical basis of significance tests.

Since it is unreasonable to suppose that the event which did in fact occur was so drastically improbable, one concludes instead that the null hypothesis must be wrong. The rationale is that it has a negligible *likelihood* of 0.01 in the light of the observed evidence. It is therefore rejected to accept the alternative hypothesis, h_A, which in the present example says that the coin is biased.[83]

A statistical significance test consists in a stringent policy of discriminating between two logically incompatible hypotheses, h_0 and h_A. It is mainly based

---

[83] Under this assumption, the anomalous behavior of the coin could have been predicted with the probability of approximately 1. Thus, the likelihood of h_A in the light of evidence '5386_heads' is very high. The experimental outcome supports h_A much better than h_0 because $h_A \mid 5386\_heads > h_0 \mid 5386\_heads$. This remark suggests that significance tests are directly related to likelihood tests that we have considered in the preceding section. They are in fact a standardized subclass thereof and should also be viewed as tests of *comparative support*.

on the identification of those possible events, i.e., the reject class R, whose occurrence is considerably less probable than results on the condition that h_A is true. The standardized probability values for members of this reject class are $p = 0.01$ and $p = 0.05$, and are called the *significance levels* 1% and 5%, respectively. If the experimental results lie in a $p = 0.01$ or $p = 0.05$ region, then they are said to be significant at the level 1% or 5%, respectively. The lower the level, the better *justified* is the acceptance of the alternative hypothesis. Obviously, this is not a proof of its truth. The outcome of our coin-tossing experiment above was significant at the 1% level.

What is evidence in medicine?

Although the phrase "evidence" is the basic notion in the justification of medical and other scientific hypotheses and knowledge, including diagnoses and prognoses, it is a polysemous and ill-defined term. As alluded to on page 370, the emergence of the myth of *evidence*-based medicine is attributable to the unclear semantics of this single word. For simplicity's sake, we have used the term until now as synonymous with *data* gathered through perception, observation, experience, experiment, surveys, interviews, etc., which increase the credibility of a statement (assumption, hypothesis). This inchoate understanding will be revised by an improved explication of the concept of evidence in the following two sections:

 ▷   What evidence is
 ▷   What evidence is not.

What evidence is

At the one extreme, empiricist philosophers in the twentieth century identified evidence with sensory data and perception. Quine, for example, said that "The stimulation of his sensory receptors is all the evidence anybody has had to go on, ultimately, in arriving at his picture of the world" (Quine, 1969b, 75). At the other extreme, proponents of approaches such as evidence-based medicine consider scientific knowledge, hypotheses, and theories as evidence. Our concept of evidence below will show why both extremes are inappropriate.

In our framework, the language of sentence probability will be used that is introduced in Section 29.3 on page 988. The term "evidence" refers to our knowledge that a particular singular *event* of arbitrary complexity has occurred. We shall use the term "event" in its most general sense as defined on page 974. It denotes spatio-temporally localizable occurrences. The entity for which an event serves as evidence, is a *hypothesis*. For example, that a patient has a severe cough and high fever is evidence for the hypothesis that she might have a respiratory disease. Evidence will be represented by its description, i.e., by a sentence such as "this man has a severe cough and high fever". It will be briefly symbolized by $e, e_1, e_2, \ldots$; and hypotheses will be represented by

$h, h_1, h_2, \ldots$ Before introducing our concept of evidence, we will discuss some important features that we want to preserve of what is usually called evidence.

Whatever else it may be, evidence is a belief-forming entity. It confers justification on a belief and makes it appear reasonable. It also can be defeated by new evidence at a later point in time. Something that is evidence for me, need not be evidence for you and vice versa. That means that evidence is something pragmatic. For example, when Elroy Fox tells us that he has recently visited Ghana and I notice that his conjunctiva is yellow, I might suspect that he contracted hepatitis in Ghana because as a physician I am aware of the association between conjunctival jaundice and hepatitis. But my son, who sees the same yellowish discoloration of Elroy Fox's conjunctiva, does not share my suspicion, because he is a mathematician and not a physician. That is, due to his lack of medical background knowledge, Elroy Fox's conjunctival jaundice is not informative for him and does not point to hepatitis.

That evidence points to something, shows that it resembles a *symptom* such that we have reason to remember now the notion of symptom that was explicated in Definition 47 on page 198. Let there be an event that is described by the sentence "e". In addition to its being a pointer to something, in order for e to be evidence for hypothesis h for an individual x, this individual must be aware of the association between e and h. With this basic feature at hand, we shall introduce two variants of evidence below: (i) *evidence for* a given hypothesis h, which increases one's belief in the hypothesis; and (ii) *evidence against* a given hypothesis h, which decreases one's belief in the hypothesis.

An additional feature of our concept of evidence will be this: We shall relativize evidence to the background context (background information, background knowledge, or simply *context*) with respect to which it is considered to be evidence for or against a hypothesis. For it may be that in another context, the same occurrence is evidence for something else or for nothing at all. In our above example, Elroy Fox's conjunctival jaundice was considered to be evidence for hepatitis because the background context was "Elroy Fox has recently visited Ghana". But if he had not visited Ghana and were an alcoholic instead, one would on the basis of the same evidence rather suspect that he has liver cirrhosis. The background context will be represented by the sentence describing it, symbolized by β.

Definition 145 (Evidence for). *An event, described by the sentence e, is in a context β evidence for a hypothesis h for an individual x, or* Evidence_for(e, β, h, x) *for short, iff:*

1. $p(h \mid \beta \wedge e) > p(h \mid \beta)$;
2. x believes that $\beta \wedge e$;
3. x believes (1).

Obviously, the term "evidence_for" is a quaternary predicate of the form Evidence_for(e, β, h, x). Note that in clauses 2–3 of its definition above we have not required that the individual x *knows that*, or *is convinced that*, something is the case because believing is implied by knowledge as well as by conviction. See Axiom KB 1 in Table 45 on page 943, and the group of sentences (242) on page 948. Consider as an example Elroy Fox's trip to Ghana referred to above, and take yourself to be the individual x. Given below is the definition for the following concept of *evidence against:*

Definition 146 (Evidence against). *An event, described by the sentence e, is in a context β evidence against a hypothesis h for an individual x, or* Evidence_against(e, β, h, x) *for short, iff:*

1. $p(h \mid \beta \wedge e) < p(h \mid \beta)$;
2. *x believes that $\beta \wedge e$;*
3. *x believes (1).*

It is worth noting that we have defined *evidence* by, but have not identified it with, the *probabilistic relevance* of the evidence e to the hypothesis h in the context β. Mere probabilistic relevance does not suffice. Evidence is embedded in an epistemic, and thus, pragmatic structure. Accordingly, an event outside of an epistemic structure lacks any evidential value. It is *evidentially neutral* or *silent*, so to speak. This was already demonstrated by my son's oversight of the evidential significance of Elroy Fox's conjunctival jaundice above. This feature is captured by the following concept:

Definition 147 (Evidential neutrality). *An event, described by the sentence e, is in a context β evidentially neutral about a hypothesis h for an individual x, or* Evidentially_neutral(e, β, h, x) *for short, iff* $\neg$Evidence_for$(e, \beta, h, x) \wedge$ $\neg$Evidence_against(e, β, h, x).

Definitions 145–147 imply the following Corollary 8 which properly explains our allusion above to the pragmatic nature of evidence: What someone considers evidence for or against something, need not be considered evidence for or against the same thing by someone else.

Corollary 8 (Evidential neutrality). *An event, described by the sentence e is, in a context β, evidentially neutral about a hypothesis h for an individual x iff:*

1. $p(h \mid \beta \wedge e) = p(h \mid \beta)$, *or*
2. *x does not believe that $\beta \wedge e$, or*
3. *x does not believe that $p(h \mid \beta \wedge e) \neq p(h \mid \beta)$.*

The negated caluses 2–3 in this definition do not mean that the agent believes the opposite. A sentence of the form "x does not believe that α" is not equivalent to "x believes that $\neg\alpha$". It only means that the agent lacks the doxastic state of believing α like your lack of belief in Sherlock Holmes's ability or inability to speak Papiamentu (see Section 27.3 on page 937).

   The concepts of evidence_for and evidence_against introduced above are based on the following two probabilistic relations, respectively:

$$p(h \mid \beta \wedge e) > p(h \mid \beta)$$
$$p(h \mid \beta \wedge e) < p(h \mid \beta).$$

One can therefore straightforwardly introduce a quantitative concept of evidence by the subtraction:

$$p(h \mid \beta \wedge e) - p(h \mid \beta)$$

to determine the *degree of evidentiality* of an event e for a hypothesis h. If the difference is $+r$, then Evidence_for(e, β, h, x) to the extent r; if it is $-r$, then Evidence_against(e, β, h, x) to the extent r; and if it is zero, then Evidentially_neutral(e, β, h, x). Such a technique has been used to introduce a quantitative concept of causality in Definition 80 on page 260. We will not here repeat that process in detail. It may only be added that with the aid of a quantitative concept of evidence, comparative concepts may also be introduced (e.g., weaker evidence for, stronger evidence against, etc.).

So far, we have seen that the content of evidence is a singular event of arbitrary complexity, i.e., an occurrence that can be localized in space and time. For example, the presence of some complaints, problems, symptoms, signs, findings, or diseases in individual human beings may serve as evidence if the background knowledge that we have required in the definitions above is available. Depending on the respective background knowledge β, such an event may serve as evidence either (i) for or against a singular hypothesis such as diagnosis and prognosis; or (ii) for or against a general hypothesis of deterministic or statistical nature which it supports or rebuts.

What evidence is not

Medical hypotheses were extensively analyzed on pages 395–399. The products of medical research are general hypotheses. Unlike a singular statement such as "Elroy Fox has conjuntival jaundice", a general hypothesis does not have a singular, spatio-temporally localizable event as its referent. For instance, the hypothesis "whoever has angina pectoris, has coronary heart disease" does not refer to a singular event, but to a general relation between angina pectoris and coronary heart disease in all human beings.

It need not be stressed that cytological or cardiological knowledge and the like are not the only general hypotheses. The results of controlled clinical trials, i.e., efficacy values, are also general hypotheses obtained by highly complex experiments and abstract statistics. Likewise, systematic reviews as well as metaanalyses yield general hypotheses. But according to our definitions in the preceding section, general hypotheses cannot serve as evidence. Consequently, one may ask the following question: When general medical knowledge is not qualified as evidence, what else counts as "the best available external clinical evidence from systematic research" required by evidence-based medicine for use in clinical practice? (See p. 369 f.)

11.1.3 Are There Justified True Beliefs in Medicine?

As we shall see below, British empiricism once propagated observation, experimentation, and induction as the only legitimate sources of empirical knowledge. Spurred on by his enthusiasm for this epistemological doctrine, the
Scottish empiricist David Hume (1711–1776) wrote in 1748 what was already
quoted in footnote 13 on page 78: "When we run over our libraries, persuaded
of these principles, what havoc must we make? If we take in our hand any
volume of divinity or school metaphysics, for instance, let us ask, *Does it
contain any abstract reasoning concerning quantity and number?* No. *Does it
contain any experimental reasoning concerning matter of fact and existence?*
No. Commit it then to the flames, for it can contain nothing but sophistry
and illusion" (Hume, 1748, [1894], 165).

If such verdicts could be taken seriously at all, Hume's stance would certainly encourage many fanatics to evaluate medical knowledge in the same
vein: "When we run over our medical libraries, persuaded of the principles
of justification and truth, what havoc must we make? If we take in our hand
any volume of a medical journal or handbook, for instance, let us ask, *Does
it contain anything justified and true?* No. Commit it then to the flames, for
it can contain nothing but sophistry and illusion".

The first problem one runs into when evaluating medical knowledge epistemologically, is the difficulty of deciding which concept of truth is to be used.
We saw earlier that there are a variety of alternative truth theories. The choice
of any particular theory will shape one's judgment accordingly. Since medicine
has a long-standing quasi-empiricist tradition, it is conceivable that most medical scientists and professionals will prefer the correspondence theory. As was
emphasized, however, this has never been a complete theory and is, therefore,
useless. Consequently, we may suppose that currently the semantic theory of
truth is better suited to guide epistemological evaluations in medicine.

From the perspective of the semantic theory of truth, however, a close
examination of the content of medical journals and textbooks, like the contents
referred to above, reveals that most of what they propound as knowledge is
not true. We discussed the reasons for this failure in earlier sections (9.3, 10.6–
10.7) when analyzing the structure of medical knowledge. There we saw that
medical knowledge almost exclusively consists of elements of the following
type:

    a. hypotheses (unbounded universal hypotheses, unbounded statistical
       hypotheses, fuzzy hypotheses),
    b. theories,
    c. practical knowledge.

We shall consider them in turn:

    a'. Due to their syntax, *unbounded universal hypotheses* can never be
       true. That does not mean that they are false. It only implies that

truth is not the appropriate measure to evaluate them. The same applies to statistical-medical knowledge. Nowadays, declarative medical knowledge consists primarily of *unbounded statistical hypotheses* based on probability theory. They cannot assume truth values. As we have seen in the preceding sections, there is simply no theory of truth that covers statistical sentences. Owing to fuzzy quantifiers such as "many", "most" and others, also *fuzzy hypotheses* like "many diabetics suffer cardio-vascular diseases" lack truth conditions because fuzzy quantifiers still need a viable semantics, although Zadeh has already made significant contributions to this desideratum (Zadeh, 1978b, 1982, 1983, 1984b, 1986).

b′. Knowledge of type (b), according to our non-statement view of theories, is neither true nor false because a theory is a conceptual structure like a building is an architectural structure. As a structure, it is void of any epistemic content.

c′. Likewise, *practical knowledge,* e.g., diagnostic and therapeutic knowledge, does not assume truth values on the grounds that according to our analyses in Sections 10.6 and 15.1, it comprises conditional imperatives and deontic rules, i.e., commands and action algorithms, but no declarative statements. They have efficacy values instead of truth values. See Section 21.5.3.[84]

The second problem that ensues in epistemological evaluation of the three knowledge types above, is the issue of the justifiedness of our belief in such knowledge:

a″. On the one hand, we saw in earlier sections that insofar as deterministic medical knowledge consisting of unbounded universal statements is concerned, there are currently no acceptable methods of deductive or inductive justification of such knowledge. On the other hand, although a considerable amount of medical knowledge is presented in statistical form today, only a fraction is tested by significance tests or methods of another type. A major part of statistical-medical knowledge is mere descriptive report on percentages, e.g., in physiology, internal medicine, or in any other clinical discipline. It is claimed, for example, "we found that 20% of patients with hepatitis C developed cirrhosis and hepatocellular carcinoma within the next twenty years". As regards fuzzy medical knowledge, we do not know what the justifiedness of belief in such knowledge looks like. Even more delicate is the issue of justification of knowledge types (b) and (c) above:

b″. It was pointed out previously that according to the non-statement view, theories do not contain information, and so they cannot be

---

[84] Summarizing, we can also say that medical *un-knowledge* is much greater than medical knowledge. The term "medical un-knowledge" denotes all medical sentences that differ from what is true. The term "un-knowledge" is borrowed from John W. Gofman (1992).

subject to empirical justification. They are *evaluated* with respect to their potential as epistemic tools for investigations.

c″. Finally, practical knowledge, e.g., diagnostic and therapeutic knowledge, which has only efficacy values and no truth values, can only be comparatively justified by demonstrating that it is *preferable* to alternative knowledge because it enables one to achieve more accurate diagnoses and more recoveries, to save more lives, etc. This, however, is not epistemic justification, but moral justification. This issue will be discussed in later chapters.

Notwithstanding the epistemological problems discussed above, all of which stem from the classical concept of knowledge as *justified true belief*, it is a commonly held view in medicine that medical knowledge represents facts in 'the world out there'. Accordingly, realism is the widespread worldview in medicine. We will examine this issue below in order to explore the relationships between medical knowledge and 'the world out there'.

11.2 Realism

Realism is a hotly debated philosophical point of view 'on what there is'. In order to analyze and evalute medical realism in Section 11.2.4 below, we shall first briefly differentiate between the following main variants of realism: *metaphysical realism, semantic realism,* and *epistemic realism*. There are also other species of realism such as *moral* realism and *modal* realism that will be considered later on in Parts IV and VI.[85]

11.2.1 Metaphysical Realism

Ontological or *metaphysical realism* in the widest sense of this term is the view that (i) there are real objects, properties, and relations. That is, the entities that we commonly talk about such as the Eiffel Tower and diseases, the colors and smells that we perceive, and all other things are not mere illusions and constructions, but exist objectively; (ii) they exist independently of whether we perceive or conceive them or not, independently of the language and concepts with which we refer to them, and independently of whether and how we think about them. The first part of this thesis will be called the *existence* claim, and its second part will be referred to as the *mind-independence* claim.

Different forms of metaphysical realism are also to be distinguished. (1) *Minimal realism* states that there exists something objectively and independently of being conceived. (2) According to the ordinary or *common-sense realism,* ordinary things like chairs, books, trees, countries, emotions, and so

---

[85] Depending on the perspective one takes, realism and its counterpart, anti-realism, may appear as epistemology or ontology. For details, see Section 11.4.1.

on really exist. It is said, for example, that what is called 'the planet Mars' really exists, and moreover, it is spherical. That it exists and is spherical is a fact, and this fact is independent of whether and what anyone of us happens to think or to say about it. (3) *Scientific realism* holds that most of the entities sciences are concerned with, exist objectively. Examples are diseases, genes, molecules, electrons, Quarks, Black Holes, etc. Regarding the two special doctrines of metaphysical realism, i.e., *Platonism* and *nominalism,* see page 694.

11.2.2 Semantic Realism

Semantic realism is directly associated with the traditional view of language and meaning. We usually believe that terms and statements have meanings in that they *refer* to something outside themselves. For example, a predicate such as "diabetic" is supposed to refer to a property (or extensionally: to a class, i.e., the class of people who have diabetes). And a statement such as "Elroy Fox has diabetes" is supposed to refer to a fact. Someone is a semantic realist if she holds that a term has a meaning because it has a referent and this referent exists; and a statement has a meaning because it refers to a fact and this fact exists when the statement is true. This view says, in essence, that meaning originates from reality and reference to it.

Semantic realism is a metaphysical doctrine based on the Aristotelean Principle of Two-Valuedness discussed on page 874. This is easily recognized by presenting a meaningful conjecture for which there is neither a proof nor a disproof. An example is the statement "every positive even number is the sum of two prime numbers". Although there is no known method to prove or disprove this statement, most people hold that it is, 'like any other statement', either true or false even though we are unable to determine which one of these truth values it has. That is, a semantic realist believes in the existence of facts which lend meaning to statements, whether they be determinate or indeterminate.

11.2.3 Epistemic Realism

Epistemic realism goes a step further. It says that science, or more generally, we humans, can get to the truth and acquire genuine knowledge and, moreover, that we actually do so. There are true statements both in science and everyday life. The truth or falsity of a statement, a hypothesis, or a whole system of hypotheses is settled by the world. It does not depend on how anybody thinks the world is. In a nutshell, epistemic realism is the doctrine according to which facts are knowable and determine the truth of our statements. Most epistemic realists also believe that there are true scientific theories. According to the non-statement view of theories sketched in an earlier section, however, theories cannot be true or false because they are not statements.

11.2.4 Medical Realism

The mainstream ontological-epistemological stance in medicine is realism, referred to here as *medical realism*. Medical realism includes all three aspects sketched above, i.e., metaphysical, semantic, and epistemic realism.

Most medical students believe that all medical objects really exist and do so independently of how we conceive them by our languages and theories. For example, viruses, bacteria, genes, nerve membrane potentials, headaches, diseases, causes of diseases, and so on all exist independently of whether we are aware of their existence or not. These medical realists obviously ignore the distinction between T-theoretical and T-non-theoretical entities. They thus entertain medical realism as a medical version of the inchoate, common-sense realism to the effect that dubious entities such as the Oedipus complex and personality disorders are taken seriously. Immature and wild theorizing is the fruit of this attitude. Some reflection on the fundamental term of ontology, i.e., "there is ...", is needed to critically examine the situation. This issue will be discussed in Part VI.

In line with the mind-independence claim of metaphysical realism sketched on page 488, a medical realist, e.g., Barry Smith (2004, 2008), believes that medical predicates that we encounter in biomedical terminologies, and disease terms such as "diabetes", "hepatitis", and "AIDS" refer to classes that exist in 'the world out there'. A medical realist further believes that the existence of such classes is independent of the specific languages used and of the culture and thought style of the users of these languages. It is supposed that the aim of medical research is to 'discover' these pre-existent classes, e.g., diseases. The efforts yield medical knowledge and theories that describe, systematize, and explain objectively existing facts. We shall see in the next sections that these views are problematic. To prepare the discussion, let us first briefly consider an example, the Helicobacter theory of peptic ulcer disease. A valuable exposition of the history and philosophy of the Helicobacter theory can be found in Paul Thagard's work, from which we shall draw in our discussion (Thagard, 1999).

Until the 1980s, it was a common belief in clinical medicine that gastritis, duodenitis, and peptic ulcer disease were psychosomatic diseases having psycho-social causes.[86] Since the publication of Sigmund Freud's *The Interpretation of Dreams* in 1900, a vast number of ideas emerged based upon the notion that the maladies above were of psycho-social origin. Many of these ideas were taught by physicians, psychologists, psychoanalysts, and psychoso-

---

[86] Gastritis, from the Greek term $\gamma\alpha\sigma\tau\acute{\eta}\rho$ (gaster) meaning "stomach", is the inflammation of the epithelium, i.e., gut lining, of the stomach. The suffix "itis" generally means "inflammation". Duodenum is the initial part of the small intestine directly following the stomach. A peptic ulcer of the stomach and duodenum is a wound in the gut lining of these organs. It occurs when the lining is eroded by the acidic digestive juices which are secreted by the stomach cells. Until the 1980s, it was believed that the inflammation and ulceration of these organs were mediated by excess acidity with psycho-social factors being its ultimate causes.

maticists, and published in medical journals and textbooks. For example, see (von Uexküll, 1985). Accordingly, many patients suffering from such gastro-duodenal diseases have been subjected to ineffective psychotherapies. This unsatisfactory situation shifted dramatically after 1983. As of 1979, the Australian pathologist Robin Warren at the Royal Perth Hospital in Perth, Western Australia, observed a new type of bacteria in the vicinity of damaged cells in the gut lining of the *pylorus* of patients with gastritis and peptic ulcer disease.[87] Warren asked the head of the gastroenterology department, Thomas Edward Waters, for collaboration to explore the clinical significance of the bacteria. Waters suggested for the job his junior physician colleague Barry Marshall, who was then a trainee. Warren agreed, and he and Marshall started collaborative research on the subject, studying the newly found bacterium and its association with stomach inflammation and ulcers (Warren and Marshall, 1983; Marshall and Warren, 1984; Marshall, 1994; Marshall, 2002a; Warren, 2002). Initially they baptized the bacterium *Campylobacter pyloridis,* but after a grammatical correction it was renamed *Campylobacter pylori.* This name too was inaccurate because they mistakenly supposed that the bacterium was a member of the known genus of Campylobacter, which was later disproved by genetic analyses. Due to its spiral form, the new bacterium was renamed Helicobacter pylori (Goodwin et al., 1989). It has since been found in more than 80% of patients with gastric and duodenal ulcers. Based on additional investigations, Warren and Marshall claimed that the bacterium was the cause of these ulcers. However, their etiologic conjecture was rejected by the medical community because the dominant view at the time held that no micro-organism could survive the strongly acidic milieu of the stomach. Marshall conducted a self-experiment to convince the skeptics. After undergoing gastroscopy to ensure that he had no stomach diseases, he swallowed a three-day culture of Helicobacter pylori. Within a week, he developed Helicobacter gastritis (Marshall et al. 1985). The growing recognition of the significance of the results increased the interest of gastroenterologists in the subject worldwide. In 1994, a *US National Institutes of Health Consensus Development Conference* evaluated the etiologic conjecture and recommended antimicrobial treatment of patients infected with Helicobacter pylori.[88]

As it turns out, the recommended antimicrobial treatment of patients suffering from peptic ulcer disease has proven extremely effective therapeutically. Note, however, that if the elimination of an event A, e.g., Helicobacter infection, prevents another event B, e.g., peptic ulcer disease, we are not allowed to say that A causes B. The prevention of B by eliminating A only says that $\neg A \rightarrow \neg B$. This statement is equivalent to $B \rightarrow A$. The latter sentence, however, means that when peptic ulcer disease is present, then Helicobacter

---

[87] For the terms "pylorus" and "Helicobacter pylori", see footnote 43 on page 222.

[88] Helicobacter pylori in peptic ulcer disease. NIH Consensus Statement 1994 Jan 7–9; 12(1) 1–23. http://consensus.nih.gov/1994/1994HelicobacterPyloriUlcer094 html.htm. Last access: October 27, 2010.

infection is present. It does not say that if Helicobacter infection occurs, then peptic ulcer disease will emerge.

Nevertheless, a *medical realist* is convinced that diseases and their causes really exist and we can acquire *knowledge* about them. For example, she believes that Warren and Marshall's Helicobacter hypothesis above is true and describes a fact in the world out there such that the bacterium Helicobacter pylori really exists and the causal *relationship* between this bacterium and peptic ulcer disease also exists. She doesn't take into account that such a hypothesis is open for discussion. She also neglects the *social fact* that it was accepted in the medical community only after the recommendation by the US National Institutes of Health Consensus Development Conference referred to above. We shall come back to this issue in Section 11.5.4 below.[89]

11.3 Anti-Realism

Non-realism or anti-realism comprises a number of arguments and doctrines opposing realism, especially its mind-independence claim. In the present section, we will discuss three of them – metaphysical anti-realism, semantic anti-realism, and epistemic anti-realism – in order to see whether there are any reasons to adopt a medical anti-realism. Our aim is to prepare an alternative medical-epistemological view that we shall refer to as technoconstructivism, discussed in Chapter 12.

11.3.1 Metaphysical Anti-Realism

Ontological or *metaphysical anti-realism* denies that there is a world of mind-independent objects, properties, and relations. A strong version of this view that has come to be known as subjective idealism was advocated by the Irish philosopher George Berkeley (1685–1753) who claimed that the world consists only of minds and their contents. A weak version of the view we find in the so-called *radical constructivism* introduced by Ernst von Glasersfeld (1987, 1995). It says that the concepts in terms of which we perceive and conceive the experiential word we live in, are generated by ourselves. In this sense, it is we who are responsible for the world we are experiencing. We have no way of checking the truth of our knowledge with the world presumed to be lying beyond our experiential interface. To do this, we would need an access to such a world that does not involve our experiencing it.[90]

---

[89] For their work on Helicobacter pylori and its role in the inflammation and ulceration of the stomach and duodenum, Warren and Marshall received *The Nobel Prize in Physiology or Medicine 2005*.

[90] Ernst von Glasersfeld, a former psychologist at the University of Georgia (USA), was born as an Austrian citizen in 1917 in Munich, Germany. He grew up in Czechoslavakia and received Czech citizenship. He also lived in North Italy and

11.3.2 Semantic Anti-Realism

Semantic anti-realism is the view that there are no referential words-to-world relationships. Language does not have a representational function, a term does not have a meaning. A predicate does not 'represent' a class, a sentence does not 'represent' a fact. A language is only used in a cultural and social context, and is a collection of culturally and socially devised and maintained practices.

A weak version of semantic anti-realism underlies the so-called Principle of Linguistic Relativity according to which worlds are relative to languages. An early expression of this doctrine is the well-known *Sapir–Whorf hypothesis:* "Human beings do not live in the objective world alone, but are very much at the mercy of the particular language which has become the medium of expression for their society. The worlds in which different societies live are distinct worlds, not merely the same world with different labels attached" (Mandelbaum, 1963, 162).[91]

A strong version of semantic anti-realism is the *semantic nihilism* advanced by Ludwig Wittgenstein and supported by Saul Kripke's interpretation (Kripke, 1982). We discussed this view in Section 2.6 on page 46. It implies that neither terms nor sentences have determinate empirical content. For this reason, we cannot say that there are classes, relations, and facts in the world out there which would lend any meaning to our terms and sentences. Thus, nature plays no role in how we use our languages, and does not place any normative constraints on which sentences we should accept as true. It is we who *construct* their meaning in that our social practices determine how to use terms and sentences.

---

was educated in a boarding school in Zuoz in the French-speaking Switzerland. Thus, as a multilingual fellow fluent in Czech, German, Italian, French, and English he recognized already in his adolescence that access to the world is different in different languages. Later he would build on this early experience to inaugurate an epistemology that has come to be termed *radical constructivism*. He based this philosophy on an epistemological theory of the Swiss developmental psychologist Jean Piaget (1896–1980) who analyzed how, by mental operations, children *construct* what they view as 'the reality' (Piaget, 1937).

[91] Edward Sapir (1884–1939), the most influential figure in American linguistics in the 20th century, was born in Lauenburg, Germany, now Lebork in Poland. He graduated from Columbia University and worked as an anthropologist and linguist. Some of his suggestions on the relationships between language, thought, and world were adopted and further developed by his student and colleague Benjamin Lee Whorf (1897–1941). Whorf was a chemical engineer and worked as a fire prevention engineer. In 1931, he began studying linguistics at Yale University under Sapir and collaborated with him later. He is therefore known as one of the creators of the Sapir–Whorf hypothesis. In his diction, the hypothesis says that "[...] users of markedly different grammars are pointed in different evaluations of externally similar acts of observations, and hence are not equivalent as observers but must arrive at somewhat different views of the world" (Whorf, 1956, 221).

11.3.3 Epistemic Anti-Realism

There is no sharp borderline between semantic anti-realism and *epistemic anti-realism*. Epistemic anti-realism is the doctrine that we cannot, and do not, gain knowledge of mind-independent facts simply because there are no such facts.

There are different species of epistemic anti-realism, e.g., empiricism, instrumentalism, conceptualism, and social constructivism. (a) *Empiricists* claim that our knowledge is confined to observable entities. Knowledge of unobservable, i.e., *T*-theoretical, entities is impossible. (b) *Instrumentalism* in its general form views knowledge as a tool used in predicting and controlling events and integrating our actions with our experiential world, but not as something capable of truth or falsity about facts. (c) According to *conceptualism*, scientific knowledge does not provide truths about a mind-independent world. Rather, it emerges on the basis of a particular conceptual system that is used in a particular community and epoch to achieve particular goals. What is called scientific knowledge, is thus relative to conceptual systems, societies, and goals. For this reason, the existence of any alleged fact that is known is dependent on these factors. (d) The most interesting and momentous species of epistemic anti-realism is the *social constructivism*. It says, in essence, that knowledge does not deal with society-independent facts and truths. It is a social construct.

Note that the afore-mentioned four species of epistemic anti-realism are not mutually exclusive. But we will not go into details here. Only the latter two positions, conceptualism and social constructivism, will be briefly illustrated below to examine whether they provide any reasons for what we will refer to as medical anti-realism.

11.3.4 Medical Anti-Realism

As was emphasized above, in the light of the evolution of medical knowledge, which demonstrates the mortality of all medical knowledge, medical realism turns out a naive epistemological stance. In this section, we will study its counterpart, i.e., medical anti-realism, which includes metaphysical, semantic, and epistemic anti-realism.

In publishing and publicizing new papers, books, or information of any other type about some medical subject, e.g., on the yield of Helicobacter pylori research sketched in Section 11.2.4 above, it is usually supposed that the authors are presenting new medical knowledge of *facts*. Medical realism claims that these 'facts', e.g., Helicobacter pylori as a new type of bacteria and its causal role in the pathogenesis of peptic ulcer disease, exist mind-independently and are 'discovered' by medical scientists. According to medical anti-realism, however, those alleged 'facts' do not exist mind-independently. They are products of society, culture, and the human mind, and thus something invented. Otherwise put, the status of their existence is relative to society, culture, and the human mind. This thesis of ontological relativity will be thoroughly analyzed in Part VI. Let us briefly consider as an example of medical anti-realism the following conceptualism:

The Hippocratic and Galenic *humoral pathology* was rooted in the pre-anatomical era of antiquity. It was based on the idea that there are four fluids or humors in human body, i.e., blood, phlegm, black bile, and yellow bile. It considered illness as an imbalance of these four humors and continued to be the core of the mainstream medicine in Europe until the eighteenth century. Things changed gradually through the arrival of the first anatomy book in the history of medicine, *De Humanis Corporis Fabrica* (Vesalius, 1543), and the then emerging early empiricism conceptualized by Francis Bacon and John Locke. A novel, empirical-anatomical system emerged within which illness appeared to have something to do with solid parts of the body. By the end of the eighteenth century, humoral pathology was replaced with macroscopic-anatomical pathology ensuing from Giovanni Battista Morgagni's *De Sedibus et Causis Morborum per Anatomen Indagatis* (Morgagni, 1761). *Tissue pathology* was soon added to this new conceptual system by Marie Francois Xavier Bichat (1771–1802). After the development of the microscope enabled Theodor Schwann to advance his animal cell theory around 1838 (Schwann, 1839), *cellular pathology* was inaugurated by Rudolf Virchow, who considered diseases the results of changes that occur in cells (Virchow, 1855, 1858). With some alterations and additions, this view dominated medicine until about the 1950s. We are currently witnessing the emergence of a competing conceptual system that interprets and treats diseases as disturbances of molecules in the body, and may therefore be termed *molecular pathology*, e.g., pathobiochemistry and gene pathology. Perhaps our descendants will encounter, learn, and employ *quantum pathology* or something like that in the near future.

We have here exemplified only a few of the numerous conceptual systems that have appeared in the history of medicine, i.e., humoral pathology, macroscopic-anatomical pathology, histopathology, cellular pathology, and molecular pathology. Each of these systems has its specific concepts, ideas, and frameworks about what disease is, what diseases exist, how they relate to one another, and how they are to be diagnosed and treated. For example, relative to humoral pathology there 'existed' a host of 'fever diseases' caused by one form of humoral imbalance or another. However, none of them survived the conceptual change from humoral pathology to cellular pathology simply because *the whole conceptual system* termed 'humoral pathology' was displaced by the successive appearances of macroscopic-anatomical pathology, histopathology, and cellular pathology. In contemporary medicine, the same is true of the so-called mental diseases and personality disorders. Many have come into being and have been included in the nosological system of psychiatry and later removed, e.g., hysteria, neurasthenia, and homosexuality. So we must ask medical realists the following question: If diseases are existing entities discovered in the real world, where do they go after they are abandoned by medicine? According to conceptualism, the assertion of their existence is relative to conceptual systems, i.e., vocabularies, systems of knowledge, and theories as frames of reference.

The ontological relativity stated above, is not confined to diseases. It concerns all of the subjects dealt with in medicine, for example, cells, genes, nerve membrane potentials, stress, etc. In talking about a particular medical subject or field, one uses a particular conceptual system consisting of a specific vocabulary. On the one hand, the use of a particular conceptual system with its specific vocabulary already shapes 'the reality' through the taxonomy it imposes thereon. On the other hand, without such a conceptual system one cannot know whether such a reality exists, and will thus be unable to talk about it at all. On this account, the supposition that something particular such as Helicobacter pylori exists in 'the reality' independently of a specific conceptual system, i.e., microbiology and cellular pathology in the present case, betrays considerable philosophical naivety. See the Principle of Linguistic Relativity mentioned on page 493.

Conceptual systems are products of the human mind, which develops and acts in human society. The dependence of knowledge and worldview upon conceptual systems implies that knowledge and worldview are dependent on the human mind and society. It is especially this dependence upon society that constitutes the subject of an alternative approach, *social constructivism*, which we shall study below.

11.4 Beyond Realism and Anti-Realism in Medicine

The debate between realistic and anti-realistic positions is as old as the history of philosophy. Its longevity is due to the persistent Aristotelean worldview referred to on page 874 and will presumably endure so long as this worldview – with its bivalent notion of truth and its Principles of Non-Contradiction and Excluded Middle – dominates human thinking. Two solutions recommend themselves, i.e., *fuzzy epistemology* and *constructivism*. They will be briefly discussed in the present section. A third one, *perspectivism*, will be advanced in Chapter 23.

11.4.1 Fuzzy Epistemology

In the debates sketched above, no clear distinction is made between an *epistemological* claim such as "the assertion that Helicobacter pylori is the cause of peptic ulcer disease is true" and an *ontological* one such as "there *exists* a causal relationship between Helicobacter pylori and peptic ulcer disease". The reason that no distinction is made is the metaphysical postulate that the truth of a sentence may be equated with the existence of a state of affairs that it denotes. So realism and its counterpart, anti-realism, may each be viewed as a coin with two equivalent sides, an epistemological side and an ontological side. For details, see page 697.

In our discussion about the relationships of medical knowledge to 'the world out there' we saw that traditionally the ontological question of whether some object or fact really exists or not, is treated as a question with only a Yes or No answer. That is, something either does or does not exist. For example, consider the debate about whether mental diseases really exist. There are those whose answer to this question is Yes, and those whose answer is No. There are no other positions *between* these two extremes. The epistemological question of whether a particular item of medical knowledge is true is treated likewise. We have frequently noted in this book that this general pattern reflects the Aristotelean bivalent tradition that allows only two options, i.e., true or false, yes or no, 1 or 0, black or white. There is no doubt that this tradition is responsible for the bivalence found in questions of ontology and epistemology, nor that it is responsible for the *realism* versus *anti-realism* debate sketched above. For instance, it is either maintained that mental diseases exist (nosological realism), or it is said that mental diseases do not exist (nosological anti-realism). Based on the critique of the Aristotelean worldview, for example on page 998, the serious question that we will now ask, is: What may happen when the Aristotelean bivalence is replaced with multivalence?

On the one hand, we can heed fuzzy logic and replace the confined system of alethic bivalence, i.e., {true, false}, with a many-valued system by treating truth as a *linguistic variable* with many fuzzy values auch as {true, fairly true, quite true, very true, extremely true, false, fairly false, quite false, very false, extremely false, ... etc. ...}. (See page 1030.)

On the other hand, we can do the same with regard to the bivalent ontology {exists, does not exist} we are accustomed to. The result will be a many-valued world in relation to which the black-or-white debate on 'the world out there' becomes obsolete. As simplistic, archaic worldviews, realism and anti-realism will vanish to clear the way for fuzzy epistemology with shades of truth of knowledge in general and scientific knowledge in particular, on the one hand; and for fuzzy ontology with shades of existence, on the other. We shall come back to this issue in Chapter 18.

11.4.2 Constructivism

Constructivism considers realism to be a naïve stance because of its mind-independence claim. It can be traced back to the Italian historian, rhetorician, and philosopher Giovanni Battista Vico (1668–1744). As an opponent of the Cartesian epistemology, he inaugurated the constructivistic *verum factum* principle *Verum ipsum factum*. The term "factum" is the past participle of the Latin verb "facere" meaning "to make", "to do". Thus, Vico's principle says that *the true is the made* such that we can acquire full knowledge of any thing only if we understand how it came to be what it is as a product of human action (Vico, 1710).

Constructivism in general claims that the respective subject of discussion is man-made, i.e., a human construct. It has assumed different shapes in different disciplines over time. Three main representatives are the following ones: (i) *radical constructivism*, which was mentioned on page 492 above; (ii) psychological or *cognitive constructivism*, which is associated with the Swiss developmental psychologist Jean Piaget (Piaget, 1937); it says that a learner does not learn by having information poured into her head. Rather, she builds her knowledge through her own experiences, beliefs, opinions, and ideas, and actively 'constructs' reality by her own mental operations. The verb "to construct" comes from the Latin preposition "cum" meaning "with", and the Latin verb "struere" meaning "to build", "to form"; and (iii) *social constructivism*, which considers much of what human beings are concerned with, as social constructs, i.e., as products of social institutions, social practices, and interactions between social groups. For example, see (Berger and Luckmann, 1966). Social constructivism has great epistemological significance in medicine, as we shall study in the next section.

11.5 Social Epistemology

It is a common belief that it is the individuals who are in possession of knowledge, and that the acquisition and justification of their knowledge are dependent upon their own, inner mental faculties. For example, Albert Einstein is considered the inventor of the two theories of relativity; the 19th century German pathologist Rudolf Virchow is considered the inventor of the theory of cellular pathology; the Austrian neurologist Sigmund Freud is considered the inventor of the theory of psychoanalysis; and so on. And anybody who is conversant with any of these theories, is supposed to have learned it personally, adding it to the private treasure of her knowledge. Let us call this traditional conception an individualistic epistemology. Its agents are individuals. In contrast to this received view, *social epistemology* is roughly the theory of knowledge as applied to groups of people. It inquires into the *social* nature, origin, and possession of epistemic attitudes such as conjectures, beliefs, and knowledge.

Social epistemology studies the relationships between social groups, roles, and institutions, on the one hand; and the genesis, development, and acquisition of epistemic attitudes, on the other. For our purposes, we are interested only in the social epistemology of scientific knowledge and methodology, especially in medicine. If it turns out true that the social relations between scientists not only shape, but literally determine the products of their cognitive pursuit, then we would have reason to believe that scientific knowledge and methodology are socially conditioned, and therefore, social entities. The doctrine of *social constructivism* referred to in the preceding section claims just that. In the present section, we will discuss the origin and justification of this view and the relevance it bears for medical knowledge production and epistemology. Our discussion divides into the following four parts:

11.5.1 Logical Empiricism and Critical Rationalism

11.5.1 Logical Empiricism and Critical Rationalism

The social epistemology of scientific knowledge emerged as a critique and refutation of the epistemological doctrines of two different, influential schools of thought, *logical empiricism* and *critical rationalism*, in the middle of the twentieth century. Below, we will briefly sketch these two doctrines in order to understand why they needed revision, how they gave rise to social epistemology, and what fundamental differences there exist between them and the latter.

Logical empiricism

Empiricism, from the Greek term εμπειρια (empeiria) meaning "experience", is an epistemological doctrine which says that knowledge comes from experience. Nearly two millennia ago the great Greek physician Galenus of Pergamum (129–199 or 200? 216? 217? AD), better known as Galen, argued that medical knowledge was a matter of experience (Galen, 1985, 24).[92] Empiricism of this form, then, has obviously played an important role in medicine since antiquity. Medicine without experience, i.e., without perception and observation, is unthinkable. But this age-old, Galenean 'medical empiricism' is both indispensable and innocent. It is only the British form of empiricism, which emerged in the seventeenth and eighteenth century, that has caused turbulences and turmoils in recent philosophy and epistemology.

Until the 17th century, experience hardly played a role in non-medical and non-astronomic areas. Scholarly discourse was based merely on book wisdom and traditionalism à la the popular slogan "As the great Aristotle said, things are such and such". This gradually changed with the British empiricism, or *empiricism* for short. Its foundations are found in Francis Bacon's work (see footnote 80 on page 447), and it was first explicitly articulated by the British philosopher John Locke (1632–1704). Opposing *rationalism*, i.e., the primacy of reason and intellect in acquiring knowledge about the world, Locke argued that nothing is knowable without experience. All knowledge is derived from sense experience and all belief is justified by sense experience. The mind at birth is a blank tablet, a tabula rasa, on which experiences leave their marks. *Nihil in mente quod non prius in sensu:* "There is nothing in the mind that was

---

[92] "We say that the art of medicine has taken its origin from experience, and not from indication. By 'experience', we mean the knowledge of something which is based on one's own perception, by 'indication', the knowledge which is based on rational consequence. For perception leads us to experience, whereas reason leads the dogmatics to indication" (Galen, 1985, 24).

not previously in the senses". Among other leading advocates of empiricism were George Berkeley and David Hume.[93]

Logical empiricism, also called logical positivism or neopositivism, was a twentieth century movement with a widespread following in Europe and the United States of America. It was a late outgrowth of British empiricism established by a small group of scholars, known as the Vienna Circle, on the basis of the philosophy of Bertrand Russell and the early work of Ludwig Wittgenstein (Russell, 1903, 1912, 1914, 1919, 1924; Wittgenstein, 1922).[94]

The aim of the movement was to bring about a scientific philosophy, epistemology, and methodology by employing methods of formal logic, introduced by Gottlob Frege and Bertrand Russell shortly before. See footnote 155 on page 845. Their work advanced the analytic philosophy enormously. Logical empiricists considered metaphysics and theology nonsense and sought linguistic criteria to distinguish between intelligible and nonsensical discourse (Carnap, 1932), so as to prevent unintelligible Heideggerean hieroglyphics such as "the nothingness nihilates" (Heidegger, 1927, 1929, 1965). The first suggestion they made was (i) the requirement of empirical *verifiability.* It says that in order for a statement to be meaningful, it must in principle be verifiable by observation and experience, i.e., it must be possible in a finite number of steps to determine whether the statement is true. However, it was soon recognized that for logical reasons most scientific statements are not verifiable in this sense. For example, we saw in Section 9.3 on page 395 that no un-

---

[93] John Locke was a British philosopher, medical researcher, government official, economic writer, opposition political activist, and finally a revolutionary. Much of his work is characterized by opposition to authoritarianism. He believed that using reason to grasp the truth and determining the legitimate functions of institutions will optimize human flourishing. This amounts to following natural law and the fulfillment of divine purpose for humanity. In his monumental book "An Essay Concerning Human Understanding", first published in 1690, in which he introduces the doctrine of empiricism (Locke, 2008), Locke concerns himself with determining the limits of human understanding in respect to God, the self, natural kinds, and artifacts. He had an enormous influence on the development of both political philosophy and the empirical sciences and has also influenced many enlightenment philosophers such as Bishop George Berkeley and David Hume (see footnote 195 on page 986).

[94] The Vienna Circle (1923–1936) was a small group of philosophers, natural scientists, social scientists, and mathematicians. It was initiated by the Austrian mathematician and philosopher Hans Hahn (1879–1934) and included such prominent scholars as Moritz Schlick, Otto Neurath, Rudolf Carnap, Friedrich Waismann, Herbert Feigl, Karl Menger, Kurt Gödel, and others. The Circle started with the doctrine that knowledge of the world was sense data plus logic (Carnap, 1928). It disintegrated after the Nazis took control of Austria in the late 1930s. Most of its members emigrated to the USA. The influence of the movement ended around 1970. Its conceptual tools and methods of philosophizing, however, have been carried on throughout the world. For details on the history of Vienna Circle and logical empiricism, see (Ayer, 1959, Hanfling, 1981; Kraft, 1953; Moulines, 2008).

bounded universal sentence of the form "all patients with pneumonia cough" is verifiable. Therefore, the unsatisfiable requirement of verifiability was replaced with (ii) the weaker requirement of *confirmability* (Carnap, 1936). It says that for a given statement in the empirical sciences, there must exist some observational evidence that supports the statement. For instance, the hypothesis that all patients with pneumonia cough receives a small degree of support from the observation that the patient Elroy Fox has pneumonia and also coughs. An increase in the number of observations of this type raises the degree of confirmation of the hypothesis. However, as we saw earlier, a universal hypothesis of the form "all patients with pneumonia cough", i.e., $\forall x(Px \rightarrow Qx)$, does not deductively follow from a finite set of observational evidence of the form $\{Pa \wedge Qa, Pb \wedge Qb, Pc \wedge Qc, \ldots etc. \ldots\}$. For this reason, the new empiricist requirement of confirmability was considered an inductive relation between evidence and hypothesis, rather than deductive, and the approach has come to be known (iii) as *inductivism*. As discussed in Section 29.2, an inductive logic is required to anchor inductive confirmation. This was one of the major aims of the prominent logical empiricist Rudolf Carnap. But he was not successful. At this time, there remains no inductive logic and no logic of confirmation.

Critical rationalism

In opposition to logical empiricism and rather than pursuing verification and inductive confirmation, the Austrian-born British philosopher Karl Raimund Popper (1902–1994) developed what would later come to be known as *critical rationalism* (Popper, 1945, 1963, 2004). He separated science from non-science by proposing that a scientific hypothesis be in principle empirically *falsifiable*. That is, it must in principle be possible to find evidence that proves the hypothesis to be false (Popper, 1963). For example, if we encounter a patient who has pneumonia and does not cough, then this evidence logically falsifies the statement that "all patients with pneumonia cough". See Proof 5 on page 473. According to Popper, scientific statements ought to behave similarly.

Following David Hume's philosophy of induction, referred to in Section 29.2, Popper held the view that no inductive inference can ever be justified. He relied completely upon deductive logic and used the following elementary fact as the basis of his falsificationism: When we have a hypothesis of the structure $\alpha \rightarrow \beta$, and its antecedent condition α is true, then we can deductively predict by Modus ponens that β will occur. In the event that $\neg\beta$ occurs, our hypothesis will be falsified because the premise $\{\alpha \rightarrow \beta, \alpha, \neg\beta\}$ implies the negation of our hypothesis, i.e., $\neg(\alpha \rightarrow \beta)$. The latter negation follows from the conjunction $\alpha \wedge \neg\beta$ via its equivalent $\neg\neg(\alpha \wedge \neg\beta)$, and then, $\neg(\neg\alpha \vee \neg\neg\beta)$. Thus, classical deductive logic is the main tool of Popper's doctrine, called *deductivism*, as opposed to the logical empiricists' failed *inductivism*.

However, real-world science is not that simple. First, scientific hypotheses and theories are much more complex than Popper's elementary hypothesis

$\alpha \rightarrow \beta$ and argument seem to suppose. Second, on his account much of what is considered science today, e.g., economics, mathematical psychology, quantum physics, biosciences, and statistics-based medicine, is not falsifiable, and thus, non-science. For instance, consider the following probabilistic hypothesis h: "The probability that a patient with bacterial pneumonia who is receiving antibiotics will recover within ten days, is 0.6". Suppose now that the patient Elroy Fox has bacterial pneumonia and receives antibiotics. His physicians will predict "the probability that Elroy Fox will recover within the next ten days, is 0.6". Elroy Fox may or may not recover within the next ten days. Neither one of these two possible events falsifies the statistical hypothesis h mentioned above. Besides probabilistic statements, there are additional types of non-falsifiable statements in science, for example, indefinite existential hypotheses such as "there are diabetics". There are even hypotheses which are neither falsifiable nor verifiable, e.g., universal-existential hypotheses such as "every cell stems from another cell" (see Section 9.3 and Table 13 on page 398).

Popper was not impressed by such counter-examples. He monotonously defended his falsificationism and deductivism until his death in 1994 by repeating that while we can never have the least reason for believing in the truth of a hypothesis, we can use a deductive argument to show that it is false. So, scientists are free to make all conjectures they like, he said. So long as a conjecture is not falsified in a test, it is, according to Popper, acceptable because it is corroborated. We can never justify anything, we merely rationally criticize and weed out unacceptable ideas and work with what is left. The method of science consists in searching for and proposing bold hypotheses and theories and trying to falsify them. Scientific endeavors thereby attain knowledge that increasingly approximates the truth, i.e., hypotheses and theories with "increasing truthlikeness or verisimilitude" (Popper, 1963, 47–52 and 329–335).

11.5.2 The Rise of Social Epistemology

The Polish physician Ludwik Fleck and the U.S.-American historian of science Thomas Kuhn didn't agree with the doctrines of logical empiricism and critical rationalism. They introduced a novel epistemology suggesting that scientific knowledge has nothing to do with truth-seeking, truth, truthlikeness, verification, confirmation, and falsification. They argued that scientific knowledge is a social product made by scientific communities in interaction with the larger society. We will sketch the essence and medical relevance of this epistemology in the next three sections:

- ▶ Ludwik Fleck
- ▶ Thomas Kuhn
- ▶ The birth of science studies.

Ludwik Fleck

In 1935, the Polish physician and bacteriologist Ludwik Fleck published a remarkable monograph in German entitled *Entstehung und Entwicklung einer wissenschaftlichen Tatsache,* i.e., the genesis and development of a scientific fact (Fleck, 1979). Like Karl Popper's influential monograph on 'The Logic of Scientific Discovery' launched in the same year (Popper, 2004), the logical-empiricist view on the nature of scientific knowledge and research was its target. Unlike Popper, however, Fleck developed an original epistemology, based on a detailed historical-philosophical study of syphilis research, that is among the most intriguing and creative epistemologies in the entire history of philosophy. Unnoticed at first, Fleck's work was rediscovered in the late 1970s.[95]

He starts his book with the question "what is a fact?", by which he meant a scientific fact. To demonstrate the intricacy of this notion, he inquires into how the clinical concept of *syphilis* emerged in a complex, historical process from the fifteenth to twentieth century, culminating in the diagnosis of the disease by a serologic test termed *Wassermann reaction,* so called after one of the bacteriologists who constructed it. Fleck traces the concept back to the end of the fifteenth century to show that at that time it encompassed a:

[...] confused mass of information about chronic diseases characterized by skin symptoms frequently localized in the genitals – diseases that sometimes assumed epidemic proportions.

Within this primitive jumble of the most diverse diseases, which crystallized during the following centuries into various entities, we can detect in addition to syphilis what we now call leprosy; scabies; tuberculosis of the skin, bone, and glands; small pox (variola); mycoses of the skin; gonorrhea, soft chancre, probably also lymphogranuloma inguinale, and many skin diseases still regarded as nonspecific today, as well as general constitutional illnesses such as gout (Fleck, 1979, 1).

How was it possible to identify and extract from "this primitive jumble of the most diverse diseases" the individual disease entity *syphilis;* to discover that it is an infectious disease caused by *Spirochaeta pallida;* to construct a serologic test called *Wassermann reaction;* and to justify the claim that a positive Wassermann reaction is diagnostically relevant to the presence of syphilis in a patient? Fleck's book aims to answer these questions. His epistemological analysis provides a complex answer revealing that the 'discovery

---

[95] Ludwik Fleck (1896-1961) lived in Lwow, Poland. In June 1941, he was deported to the Jewish ghetto in his city and later, in December 1943, to the concentration camp Buchenwald in Germany to do research on typhus serum. He survived and returned to Poland in 1945 where he held different prominent positions. In 1957, after a heart attack and the diagnosis of lymphosarcoma, he and his wife jointly emigrated to Israel to live close to their son who had been living there since the end of the war. He is widely recognized today as the founder of the social constructivist theory of science. For a comprehensive account of his life and work, see (Cohen and Schnelle, 1986).

and justification' of a 'scientific fact' is accomplished in a context that comprises historical, conceptual, administrative, political, moral, social, and many other factors the most important of which is a collaborative group of specifically trained individuals, i.e., scientists and their co-workers. The scientific fact is constructed by the direct and indirect co-operation of all of the relevant individuals, groups, and institutions. On this account, Fleck's perspective is known as *social constructivism*. Below we shall outline its essential features. To adequately understand our outline, three central notions of Fleck's framework may be sketched first: observation, fact, and cognition.

The notion of observation is commonly used as a two-place term. We usually say, for example, that doctor Smith observes the heart rate of the patient Elroy Fox, i.e., *x observes y*. That means, formally, $Obs(x, y)$ where "Obs" is the binary predicate "observes". Fleck was not trained in logic. Although from his writings it is obvious that he didn't have a deep understanding of logic, he intuitively recognized that it is more adequate to conceive the notion of observation at least as a three-place term by saying that someone, x, observes something, y, relative to an assumption z. Thus, $Obs(x, y, z)$. This is exactly the so-called theory-ladenness of observation outlined on page 403. In spite of their expertise in logic, logical empiricists overlooked this fundamental issue, believing that observation and experience were theory-neutral and independent of any background assumption and knowledge. Fleck criticized this stance, stating that "Observation and experiment are subject to a very popular myth. The knower is seen as a kind of conquerer, like Julius Caesar winning his battles according to the formula 'I came, I saw, I conquered'. A person wants to know something, so he makes his observation or experiment and then he knows" (Fleck, 1979, 84). Instead, he held the view that observation without assumption "is psychologically nonsense and logically a game" (ibid., 92).

Though he saw clearly through the myths surrounding the notion of observation, Fleck nevertheless has considerable difficulties with the second central notion of his philosophy, i.e., the notion of a scientific *fact*. Although this notion, "fact", is traditionally conceived of as denoting a state of affairs described by a true sentence (see page 19), he uses it without realizing what he actually means. With 'facts' he never means spatio-temporally localizable states of affairs such as 'the Eiffel Tower is in Paris' or 'this patient has syphilis', but universal hypotheses, ideas, conceptual systems, theories, and similar epistemic abstracta. For example, the subject of his book, i.e., the gradual formation of the entire theory of syphilis comprising the nosology, etiology, and serology of this disease, he calls "genesis and development of a scientific *fact*". However, a scientific theory is by no means a *fact*. It is a conceptual system that in the traditional sense is said to be scientific knowledge. Regardless, it is Fleck's merit to have given the first analysis of the complex context that generates such knowledge. To present his insights in a concise concept, he rejects the traditional, two-place notion of cognition, of the form "*x recognizes y*", and introduces a three-place notion in the following way:

"In comparative epistemology, cognition must not be construed as only a dual relationship between the knowing subject and the object to be known. The existing fund of knowledge must be a third partner in this relation as a basic factor of all new knowledge" (Fleck, 1979, 38; 1983). The English version of Fleck's book uses the translation "dual" to describe the relationship between the knower and the known, but this does not quite capture his critique. "Dyadic" or "binary" is a more accurate translation of the relation he rejects. What he proposes instead is cognition as a ternary relationship. We thus obtain, for the act of recognizing, a ternary relation of the type "x recognizes y on the basis of z", i.e., $Recog(x, y, z)$ for short. The third factor z Fleck calls a *thought collective*. Someone, x, recognizes something, y, as a member of a thought collective z.

Fleck understands by the term "thought collective" a community of two or more persons mutually exchanging ideas or maintaining intellectual interaction (ibid., 39 and 102). A thought collective is the communal carrier of a particular thought style. Thus, it is their manner of thinking that links the members of the collective together. However, despite his long explanations, Fleck is not precise enough about what such a thought style is. We can clarify his vague and prolix conception as the class of all conceptual, logical, and methodological tools that guide and regulate scientific research in a thought collective. Consider, for example, a psychiatric community whose members are students of psychoanalysis, and another psychiatric community whose members are behavior theorists. Thus, each of these two communities has its own thought style. When a particular patient is presented to members of both communities, her psychological state will be 'observed', characterized, and explained differently. "Even the simplest observation is conditioned by thought style and is thus tied to a community of thought. I therefore called thinking a supremely social activity which cannot by any means be completely localized within the confines of the individual" (Fleck, 1979, 98).

According to what has been stated above, Fleck argues that thinking and cognition are teamwork in a thought collective. Thus, scientific knowledge as the product of thinking is created collectively. No doubt, this creation is a *social process* such that the role of the individual scientist therein is a subordinate one. Like the performance of an orchestra cannot be regarded as the work only of individual instruments, all paths toward a fruitful understanding of scientific research and genesis of knowledge lead toward a theory of thought collectives and thought styles. A thought style predisposes the members of a thought collective to perceive, think, and act in a certain, directed fashion. It constrains the individual by determining "what can be thought in no other way" (ibid., 99). Students of different thought styles have difficulty understanding each other. What is considered meaningful according to a particular thought style, may not appear meaningful or intelligible in another thought style (ibid., 100). However, it is not possible to determine which one of them is correct because there is no absolute frame of reference. Fleck's point, otherwise put, is that distinct thought styles are incommensurable. It is this idea that later reappears in Thomas Kuhn's system as his famous incommensurability thesis (see below).

The way in which scientific knowledge develops, is also a social process. This process is not accumulative, however. It does not increase knowledge continuously. Rather, hypotheses and theories can be changed and even abandoned after a particular period of history. And they are not abandoned because they are falsified. They undergo changes according to changing thought styles. Take, for example, the successive changes in the conceptual systems of medicine, considered in Section 11.3.4 on page 494. Thus, truth in science is the solution of a problem within a particular thought style, e.g., the classification of syphilis as an infectious disease based on the view that it is caused by Spirochaeta pallida. It is neither relative nor a convention (ibid., 98–111).

Fleck divides a thought collective into two concentric circles, an esoteric circle comprising experts or 'the elite', surrounded by an exoteric circle comprising the laymen or 'the masses'. The esoteric circle consists of a hard core of *special experts* surrounded by a circle of *general experts*. The exoteric circle also includes a central group that is more interested in science than a peripheral group. A member of the exoteric circle may enter the esoteric circle by scientific education that may be considered as a process of initiation, e.g., medical education. Corresponding to these four types of persons, there are four types of scientific knowledge presented in four types of literature. First, we have the *journal science* for the special experts. Results of scientific research enter this primary source of knowledge. Scientific problem solving, theory formation, and controversies take place here. Second, *handbook science* represents for the general experts an encyclopedic condensation of the tremendous epistemic stream reported in journal science. Third, *textbook science* for the initiation of novices into the esoteric circle of experts. And fourth, *popular science* for the exoteric circle. For details, see (Fleck, 1979, 105 ff.).

Thomas Kuhn

Fleck's epistemology has served Thomas Kuhn as a major source of inspiration for the theory of science he put forward in his seminal monograph *The Structure of Scientific Revolutions*, first published in 1962 (Kuhn, 1996).[96] In

---

[96] Thomas Samuel Kuhn (1922–1996) was one of the most influential U.S.-American philosophers of science of the twentieth century. He was born in Cincinnati, Ohio, studied physics, taught history of science at Harvard from 1948 to 1956, and was professor of history and philosophy of science at the University of California at Berkeley from 1961 to 1964. He subsequently taught at Princeton until 1979 and at MIT until 1991.

Kuhn's monograph, *The Structure of Scientific Revolutions*, is the most widely read and cited book on the philosophy of science of the twentieth century. It has sold more than two million copies in about 20 languages. By contrast, Fleck's book, first published in 1935, was completely ignored by scientific communities. Of the 640 published copies, about only 200 were sold. There have only been

this popular and widely known work, Kuhn not only dealt both logical empiricism and critical rationalism a deathblow. He also popularized a new type of epistemology, inaugurated by Ludwik Fleck, that brought epistemology closer

---

five reviews in medical journals, another one in a psychology journal, and a few additional ones in popular science journals and newspapers (Fleck, 1979, xviii and 191). None of them has developed a significant effect, however. If there had not been a marginal reference to Fleck's work in a brief footnote in a monograph on epistemology by the prominent logical empiricist Hans Reichenbach, entitled *Experience and Prediction* (Reichenbach 1938, 224, note 6), it is more likely than not that his ideas would have been lost forever and the philosophy of science would not have undergone the 'Kuhnean' revolution that it has since 1962.

The author of *Experience and Prediction*, Hans Reichenbach (1891–1953), was a German-born philosopher of science. He was trained in physics and mathematics and was a student and associate of Albert Einstein. As a logical empiricist at the University of Berlin (1926–1933), he was a co-founder of the *Berlin Circle* originally called "the society for empirical philosophy". Among its members were Walter Dubislav, Kurt Grelling, Carl Gustav Hempel, David Hilbert, and Richard von Mises. In co-operation with Rudolf Carnap of the Vienna Circle, he founded in 1930 the journal *Erkenntnis*, the major journal of analytic philosophy before WW II. After the rise of Nazism, Reichenbach emigrated to Turkey in 1933 and served as the head of the philosophy department at the University of Istanbul. In 1938, he moved to the USA and was professor of philosophy at the University of California at Los Angeles until his premature death in 1953. In *Experience and Prediction*, Reichenbach included on page 224 a rather unsubstantial, brief footnote referring to Fleck's book. Prior to Kuhn's work, it was the only reference in the literature to Fleck's monograph since its publication. It was that footnote that brought Kuhn's attention to Fleck's work. He briefly acknowledges in the foreword to his acclaimed book, *The Structure of Scientific Revolutions*, that Fleck's almost unknown monograph anticipated many of his own ideas (Kuhn, 1996, viii-ix). See also Kuhn's foreword to Fleck's republished book (Fleck, 1979, vii-xi). There he says, "I have more than once been asked what I took from Fleck and can only respond that I am almost totally uncertain" (ibid., viii). Only a careful comparison of both books reveals that Fleck's theory is in fact a pretheory of Kuhn's.

In studying Reichenbach's epistemology, Kuhn's aim was to examine his differentiation between the *context of discovery* and the *context of justification* (Reichenbach 1938, 382). Reichenbach claimed that epistemology cannot be concerned with the former but only with the latter. According to him, "the analysis of science is not directed toward actual thinking processes but toward the rational reconstruction of knowledge. It is this determination of the task of epistemology which one must remember if one wants to construct a theory of scientific research" (ibid., 7 ff. and 382).

Relying on his extensive knowledge of the history of science, Kuhn did not accept Reichenbach's claim. A considerable part of *The Structure of Scientific Revolutions* is an attempt to demonstrate that in the history of science, discovery and justification have always been one and the same process. There has never been, he says, a distinction between discovering something and justifying the theory thereon.

to sociology, psychology, and the history of science. His theory is in fact a further development of Fleck's ingenious edifice enriched by many supporting examples from history of science.

As a physicist and historian of science, Kuhn had no formal training in philosophy and logic. Nevertheless, based on his knowledge of the history of science, he had good reason to criticize the logical empiricist epistemology and their distinction between the context of discovery and the context of justification (see footnote 96 on page 506). He similarly rejected Popper's critical rationalism on the grounds that "No process yet disclosed by the historical study of scientific development at all resembles the methodological stereotype of falsification by direct comparison with nature" (Kuhn, 1996, 77). Theories are not cast aside by their falsification, but by their replacement with other ones. To systematize this idea, Kuhn suggested an alternative epistemology that may be briefly sketched as follows.

According to Kuhn, science does not develop by continuous accumulation of knowledge and successful theories as it is customarily assumed. It is a discontinuous process alternating between two kinds of periods, 'normal science' and 'revolutionary science'. During a period of normal science, the members of a scientific community work within the realms of a *paradigm*, i.e., "the entire constellation of beliefs, values, techniques, and so on shared by the members of a given community" (Kuhn, 1996, 175). "A paradigm is what the members of a scientific community share, *and*, conversely, a scientific community consists of men who share a paradigm" (ibid., 176). Normal science is characterized by a sophisticated form of puzzle-solving to elaborate the paradigm. In the course of time, however, more and more puzzles arise that cannot be solved. The accumulation of such *anomalies* triggers a crisis that leads to a breakdown of the incompetent paradigm and its replacement with a new one, i.e., a *paradigm shift* or *scientific revolution*. Among the examples analyzed by Kuhn are the displacement of Aristotelean physics and geocentric astronomy by Newtonian mechanics and heliocentrism. An example in medicine that we considered on page 494, is the replacement of humoral pathology with macroscopic-anatomical and cellular pathology.

Competing paradigms, e.g., the old and the new one, are *incommensurable* because a term appearing in both of them does not have the same meaning. For example, a label such as "fever" or "apoplexia" meant in humoral pathology something completely different than in modern medicine. Other terms that constituted central concepts of humoral pathology are meaningless in modern medicine, such as "eucrasia" and "dyscrasia". The proponents of competing paradigms are like the members of different language groups. They don't understand each other and practice their trades in different worlds (Kuhn, 1996, 150 and 205). This is exactly Fleck's incommensurability thesis outlined on page 506 in the preceding section. Kuhn used the well-known duck-rabbit optical illusion to demonstrate how a paradigm shift causes one to see the same things in entirely different ways (Figure 62).

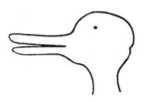

Fig. 62. Viewed from different perspectives things look different

While normal science can accumulate a growing stock of puzzle-solutions, say knowledge, revolutionary science is not accumulative, since paradigm shifts consist of revisions to existing scientific beliefs and practices. Each paradigm has its specific puzzles. So the puzzle-solutions of two incommensurable paradigms form different, incomparable sets. We pointed out on page 506 in the preceding section that Fleck also considered science to be non-accumulative.

By his monograph and jargon, Kuhn spawned the ubiquitous use and misuse of the terms "paradigm" and "paradigm shift" in almost all areas of our culture, ranging from science to politics to textile trade to cooking. This was due to the extreme vagueness of the term "paradigm" as the central notion of his epistemology. It has therefore been subject to incisive criticisms. For instance, one reviewer identified twenty-two different senses of "paradigm" in Kuhn's text (Masterman, 1970). As a reply to his critics, Kuhn tried to clarify the issue and replaced his initial label "paradigm" with two quite distinct concepts which he referred to as *disciplinary matrix* and *exemplars*. A disciplinary matrix is what he had previously called a paradigm in the strict sense of this term, i.e., the entire constellation of beliefs, values, techniques, and rules, "the common possession of the practitioners of a professional discipline". Exemplars or examples, synonymous with the Greek term "paradigm" (see page 419), are successful puzzle-solutions enabled by the disciplinary matrix. It is both the disciplinary matrix and the exemplars that are shared by a group of scientists to constitute a community (Kuhn, 1977, 463; 1996, 181–191).

Thomas Kuhn's disciplinary matrixes are analogues of Ludwik Fleck's thought styles, and his scientific communities are part of Fleck's thought collectives, i.e., their esoteric circles outlined on page 506. Like Fleck, Kuhn also regards the scientific community as the producer and validator of scientific knowledge. The community is characterized by the relative fullness of communication within the group and by the relative unanimity of the group's judgments in professional matters. Its members are responsible for the pursuit of a set of shared goals. It is exactly the disciplinary matrix that accounts for the relatively unproblematic character of their professional communication (Kuhn, 1977, 461).[97]

---

[97] Interestingly enough, Ludwik Fleck's own, revolutionary concept of *thought style* was introduced earlier by the Hungarian-born German sociologist Karl Mannheim (1893–1947) in his sociology of knowledge in 1929 (Mannheim, 1929 [1985], 7). Fleck's discovery that scientific knowledge comes from scientific communities is also found in the same work by Mannheim where he states that "knowing is fundamentally collective knowing [. . .] and presupposes a community of knowing" (ibid., 31).

With the aid of the notion of *exemplar,* Kuhn tried to introduce a novel concept of knowledge that seems related to the so-called *case-based reasoning,* well known in medical artificial intelligence and clinical decision-making, and discussed on page 639. However, his terminology is confusing because of its imprecision. For instance, he does not make explicitly clear what relationships there exist between a *disciplinary matrix* and a *theory* that is shared by the members of a scientific community. On our account, a Kuhnean disciplinary matrix may best be interpreted as a basic theory-element, discussed in Section 9.4.4 on page 429. Thus, what Kuhn calls *exemplars,* i.e., successful 'puzzle-solutions' as examples of notable scientific accomplishment, are what we have referred to as the set of actual applications of a theory on page 419, i.e., $\mathcal{I}_t$. For instance, individual diseases such as AIDS, hepatitis A-G, and measles are exemplars of the theory of infectious diseases.

The initial set of a theory's intended applications, i.e., its 'paradigmatic application' $\mathcal{I}_0$, yields the *first exemplar.* Consider, for instance, the theory of infectious diseases that started as the speculative germ theory of diseases before micro-organisms were known. After this discovery, the earliest identification of a pathogen as a definite causal agent of a disease was accomplished by Armauer Hansen in 1873. He described Mycobacterium leprae, Hansen's bacillus, that causes leprosis.[98] Leprosis, then, must be rated the initial intended application of the theory of infectious diseases, and thus, the first exemplar in the Kuhnean sense. Splenic fever, i.e., anthrax, was the second one discovered in 1876 by Robert Koch (1843–1910).

Kuhn argues that scientific knowledge is produced in scientific communities by recognizing similarities between known exemplars and other phenomena to the effect that, by puzzle-solving, scientists try to add a phenomenon to exemplars if it resembles them. So the first exemplar provides the beginning of a process of similarity recognition by the members of a scientific community. They try, according to Kuhn, to group particular situations into similarity sets, be they Newtonian physical situations or members of natural kinds. In constructing such similarity sets, explicit rules and criteria play no role. Decisive factors are neural, psychological, and social determinants of similarity recognition. The yield is scientific knowledge embedded in shared exemplars. Normal science proceeds on the basis of perceived similarity relationships between exemplars (Kuhn, 1977, 462 ff.; and 1996, 187 ff.). This Kuhnean idea is best explicable in terms of our *prototype resemblance theory of knowledge* envisaged on page 419.

Normal science is accumulative and not revisionary. By contrast, revolutionary science is revisionary and non-accumulative since a disciplinary matrix is replaced with a new one ('paradigm shift'). Due to their incommensurabil-

---

[98] Gerhard Henrik Armauer Hansen (1841–1912) was a Norwegian physician and zoologist. Note that the earliest discovery of a micro-organism (by Otto Friedrich Müller in 1773) was Trichomonas tenax. It would later be identified as a pathogen that causes pulmonary trichomoniasis.

ity, the change of disciplinary matrixes also occurs without recourse to any logic and methodology. Empirical evidence, experimental data, inductive confirmation, and falsification play no role in adjudicating between competing, incommensurable disciplinary matrixes. Conversion experiences, propaganda, authority, persuasion, beliefs, hopes, and commitment to something new are the main determinants. Kuhn quotes Max Planck who, looking back on his own scientific career, sadly remarks: "A new scientific truth does not triumph by convincing its opponents and making them see the light, but rather because its opponents eventually die, and a new generation grows up that is familiar with it" (Planck, 1949, 33–34; Kuhn, 1996, 151).[99]

The birth of science studies

Kuhn's work that has emerged on the basis of Fleck's monograph, has been extraordinarily influential both in philosophy and outside, especially in social sciences. It has significantly contributed to what has come to be known as *science studies* (Hackett et al., 2007; Sismondo, 2004). This new research area is an interdisciplinary, empirical as well as theoretical inquiry into the social, historical, psychological, and philosophical aspects and dimensions of scientific investigation and expertise. The social epistemology inaugurated by Ludwik Fleck is now part of this new endeavor.[100]

Scientific knowledge was once seen as the intellectual achievement of individual, great men or women such as Albert Einstein, Marie Curie, or William Osler working in isolation. It is difficult to understand how it was possible

---

[99] Max Karl Ernst Ludwig Planck (1858–1947) was a German physicist at the University of Berlin (1889–1928). In 1918, he received the Nobel Prize in physics for his work on black body radiation. The success of his work and subsequent developments by other physicists such as Niels Bohr, Werner Heisenberg, and Erwin Schrödinger established the revolutionary *quantum theory* of which he is regarded as the father.

[100] The earliest explicit expression of a general social epistemology is found in the works of the German political philosophers Karl Marx (1818–1883) and Friedrich Engels (1820–1895). In their joint work *The German Ideology,* written in Brussels in 1845–1846 and first published in 1932, they argued that people's social and political beliefs are rooted in the social and economic circumstances in which they live. "Consciousness can never be anything else than conscious being, and the being of men is their actual life-process [...] It is not consciousness that determines life, but life that determines consciousness" (Marx and Engels, 1975, Vol. 5, pp. 36–37). This doctrine may have given rise to the classical German sociology of knowledge that originated with the philosopher Max Scheler (1874–1928) and the above-mentioned sociologist Karl Mannheim in the 1920s (Scheler, 1924; Mannheim, 1925, 1929). The French school of the classical sociology of knowledge originated with Emile Durkheim (1858–1917) (Durkheim, 1965; Meja and Stehr, 1999). These two streams and Thomas Kuhn's epistemology contributed to the sociology of scientific knowledge represented, for example, by the *Edinburgh School* (Bloor, 1991; Barnes et al., 1996).

to overlook the intrinsically social nature of science and scientific knowledge. This fact is now being increasingly uncovered by *science studies*. In the light of these studies, we shall try to elucidate the social origin and nature of medical knowledge in what follows. It is of paramount importance to recognize that medical-scientific communities as social groups inevitably determine what is or is not medical knowledge and expertise, and thereby determine the mode and quality of clinical practice and health care.

11.5.3 Medical Knowledge is a Social Status

Our previous analyses revealed that scientific knowledge in general and medical knowledge in particular does not satisfy the strong, classical concept of knowledge to be *justified true belief*. A seemingly relaxed, common requirement is that scientific knowledge be *objective, impartial,* and *well-grounded.* "Objective" means representing 'the things as they actually are'; "impartial" means not favoring someone's opinions; and "well-grounded" means that a scientist ought to have good reasons for asserting what she asserts. Medical experts are convinced that their knowledge is in line with these quality criteria. In this section, this belief will be reconsidered in the light of a theory of knowledge according to which the knowledge of an expert may be viewed as a *social status* like being married or being a soldier, and thus, as something that by virtue of its nature cannot be subject to the quality requirements above. To present this view we must first round off the discussion we began in Section 11.5.2, i.e., the thesis that medical knowledge comes from medical communities. For details of this *commnitarian theory of knowledge* from which our analyses draw, see (Kusch, 2004; Welbourne, 1993).

It is a truism that social facilities are supportive of knowledge creation. For example, no one acquires knowledge without a socially given language. All propositional knowledge depends on conditions materially made possible by society, e.g., interpreted perception, education, communication, and reasoning. For our purposes, however, we are not concerned with ordinary knowledge, but with medical expert knowledge that for whatever reasons might deviate from that rule. So, the question we have to ask is whether medical knowledge too is socially conditioned, and if so, what the nature of this socially conditioned product is. The best way to answer these questions is to analyze the role testimony and agreement play in medical research and knowledge acquisition. We shall therefore briefly demonstrate, first, that *testimony* as a social interaction and practice is the only generative source of scientific knowledge, and second, that the primary possessors of medical knowledge are groups of medical professionals rather than individual doctors or researchers. Our discussion will be based on the notions of a *social fact, social institution* and *institutional fact*, which we shall briefly explain first. It divides into the following four sections:

▶ Social facts, social institutions, and institutional facts

- ▶ Medical knowledge by testimony
- ▶ Medical knowledge as a social institution
- ▶ Communal medical knowledge.

The first two sections introduce the auxiliary vocabulary that we shall need in the third section. For a detailed analysis of these basic notions, see (Searle, 1995; Tuomela, 2002; Grewendorf and Meggle, 2002).

Social facts, social institutions, and institutional facts

The general notion of a fact was introduced on page 19. According to that notion a fact is, relative to a particular language, a state of affairs described by a true sentence of that language. Two types of facts may be distinguished, *natural facts* and artificial or *man-made facts*, although there is no sharp dividing line between them.

Natural facts are facts occurring causally independently of human intentionality and intention. (For the notion of intentionality, see page 16.) An example is the solar eclipse that occurred in India, Bangladesh, and Nepal yesterday. A man-made fact, however, requires human intention and intentionality to occur, e.g., the fact that Elroy Fox received a heart transplant this morning. Man-made facts are also called artifacts or constructs. The category of man-made facts includes, among others, two important types of fact which are introduced in the following two sections in turn, *social facts* and *institutional facts*.

Social facts

To introduce this term, a distinction must be made between *I-intentionality* and *we-intentionality*. To this end, consider the family physician of the above-mentioned patient Elroy Fox. She believes that the patient has heart failure, and therefore describes her belief by a sentence of the form "I believe that Elroy Fox has heart failure". An attitude of this type held by an individual human being is referred to as a first person, singular attitude, I-attitude, or *I-intentionality* for short, e.g., "I am sure you will recover", "I like this book", and the like.

Suppose now that the heart of the patient must be replaced with a new one. A team of heart surgeons and assistants in an operating room are transplanting a heart into his body. The action they perform is a joint action, or teamwork, that the team may describe by a sentence of the form "we are transplanting a heart". The teamwork cannot be adequately described by the agencies of the individual team members such as:

I, Dr. Adam, am transplanting a heart   and   (124)

I, Dr. Brown, am transplanting a heart   and

I, Dr. Cohen, am transplanting a heart   and

so on because none of them is true. Rather, each member of the team is only partially contributing to the teamwork. For this reason, a correct description of their joint activity is provided only by a we-sentence of the form "we are transplanting a heart". The agent of the surgical operation is the team as a first person in the plural, "we", that cannot be split into individuals. An irreducible collective action, attitude, or intentionality of this type is referred to as a collective attitude, we-attitude, or *we-intentionality*. Thus, we distinguish between individual intentionality, I-intentionality, or I-attitude, on the one hand; and collective intentionality, we-intentionality, or we-attitude, on the other.

A community is a group of at least two individuals who have a joint intention and communicate with one another. A communal or *social fact* is a man-made fact which involves, or is produced by, a community and whose description by members of the community irreducibly contains the plural indexical "we" as its grammatical subject. Examples are facts that may be communicated by sentences of the type "we X" as exemplified above, e.g., we are transplanting a heart; we work together; we love each other; we are just leaving for a trip to Berlin; and the like. Obviously, a social fact is characterized by collective or we-intentionality. Thus it is usually represented by a sentence of the form "we X" with X being a we-verb characterizing the fact. It is an intentional we-verb like the verbs in "we are transplanting", "we do", "we love", "we believe", or "we X" in general.

A collective intentionality of a community, "we X" or "we are Xing", is not a conjunction of the intentionalities of its isolated members like in (124). Convincing examples are the surgical operation on a human heart by a team of surgeons as described above, and the cooperative execution of a symphony by an orchestra. In the latter example, only all members of the orchestra can jointly claim that "we play a symphony". No single member of the orchestra can meaningfully utter "I play a symphony". The playing of a symphony by an orchestra is a *social fact* because a symphony is a compound fact with its agent being a team, and thus a community. It is only the whole of this community, say community c, of which the sentence "a symphony is being played by c" is true. The crucial characteristic of a social fact, i.e., a collective or we-intentionality, is the fact of intending and doing something jointly, e.g., shared operating, playing a symphony, loving, knowing, etc. The agent of the fact is a community that calls itself "we".

Below, medical knowledge will be interpreted as an institutional fact. *Institutional facts* are a subcategory of social facts in the above sense. They are social facts generated not by individuals, but by *social institutions*. We therefore need to explain this basic notion of a 'social institution' first.

Social institutions

A *recurrent collective action* characterized by we-intentionality we call a *social practice*. Examples are collective rituals, rites, greeting by shaking hands, the relatively ritualized course of scientific conferences, and the more or less uniform mode of patient management in hospitals.

A *social institution* is a set of $n \geq 1$ rules or norms that are constitutive of a social practice. Thus, the institution creates that social practice. For example, rules of chess are constitutive of the chess game. Without those rules there would exist no chess game. Rules and norms of a social institution need not exist in an explicitly written form. They may also be unwritten and implicit, e.g., social positions and roles, or fragmented expectations and habits distributed over the members of the community. Familiar social institutions are schools with the roles teachers and students play; police authorities with their practice of protecting people from being deprived of their human right to life or liberty; the Church with the numerous, religious and humanitarian social practices of its believers; and the health care system with measures of clinical and preventive medicine as a complex of social practices in the above sense. Language is a social institution par excellence. Additional well-known social institutions are marriage and money. In the latter case, by virtue of communal agreement certain pieces of paper and metal qualify as currency such that people consider them valuable (cf. also Turner, 1997).[101]

Institutional facts

Social practices are generative of social facts. Such social facts are referred to as *institutional facts* because they emerge, through social practices, from and within social institutions. An example is a chant sung in a mass. Since it is a social fact generated by the institution of religion, it is an institutional fact.

To give an additional, more interesting example that will guide us in our following discussions, consider a registrar in the registry office of a city. She represents a social institution because she is empowered by the laws of the state to institute the social practice of 'marriage'. Now, she pronounces a particular couple, e.g., Ada and Basil, husband and wife by uttering the sentence "I hereby declare you as husband and wife". It is this pronouncement that *creates* Ada and Basil's new status of being married. Thus, the registrar's utterance is a performative speech act. By this act she brings into existence the state of their being married such that Ada and Basil can tell everybody "we are married to each other". Their new social status is obviously a *social fact* characterized by their collective intentionality "we are married". And since it is created by a social institution, it is an institutional fact. *As a social fact, being married is a social status, and as such, an institutional fact.*

---

[101] Note that not every joint action is a social practice. For example, a crowd of people travelling by the same train, ship, or airplane do not exercise a social practice because their travel is not based on joint intentions. Thus, it is not characterized by a we-intentionality of the sort "we are travelling from A to B". Otherwise put, the people in the crowd are not doxastically connected. We-intentionality plus recurrence are prerequisites for a social practice.

With the above notions in hand, we will now inquire into whether medical knowledge may be interpreted as an institutional fact, like the marriage between Ada and Basil mentioned above, i.e., as a social status created by a social institution. To this end, we will first analyze medical knowledge in the context of testimony. For details on knowledge by testimony, see (Welbourne, 1993, 1994; Lackey, 2010).

Medical knowledge by testimony

Most medical experts believe that medicine is primarily and exclusively an empirical science. They therefore assume that their expert knowledge stems from the following three sources: experience, memory, and reasoning. If this assumption were true, however, medicine as a scientific discipline could never exist. The assumption ignores collaboration, and hence, communication between medical experts as a source of knowledge. Yet collaboration enables testimony, and as was anticipated above, *testimony is the only generative source of scientific knowledge*. This will be demonstrated in what follows.

Our beliefs range from elementary assumptions that may be supported by direct evidence – such as the Eiffel Tower's location – to complex hypotheses and theories for which we may have only indirect evidence, e.g., the genesis of AIDS by HIV. However, most of what we know or believe, we know or believe because someone told us so, i.e., we learned it from the written or spoken words of others, from *testimony* in the widest sense. Consider, for instance, your belief that you were born on a particular date in a particular place. You believe this is true because you hold a birth certificate in your hands that originates from a particular city authority and carries your name and those data. Your belief is a *testimonial belief* on the grounds that it is based on the certificate as a written testimony. Interestingly, the testimony provided by the city authority is based itself on another testimony that stems from your parents or their proxy, or from the hospital where you may have been born, who told the city authority the story of your birth. That means that if experience, memory, and reasoning are our primary *individual* sources of knowledge, testimony is our primary *social* source of knowledge. And without this social source of knowledge, with regard to intellect human beings would not be so very distant from animals, and scientific knowledge would not exist at all. Consider the following example:

You believe that increased levels of blood cholesterol cause atherosclerosis, which may lead to diseases such as stroke and myocardial infarction, and therefore you follow, or try to follow, a particular dietary regimen to prevent high cholesterol levels in your blood and body. You yourself have not investigated the pathobiochemical effects of elevated cholesterol levels. Nor have you analyzed the metabolic advantages of the specific dietary regimen you are following. You have only been told, by written or spoken testimony, about what these effects and advantages may be.

In exactly the same manner, most of what you consider to be your knowledge and belief, you have learned from other people's words. Likewise, the author of a medical textbook draws a large amount of the information she presents to her audience, from other literature sources or persons, i.e., from testimony. This also includes the non-medical knowledge and methodology she uses that is provided by other disciplines, e.g., mathematical and statistical formulas and techniques, biological and physical theories, and the like. Even in those cases in which the author conducts primary experimental or epidemiological research, she seldom does so as an individual researcher, as an 'eyewitness' so to speak. Rather, every scientist today is part of an expert team, including technical assistants who prepare and supervise experiments, collect data, perform calculations, etc. In many cases, the team even consists of several multicenter research subteams distributed over a number of laboratories in different and distant locations. Well-known examples are the so-called multicenter studies concerned with therapy research by means of randomized clinical trials. Correspondingly, a medical journal article is usually multi-authored having two, five, ten, twenty, perhaps even a hundred or more authors. Each member of the research team is told by other members that 'things are such and such'. Thus, even in laboratory research as the allegedly primary source of scientific knowledge, there is no escape from testimony. Many of the authors of a multi-authored work will not even know how a given result or number in their work was arrived at. Interestingly enough, a member of a research team contributing to the collaborative work eventually receives a draft thereof that very often contains her own contribution integrated into the whole in a modified or corrected form as if she were being told something new, i.e., by testimony. Today medical education, medical literature, and all other sources of medical information are based on, and constitute, testimonies. Citations from, and references to, literature in a publication are also appeals to epistemic authorities, and thus, represent testimonies.

In a nutshell, medical expert knowledge is mainly *testimonial knowledge*. Testimonial knowledge cannot be reduced to non-testimonial knowledge obtained from experience, memory, and reasoning. With regard to her knowledge, a medical expert is epistemically dependent on others such that epistemic autonomy in medicine cannot and simply does not exist. And it is the testimony of others that is the basis of this epistemic dependence. In an epistemic communication, the recipient of knowledge is epistemically dependent on an *epistemic authority*, i.e., the testifier.

Testimony can exist in indefinitely long chains. As in the example above about how you came to know the date and place of your birth, a testifier herself may know something on the basis of a testimony by a third testifier, while this third party knows it on the basis of testimony by a fourth, and so on. However, the chain must start in some initial source so as to avoid both an infinite regress and a vicious circle. We shall see in the next section that this origin of the chain, i.e., the initial source of testimonial knowledge, is not 'experience, memory, and reasoning' as one would suppose, but a community, i.e., the society. To this end, we need to understand how an item of knowledge, say someone's assertion that hypercholesterolemia causes atherosclerosis, is acquired by testimony from an epistemic authority. First of all, it is important to realize that:

a. Knowledge is not simply transmitted from the testifier to the recipient like water is passed in a bucket brigade from one person to the next, or a contagious disease in a chain of infection is transmitted from one organism to another. Although testimony is a belief-forming process, the recipient's belief that hypercholesterolemia causes atherosclerosis, does not simply emerge by way of doxastic infection, i.e., not because she supposes that the testifier communicates any truth, automatically believes her, and shares her justification for what she says and believes. Concisely and in contrast to a widely accepted thesis (Welbourne, 1994, 305), it is not the testifier's belief that is transmitted in the chain;

b. Nor is it her statements, their content so to speak, which would convince the hearer that she should endorse them. This 'statement view of testimony' (Lackey, 2010, 72) presupposes that the recipient is able to adjudicate the epistemic status of the testimony. But more often than not this is not the case;

c. Rather, the recipient's belief and acceptance emerge on the basis of the information's *supposed relevance* to the context of her interests. That means that in an epistemic communication, the recipient's trust in the testifier is by no means trust in her sincerity and credibility to provide truth or reliable information, but in her *capacity and willingness to provide interest-relative, relevant information*. For a detailed analysis of the relationships between knowledge and practical interests, see (Habermas, 1968b; Stanley, 2007; Sperber and Wilson, 1995).

We saw on page 385 that according to the classical concept of knoweldge, the knowledge-conduciveness of a belief consists in its truth and justifiedness. By contrast, we are now able to recognize that both belief and knowledge as testimonial processes are dependent on the agent's interests. What she is prepared to believe and to view as knowledge, is selected and shaped by the context of her interests, and thus, by the values she holds or pursues. Our values play a central instrumental role in the formation of the web of our beliefs and knowledge. This may be viewed as *contextuality of knowledge*.

Medical knowledge as a social institution

In Chapter 8 we categorized medical diagnoses, prognoses, and treatment decisions as performatives. In the current section, we shall argue that medical knowledge also belongs to this category. The only difference is that it is a *communal performative* conducted not by an individual, but by an epistemic community. For a detailed theory of knowledge communities, see (Kusch, 2004; Welbourne, 1993).

Take, for example, a student who is told by her professor that HIV causes AIDS. Contrary to the classical conception of knowledge as justified true belief, the student receiving such testimonial expert knowledge is not supposed to possess that knowledge because she recieved from the professor a justified true belief. Rather, she is supposed to possess that knowledge because she has become a member of a group, consisting of the professor, the student and others, which constitutes an *epistemic community* possessing that knowledge. The attribution of knowledge to an individual is thus a judgment about her *social status* and is based on her membership in an epistemic community. To better understand the social character of such knowledge attribution, we will first illustrate in some detail the elementary speech act of the registrar referred to above. For the theory of speech acts, see page 53.

Two individuals, say Ada and Basil, are unmarried at time t_1. Some time later, say at time t_2, they go to the town hall that houses the registry office. This office represents the law-based social institution of marriage. There, Ada and Basil apply for marriage. After taking some preparatory steps that may need some time, the registrar eventually performs, at time t_3, the speech act "I hereby declare you husband and wife". The illocutionary act of this performative utterance generates a social fact that didn't exist before. It consists in Ada and Basil's new *social status* of being a married couple and having particular rights and duties that they didn't have before. Their assertion *"we are married to each other"* indicating a collective intentionality was not true prior to t_3. Thanks to the powers invested in the registrar by the state, it became true at t_3.

The registrar's speech act "I hereby declare you husband and wife" has three salient properties. First, it is a self-verifying utterance because it becomes true of a reality that it has created itself. Second, it is a testimony because the registrar testifies thereby that the couple is now married. So it is a performative testimony. Third, it provides knowledge in that it tells the couple and other people something new and true. Altogether, the registrar's speech act is a *performative testimony generative of knowledge*. In what follows, we shall suggest that medical knowledge may also be viewed as a performative of this type. To this end, we need to distinguish between singular and communal performatives:

A performative is a singular one if it originates with an individual, e.g., performatives made by a family doctor such as "I diagnose you as having diabetes" or "I promise to visit you at home". A communal performative, however, originates from a community, i.e., a group of at least two individuals. Its grammatical subject is the plural indexical "we" that expresses collective intentionality. Consider as an example the communal performative "we hereby declare it right to love one's neighbor like oneself". It may be conceived of as a performative spoken by an entire society which approves, and is pursuing, brotherly love.

A communal performative spoken in a society creates a *social institution* in that society. For instance, the communal performative "we hereby declare it right to love one's neighbor like oneself" creates and supports the social institution of brotherly love. Of course, this institution-creating performative is usually not brought about by the community speaking in unison. Nevertheless, it is uttered, referred to, or approved of by almost everybody in the relevant community when they talk about brotherly love, charity, and altruism; when they actually practice charity; or when they criticize someone for a lack of altruism. So, it represents a ubiquitously distributed social rule and may be regarded as an implicit communal speech act. Related communal performatives are the moral principles of benevolence and compassion which likewise create and represent social institutions. There are innumerable social institutions that owe their existence to communal performatives.

We would like to advance here the view that medical knowledge too is a social institution created by a communal performative. The performative may be conceived of as a fragmented speech act like the following, which is widely distributed over the medical community in Western cultures.

The communal performative creating the medical knowledge institution:
We hereby declare that there is a unique way of possessing the capability to cure sick people, to prevent maladies, and to promote health, and we hereby call this way *medical knowledge*.

What promises to satisfy the first part of this declaration, i.e., to cure sick people and so on, will according to its second part be called medical knowledge. In other words, whether something is medical knowledge, is determined by the communal performative testimony above. It establishes medical knowledge as a social institution, call it the *medical knowledge institution*. Astrological babble and Ayurveda, for instance, are not approved by this social institution to be medical knowledge. By contrast, other entities such as the etiology of AIDS are approved. Below, we will discuss this approval processes.

In 1983, Dr. Luc Montagnier and his team at the Pasteur Institute in Paris published a paper claiming that the retrovirus LAV played a causative role in the genesis of AIDS (Barré-Sinoussi et al., 1983). They called the accused agent *lymphadenopathy-associated virus*, LAV for short, because they had isolated it from a lymph node of a patient with lymphadenopathy, i.e., a specific disease affecting lymph nodes. It would later be renamed HIV. Let α denote the statement "LAV causes AIDS":

$$\alpha \equiv \text{LAV causes AIDS.}$$

Suppose now that at time t_1 Dr. Robert Gallo at the Institute for Human Virology in Baltimore, Maryland, studies the paper by Montagnier et al. However, he doesn't accept the etiologic claim of the authors. Rather, he prefers his own, previously published assertion that AIDS is caused by the *human T-lymphotropic virus*, HTLV for short. Some time later, at time t_2, Montagnier and two colleagues of his visit Dr. Gallo in his laboratory in Baltimore to convince him that α. They tell him that α, and show him a variety of experimental recordings substantiating their claim. After some reflection, at time

t_3, Dr. Gallo agrees with Montagnier and his colleagues that α by saying "you are right, LAV causes AIDS". This agreement with the three French testifiers indicates that a *community of knowledge* has emerged consisting of Montagnier, his two French colleagues, and Robert Gallo such that they can now jointly state their collective intentionality "we know that α". Robert Gallo who prior to the constitution of this knowledge community was ignorant of LAV's causative role, now *knows that* α because he has become a member of a knowledge community that knows that α. That is, whether an individual has acquired a particular item of medical knowledge depends on whether she has acquired *membership in an epistemic-medical community*. Thus, an individual's possession of a particular item of propositional medical knowledge is a *social status*, like being married, bestowed upon her by the social institution of 'medical knowledge'. It can also be taken away in that she may at a later time communally be judged to lack that knowledge. Examples are malpractice suits and the withdrawal of a medical license.

To summarize, medical knowledge is a social institution like money and marriage. The possession of particular items of medical knowledge by an individual is a social status obtained from an epistemic-medical community, and thus an institutional fact. There are just as few solitary medical knowers as there are married bachelors. That means that private propositional medical knowledge cannot exist, i.e., medical knowledge that has only one knower and is unknowable or unknown by others. In a nutshell, there are no epistemic monads. The possession of propositional knowledge by an individual needs to be granted by the collective intentionality, i.e., "we know", of an epistemic community that is necessarily a polyad. Thus, to understand the nature of medical knowledge is to understand epistemic-medical communities, including their social and political structures and practices. This is exactly the point made by Ludwik Fleck in 1935 (see page 503).[102]

Communal medical knowledge

We distinguish between the following three types of group knowledge: common knowledge, distributed knowledge, and communal knowledge.

---

[102] The thesis above on the impossibility of private (medical) knowledge may be referred to as the *private knowledge argument*, analogous to Ludwig Wittgenstein's well-known private language argument against the assumption that a private language could or would exist. Wittgenstein introduces in section 243 of his *Philosophical Invesigations* the notion of a private language thus: "The individual words of this language are to refer to what can only be known to the person speaking; to his immediate, private sensations. So another person cannot understand the language". He then goes on to attack this idea in sections 244–271 to the effect that such a language would be unintelligible even to its supposed originator, and thus is impossible, since meaning is something essentially social and he would be unable to establish meanings for his own, 'private' words (Wittgenstein, 1953). See also Section 2.6 on page 46.

Common knowledge in a community is knowledge that each member of the community possesses. For example, that the organism consists of cells is common knowledge in medicine: "Every physician knows that the organism consists of cells". Note, however, that in some other branches such as epistemic logic and game theory which are concerned with multi-agent systems, there is another, deviant concept of common knowledge introduced by Lewis (1969) and later formalized by Aumann (1976). The epistemic logic touched upon in Section 27.3 is a single-agent logic, concerned only with reasoning about the knowledge of single agents. Multi-agent epistemic logic in artificial intelligence, however, tries in addition to provide methods of reasoning about knowledge possessed by members of a multi-agent system, i.e., a group. A human community is a group. Let α be a sentence describing a particular state of affairs. Lewis' concept of the common knowledge of α among a group means that each member of the group knows that α, and each knows that each knows that α, and so on. This notion of common knowledge used in game theory and multi-agent epistemic logic is based on the idea of unlimited iterability and embedding of a number of n individual knowledge operators $(K_a, K_b, K_c, \dots)$ of $n > 1$ members $a, b, c, \dots$ of a group. In some circumstances, e.g., communications and games such as the muddy children puzzle, it is said that agent a knows that agent b knows that agent c knows ...that α. Thus, we have $K_a\alpha, K_aK_b\alpha, K_aK_bK_c\alpha$, and so on. This, we are told, is *common knowledge* (Gochet and Gribomont, 2006, 106 and 169 ff.). The same holds for belief. For the logic of common knowledge and belief, and mutual knowledge and belief, see (Meggle, 2002a, 2002b).

Different groups in a community, however, may know different things. For example, in a medical school housing different specialties, research teams, and specialists we find different types of expert knowledge possessed by distinct groups. While cardiologists are experts of heart diseases and may not be very conversant with theories in psychiatry, psychiatrists are knowledgeable about depression and schizophrenia, but need the assistance of a cardiologist when one of their patients has serious heart problems. Medical knowledge is thus differently distributed over different groups in the medical community. We call such knowledge *distributed knowledge*, provided that there are at least two members whose knowledge is different from one another. Distributed knowledge in a community is the union of knowledge known by all members of the community. For instance, Dr. Adam knows that HIV is a retrovirus and Dr. Brown knows that atherosclerosis is a genetic disease. So, the knowledge distributed in the dyadic community {Dr. Adam, Dr. Brown} is {HIV is a retrovirus, atherosclerosis is a genetic disease}. Distributed knowledge brings with it the following surprising phenomenon:

It has been pointed out in the literature that there may exist some knowledge that is known only by the whole of a community without being known by any one of its individual members. Suppose, for example, that Dr. Adam knows that α and Dr. Brown knows that $a \to \beta$. While none of them individually knows that β, the community {Dr. Adam, Dr. Brown} consisting of these two persons of course knows that β because β classical-logically follows from their distributed knowledge. Such knowledge we may call the implicit knowledge of a community with respect to the logic used. The epistemic subject of the implicit knowledge is the community as a whole. In our present example, only the whole is entitled to say "we know that β". So, the epistemic whole is not reducible to the set of its members because no one individual and no one individually knows that β (cf. Hardwig, 1985, 349).[103]

The union of the distributed knowledge and implicit knowledge of a community yields its total knowledge, which we may call *communal knowledge*. Note that communal knowledge is logic-relative because different logics elicit different implicit knowledge from a given distributed knowledge. It goes without saying that communal knowledge is 'greater than the sum of its parts'. This emergent surplus lends to communal knowledge an expert quality unattainable by an individual alone. We may find communal knowledge of some sort in the knowledge base of a medical expert system that is elicited from different experts. It would be interesting to inquire into whether the so-called *clinical practice guidelines* represent elements of communal knowledge (see page 581).

11.5.4 Social Constructivism

Science studies, which we touched upon on page 511, began in the early 1970s and brought a new approach to thinking about science and scientific knowledge in that the process of scientific research and reasoning became subject to microsociological investigations. Since then, a vast amount of data concerning how science is done, has been collected by sociological analyses of laboratories in diverse research centers from nuclear physics to molecular biology and genomics. Works of this type are called 'ethnographic studies of laboratory life' by a variety of sociologists of knowledge, e.g., (Knorr Cetina, 1981, 2003; Latour, 1987; Latour and Woolgar 1986; Lynch M, 1985; Pickering, 1992, 1995).

The microsociological data together with philosophical inquiries into the relationships between scientific research and its social environment suggest that scientific concepts and knowledge are *social constructs*. That means that (i) they are not prepackaged natural entities of the world; (ii) they are man-made; specifically, (iii) they are not made by individual scientists like a desk can be made by a single carpenter; rather, they are products of social groups, institutions, and practices, and of interactions and negotiations between social groups, be they research teams or larger scientific communities and associations, boards of committees, editorial boards of journals, etc. Accordingly, this

---

[103] The property of the community just described may be called its *epistemic closure* that entails the ability of an epistemic subject *to know that* β *if she knows that* α and $\alpha \rightarrow \beta$. Because of the plurality of logics, however, it is questionable whether such epistemic closure, and thus the concept of implicit knowledge, is generally acceptable. For the plurality of logics, see Section 17.1 on page 675

view of science has come to be termed *social constructivism*, sometimes also called social constructionism. The forerunners of this view are Ludwik Fleck and Thomas Kuhn, discussed in Section 11.5.2, and in addition the former Soviet developmental psychologist Lev Vygotsky (1986).[104]

Social constructivism leads to relativism, and thus, anti-realism because it implies: Since scientific concepts and knowledge are social constructs, they depend on human culture, i.e., on social, psychological, economical, religious, moral, and historical factors; as culture-dependent cognitive structures they cannot, and do not, represent an objective reality; on this account, it does not make sense to postulate and defend on the basis of scientific concepts and knowledge the 'real existence' of those entities scientific knowledge is talking about. This message of social constructivism, when it is taken seriously, would have momentous consequences for the choice of goals, morals, and methodology of doing science. But the idea causes dismay among those philosophers and scientists who advocate metaphysical, semantic, and epistemic realism and objectivism in science. For instance, Ian Hacking derisively dismisses the entire approach and accuses social constructivists of mental blindness because they would ignore real and objective facts of nature by using "the metaphor of social construction" (Hacking, 2003, 35). Its severe disparagement by such an exceptionally gifted and prominent philosopher of science demonstrates that the idea of social constructivism is not well understood in the scholarly world. This is presumably due to the lack of a clear concept of social constructivism. Since it is highly relevant to medical epistemology, we have a good reason to clearly set down the meaning of the term. To this end, we will explicate the notion of social constructivism in order to show how it may be sensibly and profitably applied to medicine.

Two versions of social constructivism may be distinguished, a weak and a strong one. The weak version holds that scientific language and knowledge are influenced by social factors. This is a truism that does not deserve further discussion. According to the strong version, however, social milieus and factors are the primary sources and forces in the genesis and development of scientific languages and knowledge. Social constructivism proper is the latter, strong version. With the aid of the terminology introduced in preceding sections it may be construed in the following way.

We have argued that what is called scientific knowledge is a social status of scientists characterized by collective intentionalities of the form "we

---

[104] Lev Semyonovich Vygotsky (1896–1934) was born in Orsha in Belarus. He studied law at Moscow University and worked as a teacher in Homel in Belarus. As of 1924, he worked at the Moscow Institute of Psychology on a couple of projects such as developmental psychology, pedagogy, linguistics, and psychopathology. Deviating from Piaget's cognitive constructivism, he held the view that learning cannot be separated from its social context, and considered learning as a social process. Until his premature death from tuberculosis in 1934, he investigated the impact of social and cultural factors on learning, language, consciousness, and thought (see Pass, 2004).

know" and "we believe". As such, it is an institutional fact, i.e., a social fact created by social institutions, especially by the institution of knowledge, and by epistemic interactions between individuals as well as communities. Based on this construal, we may explicate the concept of social constructivism by a set-theoretical predicate that may easily be applied to medical as well as other types of scientific knowledge:

Definition 148 (Social constructivism: special). ξ *is a* social-constructivistic structure *iff there are A and B such that:*

    1. $\xi = \langle A, B \rangle$,
    2. A is a set of social facts,
    3. B is set of social facts,
    4. Some elements of A cause an element of B.

That is to say: When you encounter a set of social facts, say a series X of interactions between members of a research team such that these interactions, through some publications reporting "this and that", bring about another set Y of social facts consisting of we-intentionalities of the type "we know, or we believe, that this and that is the case", then $\langle X, Y \rangle$ is a social-constructivistic structure. The case of Dr. Montagnier *vs.* Dr. Gallo sketched on page 520 is an example. What social constructivism maintains is that the production of scientific knowledge consists of such social-constructivistic structures. Since scientific knowledge as a product of such causal structures is part of the B component of the set-theoretical predicate 148, it is a social construct.

    We may generalize the definition above to also cover an additional category of objects and processes, usually called 'artifacts', as social constructs that are not knowledge, but *things* that are nevertheless constructed by we-intentions of social groups, e.g., Spacelab, the Eiffel Tower, electron microscopes, fiber endoscopes, transplants, drugs, diagnoses and recoveries through teamwork, and so on:

Definition 149 (Social constructivism: general). ξ *is a* social-constructivistic structure *iff there are A and B such that:*

    1. $\xi = \langle A, B \rangle$,
    2. A is a set of social facts,
    3. B is a set of social facts, objects, or processes,
    4. Some elements of A cause an element of B.

In light of this understanding one can see that social constructivism in fact has a firm basis and is not merely a metaphor. Contrary to some misconceptions, social constructivism does not explain "objective facts of nature in a strange fashion" since it does not explain natural facts at all. Rather, it explains man-made facts, i.e., social facts and artifacts, by other social facts as their causes. This characteristic is reflected in the two definitions above in which some social facts figure as causes, i.e., set A, having other social facts or artifacts as their effects, i.e., set B.

For instance, a social-constructivistic claim about a particular item of scientific knowledge such as the AIDS framework says that this framework is an intended application of the set-theoretical predicates above, i.e., a social-constructivistic structure. In other words, it claims that the following subjects are socially constructed: (1) the concept of AIDS; (2) the concept of HIV; (3) the assertion that there is a causal relationship between HIV and AIDS; and (4) the assertion that HIV cannot be defended against by the human organism; and so on. It does not claim that "AIDS and HIV do not exist objectively and are social fantasies". As regards our present example of AIDS, the history and current practice of AIDS research demonstrate that all investigations in this field have been conducted, and are being conducted, by communities, i.e., by national and international collaboration of numerous research teams, hospitals, patients, conferences, funding organizations, state authorities, publishers, and other groups distributed over the earth. Likewise, the results of the investigations are discussed, published, criticized, accepted, rejected, corrected, and so on by communities. This is indeed a social construction of knowledge par excellence where testimony plays a central role. The AIDS framework, say the theory of AIDS, is neither created by individuals in isolation nor is it a pure product of analyzing 'how things are' without any testimony provided by others and without any communal decisions.

To give another example, consider a social constructivist such as Andrew Pickering, whose work is also disparaged by Ian Hacking (2003, 68 ff.). Pickering claims that Quarks are social constructs. However, he is not denying the existence of Quarks. He only considers the theory of Quarks, on which the existence claim "there are Quarks" is based, as a product of particular social practices called collaborative research (Pickering, 1984).

As a final example, recall the Helicobacter theory of peptic ulcer disease sketched on pages 490–492. We may also conceive of the genesis of this theory as a social-constructivistic process. Before Robin Warren and Barry Marshall started working on the Helicobacter theory in the 1980s, spiral bacteria had already been discovered in the stomach by different scholars at least nine times since 1892 (Blaser, 2005; Konturek et al., 1996; Kidd and Modlin, 1998; Marshall, 2002b). However, their discoveries were neglected and 'forgotten' for different reasons. The primary reason for this was the lack of adequate technology, without which they were unable to directly observe peptic ulcer diseases, to take bioptic samples of the damaged gastric epithelium, and to produce cultures of the bacteria for microscopic analysis. Thanks to fiber endoscopes, gastroscopy began in the 1960s and was in general use in gastroenterology by the 1970s; this played a crucial role in the success of Warren and Marshall's collective intention to collaborate and to thereby initiate the international process of the social construction of the Helicobacter theory in the 1980s. Note that the development of fiber endoscopes and fiber gastroscopy, which made this research possible, was itself a social construction by the collaborative work of different specialties and specialists such as metallurgy, mechanics, optics, fiber optics, and medicine. See Definition 149 above. In a nutshell, fiber endoscopes and fiber gastroscopy are social constructs.

The social construction of the Helicobacter theory occurred through intense collaborative research done by a huge international network of research teams. The network started with the core group in the Royal Perth Hospital in Western Australia consisting of Robin Warren (pathologist), Barry Marshall (trainee in gastroenterology), David McGechie (microbiologist), and John Armstrong (electron microscopist). In their joint paper, Marshall and Warren thank eleven colleagues and several units for assistance and collaboration (Marshall and Warren, 1984, 1314). These persons represent different specialties such as gastroenterology, pathology, microbiology, and medical statistics. Marshall's heroic self-experiment again required the assistance and advice of several experts whom he thanks in the report (Marshall et al., 1985, 439). This latter work marks the spread of research among research teams distributed over the earth. Animal experimentation with Helicobacter is now being conducted. Biopsies are taken of almost every patient suffering from gastritis, duodenitis, and peptic ulcer disease. Therapeutic experiments with antibiotics are undertaken. Conferences are organized and take place. More and more publications on the subject appear in numerous national and international journals. Most of the papers are multi-authored, carrying the names of at least five authors. There are also publications authored by research groups rather than identified contributors, e.g., the multicenter study by EUROGAST (EUROGAST, 1993). For more details, see (Thagard, 1999).

It need not be stressed again that personal contacts and communication, conferences, journals, editors, referees, funding agencies, medical schools, hospitals, health authorities, many other institutions, and their interaction have played important roles in the generation and distribution of reports, judgments, criticisms, and hypotheses on the issues related to Helicobacter pylori and peptic ulcer disease. The brief history above vividly demonstrates how the Helicobacter theory emerged and developed by collaborative work, testimony, and agreement, i.e., in a social process essentially characterized by the collective intentionality of the participating groups in the form of "we want to know how the peptic ulcer disease develops", "we work together", "we know that hydrochloric acid is produced in the gastric epithelium", "we will analyze the bioptic material by an electron microscope", "we will find out how to inquire into the causative role of Helicobacter", and so on. All these we-intentions are social facts. They eventually generated the new social fact "we now know that Helicobacter pylori is the cause of peptic ulcer disease" expressing the researchers' collectively acquired knowledge about the causative role of Helicobacter. It is this creation of some social facts by some other social facts, i.e., a social-causal process, that we called social construction in Definitions 148–149 above. And when the construct is medical knowledge, as is the case in the present example, we are allowed to speak of its social construction.

The social-causal process of construction itself may be conceived of as a communal endeavor to search for, and to create, a *path* from an initial state of ignorance ("what are the causes of the peptic ulcer disease?") to a final state of knowing called "scientific knowledge", e.g., "peptic ulcer disease is caused by Helicobacter pylori infection". Let us call such a path over intermediate stages of the research process, that leads from ignorance to knowledge, an *epistemic path*. An epistemic path always consists of the concatenation of a number of $n > 1$ edges, $A_1 \rightarrow A_2 \rightarrow \cdots \rightarrow A_n$, leading from the initial state of ignorance, A_1, over intermediate states of partial knowledge to final knowledge, A_n. A path like this obviously does not exist 'in the world out there' prior to research. It is an artifact, and as such, contingent. In contrast to Ian Hacking's epistemology (Hacking, 2003, 31), there are no natural, inevitable, and necessary epistemic paths from ignorance to scientific knowledge. This is why epistemic paths are never discovered. They are always invented because they do not exist prior to their construction. And their invention is always a social achievement and never accomplished by individuals.[105]

In addition to research teams working on the invention of epistemic paths, there are also governmental, political, and quasi-political communities and authorities such as health departments and ministries, World Health Organization, American Medical Association, German Medical Association, and other national and international organizations that actively participate in the social construction or destruction of an epistemic artifact by partisanship. They publicly recommend either acceptance or rejection of the artifact and must therefore be viewed as social-epistemic institutions which make both *epistemological and epistemic* decisions. Most important in this respect is, for example, the role played by the U.S. National Institutes of Health (NIH), an authority of the U.S. Department of Health and Human Services located in Bethesda, Maryland. They have an "NIH Consensus Development Program" that has been operating since 1977 and has produced about 120 Consensus Statements until now concerning the management of different diseases, e.g., peptic ulcer disease, breast cancer, hepatitis, and others. Consensus Statements are produced by organizing consensus conferences. Panel members are

---

[105] What has been said above about the social nature of knowledge is confirmed by microsociological studies of scientific research. See, e.g., (Knorr Cetina, 2003, 159–191). Karin Knorr Cetina demonstrates that in high-energy physics both the individual as an epistemic subject, and individuating authorship conventions, have disappeared. Work and publication have been taken over by internationally distributed collectives. There are large-scale "mega-experiments" in high-energy physics, referred to as "post-traditional communitarian structures" by Knorr Cetina (ibid., 159 ff.), with about 2000 international participants over the course of twenty years. Papers reporting experimental results list all members of the collaboration on the first page(s) of the paper. This sometimes amounts to two or three printed pages with several hundred, alphabetically ordered names without any indication of the originators of the research or of main contributors (ibid., 166). We shall confirm this observation by our presentation of the international research project and process in the *European Organization for Nuclear Research*, CERN, in Section 12.2 on page 535.

chosen from different disciplines. For instance, regarding our present example of Helicobacter pylori, a consensus conference was organized in January of 1994 in Washington, D.C., to examine and to develop a consensus on whether or not to accept the etiologic hypothesis that Helicobacter pylori caused peptic ulcer disease. Several groups of experts were invited to present pros and cons. After twenty-two presentations the panel of the NIH Consensus Development Conference encouraged on January 9, 1994, the acceptance of the hypothesis by recommending that Helicobacter-infected patients with peptic ulcer disease should receive antimicrobial treatment (NIH, 1994).

The NIH consensus and recommendation had an enormous impact on the epistemic attitude of physicians and their professional communities worldwide. The antimicrobial treatment proved generally successful, which contributed greatly to the current opinion that Helicobacter causes peptic diseases of the stomach and duodenum. So, the nosology of peptic diseases, i.e., of the inflammation and ulcer diseases of the stomach and duodenum, has changed, moving from the psychosomatic category to the category of infectious diseases. That means, in the terminology of the structuralistic metatheory discussed in Section 9.4.2, that they have become intended applications of the theory of infectious diseases. Thus, their categorization as infectious diseases was a massive social decision. This example shows the society's impact on nosological systems.

Not only medical knowledge, but also the medium of its representation and communication, i.e., medical language, develops as a complex social construct. We saw in Section 2.1 that medical language is an extended natural language that emerges from workaday language by incorporating additional technical terms. This is achieved by introducing new, individual scientific concepts such as "membrane depolarization" and "AIDS", on the one hand; and nomenclatures and terminologies of specialties such as anatomy, clinical chemistry, pharmacology, pathology, and nosology, on the other. The latter are constructed and recommended for use by special committees and communities, e.g., the anatomical nomenclature as a system of names for use in describing the human body and its parts; and the international classification of diseases, ICD, as a system of names for codifying symptoms and diseases (FCAT, 1998; WHO, 2004). Such a system of names fixes the class of entities that are supposed to 'exist' in the respective domain (see Chapter 19). What is not included in the proposed system of names, is neither taught to nor learned by medical students, and is therefore not included in their knowledge. Knowledge is pursued and acquired only about those objects and relations that are listed in the nomenclature and terminology of a domain. Thus, medical knowledge is also conditioned by the social construction of medical language.

What the above considerations suggest, is the awareness that social constructivism is an anti-realistic epistemology insofar as it underscores the primacy of the social sphere and culture in scientific cognition and knowledge production. It is thus an anti-individualistic, i.e., social, epistemology and considers scientific language and knowledge to be *communal artifacts* and not achievements of clever individuals discovering what entities exist in 'the world out there'. In support of the constructivist view we shall demonstrate in Chapter 14 that the fundamental concept of medicine, i.e., the concept of disease, may be conceived of as a social construct. For this reason, the areas of medicine that focus on disease, such as nosology, pathology, diagnosis and therapy, turn out to be socially grounded. That means that any system of medicine practiced in a particular society and culture is something dependent on the peculiarities of that society and culture; on the complex and distinctive net of its institutions, values, religious views, political goals, and laws; and on its traditions and economic confines. Viewed from an epistemological perspective, no system of medicine will be superior to another one. They are epistemologically equivalent. Therefore, something other than epistemological criteria is needed to comparatively evaluate distinct systems of medicine.

11.6 Summary

To inquire into the semantics of medical knowledge we discussed the classical concept of knowledge, that defines knowledge as justified true belief, and its problematic character. We also briefly sketched the main theories of truth and justification to show that medical knowledge is not knowledge in the classical sense. Large parts of it are not verifiable, and there is as yet no satisfactory concept of empirical justification to characterize medical knowledge as empirically justified. Other concepts of knowledge are needed that do justice to what is called knowledge in medicine. We analyzed the question of whether medical knowledge and concepts refer to some human-independent realities, or whether they are human constructs, and as such, socially conditioned. We gave cogent arguments in support of the latter alternative based on social and communitarian epistemology. Medical knowledge turned out a social construct with the individual knowledge of a knower being a social status lent by an epistemic community. We thus showed that social constructivism may provide a viable tool for the analysis of medical-epistemological issues.

12

Technoconstructivism

12.0 Introduction

The nature of empirical-scientific knowledge in general, and of medical knowledge in particular, is currently undergoing a pervasive transformation likely to mark the end of epistemology, including the type developed in preceding chapters. In what follows, we shall outline this imminent transformation by presenting a *theory of technoconstructivism*. Because of the significance of the issue we must be painstakingly precise.

A novel conception of experimental-scientific knowledge will be advanced to argue that this type of knowledge is more and more becoming an analogue of technical products such as automobiles, shoes, and socks. Like these objects, it is increasingly being engineered by machines in specialized factories called research laboratories. Computers, artificial intelligence machinery, the Internet, and other species of machines are rapidly networking and changing our world, thereby (i) outsourcing scientists and their communities as creators of scientific knowledge, and (ii) transforming knowledge gain through scientific experimentation into a branch of technology. From this perspective, it is apparent that experimental-scientific knowledge as a technical product will need just as little epistemology as automobiles, shoes, and socks do (Sadegh-Zadeh, 2000d, 2001b–c).[106]

---

[106] The inspiration for the present theory of technoconstructivism came from my understanding of Karin Knorr Cetina's work on the sociology of scientific research in the 1980s (Knorr Cetina, 1981). I also profited from her recent work on the same topic (Knorr Cetina, 2003). However, she is not a technoconstructivist herself and would certainly not endorse my view. The following scholars have also influenced my philosophizing on the relationships between scientific experiments, human agency, and technology in one way or another since my youth: Hugo Dingler (1928), Klaus Holzkamp (1968), Jürgen Habermas (1968a, 1968b). The present framework emerged in the context of my thinking on the globalization of the machine and the emergence of Machina sapiens (Sadegh-Zadeh, 2000d, 150–158).

K. Sadegh-Zadeh, *Handbook of Analytic Philosophy of Medicine*,
Philosophy and Medicine 113, DOI 10.1007/978-94-007-2260-6_12,
© Springer Science+Business Media B.V. 2012

In preceding chapters, we studied the reasons why the classical concept of knowledge as justified true belief is problematic. To better understand the significance and peculiarities of medical knowledge, we presented alternative views such as the communitarian-performative theory of knowledge and social constructivism. Both the classical concept as well as these alternative views still rest on the assumption, however, that scientific knowledge originates with scientists and their communities. Accordingly, the prevailing view on the genesis of experimental-scientific knowledge is that scientists and their communities determine the subjects, goals, and methods of their inquiries, design scientific experiments, and thanks to their mental and intellectual capacities they are the creators of that knowledge. This age-old, basic epistemological postulate will be challenged in what follows. Specifically, we shall offer a new perspective showing that what is called experimental-scientific knowledge today, is something *produced by machines* simply because scientific experimentation has become a global technology of knowledge. We have therefore termed this view *technoconstructivism*. In this technical production process, scientists are more and more assuming the role of mere factory workers, mechanics so to speak, resembling other industrial factory workers who operate in factories that produce, for example, automobiles, shoes, or socks. Hence, experimental-scientific knowledge belongs to the category of technical products. On this account, it cannot be expected or required to possess such epistemic qualities as truth, verisimilitude, verifiability, justifiability, justifiedness, probability, plausibility, reliability, falsifiability, and the like. Rather, it has exclusively non-epistemic features such as practical value, moral value, monetary value, uselessness, harmfulness, damnableness, and others.

To propound the above conception of medical-experimental knowledge, we will now demonstrate in turn that an experimental-scientific laboratory represents a factory housing *epistemic assembly lines* and *epistemic machines* in the guise of experiments, and produces entities that carry an ancient misnomer as their name, "knowledge". Our discussion thus divides into the following five sections:

12.1 Experiments as Epistemic Assembly Lines
12.2 Epistemic Machines
12.3 Epistemic Factories
12.4 The Global Knowledge-Making Engine
12.5 The Industrialization of Knowledge.

12.1 Experiments as Epistemic Assembly Lines

To introduce a few key notations for use in our analyses below, consider first a simple biomedical experiment on the neurophysiology of epilepsy that may be roughly described as follows:

Cell cultures of the hippocampal neurons of mice or rats' brains are prepared in a particular way. Extracellular and intracellular microelectrodes are placed in these cells to examine in vitro the inhibitory effect of Gamma Amino Butyric Acid (GABA) on neuronal spikes. Different types of apparatuses are used to produce and record the brain cell spikes, e.g., an assembled open recording chamber with 64 pre-amplifiers, a 64-channel multi-amplifier, a real-time signal visualization machine, an electroencephalograph, and networked computers for graphical and statistical analyses. Hippocampal cells are stimulated and their bioelectrical activity is recorded and analyzed before and after the administration of GABA to examine the nature and extent of its inhibitory effect. The experimental data obtained are then analyzed and interpreted by the experimenter to produce a publication that represents and presents an item of epileptological knowledge.[107]

The experiment has been designed in the neurophysiology department of a medical school to investigate the neuronal and synaptic genesis of epilepsy. It will be conducted about 100 times. To explain, we shall use the following, general notations:

- the entities that enter the experiment to be analyzed, we call the set of *materials,* denoted *M;* in the present example, *M* is a set of hippocampal neurons of rats' brains;
- the EEG reading of their bioelectrical activity is referred to as the set of experimental *data,* denoted *D;*
- in order to obtain the data set *D,* the materials *M* are manipulated by performing some operations "to see how the materials react"; in the present example, hippocampal neurons are stimulated by electrical current, and their bioelectrical activity is recorded by an EEG; since by such operations data are produced, we call them data production operations, or *production operations* for short; even the simple recording of data is a production operation, i.e., the operation of recording; the

---

[107] The hippocampus is a subcortical brain part located in the medial temporal lobe in the forebrain and is considered part of the limbic system (see page 138). It plays a major role in the genesis of epileptic convulsions. A microelectrode is a thin electrode with tip dimensions of a few micromillimeters to allow nondestructive puncturing of the intra- and intercellular space for the purpose of recording electrical potentials, and measuring other parameters such as ions and pH levels of cells, etc. (A micromillimeter or nanometer is one billionth of a meter.) Pre-amplifiers and amplifiers are programmable machines for current generation and multi-electrode stimulation, and also for amplifying, filtering, sorting, and analyzing the bioelectrical signals of individual cells and cell ensembles from the brain, retina, spinal cord, heart, and muscle tissue. An *electroencephalograph,* EEG, graphically records such bioelectrical activity (from the Greek terms ἐνκέφαλος (enkephalos) meaning *brain,* and γραφή (graphe) meaning *document*). The EEG readings of animals or human beings with epilepsy or other convulsion disorders display bursts of electrical activity called *spikes.* GABA is a chemical substance that acts as a major inhibitory neurotransmitter in the central nervous system and inhibits both pre- and postsynaptic neuronal processes.

set of all *production* *o*perations performed in an experiment is denoted
PO;

- eventually the data set D is analyzed and interpreted by the experimenter; her interpretation published in articles and books is usually
viewed as experimental knowledge, denoted K. In the present example,
K describes how neuronal spikes emerge, how they cause convulsions,
how they are evoked by electrical stimuli, and are inhibited by GABA,
and so on;

- the union of data set D and knowledge K constitutes the experimental
results, denoted R; that is, $R = D \cup K$.

Customarily, an experiment is viewed as an arrangement of suitable scenarios
and devices to conduct systematic studies on objects and occurrences whose
nature is deemed to be independent of the experimenter. So, the experimenter
herself is considered an impartial observer. Experimental knowledge is thus
supposed to be something *objective* and *true* about natural phenomena that
the experimenter *discovers*. This popular view put into circulation by the
early British empiricists in the seventeenth century is terribly wrong. Recall
our concept of experiment according to which an experiment is a designed,
interventional study. On this account, we consider the experimenter not as an
uninvolved observer, but rather as an active manipulator and engineer of the
observed. For example, in the neurophysiological experiment above, the experimenter uses amplifiers to produce different types of electrical stimuli that
are presented to animal neurons by microelectrodes to evoke neuronal spikes.
It is the experimenter who has given rise to these spikes by manipulating the
electrochemical processes in the neurons under study. The phenomena that
she will write about in her publication, are not pre-existent states of affairs
that she discovered. For instance, the relationships between the frequency of
electrical stimuli and spikes, on the one hand; and the reduction of these spikes
by administering GABA, on the other, are created by the experimental setup
and production operations to the effect that experimental data as well as the
neurophysiological knowledge presented by their analysis and interpretation,
i.e., $D \cup K$, are technical artifacts *produced by conducting the very experiment.*
The possible world in which the experimental events occur is an artificially
created one.

Roughly, our thesis of technoconstructivism says that an experiment such
as the one described above is an epistemic machine that produces the experimental knowledge K. In order to detail and advance this view in the next
section, we will conceive of an experiment as a compound construction, i.e., a
system, whose constituent parts are customarily ordered in a scientific publication in the following sequence:

Objective, **materials, methods, results,** conclusion.

This array faithfully represents, or mirrors, an *assembly line* where a set of
materials, *M,* is subjected to some methods of intervention and inquiry, here

referred to as production operations PO, to yield some results, R. We have seen above that the results R are composed of (i) a data set D obtained by experimental records, and (ii) the experimental knowledge K produced by interpreting those data. Thus, $R = D \cup K$. Note that:

   a. M is a simple or compound set of materials, $M = M_1 \cup \ldots \cup M_k$,
   b. PO is a simple or compound set of production operations, $PO = PO_1 \cup \ldots \cup PO_m$,
   c. D is a simple or compound set of data, $D = D_1 \cup \ldots \cup D_n$,
   d. $R = D \cup K$ is the set of results

with $k, m, n \geq 1$. The three components of an experiment, i.e., M, PO and R, constitute an assembly line such that $R = D \cup K$. Since the assembly line supplies *knowledge, K*, we have termed it an epistemic assembly line. By virtue of this feature, an experiment will turn out an epistemic machine.

12.2 Epistemic Machines

As mentioned previously, systematic, experimental research emerged in the seventeenth century in the wake of the so-called Scientific Revolution, which would later be recognized as the commencement of British empiricism and the natural sciences. Its gradual evolution to a technology of knowledge must be considered unavoidable because we can prove that an experiment is indeed a machine in the strict sense of this term. Before we proceed to the proof, consider first as an example the Large Hadron Collider (LHC) in the European Organization for Nuclear Research, usually referred to as CERN. It is a giant particle accelerator at the Franco-Swiss border near Geneva placed in a circular tunnel with a circumference of 27 kilometers that is buried around 50 to 175 m underground (Figure 63).

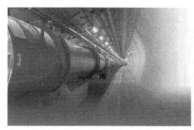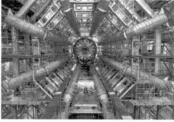

Fig. 63. Large Hadron Collider (LHC) near Geneva. How the experiment-machine produces data and knowledge is discussed in the body text. The photographs are published with the permission of CERN

LHC was built by CERN in collaboration with over 10,000 scientists and engineers from hundreds of laboratories and universities in over 100 countries.

It is an experimental setting to test some of the central predictions of particle physics (Halpern, 2009; Lincoln, 2009).[108] The experiment started on September 10, 2008. After only nine days, however, it had to be stopped due to serious faults in the machine that damaged a number of superconducting magnets. It restarted in October 2009. "It will produce roughly 15 petabytes, i.e., 15 million gigabytes, of data annually – enough to fill more than 1,7 million dual-layer DVDs a year. Thousands of scientists around the world want to access and analyze the data, so CERN is collaborating with institutions in 33 different countries to operate a distributed computing and data storage infrastructure: the LHC Computing Grid. Data from the LHC experiments is distributed around the globe, with a primary backup recorded on tape at CERN. After initial processing, these data are distributed to eleven large computer centers – in Canada, France, Germany, Italy, the Netherlands, the Nordic countries, Spain, Taipei, UK, and two sites in the USA – with sufficient storage capacity for a large fraction of the data, and with round-the-clock support for the computing grid".[109]

By visiting a laboratory of neurophysiology, hematology, pharmacology, or pathology we may easily see that a medical experiment today is also an instance of a highly sophisticated technology of knowledge production. It will be reconstructed here as an epistemic machine in two steps. First, we shall represent the epistemic assembly line, discussed in the previous section, as a *production system*. Second, we shall show that from the perspective of automata theory, such a production system is indeed a machine. Since it produces knowledge, we call it an *epistemic machine*. Thus our argument will take the following two steps:

12.2.1 An Experiment is a Production System
12.2.2 An Experiment is an Epistemic Machine.

12.2.1 An Experiment is a Production System

As defined on page 122, a production system is an ordered pair of the form $\langle \{M, R\}, PO \rangle$ such that M is a set of *materials*, R is a set of *products*, and PO is a set of *production operations* whose application to M yields R, i.e.,

---

[108] The acronym "CERN" originally stood, in French, for *Conseil Européen pour la Recherche Nucléaire* (European Organization for Nuclear Research) to refer to a European laboratory for the study of the atomic nucleus. After the CERN convention was ratified by the 12 funding Western-European countries (Belgium, Denmark, France, Federal Republic of Germany, Greece, Italy, the Netherlands, Norway, Sweden, Switzerland, United Kingdom), the *European Organization for Nuclear Research* officially came into being on September 29, 1954. The provisional CERN was dissolved but the acronym remained. Have a look at CERN here http://public.web.cern.ch/public/. Last accessed November 1, 2010.

[109] See http://public.web.cern.ch/public/en/LHC/Computing-en.html. Last accessed November 1, 2010.

$PO(M) = R$. For example, a bakery is a production system of the form $\langle\{\{flour, water\}, bread\}, bread\text{-}baking\rangle$ in which by applying specific production operations of bread-baking, bread is produced from the materials flour and water, i.e., bread-baking($\{$flour, water$\}$) = bread. In the present context, we will use biomedical experiments as our examples, although our theory covers the class of all experiments.

A biomedical experiment as an assembly line, as outlined in Section 12.1, is a production system of the form $\langle\{M, R\}, PO\rangle$ in which the set M of materials is provided by the subjects of the experiment, e.g., chemical substances, cells, tissues, animals and the like; and the set R of products is $R = D \cup K$, i.e., the data-knowledge union $D \cup K$ produced from M by the production operations PO. These production operations comprise the experimental equipment, also including the experimenters. In an experiment as a production system of the form:

$$\langle\{M, R\}, PO\rangle \tag{125}$$

the components M, R, and PO may in general be conceived of in the following fashion:

1. Materials M: The set of materials, M, consists of a number of objects or processes that enter the experiment as *input* to be analyzed, e.g., atoms, molecules, genes, cells, tissues, animals, patients, etc. In our epilepsy example above, the materials M comprised hippocampal neurons of rats or mice.

2. The product R: The product, R, consists of (i) a set D of collected data such as neuronal spikes, blood counts, heart rate, spectroscopic images, and so on obtained from the materials M by applying some of the production operations, PO; and (ii) the experimental knowledge K produced from data D by applying some additional production operations such as statistics, reflecting, and thinking to analyze and interpret the data. Thus, $R = D \cup K$. In our above epilepsy example, the data set D consisted of EEG readings of hippocampal neurons replete with spikes evoked by electrical stimulation of neurons and inhibition of spikes by administering GABA. Knowledge K was presented in several published articles on the neurophysiology of epilepsy.

3. Production operations PO: This is the experimental equipment consisting of devices and experimental techniques used, including the design of the experiment and the algorithm according to which the whole experiment is conducted. The experimenters too constitute a part of PO, be they scientists or their technical assistants. They are highly specialized operators in the production of the experimental results. In our above experiment on epilepsy, production operations comprise, among the experimenters, the application of a variety of apparatuses such as amplifiers, microelectrodes, electroencephalographs, GABA, etc. We partition the large set PO of an experiment into two subsets, PO_1 and

PO_2, such that $PO = PO_1 \cup PO_2$. The first subset, PO_1, is applied to the set of materials, M, to yield the data set D, while the second subset, PO_2, is applied to this data set itself to analyze and interpret them so as to construct the experimental knowledge, K. That is, $PO_1(M) = D$ and $PO_2(D) = K$. Thus, experimental knowledge K emerges by the application of the operation composition $PO_2 \circ PO_1$ to experimental materials: $K = PO_2 \circ PO_1(M)$. For example, PO_1 may be the employment of different devices such as instruments and machines, particular surgical operations to prepare the experimental animals, various inscription techniques such as measurements and recordings to obtain inscriptions, e.g., electroencephalographic recordings. PO_2 may consist of rule-directed procedures, the application of statistical and other mathematical methods and software, antecedently available knowledge, conceptual frameworks, theories, logics of different type, and so on.

An experiment as a production system of the form $\langle \{M, R\}, PO \rangle$ has thus been formally refined to yield the structure:

$$\langle M, D, K, PO_1, PO_2 \rangle \tag{126}$$

with $D \cup K = R$ and $PO_1 \cup PO_2 = PO$. The following definition will finalize our intuitive considerations.

Definition 150 (Experiment). *ξ is an experiment iff there are M, D, K, PO_1, and PO_2 such that:*

1. *$\xi = \langle M, D, K, PO_1, PO_2 \rangle$,*
2. *M is a non-empty set of materials;*
3. *PO_1 and PO_2 are sets of production operations;*
4. *D is a set of data obtained by applying PO_1 to M, i.e., $PO_1(M) = D$;*
5. *K is experimental knowledge obtained by applying PO_2 to D, i.e., $PO_2(D) = K$. So, $K = PO_2(PO_1(M)) = PO_2 \circ PO_1(M)$.*

This definition implies the following corollary which says that some production systems are experiments:

Corollary 9 (Some production systems are experiments). *A production system of the form $\langle \{M, R\}, PO \rangle$ is an experiment iff there is a quintuple $\langle M, D, K, PO_1, PO_2 \rangle$ such that:*

1. *$\langle M, D, K, PO_1, PO_2 \rangle$ is an experiment according to Definition 150;*
2. *$R = D \cup K$;*
3. *$PO = PO_1 \cup PO_2$.*

12.2.2 An Experiment is an Epistemic Machine

With the above considerations in mind, we may now demonstrate that an experiment in general and a medical experiment in particular is a machine.

To this end, we have to be aware that (i) an experiment can always be reconstructed as a structure of the form $\langle M, D, K, PO_1, PO_2 \rangle$; and (ii) the materials M that enter the investigation, may be interpreted as *input* into the system, e.g., the hippocampal neurons in the above-mentioned epilepsy experiment. The application of PO_1 to the input M to obtain data set D, and the application of PO_2 to data set D to obtain the experimental knowledge K, constitute the process of knowledge production by the experiment. Knowledge K produced in this way and delivered to the outside world, is the system's *output*. Thus, the whole experiment will turn out an *input-output machine* like a computer or automobile. The latter uses gasoline as input and produces kinetic energy, heat, electrical energy, and exhaust fumes as output. Since an experiment-machine supplies knowledge as its main output, it will be termed a knowledge-making machine, or an *epistemic machine* for short.

The categorization of experiments as a particular type of machine is by no means a metaphor. Our thesis says that a scientific experiment is a model for the set-theoretical predicate "ξ is a finite-state machine" or "ξ is a finite-state fuzzy machine", introduced by Definitions 29–30 on page 129. We have seen that a crisp, finite-state machine or automaton is a quintuple of the form:

$$\langle I, Z, O, S, OR \rangle$$

such that I is a finite set of *input states;* Z is a finite set of *internal states;* O is a finite set of *output states;* S is a *state-transition relation* that associates input states with internal states; and OR is an *output relation* that associates internal states with output states. In line with this concept, the five components of our quintuple:

$$\langle M, D, K, PO_1, PO_2 \rangle$$

in 126 above, which we obtained by refining an experiment $\langle \{M, R\}, PO \rangle$, is a *finite-state machine* such that we have:

- Input states: The materials, M, provide a set of *input states*. For example, the hippocampal neurons in our epilepsy experiment above are such input states.
- Internal states: The data set D obtained from M is the set of *internal states* of the whole machine, e.g., the continuing records of the bioelectrical activity of the hippocampal neurons of a rat's brain in our experiment above. The set of internal states of the machine, D, emerges and grows through the application of production operations PO_1 to elements of M during the experimentation.
- Output states: The experimental knowledge, K, is the set of *output states* that is obtained from internal states, D, by applying the production operations PO_2 to elements of D. This application of PO_2 to D consists in the analysis and interpretation of the experimental data by using scientific theories, logic, statistics, other mathematical theories, the experimenter's experience and skill, etc.

- State transition relations: Prior to the start of the experiment and the recording of experimental data, the initial internal state of the machine is $z_0 \in D$, i.e., 'the empty state'. When the experiment gets started, the application of PO_1 to the first input state i_1, e.g., a hippocampal neuron, generates, together with z_0, the next internal state $z_1 \in D$. That is, $PO_1(i_1, z_0, z_1)$ or $PO_1(i_1, z_0) = z_1$. For example, an electrical stimulus administered to a neuron generates a spike that is recorded by EEG as the first internal state of the machine. GABA application generates internal states of another type in that neuronal spikes disappear. Thus, the production operations PO_1 serve as *state-transition relations*. When applied to materials M as input and available internal states, they generate new internal states of the machine, i.e., new experimental data.
- Output relations: PO_2 is another set of production operations that serve as *output relations* transforming some internal states, i.e., elements of D, into output that is presented to the outside world as knowledge, K. This transformation consists in the analysis and interpretation of data D on the basis of background methodology and the knowledge of the experimenters.

In an experiment as a machine of the form $\langle M, D, K, PO_1, PO_2 \rangle$ such that:

$$\langle M, D, K, PO_1, PO_2 \rangle = \langle I, Z, O, S, OR \rangle$$

the state-transition relations PO_1 may be conceived of as data-making devices. Examples are pipettes, microscopes, microelectrodes, electrocardiographs, electrophoresis, sensors, computers, and so on. They will be referred to as state-transition operators or *data-makers*. They elicit data, D, from materials M. The output relations PO_2 are knowledge-making devices. They produce knowledge, K, from data D and will therefore be called output operators or *knowledge-makers*. We have thus:

$$PO_1 = \text{data-makers} \qquad \text{are state-transition relations (or operators).}$$
$$PO_2 = \text{knowledge-makers} \quad \text{are output relations (or operators).}$$

It was emphasized above that the experimenters themselves, whether they be scientists or their assistants of different specialties, are specialized technical operators and thus constituent parts of $PO_1 \cup PO_2 = PO$. Some of them may act as state-transition operators PO_1, i.e., data-makers. Examples are the biotechnical assistants who conduct the recordings. Some others may act as output operators PO_2, i.e., knowledge-makers. Examples are scientists themselves, particularly those who conduct the experiment, interpret the data, and publish the results. Four additional aspects are also worth noting:

First, since all five components of the machine $\langle M, D, K, PO_1, PO_2 \rangle$ are in fact fuzzy sets, an epistemic machine is actually an *epistemic fuzzy machine* according to the concept of fuzzy machine introduced in Definition 30 on page 130. Specifically, the input and internal states of an epistemic machine are fuzzy sets and the operators are fuzzy relations.

Second, an epistemic machine of the form $\langle M, D, K, PO_1, PO_2 \rangle$ described above may be conceived of as a compound of two interacting production systems of the following form:

$$\langle \{M, D\}, PO_1 \rangle$$
$$\langle \{D, K\}, PO_2 \rangle$$

In the first production system, the products D, i.e. data, are produced from materials M by data-makers PO_1. They then constitute the materials to be processed in the second production system. In the latter, the data D are processed by knowledge-makers PO_2 into the final product K termed "knowledge". The concatenation and interlinking of both production systems yields the machine $\langle M, D, K, PO_1, PO_2 \rangle$. By generalizing this idea, an epistemic machine may be conceived of as a collaborative interleave of more than two production systems as illustrated by the following chain with $n > 1$:

$$\langle \{M, D_1\}, PO_1 \rangle$$
$$\langle \{D_1, D_2\}, PO_2 \rangle$$
$$\langle \{D_2, D_3\}, PO_3 \rangle$$

$$\vdots$$

$$\langle \{D_n, K\}, PO_{n+1} \rangle.$$

Third, in an epistemic machine $\langle M, D, K, PO_1, PO_2 \rangle$ both data-making and knowledge-making are theory-laden. The production of data D from materials M by applying data-makers PO_1, as well as the production of knowledge K from data D by applying knowledge-makers PO_2, is based on the assumption that some other scientific knowledge is valid and some particular methods of measurement and reasoning are sound. For example, in our above-mentioned epilepsy experiment, the neurophysiologist presupposes that the physical theories of mechanics and electricity behind the electroencephalograph she uses as a PO_1 device, are something reliable so as to believe in the accurate representation of electrical neural activity by EEG waves. She uses methods of measuring temperature, length, weight, size, blood sugar concentration, and other attributes of her experimental subjects and data. So she presupposes that these background, measurement methodologies are trustworthy. She uses in addition Hodgkin and Huxley's biomedical theory of excitable membranes and additional theories from neurophysiology, physics, chemistry, and other disciplines to interpret the genesis and inhibition of neuronal spikes in the data set D. We may thus conclude that a medical experiment as well as the production of data and knowledge thereby are theory-laden. This finding is in conflict with the traditional view that experimentation enables direct and impartial observations and provides experimenter-independent, objective knowledge about facts. Obviously, facts are made by antecedent theories and methodologies, and by experimental designs and devices.

Fourth, in our discussion so far the experimenter has been actively participating in experimentation in that she has been a constituent part of data-makers and knowledge-makers. However, it will be shown below that her role is evolving such that she herself is increasingly becoming just one device among the many other devices in the epistemic machine.

12.3 Epistemic Factories

With the ideas above in hand, we may now explore further the analogies between experimental-scientific research and industry, and between experimental-scientific knowledge and industrial products. Scientific experiments are traditionally viewed as techniques to read the book of nature, to decipher and translate it, to causally analyze and explain phenomena, to test hypotheses so as to support or falsify them, and in this way to attain the truth. In contrast to this traditional view, we have reconstructed scientific experiments as epistemic machines that like other machines *produce* something as their output. Usually their output comprises a wide variety of entities, e.g., knowledge, animal cadavers, waste, revenue, academic careers, social power, etc. Depending on one's perspective, one will consider any of these outputs to be the main product of the machine. The places or plants where such epistemic machines are installed, have come to be termed research laboratories, or laboratories for short. On our view, however, laboratories are not places where the book of nature is read or translated, phenomena are causally analyzed and explained, or scientific truth is pursued and found. Rather, we consider them to be *factories* where epistemic machines are used to fabricate some products one of which is scientific knowledge. Biomedical laboratories will serve as our examples, although research laboratories of any other type would do as well, the most suitable ones being nuclear physics laboratories such as the Large Hadron Collider in CERN shown in Figure 63 on page 535.

Usually, a factory is defined as an industrial site where machines process raw materials into products, or one product into another, e.g., metal and other materials into automobiles. In complete accord with this definition, laboratories of experimental research as well as the institutions housing such laboratories turn out to be *factories,* e.g., universities and non-university research institutions, including industrial companies involved with scientific research such as the R&D departments of pharmaceutical companies. Since their main and final products are called knowledge, these knowledge factories will be referred to as *epistemic factories.* Thus, an epistemic factory is simply a site where we find one or more epistemic machines producing knowledge.

That scientific experiments are performed in a laboratory means that the laboratory houses epistemic machines. A laboratory may house a variety of epistemic machines in the same department or place, or in separate ones. For instance, in a physiology institute at a university a number of different animal experiments are carried out by distinct teams in separate rooms, e.g., experiments on the genesis of epilepsy, ventricular fibrillation, blood coagulation, insulin secretion, and so on. However, while there are many reasons that justify our categorization of such an institution as a factory, we shall confine ourselves to the discussion of these three components: materials, data, and knowledge. In the following sections, we shall demonstrate that these three components of an epistemic machine, $\langle M, D, K, PO_1, PO_2 \rangle$, are engineered entities with knowledge K being engineered in the laboratory itself:

    12.3.1   The Engineering of Materials
    12.3.2   The Engineering of Data
    12.3.3   The Engineering of Knowledge.

12.3.1 The Engineering of Materials

Consider again the epilepsy experiment described above. Mice and rats are used to investigate the genesis of brain cell spikes so as to develop antiepileptic agents. The animals that serve as materials or input, *M,* for the epistemic machine are not wild animals caught for experimental purposes. They are so-called laboratory mice, rats, or dogs which are themselves the product of other laboratories specialized in breeding mice, rats, dogs, cell lines, bacteria, and other biological organisms for research purposes. As Karin Knorr Cetina impressively describes (Knorr Cetina, 2003, 145):

[...] the warm rooms where cell lines and bacteria are cultured and grown, the rooms in which mice are raised and bred, are *production facilities.* For example, laboratory mice are today bred and put on the scientific market by special laboratories dedicated to producing stable strains that are simple to maintain, robust, free from diseases and that have certain genetic features. Once these mice have been acquired by a research lab, they are again put into isolated facilities in which the conditions for their further breeding and reproduction have been optimized. This is where breeding colonies are created, and where mice are submitted to the preparatory treatments *to condition them for their tasks* [emphasis added by the present author]. Well-kept facilities pride themselves on their fastidious record-keeping: they record the date of birth of each mouse, the mating patterns, the size of each new litter, the deaths, and the special features. They also collect aggregate data about potentially interesting variants, the number of the males that are sexually mature, of those which may serve as wet nurses, and so on. Well-kept mouse facilities are also continually reorganized; males that have reached the reproductive age are put into separate cages, males and females designated for mating are placed together, litters are separated from parents, and mice that are no longer needed and young mice that are redundant are put to death or transferred to other units. *A well-maintained, well-recorded mouse facility is a well-oiled production line. It produces and manages a steady flow of mice of the kind desired in the laboratory* [emphasis added by the present author].

    This consideration demonstrates that the input to an epistemic machine is itself something that has been produced, as an output of another machine, especially for this purpose. It is a technical product. It originates from the technology of laboratory animals that has come to be termed *laboratory animal science.* There are many institutes, both independent and university-based, that carry this title and are concerned just with this type of research. There are also national and international laboratory animal science associations, as well as journals on laboratory animals, and so on. That is, the laboratory animal is an object of research and technology dedicated to the *fabrication of laboratory animals.* Thus, the animals that are used in epistemic factories as subjects are themselves artifacts of other epistemic factories.

The engineering and industrial character of experimental-scientific research is clearly evident in disciplines such as particle physics. The objects of research, i.e., elusive elementary particles and events, are created by *machines* (cf. Knorr Cetina, 2003, 266). See, for example, the particle accelerator LHC in CERN outlined on page 535 above. What researchers investigate using this gigantic particle accelerator, is engineered and prepared beforehand. The same obtains in molecular-biological research where cells and bacteria are genetically engineered to produce DNA or RNA so as to inquire into their structure and function. In biomedical areas such as stem cell research, embryos are produced as stem cell resources. That is, to investigate into stem cells, embryos are artificially produced.

The examples above illustrate that the objects of biomedical research are no longer natural phenomena, but artifacts. Here biomedical scientists have an additional opportunity to acknowledge the fact that they do not analyze something whose existence is independent of their own research projects and facilities. They analyze what they have designed and produced themselves. They are not theoretical scientists, but engineers of biomedical knowledge and are doing technology of knowledge (see page 545 below).

12.3.2 The Engineering of Data

Once the fabricated *materials, M,* have entered an epistemic machine as input, the engineering of data starts. At this point, a number of data-making production operations, PO_1, consisting of technical devices from pipettes to electroencephalographs to nuclear magnetic resonance spectrometers to computers and the Internet are applied to materials M. However, the outcome of these operations are not yet interpreted. They are still sets of raw *data, D,* such as blood counts, records of brain cell spikes, electrophoretic diagrams, nitrogenous base profiles of DNA samples, 3-dimensional representations of electrocardiographic wave averages, ultrasonic images of the pancreas, and so on. They are obtained by manipulating the processes occurring in the input materials through administering chemical, electrical, optical, acoustic, or other stimuli and then recording the evoked responses. Thus, the process of internal state-transition and data-making in the epistemic machine is based on a sophisticated technology of intervention and recording. We saw on page 403 that in 1906, the French physicist Pierre Duhem was already aware of the multitude of scientific theories behind this data-making technology:

Go into this laboratory; draw near this table crowded with so much apparatus: an electric battery, copper wire wrapped in silk, vessels filled with mercury, coils, a small iron bar carrying a mirror. An observer plunges the metallic stem of a rod, mounted with rubber, into small holes; the iron oscillates and, by means of the mirror tied to it, sends a beam of light over to a celluloid ruler, and the observer follows the movement of the light beam on it. There, no doubt, you have an experiment; by means of the vibration of this spot of light, this physicist minutely observes the oscillation of the piece of iron. Ask him now what he is doing. Is he going to answer: "I am studying the oscillations of the piece of iron carrying this mirror"? No, he will tell you that he is measuring the electrical resistance of a coil. If you are astonished and ask him what meanings these words have, and what relation they have to these phenomena he has perceived and which you have at the same time perceived, he will reply that your question would require some very long explanations, and he will recommend that you take a course in electricity (Duhem, 1954, 145).

Thus, the technology of intervention and recording provides experimental-scientific laboratories with a host of data-making devices. The entirety of such devices used in a particular epistemic machine we will refer to as the *data-making engine*. In an epistemic machine of the form $\langle M, D, K, PO_1, PO_2 \rangle$:

- the *data-making engine* is PO_1 minus the human experimenters

who use the engine to produce the data set D from materials M. Without a data-making engine no experimental data would exist. The engine produces a *stream of data* in that it successively transforms the input states and the current internal states of the epistemic machine into new ones. The data are not simply gathered or inscribed as if they were something pre-existent. Rather, their production is in fact *data engineering*. Consider, for example, the tremendous amount of advanced mathematics, physics, and computational technology contained in a data recording device such as nuclear magnetic resonance spectrometer or Large Hadron Collider mentioned above. Although an experimenter is employing the data-maker or is interpreting the data, she is ignorant of the device's engineering and its capabilities.[110]

12.3.3 The Engineering of Knowledge

Duhem's account above reminds us of the difference between data and knowledge. Data are the uninterpreted results of recordings, e.g., waves and wavelets on the ECG chart of a patient. Someone who is not acquainted with electrocardiography will not know what these waves and wavelets mean, for instance, what a QRS complex looks like and indicates. She will be unable to identify it, to distinguish between normal and pathological QRS complexes, and

---

[110] The sociologists of science Bruno Latour and Steve Woolgar have referred to the data-making machinery used in scientific experiments as "inscription devices" (Latour and Woolgar, 1986, pp. 51, 89, 245). This well-known term is an ill-chosen expression, however, because it leaves open the misconception that experimental data mirror things that exist independently of the devices 'inscribing' them.

to recognize those pathological QRS complexes which point to, for example, 'ventricular fibrillation'.

To obtain *knowledge* from *data,* special background theories, knowledge, logic, and methodology are required to interpret the data stream, to discover significant patterns therein, and to discover any relationships between such patterns. The facilities that analyze and interpret the data stream produced in an epistemic machine, we called knowledge-makers or output operators, i.e., $PO_2 \subseteq PO$. With the advent of computers, artificial intelligence research, and the Internet a new technology of knowledge-making has emerged that more and more provides laboratories with a host of devices and software ('expert systems') that are capable of automatically managing data streams, accessing local or remote databases, and extracting knowledge therefrom. These recent computational techniques have come to be known as data mining, knowledge discovery, and knowledge extraction. See, e.g., (Cios et al., 2007; Han and Kamber, 2005; Maimon and Rokach, 2005). The entirety of such knowledge-making devices contained in the production operations of an epistemic machine will be referred to as the *knowledge-making engine.*

Laboratories have increasingly become networked institutions where almost everything is managed or facilitated by internal and external computer networks, from locally accessed intranets to worldwide access provided by the Internet. An epistemic machine of the form $\langle M, D, K, PO_1, PO_2 \rangle$ in a laboratory is usually part of this network. In such a machine:

- the *knowledge-making engine* is PO_2 minus the human experimenters

who use the engine to produce knowledge K from data D. For example, provide a statistical knowledge engine ('statistical package') with a large DNA database and ask for correlations between ten different variables therein. The results are typically returned in a few seconds or minutes. Calculation by traditional methods would require several experts and months.

Such knowledge-making engines are increasingly used in experimental-medical laboratories and will become standard in the near future. It is therefore worth noting that the *knowledge* one obtains from an experiment is relative to the *knowledge-making engine* one uses. Suppose, for example, that a particular knowledge-making engine contains a method of probabilistic-causal analysis, PO_2, whereas another knowledge-making engine contains a statistical significance test, i.e., method PO_2'. It is obvious that the application of these two engines to one and the same data stream D will yield two different items of knowledge because $PO_2(D) \neq PO_2'(D)$. Knowledge produced by the first engine will convey some causal information, knowledge produced by the second engine will not do so. That is, knowledge is knowledge-making engine relative. The knowledge you get depends on the engine you use.

Laboratories have their own histories and funding agencies or institutions. They have their caretaking personnel, their workshops and technicians, and so on. A scientist joining a laboratory will therefore have to adapt herself to the facilities she finds there. She will have to work by employing the available data and knowledge-making engines. She will have to produce the kind of knowledge that the available engines enable her to engineer. Otherwise put, she is a factory worker in the confines of the factory. In most cases she does not even clearly know how the knowledge-making engine works and attains the results it eventually supplies. Consider as an example a young scientist in the neurophysiology department described above investigating the genesis of epileptic convulsions. Suppose the knowledge-making engine that she is using, has just performed a statistical significance test and has found that the data obtained on the anti-epileptic effect of GABA are statistically significant at the 0.01 level. Now, ask the young scientist the question, "statistically significant at the 0.01 level: what does that really mean?". If you are fortunate, she may answer with some degree of clarity; however, chances are that our young scientist has not the foggiest idea.

We deliberately introduced the term "the engineering of knowledge" to clearly differentiate our subject from a recent artificial intelligence discipline called *knowledge engineering* (also called knowledge-based systems research, expert systems research, decision support systems research, and the like). In contradistinction to what we are conceptualizing as the engineering of knowledge, knowledge engineering is concerned with the development and maintenance of knowledge-based computer programs that process antecedently available knowledge. It does not produce new knowledge. See, e.g., (Buchanan and Shortliffe 1984).

However, as is the case in all instances of self-reference, a difficulty arises here, too. For there is no sharp distinction between a knowledge-making engine that produces new knowledge, and a knowledge-based system that uses available knowledge, for example, a chemical expert system like Dendral. (Dendral analyzes mass spectra of unknown molecules and makes inferences as to their chemical structure and identity.) Similarly, a knowledge-making engine is also a knowledge-based system that utilizes antecedently available knowledge to extract new knowledge from data streams. If one considers in addition the mathematical-computational capacities of most knowledge-making engines, then most can in fact be considered knowledge-based systems. These notes demonstrate anew that knowledge is self-referential in that to acquire new knowledge requires old knowledge. Otherwise put, knowledge is capable of autodetermination. It proliferates autonomously.

12.4 The Global Knowledge-Making Engine

A myriad of computers and sensors are connected to one another worldwide and constitute an earth-spanning neural network. This network will be referred to as the Global Net, or GN for short. Part of it, which is accessible to all humans by computers over public telephone networks and satellites, is the well-known Internet. In addition, the GN also includes local area networks and intranets in business, industry, and universities as well as other research institutions, clinics, administrations, authorities, and other establishments. We pointed out above that through the Internet, scientific laboratories as epistemic factories are connected to the GN. In this way a dynamic, global ocean of information, knowledge, and Web technology can be accessed and used by the knowledge-making engine of every epistemic machine $\langle M, D, K, PO_1, PO_2 \rangle$ installed in a laboratory. We may therefore conclude that the entirety of GN-enabled knowledge-making engines in laboratories around the earth constitutes a Global Knowledge-Making Engine.[111]

12.5 The Industrialization of Knowledge

We have seen above that in experimental-medical research, materials are technologically produced and data streams are automatically elicited, recorded, and managed by data-making engines. The analysis and interpretation of data is also more and more being automated. It is performed by the local and remote computational machinery and software that we have called the Global Knowledge-Making Engine. A *knowledge technology* is emerging that increasingly produces our experimental-medical knowledge. By generalizing this observation, our thesis of epistemic technoconstructivism stated on page 532 may now be concisely restated as follows:

Technoconstructivism: During the last few centuries, experimental sciences have contributed to the industrialization of experimental research to the effect that experimental-scientific knowledge has become a technological construct produced in epistemic factories by the Global Knowledge-Making Engine.

Because of its far-reaching philosophical and practical consequences, a final account of this thesis will clarify some of its additional aspects in order to further substantiate it:[112]

The industrialization of experimental research, or *epistemic industry* for short, has gradually developed over the last three centuries following the emer-

---

[111] In a wider context, this global machine was reconstructed by the present author as the *Machina sapiens* (Sadegh-Zadeh, 2000d).

[112] As discussed in Section 11.5.4 on page 523 above, social constructivism argues that scientific knowledge is socially constructed. Moreover, it has also contributed to an analogous theory on the social construction of technology (Bijker et al., 1999; MacKenzie and Wajcman, 1999). But these doctrines remain one-sided if one does not add at the same time the clause "and vice versa". That is, society as well as scientific knowledge are technologically constructed. One should be aware, however, that social constructivism and technoconstructivism are not two competing doctrines and do not contradict each other. Rather, they are complementary in that there is a hypercyclic-causal relationship between society and technology. Each of them conditions the other. For details of this hypercyclic coevolution of society and technology, see (Sadegh-Zadeh, 2000d).

gence of the natural sciences of physics and chemistry. In the wake of anatomical pathology in the late eighteenth century, medicine joined this endeavor by moving into the laboratory. See, for example, Giovanni Battista Morgagni's *De Sedibus et Causis Morborum per Anatomen Indagatis* (Morgagni, 1761) and the chemical interpretation of the organism and diseases by the French physician Jean-Baptiste Théodore Baumes in 1798.[113] Since then experimentation has been the basis of the medical sciences, leading to the development of other branches such as biochemistry, pharmacology, pharmacy, microbiology, medical physics, and others. Thus, a multitude of experimental health sciences have been established. As compared to its pre-laboratorized state in the eighteenth century, medicine today has a myriad of diagnostic, therapeutic, and preventive measures and devices at its disposal to diagnose, remedy, relieve, and prevent much suffering and to save many lives. Life expectancy has doubled. In light of our discussion, the focal epistemological question becomes: Is this impressive advancement thanks to the attainment of *truth* by experimental knowledge, or is it rather thanks to the development of efficacious remedies and efficient devices through *technoconstruction,* where truth plays no role? To answer this question, recall the term "epistemic path" introduced on page 528.

As an illustration, we will consider the epistemic path from a state of ignorance to a state of knowledge about a particular disease, say multiple sclerosis. Suppose that there is a point in time, t_1, at which a particular disease such as multiple sclerosis cannot yet be satisfactorily diagnosed and remedied. A wide variety of diagnostic and therapeutic failures may hamper the management of that disease. Medical experts may therefore be at pains to search for improvements worldwide. They may eventually succeed at a later point in time, t_2, and find both an enhanced diagnostic technique and a fairly efficacious treatment. For simplicity's sake, let us use as our example the efficacious treatment only, denoted by the acronym "ETR". We may realistically

---

[113] Jean-Baptiste T. Baumes (1756–1828) was a physician at the University of Paris, and later, in Montpellier. As a young doctor he was awarded a prize for his work on neonatal jaundice in 1785 (Baumes, 1806). With his major iatro-chemical work he contributed significantly to the emergence of medical and clinical chemistry (Baumes, 1798, 1801). In the late eighteenth and early nineteenth centuries, patient care increasingly moved, beginning in Paris, from bedside medicine at the patient's home to clinics where more and more laboratories were being established (Foucault, 1994; Cunningham and Williams, 2002). This process of laboratorization of medicine in clinics, which gave rise to the experimental-medical sciences, was particularly advanced by the discovery of the animal cell, micro-organisms, and pathogenic agents as well as by the German founder of physiology, Johannes Peter Müller (1801–1858), and his famous students such as Theodor Schwann (1810–1882) who discovered the animal cell around 1938; Friedrich Gustav Jakob Henle (1809–1885); Karl Ludwig (1816–1895); Emil du Bois-Reymond (1818–1898); Hermann Helmholtz (1821–1894); and Rudolf Virchow (1821–1902), the founder of the cellular pathology.

suppose in addition that on the way to this achievement extensive experimental investigations were carried out into the biomedical conditions of the disease, for example, into its cytology, histology, immunology, microbiology, genetics, pathology, pathophysiology, pharmacology, etc. Numerous scientific conferences may have taken place, thousands of articles and books may have been published, and finally, as a fruit of intense international collaboration, highly valuable therapeutic knowledge may have been acquired to the effect that the treatment ETR could be developed. ETR consists in administering the synthesized drug XYZ.

Thus, international collaboration led from the state of ignorance at time t_1 to the state of therapeutic knowledge at a later time, t_2. As pointed out previously, the epistemic path from ignorance at t_1 to knowledge at t_2 is an artifact, brought about by an international collaboration in the present example, whose creation depends on a multitude of accidental factors. There are no natural, pre-existing epistemic paths from ignorance to knowledge to be 'discovered'. In a nutshell, our epistemic technoconstructivism says that this path as an artifact, eventually materialized in the drug XYZ, is technologically constructed by epistemic industry. All scientific knowledge *published* along the epistemic path leading to the artifact XYZ is a mere protocol of the endeavor that soon fades away. Thus, it represents a gratuitous epiphenomenon and byproduct, a mnemonic device, so to speak, used alongside the path that could as well have been omitted. What counts is the main product of the whole process of construction, i.e., the commodity XYZ.

If there is still any doubt regarding epistemic technoconstructivism, consider experimental-medical research activities undertaken in laboratories of commercial institutions such as the pharmaceutical industry or biotech companies and centers. Today a considerable amount of biomedical publications originate from laboratories of this type as they closely cooperate with universities. But what are their researchers really doing in their laboratories? Are they really interested in the discovery of truth or truthlikeness about the world and its phenomena, or rather in something else? Organisms, cells, and viruses; their biological structure and metabolism; and chemical substances and molecules are analyzed with the intention of pursuing proprietary knowledge. This knowledge may then be used as a basis for producing new organisms, cells, viruses, substances, and molecules that can in turn be used to make money, remedy maladies, relieve pain, reduce risk, prevent harm, prolong life, and generate many more moral goods.

12.6 Summary

Scientific experiments in general and medical experiments in particular were reconstructed as production systems to show that they are models for the concept of the input-output machine introduced in Definitions 29–30 on page 129. As such, they may be categorized as machines. Since the main output of these machines is usually referred to as knowledge, we called them epistemic machines. Experimental-medical laboratories house such knowledge-producing epistemic machines. They may therefore be viewed as epistemic factories. Today an epistemic factory is networked with the Global Knowledge-Making Engine (GKME) that consists of the Internet, intranets, and local area nets. Driven by artificial intelligence, the GKME is on the verge of automating the production of knowledge in epistemic factories. Experimental-scientific research is thus becoming industrialized with its product being knowledge. In a not-too-distant future, then, it will be pointless to ask whether such an industrial product does or does not possess epistemological properties such as truth, falsehood, truthlikeness, probability, justifiedness, credibility, reliability, plausibility, etc. The product will simply be handled as a modularized, portable and copyable commodity, and applied according to its expected utility.

Part IV

Medical Deontics

13

Morality, Ethics, and Deontics

13.0 Introduction

The subject of our discussion in what follows is not medical ethics or bioethics. Rather, we shall look a bit further than usual into medical values. By so doing, to the long-standing debate over whether medicine is a science or an art, we shall add a third option. Specifically, we shall endeavor to show that medicine is a deontic discipline and therefore requires a field of inquiry which will be referred to as *medical deontics*.[114]

To lay the groundwork for our argument, we shall first clarify the differences between morality, ethics, and deontics. Subsequently, we shall show that *common morality* as shared moral beliefs of a society is a deontic-social institution and underlies the categorization of some human conditions as prototype diseases on the basis of which the fundamental concept of medicine, i.e., *disease*, emerges as a deontic construct. In this way, it generates the category of diseases and shapes nosology, diagnostics, therapy, and prevention. Finally, the deontic nature of medicine will be uncovered. Our analysis thus consists of the following three chapters:

13 Morality, Ethics, and Deontics
14 Disease as a Deontic Construct
15 Medicine is a Deontic Discipline.

To clarify the relationships between the three areas *morality, ethics*, and *deontics*, we must first note that the term "morality" is ambiguous. It means both a particular quality of human behavior as well as the moral rules governing that behavior. Depending on the context, we shall use it in both senses. It must also be noted that unfortunately, morality and theories of morality

---

[114] The new term "deontics" derives from the adjective "deontic" (see page X) that means *normative, prescriptive, directive,* and *preceptive* as opposed to *descriptive, constative,* and *assertive.*

K. Sadegh-Zadeh, *Handbook of Analytic Philosophy of Medicine,*
Philosophy and Medicine 113, DOI 10.1007/978-94-007-2260-6_13,
© Springer Science+Business Media B.V. 2012

are not always clearly distinguished in the literature. While morality is understood either as a feature of human behavior and conduct, on the one hand, or as the rules governing that behavior and conduct, on the other, a theory of morality is something said about morality. We shall therefore differentiate between these two levels, i.e., morality itself on the object-level and the theories thereof on the meta-level. The latter are also referred to as moral philosophy, which consists of *ethics* and *metaethics*. Below, we shall briefly consider ethics and metaethics in order to expand them into *deontics,* which we need for our subsequent analyses. Our discussion will presuppose the acquaintance with deontic logic outlined in Section 27.2 on page 927. It divides into the following three sections:

13.1 Morality
13.2 Ethics and Metaethics
13.3 Deontics.

13.1 Morality

The adjective "moral", from the Latin adjective "moralis, morale" derived from the substantive "mos" meaning *custom,* is a fuzzy predicate that partitions human behavior (conduct, actions) into two vague classes, the class of moral actions and that of non-moral actions. Non-moral actions are also referred to as morally neutral. A human action is moral if it affects the lives of others, morally neutral, otherwise. For example, keeping one's promise or doing harm to a patient are moral actions, whereas eating an apple and walking are none. The class of moral actions is itself partitioned into two subclasses, the subclass of right actions and the subclass of wrong actions, also called good and bad (or evil) actions, respectively (Figure 64).

Now, the following basic question arises: What actions are to be considered *moral* actions, be they right or wrong, good or bad? In other words, how is the predicate "moral" defined? What is it that characterizes the category of moral actions? What is morality? This question has already been answered above by defining a moral action as one that affects the lives of other individuals. For example, the cruel treatment of a person affects her life. Curing a cancer patient by performing surgery or chemotherapy

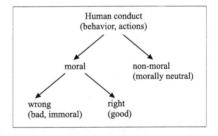

Fig. 64. Taxonomy of human conduct

does so too. Both types of action are therefore to be considered moral actions. Specifically, a moral action is said to be good when it relieves or prevents harm to others, and thereby lessens human suffering and thus contributes to human welfare. Otherwise, it is said to be bad or immoral, i.e., when it does harm to others and thereby increases suffering. We will not give an exhaustive list of the specific constituent features of the concept of morality outlined above. However, a few examples are: honesty, beneficence, and justice.

The concept of morality sketched above is obviously anthropocentric. It does not consider the harm done by human agents to non-human creatures, e.g., the cruelty, torture, and violence toward animals in agriculture and slaughterhouses, in biomedical and pharmaceutical laboratories, and in everyday life. Disregard for the man-made suffering of non-human creatures renders the ordinary, anthropocentric concepts of morality suspect and unacceptable. However, we cannot discuss the philosophical and metaphysical intricacies of this issue here. In the present context, we will consider the lessening and prevention of harm to sentient creatures as the central feature of morally good acts, and the opposite thereof as the central feature of morally bad acts. The harm referred to may consist in death, suffering, pain, discomfort, disability, loss of autonomy, or loss of pleasure (see also Gert et al., 2006, 11 f.).

The scenarios, situations, and states of affairs, or possible worlds for short, that are either pursued or avoided by moral actions are usually referred to as moral values. Positive moral values, or values for short, are those pursued by good moral actions and avoided by bad ones, e.g., assistance to those who need it. Negative moral values, or disvalues for short, are those avoided by good moral actions and pursued by bad ones, e.g., dishonesty and murder. For a precise definition and analysis of these and additional value concepts such as absolute value, relative value, intrinsic value, and extrinsic value, see (Sadegh-Zadeh, 1981a).

Morality in a human society is usually codified in a variety of ways, for example:

a. as so-called moral values in the form of a good-bad dichotomy of human conduct, e.g., *harming is bad; honesty is good; murdering is bad; assisting those who need it is good;*

b. as moral injunctions and commands in terms of imperatives such as *first do no harm; tell the truth; do not commit murder; render assistance to those who need it;* or

c. as moral norms in the form of duties or moral rules like *thou shalt not do harm; thou shalt tell the truth; thou shalt not commit murder; thou shalt render assistance to those who need it.*

The entirety of a community's (group's, society's) moral values, imperatives, and rules is referred to as its morals or its morality. We shall approach morality in terms of moral rules as in (c).

13.2 Ethics and Metaethics

Above we talked about morality and morals. Thus, we did a little bit of moral philosophy. Specifically, we did both ethics and metaethics.

The Greek term ἔθος (ethos) means the same as the Latin word "mos", i.e., "custom". *Ethics* has emerged as the science of ethos. Modern ethics is the study of moral action and is concerned with the morality and morals of human beings and societies. It seeks to identify, clarify, and represent their moral values, imperatives, and rules. It also seeks to organize those values, imperatives, and rules into a system; explain their genesis; examine their properties, adequacy, relationships, and consequences; and to justify, refute, or improve them. The emerging system is referred to as a moral system or *ethic*, or simply *morals*.

As noted above, we shall prefer to use the notion of a moral rule as in (c) in order that we can employ logic in ethics. A moral rule is usually an explicitly formulated directive to undertake a certain course of action. If the moral rules explored by ethics are antecedently available and have been used in a community or area in the past or are used in the present, the ethics is called empirical or *descriptive ethics*. A descriptive ethics is concerned with the actual moral behavior of people. Examples are medical-ethical inquiries into the moral rules that have either been operative or treated with contempt in Nazi medicine, or are operative in contemporary US health care, or any other health care system. By contrast, *normative ethics* addresses Immanuel Kant's second question: "What ought I to do?" ", or more generally, "what ought we to do?". It seeks to formulate, advance, or prescribe moral rules as norms of conduct in that it introduces, analyzes, justifies, systematizes, or refutes them to develop a particular ethic. For instance, contemporary medical-ethical discussions – about stem cell research, cloning, brain death, assisted suicide, and xenotransplantation – that aim to regulate moral issues in medicine, belong to normative ethics. The so-called "principles of biomedical ethics" discussed by Beauchamp and Childress comprising the four moral principles or rules of respect for autonomy, non-maleficence, beneficence, and justice constitute a miniature system of normative medical ethics (Beauchamp and Childress, 2001).

While descriptive ethics is void of any normative requirements, normative ethics includes in addition descriptive-ethical elements. A domain ethics or *professional ethics* is concerned with the moral system of a particular profession such as medicine. It may be purely descriptive, though it usually has both descriptive-ethical and normative-ethical components. One example is contemporary medical ethics, including the Beauchamp and Childress approach mentioned above, which has come to be known as *principlism* (Clouser and Gert, 1990; Beauchamp and DeGrazia, 2004; Gert et al., 2006, 99 ff.).

In summary, ethics is the science of morality and is concerned with both morality as a feature of human behavior and morality as a canon of rules of behavior, i.e., morals. As such, it is primarily conducted in the realm of language. A distinction is usually made between ethics and *metaethics*. This distinction, however, is artificial. Ethics and metaethics cannot be sensibly separated from one another.

Metaethics encompasses inquiries into the semantic, logical, epistemological, and ontological presuppositions and problems of moral reasoning. It is thus concerned with, for example, the concepts of morality, moral value, moral imperative, and moral rule. It is also concerned with questions of the following type: What is the subject of a moral judgment? Is it a physical object, a state of affairs, or a human action? What is an ethical theory? Does moral knowledge exist? For instance, is it knowledge when we say that something is morally good or bad? If it is, then there must be moral facts to know something about. Are there such moral facts? Can a moral judgment which says that a particular action is morally good or bad be true, or is it rather a matter of taste and labeling? How can a moral judgment be justified? And so on.

Due to the diversity of responses and approaches to these problems, there are a large number of metaethical views and theories on morality, moral judgment, moral knowledge, and moral reasoning. Examples are moral realism, moral anti-realism, moral skepticism, cognitivism, non-cognitivism, and many others. For instance, moral realism says that there are indeed moral facts, whereas moral anti-realism denies the existence of moral facts. See, for example (Fischer and Kirchin, 2006; Horgan and Timmons, 2006; Miller, 2003).

We will not go into the details of metaethical problems here. We will try to clarify only a single issue in order to use it in our discussion below, i.e., the reconstruction of morality as a normative or rule-based social institution. To this end, we will first demonstrate an analogy between ethics and law that will enable us to combine them to form what we shall refer to as *deontics*.

13.3 Deontics

Descriptive ethics informs us about the moral IS, i.e., about the actual morality in a particular community in the present or past. Its results are reports, and for that matter, not morally binding. To know that some people believe that something is morally good or bad may be interesting. But you need not share their beliefs and need not behave as they do. It is only the moral rules promulgated by the normative ethics of a given community that are morally binding on members of that community. A normative-ethical system, briefly referred to as a *normative system*, comprising moral rules is concerned with the moral OUGHT, which tells us how to live by suggesting a more or less attractive conception of a good moral agent. However, in this case it does not suffice to assert "what is morally good", e.g., *honesty is good*. Normative-ethical items are often put forward in terms of such value assertions. It is overlooked that a value assertion of this type has the syntax of a *constative* like "the Eiffel Tower is high". Therefore, it sounds rather like a descriptive report, or like empirical knowledge whose subject has a particular

property, for example, goodness, which is identified as a 'fact'. It is just this
pseudo-constative character of normative-ethical sentences that gives rise to
philosophical-metaethical debates about moral realism and anti-realism (Cuneo, 2010; Kramer, 2009; Shafer-Landau, 2005).

In order for a normative-ethical item to be discernible as something mandatory, it must place constraints on the pursuit of our own interests by prescribing what we ought to do, what we must not do, and what we may do. That is,
it must suggest a *rule* of conduct that regulates human behavior. Examples
are the following moral rules or norms:

1. Everybody *ought to* tell the truth;
2. Everybody is *forbidden* to commit murder;
3. Everybody is *allowed* to drink water.

Expressed in the terminology of deontic logic, these sentences say (see Section
27.2):

1'. For everybody x, it is obligatory that x tells the truth;
2'. For everybody x, it is forbidden that x commits murder;
3'. For everybody x, it is permitted that x drinks water.

They contain familiar deontic operators such as "it is obligatory that", "it is
forbidden that", and "it is permitted that". For natural language synonyms
of these operators, see Section 27.2.1 on page 928. Thus, moral rules are
obviously representable by deontic-logical sentences. This is why we call them
deontic rules. And since they constrain human behavior, they are also referred
to as deontic norms, or *norms* for short. The above rules are of the following
deontic-logical structure:

1''. $\forall x\, OB(Tx)$
2''. $\forall x\, FO(Mx)$
3''. $\forall x\, PE(Wx)$

where *OB*, *FO*, and *PE* are the above-mentioned deontic operators *obligatory,
forbidden,* and *permitted,* respectively; and Tx, Mx, and Wx represent the action sentences "x tells the truth", "x commits murder", and "x drinks water",
respectively. An *ethic* as a system of morality in fact consists of such deontic norms and has therefore been called a *normative system* above. Examples
are the Christian ethic, the moral codes of health care systems in Western
countries, and the medical-ethical system of Beauchamp and Childress, which
is composed of four deontic norms (respect for autonomy, non-maleficence,
beneficence, and justice).

Deontic operators also enable us to represent juridical laws, i.e., legal
norms such as "theft is forbidden", "practicing physicians must report new
cases of tuberculosis to public health authorities", or "as of age 6, children
have to be enrolled in school", as deontic rules. That is:

a. For everybody x, it is forbidden that x steals;

b. For everybody x, if x is a practicing physician, then it is obligatory that x reports new cases of tuberculosis to public health authorities;

c. For everybody x, if x is a child of age 6, it is obligatory that x is enrolled in school.

All three examples are actually German laws. Obviously, legal norms too are deontic sentences and are thus amenable to deontic logic. We may therefore treat moral as well as legal rules in medicine as deontic norms. As was pointed out above, a deontic norm is not a constative sentence like "Mr. Elroy Fox has gallstone colic". Thus, it is not a statement and does not assert something true or false. It is a prescription, a command, and as such, without empirical content. The inquiry into the syntactic, semantic, logical, and philosophical problems of deontic norms and normative systems has come to be known as deontic logic and philosophy, or deontics for short (see footnote 174 on page 930).

The above examples demonstrate that no syntactic, linguistic, or logical distinction can be drawn between the moral and the legal because both types of rules are of deontic character. Moreover, legal-normative and moral-normative systems are not disjoint. They share many rules of conduct such as, for instance, "murder is forbidden". Since the realization of any such rule usually depends on some factual circumstances, it is both philosophically and logically important to note at this juncture that many, perhaps most, deontic rules are conditional norms such as rules (b–c) above. In Section 27.2.4, they are called deontic conditionals. Rule (b) is a deontic conditional with the following syntax:

$$\forall x \big(Px \rightarrow OB(Qx) \big) \tag{127}$$

and says: For all x, if x is P, then it is obligatory that x is Q. This is a simple *conditional obligation*. Written in a generalized form and as *universal closures*, conditional obligations, prohibitions, and permissions are of the following structure (for the term "universal closure", see page 869):

$$\mathcal{Q}(\alpha \rightarrow OB\beta)$$
$$\mathcal{Q}(\alpha \rightarrow FO\beta)$$
$$\mathcal{Q}(\alpha \rightarrow PE\beta)$$

such that $\mathcal{Q}$ is the prefixed quantifier complex of the sentence, e.g., $\forall x$ in (127) above or $\forall x \forall y \forall z$ or something else, and α as well as β are sentences of arbitrary complexity. An example is the following conditional obligation: If a terminally ill patient has an incurable disease, is comatose, is dying, and has a living will that says she rejects life-sustaining treatment, then physicians and other caregivers ought not to sustain her life by medical treatment. That is:

$$\mathcal{Q}(\alpha \rightarrow OB(\neg\beta_1 \wedge \neg\beta_2)) \tag{128}$$

where:

$$\alpha \quad \equiv \quad \alpha_1 \wedge \alpha_2 \wedge \alpha_3 \wedge \alpha_4 \wedge \alpha_5 \wedge \alpha_6 \wedge \alpha_7$$

and:

$$\alpha_1 \quad \equiv \quad x \text{ is a terminally ill patient,}$$
$$\alpha_2 \quad \equiv \quad x \text{ has an incurable disease,}$$
$$\alpha_3 \quad \equiv \quad x \text{ is comatose,}$$
$$\alpha_4 \quad \equiv \quad x \text{ is dying,}$$
$$\alpha_5 \quad \equiv \quad \text{there exists a living will of } x \text{ which says that } x \text{ rejects life-sustaining treatment,}$$
$$\alpha_6 \quad \equiv \quad y \text{ is a physician,}$$
$$\alpha_7 \quad \equiv \quad z \text{ is a caregiver other than } y,$$
$$\beta_1 \quad \equiv \quad y \text{ sustains } x\text{'s life by medical treatment,}$$
$$\beta_2 \quad \equiv \quad z \text{ sustain } x\text{'s life by medical treatment,}$$
$$\mathcal{Q} \quad \equiv \quad \forall x \forall y \forall z.$$

Using these notations, we may take a look at the micro-structure of sentence (128) to understand why macro-representations such as (128) are preferred:

$\forall x \forall y \forall z (x$ is a terminally ill patient $\wedge$ x has an incurable disease $\wedge$
x is comatose $\wedge$ x is dying $\wedge$ there exists a living will of x
which says that x rejects life-sustaining treatment $\wedge$
y is a physician $\wedge$ z is a caregiver other than $y \rightarrow$
$OB(\neg\, y$ sustains x's life by medical treatment $\wedge$
$\neg\, z$ sustain x's life by medical treatment$)$.

Note, first, that the ought-not component in the consequent of (128) is formalized as $OB(\neg\beta_1 \wedge \neg\beta_2)$ and not as $\neg OB(\beta_1 \wedge \beta_2)$. The latter formulation would mean that it is not obligatory that $\beta_1 \wedge \beta_2$, whereas the rule says "it is obligatory that $\neg\beta_1 \wedge \neg\beta_2$". Note, second, that according to deontic-logical theorem 4 in Table 42 on page 934, the sentence $OB(\neg\beta_1 \wedge \neg\beta_2)$ is equivalent to $OB\neg\beta_1 \wedge OB\neg\beta_2$ such that rule (128) above and the following rule (129) are equivalent:

$$\mathcal{Q}(\alpha \rightarrow OB\neg\beta_1 \wedge OB\neg\beta_2) \tag{129}$$

Further, "ought not to γ" is the same as "it is obligatory that not γ", i.e., $OB\neg\gamma$. This is, by Definition 232 on page 929, equivalent to "it is forbidden that γ", written $FO\gamma$. Thus, the consequent of our last formulation (129) says that $FO\beta_1 \wedge FO\beta_2$. That is, "it is forbidden that a physician sustains the patient's life by medical treatment and it is forbidden that other caregivers sustain her life by medical treatment". We eventually obtain the sentence:

$$\mathcal{Q}(\alpha \rightarrow FO\beta_1 \wedge FO\beta_2). \tag{130}$$

We see that because of equivalence between $OB\neg\alpha$ and $FO\alpha$, it makes no difference whether a norm is formulated negatively as a negative obligation such as (129), e.g., "one ought to do no harm to sentient creatures", or positively as a prohibition such as (130), e.g., "it is forbidden to do harm to sentient creatures".

The discussion in the literature on the distinction between moral rules, moral norms, moral principles, moral ideals, moral commitments, virtues, and values is often misleading because all of these entities are in fact one and the same thing, i.e., deontic rules as explicated above. For instance, it was already pointed out in the preceding section that all four *principles* of Beauchamp and Childress's principlism (the principles of respect for autonomy, non-maleficence, beneficence, and justice) are deontic rules. To exemplify, the principle of autonomy says in effect "one ought to respect the autonomy of the patient". Likewise, the principle of non-maleficence says "one ought not to inflict evil or harm"; and so on. Thus, Beauchamp and Childress's principles of biomedical ethics are deontic rules of obligation (see also Beauchamp and Childress, 2001, 114 ff.).

We must be aware, however, that not every deontic sentence is a deontic rule. An example is the deontic sentence "it is obligatory that the sky is blue". Although it is a syntactically correct deontic sentence, semantically it is not meaningful. Only human actions can sensibly be qualified as obligatory, forbidden, or permitted. Whatever is outside the sphere of human action, cannot be the subject of deontics.

With the above considerations in mind, a concept of an *ought-to-do action rule* will now be introduced which we shall use below to uncover both the deontic character of the concept of disease and medicine. To this end, we shall first recursively define what we understand by the term "action sentence". A sentence of the form $P(t_1, \ldots, t_n)$ with an n-place predicate P will be called an *action sentence* if P denotes a human action such as "tells the truth" or "interviews", and each t_i is a term in logical sense, i.e., an individual variable or constant such as "x" or "Elroy Fox". Thus, sentences such as "Dr. Smith interviews Elroy Fox" and "Elroy Fox tells the truth" are action sentences, whereas "the sky is blue" is none. Our aim is to base the notion of a deontic rule on action sentences so as to prevent vacuous obligations such as "it is obligatory that the sky is blue".

Definition 151 (Action sentence).

1. *If P is an n-ary action predicate and $t_1, \ldots, t_n$ are terms – in logical sense –, then $P(t_1, \ldots, t_n)$ is an* action sentence;
2. *If α is an action sentence, then $\neg\alpha$ is an action sentence referred to as the omission of the action;*
3. *If α and β are action sentences, then $\alpha \wedge \beta$ as well as $\alpha \vee \beta$ are action sentences;*
4. *If α is any sentence and β is an action sentence, then $\alpha \rightarrow \beta$ is an action sentence, referred to as a conditional action sentence.*

For example, "Elroy Fox is ill" is not an action sentence. "Elroy Fox tells the truth" is an action sentence. And "if Dr. Smith interviews Elroy Fox, then he tells the truth" is a conditional action sentence. The notion of a *deontic rule* will now be introduced in two steps:

Definition 152 (Deontic action sentence).

1. *If α is an action sentence and ∇ is a deontic operator, then $\nabla\alpha$ is a deontic action sentence;*
2. *If α and β are deontic action sentences, then $\neg\alpha$, $\alpha \wedge \beta$, and $\alpha \vee \beta$ are deontic action sentences;*
3. *If $\alpha \rightarrow \beta$ is an action sentence, then $\alpha \rightarrow \nabla\beta$ is a deontic action sentence referred to as a* deontic conditional.

Definition 153 (Deontic rule).

1. *If α is a deontic action sentence with $n \geq 1$ free individual variables $x_1, \ldots, x_n$, then its universal closure $\forall x_1 \ldots \forall x_n \alpha$ is a deontic rule;*
2. *A deontic rule of the form $\forall x_1 \ldots \forall x_n(\alpha \rightarrow \nabla\beta)$ is called a* conditional obligation *if $\nabla \equiv OB$; a* conditional prohibition *if $\nabla \equiv FO$; and a* conditional permission *if $\nabla \equiv PE$.*

A deontic rule is also called a *deontic norm*. For example, according to part 1 of Definition 152, the sentence "it is obligatory that x tells the truth" is a deontic action sentence because its core, "x tells the truth", is an action sentence. And according to part 1 of Definition 153, its universal closure is a deontic rule, i.e.:

1. For everybody x, it is obligatory that x tells the truth.

Additional examples are:

2. For everybody x, it is forbidden that x steals;
3. For everybody x, if x is a child of age 6, it is obligatory that x is enrolled in school.

These three rules may be formalized as follows:

- $\forall x\, OB(Tx)$
- $\forall x\, FO(Sx)$
- $\forall x\big(Cx \rightarrow OB(ESx)\big)$.

The first two examples are unconditional deontic rules. The third example represents a conditional deontic rule, specifically a conditional obligation. Thus, an unconditional deontic rule is a sentence of the form:

$$\mathcal{Q}\nabla\beta$$

and a conditional deontic rule is a sentence of the form:

$$\mathcal{Q}(\alpha \rightarrow \nabla\beta),$$

where $\mathcal{Q}$ is a universal quantifier prefix $\forall x_1 \ldots \forall x_n$; ∇ is one of the three deontic operators *obligatory, forbidden,* or *permitted;* and β is an action sentence.

We know from Definition 232 on page 928 that the three deontic operators are interdefinable. Specifically, *PE* is definable by *FO*, and *FO* is definable by *OB:*

$$FO\alpha \equiv OB\neg\alpha$$
$$PE\alpha \equiv \neg FO\alpha \quad \text{and thus: } PE\alpha \equiv \neg OB\neg\alpha.$$

On this account, the obligation operator *OB* may serve as the basic and only deontic operator to formulate both types of deontic rules, moral rules and legal rules. That means that all such rules prescribe obligatory actions, i.e., ought-to-do actions, or their omissions. They may therefore be viewed as *ought-to-do action rules, ought-to-do rules*, or *action rules* for short. These terms will be used interchangeably.

According to the terminology above, an ought-to-do rule may be unconditional or conditional. An unconditional ought-to-do rule is an unconditional obligation such as "everybody ought to tell the truth". It does not require any preconditions. A conditional ought-to-do rule, however, is a conditional obligation and has a precondition. An example is the conditional obligation "a child of age 6 ought to be enrolled in school". That is, "for everybody x, *if* x is a child of age 6, then it is obligatory that x is enrolled in school". As was already pointed out, most medical-deontic rules are conditional obligations of this type and thus conditional action rules. We shall come back to this issue below to inquire into the nature of morality, disease, and medicine.

13.4 Summary

We distinguished between morality, ethics, metaethics, and deontics. By "medical deontics" we understand the deontic-logical analysis and philosophy of morality and law in medicine. It was shown that moral as well as legal rules are representable as deontic sentences in the language of deontic logic. We introduced the notion of a deontic rule to demonstrate that all deontic rules are actually ought-to-do rules. Conditional ought-to-do rules, called conditional obligations, are of particular importance not only in medical ethics and law, but also in clinical medicine. We saw in Section 10.6 on page 450 that diagnostic-therapeutic knowledge is practical knowledge consisting of conditional obligations. On this account, clinical medicine belongs to the realm of medical deontics. We shall continue this discussion in Section 21.5.3.

Disease as a Deontic Construct

14.0 Introduction

We saw on pages 174–183 that *disease,* as a resemblance category, is a social construct in that it is a society-relative category whose prototypes are established by that society. In the present chapter, we will explain and substantiate this thesis. It will be argued that prototype diseases, as focal generators of the category *disease,* are deontic-social constructs emerging from particular ought-to-do rules of a society. To this end, we shall introduce four notions upon which our conception is based, i.e., the notions of common morality, deontic institution, deontic set, and deontic-social construct. Our discussion thus divides into the following four parts:

14.1 Common Morality
14.2 Common Morality as a Deontic-Social Institution
14.3 Deontic Sets
14.4 The Deontic Construction of Prototype Diseases.

14.1 Common Morality

As Tristram Engelhardt correctly observes, "There are competing moralities. There are competing bioethics. There are those who support and those who condemn homosexual activities and marriages. There are those who support and those who condemn abortion. There are those who support and those who condemn social democratic approaches to the allocation of resources. There are those who support and those who condemn physician-assisted suicide, euthanasia, and capital punishment. There is public debate and sustained disagreement about the significance of human sexuality, reproduction, property rights, the limits of governmental authority, the allocation of scarce resources, suffering, dying, and death, as well as about the nature of the good and human flourishing" (Engelhardt, 2006, 2).

K. Sadegh-Zadeh, *Handbook of Analytic Philosophy of Medicine,*
Philosophy and Medicine 113, DOI 10.1007/978-94-007-2260-6_14,
© Springer Science+Business Media B.V. 2012

The observation above reminds us that not all moral values are universally shared. That means, in our terminology introduced in the preceding chaper, that not all human beings and not all communities subscribe to the same set of moral rules. In spite of this far-reaching diversity and difference, regarding a few basic human values there is a consensus worldwide which may be referred to as consensus morality or *common morality*. Whatever the reasons may be, whether they be biological or metaphysical, "a minimalist set of such values can be recognized across societal and other boundaries" (Bok, 2002, 13 ff.; Gert, 2004; Gert et al., 2006).[115]

A minimum set of shared values are indispensable to human coexistence. As the conditions for shared pursuit of the good, they constitute the cement of social cohesion, so to speak. Among them are, for example, the rearing of children, respecting one's parents, reciprocating aid, caring for the suffering and the weak, telling the truth, dealing fairly with others, as well as abstaining from deceit, betrayal, violence, and murder. This limited set of values may be viewed as some sort of common morality because it entails *ought-to-do rules* of the following type: one ought to render assistance to those who need it; one ought to care for the suffering; one ought not to betray other people; one ought not to commit murder; etc. Although these rules are frequently violated by some individuals in all societies, they nevertheless constitute standard basic morality at the community level in that *most,* not all, community members share and propagate them in public by agreement. Thus, by "common morality" we do not mean universal morality. We take common morality to be majority-based, group-specific, and country-specific. Also we do not consider common morality the basis of all morality.

14.2 Common Morality as a Deontic-Social Institution

Like medical knowledge, and scientific knowledge in general, whose genesis and maintenance by implicit communal speech acts – such as the communal performative on page 520 – was discussed in Section 11.5.3, the rules of common morality emerge and are maintained by communal agreement that may be viewed as an implicit communal speech act of the following form:

---

[115] "Now it is a condition of the existence of any form of social organization, of any human community, that certain expectations of behavior on the part of its members should be pretty regularly fulfilled: that some duties, one might say, should be performed, some obligations acknowledged, some rules observed. We might begin by locating the sphere of morality here. It is the sphere of the observance of rules, such that the existence of some such set of rules is a condition of the existence of a society. This is a minimal interpretation of morality. It represents it as what might literally be called a kind of public convenience: of the first importance as a condition of everything that matters, but only as a condition of everything that matters, not as something that matters in itself" (Strawson, 1970, 103).

The communal performative creating the institution of common morality: We hereby declare it right to rear our children, to have respect for our parents, to render assistance to those who need it and ... and not to commit murder.

The speech act is not made explicitly, but only implicitly in that the majority of community members approve and share the rules of common marality by obedience, talk about them positively, and criticize or even punish those who deviate from them. It is through this performative communal speech act that the common morality becomes a *social institution*.

The notion of a social institution was discussed on page 514. There we saw that a social institution is characterized by a number of rules that are constitutive of a *social practice*. In the preceding section, common morality was defined as a minimum set of ought-to-do rules in a community. These rules constitute a social institution in that they are responsible for social practices such as the rearing of children; respecting one's parents; reciprocating aid; caring for the suffering and the weak; and similar practices. Since the rules are of deontic character, the emerging social institution may be viewed as a *deontic-social institution*. Thus, common morality is a deontic-social institution constitutive of particular deontic-social practices. In what follows, it will be shown that what is called *disease* in medicine is a construct of such deontic-social practices. To this end, we need the new concept of a *deontic set*.

14.3 Deontic Sets

By bringing about deontic-social practices, the common morality of a society structures that society. The structuring consists in the partitioning of the society into different categories of individuals according to whether they obey or violate a particular rule, e.g., 'the set of criminals' and 'the set of non-criminals'; 'the set of honest people' and 'the set of dishonest people'; and others, which we call *deontic sets* because they are induced by *deontic* rules of the society.

Deontic sets are not natural kinds, but social constructs, for there are no natural deontic rules that could be obeyed or violated. For example, 'the set of criminals' is not a natural category like apple trees or the set of those with blue eyes. It comes into existence by classifying the social conduct of people in relation to deontic rules which forbid some criminal conduct. It may therefore be viewed as a deontic-socially constructed class, set, or category. This idea will be developed in the present section to show below that what is called "disease" in medicine, is such a deontic-social construct and not a natural category. To begin with, recall that deontic sentences say what one ought to do, is forbidden to do, and so on. As a simple example, consider the following sentence:

For everybody x, it is obligatory that x tells the truth.   (131)

This means, extensionally, "For everybody x, it is obligatory that x belongs to the set of those people who tell the truth". If the set of those people who tell the truth, is denoted by " T ":

$$T = \{y \mid y \text{ tells the truth}\}$$

then the deontic sentence (131) may also be represented extensionally in the language of set theory in the following way:

For everybody x, it is obligatory that x belongs to set T.

That is,

$$\forall x(\text{it is obligatory that } x \in T)$$

or more formally:

$$\forall x\big(OB(x \in T)\big)$$

where the extensionally written sentence " $x \in T$ " translates the intensionally expressed action sentence " x tells the truth". Based upon the considerations above, the notion of a deontic set may be introduced in two steps as follows (Sadegh-Zadeh, 2002).[116]

Definition 154 (Deontic subset). *If Ω is a universe of discourse, e.g., the set of human beings or a particular community, with A being any subset of it, then A is a deontic subset of Ω iff one of the following deontic norms exists in Ω :*

$$\forall x\big(OB(x \in A)\big)$$
$$\forall x\big(OB(x \in \overline{A})\big) \qquad \text{i.e., } \forall x\big(OB(x \notin A)\big)$$

where $\overline{A}$ is the complement of set A.

For instance, let Ω be the set of human beings and consider the following subsets of Ω :

---

[116] We could take all three standard deontic modalities (obligation, prohibition, and permission) into account to introduce three corresponding notions of a deontic set, i.e., the set of those who do obligatory actions, the set of those who do forbidden actions, and the set of those who do permitted actions. However, for the sake of convenience we confine ourselves to the modality of obligation only. The reason is that, as was shown in several places, e.g. in Definition 232 on page 929, the three modalities are interdefinable. We therefore chose *obligation* as our basic deontic modality by which all other deontic modalities were defined. See Definition 232 on page 929. Thus, a deontic set based on the operator OB is fundamental in that the others may be derived from it.

$P \equiv$ the set of those people who keep their promises$\qquad$(132)

$L \equiv$ the set of liars

$H \equiv$ the set of helpful people

$M \equiv$ the set of murderers

$G \equiv$ the set of gardeners.

According to Definition 154 the fifth set, G, is not a deontic subset of Ω because there is no deontic rule in the human community requiring that one ought to become a gardener or that forbids one from becoming a gardener. However, the first four sets listed in (132) are deontic subsets of Ω because the following four deontic norms are elements of common morality, and thus, exist in the human community:

You ought to keep your promises,

you ought not to lie,

you ought to be helpful,

you ought not to commit murder.

That is:

$\forall x \in \Omega (x$ ought to belong to $P)$

$\forall x \in \Omega (x$ ought to belong to $\overline{L})$

$\forall x \in \Omega (x$ ought to belong to $H)$

$\forall x \in \Omega (x$ ought to belong to $\overline{M})$.

Stated more formally, we have:

$\forall x \in \Omega \big(OB(x \in P) \big)$

$\forall x \in \Omega \big(OB(x \in \overline{L}) \big)$

$\forall x \in \Omega \big(OB(x \in H) \big)$

$\forall x \in \Omega \big(OB(x \in \overline{M}) \big)$.

Definition 155 (Deontic set). *A set A is a deontic set iff there is a base set Ω of which A is a deontic subset according to Definition 154.*

For instance, the sets T, P, L, H, and M mentioned above are deontic sets, whereas set G in (132) is none. From these considerations we can conclude that a deontic norm in a society defines, creates, or induces a deontic set (class, category). Those people who satisfy the norm are members of that deontic set, whereas those people who violate the norm stand outside of the set, i.e., are members of its complement. For instance, the deontic set of helpful people includes all those who satisfy the norm *you ought to be helpful*, whereas the deontic set of murderers includes all those who violate the norm *you ought not to commit murder.*

Although deontic sets really exist in the world out there, e.g., the inmates of prisons called "criminals", their existence depends on the norms of the social institution creating them. For this reason, we consider them as deontic-social constructs, or *deontic constructs* for short. This idea will be instrumental in demonstrating the deontic character of the concept of disease in the next section.

14.4 The Deontic Construction of Prototype Diseases

The concept of disease suggested on pages 174–183 is based on the idea that *disease* is a prototype resemblance category like the category of birds. The category emerges recursively from its best examples, called its prototypes, and a similarity relationship such that a human condition is considered a disease if it resembles a prototype disease. It is the prototypes that by similarities between them and other human conditions generate the category. According to this conception, the category is relative to a human society because its prototypical members, as its generators, are instituted by that society. Thus, the question of "what is disease?" reduces to "what is a prototype disease?" or "where do prototype diseases come from?".

We presume that some states of intense human suffering have existed for a long time in the history of mankind. Examples are human conditions such as angina pectoris, breast cancer, convulsion, and hemiplegia. They were described in Corpus Hippocraticum more than two millennia ago. As obvious states of suffering, they do not require any expert judgment to be identified as *humanitarian emergencies*. In their capacity as obvious humanitarian emergencies, they trigger ought-to-do action rules of brotherly love and charity in order to help and rescue the afflicted. We may therefore consider them *action-provoking* human conditions. Human conditions of this type have been selected by human beings in the prehistory of medicine as subjects of care to mean that the life of the afflicted person is threatened, and she is suffering and in need of assistance, advice, and any other useful aid that may relieve her pain and prevent her death, incapacitation, and continuing discomfort. It is appropriate to call the class of such provoked actions "treatment" to denote the interventions made in the afflicted persons' conditions. Terms such as "disease", and its synonyms in other languages, have been invented in later epochs of medical history to signify the subject of those action-provoking human conditions, i.e., *the subject of treatments*. Likewise, medical-scientific investigations into their nature and genesis have followed their recognition and categorization as humanitarian emergencies. To put it concisely, the afflicted person's state is *named* "disease" by the society to denote something that it finds undesirable and whose amelioration by way of a treatment it finds desirable and deontically obligatory. From the semantic point of view, this naming act is an ostensive definition of the term "disease" by members of a particular society in that they point to an action-provoking, prototype human condition such as angina pectoris and breast cancer declaring "this we name disease". Judged from an action-theoretic perspective, however, the term may be characterized as a label designating a *deontic set* in the following sense:

Viewed from the perspective of non-human, animated species themselves, i.e., plants and animals, there are no such things as 'diseases' in their world. The idea that there exist plant and animal diseases is due to our own, anthropomorphic worldview. For whatever reasons, neither a damaged plant nor an impaired animal enjoys compassion, treatment, and care by other plants and animals. They ail, suffer, fall prey to predators, or die. The opposite is the case only in the species Homo sapiens because human communities house a deontic-social institution of common morality to the effect that the impairment and suffering of an individual provoke nursing practices by others. They are action-provoking emergencies, and by virtue of the remedial and caring practices, i.e., 'treatments', that they provoke, they are experienced and categorized as something *ought-to-be-treated*, ostensively named "disease". We therefore suggest viewing a prototype disease as a scientifically-medically reconstructed property that characterizes an artificial, *deontic set* comprising ought-to-be-treated individuals. A prototype disease is thus a deontic-social construct by the institution of common morality, or a *deontic construct* for short.

A deontic construct in a society is an entity, be it an individual thing or a category, that is brought about by members of the society as a product of their ought-to-do actions. For instance, the category of 'criminals' is a deontic construct by virtue of specific deontic rules which require or prohibit particular conduct. Likewise, the category of literates in Germany is a deontic construct because school attendance is legally required in Germany: "Any child of age 6 ought to be enrolled in school". It is this legal norm and its ancillaries whose implementation and execution in Germany make the people learn and acquire literacy. A prototype disease in a society is also a deontic construct of that society because it emerges qua something ought-to-be-treated – and not qua a phenomenon or occurrence – from the norms of the deontic-social institution of common morality. As a particular human condition such as heart attack, convulsion, stroke, or breast cancer, it provokes actions of community members to rescue the afflicted, to help her, and to ameliorate her condition. Such a human condition is designated a "disease" simply to have a name for this type of action-provoking, ought-to-be-treated states of affairs. It could be, or could have been, named otherwise, e.g., "esaesid". What it has been termed is unimportant. Its primary characteristic is its being action-provoking. It is action-provoking not because it is a disease in the interpreted sense of this term, but because the majority of the community where it occurs, share basic values and attitudes such as sanctity of life, compassion, sympathy, benevolence, beneficence, love, and charity according to which rescue, relief, help, remedy, and care are deontically required in *such humanitarian emergencies*. By their recurrent remedial and preventive we-intentions, actions, and attitudes they bring about the collective act, or social practice, of treating something as a disease that without this we-act would not be a disease, but rather a state of affairs comparable to the damage and impairment in plants and animals as seen from their own perspective. It is questionable whether human monads not living in polyads, i.e., in human communities, would ever consider themselves as having any disease. That means, by analogy to the Wittgensteinean impossibility of private language, that there are no private diseases. Prototype diseases are, as deontic constructs of a society, essentially social artifacts.

As pointed out on page 568, common morality may be viewed as an implicit communal performative of the form "we hereby declare it right to rear our children, to have respect for our parents, to render assistance to those who need it and ... and not to commit murder". This social performative also includes the implicit speech act "we ... hereby declare it right to help suffering people". We may suppose that the caring reaction to action-provoking ought-to-be-treated states of affairs, called prototype diseases above, comes from this communal performative, which is entailed in the deontic-social institution of care that is based on common morality. Seen from this perspective, prototype diseases as something ought-to-be-treated are brought about by the social practice of nursing and care generated by the collective performative of common morality.

The deontic character of prototype diseases is conferred on their resemblants, i.e., on other human conditions, by the similarity relationship to form the category of *diseases*. Every new member that is added to the category as a resemblant, e.g., alopecia areata or computer-game addiction, is categorized a disease by virtue of its similarity to a prototype disease. It is then considered something ought-to-be-treated and ought-to-be-controlled. In exactly this deontic sense, the concept of disease is not descriptive, but normative. It identifies "what ought not to be" (Engelhardt, 1975, 127).

What we suggested above as the deontic origin of disease, is usually referred to in the philosophy of medicine as its value-ladenness. Although both views are virtually equivalent, we deliberately avoided the latter terminology because it is well-worn, on the one hand; and inaccessible to logical scrutiny and discourse, on the other. It is only their logical and semantic opacity that renders the traditional normativist theories open to attack by descriptivists like Christopher Boorse.

14.5 Summary

By "minimum morality" we understand a minimum collection of moral ought-to-do rules. A minimum morality shared by all or most members of a community is referred to as the common morality of that community. A human society is characterized by a specific common morality. The rules of its common morality are constitutive of particular social practices such as charity, care, prevention of criminality, etc. These deontically generated social practices structure the society in that they partition it into the set or category of those people who satisfy a particular deontic rule and the set or category of those who do not. We called such sets deontic sets or categories. A deontic set is not a natural kind. It comes into existence by compliance with, or violation of, deontic rules of the common morality in a society, e.g., the set of 'criminals' or the set of those who are 'in need of help'. It is thus a man-made entity, specifically a deontic-social construct. We showed that prototype diseases are such deontic-social constructs to the effect that the category of diseases turns out to be a deontic-social construct. Diseases are not natural phenomena. They are man-made.

Medicine is a Deontic Discipline

15.0 Introduction

Vita brevis, ars longa. This is the Latin translation of the first two lines of an aphorism by Hippocrates which reads: O βιος βραχυς, η δε τεχνη μακρη (Aphorims, section I, No. 1). It shows that in Ancient Greece medicine was viewed as an art, téchne. The view persisted in Western medicine until medical research joined the methodology of natural sciences in the late eighteenth century. The judgment soon emerged that medicine had been an unscientific endeavor in the past and had now become a scientific discipline: "Medicine will be a science, or it will not be" (Naunyn, 1909, 1348).[117] The terms "science" and "scientific" were overtly identified with natural science. Any deviant approach was considered unscientific, e.g., humoral pathology and homeopathy, and had to be banished from medicine. Since then there is, between the proponents and opponents of this view, an ongoing debate on the 'nature of medicine' concerned with whether medicine is a science or an art. We will not participate in this long-standing controversy because the very question is pointless for different reasons. For a detailed discussion on this issue, see Chapter 21 and (Marcum, 2008, 301 ff.).

On the basis of our discussions in the preceding chapters, we shall elucidate an important, additional aspect of medicine, which up to this point in time has been overlooked. Specifically, we shall argue that clinical medicine is a normative, or *deontic,* discipline like ethics and law. That is to say, it is an area where ought-to-do actions are investigated as well as performed, and ought-to-do rules are searched for. This construal is not only interesting philosophically. It is also instrumental in inquiring into the logic of medicine

---

[117] Bernhard Naunyn (1839–1925) was a German internist, pathologist and pharmacologist, and served in Dorpat, Bern, Königsberg, and Straßburg. He is remembered for introducing experimentation into clinical medicine. His dictum quoted above is often misquoted as "medicine will be a natural science, or it will not be" (see Sadegh-Zadeh, 1974).

K. Sadegh-Zadeh, *Handbook of Analytic Philosophy of Medicine,*
Philosophy and Medicine 113, DOI 10.1007/978-94-007-2260-6_15,
© Springer Science+Business Media B.V. 2012

and the methodology of clinical judgment and decision-making (see Chapter 8 and Part VI).

Medicine is concerned with the promotion, protection, and restoration of health through the prevention and treatment of maladies in individual patients as well as in communities. It accomplishes this task as clinical practice of health care, on the one hand; and as medical research, on the other, although there is no sharp boundaries between them. We shall study their deontic character in what follows. Our inquiry divides into these three sections:

15.1 Deonticity in Clinical Practice
15.2 Deonticity in Medical Research
15.3 Deontic Things in Medicine.

15.1 Deonticity in Clinical Practice

In this section, we shall advance the idea that clinical practice is a deontic domain. Specifically, it is an area where ought-to-do norms are executed, and thus, ought-to-do actions are performed, *duties* so to speak. We anticipated this view in our earlier discussions about the concept of clinical indication. It may easily be explained and confirmed by analyzing the logical structure of clinical knowledge:

In our previous discussions, we partitioned the set of sentences into declarative sentences such as "it is raining" and "AIDS is an infectious disease" on the one hand; and non-declarative sentences, on the other. In contrast to declarative sentences, non-declarative sentences do not describe any object, process, or state of affairs. They do not report on what IS. Examples are the following categories of sentences: interrogatives, requests, imperatives, expressives, and deontic sentences (see page 22).

Scientific knowledge in almost all disciplines is represented by declarative sentences, specifically by constatives. For example, anatomical knowledge describes the human body, its organs, cells, etc. Its sentences say, for instance, "the cell membrane is triple-layered, having two dark bands separated by an unstained layer". Exceptions from this merely constative style of talking are normative ethics and law. They deal with deontic sentences. We therefore combined them above to form the field of *deontics*. What we are doing here is showing that besides normative ethics and law, medicine is the third branch of deontics.

As an institution and not as the practicing of individual physicians, clinical practice is a deontic, rule-based practice of healing and may thus be considered practiced deontics, or practiced morality in a narrow sense. This is because clinical knowledge proper that is advanced and used in clinical practice, consists not of declarative sentences like in anatomy or physics, but of deontic rules. By the term "clinical knowledge proper" we understand diagnostic and therapeutic knowledge that in clinical decision-making guides the physician through the dynamic, branching clinical questionnaire discussed in Section 8.1.2 on page 283. The logical structure of diagnostic and therapeutic knowledge was already analyzed on pages 450–457. From those analyses we may conclude that a diagnostic as well as a therapeutic rule is, as an indication rule, in general an ought-to-do sentence of the following form:

$$\mathcal{Q}\Big(\alpha_1 \wedge \ldots \wedge \alpha_k \rightarrow \Big(\beta_1 \wedge \ldots \wedge \beta_m \rightarrow \tag{133}$$

$$OB\big((\gamma_1 \wedge \ldots \wedge \gamma_n)_1 \vee \ldots \vee (\delta_1 \wedge \ldots \wedge \delta_p)_q\big)\Big)\Big)$$

with $k, m, n, p, q \geq 1$, and with $\mathcal{Q}$ being the quantifier prefix that binds all free individual variables of the formula succeeding it. The sentence is a universally closed ought-to-do rule according to Definition 153 on page 564 such as, e.g., $\forall x \forall y \big(Ax \rightarrow (Bxy \rightarrow OB(Cx))\big)$. By the Importation and Exportation Rules of deduction in Table 36 on page 895, an ought-to-do sentence of the form (133) is equivalent to:

$$\mathcal{Q}\Big(\alpha_1 \wedge \ldots \wedge \alpha_k \wedge \beta_1 \wedge \ldots \wedge \beta_m \rightarrow \tag{134}$$

$$OB\big((\gamma_1 \wedge \ldots \wedge \gamma_n)_1 \vee \ldots \vee (\delta_1 \wedge \ldots \wedge \delta_p)_q\big)\Big)$$

and is obviously a conditional obligation, i.e., a genuine deontic rule as defined in Definition 153. That diagnostic-therapeutic knowledge does not consist of declarative sentences, implies that *it does not make statements* about 'the world out there'. It commands.

These considerations demonstrate that diagnostic and therapeutic decisions are reached by executing deontic rules as commands. They also explain the deontic reasons for malpractice suits. Medical malpractice is the performance of a prohibited clinical action, i.e., an action that violates the standards of clinical practice prescribed by clinical ought-to-do rules as above. This notion of malpractice includes failure as well as negligence. Consider as a simple example the following clinical situation that elucidates the deontic character of clinical medicine:

A 40-year-old male patient is complaining of acute chest pain that radiates to his left arm. His physician has the suspicion that he might either have myocardial infarction or reflux esophagitis. He asks the young patient whether he's had any health problems in the past. The patient denies. The doctor therefore rejects the supposition of myocardial infarction, administers some anti-acidic medication against reflux esophagitis, and sends the patient home. Sadly, he dies within a few hours. The autopsy reveals that he died of myocardial infarction. The physician is immediately accused of malpractice because he did not perform at least one of the following diagnostic examinations: recording an ECG or determining the concentration of heart-relevant enzymes in the patient's blood. By failing to do one of these examinations, he violated the following clinical ought-to-do rule:

- If a patient complains of acute chest pain that radiates to her left arm, then
- if you want to know whether she has myocardial infarction, then
- it is obligatory that you record an ECG or determine the concentration of heart-relevant enzymes in her blood.

To clearly demonstrate that this is a diagnostic ought-to-do rule, we will use the following predicates:

CPx $\equiv$ x complains of acute chest pain that radiates to x's left arm,
$DRyx$ $\equiv$ y is the doctor of x,
$WKyx$ $\equiv$ y wants to know whether x has myocardial infarction,
$ECGyx$ $\equiv$ y records an ECG in x,
$ENZyx$ $\equiv$ y determines the concentration of heart-relevant enzymes in x's blood.

The sentence above says:

$$\forall x \forall y \Big(CPx \rightarrow \big(DRyx \wedge WKyx \rightarrow OB(ECGyx \vee ENZyx) \big) \Big).$$

This is clearly an ought-to-do rule and deontic-logically equivalent to the obligation:

$$\forall x \forall y \big(CPx \wedge DRyx \wedge WKyx \rightarrow OB(ECGyx \vee ENZyx) \big)$$

and this to the prohibitions:

$$\forall x \forall y \big(CPx \wedge DRyx \wedge WKyx \rightarrow FO\neg(ECGyx \vee ENZyx) \big)$$
$$\forall x \forall y \big(CPx \wedge DRyx \wedge WKyx \rightarrow FO(\neg ECGyx \wedge \neg ENZyx) \big).$$

The latter contra-indication says: "If someone complains of acute chest pain that radiates to her left arm, and her physician wants to know whether she has myocardial infarction, then it is forbidden that she, the physician, omits both to perform an ECG and to determine the concentration of heart-relevant enzymes in the patient's blood". The failure to perform at least one of these two alternative diagnostic actions has caused a misdiagnosis in that the physician has overlooked the patient's myocardial infarction. The death of the patient caused by the misdiagnosis could have been avoided if the physician had performed one of the examinations. Therefore, the physician is responsible for this death due to her neglect of the ought-to-do rule above.

From the discussion above we may conclude that clinical ought-to-do rules are both clinical-practical know-how as well as deontic constraints on physician conduct. Additional deontic constraints on clinical practice are imposed by the familiar medical-ethical and legal norms that protect patient rights and human values. Examples are the principles of beneficence and non-maleficence, respect for patient autonomy, and prohibition of euthanasia.

Recent innovations in patient management that vindicate our conception of deonticity in medical practice are the so-called *clinical practice guidelines*, which are becoming widely accepted throughout health care. Although they are often presented either in the guise of "evidence-based medical knowledge" or flowcharts, they are in fact clinical *ought-to-do rules* and convey expert recommendations regarding diagnostics, therapy, prevention, and management of patients who have a particular clinical problem or condition such as angina pectoris, hypercholesterolemia, or apoplexia. A typical example is the following simple guideline: "Individuals with symptoms of cardiovascular disease, or who are over the age of 40 years and have diabetes or familial hypercholesterolemia, *should* be considered at high risk of cardiovascular events". The aim of clinical practice guidelines is to standardize health care, to assist practitioners and patients in decision-making about appropriate care in specific circumstances, and to reduce costs (Field and Lohr, 1990; ICDL, 2000).

15.2 Deonticity in Medical Research

Medical research comprises clinical research and non-clinical research. The latter has come to be termed biomedical research, biomedical sciences, or medical biosciences, and is conducted in disciplines such as anatomy, physiology, biochemistry, cytology, biophysics, and the like.

The ought-to-do rules of clinical practice discussed above originate from *clinical research*. This area is concerned with nosological, diagnostic, and therapeutic research, as well as any other malady-related issues. The goal is to acquire knowledge about the nature, genesis, diagnostics, therapy, and prevention of maladies. Accordingly, clinical research extends, without sharp boundaries, into non-clinical, biomedical research.

Deontic aspects are imported into clinical research by the concept of disease that was characterized as a deontic category on page 572. As an investigation into the diagnostics, therapy, and prevention of this deontic category, clinical research is a deontic domain like clinical practice. This may be explained with reference to diagnostic research:

Diagnostic research seeks diagnostic rules which enable the physicians to diagnose individual diseases. A diagnostic rule is either a rule for diagnosing a new disease, e.g., the diagnostic rules searched for in the 1980s for the then new disease AIDS; or a rule for diagnosing an already known disease like myocardial infarction or multiple sclerosis. In either case, the yield is a conditional obligation of the form (133–134) in the preceding section.

A second aspect of deonticity in medical research consists of deontic constraints imposed by ethics and law, for example, on human and animal experimentation. Thanks to such constraints medical researchers are not allowed to explore whatever and however they want. Medical-ethical and legal debates about what should be permitted or prohibited in medical research, e.g., embryonic research and cloning, demonstrate the genesis of such constraints.

15.3 Deontic Things in Medicine

Churchs, universities, printed love stories, and computers didn't exist prior to the emergence of Homo sapiens on earth. In other words, they didn't and do not exist outside the human world because they are not natural objects. They are man-made. Behind them lie human values, goals, and intentions. All man-made objects of this type are referred to as artifacts or constructs. Some types of constructs, e.g., money and scientific knowledge, are social facts and have their origin in social institutions. We have therefore called them social constructs (see page 523).

Depending on the type of acts, theories, and goals that play a causative role in bringing about a construct, one may classify them as follows: architectural constructs such as buildings and bridges; esthetic constructs such as paintings and symphonies; ballistic constructs such as rockets and atomic bombs; and so on. Individual, concrete constructs such as these examples may also be referred to as *things* instead of constructs, e.g., architectural things, esthetic things, ballistic things, etc. Analogously, we may presume that there are *deontic things* on earth:

The concept of deontic construct was introduced and discussed above. On the basis of that terminology, a *deontic thing* may be conceived of either (i) as a construct directly made by ought-to-do actions, or (ii) as an auxiliary construct to make some ought-to-do actions succeed, i.e., to bring about a deontic thing. For example, recovery processes brought about by therapeutic actions are deontic things on the grounds that the latter are ought-to-do actions. Likewise, artificial therapeutica such as drugs are deontic things because they are made to serve as therapeutic auxiliaries. Hospitals and doctors' offices are also deontic things. For they are artificial auxiliaries that enable clinical ought-to-do actions such as patient care and treatments.

15.4 Summary

We introduced the concept of the deontic rule to show that medical knowledge proper, i.e., clinical-practical knowledge, consists of such deontic rules. Clinical-practical knowledge is deontic-procedural knowledge concerned with diagnosis, therapy, and prevention. The term "procedural" means to know how to do something, e.g., to diagnose or treat a particular disease state. Diagnostic-therapeutic knowledge of this type is representable by conditional obligations. A conditional obligation, as an ought-to-do action rule, does not logically follow from descriptive or explanatory research that describes how things are, and explains why they occur. It is not justified by purely empirical research and evidence either. It comes from social institutions, i.e., medical communities in the present case, and is justified in comparison with alternative action rules by demonstrating that it is *better than* the latter. The comparative predicate "is better than", however, is an evaluative one and has again something to do with human values, intentions, and goals. We shall come back to this issue later on.

Based on the considerations above, medical practice and research may be viewed as deontic disciplines that necessitate appropriate methods of inquiry termed *medical deontics* in preceding sections. We exemplified the deontic character of medicine by demonstrating that prototype diseases are deontic-social constructs. They are delimited as out-to-be-treated categories of states of affairs on the basis of common morality that requires the members of a society to charitably act in humanitarian emergency situations.

Finally, a new type of social constructs were introduced that we termed *deontic things*. A deontic thing may be recursively defined as an individual object or process that (i) is brought about by deontically required actions, e.g., a recovery process brought about by therapy, as well as an individual patient's state of health at the end of such a recovery process; or (ii) is a man-made auxiliary that causally contributes to bringing about a deontic thing, e.g., a drug or a medicinal bath. A disease state ascribed to a patient by a diagnosis is also a deontic thing because according to our theory of diagnosis it is constructed by diagnostic rules as ought-to-do rules.

Like esthetic things, the genesis and handling of deontic things depends on human values, intentions, and goals materialized in deontic action rules. Analogous to esthetic things that are called artworks, deontic things may be considered *dutyworks*. The physician's achievements are such dutyworks. We shall look more closely at this point of view in Section 21.6 on page 777.

Part V

Medical Logic

16

Logic in Medicine

16.0 Introduction

Problem-solving in any domain requires adequate methods of problem-solving. For example, methods of arithmetic guide us in dealing with arithmetical problems such as "what is 4 + 5?". Arithmetical problems cannot be tackled by means of hammers or microscopes. Likewise, any issue that needs reasoning requires a particular method of reasoning, i.e., logic. Reasoning is not the art of asserting what one likes to assert. Unfortunately, philosophy of medicine has scarcely concerned itself with methods of reasoning in medicine.

The present Part V is concerned with the role that logic plays, or may play, in medicine and with its impact thereon. The question will be discussed whether medicine has a specific, inherent logic that governs medical reasoning and might be called 'the logic of medicine', or *medical logic* for short. This popular term, and consequently the question, is ambiguous, however. To clarify, we shall first examine a number of logics that are both needed and applicable in medicine.

To begin with, we have to distinguish between two issues. On the one hand, there is the issue of whether a particular system of logic, e.g., intuitionistic logic, may or may not be useful in medicine for solving medical and metamedical problems. The role that existing systems of logic may or may not play in medicine, we call *logic in medicine*. On the other hand, there is the issue of whether medicine may or may not have a 'natural', medical logic of its own that inherently governs medical reasoning. This is an altogether different issue than the former and will therefore be referred to as the *logic of medicine*. Our inquiry thus divides into the following two chapters:

16 Logic *in* Medicine
17 The Logic *of* Medicine.

Medical students are not taught logic. As a result, physicians, medical scientists, and even philosophers of medicine are usually no better acquainted

K. Sadegh-Zadeh, *Handbook of Analytic Philosophy of Medicine*,
Philosophy and Medicine 113, DOI 10.1007/978-94-007-2260-6_16,
© Springer Science+Business Media B.V. 2012

with logic than is a novelist or a grocer. The fact that modern medicine has neglected logic in medical practice, research and philosophy, is one of the reasons why the artificial intelligence of computer technology is more and more taking over the reasoning responsibility in medicine. It was not until the emergence of medical informatics in the 1960s and analytic philosophy of medicine in the 1970s that methods of logics were explicitly applied to medical and metamedical issues.[118] Since the advent of medical artificial intelligence and knowledge engineering technology in the 1970s, there has been a relatively intense application of different systems of logic for the purpose of developing logic-based computer programs to aid in clinical and non-clinical decision-making.[119] However, medical students and practicing physicians are neither sufficiently aware of this situation nor are they actively participating in its improvement. They are only consumers of its products, i.e., medical expert and decision support systems and other medical IT devices that are being produced by medical artificial intelligence technology. By this consumption, they increasingly hand over their reasoning responsibilities to machines that are steadily acquiring medical intelligence. In the current chapter, we shall shed some light on the potentials and limits of how systems of logic are, or may be, used in medicine as methods of reasoning and systematization.

From the various systems of logic considered in Part VIII we learn that the term "logic" ought to be used in the plural, i.e., *logics*. This pluralism of logical systems is also reflected in the application of logics to medicine in recent years. Logical pluralism in medicine has both its reasons and its consequences. We shall discuss them in turn to explain why a logic is no more than a mere instrument like a mathematical theory or any other theory. It can only be evaluated depending on how effectively it works in achieving some specified goals and on what drawbacks it leads to in the process.

The first reason for logical pluralism in medicine is obvious. It lies in the syntax of the sentences to which a particular system of logic can be applied. Since any logic has its own language with a specific syntax, it is not universally useful and cannot be applied to sentences whose syntax differs from its own. We shall demonstrate only a few examples. To this end, we will briefly consider the application of some classical and non-classical systems of logic in medicine. Our analysis consists of the following five sections:

16.1   Classical Logic in Medicine
16.2   Paraconsistent Logic in Medicine
16.3   Modal Logics in Medicine
16.4   Probability Logic in Medicine
16.5   Fuzzy Logic in Medicine.

---

[118] The only exception was the application of sentential logic and Boolean algebra to neural behavior by Warren McCulloch and Walter Pitts in 1943 (McCulloch and Pitts, 1943) that would decades later be rediscovered and viewed as the starting point of artificial neural networks (ANN) research and neurocomputing.

[119] See the journal *Artificial Intelligence in Medicine* (Elsevier) commenced in 1989.

16.1 Classical Logic in Medicine

When medical scholars talk about logic in medicine, they usually mean classical logic, as other types of logic are not well known in medicine. The highly developed representative of classical logic is the first-order predicate logic with identity sketched in Chapter 26. It constitutes the basic logic of classical mathematics. Insofar as the application of classical mathematics in medicine is concerned, the underlying logic is of course classical logic. Analogous applications in non-mathematical contexts are medical argumentations in research and practice. A simple example may illustrate. From the following premises:

- If someone is HIV positive, then she has AIDS,   (135)
- Anthony Perkins is HIV positive,

we can draw this conclusion: *Anthony Perkins has AIDS*. This argument is of the following form:

$$\{\forall x(Ax \to Bx), Aa\} \vdash Ba \tag{136}$$

where $A \equiv$ is HIV positive; $B \equiv$ has AIDS; $a \equiv$ Anthony Perkins. For a proof of the argument (136), see Proof 11 on page 896. The language of the argument is an extensional language of the first order. That is, quantifiers range over individual variables only, and the language contains no intensional particles, e.g., modal expressions. Deductive diagnostic-therapeutic judgment is in principle based on deductive argumentations of this and similar type. Examples are medical expert systems such as MYCIN and others that use deductive logic. See, e.g., (Buchanan and Shortliffe, 1984).

Predicate logic is used not only to prove that a particular set of premises implies a particular conclusion like in the above example. It is also used to prove (i) that a particular assertion is not true; (ii) that a particular assertion is true; and (iii) whether a particular item of knowledge is logically compatible or incompatible with a particular evidence. This will be illustrated in turn:

(i) Prove that a particular assertion is not true. Suppose someone makes an assertion and you are of the opinion that it is not true. To prove whether this is the case, you need only to demonstrate that her assertion implies a contradiction. This contradiction will automatically falsify the assertion in virtue of the rule *Reductio ad absurdum* mentioned in Table 36 on page 895. To illustrate, consider the following simple example. Suppose someone advances the two premises in (135) above and adds "Anthony Perkins does not have AIDS". Her whole assertion is inconsistent and can therefore be easily falsified. To this end, we will show that the conjunction:

(135) ∧ Anthony Perkins does not have AIDS,

that is:

$$\forall x(Ax \to Bx) \land Aa \land \neg Ba \tag{137}$$

implies a contradiction, and thus, cannot be true.

Assertion 6. $\forall x(Ax \rightarrow Bx) \wedge Aa \wedge \neg Ba$ *is false.*

Proof 6:

1.	$\forall x(Ax \rightarrow Bx) \wedge Aa \wedge \neg Ba$	Premise
2.	$\forall x(Ax \rightarrow Bx)$	$\wedge$-Elimination: 1
3.	Aa	$\wedge$-Elimination: 1
4.	$\neg Ba$	$\wedge$-Elimination: 1
5.	$Ax \rightarrow Bx$	$\forall$-Elimination: 2
6.	$Aa \rightarrow Ba$	Substitution Rule: 5
7.	Ba	Modus ponens: 3, 6
8.	$Ba \wedge \neg Ba$	$\wedge$-Introduction: 4, 7
9.	$\big(\forall x(Ax \rightarrow Bx) \wedge Aa \wedge \neg Ba\big) \rightarrow Ba \wedge \neg Ba$	Deduction Theorem 2: 1, 8
10.	$\neg\big(\forall x(Ax \rightarrow Bx) \wedge Aa \wedge \neg Ba\big)$	Reductio ad absurdum: 9. QED

(ii) Prove that a particular assertion is true. To prove that an assertion α is true, suppose it is not true, i.e., $\neg\alpha$ is true. Now, try to demonstrate, as in (i), that $\neg\alpha$ implies a contradiction, and then conduct a Reductio ad absurdum. If you succeed, you will thereby verify the assertion $\neg\neg\alpha$, i.e., α. This method is referred to as *indirect proof*. That is, the truth of something is indirectly proved by demonstrating the falsehood of its negation.

(iii) Compatibility and incompatibility between statements. Consider the AIDS example above once again where the proponent asserted the two premises in (135) and added that "Anthony Perkins does not have AIDS". This latter assertion is logically incompatible with the two premises. To demonstrate how we can prove the logical compatibility and incompatibility between sentences, we will first define these two notions.

Definition 156 (Classical-logical compatibility and incompatibility).

1. *A set of sentences,* $\mathfrak{F}$*, and* $n \geq 1$ *other sentences* $\alpha_1, \ldots, \alpha_n$ *are* logically compatible *iff* $\mathfrak{F} \cup \{\alpha_1, \ldots, \alpha_n\}$ *is consistent.*
2. *A set of sentences,* $\mathfrak{F}$*, and* $n \geq 1$ *other sentences* $\alpha_1, \ldots, \alpha_n$ *are* logically incompatible *iff they are not logically compatible, i.e., iff* $\mathfrak{F} \cup \{\alpha_1, \ldots, \alpha_n\}$ *is inconsistent.*

To prove, for instance, that the assertion "Anthony Perkins does not have AIDS" is logically incompatible with the two premises (135) above, we must demonstrate that according to Definition 156.2 the union (135) $\cup$ {Anthony Perkins does not have AIDS} is inconsistent. To this end, we proceed like in case (i) above and show that the union:

(135) $\cup$ {Anthony Perkins does not have AIDS}

that is:

$\{\forall x(Ax \rightarrow Bx), Aa\} \cup \{\neg Ba\}$

implies a contradiction. The proof is similar to lines 2–8 of Proof 6 above when we take lines 2–4 to be our premises.

As mentioned previously, many medical expert systems are based on classical logic and employ the techniques demonstrated above (see, e.g., Ligeza, 2006). Best examples are all rule-based medical expert systems written in the programming language Prolog. This language is in fact the programmed, decidable part of predicate logic (Bramer 2005; Clocksin and Mellish, 2003; Sterling and Shapiro, 1994).

In order for a medical expert system to process information about topographic, spatial, and functional relationships between body parts or bodily processes, its medical-empirical knowledge base is supplemented with some non-empirical, formal knowledge that is axiomatically-artificially constructed. A prominent example of such knowledge is *mereology*. The Greek term $\mu\varepsilon\rho o\varsigma$ (meros) and its Latin synonym "pars" mean "part". Mereology, or *partology* in Latin, is an axiomatic framework for the analysis of part-whole relationships. Its axioms and postulates are formulated in the first-order language to enable predicate-logical inferences. A few examples are given below in Table 15 in order to refer to and fuzzify them later on page 741 ff. In the table, the binary predicates *P, PP, O* and *D,* and the unary predicate *PT* are used. The first one is the primitive of the framework and all other ones are defined thereby. They read:

Pxy	$\equiv$	x is_a_part_of y	e.g., the lens is_a_part_of the eye,
$PPxy$	$\equiv$	x is_a_proper_part_of y	the lens is_a_proper_part_of the eye
Oxy	$\equiv$	x overlaps y	the eyeball overlaps the lens,
Dxy	$\equiv$	x is_discrete_from y	the lens is discrete_from the iris,
PTx	$\equiv$	x is_a_point.	

Table 15: Some mereological axioms and definitions

Axioms:

1. $\forall x Pxx$ — Every object is_a_part_of itself (i.e., parthood is reflexive),
2. $\forall x \forall y (Pxy \land Pyx \rightarrow x = y)$ — if x is_a_part_of y and y is_a_part_of x, then x and y are identical (i.e., parthood is antisymmetric),
3. $\forall x \forall y \forall z (Pxy \land Pyz \rightarrow Pxz)$ — parthood is transitive.

Definitions:

4. $\forall x \forall y (PPxy \leftrightarrow Pxy \land \neg (x = y))$ — an object is_a_proper_part_of another one if and only if it is a part thereof and different therefrom,
5. $\forall x \forall y (Oxy \leftrightarrow \exists z (Pzx \land Pzy))$ — objects with common parts overlap,
6. $\forall x \forall y (Dxy \leftrightarrow \neg Oxy)$ — an object is discrete from another one if and only if they do not overlap,

Table 15: Some mereological axioms and definitions

7. $\forall x\big(PTx \leftrightarrow \forall y(Pyx \rightarrow y = x)\big)$ an object is a point if and only if it is identical with anything of which it is_a_part.[120]

According to axioms 1–3 in Table 15 and Definition 4 on page 69, the relation of parthood is a partial ordering of the universe of discourse since it is reflexive, transitive, and antisymmetric. For instance, a human heart is part of itself (axiom 1). It is also part of the circulatory system. Since the latter is part of the human body, a human heart is part of the human body (axiom 3). It is even a proper part of the human body because it is not identical therewith (sentence 4). The mereological axioms in Table 15 imply a large number of theorems. A few examples are listed in Table 16.

Table 16: Some mereological theorems

1. $\forall x \neg PPxx$	Proper parthood is irreflexive,
2. $\forall x \forall y(PPxy \rightarrow \neg PPyx)$	proper parthood is asymmetric,
3. $\forall x \forall y \, z(PPxy \wedge PPyz \rightarrow PPxz)$	proper parthood is transitive.
4. $\forall x Oxx$	overlap is reflexive,
5. $\forall x \forall y(Oxy \rightarrow Oyx)$	overlap is symmetric,
6. $\forall x \forall y(PPxy \rightarrow Oxy)$	an object and its proper parts overlap,
7. $\forall x \forall y(Oxy \wedge Pyz \rightarrow Oxz)$	if x overlaps a part of z, then it also overlaps z.

For instance, a chromosome is a proper part of the cell nucleus because it is a part thereof and not identical therewith (Definition 4 in Table 15). Likewise, the cell nucleus is a proper part of the cell. Thus, a chromosome is a proper part of the cell (theorem 3 in Table 16). But it is not a proper part of itself (theorem 1), whereas it overlaps itself (theorem 4). According to theorems 4–5, and Definition 4 on page 69, the relation *Overlap* is a quasi-ordering of the universe of discourse.

---

[120] Edmund Husserl (1859–1938), an Austrian-born German philosopher and the founder of phenomenology, introduced in his *Logical Investigations* (Husserl, 2001), first published in 1900/01, the term "formal ontology" to analyze *parts and wholes*. Stanisław Leśniewski, a Polish logician and mathematician (1886–1939), developed a formal theory of part-whole relationships from 1916 onwards and coined the term "mereology" in 1927 (Rickey and Srzednicki, 1986). The theory was improved by his student Alfred Tarski (1927). For details on mereology, see, e.g., (Carnap, 1954; Donnelly et al., 2006; Pontow and Schubert, 2006; Simons, 2000b).

The examples we have considered thus far should not give the impression that the first-order predicate logic is sufficient for all medical purposes. All arguments whose underlying language transcends the syntactic limits of the first-order language $\mathcal{L}_1$ require other or stronger logics. For instance, the first-order predicate logic does not enable us to infer anything from the following medical premises (see also Chapter 27):

- Many diabetics are at risk of suffering coronary heart disease,
- the patient Elroy Fox is a diabetic;

or from these premises:

- Up to 20% of patients may have a relapse of diarrhea from Clostridium difficile within 1 or 2 weeks after stopping initial therapy;
- the patient Elroy Fox had diarrhea from Clostridium difficile three weeks ago;
- he had recovered; but he stopped initial therapy a few days ago.

Fuzzy quantifiers such as "many" in the first example do not belong to first-order language. The same applies to percentage in the second example because it signifies the ratio of two numbers that represent the size of two classes, for instance, the number of those in a population who have diarrhea divided by the size of the population. The term "the number of those with diarrhea" has a set as its argument, i.e., *those with diarrhea,* and is therefore not permitted for use by the syntax of a first-order language (see Section 26.2.1 on page 857). So, first-order logic cannot handle the examples above. It also cannot handle the modal parts of medical language composed of modal sentences, on the one hand; and the issue of consistency and inconsistency of medical knowledge, on the other. We now turn to these issues.

16.2 Paraconsistent Logic in Medicine

The traditional representation of medical knowledge in textbooks does not betray the fact that its application to an individual patient in diagnostic-therapeutic decision-making requires a particular logic which is capable of dealing with the syntax of that knowledge. Some physicians may believe that it is enough to possess that knowledge and to try to use it according to one's liking. The naivety of this view becomes obvious by considering the precise formal representation of the very textbook knowledge in the medical knowledge base of an expert system.

It is well known that the content of a textbook does not originate from the single brain of its individual author. Likewise, medical knowledge bases used in medical expert or decision support systems stem from various knowledge sources such as handbooks, journals, and domain experts. For instance, to build a cardiologic expert system, domain experts in cardiology are interviewed in order to compile their expert knowledge. Since different experts have different experiences during their career and often disagree with each other about states of affairs, it is conceivable that a particular medical expert system contains logically incompatible knowledge items. This situation renders the knowledge base inconsistent in terms of classical logic. It is practically difficult and sometimes even impossible to detect and localize such inconsistencies in a large knowledge base or in a hospital database used by an expert system. Suppose now that the reasoning method operative in the expert system, i.e., its *inference engine*, is based on classical logic. As outlined in Section 28.3 on page 961, the concept of inference of classical logic is explosive. That means that when set *KB* is the inconsistent knowledge base of the expert system and *D* is the set of data of an individual patient for whom a diagnosis is sought, the inference engine will infer from the inconsistent set KB ∪ *D* arbitrary statements about the patient, including false statements, because from inconsistent premises *everything* follows (see the deduction rule "Ex Contradictione Quodlibet" in Table 36 on page 895). By implying all statements of the world, the expert system becomes trivialized because it says everything, and therefore nothing about the patient. Such trivializations of knowledge bases can be prevented by using, as the underlying logic of the inference engine, *paraconsistent* logic instead of classical logic. As pointed out on page 962, paraconsistent logic is inconsistency tolerant and does not lead to inferential explosions. Outside of the logical sciences, however, this type of logic is not yet well known in the scholarly world. A few authors have recently tried to apply them in the theory of logic programming (da Costa and Subrahmanian, 1989; Blair and Subrahmanian, 1987, 1989; Grant and Subrahmanian, 1995).

16.3 Modal Logics in Medicine

We have seen in preceding chapters that medical knowledge and communication use a more comprehensive language that transcends the confines of a first-order language. Specifically, it is a multimodal language of higher order, and as such, it cannot be reduced to a first-order language. As a consequence, first-order logics are not sufficient tools of reasoning in medicine. The handling of a modal language and knowledge requires modal logics. Consider, for example, the following premises:

1. If a patient has angina pectoris, *it is possible that* she has coronary heart disease;
2. Elroy Fox has angina pectoris.

The first one of these sentences contains the alethic-modal operator "it is possible that" and is thus an alethic-modal sentence. The premises are of the following syntax (see Section 27.1.1):

1'. $\forall x (Px \rightarrow \Diamond Qx)$
2'. Pa.

Here, the predicates P and Q stand, respectively, for "has angina pectoris" and "has coronary heart disease". The individual constant "a" signifies "Elroy Fox", and "$\Diamond$" represents the modal operator *it_is_possible_that*. So, alethic modal logic is required to infer the sentence:

$$\Diamond Qa$$

which says *it is possible that Elroy Fox has coronary heart disease*. As an additional example, we will demonstrate that diagnostic decision-making requires at least deontic logic. As we saw in previous sections (10.6–10.7 and 15.1), diagnostic-therapeutic knowledge consists of deontic rules, and thus, of commitments of the form:

    a. when you are faced with a clinical situation δ_1, then
    b. if you want to reach the goal δ_2, then
    c. action α should be performed / is forbidden / is allowed.

That is:

$$\forall x_1 \ldots \forall x_n \big(\delta_1 \to (\delta_2 \to \nabla\alpha)\big)$$

or, equivalently, in virtue of the Importation Rule:

$$\forall x_1 \ldots \forall x_n (\delta_1 \wedge \delta_2 \to \nabla\alpha)$$

where δ_1 and δ_2 are statements of arbitrary complexity about the patient; α is an action sentence; and ∇ is one of the following three deontic operators: it_is_obligatory_that; it_is_forbidden_that; it_is_permitted_that. Suppose now that there is a patient with the data $\delta_1 \wedge \delta_2$. Deontic logic is needed to draw the conclusion that $\nabla\alpha$, i.e., α is obligatory, forbidden, or permitted depending on the operator ∇. For example, the following premises:

- $\forall x \big(Px \wedge Qx \to OB(Rx)\big)$
- $Pa \wedge Qa$

deontic-logically imply the sentence:

- $OB(Ra)$

that says that the individual a ought to do R. It is not possible to arrive at such a diagnostic-therapeutic ought-to-do conclusion without deontic-logical reasoning. Diagnostic-therapeutic reasoning of course requires many types of logics, but among them deontic logic is the most important. That neither real-world clinical decision-makers nor designers of clinical decision support systems are aware of deontic logic, is only proof of the importance of logical-philosophical inquiries into medicine. Such inquiries produced extensive research and discussion about the role of deontic logic in law. See, e.g., (Hage,

2005; Royakkers, 1998).[121] Based on our discussion about deontic logic in Section 27.2, one can see that since both law and medicine centrally involve deontic notions, logical-philosophical analyses of medicine will most likely produce similarly extensive results.

An important question to ask in this context is whether the deontic logic referred to above is really an appropriate logic for use in medicine. Unfortunately, as was briefly outlined in Section 27.2.3 on page 933, the available deontic logics as extensions of classical logic lead to inconsistencies. Accordingly, *paraconsistent deontic logics* seem to be a suitable alternative because they are inconsistency tolerant systems. For details, see (da Costa and Carnielli, 1986; Grana, 1990).

16.4 Probability Logic in Medicine

Medicine is essentially an uncertain endeavor. Fortunately, however, there are several tools to cope with this uncertainty. Among them are also probability theory and statistics which have a wide range of application in medicine. Without them, medical research and practice would be unfeasible today. But only three minor examples will be outlined in the present section. We shall first distinguish between *uncertainty* and *randomness* in medicine to show that the concept of probability has different meanings, and plays different roles, in these two contexts. We shall in addition introduce the method of probabilistic-causal analysis and some important types of probabilistic-causal factor. Our discussion divides into the following four sections:

16.4.1 Uncertainty and Randomness

The notions of certainty and uncertainty refer to *subjective,* epistemic states of human beings, but not to states of the external world. A particular person, say the present reader, may be subjectively certain or uncertain about whether HIV is a DNA or an RNA virus. There is no *objective* certainty or uncertainty in the world out there, but only determinacy or indeterminacy, i.e., randomness, of phenomena and events. The difference between uncertainty and randomness is this:

---

[121] In medicine, Moore and Hutchins (1980, 1981) have introduced special operators for the intuitive concepts of *certainty, demand,* and *effort,* akin to the operators of alethic-modal logic, to account for the technical and ethical limitations on human studies in medical research and practice.

Certainty and uncertainty are 'in the subjective, inner world'. Whenever a human being *knows* or *is convinced that* something is the case, then she is *certain* about it. Certainty corresponds to knowledge and conviction. Uncertainty as the lack of certainty consists in a subjective, epistemic state below the threshold of knowledge and conviction comprising subjective states of belief, conjecture, possibility considerations, and ignorance (see Section 27.3.1).

Randomness, however, is 'in the world out there'. A phenomenon or event *A* is indeterministically or *randomly* associated with another phenomenon or event *B* when there is no regularity of joint occurrence of *A* and *B* to the effect that the conditional "if *A* occurs then always *B* occurs" is not true. When *A* occurs, then only sometimes does *B* also occur. *A* is not associated with *B* in 100% of cases. For example, when someone has a cough, *A,* only sometimes does she have bronchitis, *B*. At some other time she does not have bronchitis. For whatever reasons, the association between cough and bronchitis is random. So, the deterministic conditional "if a patient coughs, then she has bronchitis" is not true.

Uncertainty about something may have different causes. On the one hand, it may be due to (i) *randomness* when our knowledge about the association between two events says that this association is indeterministic. On the other hand, it may be due to the (ii) *vagueness*, i.e., fuzziness, of a class such that we are unable to say whether a particular object is or is not a member of that class, for example, the class of diabetics. The reason is that, according to our analyses in Section 2.4.1 on page 38, vague classes have no sharp boundaries that would enable us to precisely localize an object as being either 'in' or 'outside' of the class. The objective feature *randomness* as well as the subjective feature *uncertainty* due to randomness, can be measured by probability. But the management of uncertainty due to vagueness requires fuzzy logic. We shall be concerned with this issue in Section 16.5 below and in Chapter 30.

Random as well as subjectively uncertain events are said to be likely or *probable*. We have previously distinguished between qualitative, comparative, and quantitative terms. Accordingly, randomness and uncertainty are treated as qualitative, comparative, or quantitative probabilities. Examples are:

It is *probable* that Elroy Fox has diabetes   (qualitative)
that he has diabetes is *more probable than* that he has hepatitis   (comparative)
the *probability* that he has diabetes, is 0.7   (quantitative)

The latter sentence says "the degree of probability that he has diabetes, is 0.7". The first attempts to find precise, numerical representations of *uncertainty and randomness* were made by the mathematicians Pascal and Fermat in the seventeenth century. The result of investigations since then is what we call stochastics or the theory of probability and mathematical statistics today (see footnotes 186–187 on page 970). We pointed out earlier that the quantitative notion of probability as the basic concept of probability theory is a formal, empirically uninterpreted term. Formally, it is a normalized additive measure in a mathematical sense. It can be interpreted and used differently in different contexts of application (see Section 29.1.6 on page 982):

On the one hand, in a context of human subjective uncertainty, it may be interpreted as a measure of subjective uncertainty so as to make belief states numerically representable. For example, to say that "the probability that Elroy Fox has diabetes, is 0.7" is the same as "to the extent 0.7, I believe that Elroy Fox has diabetes". Otherwise put, belief may be quantified as probability to make it amenable to probability theory. Degree of belief is degree of *subjective probability*.

On the other hand, random events and processes cannot be described by deterministic conditionals such as "if A then B". Statistics is used instead to quantify the frequency of association between A and B and to represent the indeterministic relationship between them as a degree of probability. The extent of this randomness is a degree of *objective probability*.

In the wake of the increasing probabilization of uncertainty and randomness in medicine since the eighteenth century the naked, neutral term "probability" has become a respected element of medical language, methodology, and epistemology. Unfortunately, however, the two types of probability, the subjective and the objective, are not carefully differentiated in medicine and other disciplines. For details on the philosophy of probability, see (Skyrms, 2000).

Probability theory and statistics are applied in almost all areas of contemporary medicine. Well-known examples are controlled clinical trials and expected value decision-making considered in Section 8.4. The most important significance that probability theory has in medicine, however, is its contribution to our understanding and representation of medical causality. One should only be aware that whether the term "the probability of" refers to single cases such as individual patients, or whether it refers to classes, is not typically clarified. What is meant, for example, by the statement "In Germany, the probability of suffering from schizophrenia is 0.01"? Does the number 0.01 quantify the chance that any *individual* resident in Germany will suffer from schizophrenia, or is it a *global* measure of the occurrence of the random event 'schizophrenia' in Germany? In the former case, we would have a subjective probability estimate, whereas the latter is an expression of objective probability. Specifically, the latter is a measure of the propensity of the random conditions that produce schizophrenia to occur at the population level (for the term "propensity", see page 982). The differentiation above is important for understanding the meaning of probability concepts in etiology, epidemiology, diagnostics, and therapy.

16.4.2 Probabilistic-Causal Analysis

As pointed out on page 343, it is customarily assumed that clinical diagnosis is made by means of the so-called hypothetico-deductive method of explaining the patient's suffering, referred to as *D-N explanation*. This is an unrealistic view because medical knowledge used in clinical decision-making scarcely contains deterministic-causal laws to enable causal explanations and thereby provide clinical diagnoses (see page 226).

Suppose that the patient Elroy Fox has acute fever and a cough. Thus, we have the patient data set $D = \{$Elroy fox has acute fever, Elroy Fox has a cough$\}$. The following diagnostic question arises: Why did D occur? If there are no deterministic-causal laws to causally explain the event D by a D-N explanation, we may try to answer our question by a weaker causal argument, i.e., by *probabilistic-causal analysis*. This method will be briefly outlined in the present section. We shall describe the procedure first, followed by a definition of the concept. (For details of the theory of probabilistic-causal analysis, see Stegmüller, 1973b, 339 ff.)

The procedure described

To probabilistic-causally analyze an event D such as $\{$Elroy fox has acute fever, Elroy Fox has a cough$\}$ that occurs in a reference class or population PO, (i) first the population PO must be exhaustively partitioned into mutually exclusive events such that each of these events is causally relevant to D, and then (ii) from among these causally relevant events those events must be identified that have actually occurred to cause D. We will explain:

In Section 6.5, medical etiology was based on a theory of probabilistic causality. Genuine causal structures were introduced to obtain the notions of positive cause, negative cause, and degree of causal relevance. We showed how the degree of *causal relevance* of an event A to an event B in a context or population PO, denoted $cr(A, B, PO)$, may be defined as the extent of the increase or decrease of the probability of occurrence of B conditional on A in the context PO:

$$cr(A, B, PO) = p(B \mid PO \cap A) - p(B \mid PO).$$

The expression $cr(A, B, PO)$, i.e., the degree of causal relevance of event A to event B in the context or population PO, represents the degree of causation of B by A in PO. It is a number in the interval $[-1, +1]$. For the sake of simplicity, here the temporal order of events is not considered. For details, see Section 6.5.

The conceptual framework referred to enables us to conduct probabilistic-causal analyses in medicine, especially in clinical decision-making where diagnoses are sought for a patient such as Elroy Fox above with the data $D = \{\delta_1, \ldots, \delta_m\}$. Each δ_i in this data set is a statement describing a problem, symptom, complaint, sign, or finding, e.g., $D = \{$Elroy fox has acute fever, Elroy Fox has a cough$\}$. To conduct a probabilistic-causal analysis of these data in order to find a probabilistic-causal diagnosis for the patient, we will first introduce the auxiliary notion of a *causally relevant partition:*

Let $p(D \mid PO) = r$ be the *base probability* that the patient data set D has in the reference population PO to which the patient belongs. A *causally relevant partition* of this population with respect to D is:

1. a partition π of the class PO into $n > 1$ subclasses $\{C_i, \ldots, C_n\}$, i.e., $\pi = \{PO \cap C_1, \ldots, PO \cap C_n\}$, such that:
2. each subclass C_i is causally relevant to D in PO, i.e., $p(D \mid PO \cap C_i) \neq p(D \mid PO)$, or equivalently, $p(D \mid PO \cap C_i) - p(D \mid PO) \neq 0$ for all $C_i \in \{C_i, \ldots, C_n\}$.

The partition is said to be *homogeneous* iff:

3. there is no additional, causally relevant partition of any sublasses $PO \cap C_i$ with respect to D.

The latter clause guarantees the homogeneity of the partition π by demonstrating that a further, causally relevant partition π' of a subclass $PO \cap C_i$ is not possible. An homogeneous partition provides what we have called *differential diagnoses* on page 332. Suppose, for example, that the reference population PO to which our patient Elroy Fox belongs, is the category of *men_over_60* years of age. And suppose in addition that in this population we have the following base probability of the data $D = \{$has acute fever, has a cough$\}$:

$$p(has\_acute\_fever \cap has\_a\_cough \mid men\_over\_60) = 0.003.$$

An example partition of the reference population *men_over_60* is the following set:

men_over_60 $\cap$ *has_bronchitis* $\cap$ *has_pneumonia*
men_over_60 $\cap$ *has_bronchitis* $\cap$ *has_no_pneumonia*
men_over_60 $\cap$ *has_no_bronchitis* $\cap$ *has_pneumonia*
men_over_60 $\cap$ *has_no_bronchitis* $\cap$ *has_no_pneumonia*

with supposed probabilities:

$p(D \mid men\_over\_60 \cap has\_bronchitis \cap has\_pneumonia) = 0.95$
$p(D \mid men\_over\_60 \cap has\_bronchitis \cap has\_no\_pneumonia) = 0.7$
$p(D \mid men\_over\_60 \cap has\_no\_bronchitis \cap has\_pneumonia) = 0.8$
$p(D \mid men\_over\_60 \cap has\_no\_bronchitis \cap has\_no\_pneumonia) = 0.001.$

These probabilities demonstrate that each of the four subclasses of the partition is causally relevant to D in the patient's population $PO = $ men_over_60 with the base probability $p(D \mid PO) = 0.003$. The first three are causally positively relevant, whereas the fourth one ('has no bronchitis $\cap$ has no pneumonia') is causally negatively relevant to D. Given the above partititon of the reference class, we have the following *differential diagnoses:*

Elroy Fox $\in$ *has_bronchitis* $\cap$ *has_pneumonia*
Elroy Fox $\in$ *has_bronchitis* $\cap$ *has_no_pneumonia*
Elroy Fox $\in$ *has_no_bronchitis* $\cap$ *has_pneumonia*
Elroy Fox $\in$ *has_no_bronchitis* $\cap$ *has_no_pneumonia*.

An homogeneous, causally relevant partititon of a base population PO with respect to patient data D provides a set of differential diagnoses for D. The potential diagnoses in the set are mutually exclusive and jointly exhaustive. An examination is required to identify from among these alternative classes a *causally-positively relevant* one to which the patient Elroy Fox actually belongs, e.g., "Elroy Fox has bronchitis and no pneumonia". In this case, our final diagnosis would be:

Diagnosis = {*Elroy Fox has bronchitis and no pneumonia*}

because this finding is probabilistic-causally positively relevant to patient data:

$$p(D \mid PO \cap has\_bronchitis \cap has\_no\_pneumonia) > p(D \mid PO).$$

The concept defined

To arrive at the final diagnosis above, we conducted a probabilistic-causal analysis of the state of health of the patient whose initial data is $D =$ {Elroy fox has acute fever, Elroy Fox has a cough}. In general, if there are:

- an individual a,
- her initial data set D,
- a reference class or population PO to which she belongs, and
- a base probability $p(D \mid PO)$,

then a probabilistic-causal analysis of D is a pair of the following form (for details, see Stegmüller, 1973b; Westmeyer, 1975; Sadegh-Zadeh, 1978a, 1979):

⟨Analysandum, Analysans⟩

such that:

Analysandum $= \langle p(D \mid PO), a \in D \cap PO \rangle$

and:

Analysans $= \langle \pi, KB, a \in PO \cap C_i \rangle$

with:

$$\pi = \{PO \cap C_1, \ldots, PO \cap C_n\} \quad \text{with } n > 1$$
$$(PO \cap C_i) \cap (PO \cap C_j) = \varnothing \quad \text{for } i \neq j$$
$$(PO \cap C_1) \cup \ldots \cup (PO \cap C_n) = PO.$$

Here, π is an homogeneous, causally relevant partition of PO providing an exhaustive set of mutually exclusive differential diagnoses; and KB is a knowledge base comprising a set of $n > 1$ probability statements:

$$p(D \mid PO \cap C_1) = r_1$$
$$p(D \mid PO \cap C_2) = r_2$$

$$\vdots$$

$$p(D \mid PO \cap C_n) = r_n$$

about the partition such that each $PO \cap C_i$ is an element of the partition with positive causal relevance to D, e.g.:

$$p(D \mid PO \cap \text{has\_bronchitis} \cap \text{has\_no\_pneumonia}) > p(D \mid PO).$$

See also axiom 13 in Definition 101 on page 321, and the concept of causal diagnosis on page 329.

16.4.3 Probabilistic-Causal Factors

The concept of probabilistic-causal diagnosis sketched in the preceding section may be generalized to introduce some etiologic-epidemiologic notions such as *causal factor, risk factor, preventive factor,* and *protective factor* (see Definitions 114–115 on page 378). That something, A, is a positive causal factor of something else, B, means that A is a part of a more or less complex, positive cause $X_1 \cap \ldots \cap X_n \cap A$ of B with $1 \leq i \leq n$. That is:

Definition 157 (Positive causal factor). *A is a* positive causal factor *for B in a context* $X_1 \cap \ldots \cap X_n$ *iff:*
  1. $cr(A, B, X_1 \cap \ldots \cap X_n) = p(B \mid X_1 \cap \ldots \cap X_n \cap A) - p(B \mid X_1 \cap \ldots \cap X_n),$
  2. $cr(A, B, X_1 \cap \ldots \cap X_n) > 0.$

For example, high blood pressure in diabetics is a positive causal factor for myocardial infarction. The notion of a negative causal factor may be introduced in a similar way. (For the numerical function cr of causal relevance, see Definition 80 on page 260.)

Definition 158 (Negative causal factor). *A is a* negative causal factor *for B in a context* $X_1 \cap \ldots \cap X_n$ *iff:*
  1. $cr(A, B, X_1 \cap \ldots \cap X_n) = p(B \mid X_1 \cap \ldots \cap X_n \cap A) - p(B \mid X_1 \cap \ldots \cap X_n),$
  2. $cr(A, B, X_1 \cap \ldots \cap X_n) < 0.$

For example, sports and low-fat nutrition in both males and females are negative causal factors for myocardial infarction. They decrease the probability of myocardial infarction occurring. The two definitions above are in essence the same as Definition 73 on page 255.

What is usually called a risk factor is actually a positive causal factor that contributes to the occurrence of an undesired event, e.g., a disease state. A preventive or protective factor is a negative causal factor that hinders the occurrence of an undesired event. These notions were introduced in Definitions 114–115 on page 378. It is not advisable to interpret the probability, p, in all these concepts as subjective probability. Such an interpretation would mean that the positive or negative causal effect of a factor is a degree of subjective, personal belief of an individual, e.g., of a physician or epidemiologist. Since the goal in medicine is not to establish subjective degrees of belief, it is preferable to distinguish subjective and objective probabilities as discussed in previous sections. To assert, for instance, that high blood pressure in diabetics is a risk factor for myocardial infarction, means that *the population* of diabetics with high blood pressure produces more myocardial infarctions than the population without that risk factor. This *higher incidence* of myocardial infarction in the population of diabetics with high blood pressure is not the degree of subjective belief of an individual, but a feature of 'the world out there' measured by the quantitative notion of probability, p, i.e., an objective probability. This warning notwithstanding, in decision analysis and expert systems research the so-called causal *belief networks* or causal *Bayesian networks* have become a popular tool of knowledge representation for use in probabilistic reasoning. Such networks, however, blur the significant difference between subjective and objective probability. For example, see (Cooper, 1988; Neapolitan, 1990; Pearl, 2001).

16.4.4 Bayesian Reasoning

One of the most important probabilistic tools used for reasoning purposes in medicine is Bayes's Theorem. This theorem is discussed in Section 29.1.5 on page 980. As pointed out on page 784, it was proposed for use in medicine by Ledley and Lusted in 1959 and today plays a major role in medical decision-making and clinical decision support systems (Ledley and Lusted 1959; Sadegh-Zadeh, 1980b).

16.5 Fuzzy Logic in Medicine

All of the bivalent logics considered in preceding sections require that medical statements be capable of possessing determinate truth values and be true or false. This presupposition of bivalence could be satisfied only if medical terms had precise meanings and denoted crisp sets, i.e., classical sets with sharp boundaries, so that one could determine whether a particular object does or does not fall within a particular class. We know, however, that this is not the case. Almost all medical terms are vague. The class of those people, for example, who have pneumonia or any other disease is not a crisp set, but a fuzzy set with unsharp boundaries. We are therefore not always able to say whether a particular patient such as Elroy Fox is definitely in or outside the set of those patients who have pneumonia. As a consequence, we shall not always be in the position to know whether a statement such as "Elroy Fox has pneumonia" is true or false (see Chapter 30).

Likewise, probability theory and logic can be meaningfully applied only under the assumption that the events to which probabilities are assigned are crisp events. However, due to the above-mentioned vagueness of most real-world classes, there are virtually no such events. For example, we do not know how many days 'a few days' exactly are. On this account, it does not make sense to assert a probability statement such as "the probability that the patient Elroy Fox will recover in a few days, is 0.8". For one can immediately ask what event is meant by "recovery in a few days"? When exactly could, or will, it commence? The event has no clear start and no clear finish. It is a fuzzy event. If we define the fuzzy set *few* in the following way:

$$few = \{(1,1),(2,1),(3,0.8),(4,0.6),(5,0.3),(6,0.2),(7,0.1)\},$$

it becomes apparent that the degree of probability 0.8 cannot be equally valid for all segments of the fuzzy period 'a few days'. Thus, fuzzy events make it difficult to apply the theory of quantitative probability successfully. The reason is that the basic concept of the traditional theory of probability, i.e., the concept of probability space, requires crisp events and does not hold for fuzzy events. The theory must therefore be fuzzified to be meaningfully applicable (Zadeh, 1968a; Buckley, 2006).

The only remedy to the above-mentioned difficulties is to use fuzzy logic in medicine. By so doing, a host of new philosophical and metaphysical problems of medicine will also become apparent. Indeed, fuzzy logic is increasingly employed in almost all areas of medical research and practice (Mahfouf et al., 2001; Steimann, 1997, 2001a). To demonstrate its impact on medicine and philosophy of medicine, we shall briefly discuss the following six issues:

16.5.1 Fuzzy Control
16.5.2 Fuzzy Clinical Decision-Making
16.5.3 Similaristic Reasoning in Medicine
16.5.4 Fuzzy Logic in Biomedicine
16.5.5 Fuzzy Deontics
16.5.6 Fuzzy Concept Formation in Medicine.

For additional applications, see (Barro and Marin, 2002; Mordeson et al., 2000; Steimann, 2001b; Szczepaniak et al., 2000; Sadegh-Zadeh, 2001a).

Until recently, fuzzy logic has been developed mainly by mathematically oriented engineers and scholars to the effect that like probability theory, it does not yet have a clear and perfect syntax in general use. Its syntax, and consequently its semantics, do not in general satisfy usual logical standards. To develop it to the extent necessary, however, is beyond the scope of our project. Though whenever syntactic amendments are feasible without pervasively changing the received syntax, we shall introduce them in their respective contexts.

16.5.1 Fuzzy Control

As mentioned on page IX of the Preface, medicine is a science and practice of intervention, manipulation, and *control* in the area of health and malady. In this capacity, it is more and more becoming a branch of technology to the effect that the division between health care and health engineering is gradually disappearing. Fuzzy automata that monitor and control disease states, as well as treatment and recovery processes, play increasingly important roles in intensive care units, anesthesia, surgery, cardiology, pharmacological therapy, and other medical domains. Their areas of application range from those that involve simple tasks, such as dosing and administering insulin, to those that involve highly sophisticated control devices, such as adaptive cardiac pacemakers, smooth surgical robots, and even artificial hearts (Hsu, 2004). Correspondingly, a greater amount of research in medicine is dedicated to developing machines that undertake more and more life and death decisions. The automation of diagnostic-therapeutic judgment by medical expert systems also belongs to this long-term enterprise. In what follows, the logic behind this innovative technology will be briefly explained to show its philosophical, moral, and social consequences. Our discussion divides into the following two sections:

▶ The concept of control
▶ Fuzzy controllers.

For the notion of fuzzy automata, see Definitions 29–30 on page 129. For a survey of the use of fuzzy automata in medicine, see (Mahfouf et al., 2001).

The concept of control

To control a system means to intervene in its functioning by changing some of its basic parameters so as to perturb it into some desired state. For example, economic systems are controlled by increasing or decreasing the credit rates or taxes. Ecosystems are controlled by afforesting or deforesting. Just as tax reduction and deforestation are controls, so are anesthesia, surgical operations, and drug therapy. In these cases, medical personnel control patients by manipulating some parameters of their organism and psyche.

In engineering as the science and practice of automated control, a system that is controlled is called a plant. But we shall here prefer the term *"the controlled system"* because in medicine it sounds strange to refer to patients as plants. Accordingly, a system that controls another one is called a *controller*. Through commands and control actions, a controller regulates or alters the controlled system so that it exhibits certain desired properties. Thus,

we should be aware that physicians are controllers. Upon measuring a patient's blood sugar level and finding it to be too high, a physician may decide
to inject the patient with insulin, and by this control command reduce her
blood sugar. In this example, the physician is a controller of the patient's
blood sugar level and metabolism.

The controller and the controlled system constitute a control loop that
arises in the following way. Like in any other system, two key features of a
controlled system are its inputs and outputs. Some of its outputs serve as
inputs to the controller. This, then, measures them by a sensor, evaluates the
measurements, and transforms the result into outputs that by modifying the
controlled system's inputs, control this system (Figure 65).

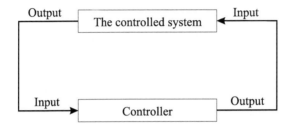

Fig. 65. The control loop. Some of the controlled system's outputs are used by the
controller as input to transform them into its own outputs. These outputs of the
controller serve as control actions or commands, e.g., a drug injection, that are used
by the controlled system as input. The controlled-controller loop is thus a feedback
system. For example, the measurement of the blood sugar of a patient (her output)
is evaluated by a controller (as its input) to conclude that the patient needs 0.5 mg
insulin (the controller's output). The injection of 0.5 mg insulin then constitutes a
new input to the controlled system

A parameter that is controlled in a controlled system, is called a *variable*
because its values may vary. For example, the blood sugar level of the above-
mentioned patient is a variable that is measured and controlled by her physician through the injection of insulin. Other controlled variables might be
the patient's blood pressure, appetite, blood cholesterol, or the disease state
from which she suffers, e.g., pneumonia. We will now briefly study how fuzzy
logic-based, automated controllers accomplish such control tasks today.

Different types of devices and machines have served as traditional controllers for centuries. After the advent of mathematical control theory in the
1950s, they could be made considerably more sophisticated through the introduction of the so-called PID controllers (Proportional Integral Derivative).
The main drawback of these traditional controllers is that they require too
much mathematics. But even more importantly, they require precise knowledge of the relationships between input and output variables expressed by
means of highbrow mathematical formalism such as differential equations,
and thus, require precise measurements of the variables to be controlled (En-

gelberg, 2005; Zabczyk, 2007). However, with the increasing complexity of a system, its precise analysis and description become incresingly less feasible and ultimately futile. This is particularly true for the human organism in health and disease. The inventor of fuzzy logic put it convincingly as follows:

"Given the deeply entrenched tradition of scientific thinking which equates the understanding of a phenomenon with the ability to analyze it in quantitative terms, one is certain to strike a dissonant note by questioning the growing tendency to analyze the behavior of humanistic systems as if they were mechanistic systems governed by difference, differential, or integral equations. [. . .] Essentially our contention is that the conventional quantitative techniques of system analysis are intrinsically unsuited for dealing with humanistic systems or, for that matter, any system whose complexity is comparable to that of humanistic systems. The basis for this contention rests on what might be called the *Principle of Incompatibility*. Stated informally, the essence of this principle is that as the complexity of a system increases, our ability to make precise and yet significant statements about its behavior diminishes until a threshold is reached beyond which precision and significance (or relevance) become almost mutually exclusive characteristics. It is in this sense that precise quantitative analyses of the behavior of humanistic systems are not likely to have much relevance to the real-world societal, political, economic, and other types of problems which involve humans as individuals or in groups" (Zadeh, 1973, 28).

"In short, I believe that excessive concern with precision has become a stultifying influence in control and system theory, largely because it tends to focus the research in these fields on those, and only those, problems which are susceptible to exact solution. As a result, the many classes of important problems in which the data, the objectives, and the constraints are too complex or too ill-defined to admit of precise mathematical analysis have been and are being avoided on the grounds of mathematical intractability" (Zadeh, 1972b, 3).

These considerations and insights led Lotfi Zadeh to conceive *fuzzy control* as a replacement for traditional control in the early 1970s. Since in medicine the significance of research and practice is highly desired, precision is to be reduced in favor of significance. Employing a fuzzy language of medicine accomplishes this goal. Such a language is more instrumental than a mathematical language because medical subjects such as pathological processes, treatment efficacy, recovery, and everything else concerning health and disease are vague objects and events whose precise measurement does not necessarily produce significance. For example, a vague norm such as "high blood sugar levels ought to be reduced" is preferable to the precise norm "blood sugar levels above 160 mg% ought to be reduced to 100 mg%". This idea of replacing precision with vagueness is central to fuzzy control, which is discussed below. For details on the theory and practice of fuzzy control, see (Hampel et al., 2000).

Fuzzy controllers

During only a short period of time fuzzy control has become an advanced area of research and practice in medicine. Roughly, it may be characterized as control by means of simple fuzzy sentences rather than by complicated mathematical equations. It rests on the ingenious idea that a small number of very simple *fuzzy rules* on a variable yield a fuzzy algorithm to smoothly control that variable (Zadeh, 1968b, 1972b, 1994, 1996b, 2009).[122] The smoothness and efficiency of fuzzy control by fuzzy rules is highly remarkable and unrivalled. The rules may be elicited from experts of the respective domain, or they may be novel or even ad hoc ones. In any event, they are fuzzy sentences such as "if the blood sugar level is moderately high, then inject a medium dose of insulin". They need not express precise, mathematical relationships such as "if the blood sugar level is 400 mg%, then inject 1.8 mg insulin". To explain, we shall exemplify an automated fuzzy controller of blood sugar level in diabetics. To this end, we need to introduce the basic notion of fuzzy control, i.e., the term "fuzzy rule". We will do so intuitively and stepwise with a view to applying it to other subjects too. Consider first the following clinical truism:

Acute bronchitis is associated with a severe cough.

This example demonstrates how elliptical natural language sentences usually are. Actually, the sentence is an if-then sentence on the relationship between acute bronchitis and severe cough with the following deep structure:

If an individual has acute bronchitis, *then* she has a severe cough.   (138)

To show that such seemingly plain natural language conditionals are powerful fuzzy tools, the syntax of (138) will be slightly enhanced. By means of fuzzy logic, its vague expressions "has acute bronchitis" and "has a severe cough" are reconstructible as equations in the following way. By introducing two new words, "the state of bronchitis" and "the state of cough", sentence (138) may be rewritten as:

If the *state of bronchitis* of an individual is acute, then her *state of cough* is severe.   (139)

In the antecedent of this conditional, the italicized new word *"state of bronchitis"* is a linguistic variable. Therefore, we will write it with capital initials as "State_Of_Bronchitis". And "acute" is the linguistic value or term it has taken from among its term set. Its term set, $T(State\_Of\_Bronchitis)$, may be conceived of as something like the following collection:

$$T(State\_Of\_Bronchitis) = \{peracute, acute, subacute, fulminant,$$
$$chronic, subchronic, \dots\}.$$

---

[122] For the concept of algorithm, see footnote 9 on page 47. A *fuzzy algorithm* is an ordered set of instructions some or all of which are fuzzy. Fuzzy algorithms pervade much of what we do, for example, when we walk, drive or park a car, tie a knot, search for a telephone number in a telephone directory, etc. They are also employed in many areas such as programming, management science, medical diagnostics and therapy, and others (Zadeh, 1968b, 1973).

Similarly, the italicized new word "state of cough" in the consequent of (139), which we will write as "State_Of_Cough", is a linguistic variable having "severe" as its linguistic value or term in the present example. It may have a term set, $T(State\_Of\_Cough)$, like the following one:

$$T(State\_Of\_Cough) \ = \ \{mild, \ moderate, \ severe, \ very \ severe, \ \dots \}.$$

To easily distinguish linguistic variables from numerical variables, we will write the former always with initial capital letters as above, while the latter will be written with lower-case initials. A bit more formalized with the aid of the amended terminology, the statement (139) says that for every human being x:

$$\text{If } State\_Of\_Bronchitis(x) = acute, \tag{140}$$
$$\text{then } State\_Of\_Cough(x) = severe.$$

As pointed out in Section 30.4.1, from a syntactic point of view the linguistic variables State_Of_Bronchitis and State_Of_Cough are functions that may be written "f" and "g", respectively. Accordingly, the sentence (140) is of the following form:

$$\text{If } f(x) = A, \ then \ g(x) = B \tag{141}$$

where:

$$f \equiv State\_Of\_Bronchitis$$
$$g \equiv State\_Of\_Cough$$
$$A \equiv acute \quad \text{with } A \in T(State\_Of\_Bronchitis)$$
$$B \equiv severe \quad \text{with } B \in T(State\_Of\_Cough)$$

such that in the present example regarding the patient x, the functions f and g take, respectively, the values $A \in T(State\_Of\_Bronchitis)$ and $B \in T(State\_Of\_Cough)$, i.e., "acute" and "severe".

It has become customary in fuzzy logic to symbolize linguistic variables by capitals like X and Y, and to refer to them simply as *variables*. The functional expression "$f(x)$" in the antecedent of (141) is usually written X and called variable X, and the functional expression "$g(x)$" in the consequent is written Y and called variable Y. Thus, a sentence of the form (139–141) may in a simple fashion be represented as follows:

$$\text{If } X \text{ is } A, \ then \ Y \text{ is } B \tag{142}$$

where X and Y are linguistic variables with A and B being their respective linguistic values: "If bronchitis is acute, then cough is severe", so to speak. According to the theory of linguistic variables discussed in Sections 30.4.1, the linguistic values A and B in the antecedent and consequent of the conditional

(142), i.e., the values *acute* and *severe* in the present example, are fuzzy sets. The whole sentence turns out a *fuzzy conditional*. On page 1037, a sentence is defined to be a fuzzy conditional if and only if (i) it is a conditional $\alpha \to \beta$ and (ii) contains fuzzy terms in its atecedent α, consequent β, or both. Fuzzy conditionals are powerful tools for summarizing and compressing information through the use of granulation; they demonstrate the useful service of fuzzy expressions (see page 1029).

Definition 159 (Fuzzy rule). *A sentence is referred to as a* fuzzy conditional command, fuzzy conditional rule, *or* fuzzy rule *for short, iff it is a closed fuzzy conditional* $\mathcal{Q}(\alpha \to \beta)$ *whose consequent* β *is a command of the form "do such and such!" or an action sentence of another type as defined in Definitions 151–152 on page 563.*

A typical category of fuzzy rules is provided by those fuzzy conditionals which associate one or more *linguistic variables* in their antecedents with one or more *linguistic variables* in their consequents. A simple example is the following fuzzy rule:

> If the *blood sugar level* of the patient is *moderately high*, then *inject a medium dose* of insulin.

That is, in formal analogy to our previous example:

> If X is A, then Y (i.e., the dose of insulin injection) is B.

In this example, X represents the linguistic variable *blood sugar level* of an individual x; and Y is the linguistic variable *dose of insulin injection* as a recommended action. As pointed out above, a number of fuzzy rules of this type about a variable X provide a fuzzy algorithm to control that variable. For instance, the following five simple fuzzy rules compose a fuzzy algorithm and are able to control the variable *blood sugar level* in adult, type 1 diabetics:

1. If the *blood sugar level* of x is *low*,   (143)

          then *do not* inject insulin;

2. If the *blood sugar level* of x is *normal*,

          then *do not* inject insulin;

3. If the *blood sugar level* of x is *slightly high*,

          then inject a *low* dose of insulin;

4. If the *blood sugar level* of x is *moderately high*,

          then inject a *medium* dose of insulin;

5. If the *blood sugar level* of x is *extremely high*,

          then inject a *high* dose of insulin.

By making explicit the linguistic variables *"Blood_Sugar_Level"* and *"Dose_Of_Insulin_Injection"* contained in these rules, they read:

1′. If Blood_Sugar_Level(x) = low,
             then Dose_Of_Insulin_Injection(x) = none;
2′. If Blood_Sugar_Level(x) = normal,
             then Dose_Of_Insulin_Injection(x) = none;
3′. If Blood_Sugar_Level(x) = slightly high,
             then Dose_Of_Insulin_Injection(x) = low;
4′. If Blood_Sugar_Level(x) = moderately high,
             then Dose_Of_Insulin_Injection(x) = medium;
5′. If Blood_Sugar_Level(x) = extremely high,
             then Dose_Of_Insulin_Injection(x) = high.

In other words:

1″. If X is A_1, then Y is B_1
2″. If X is A_2, then Y is B_2
3″. If X is A_3, then Y is B_3
4″. If X is A_4, then Y is B_4
5″. If X is A_5, then Y is B_5

with $T(X) = \{A_1, A_2, \ldots, A_5\}$ and $T(Y) = \{B_1, B_2, \ldots, B_5\}$. Such a set of $k \geq 1$ fuzzy rules constitutes the *rule base* of a fuzzy controller. The present five rules, for instance, may guide a fuzzy blood sugar level controller, i.e., a so-called 'insulin pump' or 'continuous subcutaneous insulin infusion device' as an alternative to the traditional method of multiple daily injections. The pump executes the rule base and administers the prescribed doses of insulin depending on the fluctuations of blood sugar level measured by the sensor of the pump. To generalize the complexity of the rules of such a rule base, any ith rule with $i \geq 1$ may be of the following structure to include in its antecedent $m \geq 1$ linguistic variables $X_{i_1}, \ldots, X_{i_m}$, and in its consequent $n \geq 1$ other linguistic variables $Y_{i_1}, \ldots, X_{i_n}$ with their respective terms:

IF X_{i_1} *is* A_{i_1} *and* ... *and* X_{i_m} *is* A_{i_m} (144)
THEN Y_{i_1} *is* B_{i_1} *and* ... *and* Y_{i_n} *is* B_{i_n}

An example is provided in (145) from automated fuzzy anesthesia control with three variables in the antecedent and four variables in the consequent (adapted from Huang et al., 1999, 331):

IF   the *mean arterial pressure* is moderately high AND   (145)
                 is getting higher very fast AND
       the *cardiac output* is sufficient AND
                 is not changing AND
       the *mean pulmonary arterial pressure* is slightly low AND
                 is getting lower slowly,

THEN   increase the *infusion of sodium nitroprusside* moderately AND

decrease *dopamine* slightly AND

do not change *nitroglycerin* AND

decrease *phenylephrine* slightly.

A small number of such fuzzy rules constitute an outstanding algorithm for use as a *rule base* by an automated fuzzy anesthesia controller. Presumably, the proponents of precisionism will suppose that vague terms such as "high", "sufficient", "slightly", "low", and the like are not suitable tools to enable meaningful, science-based actions in medicine and elsewhere. However, the practice falsifies their supposition. We shall show below how a fuzzy algorithm works in practice, supporting our confidence that fuzzy medical language need not fear the Humean verdict referred to on page 486. To this end, we will first describe and explain the architecture of a fuzzy controller. A fuzzy controller consists of the following five modules: a *sensor*, a *fuzzifier*,

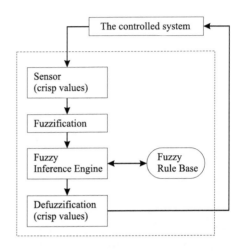

Fig. 66. The general scheme of a fuzzy controller consisting of the modules sensor, fuzzifier, rule base, inference engine, and defuzzifier. See body text

a *fuzzy rule base* as above, a *fuzzy inference engine,* and a *defuzzifier.* In what follows, these modules will be briefly outlined in turn (Figure 66).

The sensor

This is the measurement module of the fuzzy controller. It monitors and measures the variables that are to be controlled, e.g., the blood sugar level or the blood pressure, and transmits the measurement data to the next, fuzzifier module.

There are two types of sensors. The first type measures the data precisely and provides crisp data such as, for example, "320 mg%" in the case of blood sugar level. The second type provides fuzzy data such as, for example, "about 320 mg%" in a similar case. In our example, we will address the control of crisply measured variables only. For fuzzy sensors, see (Mauris et al., 1996).

The fuzzifier

We saw in our generalization (144) above that the *antecedent* of a fuzzy rule includes $m \geq 1$ linguistic variables $X_1, \ldots, X_m$ that the rule is designed to control, e.g., Blood_Sugar_Level, Systolic_Blood_Pressure, Blood_Uric_Acid_Level, etc. For each of these variables a particular set of linguistic terms, i.e., linguistic values A_1, A_2 and so on, are used in the rule base. For instance, in our above-mentioned rule base we had the variable "Blood_Sugar_Level" with the following fuzzy sets as its linguistic values:

$$T(Blood\_Sugar\_Level) = \tag{146}$$
$$\{\text{low, normal, slightly high, moderately high, extremely high}\}$$

As outlined on page 1028, such linguistic values partition the universe of discourse Ω that is represented by the values of the *numerical* base variable, into triangular, trapezoidal, bell-shaped, S-shaped, or other types of fuzzy sets. Our present linguistic values listed in (146) partition the quantitative *blood sugar level* into five trapezoidal fuzzy sets (Figure 67).

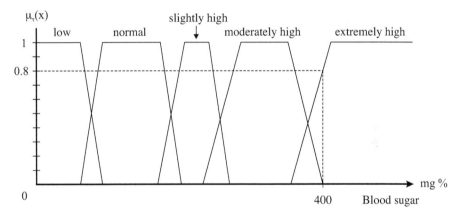

Fig. 67. The five fuzzy granules (low, normal, slightly high, moderately high, extremely high) over the blood sugar concentration values as our universe of discourse

Let X be a linguistic variable in the antecedent of a fuzzy rule, such as *Blood_Sugar_Level* with linguistic values $A_1, \ldots, A_n$ like in (146), and let Ω be a universe of discourse such as the measurement of the patients' blood sugar level on which $A_1, \ldots, A_n$ are fuzzy sets; then the *fuzzification* of an element y of the crisp universe of discourse, $y \in \Omega$, with respect to the linguistic variable X is the determination of its membership degree in each of the fuzzy sets $A_1, \ldots, A_n \in T(X)$, i.e., the determination of its membership vector:

$$\big(\mu_{A_1}(y), \ldots, \mu_{A_n}(y)\big) \qquad \text{with } A_1, \ldots, A_n \in T(X) \qquad (147)$$

referred to as the *fuzzification vector of y with respect to the linguitsitic variable X* and written $fv_X(y)$. For example, the fuzzification of a blood sugar level of 400 mg% with respect to the linguistic variable Blood_Sugar_Level in (146) above yields the fuzzification vector (0, 0, 0, 0, 0.8) that means that:

$$
\begin{aligned}
\mu_{low}(400) &= 0 \\
\mu_{normal}(400) &= 0 \\
\mu_{slightly\text{-}high}(400) &= 0 \\
\mu_{moderately\text{-}high}(400) &= 0 \\
\mu_{extremely\text{-}high}(400) &= 0.8
\end{aligned}
$$

We have thus $fv_{Blood\_Sugar\_Level}(400) = (0,0,0,0,0.8)$. Such a fuzzification is conducted by the fuzzifier module in a fuzzy controller. The fuzzifier examines to what extent a crisp data such as 400 mg% that it receives from the sensor, is a member of any fuzzy set A_i in the term set $T(X)$ of the linguistic variable X the controller is designed to control. In line with (147), the fuzzifier in our example has provided the following result:

$$
\begin{aligned}
fv_{Blood\_Sugar\_Level}(400) = \big(&\mu_{low}(400), \mu_{normal}(400), \mu_{slightly\text{-}high}(400), \\
&\mu_{moderately\text{-}high}(400), \mu_{extremely\text{-}high}(400)\big) \\
= (&0,0,0,0,0.8).
\end{aligned}
$$

Thus, the fuzzifier transforms the crisp input data into a vector of real numbers in [0, 1] by using the inference engine that includes, among other things, also the definition of the fuzzy sets involved, especially of those in the term set $T(X)$. What the purpose of this fuzzification is, will be discussed after the next module.

The rule base

The rule base contains a number of fuzzy rules about the variables to be controlled. In our example, we use rules 1–5 listed in (143) on page 610 to guide the blood sugar controller. The rule base of a fuzzy controller is its knowledge base, so to speak. Thus, a fuzzy controller belongs to the class of rule-based or knowledge-based fuzzy machines. (For the concept of a fuzzy machine, see Definition 30 on page 130.)

The inference engine

The crisp inputs to a controller are fuzzified by its fuzzification module. In our example above, we obtained the fuzzification vector (0, 0, 0, 0, 0.8) which said that the patient's blood sugar level, 400 mg%, is *extremely high* to the extent 0.8, i.e., $\mu_{extremely\text{-}high}(400) = 0.8$. Such a fuzzified input must be properly evaluated and transformed to an output, i.e., to a reaction of the controller. This task is accomplished by the inference engine. It uses the rule base of the controller and the generalized Modus ponens of fuzzy logic (see page 1040) to map the fuzzification vector of the current input, by means of specific methods that cannot be discussed here, onto the linguistic values of the linguistic variables involved in the *consequents* of the rules. In our present example, the following linguistic values of the linguistic variable *Dose_Of_Insulin_Injection* are involved in the consequents:

$$T(Dose\_Of\_Insulin\_Injection) = \{none, low, medium, high\}.$$

The mapping of the fuzzified input $(0, 0, 0, 0, 0.8)$ onto {none, low, medium, high} values of insulin dose yields:

$$(0, 0, 0, 0.8).$$

This order of fuzzy set membership is the result of applying rule No. 5 in (143) on page 610 for fuzzifying the crisp input, which gives us the following conditional:

- If the Blood_Sugar_Level is extremely high, then inject a *high* dose of insulin

or equivalently:

- If X is extremely high, then Y is *high*

with the linguistic value *high* included in its consequent. Thus, the insulin dose x that is to be injected, must have a membership degree $\mu_{high}(x) = 0.8$. See next section.

The defuzzifier

This final module converts the fuzzified result, that is provided by the inference engine, into crisp values and passes them as commands to the controlled system. In our example above, the result obtained was $\mu_{high}(x) = 0.8$. The tentative Figure 68 shows that this membership degree belongs to an insulin dose of 9 units.

By and large, using the five vague sentences listed in (143) on page 610 above as the rule base of a fuzzy controller will enable smooth, automated control of an adult diabetic's blood sugar level. However, we used an oversimplified example that covers just the basics of fuzzy control because that level of clarification is sufficient for us to deal with some metaphysical problems of medicine in Part VI. For detailed analyses of the fuzzification-inference-defuzzification process within a fuzzy controller, see (Hampel et al., 2000; Jantzen, 2007; Michels et al., 2006).

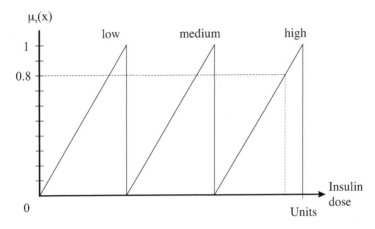

Fig. 68. The insulin doses required by different blood sugar levels. The three triangular values partition the admissible insulin doses into triangular fuzzy sets. The process of fuzzification, fuzzy inference, and defuzzification in our example above yields the command: Inject 9 units insulin (a speculative value)

16.5.2 Fuzzy Clinical Decision-Making

Since most clinical issues and decision environments are characterized by vagueness, we may ask whether fuzzy methodology is an appropriate tool for managing the uncertainty problems associated with vagueness. In the present section, we will inquire into its practical relevance to clinical medicine by means of elementary examples from *possibility theory* and its application in clinical decision-making. Our aim is to point out some philosophical problems that are central to this *possibilistic approach* in medicine. To this end, some basic terminology will be introduced below. Our discussion consists of the following three parts:

▶ Possibility theory
▶ Possibilistic diagnostics
▶ Fuzzy therapeutic decision-making.

Possibility theory

The randomness of events as an objective feature of the world and the uncertainty about their occurrence as a subjective feature of human beings create practical as well as philosophical challenges in medicine. Fortunately, there are various conceptual tools and methods to cope with the problems they cause. Among those that play a predominant role in science, are probability and statistics. However, as frequently emphasized in previous chapters, the statistical information and numerical probabilities required to use such methods, are often missing in medicine. More importantly, vague events do not sensibly assume precise probabilities. For example, it is meaningless to assert that "the probability of good weather tomorrow is 0.8". What exactly is 'good weather tomorrow' to which the probability 0.8 is assigned? What degree of temperature, what amount of sun, and what amount of wind must it, or is it allowed to, have? There are no precise answers to this question because 'good weather' is a vague, or fuzzy, event. Therefore, no precise degree of probability can be assigned to it. The vagueness that exists in medicine concerning health, disease, and recovery events, states, and processes is comparable to the vagueness in our example above, which severely limits the use of probability theory as a conceptual tool in medicine. A viable alternative to probability theory that can overcome problems of vagueness is *possibility theory,* which was introduced in 1978 by Lotfi A. Zadeh as one of the fruits of his fuzzy set theory and logic. Possibility theory handles a vague event by assigning to it a *degree of possibility.* This notion will be briefly sketched below in order to judge the value of its application in medicine. For more details of the theory and its application, see (Zadeh, 1978a–b, 1981; Dubois and Prade 1988; Dubois et al., 2000).

It should be noted at the outset that possibility and probability are completely different from one another. They are not equivalent terms and cannot be used interchangeably. However, like the theory of probability, the theory of possibility is an uninterpreted, formal theory. And like the concept of probability, the concept of possibility may also be interpreted in practice in several ways. Some of its interpretations are mentioned in footnote 169 on page 914. The concept of possibility considered in the present section allows at least for two interpretations: physical possibility and epistemic possibility (for other kinds of possibility, see Hacking, 1975b):

As an objectivist interpretation of the term, on the one hand, *physical possibility* refers to features of the physical world and means the ease with which an event may occur or an action may be performed, e.g., jumping two meters high as asserted by the statement "it is possible for Elroy Fox to jump two meters high on earth". That is, he *can* do so. As a subjectivist interpretation of the term, on the other hand, *epistemic possibility* refers to epistemic states of human beings and means considering something possible, e.g., "it is possible that Elroy Fox has diabetes". In other words, "I consider it possible that he has diabetes". Considering something possible is the weakest epistemic modality discussed in Section 27.3 on page 937. At this semantic point, possibility theory touches the epistemic logic, although they are two totally different approaches. While epistemic logic as an extension of classical logic is a qualitative theory, possibility theory is a quantitative extension of fuzzy set theory.

Possibility theory also deals with the concept of necessity and yields, in conjunction with fuzzy logic, a *possibilistic logic* that promises a wide application in medicine. Note that possibilistic logic differs from alethic-modal logic, studied in Section 27.1. While the latter is a qualitative theory of reasoning with possibility and necessity, possibility theory provides a quantitative theory of these concepts. Their quantification, which will be outlined in what follows, is the foundation of possibility theory.

To demonstrate the applicability of possibility theory in medicine, we shall undertake a brief possibilistic analysis of diagnosis below. To this end, we shall need the following three notions, which will be introduced in the next three sections:

▷ Degrees of possibility
▷ Possibility distributions
▷ Joint possibility distributions.

Degrees of possibility

The concepts that we shall introduce in what follows are demanding. Details, elaborate definitions, and other technicalities will therefore be avoided. To keep their presentation as uncomplicated as possible, we will first briefly summarize our discussion of linguistic variables and our notational conventions.

Recall from previous chapters that we differentiate between linguistic variables and numerical variables by capitalizing the former, as in *Heart_Rate*, and using lower-case letters for the latter, as in *heart_rate*. Recall also that a linguistic variable v such as the Heart_Rate of a patient takes linguistic values such as *slow, rapid, very rapid, etc.*, symbolized by A, B, C, etc. The set of linguistic values that a linguistic variable v can take, constitutes its *term set*, written $T(v)$. We have, for example, $T(Heart\_Rate) = \{slow, rapid, very\ rapid, \ldots\}$. By contrast, a numerical variable is a numerical function and takes values from among a particular set of numbers called its range, denoted Ω. For instance, the range of the numerical variable *heart_rate* is an open set of positive integers $\Omega = \{0, 1, 2, \ldots, 50, \ldots, 300, \ldots\}$ used to indicate the number of heart beats of an individual per minute. An example is the statement "the heart_rate of Elroy Fox is 50". We saw earlier that both types of variables are in fact functions such that their correct syntax would be:

1. $f(x) = A$ the Heart_Rate of Elroy Fox is slow (linguistic variable),
2. $g(x) = z$ the heart_rate of Elroy Fox is 50 (numerical variable).

Unfortunately, the customary notation of linguistic and numerical variables deviates considerably from this traditional, logical syntax such that the compound terms $f(x)$ and $g(x)$ above are represented by single capitals such as X and Y, respectively. Accordingly, the statements 1–2 above are usually written:

1′. X is A verbally described by: "Heart_Rate is A",
2′. $Y = z$ "heart_rate is z",

where X is read "Heart_Rate" and Y is read "heart_rate". A linguistic variable X operates on the values of a numerical variable Y as its universe of discourse, and transforms subsets thereof into fuzzy sets such as SLOW, RAPID, etc. So we may easily recognize that a term such as "slow" has a fuzzy set as its denotation, it will be written in capitals as SLOW. That is, a linguistic value written in capitals indicates that the term is exclusively used extensionally and represents the fuzzy set it denotes. With this brief review in mind, the basic concepts of possibility theory are introduced below, so that we may apply them to clinical decision-making.

Suppose that a patient suffering from lower abdominal pain has just been admitted to a surgical hospital ward. The ward doctor has not met the patient yet and doesn't know anything about her. To inform himself about the patient, he asks the nurse some questions. In order not to unduly complicate our analysis, we do not use a medical example and do not suppose that for the sake of diagnostic hypothesizing he asks her after the patient's complaints. Rather, we use a much simpler, well-structured, and transparent example: He asks the nurse for the age of the patient. She replies:

Mrs. Amy Fox is young. (148)

The doctor is disappointed because this statement does not provide precise information about the age of the new patient. It only suggests that her numerical age lies in the fuzzy set YOUNG that constitutes one of the granules over the universe of discourse, i.e., over the set $\Omega = \{1, 2, 3, \ldots, 100, \ldots\}$ of numerical ages (Figure 69).

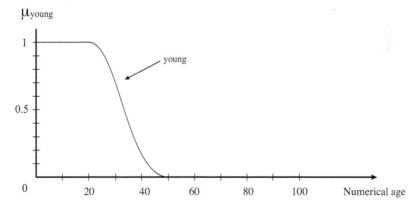

Fig. 69. The fuzzy set YOUNG. The graph of its function, μ_{YOUNG}, represents a granule over the values of the numerical variable *age*

The ward doctor is interested in the precise age of the patient and starts hypothesizing about it. That she is young means that the linguistic variable

Age takes the value YOUNG. The doctor knows that YOUNG is a fuzzy set that has no sharp boundaries, and thus, imposes a fuzzy restriction on numerical ages so that they fall within the fuzzy set YOUNG to different extents. From this knowledge he concludes that only a particular subset of Ω, i.e., a group of numerical ages, are possible candidates to precisely characterize the young patient's age. For example, given the information (148) and Figure 69, Amy Fox cannot be 50 years old or older. Her age must lie somewhere between 1 and 49 years. So, the doctor has good reason to assume:

> It is possible that the young patient is 1 year old,
> It is possible that the young patient is 10 years old,
> It is possible that the young patient is 20 years old,
> It is possible that the young patient is 30 years old,
> It is possible that the young patient is 40 years old,
> It is not possible that the young patient is 50 years old.

He asks himself how to assign a number to each of these possibilities as a degree of its strength so that they can be quantitatively compared with one another. Let the membership function of the fuzzy set YOUNG be symbolized by μ_{YOUNG}. According to Figure 69 we have, for instance, $\mu_{YOUNG}(30) = 0.7$. That is, a person aged 30 years is *young* to the extent 0.7. Since the ward doctor has no information available on the age of the new patient other than that she is young, he decides to interpret 0.7 as the *degree of possibility* that she is 30 years old. As a justification of his decision, he refers to the following *possibility postulate* introduced by Lotfi Zadeh that relates the value x of a numerical variable Y with the degree of x's membership in a fuzzy set (Zadeh, 1978a–b, 1981):[123]

Possibility Postulate: Let X be a linguistic variable and Y be a numerical variable such as *Age* and *age*, respectively. Suppose that X is A, e.g., "Age is YOUNG" as in (148) and Figure 69. In the absence of any information about the value of the numerical variable Y other than that X is A, the possibility that in fuzzy set A the variable Y takes the value x, written *possibility*$(Y = x, A)$, is numerically equal to the grade of membership of x in A. That is:

$$possibility(Y = x, A) = \mu_A(x) \qquad \text{[Possibility Postulate]} \quad (149)$$

Since our present example in (148) above says that "Age is YOUNG", we obtain according to the Possibility Postulate the following statement:

---

[123] The syntax of the concepts introduced in what follows will slightly deviate from the common usage of these terms in the literature because the 'common usage' is in need of improvement. For example, our concepts of *possibility function* and *possibility distribution* will be binary functions, whereas they are usually handled as unary ones. We shall use an amended syntax beginning with the notion of possibility postulate.

$$possibility(age = 30, YOUNG) = \mu_{YOUNG}(30) = 0.7 \qquad (150)$$

which says: *The possibility that the young patient Amy Fox is 30 years of age, is 0.7.* If the nurse had said that "Mrs. Amy Fox is very young", then in this new fuzzy set ('very young') age 30 would have received another degree of possibility:

$$possibility(age = 30, VERY\_YOUNG) = \mu_{VERY\_YOUNG}(30) = 0.7^2 = 0.49.$$

That is, the possibility that the very young patient Amy Fox is 30 years of age, is 0.49. As is obvious from the above considerations, we are conceiving a quantitative concept of possibility, referred to as *degree of possibility,* that relativizes the grade of possibility of an event such as "Amy Fox is 30 years of age" to a particular fuzzy set A. An event such as "Amy Fox is 30 years of age" may have different degrees of possibility in different fuzzy sets, e.g., in YOUNG, VERY_YOUNG, etc. Thus, our quantitative possibility concept is a binary function of the following form:

> The degree of possibility, or the possibility, that the variable Y takes the value x in fuzzy set A is r,

symbolized by:

$$\pi(Y = x, A) = r$$

and abbreviated to the pseudo-unary function:

$$\pi_{Y/A}(x) = r.$$

For instance, in our above examples we had:

$$\pi_{age/YOUNG}(30) = 0.7$$
$$\pi_{age/VERY\_YOUNG}(30) = 0.49.$$

We will now define the function $\pi_{Y/A}$. It is usually called "the possibility distribution function". But we may also refer to it simply as the *possibility function.*

Definition 160 (Possibility function). *If (i) X is a linguistic variable such as Age with $T(X)$ being its term set; (ii) Y is a numerical variable such as age that takes values in the universe of discourse Ω; (iii) X operates upon the values of Y to generate fuzzy sets contained in $T(X)$ such as YOUNG, VERY_YOUNG, etc.; and (iv) $A \in T(X)$ is any of these fuzzy sets with μ_A being its membership function, then:*

$$\pi_{Y/A}(x) = \mu_A(x) \qquad \text{for all } x \in \Omega. \qquad \text{(Possibility Postulate)}$$

Thus, the degree of possibility of an event in a fuzzy set A is defined by means of the membership function of this fuzzy set. Therefore, the range of the function π is the unit interval $[0, 1]$. That means that it maps the universe of discourse Ω to $[0, 1]$:

$$\pi_{Y/A} \colon \Omega \mapsto [0, 1] \qquad \text{with } A \in T(X)$$

to take values between 0 and 1, inclusive, called degrees of A-possibility or simply degrees of possibility. We have, for instance (see Figure 69 on page 619):

$$\pi_{age/YOUNG}(20) = 1$$
$$\pi_{age/YOUNG}(30) = 0.7$$
$$\pi_{age/YOUNG}(40) = 0.17$$
$$\pi_{age/YOUNG}(50) = 0.$$

Possibility distributions

Informally, let Y be a variable that in a set A receives particular values. Then, the possibility distribution of Y in A is the fuzzy set of possible values of Y in A. This notion will be made precise in what follows with a view to making use of it in our concept of fuzzy clinical judgment below.

By virtue of Definition 160, the ward doctor above can now put forward the following set of possibility considerations. To limit the set, we will consider only some integer values up to 50, as the set of ages in reals is infinite:

{The possibility that the young patient is 1 year of age is 1, (151)

the possibility that the young patient is 10 years of age is 1,

the possibility that the young patient is 20 years of age is 1,

the possibility that the young patient is 30 years of age is 0.7,

the possibility that the young patient is 40 years of age is 0.17,

the possibility that the young patient is 50 years of age is 0}.

The set (151) represents a *possibility distribution* of numerical ages in the fuzzy set YOUNG induced by the vague information (148) that the patient is young, and by Definition 160. This heuristic impact of the vague information (148) may be summarized by the following decision:

If Age is young, then (151). (152)

By tabulation, the possibility distribution (151) may be represented as shown in Table 17. Ages above 50 are not included in the table because their values are 0. The distribution is obviously a collection of number pairs such that in the second row a real number from the unit interval $[0, 1]$ is attached to

Table 17. The patient's possible ages with their degrees of possibility

Possible ages of the young patient:	1	10	20	30	40	50
degree of possibility:	1	1	1	0.7	0.17	0

a numerical age in the first row as its *degree of possibility* in the fuzzy set YOUNG. The presentation of the collection of number pairs in set notation yields the following *fuzzy set* that is called "the possibility distribution of the numerical variable *age* in the fuzzy set YOUNG", conveniently written:

$$\Pi(age,\ YOUNG) \tag{153}$$

and abbreviated to $\Pi_{age/YOUNG}$:

$$\Pi_{age/YOUNG} = \{(1,1),(10,1),(20,1),(30,0.7),(40,0.17),(50,0)\}. \tag{154}$$

The Greek capital Pi used in this fuzzy set, Π, stands for the term "the possibility distribution of". A number pair of the form "(x,a)" such as (40, 0.17) comprises a numerical age x as its first element, while its second element is the *degree of possibility* of that age in the fuzzy set YOUNG. For example, (20, 1) means that the degree of possibility that the above-mentioned patient Amy Fox is 20 years of age, is 1, whereas (40, 0.17) means that the degree of possibility that she is 40 years of age, is 0.17. It is worth noting that (i) the assignment of real numbers from the unit interval [0, 1] to ages is conducted by the *possibility function* $\pi_{Y/A}$, i.e., by $\pi_{age/YOUNG}$ in the present example; and (ii) due to Definition 160, the emerging *possibility distribution* $\Pi_{Y/A}$, i.e., the set $\Pi_{age/YOUNG}$ in (154), is indeed a *fuzzy set* of possibilities. Specifically, the possibility distribution (154) is the following fuzzy set:

$$\Pi_{age/YOUNG} =$$
$$\left\{\left(1,\pi_{age/YOUNG}(1)\right),\ \left(10,\pi_{age/YOUNG}(10)\right),\ \left(20,\pi_{age/YOUNG}(20)\right),\right.$$
$$\left.\left(30,\pi_{age/YOUNG}(30)\right),\ \left(40,\pi_{age/YOUNG}(40)\right),\ \left(50,\pi_{age/YOUNG}(50)\right)\right\}$$

or to present it completely:

$$\Pi_{age/YOUNG} = \{(x,\pi_{age/YOUNG}(x)) \mid x \in \Omega\}.$$

For the intuitive considerations above to be applicable in medicine, we must conceptualize them more precisely. A closer look at the possibility distribution (154) reveals that the distribution is equal to fuzzy set YOUNG itself as depicted in Figure 69 on page 619:

$$YOUNG = \{(1, 1), (10, 1), (20, 1), (30, 0.7), (40, 0.17), (50, 0)\}$$

such that we have:

$$\Pi_{age/YOUNG} = \{(1,1),(10,1),(20,1),(30,0.7),(40,0.17),(50,0)\} \qquad (155)$$
$$= \text{YOUNG}.$$

That the possibility distribution of numerical ages in the fuzzy set YOUNG equals the fuzzy set YOUNG itself, is a consequence of Definition 160 which, on the basis of Zadeh's Possibility Postulate on page 620, defines the possibility function $\pi_{Y/A}$ by the membership function of fuzzy set A. Thus, we may equate the *degree of possibility* that a young individual is x years of age, with the degree of that individual's membership in the fuzzy set YOUNG. But some additional syntax is needed to assess the practical-medical significance of this framework. As the example (153) on page 623 demonstrates, the Greek capital Π represents a binary, set-valued function with the general syntax:

$$\Pi(Y, A) = P$$

abbreviated to:

$$\Pi_{Y/A} = P$$

that reads "the possibility distribution of the numerical variable Y in the fuzzy set A is P" such that (i) its first argument Y is a numerical variable such as *age;* (ii) its second argument A is a fuzzy set of values for that variable such as YOUNG; and (iii) its value is a *set P*. Due to the definition of the possibility function $\Pi_{Y/A}$ in Definition 160 on page 621, it will turn out below that $P = A$, i.e., $\Pi_{Y/A} = A$ such that the fuzzy set A itself constitutes the possibility distribution of Y in A. See the example $\Pi_{age/YOUNG} = \text{YOUNG}$ in (155) above. The function Π can now be defined as follows:

Definition 161 (Possibility distribution). *If* (i) *X is a linguistic variable such as* Age *with $T(X)$ being its term set;* (ii) *Y is a numerical variable such as* age *that takes values in the universe of discourse Ω;* (iii) *X operates upon the values of Y to generate fuzzy sets contained in $T(X)$ such as YOUNG, OLD, etc.; and* (iv) *$A \in T(X)$ is any of these fuzzy sets with μ_A being its membership function, then:*

$$\Pi_{Y/A} = P$$

iff there is a function $\pi_{Y/A}$ such that:

1. $\pi_{Y/A} : \Omega \mapsto [0,1]$
2. $\pi_{Y/A}(x) = \mu_A(x)$ for all $x \in \Omega$
3. $P = \{(x, \pi_{Y/A}(x)) \mid x \in \Omega\}$.

Clause 2 is Definition 160 based on the Possibility Postulate. The possibility function $\pi_{Y/A}$ is usually referred to as the *possibility distribution function* associated with the distribution $\Pi_{Y/A}$. The definition above implies the following relationship called the *Possibility Assignment Equation* (Zadeh, 1978a, 7):

$$\text{If } X \text{ is } A, \text{ then } \Pi_{Y/A} = A \qquad \text{[Possibility Assignment Equation]} \quad (156)$$

because the set P in clause 3 is, due to clause 2, just the fuzzy set A. Thus, we may conclude from Definition 161 that the possibility distribution of the variable Y in a fuzzy set A is identical with A. We are now able to easily observe that a figure auch as Figure 109 on page 1027 depicts the possibility *distributions* of the numerical *age* in the linguistic *Age*, i.e., its granulation in terms of *young, old, very old,* etc.

In closing this section, we will show that possibility and probability are not identical, and therefore, must be clearly distinguished from one another. To do so, we will again use our example statement (148) on page 619 in which the nurse reports to the ward doctor: "Mrs. Amy Fox is young". We saw that based upon this information and through the decision (152), which was motivated by the Possibility Postulate, the doctor correctly arrived at the following, shortened possibility distribution of ages concerning the young patient:

$$\Pi_{age/YOUNG} = \{(1,1),(10,1),(20,1),(30,0.7),(40,0.17),(50,0)\} \quad (157)$$

The *probability distribution* regarding this new patient's age that the doctor may also consider, will now be added to present the set in tabular form and to make the differences apparent (Table 18):

Table 18. Differences between possibility and probability

The possible age of the young patient	1	10	20	30	40	50
degree of its possibility		1	1	1	0.7	0.17	0
degree of its probability		0	0	0.2	0.3	0.5	0

The hospital has a specialist, pediatric surgery ward. So, the doctor knows that usually no patient younger than 16 years old is admitted to the adult surgical ward in which he works. He therefore assigns to the ages 1 to 10 the probability degree 0. Most patients of the ward are usually middle-aged. Their number decreases the younger they are. For this reason he assigns, according to his experience, suitable probability estimates to the ages 20 to 40. Age 50 gets assigned probability 0 because the young patient cannot be 50 years old.

Besides the obvious numerical differences between the possibility and probability degrees that Table 18 demonstrates, the following characteristic is the critical one. According to Kolmogorov Axioms 2–3 of probability calculus introduced in Definition 237 on page 975, the probabilities of disjoint events add up. Since the numerical ages in Table 18 above are disjoint, we have the probability degrees $0 + 0 + 0.2 + 0.3 + 0.5 + 0 = 1$. But the sum of possibility degrees is $1 + 1 + 1 + 0.7 + 0.17 + 0 = 4.87$ and exceeds 1. They do not add up. Thus, possibility is *not* probability and vice versa. What is possible, e.g., age 10, may not be probable. And what is improbable, e.g., age 1, need not be impossible. A high degree of probability does not imply a high degree of possibility. Nor does a low degree of probability imply a low degree of possibility. Possibility and probability characterize randomness of events and our uncertainties about them from two different perspectives. They are independent of each other in that from a possibility distribution of a variable Y no probability distribution of that variable can be deduced and vice versa. For details, see (Zadeh, 1978a, 1978b, 1981).[124]

Joint possibility distributions

With the aid of the framework above, we shall develop a method of possibilistic diagnostics in the next section, which will enable us to calculate the degree of possibility – not probability – of one or more diseases in a patient. In our analyses, we shall be simultaneously concerned with a number of symptoms, signs, and findings that the patient may have, i.e., with values of several variables such as age, body temperature, blood sugar level, cholesterol level, and others, each of which ranges over a specific universe of discourse. To tackle this complex task of examining the interaction of multiple variables at a time, we shall need their *joint possibility distribution*. This key notion is briefly introduced in the present section. For more details, see (Zadeh, 1978a, 1978b, 1981).

Let $X_1, \ldots, X_n$ be $n > 1$ linguistic variables such as *Age, Body_Temperature, Blood_Sugar_Level,* and others with their term sets being $T(X_1), \ldots, T(X_n)$, respectively. And let $Y_1, \ldots, Y_n$ be $n > 1$ numerical variables such as *age, body_temperature, blood_sugar_level,* and others, each of which takes values in one of the universes of discourse $\Omega_1, \ldots, \Omega_n$, respectively. That is, variable Y_i takes values in the universe Ω_i. Finally, let $A_1, \ldots, A_n$ be $n > 1$ fuzzy sets such as YOUNG, LOW, EXTREMELY_HIGH, and the like such that the ith fuzzy set, A_i, is an element of $T(X_i)$, i.e., a fuzzy restriction on a universe of discourse $\Omega_i \in \{\Omega_1, \ldots, \Omega_n\}$ generated by the linguistic variable X_i. This terminology may be briefly illustrated by the following examples:

- The fuzzy set YOUNG, A_1, may be generated by the linguistic variable *Age* that operates on numerical ages $= \{1, 2, 3, \ldots, 100, \ldots\}$ as the universe of discourse of the numerical variable *age*. Thus, $A_1 \in T(X_1)$;
- The fuzzy set LOW, A_2, may be generated by the linguistic variable *Body_Temperature* that operates on numerical body temperatures $= \{\ldots, 35, 36, \ldots, 41, 42, \ldots\}$ °C as the universe of discourse of the numerical variable body_temperature. Thus, $A_2 \in T(X_2)$;

---

[124] Numerical variables used in possibility theory correspond to random variables in probability theory. And possibility distribution functions correspond to probability distribution functions (see footnote 190 on page 977).

and so on such that $A_n \in T(X_n)$. Now, the assortment of variables and values characterized above may be amalgamated in the following way:

A number of $n > 1$ linguistic variables $X_1, X_2, \ldots, X_n$ may be conceived of as a composite, n-ary variable $X = \langle X_1, X_2, \ldots, X_n \rangle$. A number of $n > 1$ numerical variables $Y_1, Y_2, \ldots, Y_n$ may be conceived of as a composite, n-ary variable $Y = \langle Y_1, Y_2, \ldots, Y_n \rangle$. And likewise, their ranges $\Omega_1, \Omega_2, \ldots, \Omega_n$ may be conceived of as a Cartesian product, i.e., as an n-ary relation, $\Omega = \Omega_1 \times \cdots \times \Omega_n$ with the composite, numerical variable Y taking values in Ω. The composite linguistic variable X operates on the values of the composite numerical variable Y as its universe of discourse, generating the fuzzy relation $A = A_1 \times \cdots \times A_n$ in Ω. Under these circumstances, the information:

$$X_1 \text{ is } A_1 \ \& \ X_2 \text{ is } A_2 \ \& \ \cdots \ \& \ X_n \text{ is } A_n \tag{158}$$

such as, for example, "Age is YOUNG & Body_Temperature is LOW & $\cdots$ & Blood_Sugar_Level is EXTREMELY_HIGH", is represented simply by:

$$X \text{ is } A.$$

It induces, in terms of (156), the possibility assignment equation:

$$\Pi_{Y/A} = A \tag{159}$$
$$= A_1 \times \cdots \times A_n$$

which says that the possibility distribution of the composite numerical variable Y in the fuzzy set A is the fuzzy set A itself that represents the fuzzy relation $A_1 \times \cdots \times A_n$. Furthermore, because $Y = \langle Y_1, Y_2, \ldots, Y_n \rangle$, the possibility distribution $\Pi_{Y/A}$ in (159) is the n-ary or *joint possibility distribution* of the n numerical variables $Y_1, Y_2, \ldots, Y_n$ such that:

$$\Pi_{Y/A} = \Pi_{Y_1/A_1} \times \cdots \times \Pi_{Y_n/A_n}.$$

It decomposes into a system of unary possibility distributions Π_{Y_i/A_i}:

$$\Pi_{Y_1/A_1}$$
$$\Pi_{Y_2/A_2}$$
$$\vdots$$
$$\Pi_{Y_n/A_n}.$$

Correspondingly, the *joint possibility distribution function* of the joint possibility distribution $\Pi_{Y/A}$ as a fuzzy set is $\pi_{Y/A}(x)$ given by:

$$\pi_{Y/A}(x) = \pi_{(Y_1, \ldots, Y_n)/(A_1, \ldots, A_n)}(x_1, \ldots, x_n)$$

with $x = (x_1, \ldots, x_n) \in \Omega$ and $x_i \in \Omega_i$. If F and G are fuzzy sets in the universes of discourse V and W, respectively, their Cartesian product $F \times G$ is a fuzzy relation such that its membership function $\mu_{F \times G}$ is given by:

$$\mu_{F \times G}(x) = min\big(\mu_F(v), \mu_G(w)\big)$$

with $v \in V$ and $w \in W$. According to this fuzzy set-theoretical definition and the Possibility Postulate (149), we have for any $x \in \Omega$ the following *joint possibility degree:*

$$\pi_{Y/A}(x) = \pi_{(Y_1, \ldots, Y_n)/(A_1, \ldots, A_n)}(x_1, \ldots, x_n) \tag{160}$$
$$= min\big(\pi_{Y_1/A_1}(x_1), \ldots, \pi_{Y_n/A_n}(x_n)\big)$$

where *min* is the generalized minimum operator for more than two arguments, introduced in Definition 38 on page 177.

Possibilistic diagnostics

In determining the medical-practical significance of our considerations above, we must disregard the value distinction that is customarily made in medicine between soft data and hard data. Recall that the former are simply qualitative and vague, e.g., "the patient's blood sugar level is *extremely high*", while the latter are quantitative such as "the patient's blood sugar level is *500 mg/dl*". It is generally believed in natural sciences that soft data are useless in research and practice because they are not amenable to exact reasoning. Hard data are therefore preferred to soft data. This dogmatic preference as one of the basic attitudes of natural scientists constitutes a target of enduring criticism in the humanistic philosophy of medicine. For example, see (Marcum, 2008).

Most parts of medical knowledge and data, particularly in clinical medicine, count as soft data and knowledge because of their vague character. Examples are statements of the following type: the patient has *severe* headaches; she is *icteric;* she complains of *sleeplessness;* her blood sugar level is *extremely high;* she has *moderate* tachycardia; angina pectoris is *often* associated with *shortness* of breath; and so on. Their vagueness is indicated by the italicized words. In previous chapters we were frequently concerned with the question of what doctors and scientists may infer from such soft data and knowledge when they are used in clinical reasoning and research, and what methods of inference are to be used. The present section provides an answer to this question by demonstrating that possibility theory is a useful tool for handling vague and incomplete information when, for example, the available data on a patient are neither precise nor sufficient to make a firm clinical decision. We shall use a diagnostic example to illustrate. Similar approaches which have been a source of inspiration for the present author may be found in (Mordeson et al., 2000, ch. 5; Sanchez and Pierre, 2000).

In dealing with problems of the type we shall be considering below, possibility theory is preferable to probability theory and statistics for at least the following reason. Probability is concerned with *randomness* of crisp events and with our uncertainty about their occurrence caused thereby or by incomplete knowledge, whereas possibility deals with *vagueness* and our uncertainty caused thereby. Probability measures randomness or subjective belief. It does not measure vagueness. It will be shown below that soft medical knowledge and data consisting of vague statements of the following type are very valuable information from which we can indeed infer diagnoses without recourse to probability and statistics:

IF   Body_Temperature is *low* AND   (161)

           Blood_Sugar_Level is *extremely high* AND

           Heart_Rate is *rapid* AND

           Systolic_Blood_Pressure is *very low* AND

           Cholesterol_Level is *slightly increased* AND

           Leucocyte_Count is *decreased,*

THEN   Morbus NN is *present.*

We now refer to the fuzzy-logical method of representing medical knowledge by applying the theory of linguistic variables. In natural languages, a term such as "temperature" is used ambiguously in that it refers to soft data such as "warm" and "cold", on the one hand; and to hard data such as "36 °C", on the other. To prevent the problems caused by such ambiguities, we shall use linguistic as well as numerical variables. The soft knowledge mentioned in (161) above was formulated by means of linguistic variables such as "Body_Temperature", "Blood_Sugar_Level", etc. As before, we shall capitalize variables of this type so as to clearly distinguish them from numerical variables which will be represented by lower case letters such as "body_temperature" in the statement "body_temperature is 36 °C".[125]

Let there be $n \geq 1$ linguistic variables $X_1, X_2, \ldots, X_n$ signifying symptoms, complaints, problems, signs, or findings. Examples are the following six linguistic variables used above: Body_Temperature, Blood_Sugar_Level, Heart_Rate, Systolic_Blood_Pressure, Cholesterol_Level, and Leucocyte_Count. The term set of a linguistic variable X_i may be written $T(X_i)$ such as, for instance, $T(Body\_Temperature) = \{$extremely low, low, normal, slightly high, moderately high, extremely high$\}$. A qualitative statement of the form "Body_Temperature is low" will in general be symbolized by:

X_i is A_i

where $X_i \in \{X_1, X_2, \ldots, X_6\}$ and $A_i \in T(X_i)$. Furthermore, let there be $n \geq 1$ numerical variables $Y_1, Y_2, \ldots, Y_n$ which correspond to the linguistic

---

[125] Unfortunately, the syntactic and semantic distinction noted above between these two types of variables is generally neglected in the literature, an omission that may give rise to technical and philosophical misinterpretations and misunderstandings. For example, a word such as "temperature" can cause confusion when it is used in the same context both as a linguistic variable with values such as "warm" and "cold", and as a numerical variable with values such as "36 °C". A qualitative function is not identical with a quantitative one.

variables above, respectively. A numerical variable Y_i takes values in a set Ω_i with the generic element of Ω_i denoted x_i. Examples are:

body_temperature measured in °C or °F: $\quad \Omega_1 = \{0, 1, 2, \ldots, 37, \ldots\}$,
blood_sugar_level measured in mg/dl: $\quad \Omega_2 = \{0, 1, 2, \ldots, 300, \ldots\}$,
heart_rate measured in frequency per minute: $\Omega_3 = \{0, 1, 2, \ldots, 150, \ldots\}$,
systolic_blood_pressure measured in mm Hg: $\quad \Omega_4 = \{0, 1, 2, \ldots, 150, \ldots\}$,
cholesterol_level measured in mg/dl: $\quad \Omega_5 = \{0, 1, 2, \ldots, 250, \ldots\}$,
leucocyte_count measured in mm³ blood: $\quad \Omega_6 = \{0, 1, 2, \ldots, 6000, \ldots\}$.

A quantitative statement of the form "body_temperature is 36 °C" will in general be symbolized by:

$$Y_i = x_i$$

where $Y_i \in \{Y_1, Y_2, \ldots, Y_6\}$ and $x_i \in \Omega_i$. A linguistic variable X_i operates on the values of a numerical variable and produces fuzzy sets thereof as granulations of information such as LOW, NORMAL, SLIGHTLY_HIGH, etc. Thus, each granule $A_i \in T(X_i)$ is a fuzzy subset of Ω_i. For instance, the linguistic variable Body_Temperature, X_1, operates on the values of the numerical variable body_temperature, i.e., $\Omega_1 = \{0, 1, 2, \ldots, 37, \ldots\}$, and generates triangular and trapezoidal fuzzy sets depicted in Figure 70.

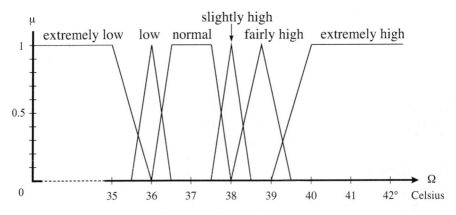

Fig. 70. The linguistic variable Body_Temperature has 3 triangular and 3 trapezoidal linguistic values. It acts on the numerical variable *body_temperature* as our universe of discourse $\Omega_1 = \{0, 1, 2, \ldots, 37, \ldots\}$ °C. A body temperature of 37 °C, for example, is *normal* to the extent 1. A body temperature of 39,1 °C is *fairly high* to the extent 0.4, and son on

Obviously, soft medical knowledge has not become useless by the association of medicine with natural sciences. On the basis of the terminology above, it may be represented by means of linguistic variables to serve practical purposes in clinical judgment. This will be shown by an example (Figure 71).

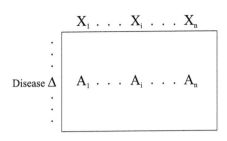

Fig. 71. Clinical knowledge, provided as a matrix, about a group of diseases defined by linguistic variables. A disease such as Disease Δ is defined by a conjunction consisting of $n \geq 1$ statements of the form "X_i is A_i" with $1 \leq i \leq n$, for instance, "X_1 is A_1 AND X_2 is A_2 AND ... AND X_n is A_n". Adapted from (Sanchez, 2000, 208)

	Body_Temperature	Blood_Sugar_Level	Heart_Rate	Systolic_Blood_Pressure	Cholesterol_Level	Leucocyte_Count
Morbus NN	low	extremely high	rapid	very low	slightly increased	decreased

Fig. 72. A group of diseases defined by six linguistic variables X_1 to X_6 and their term sets. The definition of the disease Morbus NN is explicitly given

Suppose now there are a group of maladies, say diseases, about which we have a knowledge base as displayed in Figure 72. Elements of this knowledge base may be exemplified by Morbus NN that is represented as follows:

A patient has Morbus NN iff: Body_Temperature is *low* AND

Blood_Sugar_Level is *extremely high* AND

Heart_Rate is *rapid* AND

Systolic_Blood_Pressure is *very low* AND

Cholesterol_Level is *slightly increased* AND

Leucocyte_Count is *decreased.*

Formally, it says that:

A patient has Morbus NN iff X_1 is A_1 AND ... AND X_6 is A_6

where:

$X_1 \equiv$ Body_Temperature $\qquad A_1 \equiv$ LOW $\in T(X_1)$
$X_2 \equiv$ Blood_Sugar_Level $\qquad A_2 \equiv$ EXTREMELY_HIGH $\in T(X_2)$
$X_3 \equiv$ Heart_Rate $\qquad A_3 \equiv$ RAPID $\in T(X_3)$
$X_4 \equiv$ Systolic_Blood_Pressure $A_4 \equiv$ VERY_LOW $\in T(X_4)$
$X_5 \equiv$ Cholesterol_Level $\qquad A_5 \equiv$ SLIGHTLY_INCREASED $\in T(X_5)$
$X_6 \equiv$ Leucocyte_Count $\qquad A_6 \equiv$ DECREASED $\in T(X_6)$.

If a patient, say Elroy Fox, presents some particular soft data, they may be analyzed to inquire into whether there is a disease in the knowledge base that with the highest *degree of possibility* fits the patient's data. The analysis and calculation is performed in the following way. Let us suppose that the examination of the patient yields these results:

body_temperature = 36 °C;   (162)

blood_sugar_level = 400 mg/dl;

heart_rate = 140;

systolic_blood_pressure = 80 mm Hg;

cholesterol_level = 230 mg/dl;

leucocyte_count = 3000.

Like the fuzzifier of a fuzzy controller discussed on page 613, we can now fuzzify these findings by determining for each of them the degree of its membership in the corresponding fuzzy set A_i, for example, the extent to which a cholesterol level of 230 mg/dl fits the fuzzy set SLIGHTLY_INCREASED. See Figure 73.

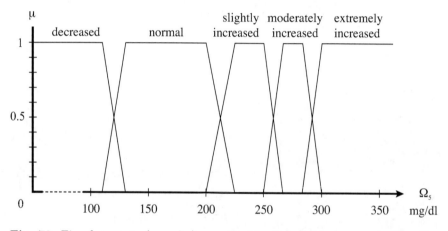

Fig. 73. Five fuzzy sets (granules) over the blood cholesterol concentration. For each numerical concentration x, e.g., 230 mg/dl, we can determine the extent to which it is a member of any of these five granules. For example, 230 mg/dl is *slightly increased* to the extent 1

It turns out that $\mu_{SLIGHTLY\_INCREASED}(230) = 1$. According to Definition 160, the degree of possibility that a cholesterol level of 230 mg/dl fits the fuzzy set SLIGHTLY_INCREASED, equals its degree of membership in that set:

$$\pi_{colesterol\_level/SLIGHTLY\_INCREASED}(230) =$$
$$\mu_{SLIGHTLY\_INCREASED}(230) = 1.$$

The same method is applied to other findings of the patient listed in (162) above. As a result, we obtain these six possibility degrees:

$$\pi_{Y_1/A_1}(36) \tag{163}$$
$$\pi_{Y_2/A_2}(400)$$
$$\pi_{Y_3/A_3}(140)$$
$$\pi_{Y_4/A_4}(80)$$
$$\pi_{Y_5/A_5}(230)$$
$$\pi_{Y_6/A_6}(3000).$$

The smallest one of these numbers will provide, according to (160) on page 628, the *joint possibility degree* we are searching for. We will now describe the procedure. The results of the patient examination (162) above may be formalized as follows:

$$Y_1 = x_1 \text{ AND} \ldots \text{ AND } Y_6 = x_6 \qquad \text{with } x_i \in \Omega_i$$

If we consider our six linguistic variables $X_1, X_2, \ldots, X_6$ as a composite variable $X = \langle X_1, X_2, \ldots, X_6 \rangle$; our six numerical variables $Y_1, Y_2, \ldots, Y_6$ as a composite variable $Y = \langle Y_1, Y_2, \ldots, Y_6 \rangle$; the six universes of discourse $\Omega_1, \ldots, \Omega_6$ as the Cartesian product $\Omega = \Omega_1 \times \cdots \times \Omega_6$; and the six fuzzy granules $A_1, \ldots, A_6$ as a fuzzy relation $A = A_1 \times \cdots \times A_6$ in Ω; then we can employ the concept of *joint possibility distribution* in the following way:

If X is A, then $\Pi_{Y/A} = A = A_1 \times \cdots \times A_6$.

This basic possibility assignment equation is, according to our presuppositions above, composed of six such equations:

If X_1 is A_1, then $\pi_{Y_1/A_1} = A_1$
If X_2 is A_2, then $\pi_{Y_2/A_2} = A_2$

$$\vdots$$

If X_6 is A_6, then $\pi_{Y_6/A_6} = A_6$.

That is:

If Body_Temperature is low, then $\Pi_{body\_temperature/LOW} = LOW$

$$\vdots$$

If Heart_Rate is rapid, then $\Pi_{heart\_rate/RAPID} = RAPID$.

Correspondingly, we have the following six unary or *single* possibility degrees listed in (163) above:

$$\pi_{Y_i/A_i}(x_i) = \mu_{A_i}(x_i) \qquad x_i \in \Omega_i \text{ with } 1 \le i \le 6$$

and one n-ary or *joint* possibility degree

$$\pi_{Y/A}(x) = \pi_{(Y_1, \dots, Y_6)/(A_1, \dots, A_6)}(x_1, \dots, x_6) \qquad \text{with } x = (x_1, \dots, x_6) \in \Omega$$

such that:

$$\pi_{Y/A}(x) = \pi_{(Y_1, \dots, Y_6)/(A_1, \dots, A_6)}(x_1, \dots, x_6)$$
$$= min\big(\pi_{Y_1/A_1}(x_1), \dots, \pi_{Y_6/A_6}(x_6)\big).$$

The joint possibility degrees of the compound variable $Y = \langle Y_1, Y_2, \dots, Y_6 \rangle$ with respect to *five diseases* are listed in Figure 74. Each joint possibility, being the minimum of a 6-ary possibility of 6 *findings* in any of the diseases, provides a degree of possibility that the respective disease is present in the patient. Now the *maximum of the minima* is determined. The disease with the highest degree of joint possibility can be identified to obtain a possibilistic diagnosis. This is, in the present example, Morbus NN.

Findings and their possibilities

		Y_1	Y_2	Y_3	Y_4	Y_5	Y_6
Disease D_1	0.00	0.00	0.8	1	0.0	1	0.00
Disease D_2	0.00	0.00	0.00	0.00	0.00	0.00	1
Morbus NN	0.8	1	0.8	1	1	1	1
Disease D_3	0.00	1	0.00	0.00	0.00	0.00	0.00
Disease D_4	0.00	0.00	0.00	1	1	0.00	0.00

Degrees of joint possibility. Each degree provides the degree of possibility of the respective disease.

Fig. 74. Degree of possibility of a disease as the joint possibility of the variables $Y_1, Y_2, \dots, Y_6$ in that disease. See Figure 71 once again. In each line of the in-box, the degree of possibility of each finding is determined via its degree of membership in the respective fuzzy granule. Each line thus contains six single possibility degrees whose minimum provides the joint possibility of the compound variable $Y = \langle Y_1, Y_2, \dots, Y_6 \rangle$ in the compound fuzzy set $A = A_1 \times \cdots \times A_6$. This joint possibility reflects the possibility of the disease in question. Now the maximum of the minima can be determined, i.e., $max(min_1, \dots, min_6) = 0.8$ in the present example

There are also many other fuzzy-theoretic approaches to diagnostics. Among the interesting ones are Adlassnig and his collaborators' CADIAG project where the authors introduce a new, fuzzy-theoretic method of medical knowledge representation by fuzzifying frequency notions such as "frequently", "seldom", "never" and others, and temporal notions such as "a few days", "more than four weeks", etc. See Section 9.2.5 on page 391 and (Adlassnig, 1980, 1986; Adlassnig and Akhavan-Heidari, 1989; Boegl et al., 2004).

Fuzzy therapeutic decision-making

As was pointed out in previous chapters, we must clearly distinguish between uncertainty that is due to randomness of events, on the one hand; and uncertainty arising from vagueness of classes, on the other. In the former case, we don't know whether a particular token event will occur, e.g., whether a cancer patient will survive the next six months, because we do not have a sufficiently efficacious treatment at our disposal. In the latter case, we do not know whether a particular token event will occur because it is a vague, fuzzy, event without sharp boundaries, making a precise categorization impossible. "Good weather" is an example of a fuzzy event because of the uncertainty one faces when determining precisely what good weather is. When a decision has a fuzzy goal like "good weather" above, and must be made under fuzzy constraints, classical decision theory based upon probability will not help. The theory of fuzzy decision-making is a more useful tool in such circumstances (Bellman and Zadeh, 1970; Klir and Yuan, 1995; Dompere, 2010).

Most, perhaps all, therapeutic decisions are made in fuzzy environments in that the goals they pursue as well as the measures they apply are fuzzy. To explain, consider a 'long survival period' that a physician and a cancer patient want to attain as the treatment goal. How long is a *long survival period?* Even without speculating about possible answers, it is obvious that a long period is a fuzzy set of time intervals. One year is a long period to a particular extent; two years are long to a greater extent; three years are long still to a greater extent; and so on. Here we will not develop a theory of fuzzy therapeutic decision-making. As a supplement to our discussions in Section 8.4 on page 353, we shall present only a simple example to illustrate the basic idea of a fuzzy therapeutic decision and its relevance to the philosophy of medical practice. Our example will demonstrate an instance of individual, single-stage therapeutic decision-making with simple optimization. These notions were introduced on page 356. We shall discuss in turn the following four main components involved in fuzzy decision-making:

▷   A set of *alternative actions* to attain the goal
▷   the *goal* of the decision
▷   the *constraints* under which the goal is pursued
▷   the optimal action to perform referred to as the *decision*.

Alternative actions

Let $A = \{a_1, \ldots, a_n\}$ with $n \geq 1$ be a set of alternative actions, *alternatives* for short, such that each a_i is a particular action by which to attain the goal.

Goals, constraints, and decisions are construed as fuzzy sets on the set A of alternatives as the base set in what follows.

Suppose, for example, that our patient Elroy Fox is suffering from a life-threatening disease, say prostate cancer. Using fuzzy decision analysis, we will seek a therapeutic decision from among four candidate treatments, i.e., $A = \{$surgical operation, radiotherapy, chemotherapy 1, chemotherapy 2$\}$. This set of available alternative treatments will be symbolized by $A = \{T_1, T_2, T_3, T_4\}$. In this situation, the basic question of fuzzy therapeutic decision-making is: Which of the treatments T_1, T_2, T_3, T_4 is to be chosen? To give an answer, we must know the goal and the constraints of our decision-making.

The goal

A goal, G, in a fuzzy decision-making environment is a more or less complex event or situation that the decision-maker plans to attain by performing a particular action. It may be viewed as a set such that the decision-maker's aim is to act in a way that will render the patient a member of that set. For instance, when a physician says to a patient "I shall do my best to cure you", she means "I shall do my best to render you a member of the set of the cured". The goal in this case is to attain the patient's membership in the set of the cured. There may exist $m \geq 1$ goals $G_1, \ldots, G_m$ in a decision-making situation.

The set of alternatives, $A = \{a_1, \ldots, a_n\}$, provides different actions by each of which a goal G can be attained to a particular extent. An action may be more efficacious than another one. Thus, the goal G may be conceived of as a fuzzy set over the set A of alternatives in the following way. To each alternative a_i we assign the extent to which it enables us to attain a goal G, i.e., the membership grade $\mu_G(a_i)$. We thus obtain the following fuzzy set as the goal G:

$$G = \{(a_1, \mu_G(a_1)), \ldots, (a_n, \mu_G(a_n))\}.$$

In our present example, the goal of decision-making is simply to attain a *long survival period after the treatment* of the patient. Among the four alternatives that are being considered, for instance, radiotherapy may guarantee a long survival period to the extent 0.2. In this case, we would have the fuzzy goal $G = \{\ldots, (\text{radiotherapy}, 0.2), \ldots\}$ where the ellipses are placeholders for the other three treatments. Assume that on the basis of available therapeutic knowledge acquired by controlled clinical trials, the physician and the patient jointly assign to the four treatments $A = \{T_1, T_2, T_3, T_4\}$ the following membership grades in the fuzzy set of *long survival period after the treatment* (Figure 75):

$$G = \{(T_1, 0.6), (T_2, 0.2), (T_3, 0.8), (T_4, 1)\}.$$

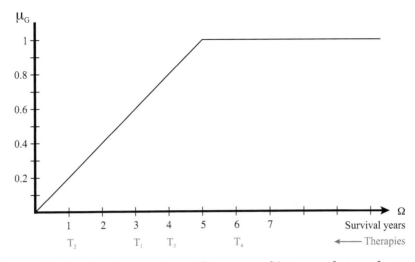

Fig. 75. The length of a survival period is expressed in terms of years after treatment. Treatments are assigned to periods

The constraints

A constraint, C, in a fuzzy decision-making environment is a requirement that imposes some restriction upon decision-making. An example is the following constraint that our patient Elroy Fox might put: "If there is pain as a consequence of the treatment, then it should be tolerable". There may be many such constraints in a decision-making situation. Analogous to a goal, a constraint is also conceived of as a fuzzy set, C, on the set of alternatives in the following way:

$$C = \{(a_1, \mu_C(a_1)), \ldots, (a_n, \mu_C(a_n))\}.$$

with μ_C as its membership function such that a pair of the form $(a_i, \mu_C(a_i))$ says that action a_i satisfies constraint C to the extent $\mu_C(a_i)$. For instance, radiotherapy may satisfy the patient Elroy Fox's constraint "tolerable pain" to the extent 0.7. In this case, we would have the fuzzy constraint $C = \{\ldots, (\text{radiotherapy}, 0.7), \ldots\}$ where the ellipses are placeholders for the other three treatments.

In our present example, we have these two constraints: "If there is pain as a consequence of the treatment, then it should be tolerable", and "if there is incapacitation, it should be mild". They may be represented as follows:

$C_1 = $ tolerable pain
$C_2 = $ mild incapacitation.

The physician and the patient may jointly assign to the four treatments $A = \{T_1, T_2, T_3, T_4\}$ the following grades of membership over the set A of alternatives, respectively, to produce the two new fuzzy sets C_1 and C_2:

$$C_1 = \{(T_1, 0.9), (T_2, 0.7), (T_3, 0.5), (T_4, 0.4)\}$$
$$C_2 = \{(T_1, 0.8), (T_2, 0.6), (T_3, 0.8), (T_4, 0.6)\}.$$

The decision

A decision, D, in a fuzzy decision-making environment is a fuzzy set that contains all actions from among the alternatives $A = \{a_1, \ldots, a_k\}$ with the degrees of their efficacy for both attaining the goals and satisfying the constraints. Thus, if there are $m \geq 1$ goals $G_1, \ldots, G_m$ and $n \geq 1$ constraints $C_1, \ldots, C_n$, a decision D in this situation is defined as the following fuzzy set:

$$D = G_1 \cap \ldots G_m \cap C_1 \cap \ldots \cap C_n.$$

That is, D is defined as the intersection of goals and constraints, and thus, by its membership function that assumes as its value, for each action a_i, the minimum of that action's membership degrees in the constituent fuzzy sets of the decision. Since we are here concerned with finite sets only, the membership function of the intersection D is defined as follows:

If we symbolize $G_1 \cap \ldots \cap G_m \cap C_1 \cap \ldots \cap C_n$ by X, then

$$\mu_D(a_i) = \mu_X(a_i) = min(\mu_{G_1}(a_i), \ldots, \mu_{C_n}(a_i)) \qquad \text{for all } a_i \in A.$$

Regarding our example, we have:

$$\begin{aligned}
D &= G \cap C_1 \cap C_2 \\
&= \{(T_1, 0.6), (T_2, 0.2), (T_3, 0.8), (T_4, 1)\} \cap \\
&\quad \{(T_1, 0.9), (T_2, 0.7), (T_3, 0.5), (T_4, 0.4)\} \cap \\
&\quad \{(T_1, 0.8), (T_2, 0.6), (T_3, 0.8), (T_4, 0.6)\}. \\
&= \{(T_1, 0.6), (T_2, 0.2), (T_3, 0.5), (T_4, 0.4)\}.
\end{aligned}$$

Set D is a fuzzy characterization of the concept of *desirable treatment*. The most desirable treatment to be chosen, i.e., the optimal decision D^{opt}, is the treatment option with the maximum value. That is:

$$D^{opt} = max(\mu_D(a_1), \ldots \mu_D(a_n)) \qquad \text{for all } a_i \in A.$$

In our above example we have $D^{opt} = \{(T_1, 0.6)\}$. Thus, the choice of treatment T_1 with a survival period of 3 years is the optimal decision. Note, however, that for the sake of simplicity we have tacitly assumed that all goals and constraints are of equal importance and have also neglected treatment costs. In real-world decision-making situations, these aspects have to be considered. For details, see (Bellman and Zadeh, 1970; Dompere, 2010).

16.5.3 Similaristic Reasoning in Medicine

More often than not there is no sufficient domain knowledge available to understand and manage a particular clinical problem, e.g., a patient's suffering. In such circumstances of 'incomplete domain knowledge', knowledge of another type will be needed to solve the problem. For instance, the patient data at hand may indicate similarities between the current case and some previous cases that have already been successfully resolved in the past. Using such similarities to reason about, and manage, a present problem situation by reusing previous experiences, we shall refer to as analogical or *similaristic reasoning*. For details of the theory and methodology of this technique, see (Hüllermeier, 2007; Leeland, 2010; Pal and Shiu, 2004).

Similaristic reasoning is a salient characteristic of natural human problem solving. It has been known as *casuistry* in the history of ethics and theology, and as *casuistics* in the history of medicine. A sophisticated type of these similaristic methods, the so-called instance-based or *case-based reasoning*, was born in the 1980s (Bareiss and Porter, 1987; Kolodner and Kolodner, 1987; Koton, 1988; Turner, 1989). It has been attracting research interests in computer science and artificial intelligence since then. To inquire into its clinical applicability, this new approach will be briefly outlined in the following two sections:

- ▶ Case-based reasoning
- ▶ case-based diagnostics.

Case-based reasoning

Case-based reasoning, or CBR for short, is a method for solving a current problem by reusing experience on previously solved problems, called cases. It is increasingly becoming an important subject of research in medical artificial intelligence and clinical decision-making. Although it is often viewed as a recent brainchild of Janet Kolodner (Kolodner, 1993), it does not represent a novel approach. Rather, it is rooted in the so-called *casuistry*, a case-based moral judgment that had its origin in Stoicism and in the writings of Cicero (106–43 BC), and was used as a method of moral reasoning in the Catholic Church in the early modern period. Contemporary bioethics research is also devoting attention to casuistry as a method of moral decision-making (Boyle, 2004; Hanson, 2009; Strong, 1999). Casuistry flourished during the sixteenth and seventeenth centuries in the Roman Catholic Church (Jonsen and Toulmin, 1988; Keenan and Shannon, 1995), and was also used in medicine in the eighteenth and nineteenth centuries giving rise to the well-known case reports or *casuistics*. However, as a moral-philosophical and medical-casuistic approach, it lacked a formal methodology. This facility was provided by, and after, Janet Kolodner's pioneering work on CBR mentioned above.

As a revival of casuistry, CBR is an empirical approach in that it exploits previous experiences to find solutions for present cases. Previous experiences on individual cases are stored in the memory of a CBR system referred to as its *case base*. Facing a new problem, e.g., a new patient with a particular state of suffering, it retrieves *similar cases* from its case base and adapts them to fit the problem at hand and to provide a solution for it (Jurisica et al., 1998). It thus rests on the basic CBR axiom that *similar problems have similar solutions*. It should not be overlooked, however, that this view is reminiscent of homeopathy, which relies on Samuel Hahnemann's esoteric *law of similars*, i.e., "similia similibus curentur", *like cures like,* conceived by Hahnemann in 1796 and first formulated in Latin in 1810 (Jütte, 1996, 23 and 181). In order for CBR to be distinguishable from such speculative conceptions, therefore, it must be based on a framework with efficient methods of case representation and a clear notion of case similarity.

Usually CBR is contrasted with the so-called 'model-based reasoning'. The latter term, popular in artificial intelligence research, is inappropriate, however, and ought to be avoided. It is a poorly chosen label used to designate the knowledge-based, or knowledge-guided, approach that uses general, scientific knowledge in the premises of arguments, e.g., so-called *rule-based* clinical expert systems such as MYCIN and others. In contrast, the knowledge contained in the case base used in CBR is merely the description of some individual cases without any generalization or statistical surveys. The expertise that is used as 'knowledge' in a CBR system simply consists of narrations on specific problems embodied in a *library* about single cases, for example, about (i) the patient Elroy Fox who had had symptoms *A, B* and *C,* and had received the drug *D* to the effect E; (ii) the patient Joseph K who had had symptoms *F, G* and *H,* and had received the drug *I* to the effect *J;* and so on. A current case is matched against such exemplars in the case base to make a judgment and decision. How is the comparison to be made, and the judgment and decision to be attained? Otherwise put, how is information on previous cases to be used so as to manage a present case? This is the central methodological question CBR is concerned with. The first answer it provides is that there must be some similarity between the present case and one or more cases in the case base. Such inter-case similarities are utilized in judging and decision-making by CBR. As an example of CBR, we will briefly discuss case-based diagnostics to make some suggestions regarding the similarity search.

Case-based diagnostics

The case base of a CBR system for diagnosis contains records detailing the making of the diagnosis for each individual case. The records include information of the following type: (i) every individual case's initial data, i.e., initial patient complaints, symptoms, signs, and findings; (ii) the course of diagnostics, i.e., the diagnostic examinations performed at each diagnostic stage and the data gathered; (iii) final patient data; (iv) the set of patient data used in making the diagnosis; (v) the diagnosis; and (vi) whether the diagnosis was confirmed or disconfirmed by biopsy, operation, autopsy, or controls of another type.

Suppose there is a particular patient, say Elroy Fox, with a set D of initial data. To solve the diagnostic problem for this patient by CBR, set D is matched with all initial data sets in the case base to retrieve a number of sufficiently similar cases, given a similarity threshold of some kind. In order for data set D to be comparable to a data set D' of a case in the case base, both data sets must be represented as fuzzy sets. For example, suppose D and D' are the following fuzzy data sets:

$$D = \{(\text{fever, } 1), (\text{vomiting, } 0.7), (\text{tachycardia, } 0.5)\}$$
$$D' = \{(\text{fever, } 0.8), (\text{vomiting, } 1), (\text{tachycardia, } 0.5)\}.$$

By Similarity Theorem on page 173, we obtain the following degree of similarity between these two data sets:

$$simil(D, D') = \frac{(0.8 + 0.7 + 0.5)}{(1 + 1 + 0.5)} = 0.8.$$

From among the retrieved set of cases, by applying the Similarity Theorem, the best case is selected, i.e., the case whose initial data set has the maximum similarity to D, and the patient Elroy Fox is examined like that case. The same procedure is followed in making the diagnosis on the basis of the final patient data set. When more than one case is retrieved, the solution must be transformed into a solution for the current patient, Elroy Fox. This adaptation process is the most important and difficult step of CBR and cannot be discussed here. For details, see (Hüllermeier, 2007; Pal et al., 2001; Pal and Shiu, 2004).

16.5.4 Fuzzy Logic in Biomedicine

The term "biomedicine" denotes the category of so-called medical biosciences comprising anatomy, physiology, biochemistry, genetics, microbiology, and similar disciplines concerned with biological objects and issues in medicine. Biomedicine is also a fruitful domain for the application of fuzzy logic. In the present section, an interesting example will be demonstrated that deals with the fuzzification of biopolymers so as to render them amenable to fuzzy logic. To this end, biopolymers are represented as ordered fuzzy sets. In this way, they can be treated as points in n-dimensional unit hypercubes and subjected to n-dimensional geometric analyses and calculations. The concept of the unit hypercube was discussed on page 207.

A biopolymer is a linear macromolecule consisting of a large number of identical or similar building blocks, called its *monomers* (from the Greek term "meros" meaning part. See page 591). They are linked by bonds to form a chain. The most important biopolymers are nucleic acids, i.e., DNA and RNA, and proteins. We shall here confine ourselves to nucleic acids. They constitute the genetic material of organisms and viruses.[126]

Sequence analysis or sequencing aims at determining the building blocks of a nucleic acid, i.e., its monomeric units called nucleotides, and their order in the molecular chain of the acid. It commenced in the early 1960s with the deciphering of the genetic code. *Sequence comparison,* by contrast, is a pat-

---

[126] There are two types of nucleic acids, deoxyribonucleic acid (DNA) and ribonucleic acid (RNA). DNA is the genetic material that all single-cell and multiple-cell *organisms* and some types of *viruses* (DNA viruses) inherit from their parents (recall the 'double helix'). Some other viruses, e.g., HIV, bear RNA as their genetic material and are therefore called RNA viruses. Both DNA and RNA govern, among other things, the production of proteins in organisms and viruses, and thus their life and death affairs.

As a linear polymer, a DNA and RNA molecule is a sequence of smaller molecules called its monomeric units. Chemically, these monomeric units belong to the category of nucleotides. A number of $n > 1$ nucleotides are linearly linked by bonds to form a chain that is called a trinucleotide or *triplet* if $n = 3$; an *oligonucleotide* if 'n is small'; and a *polynucleotide* if 'n is large'; A mononucleotide is a single nucleotide molecule. We shall use "polynucleotide" as an umbrella term. For example, the genetic material of the tiny RNA virus HIV consists of about 10,000 nucleotide monomers. The human genome has a billion-long code of DNA information.

A mononucleotide is itself composed of three smaller molecular building blocks: a five-carbon sugar, a phosphate group, and a nitrogenous base. In a DNA and RNA polynucleotide chain, a nucleotide monomer has its phosphate group bonded to the sugar of the next nucleotide link. So the chain has a regular sugar-phosphate backbone with variable appendages. These appendages are *four* possible nitrogenous bases called *Adenine* = A; *Cytosine* = C; *Guanine* = G; and *Thymine* = T in DNA, but in place of the latter, *Uracil* = U in RNA. The specific sequence of these base appendages in a polynucleotide is characteristic of the molecule and is referred to as its *base sequence*. Whereas a particular polynucleotide may have the base sequence GUAUACUGU ... etc., another one may have the base sequence GTTTACACT... etc. So, in discussions about polynucleotides they are identified with their base sequences.

In a cell's chain of command, instructions for protein synthesis flow from DNA to RNA (i.e., messenger RNA = mRNA) to protein. In the latter step, the genetic message encoded in an mRNA base sequence such as GUAUACUGU... orders amino acids into a protein of specific amino acid sequence. The mRNA message is read in the cell as a sequence of base triplets XYZ, analogous to three-letter code words. An mRNA base triplet XYZ is therefore called a *codon*. A triplet codon XYZ along an mRNA sequence specifies which one of the 20 existing amino acids will be inserted in the appropriate site of a protein chain. For example, the codon GUA is responsible for the amino acid valine. Since there are four bases for mRNA, there are $4 \cdot 4 \cdot 4 = 64$ such codons making up the dictionary of the *genetic code*. The dictionary is redundant because $64 > 20$. It is not one-to-one, but many-to-one. For instance, the four codons GUA, GUC, GUG, and GUU stand for the amino acid valine, and thus you get from the above mRNA segment GUAUACUGU$\cdots$ the protein chain valine-tyrosine-cysteine-$\cdots$ etc.

tern matching task to determine the structural relationships such as identity, similarity, and dissimilarity between chains of nucleic acids whose sequences have already been analyzed and are known. It deals with taxonomic and diagnostic questions such as, for example, "is this sample of RNA before my eyes an HIV or something else?" and "how similar or dissimilar is the human genome with that of chimpanzee?". To answer questions of this type requires reliable techniques of sequence comparison between chains of nucleic acids. As an exercise of applying fuzzy logic in biomedicine, we shall briefly address this problem in the following six sections to sketch an abstract geometry of polynucleotides that may be used for diagnostic purposes in genetic sciences:

- ▶ Polynucleotides
- ▶ Fuzzy polynucleotides
- ▶ Polynucleotides as points in the fuzzy hypercube
- ▶ The genetic code is 12-dimensional
- ▶ The fuzzy genetic space
- ▶ Fuzzy linear polymers.

In the final section, the approach will be generalized by introducing the concept of *fuzzy linear polymer*. Due to the bio-informational facts sketched above and in footnote 126 on page 642, the focus of our concern in what follows will be the *base sequence* of polynucleotides in that we shall translate it into an ordered fuzzy set. The idea behind this plan is the recognition that by translating a subject into a fuzzy set the constructs of fuzzy set theory and logic become accessible to that subject domain. For details of the theory, see (Sadegh-Zadeh, 2000b; 2007).

Polynucleotides

A DNA and RNA molecule is called a polynucleotide because it consists of many monomeric units from the chemical class of nucleotides. As is usual, we will here formally represent the monomers of a polynucleotide by their nitrogenous bases, and thus, a polynucleotide itself by its base sequence such as GTTTACGAA. We may in this way conceive a polynucleotide as a sequence of letters, i.e., as a word over a particular alphabet.

An alphabet is an ordered n-tuple of prototypical signs, characters, or *letters*, $\langle L_1, \ldots, L_n \rangle$, with $n \geq 1$ being its length. So, it is called an n-ary alphabet. For example, the English alphabet $\langle A, B, C, \ldots, Z \rangle$ is 26-ary because its length is 26. We distinguish between:

DNA alphabet $= \langle T, C, A, G \rangle$ and
RNA alphabet $= \langle U, C, A, G \rangle$.

Both are quaternary. Their letters are the initials of the names of nitrogenous bases (Thymine, Cytosine, Adenine, Guanine, Uracil) contained in the five different monomers of polynucleotides. As outlined in footnote 126 on page

642, we shall call every word over these alphabets a *polynucleotide,* including mononucleotides, triplets, oligonucleotides, and genuine polynucelotides. Words are formed over both alphabets according to the following recursive definition:

Definition 162 (Words).

1. *If the n-tuple $\langle L_1, \ldots, L_n \rangle$ consisting of the $n \geq 1$ letters $L_1, \ldots, L_n$ is an n-ary alphabet of a language $\mathcal{L}$, then an instance of a letter $L_i \in \langle L_1, \ldots, L_n \rangle$ is called* a word over $\langle L_1, \ldots, L_n \rangle$ *of length 1;*
2. *If w_1 and w_2 are words over $\langle L_1, \ldots, L_n \rangle$ of length p and q, respectively, then their concatenation $w_1 w_2$ is a word over $\langle L_1, \ldots, L_n \rangle$ of length $p + q$.*

While, for instance, "BOOK" is a word of length 4 over the English alphabet, the sequence GTTTACGAA is a word of length 9 over the DNA alphabet $\langle$T, C, A, G$\rangle$, and the sequence UGGAAC is a word of length 6 over the RNA alphabet $\langle$U, C, A, G$\rangle$. We shall use RNA words only. Our analyses also hold for DNA words. The terms "word", "string", and "sequence" are used as synonyms.

Fuzzy polynucleotides

A fuzzy polynucleotide is a polynucleotide represented as a *fuzzy sequence.* To demonstrate, we first introduce the notion of a fuzzy sequence. A fuzzy sequence is simply an *ordered fuzzy set,* i.e., a fuzzy set over an ordered universe of discourse $\Omega = \langle x_1, \ldots, x_n \rangle$, for example, $\langle (x_1, 0.8), (x_2, 1), \ldots, (x_n, 0.4) \rangle$. An ordinary polynucleotide is representable as such an ordered fuzzy set. This is the basic idea of our theory. For details, see (Sadegh-Zadeh, 2000b).

To begin with, we consider the alphabet, over which a polynucleotide is a word, as our ordered universe of discourse, e.g., the RNA alphabet $\langle$U, C, A, G$\rangle$, and fuzzify this universe. We thereby obtain an alphabet of fuzzy letters over which a polynucleotide turns out a fuzzy word. For example, let μ_U, μ_C, μ_A, and μ_G be four different functions each of which in a particular way maps the RNA alphabet $\langle$U, C, A, G$\rangle = \Omega$, as our universe, to unit interval $[0, 1]$:

$$\mu_U \colon \langle U, C, A, G \rangle \mapsto [0,1] \quad \text{with } \mu_U(\langle U, C, A, G \rangle) = \langle (U, \mathbf{1}), (C, 0), (A, 0), (G, 0) \rangle$$
$$\mu_C \colon \langle U, C, A, G \rangle \mapsto [0,1] \quad \text{with } \mu_C(\langle U, C, A, G \rangle) = \langle (U, 0), (C, \mathbf{1}), (A, 0), (G, 0) \rangle$$
$$\mu_A \colon \langle U, C, A, G \rangle \mapsto [0,1] \quad \text{with } \mu_A(\langle U, C, A, G \rangle) = \langle (U, 0), (C, 0), (A, \mathbf{1}), (G, 0) \rangle$$
$$\mu_G \colon \langle U, C, A, G \rangle \mapsto [0,1] \quad \text{with } \mu_G(\langle U, C, A, G \rangle) = \langle (U, 0), (C, 0), (A, 0), (G, \mathbf{1}) \rangle$$

to yield the following four different *fuzzy letters* as ordered fuzzy sets:

Letter U	$\equiv \langle (U, 1), (C, 0), (A, 0), (G, 0) \rangle$	read 'U'	(164)
Letter C	$\equiv \langle (U, 0), (C, 1), (A, 0), (G, 0) \rangle$	read 'C'	
Letter A	$\equiv \langle (U, 0), (C, 0), (A, 1), (G, 0) \rangle$	read 'A'	
Letter G	$\equiv \langle (U, 0), (C, 0), (A, 0), (G, 1) \rangle$	read 'G'	

Note that a fuzzy letter is expressed by means of the entire alphabet and weighting the characters therein. By employing fuzzy letters we may reconstruct, for example, the RNA sequence UGG as the ordered fuzzy set:

⟨Letter U, Letter G, Letter G⟩,

that is:

⟨(U, 1), (C, 0), (A, 0), (G, 0), (U, 0), (C, 0),
(A, 0), (G, 1), (U, 0), (C, 0), (A, 0), (G, 1)⟩.

This ordered fuzzy set is a *fuzzy polynucleotide*, i.e., our RNA triplet UGG as a fuzzy sequence. To simplify the representation of the four fuzzy letters in (164) above, we may use only their membership vectors. By so doing, we obtain the following four simplified *fuzzy letters in vector notation* or 'quaternary numbers':

$$\text{Letter U} = \quad (1, 0, 0, 0) \tag{165}$$
$$\text{Letter C} = \quad (0, 1, 0, 0)$$
$$\text{Letter A} = \quad (0, 0, 1, 0)$$
$$\text{Letter G} = \quad (0, 0, 0, 1).$$

With the help of this vector notation, our fuzzy RNA sequence UGG above is simplified thus:

$$\underbrace{(1, 0, 0, 0,}_{U} \underbrace{0, 0, 0, 1,}_{G} \underbrace{0, 0, 0, 1)}_{G}.$$

This 12-dimensional vector represents our example, i.e., the triplet codon UGG. Analogously, the following 24-dimensional vector is the polynucleotide UGGAAC consisting of two triplet codons, i.e., UGG and AAC:

$$(1, 0, 0, 0, 0, 0, 0, 1, 0, 0, 0, 1, 0, 0, 1, 0, 0, 0, 1, 0, 0, 1, 0, 0).$$

These examples demonstrate that a polynucleotide of length $n \geq 1$ is a fuzzy polynucleotide of length $4n$. It has a vector of length $4n$ because each fuzzy letter is of length 4. The vectors of our example fuzzy polynucleotides above were composed of the bivalent set $\{0, 1\}$. We therefore call a fuzzy polynucleotide of this type *bivalent*. However, a fuzzy polynucleotide is not necessarily bivalent. It may also be *multivalent* since the membership function of a fuzzy set has the entire unit interval $[0, 1]$ as its range. Thus, the set of *all* fuzzy sets over the RNA alphabet ⟨U, C, A, G⟩, i.e., the fuzzy powerset $F(2^{\langle U, C, A, G \rangle})$, is infinite such that every element of $F(2^{\langle U, C, A, G \rangle})$ is a fuzzy letter. A polynucleotide that contains at least one such genuinely fuzzy letter, is a multivalent sequence. A simple example is the following mononucleotide consisting of only one fuzzy letter:

$\langle (U, 0.4), (C, 0.2), (A, 0), (G, 0.8) \rangle$

that is, the vector:

$(0.4, 0.2, 0, 0.8)$.

The components of this sequence are not limited to the bivalent set $\{0, 1\}$. So, it is a multivalent sequence. There may exist circumstances, e.g., an experiment or a genetic examination, in which we are not certain whether the third site (marked here with an 'X') on a particular triplet such as UGX bears a U, a C, an A, or a G. In such cases, we may hypothesize about the biochemical nature of the site X by supposing a *degree of possibility* – or, alternatively, a degree of probability – to which any of the four bases may be present at that site to obtain, for example, the following vector:

$$\underbrace{(1, 0, 0, 0,}_{\text{First}} \underbrace{0, 0, 0, 1,}_{\text{second}} \underbrace{0.4, 0.2, 0, 0.8)}_{\text{third base}}.$$

Note that this is not a probabilistic vector because the sum of its components exceeds 1. Rather, it is a possibilistic one. A probabilistic vector will be given below. To explain, the vector says that:

1. the first base is a U with possibility 1, a C with possibility 0, an A with possibility 0, and a G with possibility 0,
2. the second base is a U with possibility 0, a C with possibility 0, an A with possibility 0, and a G with possibility 1,
3. the third base is a U with possibility 0.4, a C with possibility 0.2, an A with possibility 0, and a G with possibility 0.8.

Summarizing, if $(a_1, \ldots, a_n)$ is a fuzzy polynucleotide in vector notation as our examples above, it is bivalent if each $a_i \in \{0, 1\}$; and multivalent if at least one $a_i \in [0, 1]$. By distinguishing between these two types of fuzzy polynucleotide sequences, we may interpret a fuzzy polynucleotide (i) possibilistically to open thereby a door to the application of the theory of possibility in genetic structures; or (ii) probabilistically to open the door to the application of the theory of probability in genetic structures. In any case, a polynucleotide of length $n \geq 1$ is a fuzzy polynucleotide of length $4n$ and thus representable by a real-valued vector $(r_1, r_2, \ldots, r_{4n})$ of length $4n$ such that each component r_i of the vector is an element of $[0, 1]$. In such vectors, symbol "r" is reminiscent of "real number" $r \in [0, 1]$.

Polynucleotides as points in the fuzzy hypercube

We saw on page 211 that a fuzzy set $\{(x_1, r_1), (x_2, r_2), \ldots, (x_n, r_n)\}$ of length n represents a point in an n-dimensional unit hypercube $[0, 1]^n$. The objects $(x_1, x_2, \ldots, x_n)$ are conceived of as the axes of the cube, and on these axes the n-dimensional membership vector $(r_1, r_2, \ldots, r_n)$ of the set is interpreted as the coordinates of the point in the cube such that a component r_i belongs to the axis x_i with $n \geq 1$. In the same fashion, a fuzzy polynucleotide as a fuzzy sequence $\langle (x_1, r_1), (x_2, r_2), \ldots, (x_n, r_n) \rangle$ over an alphabet presents itself as a point in an n-dimensional unit hypercube $[0, 1]^n$ when a nitrogenous base at position i of the sequence, x_i, is assigned to the axis i of the cube, and the membership vector $(r_1, r_2, \ldots, r_n)$ of the sequence is taken to represent the coordinates of the point within the cube. For example, the 4-dimensional vector $(0.4, 0.2, 0, 0.8)$ is the membership vector of the above-mentioned fuzzy mononucleotide $\langle (U, 0.4), (C, 0.2), (A, 0), (G, 0.8) \rangle$. Thus, it is a point in the 4-dimensional unit hypercube $[0, 1]^4$ with the axes U, C, A, and G, respectively. Since a polynucleotide of length n is a fuzzy polynucleotide of length $4n$, it is a point in the $4n$-dimensional unit hypercube $[0, 1]^{4n}$. For instance, HIV with its about 10,000 nucleotides is a point in the 40,000-dimensional cube $[0, 1]^{40,000}$. An example is depicted in Figure 76.

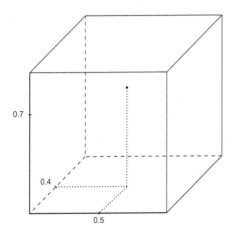

Fig. 76. Because of the high dimensionality of polynucleotides they are points in cubes higher than 3 dimensions, and thus, graphically not representable. This is merely an illustration. The dot in the cube is the fuzzy set $\{(x_1, 0.5), (x_2, 0.4), (x_3, 0.7)\}$ with its fuzzy vector being $(0.5, 0.4, 0.7)$. For additional examples, see pages 207–217

By supplementing an n-dimensional cube $[0, 1]^n$ with a distance measure $dist$ over $[0, 1]^n$, we obtain an n-dimensional metric space $\langle [0, 1]^n, dist \rangle$. For the notion of a metric space, see Definitions 55–56 on page 212. In a metric space $\langle [0, 1]^n, dist \rangle$ we can determine how distant from, and thus how close and similar to, one another two points of the space are. The function $diff$ introduced in Definition 34 on page 172 to measure the difference between two fuzzy sets, may serve as such a distance function to yield the metric space $\langle [0, 1]^n, diff \rangle$ for fuzzy polynucleotides. This metric space enables us to determine the distance and proximity, i.e., dissimilarity and similarity, between polynucleotides. Here is a simple example. We will compute the difference, proximity, and similarity between the following three RNA sequences, s_1 through s_3:

$$s_1 \equiv \text{AAAGGG} \qquad \text{codes for amino acids: lysine / glycine}$$
$$s_2 \equiv \text{AGUCUG} \qquad \text{codes for amino acids: serine / leucine}$$

$s_3 \equiv$ AUACGG   codes for amino acids: isoleucine / arginine.

They consist of six triplet codons listed in Table 19 and have obviously the following 24-dimensional membership vectors, respectively:

$s_1 \equiv$ $(0,0,1,0,0,0,1,0,0,0,1,0,0,0,0,1,0,0,0,1,0,0,0,1)$
$s_2 \equiv$ $(0,0,1,0,0,0,0,1,1,0,0,0,0,1,0,0,1,0,0,0,0,0,0,1)$
$s_3 \equiv$ $(0,0,1,0,1,0,0,0,0,0,1,0,0,1,0,0,0,0,0,1,0,0,0,1)$.

Table 19. Six triplets, their membership vectors, and the amino acids they code for

Codon:	its membership vector:	the coded amino acid:
AAA	(0, 0, 1, 0, 0, 0, 1, 0, 0, 0, 1, 0)	lysine
GGG	(0, 0, 0, 1, 0, 0, 0, 1, 0, 0, 0, 1)	glycine
AGU	(0, 0, 1, 0, 0, 0, 0, 1, 1, 0, 0, 0)	serine
CUG	(0, 1, 0, 0, 1, 0, 0, 0, 0, 0, 0, 1)	leucine
AUA	(0, 0, 1, 0, 1, 0, 0, 0, 0, 0, 1, 0)	isoleucine
CGG	(0, 1, 0, 0, 0, 0, 0, 1, 0, 0, 0, 1)	arginine

According to our previous definitions of difference, similarity, and proximity on pages 172 and 216, we obtain the following degrees of difference, similarity, and proximity between the first and the other two RNA sequences:

$$diff(s_1, s_2) = \frac{8}{10} = 0.8$$

$$diff(s_1, s_3) = \frac{4}{8} = 0.5$$

$$simil(s_1, s_2) = 1 - 0.8 = 0.2$$
$$simil(s_1, s_3) = 1 - 0.5 = 0.5$$

$$prox(s_1, s_2) = 0.2$$
$$prox(s_1, s_3) = 0.5.$$

Distance and proximity between two polynucleotides are spatial relations between two points of the unit hypercube representing those polynucleotides. This makes it possible to develop an abstract geometry of polynucleotides, and of biopolymers in general. We sketched this geometry earlier on pages 212–217. For an example, see Figure 77.

In our framework sketched above, only polynucleotide sequences of equal length can be compared with one another because polynucleotide sequences of *unequal* length cannot be represented as points in the same n-dimensional hypercube $[0, 1]^n$. This is a disadvantage, as it would be interesting to know whether there is any similarity or dissimilarity between sequences of unequal length such as, for example, CUAAGGAUG and CUAAGG, or genomes of unequal length in general. So, unlike our framework sketched above, in what follows we shall introduce an alternative, 12-dimensional, standard metric space which is general enough to cover polynucleotides of arbitrary length.

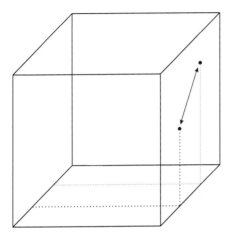

Fig. 77. The double arrow between the two points in the cube reflects their spatial distance. This distance may be measured by different Minkowski metrics, e.g., Hamming distance, Euclidean distance, etc. Our metric is the difference function *diff* given in Definition 34 on page 172

The genetic code is 12-dimensional

Recall that a base sequence consisting of only one single base $X \in \langle U, C, A, G \rangle$ is a four-dimensional fuzzy sequence because each of our fuzzy letters over $\langle U, C, A, G \rangle$ is 4-dimensional. Any additional base in the sequence adds four dimensions. Thus, a base sequence $s = X_1 \ldots X_n$ of length n is a point of the $4n$-dimensional unit hypercube $[0, 1]^{4n}$.

The physical space can be, and is, treated as an interpretation of the three-dimensional real space $[0, +\infty]^3$ and is therefore considered three-dimensional. By adding the time as a fourth dimension, Einstein's four-dimensional universe is obtained as an interpretation of the four-dimensional real space $[0, +\infty]^4$. The objects that are dealt with in the former space are three-dimensional *because* they are points of a three-dimensional space. The objects that are dealt with in the latter space are four-dimensional *because* they are points of a four-dimensional space.

Similarly, in our framework the *genetic code* is twelve-dimensional because a triplet codon XYZ has a $3 \cdot 4 = 12$-dimensional membership vector $(r_1, \ldots, r_{12})$ and is thus a point in the 12-dimensional unit hypercube $[0, 1]^{12}$ as a subspace of the real space $[0, +\infty]^{12}$. Each of the bivalent 64 codons of the genetic code is located at one of the $2^{12} = 4096$ corners of this 12-dimensional unit cube. The examples in Table 20, taken from Table 19 above, may illustrate:

Table 20. The 12-dimensionality of triplet codons

Codon:	its membership vector:	the coded amino acid:
AUA	(0, 0, 1, 0, 1, 0, 0, 0, 0, 0, 1, 0)	isoleucine
CGG	(0, 1, 0, 0, 0, 0, 0, 1, 0, 0, 0, 1)	arginine

We should be aware, however, that a triplet codon need not necessarily reside at a corner of the cube $[0,1]^{12}$. It can reside within the cube as well when it is a multivalent triplet, because in this case the components of its membership vector are not confined to 0 and 1, but also include membership degrees between 0 and 1 such as, for example:

$$(0.3, 0.1, 0.4, 0.2, 1, 0, 0, 0, 0, 0, 1, 0). \tag{166}$$

This is the vector of a mutant of the triplet AUA in Table 20 which differs from AUA in that its first letter consists of:

U to the extent 0.3
C to the extent 0.1
A to the extent 0.4
G to the extent 0.2.

How is this possible? This four-dimensional possibility reflects states of our uncertainty where no sufficient knowledge about the chemical structure of a sequence is available, e.g., due to poor sequencing. Probabilistic predictions in experiments of the outcome of replications may be considered as additional examples. In an experiment of this kind the vector (166) may predict the copy of the segment AUA of a replicating virus. This hypothetical, multivalent triplet is a probabilistic one because $0.3 + 0.1 + 0.4 + 0.2 = 1$. It is not located at a corner of the cube, but is a point inside the cube. As our information about the outcome changes during the experimentation, the vector (166) also changes due to the fluctuating probability distribution. A vector of the form $(r_1, \ldots, r_{12})$ at a particular time may thus change into $(r'_1, \ldots, r'_{12})$ at a later time such that $r_i \neq r'_i$ for any $i \geq 1$. Temporal fluctuations of these vectors represent the trajectory of a moving point in the cube $[0,1]^{12}$, its dynamic or history so to speak. Suppose now that in our experiment regarding the triplet AUA above:

- the initial triplet AUA is the point A,
- the predicted, hypothetical triplet (166) is the point B,
- and the actually emerging copy is the point C

of the cube (Figure 78). What spatial relationships exist between these three points? Is it possible to conclude from the distance between the final point C and the hypothesized point B how accurate our prediction has been?

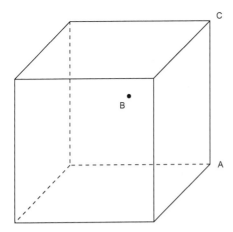

Fig. 78. For illustration purposes, a three-dimensional hypercube is used instead of a twelve-dimensional one because the latter is not representable graphically. The initial, bivalent triplet codon AUA may reside at the corner A. Point B is the predicted state of its multivalent mutant (166). The actually emerging bivalent mutant resides at the corner C. What is the distance between A and B and between B and C? How close to the target C was the prediction of point B? Similar problems concerning the geomrtry of diseases have been dealt with on page 212

The fuzzy genetic space

As was shown above, the 12-dimensional unit hypercube $[0,1]^{12}$ is the 'house of the genetic code'. By providing it with our difference function *diff* as a metric, a 12-dimensional metric space $\langle [0,1]^{12}, diff \rangle$ emerges. We dubb this metric space *the fuzzy genetic space* for the following reason:

Sequence comparison in genetic sciences serves both diagnostics and taxonomy, for example, to inquire into whether there is any ancestral relationships (homology) between two species, e.g., man and ape; ape and earthworm; etc. It is carried out mainly by analyzing the structural differences and similarities between polynucleotide chains. The fuzzy genetic space $\langle [0,1]^{12}, diff \rangle$ will provide an ideal tool for analyses of this and similar type. To this end, we will now introduce a second method of fuzzification of polynucleotides that differs from the one used above. Data compression enables us to map any polynucleotide of arbitrary length into the 12-dimensional unit cube $[0,1]^{12}$ such that it becomes a point of this small space. That is, the fuzzy genetic space $\langle [0,1]^{12}, diff \rangle$ will house *all* polynucleotides of all species. In this way two arbitrarily chosen polynucleotides of equal or unequal length, e.g., of man and mouse, may be compared with one another to determine their distance and proximity, similarity and dissimilarity. As before, we shall confine ourselves to RNA molecules. DNA molecules can be treated in the same fashion.

The universe of our discourse is the set of all RNA chains consisting of $n \geq 1$ triplet codons, conveniently denoted $\mathbb{RNA}$. That is, $\mathbb{RNA} = \{s \mid s$ is an RNA sequence consisting of $n \geq 1$ triplet codons$\}$. In the next section, we shall map this universe to the unit hypercube $[0,1]^{12}$ by constructing a function, symbolized by the acronym *"bp"*, that determines the *base profile* of any RNA sequence. If $s \in \mathbb{RNA}$ is such a sequence, we shall write:

$$bp(s) = (r_1, r_2, \ldots, r_{12})$$

to say that:

the base profile of sequence s is $(r_1, r_2, \ldots, r_{12}) \in [0,1]^{12}$

with each $r_i \in [0,1]$. The base profile of a polynucleotide will thus be a 12-dimensional multivalent vector. This vector is determined by the function bp defined in the next section and applied thereafter. Our analysis consists of the following two sections. Readers not interested in the definition of the function bp may skip the first one:

▷   The base profile of a polynucleotide
▷   The geometry of polynucleotides.

The base profile of a polynucleotide

To render every polynucleotide a point of the 12-dimensional hypercube $[0,1]^{12}$, it must be transformed to a 12-dimensional vector $(r_1, r_2, \ldots, r_{12})$. This is accomplished by the function bp that maps all RNA chains to $[0,1]^{12}$:

$$bp\colon \mathbb{RNA} \mapsto [0,1]^{12}.$$

This function works as follows. Roughly, in a polynucleotide sequence s the absolute frequency of a nitrogenous base at any of the three sites of all triplets XYZ is determined and then divided through its weighted frequency to obtain a real number $r_i \in [0,1]$. For every sequence s there are 12 such values because there are 4 bases and 3 triplet sites such that $4 \cdot 3 = 12$. The result is a 12-dimensional vector $(r_1, r_2, \ldots, r_{12})$ as the weighted base profile, bp, of the sequence s.

To construct the function bp, we enumerate the triplets in an RNA sequence according to their location order in the chain as triplet number 1, triplet number 2,..., triplet number n such that if s is an RNA sequence with $n \geq 1$ triplets and t denotes "triplet", then s is the string $t_1 t_2 \ldots t_n$ consisting of the concatenated triplets $t_1, t_2, \ldots, t_n$. For example, in the base sequence CUAAGGAUG we have $t_3 = \text{AUG}$. The positions of the three nitrogenous bases in a triplet codon XYZ are referred to as site 1, site 2, and site 3. For instance, the base at site 2 of the triplet AUG is U. We will now assemble three auxiliary functions by which the function bp will be defined. In these functions, we shall use the following symbols:

- B is a variable ranging over the alphabet $\langle \text{U, C, A, G} \rangle$ and denoting any of the four *bases*;
- $s \in \mathbb{RNA}$ is any RNA sequence $t_1 t_2 \ldots t_n$ with $n \geq 1$ triplets $t_1, t_2, \ldots, t_n$; and
- i is a variable ranging over the three sites $\{1, 2, 3\}$ of a triplet codon XYZ of such a sequence, i.e., $i = 1, 2, 3$.

The three auxiliary function symbols that we shall use, read as follows:

$af \equiv$ "absolute frequency";
$wf \equiv$ "weighted frequency";
$wrf \equiv$ "weighted relative frequency".

The syntax of these three functions is:

$af(B, i, s) = x$ means: the *absolute frequency* of base $B \in \langle$U, C, A, G$\rangle$ at site $i \in \{1, 2, 3\}$ of all triplets of the sequence s equals x. For example, in the RNA sequence $s \equiv$ CUAAGGAUG, base G is present at site 3 of all triplets two times, i.e., $af(\text{G}, 3, s) = 2$.

$wf(B, i, s) = y$ means: the *weighted frequency* of base $B \in \langle$U, C, A, G$\rangle$ at site $i \in \{1, 2, 3\}$ of all triplets of the sequence s equals y. It is defined as follows:

If $a, b, c, \ldots, m$ are the location numbers of those triplets at whose site $i \in \{1, 2, 3\}$ the base B is present, then $wf(B, i, s) = a + b + c + \cdots + m$.

That is, $wf(B, i, s)$ is simply the arithmetical sum of the location numbers of those triplets whose site i contains base B. For example, if a base $B \in \langle$U, C, A, G$\rangle$ appears at site i of the triplets number 1, 4, 7, and 11 of a sequence, then its weighted frequency in the sequence is $1+4+7+11 = 23$. Regarding the sequence $s \equiv$ CUAAGGAUG, for instance, we have $wf(\text{U}, 2, s) = 1 + 3 = 4$.

$wrf(B, i, s) = z$ means: the *weighted relative frequency* of base $B \in \langle$U, C, A, G$\rangle$ at site $i \in \{1, 2, 3\}$ of all triplets of the sequence s equals z. This weighted relative frequency is obtained simply by dividing $af(B, i, s)$ through $wf(B, i, s)$. Thus, it is defined as follows:[127]

Definition 163 (Weighted relative frequency).

$$wrf(B, i, s) = \begin{cases} 0 & \textit{iff } af(B, i, s) = 0 \\ \frac{af(B,i,s)}{wf(B,i,s)} & \textit{otherwise.} \end{cases}$$

To give a complete example, let s_4 be the RNA sequence CUAAGGAUG. The weighted relative frequencies of its bases are displayed in Table 21. What is needed for the calculation, are the *wrf* values. For every RNA sequence $s \equiv t_1 t_2 \ldots t_n$ with $n \geq 1$ triplets t_i, there are 12 *wrf* values because there are 4 bases $\langle$U, C, A, G$\rangle$ each of which may appear at any of the 3 sites of a triplet codon $t_i \equiv$ XYZ. So, we have $4 \cdot 3 = 12$ dimensions. We are now able to define the function bp, base profile:

---

[127] The inspiration to weight relative frequency this way, came from (Georgiou et al., 2008).

Table 21. The base profile of the sequence CUAAGGAUG $\equiv s_4$

Absolute frequencies, af	Weighted frequencies, wf	Weighted relative frequencies, wrf
$af(\text{U}, 1, s_4) = 0$	$wf(\text{U}, 1, s_4) = 0$	$wrf(\text{U}, 1, s_4) = 0$
$af(\text{C}, 1, s_4) = 1$	$wf(\text{C}, 1, s_4) = 1$	$wrf(\text{C}, 1, s_4) = 1$
$af(\text{A}, 1, s_4) = 2$	$wf(\text{A}, 1, s_4) = 2 + 3 = 5$	$wrf(\text{A}, 1, s_4) = \frac{2}{5} = 0.4$
$af(\text{G}, 1, s_4) = 0$	$wf(\text{G}, 1, s_4) = 0$	$wrf(\text{G}, 1, s_4) = 0$
$af(\text{U}, 2, s_4) = 2$	$wf(\text{U}, 2, s_4) = 1 + 3 = 4$	$wrf(\text{U}, 2, s_4) = \frac{2}{4} = 0.5$
$af(\text{C}, 2, s_4) = 0$	$wf(\text{C}, 2, s_4) = 0$	$wrf(\text{C}, 2, s_4) = 0$
$af(\text{A}, 2, s_4) = 0$	$wf(\text{A}, 2, s_4) = 0$	$wrf(\text{A}, 2, s_4) = 0$
$af(\text{G}, 2, s_4) = 1$	$wf(\text{G}, 2, s_4) = 2$	$wrf(\text{G}, 2, s_4) = \frac{1}{2} = 0.5$
$af(\text{U}, 3, s_4) = 0$	$wf(\text{U}, 3, s_4) = 0$	$wrf(\text{U}, 3, s_4) = 0$
$af(\text{C}, 3, s_4) = 0$	$wf(\text{C}, 3, s_4) = 0$	$wrf(\text{C}, 3, s_4) = 0$
$af(\text{A}, 3, s_4) = 1$	$wf(\text{A}, 3, s_4) = 1$	$wrf(\text{A}, 3, s_4) = 1$
$af(\text{G}, 3, s_4) = 2$	$wf(\text{G}, 3, s_4) = 2 + 3 = 5$	$wrf(\text{G}, 3, s_4) = \frac{2}{5} = 0.4$

Definition 164 (Base profile). *If s is an RNA sequence consisting of $n \geq 1$ triplet codons, then $bp(s) =$*

$$\langle wrf(\text{U}, 1, s), wrf(\text{C}, 1, s), wrf(\text{A}, 1, s), wrf(\text{G}, 1, s),$$
$$wrf(\text{U}, 2, s), wrf(\text{C}, 2, s), wrf(\text{A}, 2, s), wrf(\text{G}, 2, s),$$
$$wrf(\text{U}, 3, s), wrf(\text{C}, 3, s), wrf(\text{A}, 3, s), wrf(\text{G}, 3, s)\rangle.$$

For our example sequence CUAAGGAUG analyzed above, we have obtained the following base profile:

$$bp\,(\text{CUAAGGAUG}) = (0, 1, 0.4, 0, 0.5, 0, 0, 0.5, 0, 0, 1, 0.4).$$

The geometry of polynucleotides

As we saw above, the base profile of an RNA sequence is a 12-dimensional vector of the form:

$$(r_1, r_2, \ldots, r_{12}) \in [0, 1]^{12}$$

provided by the weighted relative frequencies of the nitrogenous bases $\langle$U, C, A, G$\rangle$ in that RNA sequence. Even had our example been a virus of length 10,000 such as HIV or a longer polynucleotide chain, we would still have obtained a 12-dimensional vector as above. Thus, bp is indeed a function such that $bp \colon \text{RNA} \mapsto [0, 1]^{12}$. In this way, *all* RNA sequences become unique points in the unit cube $[0, 1]^{12}$. By providing the cube with a distance function such as our difference function $diff$, we obtain the metric space $\langle [0, 1]^{12}, diff \rangle$, which we dubbed *the fuzzy genetic space* above. It enables us to analyze the distance and proximity, similarity and dissimilarity between its points, i.e., between any two RNA chains of arbitrary length and source. To demonstrate an example, we will now add to the sequence:

$s_4 \equiv$ CUAAGGAUG   codes for amino acids: leucine, arginine, methionine

that we analyzed above, the following two sequences for comparison with one another in the fuzzy genetic space $\langle [0,1]^{12}, \mathit{diff} \rangle$:

$s_5 \equiv$ AUGAGGCUA   codes for amino acids: methionine, arginine, leucine
$s_6 \equiv$ GUCAGC   codes for amino acids: valine, serine.

The weighted relative frequencies of nitrogenous bases of the latter two sequences, and thus their base profiles, are displayed in Table 22. We have thus the subsequent three 12-dimensional vectors of our three RNA sequences above, although these RNA chains are of unequal length.

Table 22. The base profiles of the sequences AUGAGGCUA and GUCAGC

Absolute frequencies, af	Weighted frequencies, wf	Weighted relative frequencies, wrf
	AUGAGGCUA $\equiv s_5$	
$af(\text{U}, 1, s_5) = 0$	$wf(\text{U}, 1, s_5) = 0$	$wrf(\text{U}, 1, s_5) = 0$
$af(\text{C}, 1, s_5) = 1$	$wf(\text{C}, 1, s_5) = 3$	$wrf(\text{C}, 1, s_5) = \frac{1}{3} = 0.33$
$af(\text{A}, 1, s_5) = 2$	$wf(\text{A}, 1, s_5) = 1 + 2 = 3$	$wrf(\text{A}, 1, s_5) = \frac{2}{3} = 0.66$
$af(\text{G}, 1, s_5) = 0$	$wf(\text{G}, 1, s_5) = 0$	$wrf(\text{G}, 1, s_5) = 0$
$af(\text{U}, 2, s_5) = 2$	$wf(\text{U}, 2, s_5) = 1 + 3 = 4$	$wrf(\text{U}, 2, s_5) = \frac{2}{4} = 0.5$
$af(\text{C}, 2, s_5) = 0$	$wf(\text{C}, 2, s_5) = 0$	$wrf(\text{C}, 2, s_5) = 0$
$af(\text{A}, 2, s_5) = 0$	$wf(\text{A}, 2, s_5) = 0$	$wrf(\text{A}, 2, s_5) = 0$
$af(\text{G}, 2, s_5) = 1$	$wf(\text{G}, 2, s_5) = 2$	$wrf(\text{G}, 2, s_5) = \frac{1}{2} = 0.5$
$af(\text{U}, 3, s_5) = 0$	$wf(\text{U}, 3, s_5) = 0$	$wrf(\text{U}, 3, s_5) = 0$
$af(\text{C}, 3, s_5) = 0$	$wf(\text{C}, 3, s_5) = 0$	$wrf(\text{C}, 3, s_5) = 0$
$af(\text{A}, 3, s_5) = 1$	$wf(\text{A}, 3, s_5) = 3$	$wrf(\text{A}, 3, s_5) = \frac{1}{3} = 0.33$
$af(\text{G}, 3, s_5) = 2$	$wf(\text{G}, 3, s_5) = 1 + 2 = 3$	$wrf(\text{G}, 3, s_5) = \frac{2}{3} = 0.66$
	GUCAGC $\equiv s_6$	
$af(\text{U}, 1, s_6) = 0$	$wf(\text{U}, 1, s_6) = 0$	$wrf(\text{U}, 1, s_6) = 0$
$af(\text{C}, 1, s_6) = 0$	$wf(\text{C}, 1, s_6) = 0$	$wrf(\text{C}, 1, s_6) = 0$
$af(\text{A}, 1, s_6) = 1$	$wf(\text{A}, 1, s_6) = 2$	$wrf(\text{A}, 1, s_6) = \frac{1}{2} = 0.5$
$af(\text{G}, 1, s_6) = 1$	$wf(\text{G}, 1, s_6) = 1$	$wrf(\text{G}, 1, s_6) = 1$
$af(\text{U}, 2, s_6) = 1$	$wf(\text{U}, 2, s_6) = 1$	$wrf(\text{U}, 2, s_6) = 1$
$af(\text{C}, 2, s_6) = 0$	$wf(\text{C}, 2, s_6) = 0$	$wrf(\text{C}, 2, s_6) = 0$
$af(\text{A}, 2, s_6) = 0$	$wf(\text{A}, 2, s_6) = 0$	$wrf(\text{A}, 2, s_6) = 0$
$af(\text{G}, 2, s_6) = 1$	$wf(\text{G}, 2, s_6) = 2$	$wrf(\text{G}, 2, s_6) = \frac{1}{2} = 0.5$
$af(\text{U}, 3, s_6) = 0$	$wf(\text{U}, 3, s_6) = 0$	$wrf(\text{U}, 3, s_6) = 0$
$af(\text{C}, 3, s_6) = 2$	$wf(\text{C}, 3, s_6) = 1 + 2 = 3$	$wrf(\text{C}, 3, s_6) = \frac{2}{3} = 0.66$
$af(\text{A}, 3, s_6) = 0$	$wf(\text{A}, 3, s_6) = 0$	$wrf(\text{A}, 3, s_6) = 0$
$af(\text{G}, 3, s_6) = 0$	$wf(\text{G}, 3, s_6) = 0$	$wrf(\text{G}, 3, s_6) = 0$

$$s_4 \equiv (0, 1, 0.4, 0, 0.5, 0, 0, 0.5, 0, 0, 1, 0.4)$$
$$s_5 \equiv (0, 0.33, 0.66, 0, 0.5, 0, 0, 0.5, 0, 0, 0.33, 0.66)$$
$$s_6 \equiv (0, 0, 0.5, 1, 1, 0, 0, 0.5, 0, 0.66, 0, 0).$$

In the fuzzy genetic space $\langle [0, 1]^{12}, \mathit{diff} \rangle$, we obtain the following differences, dissimilarities, similarities, and proximities between them:

$$\mathit{diff}(s_4, s_5) = \mathit{dissimil}(s_4, s_5) = 0.426$$
$$\mathit{diff}(s_4, s_6) = \mathit{dissimil}(s_4, s_6) = 0.823$$
$$\mathit{diff}(s_5, s_6) = \mathit{dissimil}(s_5, s_6) = 0.7$$

$$\mathit{simil}(s_4, s_5) = \mathit{prox}(s_4, s_5) = 1 - 0.426 = 0.574$$
$$\mathit{simil}(s_4, s_6) = \mathit{prox}(s_4, s_6) = 1 - 0.823 = 0.172$$
$$\mathit{simil}(s_5, s_6) = \mathit{prox}(s_5, s_6) = 1 - 0.7 = 0.3$$

In our brief discussion above we demonstrated that the fuzzy genetic space is indeed an ideal metric space for quantitative analyses of relationships between all types of RNA sequences. The same metric space may be used for analogous analyses of DNA chains.

Fuzzy linear polymers

Our approach outlined in the preceding sections may easily be generalized to cover all types of sequences, and thus, all types of sequential structures including natural as well as synthetic proteins. This will be briefly sketched in the following two paragraphs:

▷ Fuzzy alphabets
▷ Fuzzy biopolymers.

Fuzzy alphabets

In Definition 162 on page 644, we defined a word over an alphabet to be a sequence of $n \geq 1$ letters of this alphabet. Using the RNA alphabet $\langle$U, C, A, G$\rangle$ as an example, we showed that by fuzzifying this alphabet we obtain fuzzy letters. Their concatenation yields fuzzy words. Fuzzy polynucleotides were such fuzzy words over the fuzzified RNA and DNA alphabets. This idea may be generlized to construct the notion of a *fuzzy linear polymer* in what follows.

Definition 165 (Fuzzy letters). *Let the n-tuple* $\langle L_1, \ldots, L_n \rangle = \mathcal{A}$ *be an n-ary alphabet of a language* $\mathcal{L}$ *with* $n \geq 1$ *letters* $L_1, \ldots, L_n$. *Then* $\widetilde{L}$ *is a fuzzy letter over* $\mathcal{A}$ *iff there is a function* $\mu_{\widetilde{L}}$ *such that:*

1. $\mu_{\widetilde{L}} : \mathcal{A} \mapsto [0, 1]$
2. $\widetilde{L} = \left\{ \langle L_i, \mu_{\widetilde{L}}(L_i) \rangle \mid L_i \in \mathcal{A} \right\}$ *for all* $L_i \in \mathcal{A}$ *with* $1 \leq i \leq n$.

That is, a fuzzy letter $\tilde{L}$ over an alphabet $\mathcal{A}$ is a fuzzy set over the base set $\mathcal{A}$ consisting of the *ordered sequence* of all letters of $\mathcal{A}$ weighted in the unit interval $[0, 1]$. For example, the following three sequences are three different fuzzy letters over the ternary alphabet $\langle$A, C, T$\rangle$:

- $\langle$(A, 0.6), (C, 0.2), (T, 1)$\rangle$
- $\langle$(A, 1), (C, 0.8), (T, 0)$\rangle$
- $\langle$(A, 0), (C, 1), (T, 0)$\rangle$.

Obviously, a fuzzy letter is a letter that is represented by the entire alphabet with weighted presence of its own individual letters in the fuzzy letter. Note that the third fuzzy letter above entails C completely, while lacking both A and T. That is, it is just identical with the crisp leter C. Note, in addition, that any crisp letter L_i of an alphabet $\mathcal{A}$ has an infinite number of fuzzy counterparts because $\mathcal{A}$ can be mapped to $[0, 1]$ in infinitely many ways. For instance, here are additional three fuzzy letters over the same alphabet $\langle$A, C, T$\rangle$:

- $\langle$(A, 1), (C, 0), (T, 0)$\rangle$
- $\langle$(A, 0), (C, 1), (T, 0)$\rangle$
- $\langle$(A, 0), (C, 0), (T, 1)$\rangle$.

Using the latter fuzzified alphabet, the word "CAT" is representable as a fuzzy word, or fuzzy sequence, in the following way:

$$\text{CAT} = \langle (A, 0), (C, 1), (T, 0), (A, 1), (C, 0), (T, 0), (A, 0), (C, 0), (T, 1) \rangle.$$

In order to save space, we will write only the fuzzy vector of such a word omitting Cs, As, and Ts. By so doing, the words "ACT", "TAT", and "TACT" turn out to be the fuzzy sequences:

$$
\begin{aligned}
\text{ACT} \;\; &= (1, 0, 0, 0, 1, 0, 0, 0, 1) \\
\text{TAT} \;\; &= (0, 0, 1, 1, 0, 0, 0, 0, 1) \\
\text{TACT} &= (0, 0, 1, 1, 0, 0, 0, 1, 0, 0, 0, 1).
\end{aligned}
$$

Other, genuinely fuzzy words over the same alphabet $\langle$A, C, T$\rangle$ would be, for instance, the following two sequences. They have no equivalents in our natural languages, but may represent damaged words:

$(1, 0.7, 0.3, 0.9, 0, 0.2, 0.5, 1, 0.8, 1, 0.7, 0)$
$(0.2., 0.8., 1, 1, 0, 0, 0.6, 0, 1)$.

Like the example alphabet $\langle$A, C, T$\rangle$ above, every alphabet $\mathcal{A} = \langle L_1, \ldots, L_n \rangle$ can be fuzzified to yield fuzzy letters and fuzzy sequences over $\mathcal{A}$, e.g. the alphabets of natural or formal languages; Morse Code; the ten digits from 0 to 9; and many others. For instance, the Latin Alphabet $\langle$A, B, C, $\ldots$, Z$\rangle$ of the English language is fuzzifiable. Each emerging fuzzy letter has a 26-ary vector. English words and sentences can thus be written as fuzzy sequences. We know that each of such fuzzy sequences is a point in a corresponding fuzzy hypercube to the effect that the abstract geometry we have developed previously may be applied to natural language words and sentences; to the information communicated via Morse Code; to numbers, etc.

What is important to emphasize is that since any letter L_i of an alphabet $\mathcal{A} = \langle L_1, \ldots, L_n \rangle$ is fuzzifiable in infinitely different ways, the set of all fuzzy letters $\tilde{L}_i$ over $\mathcal{A}$, i.e., the fuzzy powerset $F(2^{L_i})$, is infinitie. The fuzzification of the entire alphabet $\mathcal{A} = \langle L_1, \ldots, L_n \rangle$ therefore yields a *fuzzy alphabet* of the following form: $\tilde{\mathcal{A}} = \langle F(2^{L_1}), \ldots, F(2^{L_n}) \rangle$.

Fuzzy biopolymers

It has already been pointed out earlier that a linear polymer is a linear macro-molecule consisting of a large number of identical or similar monomers as its building blocks. A *fuzzy linear polymer* is simply a linear polymer fuzzified using the methods described in the preceding sections.

Biopolymers are linear polymers produced and used by biological organisms. The most important biopolymers are RNA, DNA, proteins, and polysaccharides such as glycogen. After we have demonstrated in the preceding sections that RNA and DNA are fuzzy biopolymers, it will be briefly shown below that what is called a protein, is in fact a fuzzy protein, and thus a fuzzy biopolymer. (Polysaccharides will not be considered because they are homogeneously composed of sugar molecules and are, therefore, fuzzy-theoretically less interesting.)

A protein molecule consists of one or more polypeptide chains, *polypeptides* for short. A polypeptide is a linear chain of *amino acids* as its monomers. The alphabet of proteins, $\mathcal{AP}$, is thus the set of amino acids. It is a 20-ary alphabet consisting of the following letters:

$$\mathcal{AP} = \langle G, P, A, V, L, I, M, C, F, Y, W, H, K, R, S, T, N, Q, D, E \rangle.$$

The constants signify the following twenty amino acids: ⟨Glycine, Proline, Alanine, Valine, Leucine, Isoleucine, Methionine, Cysteine, Phenylalanine, Tyrosine, Tryptophan, Histidine, Lysine, Arginine, Serine, Threonine, Asparagine, Glutamine, Aspartic acid, Glutamic acid⟩. For instance, the word "GIVEQ" over $\mathcal{AP}$ is a short initial segment of the A strand of the polypeptide *insulin*, i.e., the segment Glycine-Isoleucine-Valine-GlutamicAcid-Glutamine.

In the light of the methods we have constructed in the preceding sections, it is obviously not difficult to fuzzify the alphabet $\mathcal{AP}$ above. By so doing, a polypeptide becomes representable as a fuzzy polypeptide. Like fuzzy polynucleotides, fuzzy polypeptides are points of unit hypercubes and may thus be subjected to the abstract geometry of fuzzy biopolymers that we have demonstrated in the preceding sections regarding fuzzy polynucleotides.

16.5.5 Fuzzy Deontics

In Part IV we concerned ourselves with two-valued, crisp deontics only and considered a deontic rule an all-or-nothing norm. So conceived, a deontic rule categorically declares an action either as obligatory or not obligatory, forbidden or not forbidden, permitted or not permitted. Based on what we have seen so far regarding classical logics, we have good reason to question the adequacy of a deontic logic built upon this traditional dichotomy and bivalence. We shall address that question in the following two sections:

▶ Quantitative and comparative deonticity
▶ Qualitative deonticity.

In so doing, we will extend our conception of deontics to a gradualistic, fuzzy deontics that considerably increases the practical relevance of our previous deontic-medical analyses.

Quantitative and comparative deonticity

To motivate our task, consider the following case report. The question was posed in a recent medical-ethical publication whether truth is a supreme value (Peleg, 2008, 325). It had been prompted by the conduct of a doctor, who at the request of a Muslim patient, had attested that she was not pregnant, even though she was. The physician's aim at hiding and reversing the truth had been to prevent the divorced, pregnant woman from being killed by her relatives to maintain "the honor of the family". The doctor's preference for saving the patient's life over telling the truth had later been supported by a medical ethicist who had confirmed that "truth is not the supreme value. [...] the potential saving of life is more important and takes precedence to the truth" (ibid., 325). The author of the article, however, had moral problems with this assessment.

According to our concept of a deontic rule or deontic norm introduced in Definition 153 on page 564, both telling the truth and saving life are required by the deontic norms of common morality and medical ethics:

1. For everybody x, it is obligatory that x tells the truth,   (167)
2. For everybody x, if x is a doctor, it is obligatory that x saves the life of her patients.

The quotation above demonstrates that there are situations in medicine where a deontic norm such as the second one in (167) is given precedence over another deontic norm like the first one. Analogous examples are clinical settings where a diagnostic or therapeutic action A is to be preferred to another one, B, although both actions are declared as obligatory: "You ought to do A and you ought to do B". Observations of this type give rise to the question of how the legitimacy of norm precedence and preference may be conceptualized. We shall suggest a comparative notion of obligation, "it is more obligatory to do A than to do B", which we shall base upon a fuzzy concept of obligation. By fuzzifying the concept of obligation, we shall pave the way for fuzzy deontics, in which norms may be ranked according to the degree of obligatoriness of what they prescribe. The approach may be instrumental in medical decision-making, medical ethics, and other disciplines.

Our first step is to introduce the notion of a *fuzzy deontic set* by generalizing the notion of a deontic set, introduced in Definition 155 on page 571. To this end, recall that a deontic sentence of the form (167) above, e.g., "one ought to tell the truth", is representable in the following way:

$$\forall x \big(OB(x \in A) \big) \tag{168}$$

where $A = \{y \mid y \text{ tells the truth}\}$ is the set of those people who tell the truth. Note that the sentence (168) above may be rewritten as $\forall x((OB\in)(x, A))$ where the amalgamated binary predicate "$(OB\in)$" reads "ought to belong to". We will conceive this predicate as a compound deontic predicate and will introduce below its characteristic function that will be symbolized by $\omega(x, A)$ to read "the extent to which x ought to belong to set A". (For the term "characteristic function of a set", see page 998.)

Let us abbreviate the binary function symbol ω in $\omega(x, A)$, a lower case omega, to the pseudo-unary function symbol ω_A with the following syntax:

$$\omega_A(x) = r \quad \text{i.e., "the extent to which } x \text{ ought to belong to set } A \text{ is } r\text{".}$$

In other words: "The degree of deontic membership of x in set A is r", or "the obligatory A-membership degree of x is r". On the basis of our terminology, we can define this crisp deontic membership function ω_A as follows:

Definition 166 (Deontic membership function). $\omega_A(x) = \begin{cases} 1 & \textit{iff } OB(x \in A) \\ 0 & \textit{otherwise.} \end{cases}$

Consider, for example, the following deontic norms from page 571:

You ought to keep your promises,
you ought not to lie,
you ought to be helpful,
you ought not to commit murder,

and these sets, which were used in the same context:

$P \equiv$ the set of those people who keep their promises,
$L \equiv$ the set of liars,
$H \equiv$ the set of helpful people,
$M \equiv$ the set of murderers.

Then the four deontic norms above may be rewritten as follows:

$$\omega_P(x) = 1 \qquad \text{i.e.,} \qquad \text{to the extent 1, } x \text{ ought to keep her promises,}$$
$$\omega_L(x) = 0 \qquad \qquad \qquad \text{to the extent 0, } x \text{ ought to lie,}$$
$$\omega_H(x) = 1 \qquad \qquad \qquad \text{to the extent 1, } x \text{ ought to be helpful,}$$
$$\omega_M(x) = 0 \qquad \qquad \qquad \text{to the extent 0, } x \text{ ought to commit murder.}$$

For instance, like everybody else Mr. Elroy Fox ought to keep his promises, i.e., $\omega_P(\text{Elroy Fox}) = 1$. But he ought not to lie, and thus, $\omega_L(\text{Elroy Fox}) = 0$. In all of our examples so far, the deontic membership function ω has taken values in the bivalent set $\{0, 1\}$. It is a bivalent function and partitions by the following mapping:

$$\omega \colon \Omega \mapsto \{0, 1\}$$

the base set Ω of human beings into pairs of crisp deontic subsets, e.g., L and $\overline{L}$, liars and non-liars. A deontic set of this type with its all-or-nothing characteristic either includes an individual totally or excludes her totally. Someone is either a liar or a non-liar; a Samaritan or none; a murderer or none; and so on. There is no gradualness in deontic behavior, i.e., no degrees of deonticity. In the real world of medicine, however, we often have difficulties in determining whether someone does or does not definitely belong to a particular deontic class such as, for example, the class of those who tell the truth. Like a vague, non-deontic class such as that of diabetics or schizophrenics, the class of honest people, the class of murderers, and other deontic classes are also vague and lack sharp boundaries. It is to our advantage, then, to fuzzify the notion of a deontic set, which we may do by fuzzifying the deontic membership function. We thereby obtain the notion of a *fuzzy deontic set* in two steps as follows:

Definition 167 (Fuzzy deontic subset). *If Ω is the set of human beings or a particular community, then A is a fuzzy ε-deontic subset in Ω iff there is a deontic membership function ω_A such that:*

1. $\omega_A \colon \Omega \mapsto \{0, 1\}$,
2. $A = \{(x, \omega_A(x)) \mid x \in \Omega\}$,
3. $\varepsilon \in [0, 1]$,
4. $\omega_A(x) \geq \varepsilon \qquad$ for all $x \in \Omega$.

For instance, in a family consisting of the members {Amy, Beth, Carla, Dirk} the following set is a fuzzy 0.8-deontic subset: HONEST = {(Amy, 0.8), (Beth, 0.8), (Carla, 0.8), (Dirk, 0.8)}. We have, for example, $\omega_{\text{HONEST}}(\text{Beth}) = 0.8$. At least to the extent 0.8, Beth ought to tell the truth. Note that all members have the same minimum degree of ε-deontic membership in the set (clause 3).

Definition 168 (Fuzzy deontic set). *A is a fuzzy deontic set iff there is a base set Ω and an $\varepsilon \in [0, 1]$ such that A is a fuzzy ε-deontic subset of Ω according to Definition 167.*

Using fuzzy-deontic sentences on the basis of fuzzy-deontic sets, it becomes possible to compare the deontic strength of different norms, for example, of telling the truth and saving the life of a patient. Let T be the set of those people who tell the truth, and let S be the set of those who save other people's lives. Then the following sentence says that for Dr. You, it is more obligatory to save other people's lives than to tell the truth:

$$\omega_S(Dr.\ You) > \omega_T(Dr.\ You). \tag{169}$$

No doubt, this lowbrow example is not acceptable at first glance and per se. It only serves to show the way comparative deontic norms may be formulated. Surprisingly, however, the unconditional comparative norm (169) appears to be a meaningful constituent part of a *comparative conditional norm*. Consider, for instance, this comparative conditional norm: If the life of a patient is endangered, as was the case with the Muslim woman at the beginning of this section, then it is more obligatory that her doctor saves her life than tells the truth. That is:

The life of the patient is endangered $\rightarrow \omega_S(Dr.\ You) > \omega_T(Dr.\ You)$.

To keep it readable, we avoided completely formalizing this example. Nevertheless, it demonstrates how the moral dilemma that was quoted at the beginning of the present section, may be resolved by fuzzy deontics. Our considerations provide the nucleus of an approach to fuzzy deontics both in ethics and clinical methodology, including novel areas such as fuzzy ethics, fuzzy bioethics, fuzzy medical ethics, and other fuzzy domain ethics (Sadegh-Zadeh, 2002).

To assess the usefulness of fuzzy deontics in clinical methodology, recall the concept of differential indication introduced in Section 8.2.4 on page 310. There we distinguished between well-ordered indication structures and well-ordered differential indication structures. Both structures, introduced in Definitions 99–100, are based on a comparative relation $\succ$ of performance order for actions. Such ordering determines the temporal sequence in which clinical actions are to be performed in diagnostic-thereapeutic decision-making and patient management. The concept of graded obligation above enables such a comparative relation $\succ$. It also enables a method by which to interpret and reconstruct situations concerning the superiority of one legally protected interest over another by introducing a rank order of norms that are relevant in a given circumstance.

Qualitative deonticity

As we observed on several occasions, the notion of *circumstance,* situation, or condition plays a central role in clinical decision-making in that the making of a particular clinical decision depends on a given circumstance, e.g., the patient's specific disease state. Accordingly, we reconstructed deontic rules as deontic conditionals, for example, (i) if the patient has disease X, then you ought to do Y; or (ii) if the life of the patient is endangered, then saving her life is more obligatory than telling the truth. The *if*-component of such a rule indicates the circumstance under which its consequent is obligatory, forbidden, or permitted. We know, however, that circumstances are vague states of affairs and admit of degrees to the effect that there is a gradualness between their presence and absence. For instance, the pneumonia of a patient may be mild, moderate, or severe. The lower the degree of existence of such a state of affairs X, the higher that of its complement *not-X*, and vice versa. X and not-X co-exist to particular extents, as we saw in previous chapters. This brings with it that if under the circumstance X an action Y is obligatory (forbidden, or permitted) to a particular extent r, then it is not obligatory (not forbidden, not permitted) to the extent $1 - r$, respectively. Thus, an action may be obligatory (forbidden, or permitted) and not obligatory (not forbidden, not permitted) at the same time, respectively. We will capture this deontic peculiarity in the following way.

A concept of qualitative deonticity will be briefly outlined with hopes of stimulating further discussion and research on this subject. Our sketch will be limited to a qualitative concept of obligatoriness only. The other two deontic modalities may be treated analogously. To achieve our goal, we will first introduce the notion of a *fuzzy deontic rule*.

Definition 169 (Fuzzy deontic rule). *A deontic rule, as defined in Definition 153 on page 564, is said to be a fuzzy deontic rule iff it is a fuzzy conditional. (For the notion of a fuzzy conditional, see page 1037.)*

To illustrate, let OBL be a linguistic variable that ranges over actions, and let Y be an action. The sentence:

$$OBL(Y) = B$$

reads "the obligatoriness of Y is B", or "Y is obligatory to the extent B". For example, "the obligatoriness of antibiotic treatment is weak", or "antibiotic treatment is weakly obligatory". The term set of the linguistic variable OBL may be conceived as something like:

$$T(OBL) = \{\text{very weak, weak, moderate, strong, very strong, extremely strong}\}.$$

Let X be a linguistic variable that ranges over circumstances and takes values auch as A, A_1, A_2, etc. For example, X may be a patient's disease state *bacterial pneumonia* that takes values such as *mild, moderate,* and *severe:*

$$T(\text{bacterial pneumonia}) = \{\text{mild, moderate, severe}\},$$

e.g., 'Mr. Elroy Fox's bacterial pneumonia is mild'. That is, Mr. Elroy Fox has mild bacterial pneumonia. And let Y be an action as above. A fuzzy conditional of the following form is obviously a fuzzy deontic rule:

If X is A, then $OBL(Y) = B$

where $A \in T(X)$ and $B \in T(OBL)$. Some examples are:

   a. If the patient has mild bacterial pneumonia, then antibiotic therapy is moderately obligatory,

   b. If the patient has moderate bacterial pneumonia, then antibiotic therapy is strongly obligatory,

   c. If the patient has severe bacterial pneumonia, then antibiotic therapy is very strongly obligatory.

We have thus three related fuzzy deontic rules that regulate the treatment of bacterial pneumonia. A closer look reveals that they constitute a small algorithm that in terms of the theory of fuzzy control, discussed in Section 16.5.1, enable the deontic control of the variable *bacterial pneumonia*. The general structure of such fuzzy deontic algorithms may be represented as follows (see also page 611):

$$X_{1_1} \text{ is } A_{1_1} \text{ and } \ldots \text{ and } X_{1_k} \text{ is } A_{1_k} \to$$
$$OBL(Y_{1_1}) \text{ is } B_{1_1} \text{ and } \ldots \text{ and } OBL(Y_{1_p}) \text{ is } B_{1_p}$$

$$\vdots$$

$$X_{m_1} \text{ is } A_{m_1} \text{ and } \ldots \text{ and } X_{m_n} \text{ is } A_{m_n} \to$$
$$OBL(Y_{m_1}) \text{ is } B_{m_1} \text{ and } \ldots \text{ and } OBL(Y_{m_q}) \text{ is } B_{m_q}$$

with $k, m, n, p, q \geq 1$. Considering the concept of *indication*, introduced in Definition 96 on page 313, we may observe that our present analyses extend that concept to yield a concept of *fuzzy indication*. By means of this amended terminology, it is possible to introduce fuzzy indication and fuzzy differential indication structures that would parallel their crisp counterparts discussed previously. Clinical indication thereby becomes subject to fuzzy deontics.

16.5.6 Fuzzy Concept Formation in Medicine

Real-world categories do not have sharp boundaries like the crisp sets in mathematics such as the set of even numbers. Neither mountains and hills nor trees and bushes are separated from one another by a sharp dividing line. Also light and dark, day and night, alive and dead, wet and dry, healthy and not healthy are continuous categories characterized by the smoothness of transition between them. Fuzzy logic enables us to do justice to this ubiquitous feature of real-world objects, classes, and relations by reconstructing them as fuzzy sets. Medicine has not largely taken advantage of this fact. Surprisingly, most categories in medicine are still conceived as crisp, discontinuous entities. As an example, consider the disease *hypertension*, i.e., high blood pressure. It is customarily assumed that an individual either has or does not have hypertension. A third option does not exist. Accordingly, hypertension in adults is currently defined in medicine, based on WHO recommendations, as shown in Table 23.

Table 23. The WHO-based, current definition of hypertension

Blood pressure quality	Systolic pressure		Diastolic pressure
optimal	120 mm Hg		80 mm Hg
normal	< 130		< 85
high normal (prehypertension)	130–139		85–89
mild hypertension	140–159	and/or	90–99
moderate hypertension	160–179	and/or	100–109
severe hypertension	180 or higher	and/or	110 or higher

This multiple definition partitions the blood pressure scale into six crisp sectors and offers a conspicuously problematic concept. Three drawbacks strike one immediately. *First,* there are gaps between the last three sectors both in the systolic as well as diastolic pressure. *Second,* the partition of the blood pressure scale into the six crisp sectors above is inadequate. It is unintelligible why an individual with a blood pressure of 160/100 mm Hg is to be categorized as having moderate hypertension, while another individual whose blood pressure is only 1 degree less than that is said to have a mild hypertension. *Third,* the WHO-based concept of hypertension is ambiguous in that, for example, to an individual with a systolic blood pressure of 185 and a diastolic blood pressure of 95 mm Hg we must simultaneously attribute severe hypertension and mild hypertension (Figure 79).

In addition to these three disadvantages, crisp concepts in medicine are impractical because most cases involve vagueness such that one cannot justifiably decide whether a particular case is or is not an instance of the concept. We may avoid these disadvantages using the methods of fuzzy concept formation that we have frequently applied in preceding chapters. Examples that were graphically represented as well are the concepts of health and illness in Figures 31–32 (p. 190); blood sugar level in Figure 67 (p. 613); body temperature in Figure 70 (p. 630); blood cholesterol level in Figure 73 (p. 632); heart rate in Figure 111 (p. 1029); and others. In the same fashion, we shall try to present as an example in detail a fuzzy concept of normal and high blood pressure in the following two sections:

▶ Fuzzy blood pressure
▶ Fuzzy hypertension.

Fuzzy blood pressure

We should be aware at the outset that what is traditionally called *blood pressure* is a two-dimensional vector (x, y) such as "(185, 95) mm Hg" with x being its systolic and y being its diastolic dimension. For this reason, a many-dimensional concept of hypertension that considers the quality of both dimensions, x and y, is more adequate than the common, one-dimensional one

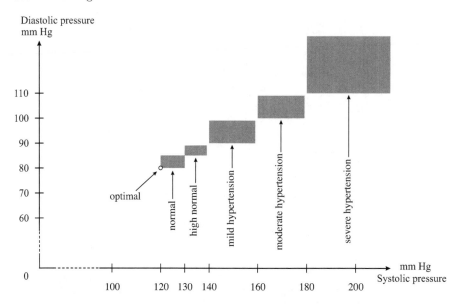

Fig. 79. Two-dimensional representation of the AND-part of the current concept of hypertension in adults shown in Table 23. The blood pressure "optimal" is only a dot. The entire partitioning of the blood pressure scale provides a crisp, step function. (A step function is a piecewise constant, discontinuous function having only finitely many pieces.) If the tuple (x, y) is the vector of a hypertensive individual's blood pressure with x being the systolic and y the diastolic component, then her blood pressure is a point in a corresponding grey area in the graph. The salient shortcomings of this concept are the three gaps mentioned in the body text, i.e., between high normal and mild hypertension, mild hypertension and moderate hypertension, and moderate hypertension and severe hypertension. For example, a patient with a systolic blood pressure of 159.5 and a diastolic pressure of 99.5 falls in the second gap. Does she have high blood pressure or not?

if it represents in its first dimension the quality of the systolic and in its second dimension the quality of the diastolic blood pressure. For example, an individual may have:

(moderate systolic hypertension, normal diastolic blood pressure)

or:

(severe systolic hypertension, mild diastolic hypertension)

or:

(moderate systolic hypertension, moderate diastolic hypertension)

and so on. We shall first introduce a many-dimensional concept of hypertension that yields such diagnoses, and then simplify it to a one-dimensional concept of hypertension in a second step. To this end, we introduce the following two numerical variables:

1. *systolic_blood_pressure* that quantitatively measures, in mm Hg, the systolic blood pressure,
2. *diastolic_blood_pressure* that quantitatively measures, in mm Hg, the diastolic blood pressure;

and the following two linguistic variables:

a. *Systolic_Blood_Pressure* with the linguistic term set {very low, low, optimal, normal, high normal, mild hypertension, moderate hypertension, severe hypertension} that operates on the first numerical variable, *systolic_blood_pressure*, transforming sets of its values into fuzzy granules such as *very low, low*, etc.,
b. *Diastolic_Blood_Pressure* with the same term set {very low, low, optimal, normal, high normal, mild hypertension, moderate hypertension, severe hypertension} that operates on the second numerical variable, *diastolic_blood_pressure*, transforming sets of its values into fuzzy granules such as *very low, low*, etc.

To simplify our analyses, we shall concentrate on those values of blood pressure which are relevant to the concept of *hyper*tension and will therefore not consider the granules *very low* and *low*. Thus, the linguistic term set that we shall use for the granules of both dimensions of blood pressure will consist of only six terms:

- T(Systolic_Blood_Pressure) = T(Diastolic_Blood_Pressure) = {optimal, normal, high normal, mild hypertension, moderate hypertension, severe hypertension}.

The six terms in the term set T(Systolic_Blood_Pressure) denote six fuzzy sets over the quantitative values of the numerical variable *systolic_blood_pressure* as our universe of discourse, $\Omega_{systolic} = [0, 300]$ mm Hg. And the six terms in the term set T(Diastolic_Blood_Pressure) denote six fuzzy sets over the quantitative values of the numerical variable *diastolic_blood_pressure* as our universe of discourse, $\Omega_{diastolic} = [0, 300]$ mm Hg. Their membership functions may be symbolized as follows:

systolic:

$\mu_{systolic\text{-}optimal}$
$\mu_{systolic\text{-}normal}$
$\mu_{systolic\text{-}high\text{-}normal}$
$\mu_{systolic\text{-}mild\text{-}hypertension}$
$\mu_{systolic\text{-}moderate\text{-}hypertension}$
$\mu_{systolic\text{-}severe\text{-}hypertension}$

diastolic:

$\mu_{diastolic\text{-}optimal}$
$\mu_{diastolic\text{-}normal}$
$\mu_{diastolic\text{-}high\text{-}normal}$
$\mu_{diastolic\text{-}mild\text{-}hypertension}$
$\mu_{diastolic\text{-}moderate\text{-}hypertension}$
$\mu_{diastolic\text{-}severe\text{-}hypertension}$

By defining these membership functions, we delineate the granules in $\Omega_{systolic}$ and $\Omega_{diastolic}$, i.e., blood pressure qualities such as "moderate systolic hypertension", "optimal diastolic pressure", etc. Definition 170 shows in its twelve parts a technique that is more transparent and applicable than the WHO-based procedure shown in Table 23 on page 665. The fuzzy granules emerging in this way are graphically represented in Figures 80–81 on page 670.

Definition 170 (Systolic and diastolic blood pressure).

A. Systolic:

1. $\mu_{systolic\text{-}optimal}(x) = \begin{cases} 0 & \text{if } x \leq 110 \text{ or } x > 120 \\ \frac{1}{5}(x - 110) & \text{if } 110 < x \leq 115 \\ -\frac{1}{5}(x - 120) & \text{if } 115 < x \leq 120 \end{cases}$

2. $\mu_{systolic\text{-}normal}(x) = \begin{cases} 0 & \text{if } x \leq 115 \text{ or } x > 125 \\ \frac{1}{5}(x - 115) & \text{if } 115 < x \leq 120 \\ -\frac{1}{5}(x - 125) & \text{if } 120 < x \leq 125 \end{cases}$

3. $\mu_{systolic\text{-}high\text{-}normal}(x) = \begin{cases} 0 & \text{if } x \leq 120 \text{ or } x > 140 \\ \frac{1}{5}(x - 120) & \text{if } 120 < x \leq 125 \\ -\frac{1}{5}(x - 140) & \text{if } 135 < x \leq 140 \\ 1 & \text{if } 125 < x \leq 135 \end{cases}$

4. $\mu_{systolic\text{-}mild\text{-}hypertension}(x) = \begin{cases} 0 & \text{if } x \leq 135 \text{ or } x > 160 \\ \frac{1}{5}(x - 135) & \text{if } 135 < x \leq 140 \\ -\frac{1}{5}(x - 160) & \text{if } 155 < x \leq 160 \\ 1 & \text{if } 140 < x \leq 155 \end{cases}$

5. $\mu_{systolic\text{-}moderate\text{-}hypertension}(x) = \begin{cases} 0 & \text{if } x \leq 155 \text{ or } x > 180 \\ \frac{1}{5}(x - 155) & \text{if } 155 < x \leq 160 \\ -\frac{1}{5}(x - 180) & \text{if } 175 < x \leq 180 \\ 1 & \text{if } 160 < x \leq 175 \end{cases}$

6. $\mu_{systolic\text{-}severe\text{-}hypertension}(x) = \begin{cases} 0 & \text{if } x \leq 175 \\ \frac{1}{5}(x - 175) & \text{if } 175 < x < 180 \\ 1 & \text{if } x \geq 180 \end{cases}$

B. Diastolic:

7. $\mu_{diastolic\text{-}optimal}(x) = \begin{cases} 0 & \text{if } x \leq 70 \text{ or } x > 80 \\ \frac{1}{5}(x - 70) & \text{if } 70 < x \leq 75 \\ -\frac{1}{5}(x - 80) & \text{if } 75 < x \leq 80 \end{cases}$

8. $\mu_{diastolic\text{-}normal}(x) = \begin{cases} 0 & \text{if } x \leq 75 \text{ or } x > 85 \\ \frac{1}{5}(x - 75) & \text{if } 75 < x \leq 80 \\ -\frac{1}{5}(x - 85) & \text{if } 80 < x \leq 85 \end{cases}$

9. $\mu_{diastolic\text{-}high\text{-}normal}(x) = \begin{cases} 0 & \text{if } x \leq 80 \text{ or } x > 90 \\ \frac{1}{5}(x - 80) & \text{if } 80 < x \leq 85 \\ -\frac{1}{5}(x - 90) & \text{if } 85 < x \leq 90 \end{cases}$

10. $\mu_{diastolic\text{-}mild\text{-}hypertension}(x) = \begin{cases} 0 & \text{if } x \leq 85 \text{ or } x > 100 \\ \frac{1}{5}(x - 85) & \text{if } 85 < x \leq 90 \\ -\frac{1}{5}(x - 100) & \text{if } 95 < x \leq 100 \\ 1 & \text{if } 90 < x \leq 95 \end{cases}$

11. $\mu_{diastolic\text{-}moderate\text{-}hypertension}(x) = \begin{cases} 0 & \text{if } x \leq 95 \text{ or } x > 110 \\ \frac{1}{5}(x - 95) & \text{if } 95 < x \leq 100 \\ -\frac{1}{5}(x - 110) & \text{if } 105 < x \leq 110 \\ 1 & \text{if } 100 < x \leq 105 \end{cases}$

12. $\mu_{diastolic\text{-}severe\text{-}hypertension}(x) = \begin{cases} 0 & \text{if } x \leq 105 \\ \frac{1}{5}(x - 105) & \text{if } 105 < x < 110 \\ 1 & \text{if } x \geq 110 \end{cases}$

Figures 80–81 demonstrate that according to these definitions a systolic blood pressure of 158 mm Hg is a moderate systolic hypertension to the extent 0.6, and a diastolic blood pressure of 96 is optimal to the extent 0. Note that the adjacent diastolic as well as systolic intervals overlap. They may therefore at first glance not seem to provide reasonable partitions of the base, numerical variables. But this false impression is due to our tendency toward bivalence. It disappears by considering the fact that the linguistic values {optimal, normal, high normal, mild hypertension, moderate hypertension, severe hypertension} defined above engender granulations of blood pressure, and thus a hexatomous *fuzzy partition* of the universe of discourse (see fuzzy taxonomy on page 64).

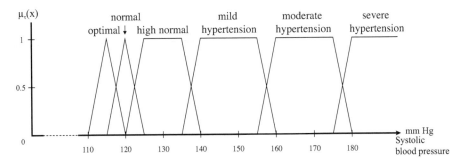

Fig. 80. The numerical variable *systolic_blood_pressure* serves as the base variable. It takes values in the universe of discourse [0, 300] mm Hg. The linguistic variable *Systolic_Blood_Pressure* acts on the values of this base variable, i.e., systolic blood pressure readings. The triangular and trapezoidal linguistic values {optimal, normal, high normal, mild hypertension, moderate hypertension, severe hypertension} granulate the values of the base variable producing fuzzy sets of people who to different extents have optimal systolic blood pressure, normal systolic blood pressure, high normal systolic blood pressure, mild systolic hypertension, moderate systolic hypertension, or severe systolic hypertension, respectively

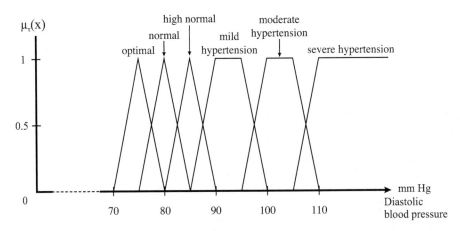

Fig. 81. The numerical variable *diastolic_blood_pressure* serves as the base variable. It takes values in the universe of discourse [0, 300] mm Hg. The linguistic variable *Diastolic_Blood_Pressure* acts on the values of this base variable, i.e., diastolic blood pressure readings. The triangular and trapezoidal linguistic values {optimal, normal, high normal, mild hypertension, moderate hypertension, severe hypertension} granulate the values of the numerical variable producing fuzzy sets of people who to different extents have optimal diastolic blood pressure, normal diastolic blood pressure, high normal diastolic blood pressure, mild diastolic hypertension, moderate diastolic hypertension, or severe diastolic hypertension, respectively

In closing this section, the structure of the concepts introduced thus far will be made explicitly clear. What we have suggested are two linguistic variables of the following form according to Definition 253 on page 1023:

$$\langle v, T(v), \Omega, M \rangle.$$

This may be exemplified by the structure of the variable *Systolic_Blood_Pressure:*

⟨ Systolic_Blood_Pressure, {optimal, normal, high normal, mild hypertension, moderate hypertension, severe hypertension}, RR, Definition 170⟩,

such that:

1. v is the name of the variable, i.e., "Systolic_Blood_Pressure" in the present example;
2. $T(v)$ is its term set;
3. Ω is the universe of discourse, i.e., the open, Riva-Rocci set of blood pressures RR = {0, 1, 2, ..., 200, 250, ...}, here replaced with the definite, real interval [0, 300] mm Hg, upon which the terms of the term set $T(v)$ are interpreted as fuzzy sets;
4. M is a method that associates with each linguistic value $\tau_i \in T(v)$ its meaning, i.e., a fuzzy set over the universe Ω denoted by τ_i. In the present example, method M is our Definition 170 on page 668. See also the visualization of the definition in Figures 80–81 above.

These well-structured linguistic variables and the 12 concepts based thereon enable a three-dimensional representation of the considered range of blood pressure, optimal through severe hypertension, as a landscape (Figure 82).

Fuzzy hypertension

Based on our considerations above, we may introduce concepts of fuzzy hypertension in different ways. The most adequate one of them will be sketched in what follows. To this end, suppose an individual a's blood pressure is represented as an ordered pair of the form ⟨*systolic_blood_pressure of a, diastolic_blood_pressure of a*⟩. For example, the blood pressure of the patient Elroy Fox may be written:

$$\langle 158, 96 \rangle \text{ mm Hg.} \tag{170}$$

Now, each of these two dimensions of blood pressure has a particular quality, e.g., "optimal", "severe hypertension", etc. We gave a fuzzy taxonomy of these qualities above to the effect that some numerical blood pressure values fall in two overlapping granules or taxa. For instance, a systolic blood pressure of 158 mm Hg is a moderate systolic hypertension of degree 0.6 and a mild systolic

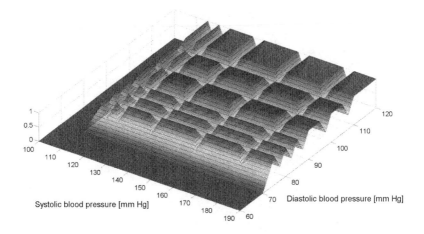

Fig. 82. A 3D representation of blood pressure based on the fuzzy concept of hypertension sketched above

hypertension to the extent 0.4 at the same time. See Figure 80 on page 670. It is therefore advantageous to *fuzzify* crisp blood pressure values in terms of fuzzy control, discussed on page 613. With respect to the six granules of each blood pressure dimension, one would obtain six distinct membership degrees. For example, the patient Elroy Fox's blood pressure presented in (170) above has the following qualities:

$$\mu_{systolic\text{-}optimal}(158) = 0 \qquad \mu_{diastolic\text{-}optimal}(96) = 0$$
$$\mu_{systolic\text{-}normal}(158) = 0 \qquad \mu_{diastolic\text{-}normal}(96) = 0$$
$$\mu_{systolic\text{-}high\text{-}normal}(158) = 0 \qquad \mu_{diastolic\text{-}high\text{-}normal}(96) = 0$$
$$\mu_{systolic\text{-}mild\text{-}hypertension}(158) = 0.4 \qquad \mu_{diastolic\text{-}mild\text{-}hypertension}(96) = 0.8$$
$$\mu_{systolic\text{-}moderate\text{-}hypertension}(158) = 0.6 \qquad \mu_{diastolic\text{-}moderate\text{-}hypertension}(96) = 0.2$$
$$\mu_{systolic\text{-}severe\text{-}hypertension}(158) = 0 \qquad \mu_{diastolic\text{-}severe\text{-}hypertension}(96) = 0.$$

Thus, the blood pressure of a patient is representable by two 6-dimensional *fuzzification vectors*, a systolic and a diastolic one. In the present example, we have:

systolic fuzzification vector $= (0, 0, 0, 0.4, 0.6, 0)$
diastolic fuzzification vector $= (0, 0, 0, 0.8, 0.2, 0)$.

For the term "fuzzification vector", see page 614. To facilitate communication about the blood pressure of individuals, one could proceed as follows: Take the maximum component of each of the two fuzzification vectors above to compose a two-dimensional blood pressure diagnosis, $\langle x, y \rangle$, of the following type:

$\langle$moderate systolic hypertension 0.6, mild diastolic hypertension 0.8$\rangle$

That means that regarding Elroy Fox, say patient a, we have:

$$\langle \mu_{systolic\text{-}moderate\text{-}hypertension}(a) = 0.6,\ \mu_{diastolic\text{-}mild\text{-}hypertension}(a) = 0.8 \rangle$$

Elroy Fox has moderate systolic hypertension to the extent 0.6, and mild diastolic hypertension to the extent 0.8. If the values in two adjacent granules are equally strong, take the graver one. For example, if the above vectors were of the form:

systolic fuzzification vector $= (0, 0, 0, 0.4, 0.6, 0)$
diastolic fuzzification vector $= (0, 0, 0, 0.5, 0.5, 0)$,

then the patient Elroy Fox would be diagnosed as having moderate systolic hypertension to the extent 0.6, and moderate diastolic hypertension to the extent 0.5. That is, his two-dimensional blood pressure diagnosis would be ⟨*moderate systolic hypertension to the extent 0.6, moderate diastolic hypertension to the extent 0.5*⟩.

It is worth noting that the fuzzy concept of hypertension introduced above allows more appropriate treatment of patients because the dosage of the anti-hypertensive therapeutica to be administered may now be precisely adjusted to the degree of their disorder like a fuzzy insulin pump does in diabetics. That is, hypertension also becomes a domain of fuzzy control in medicine that was discussed on pages 605–615.

16.6 Summary

We examined the following logics for application in medicine: classical logic, paraconsistent logic, alethic and deontic modal logics, probability logic, and fuzzy logic. The examples given demonstrate that the language of medicine has many syntactic and semantic particularities the most salient ones being that (i) as an extended natural language it has a variety of modal operators and is thus a multimodal language, and (ii) is highly vague. Each of its peculiarities requires a suitable logic capable of handling the specific problems associated with that particularity. In consequence medicine needs a variety of logics, as an all-embracing multilogic suitable for logical problems of any kind in medicine does not yet exist. So, just as any scientific domain is amenable to a variety of mathematical theories – from algebra to non-Euclidean geometries to stochastics to chaos theory –, medicine will remain a domain of application of many different types of logics. This is what we call *logical pluralism* in medicine. Simply put, there exists no 'one true logic'. However, because vagueness is ubiquitous in medicine, fuzzy logic is a promising candidate for wide-ranging use. A logic is applied in medicine whenever it is capable of assisting in practical problem-solving. It has only instrumental value. Fuzzy logic seems to have the highest instrumental value in medicine because it is both an inconsistency-tolerant method of reasoning and a powerful, versatile methodology.

The Logic of Medicine

17.0 Introduction

In discussions about reasoning in medical research and practice, we often encounter the label "the logic of medicine". There are those who believe that medicine has indeed a logic of its own like, for example, quantum mechanics supposedly rests upon a so-called 'quantum logic' in which the Distributive Laws of classical logic, listed in Table 37 on page 898, are not valid (Birkhoff and von Neumann 1936; Dalla Chiara and Giuntini, 2002). Several special treatises have also been published under the metaphoric title "the logic of medicine" (Blane, 1819; Bieganski, 1909; Oesterlen, 1852; Murphy, 1997). They use the word "logic" not in the strict sense of this term, but with a loose meaning related with the analysis of medical concepts, ideas, hypotheses, theories, methods, and decisions. They do not reveal whether medicine has its own specific, 'medical logic'. To determine whether there is such a logic of medicine or not, we shall first clarify what is meant by the term "logic". We shall then introduce some auxiliary notions to aid us in answering our question. The discussion divides into the following three sections:

    17.1 What is Logic?
    17.2 Implication Structures
    17.3 On the Logic of Medicine.

17.1 What is Logic?

Logic is usually defined as the science of reasoning, argumentation, and proving. As has been pointed out in Part VIII, however, today logic has become a science of formal languages. Only a minor part of this multifarious endeavor can be identified with the "good old science of reasoning". In this formal languages approach, inquiries into reasoning produce a variety of individual logic systems, the so-called *logics,* a few of which are outlined in Part VIII. The

K. Sadegh-Zadeh, *Handbook of Analytic Philosophy of Medicine,*
Philosophy and Medicine 113, DOI 10.1007/978-94-007-2260-6_17,
© Springer Science+Business Media B.V. 2012

only common feature of these different logics is that each one of them has a concept of inference, $\vdash$. A concept of inference in a logic L regulates whether a set of premises, A, implies a particular conclusion, α. It is therefore referred to as the inference relation, the consequence relation, or the implication relation of that logic L, denoted $\vdash_L$. Distinct logics have distinct implication relations. We distinguish between *crisp logics* such as all bivalent traditional logics of classical and non-classical type as well as traditional many-valued logics, on the one hand; and *fuzzy logic*, on the other.

By defining its characteristic function, the implication relation $\vdash_L$ of a crisp logic L may be transformed into a bivalent *implication operator*, $\Rightarrow_L$, in the following way. If A is a set of sentences and α is a single sentence, then:

$$\Rightarrow_L(A, \alpha) = \begin{cases} 1 & \text{iff } A \vdash_L \alpha \\ \\ 0 & \text{iff } A \nvdash_L \alpha, \text{ i.e., not } A \vdash_L \alpha. \end{cases} \tag{171}$$

What a logic is, may now be easily defined. A pair of the form $L = \langle S, \Rightarrow_L \rangle$ is a *crisp logic* if and only if there is a language such that S is the set of its sentences and $\Rightarrow_L$ is an implication operator over S. On this account, a crisp logic is a bivalent mapping of the form:

$$\Rightarrow_L: 2^S \times S \mapsto \{0, 1\}$$

with 2^S being the ordinary powerset of S. As defined in (171), the operator $\Rightarrow_L$ assigns to a pair (A, α) the number 1 or 0 depending on whether A does or does not imply α. Note that A is an element of the powerset 2^S, i.e., a *set of sentences*, while α is a single element of S. For example, if PL_1 is the classical predicate logic of the first order, we have:

$$\Rightarrow_{PL_1}(\{\text{Elroy Fox has hepatitis, he is icteric}\}, \text{Elroy Fox is icteric}) = 1$$
$$\Rightarrow_{PL_1}(\{\text{Elroy Fox has hepatitis, he is icteric}\}, \text{Elroy Fox coughs}) = 0.$$

Like most logics, PL_1 is a crisp logic because its implication operator $\Rightarrow_{PL_1}$ is bivalent and takes only the values $\{0, 1\}$. Even the so-called many-valued logic, outlined in Section 28.5 on page 964, is such a crisp logic with a bivalent implication operator. By contrast, a fuzzy logic, FL, is a generalized mapping of the form:

$$\Rightarrow_{FL}: F(2^S) \times S \mapsto [0, 1]$$

such that $F(2^S)$ is the fuzzy powerset of S, and $\Rightarrow_{FL}(A, \alpha) = r$ says that according to logic FL the premises A imply the sentence α to the extent $r \in [0, 1]$. Thus, $\Rightarrow_{FL}$ is a generalized, multivalent implication operator with this operator being a numerical variable (function).

A *qualitative* fuzzy logic deviates from such a quantitative one in that its implication operator $\Rightarrow_{FL}$ is a linguistic variable of the form $Implies(A, \alpha)$ whose term set may be something like:

$$T(\text{Implies}) = \{\text{weakly, moderately, strongly, very srongly, } \dots \}$$

such that a statement of the form:

$$\text{Implies}(A, \alpha) = \text{strongly}$$

says: The set A of sentences strongly implies the sentence α. For example, if $A = \{$most patients with angina pectoris have coronary heart disease, Elroy Fox has angina pectoris$\}$, and $\alpha \equiv$ "it is likely that Elroy Fox has coronary heart disease", then we have $\textit{Implies}(A, \alpha) = \textit{strongly}$. That means that the premises strongly imply the conclusion. For details, see (Sadegh-Zadeh, 2001a).

17.2 Implication Structures

To determine whether medicine is something logical in any sense or has any particular logic, requires that we be more specific about that aspect of medicine which characterizes its logicality. No doubt, it is the relation between sentences (statements, assertions, hypotheses, theories, etc.) that may or may not be logical according to a particular logic L. An example is the relation between an item of medical knowledge and patient data, on the one hand; and the prognosis for this patient concluded therefrom by a physician, on the other. To reconstruct the general structure of the relation under discussion, we introduce the notion of an implication structure.

Definition 171 (Implication structure). ξ *is an L-logical implication structure iff there are A, B, and $\Rightarrow_L$ such that:*

1. *$\xi = \langle A, B, \Rightarrow_L \rangle$;*
2. *A and B are non-empty sets of sentences;*
3. *there is a logic L such that $\Rightarrow_L$ is its implication operator;*
4. *$\Rightarrow_L(A, \alpha) \neq 0$ for every $\alpha \in B$.*

This definition says, in essence, that each statement in set B is to a particular extent L-logically implied by set A. For example, the following triple is a PL_1-logical implication structure, i.e., an implication structure according to classical predicate logic of the first order, PL_1:

$\langle\{$All human beings with acute pneumonia have fever and cough;
  Elroy Fox is a human being; he has acute pneumonia$\}$;
  $\{$Elroy Fox has fever, Elroy Fox coughs$\}$; $\Rightarrow_{PL_1}\rangle$.

For we have:

$A \quad = \{$All human beings with acute pneumonia have fever and cough;
        Elroy Fox is a human being; he has acute pneumonia$\}$
$B \quad = \{$Elroy Fox has fever, Elroy Fox coughs$\}$
$\Rightarrow_L = \quad \Rightarrow_{PL_1}$
$\Rightarrow_{PL_1}(A, \alpha) = 1$ for every $\alpha \in B$.

However, the following triple is not an implication structure:

$$\langle A, B, \Rightarrow_{Sentential\_Logic} \rangle$$

because $\Rightarrow_{Sentential\_Logic}(A, \alpha) = 0$ for every $\alpha \in B$. This is no surprise. In Part VIII it is shown how different systems of logic are. Due to differences between their syntax and semantics, they handle sentences differently.

17.3 On the Logic of Medicine

In analyzing whether there is a specific logic of medicine, we shall confine ourselves to medical practice, especially medical diagnostics, because the diagnostic process is the prominent place where a possibly existing logic of medicine would or could manifest itself as a means of diagnostic reasoning.

We saw in Section 8.2.9 that from a descriptive point of view, medical diagnostics may be categorized as a human social practice. Therefore, it cannot have a logic because human beings and the actions they perform to manage expected and unexpected social situations, are inherently illogical. To confirm this claim, examine the logical knowledge and skill of 100 physicians to see how much they understand of logic, and thus, 'how logical' in diagnostics they are able to be. You will be surprised.

Viewed from a normative perspective, however, without any doubt it is possible to regulate the process of clinical decision-making by algorithms to guide and control clinical pathfinding so as to render clinical decision-making computable. We discussed this possibility on page 316. As far as diagnostic reasoning is concerned, logic will automatically come into play whenever a diagnostician examines whether or not a particular diagnosis is justified on the basis of the available patient data and diagnostic knowledge used. Medical data and knowledge engineering including medical knowledge-based systems, decision support systems, and hospital information systems research have been creating such facilities since the 1970s. As emphasized on several occasions in preceding chapters, they are transforming clinical decision-making into an engineering science and technology of *clinical reasoning by machines*, CRM for short. The cost of this transformation in the long run is the gradual elimination of the doctor from clinical judgment and diagnostic-therapeutic decision-making. We shall come back to this issue in Section 21.7. At this time we may state that for the reasons above the application of logic in diagnostics is, and will remain, the task of the emerging CRM. As we saw previously, a clinical operator constructed and executed by CRM has a diagnostic component of the following form:

$$diag(p, D, KB \cup M) = \Delta$$

such that Δ is the diagnostic set $\{\alpha_1, \ldots, \alpha_n\}$ consisting of $n \geq 1$ statements about the patient such as {Elroy Fox has diabetes, he does not have hepatitis}. There are a variety of different logics that can be used by the methods component, M, of such a diagnostic operator to draw diagnostic conclusions from the union of patient data and knowledge base, $D \cup KB$, and to produce the diagnostic set Δ. Which one of these logics will actually be used, depends on the syntax and semantics of $D \cup KB$ because that logic, L, has to be syntactically and semantically capable of dealing with $D \cup KB$ to yield an implication structure of the form $\langle D \cup KB, \Delta, \Rightarrow_L \rangle$. The logic L will or may be, for instance:

- predicate logic   if $D \cup KB$ satisfies the syntax of predicate logic,
- probability logic   if $D \cup KB$ contains probability sentences,
- temporal logic   if $D \cup KB$ deals with time periods and series,
- deontic logic   if $D \cup KB$ contains deontic sentences,
- alethic modal logic if $D \cup KB$ talks of possibility and necessity,

and so on. In discussions about 'the logic of medicine', what people usually have in mind is a traditional bivalent logic. However, apart from the above aspects, there are two additional problems that reduce the applicability of traditional logics in medicine. The first one is the inconsistency of medical knowledge and data that requires the application of an inconsistency tolerant logic. This problem was discussed in Section 16.2 above.

A second problem that makes traditional logics almost useless in medicine, is the irremediable vagueness of medical language. As we frequently pointed out in previous chapters, basic concepts of clinical medicine such as "health", "illness" and "disease", almost all nosological predicates such as "pneumonia" and "myocardial infarction", and symptom names such as "pain", "icterus", "high blood pressure", and so on denote fuzzy categories and are thus fuzzy predicates. As fuzzy predicates, they violate central principles of classical, two-valued logic, specifically the Principles of Excluded Middle and Non-Contradiction, rendering clinical knowledge inconsistent. Consequently, traditional, consistent logics cannot be the appropriate logics to use in diagnostic reasoning. Fuzzy logic will be indispensable.

Our analyses in previous chapters have demonstrated that clinical knowledge is not a declarative, but primarily a procedural one whose sentences prescribe actions, i.e., procedures. For example, "if a patient has a cough with or without sputum, has an acute or subacute fever and has dyspnea, then, if you want to know whether she has community acquired pneumonia, then *you ought to* examine her chest and search for altered breath sounds and rales, and perform chest radiography and search for opaque areas in both lungs". In a more general form, such procedural sentences say:

- If the patient presents the data set D and
- you want to know whether she has disease X,
- then *you ought to do* $Y_1, \ldots, Y_n$ and
- examine if the outcome of Y_1 is Z_1 and $\ldots$ and the outcome of Y_n is Z_n.

(See Sections 10.6 and 10.7). Due to the fuzziness of patient data D, disease X, and test results $Z_1, \ldots, Z_n$ on the one hand; and to the deontic nature of the command "you ought to do $Y_1, \ldots, Y_n$,", on the other, the appropriate logic of diagnostics will at least be a fuzzy deontic logic or another system of paraconsistent deontic logic. We took the first steps toward the application of a logic of the former type in previous sections. For logics of the latter type, see (da Costa and Carnielli, 1986; Grana, 1990). However, many additional logics will also be needed on the grounds that a variety of knowledge types from anatomy to biochemistry to surgery to epidemiology are used in diagnostic reasoning. As was mentioned above, each of them uses sentences of different syntax and semantics, e.g., probability sentences, temporal sentences, and others.

Thus far there is convincing evidence that, on the one hand, clinical diagnostics has no inherent logic; and on the other hand, it requires a variety of different logics to manage diagnostic reasoning. No single and particular system of logic will suffice. This conclusion can be generalized with regard to medicine as a whole. The situation is comparable to the use of mathematics in medicine. A large number of mathematical theories are needed and used in medical research and practice. Like this mathematical pluralism in medicine, logical pluralism is the only solution to logical problems in medicine because there is no specific *medical logic* (Sadegh-Zadeh, 1980a, 7).

A final remark may be in order to stimulate research on a particular aspect that deserves attention and interest. In informal contexts where no rigorous measures are required or used, the term "the logic of ..." is usually understood as meaning "the rationale behind ...". For example, the question "what is the logic of your decision to do *X?*" asks "what is the rationale behind your decision to do *X?*". In this sense, and only in this sense, a collection of well-known, age-old principles of conduct in medicine that usually count as medical-ethical principles, may be considered *the logic of medicine* by which medical actions are guided as well as justified. They comprise the following basic moral maxims, axioms, or principles:

- Primum non nocere (above all do no harm),
  ≡ Principle of Non-Maleficence;
- Salus aegroti suprema lex (the patient's well-being is the highest law),
  ≡ Principle of Beneficence;
- The patient's dignity ought not to be violated,

and similar ones such as principles of autonomy, confidentiality, truthfullness, and others. Concisely, *the common morality of medicine constitutes its specific logic*. According to our analyses in Section 16.5.5 on fuzzy deontics, the question should be examined whether it is preferable to conceive a fuzzy-deontic medical logic by fuzzifying the moral principles above and establishing a fuzzy medical ethics (see *fuzzy deontics* in Section 16.5.5 on page 659).

17.4 Summary

To inquire into whether there is a specific medical logic, we first explicated the concept of logic. We found that a logic is an inference system built around a particular implication operator, and distinguished a bivalent implication operator from a multivalent, fuzzy one. The latter is general enough to also include the former. On this basis, we introduced a concept of implication structure. In order for medicine to have a specific logic, a specific medical implication operator, MIO, would be needed to render medical reasoning implication structures according to MIO. However, there is no such MIO. A variety of existing, non-medical logics each with their specific implication operators are, or may be, used in medicine. Logical pluralism and instrumentalism is the only 'medical logic' in the narrow sense of this term.

It may be objected that in medicine the subject of reasoning consists in actions, not in statements. Thus, the physician has to justify why she acts in a particular way and not why she believes that something is the case. So, in discussing medical logic, inferential logics are irrelevant.

This objection is not well-substantiated. First, medicine is something more than the physician's actions. Second, in a clinical setting the physician acts in a particular way because in the process of clinical decision-making she has decided to act in that way. Therefore, she needs to reason about this decision and not about the act itself. Why did she make the decision A and not the decision B? It is her preference of A over B that she has to justify. Justification of preference behavior is always *practical reasoning* on the basis of knowledge, data, and goals. And such reasoning requires a method of reasoning usually called logic. The common morality of medicine seems to provide such a specific medical logic.

Part VI

Medical Metaphysics

On What There Are

18.0 Introduction

Medicine and philosophy of medicine confront a variety of specific metaphysical problems whose analysis and solution have significant theoretical and practical consequences. Among them are questions of the following type: Do diseases really exist or are they mere inventions? Are there really pathological processes of the type X, e.g., autoimmune reactions, or are they mere hypothetical constructions? What is the nature of human mind? Does psychosomatic causation really exist? Is medical knowledge true or is it only useful without being true? Does medicine belong to the humanities or is it a natural science, an applied science, or something else?

In the preceding five parts of the book, we gathered the necessary tools to answer such medical-metaphysical questions. In the present part, we shall put those tools to use. Our discussion is organized in these four chapters:

As in our previous discussions, we shall start with a brief introduction to some auxiliary notions that will provide us with some grounding in theory and methodology. We shall first briefly explain what we understand by the terms "metaphysics" and "ontology". To begin with, metaphysics is a branch of philosophy, and ontology is a part of metaphysics.

Like any other philosophical term, "metaphysics" is a vague phrase. As a result, virtually all themes ranging from language to knowledge to reality to free will to love to death to God are considered to belong to the realm of metaphysics. A quick look at the etymology of the term guards against such unhelpful semantic distension:

The term "metaphysics" derives from the Greek expression $\tau \alpha \ \mu \varepsilon \tau \alpha \ \tau \alpha \ \varphi \upsilon \sigma \iota \kappa \alpha$ ("ta meta ta phusika") and means *the things after the nature*. It was

K. Sadegh-Zadeh, *Handbook of Analytic Philosophy of Medicine*,
Philosophy and Medicine 113, DOI 10.1007/978-94-007-2260-6_18,
© Springer Science+Business Media B.V. 2012

coined, more than 200 years after Aristotle's death, by the Aristotelean editor Andronicus of Rhodes who lived in the first half of the first century BC. The term was to denote a single volume collection of some notes by Aristotle which in the catalogue of his works came after the material subsumed under the title "ta phusika", *The Nature*. This one volume collection, *Metaphysics* ≡ 'after the nature', comprises Aristotle's unsystematic writings on different topics and is the first work in the history of philosophy bearing this new title. Aristotle himself didn't know the term. We may therefore consider it to have been ostensively defined as a name for that single volume book, like the name "The Eiffel Tower" is ostensively defined by reference to the well-known iron tower on the Champ de Mars beside the River Seine in Paris. There is thus no need for speculation on metaphysics and its subject matter, scope, tasks, and divisions.[128]

As a collection of Aristotle's notes, the world's first Metaphysics deals with a number of unrelated philosophical and logical issues. They include a "science of first principles and causes" that the author calls the "first philosophy" (Metaphysics, Book I 982b 9); logical foundations of philosophy and other sciences (ibid., Book IV), e.g., the three Aristotelean principles mentioned on page 874; and some chapters on matter, change, movement, wisdom, theology, and many other themes. This group of wide-ranging subjects was called "metaphysics". Conceived as such, however, the field becomes co-extensive with philosophy rendering the term "metaphysics" a superfluous phrase.

Rather, we consider metaphysics to be, like epistemology, a special branch of philosophy consisting of inquiries into *proto*- and *meta*scientific issues and problems that are not, or cannot be, dealt with by scientists themselves in their scientific disciplines. For instance, conceptual issues surrounding themes such as "what is time?", "what is a person?", and the mind-body problem are metaphysical subjects. On this account, Aristotle's 'first philosophy' as a *protoscience* is indeed metaphysics. The prefix "proto" means "first" and "before". *Before* doing research involving certain concepts that emerge from ordinary language, the concepts of time and malaise, for instance, one first needs to know some properties of these concepts. Consider research in physics as an example, where one must determine whether time is to be treated as something discrete or as something continuous. Based on knowledge of the properties of such concepts, one could distinguish, for example, between *protophysics* that analyzes protophysical concepts of time, space, matter, and related issues; *protobiology* that inquires into what should be viewed as a living thing; *protomedicine* that is concerned with protomedical concepts of well-being, malady, illness, disease, healing, life, and death; and so on.

---

[128] See, for example, the German philosopher Martin Heidegger's strange language twists in his "What is metaphysics?" (1929), which provoked logical empiricists such as Rudolf Carnap to claim that metaphysics was nonsense because metaphysical questions would arise from the abuse of language and the violation of its grammar (Carnap, 1932).

A major metaphysical issue dealt with by Aristotle in his Metaphysics is *being as being*. According to him, "There is a science which investigates being as being and the attributes which belong to this in virtue of its own nature. Now this is not the same as any of the so-called special sciences; for none of these others deals generally with being as being. They cut off a part of being and investigate the attributes of this part" (ibid., Book IV 1003a 20–25). Such an inquiry Aristotle explicitly calls "the science of being as being", which he expounds in several Books of his Metaphysics. The endeavor he refers to originated with Greek philosophers preceding him such as Heraclitus, Parmenides, and Plato, and was termed *metaphysica generalis* by medieval philosophers, while metaphysica specialis in their view dealt with all of the other problems mentioned above. The term "ontology" is just another name for *metaphysica generalis* coined in the early seventeenth century, i.e., "the science of being as being".

In the next chapter, Chapter 19, we shall discuss the ontological problems of medicine. To prepare our discussion, in the current chapter we shall briefly look at the concept of ontology itself. Our inquiry divides into the following three sections:

18.1 Ordinary Ontology
18.2 Fuzzy Ontology
18.3 Vague, Fictional, and Non-Existent Entities.

We deliberately entitled the present chapter "On what there are" so as to counter the philosopher Willard Van Orman Quine's famous and influential doctrine "On what there is". Our aim is to show that *there are* many more things in heaven and earth than Quine dreamt of in his ontology (Quine, 1948).

18.1 Ordinary Ontology

Many of us are aware of the controversial debates in medicine *on what there are*: Do diseases exist? Are there mental diseases? Do human beings have a psyche? For example, while scores of human beings are diagnosed as suffering from mental diseases and treated accordingly by psychiatrists and other specialists, the so-called antipsychiatrists argue that there are no such things as mental diseases. We shall therefore inquire into whether, and how, it is possible to distinguish between existent entities in medicine such as the patient Elroy Fox's *liver* and his token disease state *diabetes mellitus,* on the one hand; and non-existent entities such as the type disease *drapetomania,* on the other. To begin, we will take a closer look at the term "ontology".

Roughly, ontology is the study of what there is. As noted above, the term "ontology" first appeared in the literature in the early seventeenth century as a synonym of "metaphysica generalis". Its initial particle "ont" comes from the Greek το ον for *being.* Thus, the term "ontology" means *the science of being* or the theory of existence. For details on this branch of philosophy, see (Burkhardt and Smith, 2002; Loux and Zimmermann, 2005).[129]

The term "ontology" is one of the many vague phrases in philosophy. Most ontologists consider ontology to be "the science of what is, of the kinds and structures of objects, properties, events, processes, and relations in every area of reality". Thus, all of reality seems to be considered its subject matter. However, such a broad construal is inadequate and useless. The analysis of the kinds and structures of objects, properties, events, processes, and relations in every area of reality is incumbent upon empirical disciplines such as chemistry, physics, biology, archeology, cosmology, medicine, and others, but not upon a philosophical, non-empirical research field called *ontology*. We are therefore concerned here with ontology in the narrowest, original sense of the term as a theory of being, and distinguish between pure ontology, applied ontology, and formal ontology, which we shall briefly consider in turn in the following sections.

18.1.1   Pure Ontology
18.1.2   Applied Ontology
18.1.3   Formal Ontology.

18.1.1 Pure Ontology

Pure, or philosophical, ontology is a theoretical inquiry into what it means to say that something exists or is; why does anything exist rather than nothing; and what kinds of entities, called ontological categories, are the most general ones of which the world is composed.

The first question is the basic one and of great significance for all sciences as well as everyday life. We need to understand the concept of existence before we can reasonably claim that some particular things exist, e.g., the Eiffel Tower, a particular disease such as Alzheimer's, genes, the unconsciousness, electrons, Black Holes, witches, and the like. For our medical-ontological purposes, we shall briefly discuss this issue and sketch the main ontological positions to which we shall refer later on. Our discussion divides into the following four parts:

---

[129] The oldest record of the term "ontology" is the phrase "ontologia" found in Jacobus Lorhardus' *Ogdoas scholastica* (1606) and in Rudolphus Goclenius' *Lexicon Philosophicum* (1613). Jakob Lorhard or Jacobus Lorhardus (1561–1609) was born in Münsingen in South Germany and studied at the German University of Tübingen. As of 1602, he was a teacher and preacher in St. Gallen, Switzerland. His *Ogdoas scholastica* was concerned with 'Grammatices (Latinae, Graeca), Logices, Rhetorices, Astronomices, Ethices, Physices, Metaphysices, seu Ontologia'. Rudolf Göckel or Rudolphus Goclenius (1547–1628) was a professor of physics, logic, and mathematics at the German University of Marburg. He first learned about the term "ontology" from Lorhard himself. Ontology gained currency first of all by the German philosopher Christian Wolff (1679–1754) (Wolff, 1730).

▶ Existence and being
▶ Nominalism and Platonism
▶ Trope theory
▶ Ontological realism and anti-realism.

Existence and being

Seen from a semantic point of view, the ontological question of what it means to say that something exists, or is, is a linguistic concern that seeks an explication of the terms "exists" and "is". Although the search has been ongoing for the last 2300 years since Aristotle, it has not been very successful. The failure may be attributed mainly to the circumstance that the two terms are ambiguously and inconsistently used in natural languages. The problems arise when philosophers contend with such uses and cultivate, instead of correcting or discarding, them. We shall shed some light on this issue and suggest a solution in the following four paragraphs:

▷ Existence and being ≠ reality
▷ Quine's simplicism
▷ Existence and being = causal entrenchment
▷ Existence is a relation.

Existence and being ≠ reality

An adequate understanding as well as an adequate treatment of the terms "exists" and "is" are hampered by the naïve realism that our species has biologically inherited from its ancestors. Since perceiving automatically triggers believing in the existence of the perceived, human beings as perceiving creatures are can't-help-it realists supposing that "percipi est esse", to invert Bishop George Berkeley's well-known doctrine "esse est percipi": see also page 499. An individual who has a perception of something, believes that the thing she perceives exists. Not everybody is capable of resisting the biologically-based, belief-inducing force of her perceptions and to exclaim "I see it but I don't believe that it exists". It is a truism that the human perceptual and cognitive system is prone to error, illusion, hallucination, and even delusion. This is a warning not to try to explicate or define the two terms "exists" and "is" by recourse to sense perception, observation, or evidence; by saying, for example, "an object exists when people can directly or indirectly perceive it; otherwise, it does not exist". Nor do terms such as "actual", "real", and "fact" provide any definitional assistance, for they are used as odd synonyms of "is" and "exists". It would only be circular to say, for instance, that "an object exists when it is real". What does the word "real" mean? Members of different species perceive different 'realities'. The frog perceives temperature as pressure; the bee can see ultraviolet light; the bat can hear, or perceive, ultrasonic waves; birds can see the earth's magnetic field; as human beings, we inhabit a different reality; color-blind persons inhabit still another reality; and so on. So, to adequately understand "existence" and "being", other approaches are needed that require no recourse to perceptions and realities.

Quine's simplicism

A syntactic-semantic solution was proposed by the influential philosopher and logician Willard Van Orman Quine, whose famous doctrine says that "to be is to be the value of a variable" (Quine, 1948, [1963] 13 and 15). Quine means "variable" in logical sense. For example, if it is asserted that $\exists x P x$, and someone encounters an object, say a, which has the property P, then according to Proof 7 on page 893, this evidence Pa classical-logically implies the existence claim $\exists x P x$. Consequently, the object a is able to serve as a value of the variable x bound by the existential quantifier in $\exists x P x$. By virtue of Quine's thesis, then, it exists.

However, things are not that easy. For instance, we know that Sherlock Holmes is a detective. From this knowledge we may conclude the sentence that "there exists someone who is a detective", i.e., $\exists x P x$ with Px denoting "x is a detective". Thus, *Sherlock Holmes* is a value of the variable x in "$\exists x$ such that x is a detective". Consequently, he exists. This correct logical proof with the metaphysical qualms it gives rise to, is reason enough to ask how we could distinguish between imaginary and fictional entities such as Sherlock Holmes, on the one hand; and 'really' existing entities such as your heart beating in your chest, on the other.

Existence and being = causal entrenchment

Of the many stubborn ontological problems arising from the attempt to distinguish between existent and imaginary entities, the most prominent is the issue of whether existence and being are *properties* ascribed to entities, i.e., the issue of whether the terms "exists" and "is" are predicates (Moore, 1936). To elucidate, consider the following sequences:

> Your heart exists,
> your heart is.

Are these sequences grammatically correct sentences and meaningful at all? If so, are they subject-predicate sentences like the sentence "your heart beats"? If they are, are the phrases "exists" and "is", which they contain, predicates representing a *property* of your heart like the predicate "beats" does? Would your heart lack *that* property if it didn't exist? Some philosophers affirm this view, while others deny it, the most famous among the latter being David Hume and Immanuel Kant. According to Kant, for example, "By whatever and by however many predicates we may think a thing – even if we completely determine it – we do not make the least addition to the thing when we further declare that this thing is" (Kant, 2003, B 627). In contrast to such prominent denials, in the present section it is shown that whatever else the words "exists" and "is" may mean, they may also be sensibly conceived of as predicates. This conception does justice to robust natural language usages such as "your heart exists" and "your heart is". Our deviation from Kant and Hume's positions is based on our view that a word need not have only one meaning. It may have a hundred different meanings in different contexts, i.e., it may play a hundred different roles. The words "exists" and "is" are good examples. See Figure 3 on page 25.

To begin with, we should be aware that existence and being are by no means identical. Something can *be,* even though it does *not* exist. We owe this insight to Bertrand Russell, who recognized that "what does not exist must be something, or it would be meaningless to deny its existence" (Russell, 1903, 450). For instance, Pegasus *is* a winged horse, but it *does not exist.* This example clearly demonstrates that in natural languages, "exists" and "is" are not completely synonymous. While "exists" has only two meanings, the small word "is" enjoys a dozen of disjoint meanings. We already mentioned five of its different meanings in Section 5.4.2 on page 105. The term "exists" possesses none of those five meanings. It shares only the following, sixth meaning of "is". When it is said, for example, that:

The Eiffel Tower is,
the Eiffel Tower exists,

this usage is best understood as the *predication* of a property, i.e., being and existence, to an object that is known as *the Eiffel Tower* in Paris. Analogously, the following negations are denials of the same property:

Pegasus is not,
Pegasus does not exist.

In what follows, the specific role that both terms, "is" and "exists", play in predicating existence, will be represented by an easily recognizable *existence predicate*. First, however, we should be aware of an additional, seventh meaning of "is" that is shared by "exists". This is the role it plays in logic, specifically in the existence *operator* "there is an x such that ..." that is synonymous with "there exists an x such that ...". This operator is the usual existential quantifier symbolized by $\exists$ and introduced in Part VIII. Thus, both of these sentences:

There *is* an x such that x = the Eiffel Tower,
there *exists* an x such that x = the Eiffel Tower

say that $\exists x(x =$ the Eiffel Tower$)$. This operator is defined, for use in first-order languages, by its semantics presented in Definition 219.3 on page 883. There is an analogous existence operator in higher-order languages. The *existence predicate* announced above will be defined by recourse to this higher-order existence operator, also symbolized by $\exists$, because in our definitions we shall use a second-order language. To this end, we shall employ the auxiliary notion of a "causal predicate" explained below.

We must first observe that in contrast to imaginary entities such as Sherlock Holmes, Pegasus, and drapetomania, a characteristic feature of 'really' existing entities is their embeddedness in the causal context of the world in which we live. An object or a state of affairs such as a celestial body, an electron, money, unemployment, suffering, happiness, television, a geyser, a virus, a brother or aunt is embedded in the causal context of this world in that it is either (i) causally effective and develops causally positively or negatively relevant effects, or (ii) suffers such effects caused by other objects or states of affairs. For the notion of causal relevance, see Definition 80 on page 260.

That an entity x develops or suffers causally relevant effects, means that there is at least one predicate, P, such that P denotes a causally relevant property, and the behavior of the entity x is describable by the sentence Px. Simple examples are the following entities a, b, c, and d:

- a emits gamma-rays   (is causally effective)
- b congeals   (suffers a causal effect)
- c infects a patient   (is causally effective)
- d has caught a cold   (suffers a causal effect).

For simplicity's sake, a predicate P of this type will be referred to as a causal predicate. Causal predicates contained in the examples above are: *emitting gamma rays, congealing, infecting a patient,* and *catching a cold.* A causal context is described by a number of such causal predicates.

For generality's sake, we conceive a causal predicate P to be a many-place predicate that represents a causal relation between an object x and n other objects $y_1, \ldots, y_n$, i.e., $P(x, y_1, \ldots, y_n)$ where $n \geq 0$. For instance, in the statement "the sun attracts the earth" the predicate "attracts" is a binary causal predicate with the syntax $attracts(\text{sun, earth})$. Behind the condensed example "x infects a patient" above, lies the complete description "x infects $y \wedge y$ is a patient" that contains a binary causal predicate: $infects(x, y)$.

We may now introduce an existence predicate that proves false Hume's and Kant's denial that existence is a predicate. For reasons to be discussed below, we shall first introduce a binary existence predicate from which a unary existence predicate of the form "x exists" will be easily obtained.

Let $\mathcal{L}$ be a variable ranging over the set of all languages. That is, $\mathcal{L}$ may be any particular language, e.g., German, English, Papiamentu, etc. The phrase "$\mathbb{E}(x, \mathcal{L})$" reads "$x$ *exists with respect to* $\mathcal{L}$". For instance, $\mathbb{E}(\text{the\_Eiffel\_Tower, English})$. That is, the Eiffel Tower exists with repect to English language. This deliberately chosen syntax of the predicate $\mathbb{E}$ indicates that existence and being will be relativized to a particular language $\mathcal{L}$.

Definition 172 (Existence predicate, binary). *For all x and all $\mathcal{L}$, $\mathbb{E}(x, \mathcal{L})$ iff $\exists y_1 \ldots y_n \exists P$ such that:*

1. $\mathcal{L}$ is a language,

2. *P is an $(n+1)$-ary causal predicate of $\mathcal{L}$,*
3. $P(x, y_1, \ldots, y_n)$,
4. $n \geq 0$.

This definition mirrors the embeddedness of an existent in the causal context of the world, referred to as its *causal entrenchment*. It permits the causal predicate P to be unary if $n = 0$ such that $P(x, y_1, \ldots, y_n)$ becomes Px. Accordingly, an object exists, with respect to a particular language, if at least one causal property can be ascribed to it using that language. On this account, it is possible that an entity exists with respect to a language $\mathcal{L}_1$ such as German, whereas it does not exist with respect to another language $\mathcal{L}_2$ such as Cashinahua or Persian, and vice versa. This will be the case when the latter languages lack any equivalent of the causal predicate P used in German to identify the causally relevant event $P(x, y_1, \ldots, y_n)$, i.e., when the event is not expressible in those languages. Wittgenstein's often criticized Tractarian view, where he states that "The limits of my language mean the limits of my world", can be understood in exactly this sense (Wittgenstein, 1922, 5.6).

In order for an entity to exist in a world, its causal entrenchment in that world is a prerequisite because only through such an entrenchment can it be said to be ontically accessible to at least one inhabitant of that world. An entity that is ontically inaccessible to everybody cannot be ontologically transparent. We cannot know or conjecture whether it exists or not. (For the adverb "ontically", see page 44.)

Existence is a relation

According to Definition 172 above, existence – and being – is a two-place *relation*, represented by the binary predicate $\mathbb{E}(x, \mathcal{L})$, in which a causal language $\mathcal{L}$ plays a pivotal role. This is the basic idea of our theory of the relativity of existence, or *ontological relativity* for short.

Note that the ontological relativity reflected by our existence predicate is in fact a three-fold relativity. In addition to the explicit relativity of existence to a particular language $\mathcal{L}$, two implicit relativities are also involved. The first one is that the existential quantifier $\exists$, by which it is introduced, is relative to the logic used in the definiens of the predicate. The second one is that the predicate is relative to the concept of causality underlying the language $\mathcal{L}$, as it is this language that provides the causal predicate P required in the definition. In the present context, the term "language" is to be understood in its widest sense to also include the scientific theories that underlie an ontological inquiry. The reason is that a scientific theory brings with it a specific vocabulary. For example, the theory of autoimmune diseases has its own vocabulary not to be found in the theory of, say, psychoanalysis and vice versa.

We may thus conclude that assumptions about what exists or not, are relative to languages and logics. Although it may be true in German that there are electrons and mesons, these very facts may not be true, even not expressible

at all, in another language such as Cashinahua. The same holds true for the
ontological roles of logics. For example, when viewed from the perspective of
paraconsistent logic, the world contains many more entities than when viewed
from the perspective of classical logic because, in contrast to the former, the
latter precludes inconsistent objects and states of affairs. In a nutshell, an
ontology is shaped by the language and logic that it uses. In further support
of this view, we shall see in Section 18.2 below that existence and being are
not translinguistic and translogical realms. "Change your language or logic,
and you will see another world" (Sadegh-Zadeh, 1982a, 171).[130]

To simplify our notation, the binary existence predicate $\mathbb{E}(x, \mathcal{L})$ may be
written as a pseudo-unary predicate, $\mathbb{E}_{\mathcal{L}}$, such that the phrase $\mathbb{E}_{\mathcal{L}}(x)$ shortens
the sentence $\mathbb{E}(x, \mathcal{L})$. The shorthand $\mathbb{E}_{\mathcal{L}}(x)$ may even be further simplified
to obtain a genuinely unary existence predicate, which mirrors the ordinary
existence predicate "x exists" or "x is", in the following way: An entity exists
if and only if there is a language $\mathcal{L}$ such that $\mathbb{E}(x, \mathcal{L})$. That is:

Definition 173 (Existence predicate, unary). $\forall x \big(x \ exists \leftrightarrow \exists \mathcal{L} \ such \ that \ \mathcal{L}$
$is \ a \ language \land \mathbb{E}(x, \mathcal{L}) \big)$.

Nominalism and Platonism

One of the basic ontological problems concerns the type of entities that exist
in the world. Are they *concrete,* individual, spatio-temporal objects such as
Elroy Fox and the book in front of you; or can *abstract* objects without any
spatio-temporal location, such as properties, also exist? To understand this
question adequately, consider simple predications such as:

a. Elroy Fox is ill,   (172)

b. he has myocardial infarction,

c. his wife is sad.

Predications of this type are used to transmit information between agents.
They constitute an important part of our communications both in science and
everyday life. Let us abbreviate a predication of the form (172) above simply
by "Px". For example, $x \equiv$ Elroy Fox, and $P \equiv$ is ill. We need criteria that
enable us to distinguish a predication Px, that purportedly reports a fact,
from fiction. We may without much difficulty come to an agreement about
whether or not the subject x of such a predication Px exists, i.e., the *individual*
objects Elroy Fox and his wife in the present examples (172). However, do the
denotations of the predicates contained in the very same statements also exist
as independent entities, i.e., illness, myocardial infarction, and sadness? If so,

---

[130] In developing my present theory of the relativity of existence over the years,
I have profited from discussions with my Brazilian friend Professor Newton C.
Affonso da Costa, then University of Sao Paulo, and from his publications and
manuscripts, e.g., (da Costa, 1982).

how are we to understand the existence of such abstract entities? If they exist, are they located somewhere in time and space in order for us to be able to encounter them, or do they have no location? And if they do not exist, how are we to justify the claim that by predicating a non-existent entity – such as illness, myocardial infarction, and sadness – we are reporting facts? The three main ontological responses given to these questions in the history of philosophy will be briefly outlined here: Nominalism, Platonism, and trope theory.

Nominalism is an ontological position, originating from the philosophy of the Roman philosopher and theologian Anicius Manlius Severinus Boethius (about 480–526), which says that only individual objects exist, that is, objects which have a definite location in space and time such as your heart, the patient Elroy Fox, single books, chairs, molecules, atoms, celestial bodies, and the like. They are called *particulars*. Linguistically, a particular is the referent of a proper name, i.e., of an individual constant. Thus, it does not have instances. According to nominalism, there exists nothing else beyond particulars, e.g., classes (intensionally speaking: properties) and relations such as illness, tachycardia, sadness, redness, and so forth. As supra-individual and abstract entities, properties and relations are called *universals*. They are the referents of predicates. In contrast to a particular, a universal is an entity that has instances.

The opposite position is Platonic realism, or Platonism for short, which originated with Plato (427–347 BC). In contrast to nominalists, Platonists hold that in addition to particulars, universals such as illness, tachycardia, sadness, redness, numbers, and the like also exist. They are intrinsically immutable, eternal, invariants in reality, mind-independent, and non-spatial.[131]

Platonists need the belief in the existence of universals, e.g., *diabetes mellitus* as an abstract property, in order to explain individual cases such as "Elroy Fox has the property of being a diabetic". The nominalists counter that we should not postulate the existence of such abstract entities like diabetes mellitus on the basis of overloaded predications such as "Elroy Fox has the property of being a diabetic". Elroy Fox is simply a diabetic. Such are the data. Occam's razor requires one *not to postulate more entities than are necessary to explain the data.*[132]

Using our existence predicate $\mathbb{E}_{\mathcal{L}}$, it should not be difficult to adjudicate on the two positions above. While a nominalist may easily demonstrate that according to Definition 172 on page 692 individual objects may have causal

---

[131] For the presumed origin of nominalism in Bocthius' skeptical attitude toward universals, see (Kneale and Kneale, 1968, 196).

[132] *"Entia non sunt multiplicanda praeter necessitatem"*. This well-known ontological maxim is attributed to the medieval English Franciscan friar William of Ockham (about 1285–1347) who was a logician and philosopher, known as Occam. It has come to be known as Occam's razor. We are told that the commonly quoted wording of the maxim is not to be found in Occam's own writings (Thorburn, 1918).

properties, a Platonist will encounter difficulties ascribing causal properties to abstract entities such as relations and properties themselves. However, in deciding the dispute between Platonism and nominalism, one should be aware that what is a universal and what is a particular is relative to the language that is used as the frame of reference, and to the context of discourse. For example, an organism at the macro-level is an individual object, and thus, a particular. Considered at the cellular level, however, it is a huge class of cells.

Trope theory

Suppose that an object or person has a particular property such as pain, illness, or the color red. Try now to imagine that this particular property, e.g., the color of a red rose, is not the instantiation of a universal such as redness by the object or person under discussion, but a distinct individual itself, i.e., a *particular* that we encounter in a spatio-temporal zone. Such a located property or relation is called a *trope*. This term has no profound philosophical background or content, and particularly it has nothing to do with the rethoric figure of speech known as *trope*, like metaphor, metonymy, irony, synecdoche, etc. It was coined as a sort of philosophical joke by the inventor of trope theory, Donald Cary Williams (1899–1983) (Williams, 1953).[133]

Trope theorists take an intermediate position between nominalism and Platonism in that they consider individual objects, including events, as bundles of tropes. The color of the red rose above is a trope. The pain that a person has is a trope. Beyond the token red color of the individual rose there is no redness as a universal, and beyond pain-tokens of individual human beings or animals there is no other, independent pain universal. Each red rose has its own local-individual color, and each pain-individual has her own pain. The same holds for other properties and relations. The myocardial infarction of Mr. Elroy Fox, his wife's sadness about that, and similar particulars are all we can have and think about. There are no universals.

Trope theory heeds Occam's razor absolutely. It is a maximally frugal, one-category ontology. There are no other basic entities than tropes, and the reality consists in nothing but tropes. As localized, individuated properties and relations, they are, according to Williams, the 'alphabet of being'. Any object is considered to be a cluster of tropes. Tropes are connected with one another in two ways to constitute the world, by location and similarity. For details of this theory, see (Campbell, 1990; Maurin, 2002; Simons, 2000a).[134]

---

[133] With reference to George Santayana's works (Santayana, 1937), Williams says: "Recalling, however, that Santayana used 'trope' to stand for the essence of an occurrence, I shall divert the word, which is almost useless in either his or its dictionary sense, to stand for the abstract particular which is, so to speak, the occurrence of an essence" (ibid., 6).

[134] The notion of similarity in the present context provides an opportunity to interpret tropes in the light of our prototype resemblance theory, introduced on pages

Trope theory is also referred to as *tropism*. Rather than being a nominalism in the traditional sense, trope theory is a strict particularism. In Chapter 19 on page 711, we shall examine whether this ontological position may be utilized in the philosophy of medicine.

Ontological realism and anti-realism

There is a remarkable correspondence between ontology and epistemology in that in order for an object x to exist, there must be a *true* statement of the form:

$$\exists P \exists y_1 \ldots y_n P(x, y_1, \ldots, y_n) \tag{173}$$

that contains a causal predicate P and causally characterizes that object x. See Definitions 172–173 of the existence predicate on pages 692 and 694. That is, the assertability of an existence claim of the form "x exists", such as "mental illness exists", requires the truth of an $\exists$-assertion of the form (173) above. So, in an ontological debate the epistemological question will always play a central role concerning whether the corresponding $\exists$-assertion (173) is true or false. This brings with it at least two consequences:

First, ontology cannot be independent of epistemology. The quality of an epistemology will influence, via the knowledge it approves or refutes, the quality of the corresponding ontology. For example, compare the world of an astrologer with that of a physiologist. Second, an epistemic realist will be an ontological realist; an epistemic anti-realist will be an ontological anti-realist; and an epistemic constructivist will be an ontological constructivist.

Ontological realism and ontological anti-realism were outlined, respectively, as metaphysical realism and metaphysical anti-realism on pages 488 and 492, respectively. They can be differentiated by the following test: Consider the basic question of ontology, i.e., what is there? Are there objective and determinate answers to this question? Whoever says Yes, is an ontological realist, while an ontological anti-realist will say No. For instance, a nominalist is an ontological realist with respect to individual objects, while being an ontological anti-realist with respect to classes. By contrast, a Platonist is an ontological realist with respect to both types of entities. In Chapter 19, we shall concern ourselves with varieties of ontological realism and anti-realism in medicine, for example, concerning the question of whether there are mental states and diseases.

18.1.2 Applied Ontology

Applied ontology, also called domain ontology, is concerned (i) with the question of what entities exist in a particular domain, for example, in the domain

---

174–183 to construct a concept of disease. A possible approach is to postulate a variety of prototype tropes which in association with our concept of similarity yield all factual and imaginable objects.

of a scientific branch such as biology, or even in the more specialized domain of a scientific theory such as the theory of active immunity; and (ii) with their formal taxonomy. Until now, ordinary taxonomy dominates. Ordinary taxonomy is classification based on the classical subsethood relation ⊂ between classes, expressed by the binary subsumption predicate "*is_a*" such as "pneumonia is_a respiratory disease" (see page 60).

For instance, someone may be interested in a domain-ontological question such as "what is there in the world of obstetrics?". In the world of obstetrics there are, for example, human bodies, married and unmarried couples, reproductive organs, gametes, copulations, artificial inseminations, pregnancies, abortions, embryos, obstetricians, midwives, midwifery forceps, delivery rooms, deliveries, newborns, puerperal fever, and many other things.

Domain ontology is currently undergoing a significant metamorphosis. Specifically, due to a semantic shift of the term "ontology" in the computer and information sciences, a new field of research has emerged called *ontology engineering* that has also entered into medicine in the meantime (Gómez-Pérez et al., 2004; Staab and Studer, 2004; Calero et al., 2006). Ontology engineering is meant to be a domain-specific activity as defined above. It provides structured vocabularies that serve both data analysis and computation in particular domains such as bioinformatics, anatomy, obstetrics, cardiology, or software development. However, a closer look at what ontology engineers actually do and produce, shows that they are not conducting ontology in the proper sense of this term. We shall come back to this issue in Section 19.4 on page 735.

18.1.3 Formal Ontology

Once pure ontology has determined what kind of entities in general exist, and applied ontology has determined what entities exist in particular domains such as physics, anatomy, internal medicine, and others, one can analyze whether there are any formal relationships between any of these entities. For example, is the left ventricle of the heart part of the heart? Yes. Is the human heart part of the human body? Yes. Then the left ventricle is part of the human body. Such formal analyses are the subject matter of formal ontology, which constructs axiomatic frameworks by means of formal logic to study formal relationships between all types of ontological categories and all types of entities existing in specific domains. Mereology, briefly sketched on pages 591–592, is a prominent example of a formal-ontological inquiry. There we saw that it is axiomatically concerned with part-whole relationships. We shall come back to this topic in Section 19.5 on page 738.

18.2 Fuzzy Ontology

Ontological debates in medicine over whether some particular entities, e.g., mental diseases, exist or not, cannot be settled without consensus on the virtues of the ontology one uses. For, an opponent may always ask what exactly the ontology looks like to which the proponent adheres. Metaontological inquiries of this type will reveal the following peculiarity that requires remedy:

Human reason seems to hold a two-valued ontology reflected in the common belief that "an entity is or is not, there are no intermediates between being and non-being". As pointed out on page 998, this simplistic feature of the early human intellect was perpetuated by Aristotle's two-valued, only-two-options perspective, which Western culture and science have inherited from his philosophy. As a result, ontology since Aristotle has been two-valued: An object either exists or it doesn't exist; a third option is excluded. Aristotle explicitly precludes such a third possibility in many places in his *Metaphysics*. See, for example (ibid., Book IV 1011 23–24, 1011 b 29–32, 1012 a 5–11).

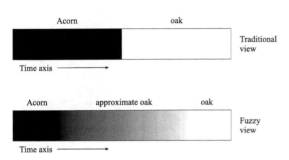

What we outlined in preceding sections, is in line with the traditional, Aristotelean, two-valued ontology mentioned above that we referred to as *ordinary ontology*. However, this ordinary ontology rests on, and generates, a highly confined worldview because it fades out major parts of the literally infinite world of existents and non-existents, for example, (i) those entities of which we do not or cannot know with certainty whether they exist or not, and (ii) those entities which only approximately exist. Consider, for instance, the long-standing

Fig. 83. In contrast to the traditional view, from the fuzzy perspective oakness does not have an abrupt beginning. Becoming an oak is something continuous, as is being an oak. Human beings and persons are, ontologically, analogs of oak trees. They have no abrupt beginnings and ends. They are vague entities (see Section 18.3.1 on page 705)

controversy in medicine and bioethics about questions such as "when does human life begin and when does it end?", or "when does the fetus become a person?" (Penner and Hull, 2008). The prototype of such queries is "when does the outgrowth of an acorn become an oak tree?". It is not difficult to discern the impossibility of drawing a sharp dividing line between the time t_1 at which "the *oak tree* does not yet exist" and the later time t_2 when "the oak tree now exists". Likewise, regarding a human fetus, no sharp dividing line can be drawn between the time at which "the person is not yet" and the later time when "the person now is". In all these and related cases, the borderline between the black period of *not-yet-an-oak-tree* and the white period of *now-an-oak-tree* is not a sharp dividing line, but a more or less wide grey area to the effect that the transition from black to white is gradual rather than abrupt. The continuous grey area of gradual transition between them is a region of partial being or approximate existence of the oak. Otherwise put, within the grey area an object under discussion only *partially is* and only *approximately exists*. See Figure 83 on page 699 and (Sadegh-Zadeh, 2001a).

The examples above demonstrate that some bioethical problems are ontological problems and may more adequately be treated using a theory of partial being and approximate existence. The prevailing insusceptibility in ontology to this issue is due to the underdeveloped state of human languages in which, among many other crisp words, the verbs "is" and "exists" are handled unimaginatively as all-or-nothing labels. To ameliorate this deficiency by creating a theory of approximate existence, we will first ask a surprising question: What may happen if we change the bivalent semantics of the two ontological verbs "is" and "exists" so they become multivalued and thereby enable ontological and ontic access to the grey areas shown in Figure 83? May we then make fuzzy ontological statements like those in Table 24?

Table 24. Basic sentences in fuzzy pure ontology

Qualitatively

  object x strongly exists (is),
  object y weakly exists (is),
  object z very weakly exists (is).

comparatively

  object x exists as strongly as object y,
  object x exists stronger (more) than object y,
  object x exists weaker (less) than object y.

quantitatively

  object a exists (is) to the extent 1,
  object b exists (is) to the extent 0.9,
  object c exists (is) to the extent 0.4,
  object d exists (is) to the extent 0.1,
  object e exists (is) to the extent 0.

What we will endeavor now is just such a semantic intervention by fuzzifying the set of all existents and that of all non-existents to demonstrate that there are no sharp boundaries between being and nothingness. To this end, we shall introduce a degree of fuzzy existence, denoted by the ternary function:

$\varepsilon(x, P, \mathcal{L})$ reads: the degree of existence of object x relative
to the causal predicate P of language $\mathcal{L}$

abbreviated to the pseudo-unary function:

$\varepsilon_{P\mathcal{L}}(x)$.

This degree of fuzzy existence will be defined by the usual membership function $\mu_P(x)$ that signifies "the degree of membership of x in fuzzy set P". Likewise, if P is an n-ary fuzzy causal relation, the expression "$\mu_P(x_1, \ldots, x_n)$" represents the membership degree of the n-tuple $(x_1, \ldots, x_n)$ in fuzzy relation P. For example, the sentence "$\mu_{infects}(Amy, Elroy\ Fox) = 0.7$" means that Amy *infects* Elroy Fox to the extent 0.7. The intended concept of approximate existence will be formed in two steps. We start with introducing the degree of existence $\varepsilon_{\mathcal{PL}}(x)$ announced above:

Definition 174 (Fuzzy existence: $\varepsilon_{\mathcal{PL}}$). *If Ω is the set of all imaginable objects with respect to language $\mathcal{L}$, then $\mathcal{PL}$ is the set of all existents with respect to the predicate P of language $\mathcal{L}$ iff:*

1. *P is an $(n+1)$-ary causal predicate with $n \geq 0$,*
2. *there is a function $\varepsilon_{\mathcal{PL}}$ that maps Ω to $[0,1]$,*
3. *$\exists y_1 \dots y_n$ such that $\varepsilon_{\mathcal{PL}}(x) = \mu_P(x, y_1, \dots, y_n)$,*
4. *$\mathcal{PL} = \{(x, \varepsilon_{\mathcal{PL}}(x)) \mid x \in \Omega\}$.*

Set $\mathcal{PL}$ is the fuzzy set of all objects each of which to a particular extent between 0 and 1 inclusive is a member of the set, and this extent is the degree of its existence with respect to the causal predicate P of language $\mathcal{L}$, denoted $\varepsilon_{\mathcal{PL}}(x)$. Thus, $\mathcal{PL}$ is the set of all fuzzy existents relative to the causal predicate P of the language $\mathcal{L}$. This concept says that to the extent $r \in [0,1]$ an entity x is a member of fuzzy set $\mathcal{PL}$, i.e., exists relative to a causal predicate P of language $\mathcal{L}$, if and only if there are $n \geq 0$ other entities $y_1, \dots, y_n$ such that to the extent r the objects $x, y_1, \dots, y_n$ stand in the causal relation P to each other, i.e., P-causally interact. For instance, if it is true that to the extent 0.7 an entity x infects Mr. Elroy Fox, then to this extent object x is a member of the fuzzy set *infects-English*.

Otherwise put, relative to the predicate "infects" of the language *English*, x exists to the extent 0.7. In the next step, the predicate P will be stripped from the realtive existence degree $\varepsilon_{\mathcal{PL}}$. Only the global relativity to language $\mathcal{L}$ will remain. But we must be aware that a language $\mathcal{L}$ will usually contain a number of causal predicates $P_1, \dots, P_n$ with $n > 1$ relative to which an object x may exist to different extents such that it will get assigned different degrees of existence, $r_1, \dots, r_n$, with $r_i \neq r_j$ for each two degrees. To prevent such inconsistent situations, these different degrees will be collected in a set, and their maximum $max(r_1, \dots, r_n)$ will be considered the degree of existence of that object x:

Definition 175 (Fuzzy existence: $\varepsilon_{\mathcal{L}}$). *For all x, for all $\mathcal{L}$, and for all $r \in [0,1]$,*

$$\varepsilon_{\mathcal{L}}(x) = r$$

iff:

1. *$\mathcal{L}$ is a language,*
2. *$\exists P_1 \dots P_n$ such that each P_i is a causal predicate of $\mathcal{L}$,*
3. *$\varepsilon_{P_i \mathcal{L}}(x) = r_i \quad$ for all $1 \geq i \geq n$,*
4. *$r = max(r_1, \dots, r_n)$.*

Note that this new, simplified, binary fuzzy existence function $\varepsilon(x, \mathcal{L})$, written $\varepsilon_{\mathcal{L}}(x)$, was defined by the previous existence function $\varepsilon_{\mathcal{PL}}(x)$ introduced in Definition 174 above. For instance, if a supposed bunch of germs, x, infects Mr. Elroy Fox to the extent 0.7 and shows, in a Petri dish, the growth factor 0.4, then we have the following two degrees of existence:

$$\varepsilon_{infects\text{-}English}(x) = 0.7$$
$$\varepsilon_{grows\text{-}English}(x) = 0.4.$$

This implies by Definition 175 the existence claim:

$$\varepsilon_{English}(x) = 0.7$$

which says that relative to the English language, the bunch x exists to the extent 0.7. For $max(0.7, 0.4) = 0.7$.

The two definitions above improve upon the one suggested in (Sadegh-Zadeh, 2001a, 7). They say, in essence, that being is a matter of degree and relative to a particular language. Relative to that language, an object exists to an extent between 0 and 1 inclusive if to this extent the object is a member of the fuzzy set $\mathcal{PL}$ introduced in Definition 174 above. To put it concisely, an object exists, with respect to a causal predicate P of a language $\mathcal{L}$, to the extent to which it exerts or suffers a P-causal impact. If a supposed entity is neither causally effective nor suffers causal effects of other entities to an extent greater than 0, then there is no such entity. As an example, consider a microbiologist who is examining whether there are bacteria or viruses in the specimen a that she has taken from a patient. She finds in the Petri dish some particular molecules she assumes have been produced by bacteria with a probability of 0.8, and by viruses with a probability of 0.2. On this account, she argues that to the extent 0.8 the specimen a in the Petri dish is a member of the class of bacterial producers. That is, $\mu_{bacterial\text{-}producer}(a) = 0.8$. The predicate "bacterial producer" is a causal predicate of microbiological language. She thus concludes, on the basis of the above definitions, that to the extent 0.8 there exist bacteria in the Petri dish.

Suppose the so-called *world* is a large Petri dish. Then an ontologist may, like in our example above, speculate "on what there is to some extent" in that extended Petri dish. By so doing, she becomes able to do fuzzy ontology by asking whether an object exists:

to the extent 0	($\equiv$ total non-existence)
to the extent 1	($\equiv$ total existence)
to an extent greater than 0 and less than 1	($\equiv$ partial existence).

The basic idea of our fuzzy ontology is the tenet that being does not accord with Hamlet's bivalent soliloquy "to be or not to be: that is the question". Rather, it is a matter of degree consisting in the extent of the causal entrenchment of an entity in a world. The transition from being to non-being and vice versa is gradual rather than abrupt. In a more general sense, Heraclitus of Ephesus (≈ 535–475 BC) once contended that $\Pi \acute{\alpha} \nu \tau \alpha$ $\rho \varepsilon \iota$, "everything flows". We may therefore call the fuzzy existence operator that we have introduced, $\varepsilon_{\mathcal{L}}(x)$, the *Heraclitean operator*. Its message is that everything exists to an extent $r \leq 1$. If relative to a language $\mathcal{L}$ this extent r equals 1, then to the extent 1 the entity exists with respect to that language. If relative to $\mathcal{L}$ the extent r equals 0, then the entity does not exist with respect to language $\mathcal{L}$. However, it may exist with respect to another language $\mathcal{L}'$. That means, first, that a language induces a specific ontology, and second, that it has now become possible to conduct fuzzy ontology by employing linguistic variables. For instance, let the infinite-valued existence of an entity be characterized by the linguistic variable *Existence_State*. To this variable may be assigned a term set, $T(Existence\_State)$, such as the following one:

$$T(Existence\_State) = \{\text{weak, very weak, medium, strong, fairly strong,}$$
$$\text{very strong, existent, non-existent, } \dots \text{ etc. } \dots \}.$$

We are obviously justified in saying, e.g., that *Existence_State*(Sherlock Holmes) = non-existent, while the bacteriologist above may assert that *Existence_State*(bacteria in this Petri dish) = strong; and you may be convinced that *Existence_State*(present book) = existent. See Figure 84.

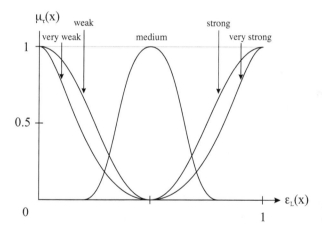

Fig. 84. Each element τ of the term set $T(Existence\_State)$ denotes a fuzzy set over the base set of the numerical existence degrees, $\varepsilon_{\mathcal{L}}(x)$. The figure tentatively illustrates the following fuzzy sets: very weak existence, weak existence, medium existence, strong existence, very strong existence

Now that we have the Heraclitean operator $\varepsilon_{\mathcal{L}}(x)$ at our disposal, we can apply all fuzzy set operations to both being and non-being. For example, if $\varepsilon_{\mathcal{L}}(x) = r$, then relative to language $\mathcal{L}$ the entity x does not exist to the extent $1 - r$. That is, an object may exist and fail to exist at the same time. "To be *and* not to be: that is the solution" for Hamlet's question. Going back to the basic operator $\varepsilon_{\mathcal{PL}}$, let P and Q be two different causal predicates of a language $\mathcal{L}$. An interesting finding is that due to the relationship:

$$\varepsilon_{\mathcal{PL} \cup \mathcal{QL}}(x) = max(\varepsilon_{\mathcal{PL}}(x), \varepsilon_{\mathcal{QL}}(x))$$

which holds between all causal predicates of language $\mathcal{L}$, the degree of existence of an object x relative to the whole of a language $\mathcal{L}$ equals the maximum degree of its existence relative to all causal predicates of $\mathcal{L}$. This is the reason why in Definition 175 we used the operator max to define the predicate-free Heraclitean operator $\varepsilon_{\mathcal{L}}(x)$. That is, when we know that something certainly exists, e.g., the Eiffel Tower, and therefore attach to it 1 as the degree of its existence, this extent will not be affected if relative to a particular causal predicate it exists to a lesser extent than 1. Thus, the traditional, crisp, pure ontology is preserved in our fuzzy pure ontology. An additional stimulating result is also worth mentioning. Let P be a causal predicate of language $\mathcal{L}_1$ and let Q be a causal predicate of another language $\mathcal{L}_2$. Then a bilingual person accomplished in both languages will be able to argue in the following way to what extent an object x exists relative to both languages:

$$\varepsilon_{\mathcal{PL}_1 \cap \mathcal{QL}_2}(x) = min(\varepsilon_{\mathcal{PL}_1}(x), \varepsilon_{\mathcal{QL}_2}(x)).$$

By means of graded, partial existence, comparative ontology also becomes possible. For instance, relative to the English language an entity x exists more, or stronger, than an entity y if $\varepsilon_{English}(x) > \varepsilon_{English}(y)$. Our considerations above demonstrate how ontology, and thus the world, becomes enriched by fuzzy logic.

A language may be associated with different logics. For example, English may be used in association with classical logic, or paraconsistent logic, or fuzzy logic, etc. Let $\mathcal{L}_i \cup L_j$ be a language $\mathcal{L}_i$ with an associated logic L_j, e.g., "English and classical logic", "German and paraconsistent logic", or "Chinese and fuzzy logic". A language with its associated logic seems to create a specific world of its own. Comparable to gravitation fields, it induces ontic fields, an ontic field being a world with the specific ensemble of its entities. To different languages and logics correspond different ontic fields such that if w_1 is the ontic field created by $\mathcal{L}_i \cup L_j$, and w_2 is the ontic field created by $\mathcal{L}_k \cup L_m$, then $w_1 \neq w_2$ if $\mathcal{L}_i \neq \mathcal{L}_k$ or $L_j \neq L_m$. Again, "Change your language or logic, and you will see another world" (Sadegh-Zadeh, 1982a, 171).

In his John Dewey Lectures presented in March 1968 at Columbia University, Quine analyzed the linguistic relativity of reference that he called *ontological relativity* (Quine, 1969a). Note that our theory of the relativity of existence suggested above is something different than Quine's ontological relativity, the most salient difference being that his theory is a semantic, while ours is a genuinely ontological framework.

18.3 Vague, Fictional, and Non-Existent Entities

There is an ongoing controversial debate about whether medical entities such as diseases and psychosomatic relationships and disorders really exist or are only fictitious. This issues will be addressed below. First, however, we shall need the basic terminology introduced in the following three sections:

18.3.1   Vague Entities
18.3.2   Fictional Entities
18.3.3   Non-Existent Entities.

18.3.1 Vague Entities

The objects we usually deal with in everyday life, which we commonly suppose exist and have definite boundaries, we refer to as standard or ordinary entities. Example are the book in front of you, square figures, and the Eiffel Tower in Paris. They belong to the extensions of *clear-cut terms,* discussed on page 35.

There are also entities, however, whose existence is uncertain or whose location, size, or boundaries cannot be definitely determined. As an example, consider the Pacific Ocean and an island therein, e.g., Hawaii. What exactly is the area occupied by the ocean? And what exactly is the area occupied by the island? Because the water fluctuates at the borders, both areas expand and shrink by turns such that it is impossible to determine their borderlines definitely. Both are vague objects. It is worth noting that this vagueness is to a great extent a permanent aspect of the circumstances, for it is an effect of tidal forces of the moon and sun, of climatic forces, and other cosmic factors.

The result above also holds for most of what are usually considered ordinary entities . For example, as mentioned on page 44, a frog is not a clear-cut, but a vague animal because it is impossible to determine when it emerges from a tadpole. There is no clear end to being a tadpole and no clear beginning to being a frog. Similarly, the human organism is a vague entity. Its external boundaries, i.e., the boundaries between the organism and external environment, as well as its internal boundaries, i.e., the boundaries between the organism and its internal environment in the bowels, are blurred. The same applies to human beings as both living things and persons. We don't know when an individual human being begins or ceases to exist as a living human organism. Nor do we know when her personhood begins or ceases to exist. All these entities are characterized by ontic indefiniteness as discussed on page 44.

One might take the position that it is not the objects, but the terms denoting them which are vague. However, this objection is misguided. Although it is true that many linguistic expressions such as "human being", "person", and "disease" arc in need of clarification and should be made precise, it is equally true that not all expressions can successfully be made precise. Try, for example, to make fuzzy terms such as "tall" and "young" precise. Of course, this is in principle possible by transforming them into quantitative terms such as "height measured in centimeters" and "age measured in years, months, etc.". However, saying that someone is 190.23 cm high or that she is 20 years and 11 seconds old is not the same as saying that she is tall or she is young, respectively. In addition, without measuring the precise height of someone and without possessing precise knowledge about her birth date we cannot say any-thing quantitative about her height and age, whereas we can directly *see* that she is tall or young. Coping with such vagueness is a normal part of human life; it is not advisable to reduce our ordinary perceptions to the Heisenberg Uncertainty level (Heisenberg, 1958). Thus, precision and vagueness must be judged from a pragmatic point of view. This is the wisdom behind Zadeh's *Principle of Incompatibility,* discussed on page 607.

18.3.2 Fictional Entities

Fictional entities are those objects featured in works of fiction such as stories, plays, operas, myths, and legends. In this section, the ontological status of these entities will be considered, as there is a surprising similarity between medical entities such as diseases and genes, on the one hand; and fictional entities such as Sherlock Holmes, Pegasus, and Superman, on the other.

The term "fiction" derives from the Latin *fingere* meaning "to form" and "to construct". A fictional entity is one created by an author in an explicit fiction. It may be a fictional object, a fictional character, a fictional event, and the like. Examples are Hamlet created by William Shakespeare (1564–1616), Sherlock Holmes created by the Scottish physician Arthur Conan Doyle (1859–1930), and the Nautilus, a fictional submarine featured by Jules Verne (1828–1905). Fictional entities, sometimes also called fictitious or imaginary entities, are to be distinguished from non-existent entities. The question of whether they exist is controversial. For details on the metaphysics of fictional entities, see (Thomasson, 1999; Everett and Hofweber, 2000; van Inwagen, 2005; Woods, 2007; Priest, 2007; Sainsbury, 2010).

We saw previously that it is not easy to deny the existence of a fictional entity such as the fictional character Sherlock Holmes. He is known to be a detective in the detective stories of Arthur Conan Doyle. The statement "Sherlock Holmes is a detective" classical-logically implies "there is someone who is a detective". To avoid such consequences one would either have to change the logic or invent a method that enables us to distinguish between those names that denote fictional entities and those denoting "real" entities. But this just refocuses the problem: what does "real" mean?

A fictional entity is brought into existence at a certain time and may cease to exist at a later point in time. As an abstract, cultural artifact it is an actually existent entity like any other artifact from furniture to sculpture. However, the existence of a fictional entity such as Sherlock Holmes differs from that of natural human beings in that it is a dependent one. If all human beings cease to exist, the fictional entity also will die, just as a language dies out when it is no longer used and understood.

Nevertheless, there is a problem with the claim that fictional entities actu-ally exist. We are told, for example, that Sherlock Holmes's place of residence is 221B Baker Street in London. If this is true of Sherlock Holmes, is it also true of London? Does London have the property of having Sherlock Holmes among its residents? A thorough examination of Baker Street would show no trace of Sherlock Holmes (Routley, 1981, 563). There is thus a break between the being of a fictional entity and *this* world where we live. To cast the break in a clear criterion, we will advance a modal approach to ontology which we shall later use in our ontology of disease and other medical entities. Specifically, a distinction will be made between two modalities of existence: existence *de dicto* versus existence *de re*. Similar approaches are to be found in (Routley, 1981, 569; Woods, 2007, 1072).[135]

We explained the difference between *de dicto* and *de re* modalities in Chapter 27, discussed several types of them, and demonstrated the general method of how to syntactically distinguish between de dicto and de re. As an analog of those modalities, we will introduce a new modality of *asserted truth*, which we will represent by the following binary assertion operator (for the unary assertion operator "it is asserted that ...", see page 911):

- It is asserted in story S that α or equivalently:
- It holds in story S that α or equivalently:
- According to story S it is true that α

symbolized by:

$$\mathcal{A}(S, \alpha)$$

where $\mathcal{A}$ connotes "it is asserted in"; S is any story, text, context, etc.; and α is any sentence of arbitrary complexity describing a state of affairs. A simple example is:

It is asserted in Shakespeare's Hamlet that Hamlet is the Prince of Denmark.

That is:

$\mathcal{A}$(Shakespeare's Hamlet, Hamlet is the Prince of Denmark).

For notational convenience, the binary operator above will be transformed into a pseudo-unary one by attaching the story variable S to it as a subscript and writing $\mathcal{A}_S$ such that instead of $\mathcal{A}(S, \alpha)$ we may conveniently write:

$$\mathcal{A}_S(\alpha)$$

or simply:

$$\mathcal{A}_S\alpha.$$

For instance:

---

[135] The inspiration for introducing the assertion operator below and the differentiation between existence *de dicto* and existence *de re* came from John Woods (2007, 1072 ff.).

$\mathcal{A}_{Shakespeare's-Hamlet}$(Hamlet is the Prince of Denmark).

Consider now the following two sentences (for the definition of "de dicto" and "de re", see page 925):

de dicto: It is asserted in Arthur Conan Doyle's story *A Study in Scarlet* that there is someone called Sherlock Holmes who is a detective and his place of residence is 221B Baker Street in London.

de re: There is someone of whom it is asserted in Arthur Conan Doyle's story *A Study in Scarlet* that he is called Sherlock Holmes and is a detective and his place of residence is 221B Baker Street in London.

The first sentence is an assertion of existence *de dicto* and the second one is an assertion of existence *de re*. They are completely different. This becomes obvious by formalizing them. Let the subscript S in the operator $\mathcal{A}_S$ denote Arthur Conan Doyle's story *A Study in Scarlet*, then we have:

de dicto: $\mathcal{A}_S \exists x(x = \text{Sherlock Holmes} \land x \text{ is a detective} \land x\text{'s}$ (174)
place of residence is 221B Baker Street in London).

de re: $\exists x \mathcal{A}_S(x = \text{Sherlock Holmes} \land x \text{ is a detective} \land x\text{'s}$ (175)
place of residence is 221B Baker Street in London).

In a *de dicto* existence sentence such as (174) that is of the general form $\mathcal{A}_S \exists x \alpha$, the modal operator $\mathcal{A}_S$ precedes the existential quantifier, whereas in a *de re* existence sentence such as (175) that is of the general form $\exists x \mathcal{A}_S \alpha$, the modal operator $\mathcal{A}_S$ lies in the scope of the existential quantifier to the effect that *quantifying in* occurs. For the notion of quantifying in, see page 926. We know from Chapter 27 that the two statements above, (174) and (175), are not equivalent.

The claim that a particular fictional entity actually exists, is an existence claim de re. Whoever denies the actual existence of that fictional entity, however, affirms the de dicto existence sentence. Thus, ontological affirmation and denial of fictional entities correspond to de dicto and de re existence, respectively. We shall come back to this issue in Section 19.6 on page 753 when we look into whether medical entities such as diseases, genes, and similar things actually exist or whether they are fictional.

18.3.3 Non-Existent Entities

It is usually said that impossible objects do not exist. However, as we saw in Section 6.3.4, there exist some contradictory states of health and illness, although they are deemed impossible and thus non-existent.

If asked whether there are non-existent entities, one would presumably accuse the questioner of not understanding her own question. For the term "non-existent entities" obviously denotes non-existents and thus seems to imply that they do not exist. But it is not that easy. Maybe they do:

A non-existent entity need not be a mythical object such as the winged horse Pegasus in Greek mythology; or Vulcan, the Roman god of fire and volcanoes in Roman mythology. We are frequently told that many other objects also do not exist, for example, round squares and even prime numbers beyond 2. Hence, *there are* entities that do not exist, e.g., round squares, even prime numbers beyond 2, Pegasus, Vulcan, and many others. This seeming paradox originated with the Austrian psychologist and philosopher Alexius Meinong (1853–1920). He developed a highly original, speculative, and controversial ontology that he called the *theory of objects* (Meinong, 1904). According to his theory, "There are objects of which it is true that there are no such objects". Some instances have been mentioned above, i.e., {Pegasus, Vulcan, round squares, even prime numbers beyond 2, etc. ...}. Every such object may be referred to and described nonetheless. For example, something is a round square if it is round and if it is square. If it is round, it is not square. Thus, it is square and it is not square, a contradictory object. We will not here go into the details of Meinong's ontology. Suffice it to note that it contributed to the development of an interesting logic of non-existent objects which may be useful in ontological inquiries, especially in the ontology of fictional entities (Parsons, 1980; Perszyk, 1993; Jacquette, 1996).[136]

A Meinongian object is anything that might be the object of our thought. Thus, the category of Meinongian objects includes both existent and nonexistent entities. Among the latter, two types of entities deserve particular attention, first, the so-called impossible entities; and second, the incomplete entities (da Costa et al., 1991, 121):

An *impossible object* is one that violates the classical Law or Principle of Non-Contradiction $\neg(\alpha \wedge \neg\alpha)$, e.g., a round square. It is worth noting, however, that impossibility is relative to logics. For instance, something that is impossible with respect to classical logic need not be impossible with respect to paraconsistent logic because in the latter logic contradictions are permitted. For this reason, a paraconsistent world is much richer than a classical-logical world and contains more existents.

An *incomplete object* is one that violates the classical Law or Principle of Excluded Middle $\alpha \vee \neg\alpha$. For example, Sherlock Holmes is an incomplete

---

[136] The paradox of non-existence was noted by David Hume. According to him, the paradox arises because to think of an object is subjectively the same as to think of an existent object. This brings with it that a non-existent entity is thought of as if it were existent (Hume, 2000, Book 1, Part 2, Section 6). The Humean idea led to Immanuel Kant's denial of existence as a predicate, which we referred to on page 690. If being existent is not considered a predicate, being non-existent cannot be considered either. Thus, one cannot talk of the class of non-existents to postulate of its elements that "they are ..." giving rise to a paradox thereby.

object because it is not the case that he speaks Papiamentu or doesn't do so. The latter assertion is true because we simply do not, and will never be able to, know whether he does or does not speak Papiamentu.

18.4 Summary

We discussed the basic question of ontology, identified seven different meanings of "is", and two meanings of "exists". To do justice to common sense, we introduced an *existence predicate* in terms of causal entrenchment. The main ontological positions were briefly outlined: nominalism, Platonism, tropism, ontological realism and anti-realism. After distinguishing between pure and applied ontology, we made a first attempt toward a fuzzy ontology, which enables us to talk about partial being. To this end, we fuzzified the existence predicate to introduce grades of being. This approach seems to open up promising and novel ontological perspectives and may eventually lead to a general theory of the relativity of existence. Finally, vague, non-existent, and fictional entities were briefly considered with the latter being the reason for distinguishing between ontology *de re* and ontology *de dicto*. This interesting and useful method may allow us to settle many ontological debates in medicine which appear to be unresolvable in traditional ways.

Medical Ontology

19.0 Introduction

Due to the intricate nature of its subject matter, medicine is always threatened by speculations and disagreements about which among its entities exist, e.g., any specific biological structures, substructures or substances, pathogenic agents, pathophysiological processes, diseases, psychosomatic relationships, therapeutic effects, and other possible and impossible things. To avoid confusion, and to determine what entities an item of medical knowledge presupposes to exist if it is to be true, we need medical ontology. The term "medical ontology" we understand to mean the study that seeks to ascertain what entities exist in the *world of medicine*, which formal relations hold between them, and whether there are any relatioships between types of medical research and practice, on the one hand; and the new worlds they create, on the other.

According to the terminology introduced in Section 18.1 on page 687, medical ontology is to be considered an applied or domain ontology. As yet no such discipline and systematic research has been established. Although physicians and medical researchers have always been unsystematically concerned with ontological problems associated with their work, only recently have first attempts been made toward an "advertisement for the ontology for medicine" (Simon, 2010). To separate the wheat from the chaff in this endeavor requires some methodological rigor. In what follows, we shall exemplify some central medical-ontological issues to show how research in this field may productively move forward, and to discuss some relationships between medical ontology and epistemology. Our discussion divides into the following six sections:

19.1 The Ontology of Medical Knowledge
19.2 Clinical Ontology
19.3 The Ontology of Psychiatry and Psychosomatics
19.4 Biomedical Ontology Engineering
19.5 Formal Medical Ontology
19.6 Medical Ontology *de re* and *de dicto*.

K. Sadegh-Zadeh, *Handbook of Analytic Philosophy of Medicine*,
Philosophy and Medicine 113, DOI 10.1007/978-94-007-2260-6_19,
© Springer Science+Business Media B.V. 2012

19.1 The Ontology of Medical Knowledge

Among the infinitely many possible worlds there is one which is the subject of medicine. This possible world we call *the world of medicine*. The world of medicine is identified by doing ontology of medical knowledge. What an item of medical knowledge such as a clinical statement or hypothesis presupposes to exist in the world of medicine if it is to be true, is referred to as its *ontological commitment*. In order to find out what the world of medicine looks like, medical ontology will be advanced as a study of the ontological commitments of medical knowledge in the following three sections:

> 19.1.1 Ontological Commitments of Medical Knowledge
> 19.1.2 Medically Relevant Ontological Categories
> 19.1.3 Models for Medical Knowledge.

We should therefore state at the outset what we understand by the term "ontological commitment" (Quine, 1948).

19.1.1 Ontological Commitments of Medical Knowledge

An item of knowledge is presumed, and used, to transmit some information. For example, a medical statement such as "AIDS is caused by HIV" informs us about how a human individual becomes afflicted with AIDS. In order for such a statement to be true, some truth conditions need to be fulfilled. Specifically, the world of medicine must include some objects with some properties and relations such that they make the statement true. Regarding our present example, there must be human beings as well as particular viruses called HIV such that if viruses of this type infect a human being, then she develops AIDS. Thus, the sentence as an assertion implicitly imposes some demands on the world. It demands that the following entities exist:

1. Human beings,
2. HIV,
3. the infection of a human being with HIV at a particular time,
4. the disease state AIDS that an HIV-infected individual develops at a later time.

As far as such requirements of an item of knowledge are existence assumptions, like in the present example, they are referred to as its *ontological commitment*. An ontological analysis of that knowledge, then, requires no metaphysical speculations. It simply consists in making explicit the implicit ontological commitment of that item of knowledge. This is achieved by analyzing its conceptual structure to lay bare its descriptive vocabulary and to answer the following two questions:

- What individual signs, i.e., individual constants and variables, does that knowledge contain?

- what n-ary predicates, and possibly functions, does it contain?

Its individual signs reveal what individual objects it refers to, while its predicates and functions further specify sets of these objects and the relations between them. The conceptual structure of an item of knowledge can best be analyzed by formalizing it. To elucidate, we will in a simplified way formalize our example "AIDS is caused by HIV" to make explicit its ontological commitment. The statement has the following structure of a generalized temporal conditional. For the translation of the predicate "causes" into a generalized temporal conditional, see Section 6.5.2 on page 226:

"AIDS is caused by HIV" means:
- For all x, for all y, for all t_1, for all t_2:

IF	1.	x is a bunch of HIV and
	2.	y is a human being and
	3.	t_1 and t_2 are points in time such that t_2 is later than t_1 and
	4.	x at time t_1 infects y
THEN	5.	there is a state z of y such that: z is AIDS and y at time t_2 develops z.

The sentence does not contain individual constants. That is, it does not refer to particular individuals such as the patient Elroy Fox or the Eiffel Tower. It contains the individual variables x, y, z, t_1 and t_2, and the predicates listed in Table 25.

Table 25. The descriptive vocabulary of, i.e., the individual signs and the predicates contained in, the sentence "AIDS is caused by HIV", and the entities whose existence it presupposes when it is to be a true statement

Predicate:	symbolized by:	arity:	denotation:
x is a bunch of HIV	$\mathrm{HIV}(x)$	unary	a set of HIV
y is a human being	$\mathrm{HUMAN}(y)$	unary	a set of human beings
t is a time point	$\mathrm{T}(t)$	unary	a set of time points
t_2 is later than t_1	$\mathrm{LATER}(t_2, t_1)$	binary	an ordered set of time points
x at t_1 infects y	$\mathrm{INFECTS}(x, t_1, y)$	ternary	an ordered set of viruses, time points, and infected human beings
z is a state of y's organism	$\mathrm{STATE\_OF\_}$ $\mathrm{ORGANISM}(z, y)$	binary	a set of states of the human organism
z is AIDS	$\mathrm{AIDS}(z)$	unary	a set of disease states
y at t_2 develops z	$\mathrm{DEVELOPS}(y, t_2, z)$	ternary	an ordered set of human beings with time points and states

The statement is of the following deep structure:

- $\forall x \forall y \forall t_1 \forall t_2 \big(\text{HIV}(x) \wedge \text{HUMAN}(y) \wedge T(t_1) \wedge T(t_2) \wedge \text{LATER}(t_2, t_1) \wedge$
  $\text{INFECTS}(x, t_1, y) \rightarrow \exists z \big(\text{STATE\_OF\_ORGANISM}(z, y) \wedge \text{AIDS}(z) \wedge$
  $\text{DEVELOPS}(y, t_2, z) \big) \big).$

The above analysis shows that:

- the individual variable x ranges over the set HIV,
- the individual variable y ranges over the set HUMAN,
- the individual variable z ranges over the set STATES_OF_ORGANISM including AIDS states,
- t_1 and t_2 range over the set T of time points linearly ordered by the relation later-than, written LATER,
- $\langle x, t_1, y \rangle$ ranges over the Cartesian product HIV $\times$ HUMAN $\times T$ (i.e., INFECTS),
- $\langle y, t_2, z \rangle$ ranges over the Cartesian product HUMAN $\times T \times$ STATES_OF_ORGANISM (i.e., DEVELOPS AIDS).

It is obvious that the truth or empirical significance of the seemingly simple statement "AIDS is caused by HIV" is committed to the existence of a number of entities, which are listed in the right-hand column of Table 25 above as the denotations of its predicates and the domains of its individual variables. The entities are a set of particular viruses, a set of human beings, a set of states of their organisms, a set of linearly ordered time points, a set of HIV-infected human beings, and a set of diseased human beings who have AIDS. Putting them all together, the ontological commitment of the sentence is the following structure:

⟨HIV, HUMAN, STATES_OF_ORGANISM, T, LATER, INFECTS,
AIDS_STATES, DEVELOPS⟩.

It is this structure in which the sentence "AIDS is caused by HIV" is to be interpreted to determine whether it is true. As outlined on page 886, a structure that makes a sentence true is said to be a *model* for that sentence. By analyzing our example sentence above and revealing its model, we did a bit of medical ontology to show what entities need to exist as preconditions of the truth of the sentence. However, we didn't delve deeply enough to ask whether the constituents of the model, e.g., HIV and AIDS states, "really exist" or are mere conceptual constructions of medicine. We shall come back to this core issue later on.

19.1.2 Medically Relevant Ontological Categories

In asking questions of the type just posed, which help determine the ontological status of a medical entity such as HIV, AIDS, dissociative identity disorder, gene, recovery, and the like, it is an advantage if one knows under what ontological category that entity falls.

What is an ontological category? Simply put, it is a most general class of entities that in the ontological taxonomy of all existents is not subordinate to another class of higher order. The term originated with Aristotle. With his work *Categories*, he founded the theory of ontological categories, postulating the following ten as the fundamental categories that constitute the world: substance, quantity, quality, relation, place, date, posture, state, action, and being acted upon. Since this early work, there has been no general agreement among philosophers about what kinds of entities count as the fundamental constituents of the world. We will not here participate in this speculative debate (Aristotle, 1963; Ackrill, 1963; Grossmann, 1983; Chisholm, 1996]).[137]

An ideal ontological categorization in terms of ordinary taxonomy of entities requires that the categories be exhaustive and mutually exclusive. Without going into details, it may be noted that the formal logic and ontology of the twentieth century superceded the above-mentioned ten Aristotelean categories by revealing that the following two categories are sufficient to reconstruct the ontology of all human knowledge and theorizing: *individual objects* and *sets*, i.e. classes, the latter of which also includes relations – and functions – as subsets of their Cartesian products. However, due to the fuzziness of real-world categories their ontological taxonomy may not be ideally feasible (see Section 19.4 on page 735).

In doing medical ontology, individual signs, predicates, and functions are sufficient to analyze the ontological commitment of medical knowledge. Thus, 'the world' needs to include only their extensions as categories, i.e., individual objects and classes. This was demonstrated by the analysis of our example "AIDS is caused by HIV" in the preceding section. Entia non sunt multiplicanda praeter necessitatem (see footnote 132 on page 695).

19.1.3 Models for Medical Knowledge

What is referred to in philosophy as the *ontological commitment* of an item of knowledge, is simply what is known in logic sciences as the *model* for that knowledge. In order for a statement to be true, it must have a model. As discussed on page 886, a model for an item of knowledge is a generalized relational structure $\langle \Omega_1, \ldots, \Omega_m; R_1, \ldots, R_n; a_1, \ldots, a_p \rangle$ such that $\Omega_1, \ldots, \Omega_m$ are $m \geq 1$ sets of objects called its domains or universes of discourse;

---

[137] There are proponents of the Aristotelean categories still today. The posthumous compilers of his works have erroneously included his highly speculative treatise *Categories* in his book on logic, *Organon*, although it does not deal with logic. This random act of compiling "has ensured that it has been discussed in almost every textbook of logic until very recent times [...] and has had considerable influence on logic, and that not entirely good" (Kneale and Kneale, 1968, 25). This disadvantageous influence is being revived in current biomedicine. For example, see (Jansen and Smith, 2008).

$R_1, \ldots, R_n$ are $n \geq 1$ subsets, i.e., relations or functions, over those domains or their Cartesian products; and $a_1, \ldots, a_p$ are $p \geq 0$ particular individual objects originating from those domains. An example is provided by the following relational structure (176):

$$\langle \text{HIV, HUMAN, STATES\_OF\_ORGANISM, } T, \text{ LATER, INFECTS,} \qquad (176)$$
$$\text{AIDS\_STATES, DEVELOPS} \rangle$$

presented on pages 714 as a model for the statement "AIDS is caused by HIV". Seen from this perspective, what is called *model theory* in logic and mathematics is in fact mathematical ontology, i.e., ontology of mathematical sciences. See, for instance (Hodges, 2008; Bell and Slomson, 2006).

It is conceivable, and to be hoped as well, that the first steps we are here taking will contribute to the emergence of a sophisticated medical ontology in analogy to mathematical model theory. In such a *medical model theory,* relationships between models of different items of medical knowledge, including theories, could be precisely analyzed. Consider, for instance, the relationship that exists between the model (176) above of "AIDS is caused by HIV" and the following structure:

$$\langle \text{HIV, HUMAN, STATES\_OF\_ORGANISM, } T, \text{ LATER, INFECTS} \rangle. \qquad (177)$$

It is obvious that the structure (177) is a subset of the model (176) above and provides a model for any group of "human beings who are infected with HIV" without any sign of manifest AIDS. It is not yet clear whether or not these HIV-infected people will develop AIDS at a later point in time. Maybe they will do so. In that case, the structure (177) will be extendible to a model such as (176). Thus, the structure (177) is a *potential model* for "AIDS is caused by HIV". We anticipated this terminology in Section 9.4.2. This further demonstrates the close ties between ontology and epistemology.

19.2 Clinical Ontology

Our subject in this section is not the ontology of clinical knowledge in general, as we employed this type of ontology in preceding sections. In the discussion that follows, we shall instead look at the ontology that is central to clinical medicine – the ontology of nosology or 'nosological ontology'.

There was a time when suffering human beings were diagnosed with diseases such as cacochymia, leucophlegmatia, dyscrasia, or melancholia. Doctors today do not learn about such diseases. Yet they were, among many others, diseases in the conceptual system of medicine that up until the eighteenth century was based on the theory of humoral pathology. See, e.g., (Blancard, 1756, 172 and 558). The question is whether they continue to exist. The answer is that of course they don't. The theory of cellular pathology, being one of the basic theories of current medicine, succeeded humoral pathology in the 1850s and does not contain such nosological predicates or equivalents thereof. Obviously, diseases can simply die out when the conceptual system of medicine within which they are considered diseases, is displaced, in a Kuhnean fashion, by another conceptual system or disciplinary matrix. As mentioned in Section 11.3.4 on page 494, similar nosological revolutions have frequently occurred during the history of medicine. They may serve as warnings to those new to the ontology of medicine who, overlooking such evidence, proclaim the existence of everything that a physician, a medical researcher, or a medical community talks about and gives names to such as "Morbus meus". We encounter this type of naïve realism in the so-called biomedical ontology engineering, which we shall discuss in Section 19.4 below.

Another extreme is a standpoint that we termed *fictionalism* and outlined on page 150. Nosological fictionalists are skeptics. They plainly deny that there are any diseases. A well-known representative is Richard Koch, a German physician and historian of medicine in the early twentieth century, who said that "the concept of disease is a fiction. In diagnosing a disease, a fictitious entity is recognized. In contrast to its constituents, a disease is a genuine fiction" (Richard Koch, 1920, pp. 130–131).

In addition to *naïve nosological realism* and the *nosological skepticism* mentioned above, we also encounter *nosological relativism* in medicine which says that diseases are relative to conceptual systems. We touched upon such issues of disease ontology on several occasions in previous chapters.

When an entity such as AIDS or computer game addiction is added to the nosological system of medicine as a new disease, or another disease such as drapetomania, hysteria, or neurasthenia is declared non-existent and its name is discarded from the nosological system, the question arises what it means to say that (i) a disease exists or does not exist. The same question applies to (ii) symptoms, complaints, signs, and findings through which diseases are defined, described, classified, and diagnosed. What does it mean, for instance, to say that there exists a symptom such as icterus, leucocytosis, headache, or delusion? Other ontologically relevant entities in clinical medicine are (iii) processes, e.g., pathological processes which are supposed to occur between two stages A and B in the development of a disease, or recovery processes. What does it mean to say that specific processes such as the pathogenesis of Alzheimer's disease or that of bronchial carcinoma exist? To address such clinical-ontological issues, we will use disease ontology as an example.

The use of unrefined natural language in medicine brings with it an ambiguous disease ontology that originates from sloppy abstract statements such as "Acute myocardial infarction causes elevation of the concentration of the enzyme CK in blood ... and so on". Statements of this type do not betray the ontological category to which an entity such as "acute myocardial infarction" is supposed to belong. Is it a property of *individuals* or does it exist as something independent of individuals, e.g., as a *class?* In the discussions below, we shall therefore have to differentiate between at least the following nosological ontologies, or *disease ontologies*, which we will look at in turn:

19.2.1 Disease Nominalism

The French physician Armand Trousseau (1801–1867) is attributed a famous slogan that says "there are no diseases, there are only sick people". This somewhat cryptic ontological position seems convincing at first glance and has many advocates. According to it, there are only individual patients. Diseases do not exist. This is the core postulate of a position in disease ontology which we shall refer to as disease nominalism.

In line with the general concept of nominalism discussed on page 694, disease nominalism is the view according to which only individual human beings who have a disease D, e.g. 'diabetes mellitus', exist. The disease D itself as an abstract entity does not exist. This ontological thesis and its meaning and consequences are analyzed in the present section.

When introducing the notion of medical ontology on pages 711–712 above, we pointed out that the ontological analysis of an item of medical knowledge requires the dissection of its conceptual structure to reveal its ontological commitment. As an example in disease ontology we will examine the following item of clinical knowledge about a particular disease, i.e., myocardial infarction:

> In human beings with acute myocardial infarction, the concentration of the enzyme CK (i.e., creatin kinase, also called creatin phosphokinase, CPK) in their blood is elevated. But CK is not specific for acute myocardial infarction because it is also elevated when skeletal muscle is damaged or destroyed. It has three different fractions: CK_MM, CK_BB, and CK_MB (MB = muscle-brain type). The fraction CK_MB rises in their blood within 2 to 8 hours of onset of acute myocardial infarction and is highly specific. It is therefore a very good marker for acute myocardial infarction. A useful indicator for acute myocardial infarction is the so-called cardiac index. This is the ratio of total CK to CK_MB and is a sensitive indicator of acute myocardial infarction when CK_MB is elevated.

We need not formalize all of these statements in detail. Only their following core will be considered to determine their ontological commitment:

> In human beings with acute myocardial infarction, the concentration of the enzyme CK in their blood is elevated. While CK is not specific for acute myocardial infarction, its fraction CK_MB is highly specific (for the notion of specificity, see Definition 49 on page 199).

Formulated a bit more clearly, these statements say:

1. If an object x is a human being and has acute myocardial infarction, then it has elevated CK. (178)

2. The probability that a human being with no acute myocardial infarction has no elevated CK, is low (i.e., "elevated CK is not specific for acute myocardial infarction": See Definition 49 on page 199).

3. The probability that a human being with no acute myocardial infarction has no elevated CK_MB, is high (i.e., "elevated CK_MB is highly specific for acute myocardial infarction").

These core statements of our example contain the following predicates and functions:

- is a human being   symbolized by: H
- has acute myocardial infarction   AMI
- has *ele*vated CK   ELCK
- has *ele*vated CK_MB   ELCK_MB
- probability as a linguistic variable p

and are of the following form:

1. $\forall x (Hx \wedge AMIx \rightarrow ELCKx)$ (179)

2. $p(\overline{ELCK} \mid H \cap \overline{AMI}) = low$

3. $p(\overline{ELCK\_MB} \mid H \cap \overline{AMI}) = high.$

Here, a symbol $\overline{X}$ signifies the complement of a set X. To represent the qualitative notion of specificity that is used in the original characterization of the disease AMI above, we have used the methodological probability function p as a linguistic variable with values such as {low, medium. high, ... etc. ...}. It will not be further considered here. The ontologist has the freedom to interpret the predicates intensionally or extensionally. In the former case, they designate properties which an individual may have. We prefer to consider the predicates extensionally. According to the formalized version (179) of our clinical knowledge given in (178), this knowledge is concerned with the following predicates and their denotations:

- H   denotes: the set of human beings,
- AMI   a subset of H with acute myocardial infarction,
- $\overline{AMI}$ a subset of II without acute myocardial infarction,
- ELCK   a subset of H with elevated CK,
- $\overline{ELCK}$ a subset of H without elevated CK,
- ELCK_MB   a subset of H with elevated CK_MB
- $\overline{ELCK\_MB}$ a subset of H without elevated CK_MB.

Obviously, the cardiological knowledge quoted above presupposes that in the world of medicine, seven types of *individual* objects exist respectively belonging to the seven sets listed above. Thus, the ontological commitment of, or model for, that knowledge is the following structure:

$$\langle H, AMI, \overline{AMI}, ELCK, \overline{ELCK}, ELCK\_MB, \overline{ELCK\_MB}\rangle. \tag{180}$$

The focus of our present interest is the question of what it means to say that the disease *acute myocardial infarction,* AMI, exists. By virtue of our reformulation (179) above, this ontological question reduces to the question whether there are individual human beings who constitute the set AMI, i.e., the set of those who have acute myocardial infarction. Do such individuals exist or not? In order to answer this question, we must know *how* the nosological predicate AMI, i.e., "acute myocardial infarction", is defined. Thus, the affirmation as well as the denial of the existence of a particular disease D presuppose that:

1. we have a *nosological predicate P* whose denotation is the disease D and
2. we have a *definition* of that predicate at our disposal.

Whenever these two conditions are satisfied, the disease D exists relative to the language that contains the predicate P *if there are* human beings who are correctly diagnosed with the disease, i.e., who belong to that class. For instance, if you have clearly defined your predicate "acute myocardial infarction" and you have $n \geq 1$ patients each of whom you have correctly diagnosed with acute myocardial infarction as defined, then relative to your medical language this disease exists. Otherwise, you would not encounter the class of those $n \geq 1$ patients with the disease. That means that independently of whether or not disease nominalism is an acceptable clinical-ontological position, disease hypernominalism a lá Armand Trousseau is not quite right.

We have frequently deplored in the course of our studies that the second condition above is seldom satisfied. Most nosological predicates are not defined in medical literature, and in addition, they are differently presented in different sources. It is difficult in such a situation to clearly decide whether a particular disease exists or not.

19.2.2 Disease Platonism

We demonstrated disease nominalism in the preceding section by formulating an example about acute myocardial infarction in a first-order language in (178). Using this language we talked about, and quantified over, individual objects, i.e., human beings in the present case, in that we said: "In human beings with acute myocardial infarction, the concentration of the enzyme CK is elevated ... and so on". In languages of this type, what is usually called 'disease' is ascribed to a patient as a feature or *property of individuals* like an eye color is such a property. A closer look at medical literature shows, however, that in presenting medical knowledge higher-order languages are often used, thereby giving rise to unnecessary and undesirable metaphysical problems and controversies. In these languages, a disease is dealt with in a way as if it were an independent entity and not a dependent property of individuals. Consider the following reformulation of our current example in a second-order language:

Acute myocardial infarction causes elevation of the concentration
of the enzyme CK in blood. But elevation of CK is not specific for
myocardial infarction because it also occurs when skeletal muscle   (181)
is damaged or destroyed ... and so on.

This text reflects the usual presentation of disease states and pathological
processes in medicine. Accordingly, we must determine what such a causal
relationship looks like that is claimed to hold between acute myocardial infarction and elevation of CK. What kind of entities must *acute myocardial
infarction* and *elevation of CK in blood* be in order for the former to cause
the latter? This question may be answered in two ways. We will consider them
in turn.

We have seen that the language of a statement can be interpreted intensionally or extensionally. The use of a first-order language in our formulation
(178) on page 719 enabled us to use the extensional approach. However, nosological predicates such as the predicate "acute myocardial infarction" in the
statement (181) above, that hides its individual variables, encourage some
scholars to consider them intensionally as higher-order *properties* like redness, albeit compound ones, that exist as supra-individual universals. Thus,
the statement (181) is usually understood as a second-order statement of the
following form:

$\forall P \forall Q$ (if P is *acute myocardial infarction* and Q is *elevation of CK
in blood,* then P causes Q) ... and so on.

Here, P and Q are predicate variables that range over properties. This is just
the type of language that gives rise to Platonism. The ontological commitment
of the statement includes the independent existence of the properties *acute
myocardial infarction* and *elevation of CK*. From this perspective, diseases are
viewed to exist as entities in themselves, and thus, independently of particular
patients. After medicine had joined the natural sciences in the late eighteenth
and early nineteenth centuries, disease Platonism was erroneously called "the
ontological view of disease".

Our examples in this section and the preceding one show that in presenting medical knowledge, one's choise of language has an ontological impact.
Nevertheless, we may ask whether there is any grain of truth in disease Platonism, as some diseases are species-specific. For example, avian influenza is a
disease caused by highly pathogenic Influenza A virus subtype H5N1 that infects birds only. Analogously, smallpox is a disease unique to humans. These
two well-known examples suffice to argue that there are diseases which are
associated with distinct species. Since a species as a whole is superordinate
to its individual members, is it conceivable that the disease is something similar and also exists as a supra-individual property of the species, for example,
as a supra-individual *natural kind* and historical process that even has its
specific natural history? There are indeed adherents of this natural kind hypothesis, e.g., (Cooper R, 2005; Dragulinescu, 2010). But it seems difficult to
defend such a Platonistic view of diseases because the pathogenesis as well

as the natural history of species-specific diseases are genetically determined. The species specificity of a disease thus has other sources. Specifically, the genetic makeup of the respective members of the species is causally responsible for rendering them susceptible to that disease. However, this reasoning may itself be used in favor of disease Platonism by arguing that genetic diseases are supra-individual entities because they affect classes of human beings, i.e., those who have the respective genetic structure. This argument is wrong on the grounds that a genetic disease is not something that affects a particular class of human beings. It is a hereditary property of individuals like their eye color, and alters their metabolism in particular directions. On this account, it may be conceived of as a biological feature of an individual human being, i.e., as a particular. This leads us to our discussion in the next section about a second approach to analyzing the ontological commitments implied by our example above.

19.2.3 Disease Tropism

Diseases may be ontologically analyzed in a second way by recourse to trope theory, which was sketched on page 696. We may therefore call this novel approach disease tropism.

Genetic diseases are not the only diseases that may be conceived of as individual conditions of human beings, and thus as *particulars*. Any other disease, including the acute myocardial infarction in our examples above, is representable as a spatio-temporally localized state of an individual referred to as her *disease state*. We previously termed such an individual disease state a *token disease*. To avoid the impression that the analysis of the ontological commitments of medical knowledge is a matter of taste, it is worth noting that the ascription of a disease by a diagnosis like "Elroy Fox has acute myocardial infarction" requires that what is diagnosed, is a state of affairs in an individual. See Section 8.2.7 on page 325.

A disease state of a patient designated by a diagnosis such as "Elroy Fox has acute myocardial infarction" is usually a compound state of affairs or property that consists of a bundle of elementary properties, i.e., its defining features, such as coronary occlusion and myocardial necrosis. Formally, a compound feature manifested by an individual is also a *particular* like the patient's individual eye color since its constituents are particulars, e.g., the particular coronary occlusion and myocardial necrosis *of this patient Elroy Fox*. If in this fashion a disease token is interpreted as a bio-psycho-social state of an individual patient, we may consider a patient's disease state as a trope or a bundle of tropes (see Section 18.1.1 on page 696).

Disease tropism says that diseases can exist. If a disease exists, then that means that it exists as tokens, i.e., single tropes, in individual patients. For instance, a disease such as acute myocardial infarction exists as a myriad of distinct tropes in the myriad of patients suffering from acute myocardial infarction. It is obvious that a trope in patient x is not the same trope as in patient y. For tropes have distinct locations and, moreover, their constituent tropes such as coronary occlusion, myocardial necrosis, and other features will have individual shapes. According to disease tropism, disease tropes in individual patients are not instantiations of a universal disease because such a universal does not exist. According to the definition of the existence predicate in Definition 172 on page 692 and of degree of existence in Definitions 174–175 on page 701, a disease trope is an existent entity because as an individual, spatio-temporally localized disease state it is (i) causally effective relative to a particular language that contains the corresponding causal predicates, and (ii) suffers causal effects in that it disappears by therapy.

This disease ontology is in line with the concept of fuzzy disease introduced in Definition 40 on page 178. Distinct patients have distinct fuzzy tokens of the same disease such as acute myocardial infarction. Their individual disease states are not identical because a fuzzy set such as $\{(A, 0.6), (B, 1)\}$ representing the disease state of a patient x is different from the fuzzy set $\{(A, 0.4), (B, 0.8)\}$ that represents the disease state of another patient y. The two disease states are two distinct points in the fuzzy hypercube discussed in Section 6.4.4. They only resemble each other to a particular extent. Thus, the ontological commitment of our prototype resemblance theory of disease entails disease tropism. The disease states of individual patients are spatio-temporally localized particulars without any disease universal beyond them.

19.2.4 Disease Realism

Disease realism or nosological realism is the position that diseases, as they are taught, diagnosed, and treated in medicine, "really" exist. They are something natural and independent of human beings, their values, intentions, and conceptual systems. They are *discovered* by nosologists and are not invented, as nosological anti-realists maintain. According to our discussions in preceding sections, nosological Platonists are nosological realists, while a nosological nominalist or tropist may be a nosological realist or anti-realist depending on the particular disease D, e.g., 'acute myocardial infarction', whose existence is under discussion.

Although material artifacts such as desks and computers are human constructs, they exist nonetheless. On this account, nosological constructivism which says that diseases are human constructs, and nosological realism are not incompatible. A nosological constructivist, for example, who holds the view that diseases are socially constructed, may also believe that what she calls a disease, exists in the world out there. However, this existence is not a natural one like mountains come into being and exist. Like the existence of a desk or a computer, a disease's existence is constructed and depends on the human mind, intentions, and values. This latter observation is a warning to all of those concerned with disease ontology. As in our earlier discussions, we carefully distinguished between disease *in the singular* as a general category, and individual diseases *in the plural* as members of that category, so we ought to differentiate between ontological claims about *disease* from ontological claims about *diseases*. The existence of the latter depends on the general concept of disease as a deontic construct that picks out particular classes of individuals (see Chapter 14).

19.3 The Ontology of Psychiatry and Psychosomatics

A considerable part of clinical medicine consists of psychiatry and psychosomatics, which deal with mental diseases and psychosomatic disorders, respectively. The latter are also called psychophysiological disorders. Examples are socially deviant behaviors such as schizophrenia and depression as well as psychosomatic disorders such as asthma bronchiale, and until recently, peptic ulcer disease. Many patients are diagnosed with such ailments and treated accordingly. In what follows, we will focus on the ontology of these ailments rather than on psychiatric and psychosomatic knowledge in general.

Mental diseases and psychosomatic disorders deserve particular medical-ontological attention because the number of conflicting schools and theories concerned with their nosology, etiology, and treatment is literally countless. This justifies the supposition that something in the conceptual bases of psychiatry and psychosomatics must be defective. For our diagnosis of this defectiveness, see page 733. In the present section, we will conduct an ontological analysis of this issue. In preparation for the anaylsis, we shall start with a brief discussion of the mind-body problem that infiltrates all psychiatric and psychosomatic theorizing. Our inquiry divides into the following four parts:

19.3.1 The Mind-Body Problem
19.3.2 Mental States
19.3.3 The Ontology of Mental Diseases
19.3.4 The Ontology of Psychosomatic Diseases.

19.3.1 The Mind-Body Problem

For simplicity's sake, we consider the terms "mind" and "psyche" as synonymous designators of a category of capacities, properties, states, and processes which are described by predicates such as "mental" and "psychic". Examples are thinking, believing, hoping, deciding, and dreaming as well as consciousness, emotions, sensations, and the like.

The philosophy of mind is characterized by a plethora of *isms*. The belief that beyond body there exists a mind is referred to as *mentalism*, from the Latin term "mens" for *mind*. The opposite position has come to be termed *materialism* or physicalism. *Dualism* is a metaphysical position that allows for the existence of both mind and body. *Monism*, by contrast, affirms the existence of only one of them.[138]

---

[138] The term "physicalism" is ambiguous. On the one hand, it denotes a semantic doctrine referred to as *semantic physicalism* which says that all non-physical terms,

The belief in the existence of mental diseases and psychosomatic disorders is based, respectively, on the assumption that (i) there are minds and mental states that become afflicted with mental diseases; and (ii) there exist mind-body relationships and they give rise to psychosomatic disorders. Behind this mentalistic assumption is the *Cartesian dualism* of the French mathematician and philosopher René Descartes (Renatus Cartesius: 1596–1650). Descartes held that the terms "mental" and "physical" designate two different *substances* such that mind is wholly distinct from the body and any other physical object. According to him, mind does not depend for its existence on the body. In contrast to the body, it is an immaterial and non-spatial, 'unextended', substance and therefore without weight, size, and other physical properties. Given this Cartesian dualism, the problem is how the mind is attached to the body, and whether there are any relationships between the two, including causal ones. This is the well-known, post-Cartesian mind-body problem that constitutes one of the most stubborn issues in philosophy, medicine, and psychology. A large number of solutions, labeled *theories of mind*, have been suggested. They cannot be discussed in detail here. Only the following main umbrella terms under which they are grouped, will be sketched. For details, see (Braddon-Mitchell and Jackson, 2007; Chalmers, 2002; Kim, 2006):

- ▶ Psychophysical interactionism
- ▶ Psychophysical parallelism
- ▶ Epiphenomenalism
- ▶ Eliminative behaviorism
- ▶ Eliminative materialism
- ▶ Psychoneural identity
- ▶ Functionalism
- ▶ Emergentism.

Psychophysical interactionism

This is a dualistic position according to which the mind exists as an entity separate from the body. It causally interacts with the body and vice versa. In Descartes' view, the two parts of this interaction meet in the pineal gland in

---

including biological and mental ones, are definable by physical terms such that the language of physics is the universal language of science (Carnap, 1931). This doctrine originating from logical empiricism certainly is wrong. On the other hand, it denotes a metaphysical thesis on the nature of existing entities. This second thesis, referred to as *pure physicalism,* originates from Greek antiquity (Democritus, Epicurus) and says that everything is ultimately physical. We shall use the term in this latter sense. Pure physicalism is what is usually called materialism. Semantic physicalism and pure physicalism constitute *reductive physicalism*, i.e., reducing something to physics. For example, someone is a reductive physicalist when she believes that biology or psychology is reducible to physics. There is also a *non-reductive physicalism*. See Section 'Emergentism' on page 728.

the brain. Modern mind-body interactionists are the philosopher Karl Popper, the neurophysiologist John Eccles, and the mathematical physicist Roger Penrose. They assert that quantum-mechanical indeterminacies in the brain make the interaction possible (Popper and Eccles, 1985; Penrose, 1996, 2002).

Psychophysical parallelism

The German philosopher Gottfried Wilhelm Leibniz (1646–1716) rejected Descartes' interactionism. Causal interaction between mind and body is not necessary, he said, because the two have been synchronized by God and always do the same things ('pre-established harmony'). A sort of modern, partial parallelism was advocated by Karl Eduard Rothschuh (1908–1984), a German historian and philosopher of medicine and biology, in his theory of organism (Rothschuh, 1963).

Epiphenomenalism

Another dualistic, non-interactionist position is epiphenomenalism, which originated with the British biologist Thomas Henry Huxley, who lived from 1825 to 1895 (Huxley, 1904). It argues that mental phenomena are caused by bodily events, but they are causally inert epiphenomena, like the smoke coming from a factory. A pain, for example, may be caused by an injury. However, it cannot be the cause of our wincing (Campbell, 1984).

Eliminative behaviorism

The introspective school of psychology, founded in the late nineteenth century by the German physiologist, philosopher, and psychologist Wilhelm Maximilian Wundt (1832–1920), considered the subject matter of psychology to be consciousness as explored through introspection (Wundt, 1874). Introspection provides first-person reports such as "I am in pain" and ""I am sad". Against this first-person perspective and Cartesian dualism, the U.S.-American psychologists John Broadus Watson (1878–1958) and Burrhus Frederic Skinner (1904–1990) argued that only directly observable *behavior* could be scientifically studied (Watson, 1919; Skinner, 1938, 1953). Highly influenced by this *behaviorism,* philosophers such as Willard Van Orman Quine and Gilbert Ryle developed a behavioristic philosophy of mind that denied the existence of common-sense psychological entities such as conscious states, experience, beliefs, sensations, emotions, and any other similar episodes taking place within an individual (Quine, 1953b; Ryle, 1949). According to Ryle, mental terms are dispositional terms denoting modes of behavior, and mentalism is due to a *category mistake*. Imagine, for instance, that a foreigner is visiting your university for the first time, he said. You show her the departments of philosophy, pathology, mathematics, archeology, bioethics, and all other units and sections. You show her all classrooms, laboratories, libraries, administrative buildings, and all other facilities. On finishing the tour through the university, your visitor comments: "That is all very nice. But now please show me your university!". Obviously she doesn't understand that your university is the whole, composed of what you have already shown her, and that there exists nothing separate to be called your "university". The mind is similarly non-existent beyond the body, "the ghost in the machine". There is no sharp dividing line between this position and the one considered next.

Eliminative materialism

This school of thought encompasses an heterogeneous group of philosophers and cognitive scientists who consider all the talk about mind and mental states as outdated, common-sense psychology, deserving of the same fate as alchemy. They deny the existence of mental states and processes and view neuroscience as an ideal framework to replace the meaningless terminology of common-sense psychology. Their doctrine is of course incoherent simply on the grounds that while they deny epistemic states such as *beliefs* because these are mental states, they *believe* nonetheless that their own theories are correct and the brain is the organ for what is erroneously called the mind. Prominent contemporary eliminativists are the husband-wife team of Paul and Patricia Churchland and Richard Rorty (1931–2007) (Rorty, 1965; Paul Churchland, 1981, 1988; Patricia Churchland, 1986; Dennett, 1987, 1991; Armstrong, 1993b, 1999).[139]

Psychoneural identity

The advent of neuroanatomy and neuropathology in the second half of the nineteenth century enabled some philosophically momentous discoveries about brain function. They included the discovery by the French physician and anatomist Paul Broca (1824–1880) of the motor speech center located in the ventro-posterior region of the frontal lobe of the brain (Broca's area); and the discovery by the German physician and neuropathologist Carl Wernicke (1848–1905) of the sensory speech center located in the posterior superior temporal gyrus (Wernicke's area). This and similar research contributed to the insight that different parts of the brain were associated with different mental abilities. In the course of the philosophical analysis and evaluation of this insight, a monistic thesis emerged in the 1950s that has come to be termed *the identity theory* of mind (Place, 1956; Feigl, 1958; Smart, 1959; Lewis, 1966). It says that mind and brain are identical, i.e., mental states are identical with

---

[139] Eliminative materialism is often categorized as reductive materialism or physicalism (see footnote 138 on page 724). However, this categorization is pointless because the adherents of the theory clearly deny the existence of mind. So, there is nothing to reduce to physics.

neural states like heat in gases is identical with the average kinetic energy of molecules. Thus, it falls under reductive physicalism (see footnote 138 on page 724). As a result, no interaction between mind and body is needed because there are no mental states separate from neural states. Without going into details, it should be mentioned here that for different reasons the identity theory is rife with difficult problems. Advocates of this view have distinguished token identity and type identity between mental and physical states as an attempt to resolve such problems. Token identity is the identity of a token mental state in an individual, such as a particular pain, with a particular neural state in that individual. Type identity concerns the identity of a type of mental state, such as pain in general, with a type of neural state such as the firing of a particular type of neurons. While token identity seems to be acceptable, type identity does not seem to hold (Borst, 1970; Kripke, 1980; Place, 2004; Rosenthal, 1991).

Functionalism

This is a dualistic doctrine according to which the mental is distinct from the physical. It originated with Hilary Putnam and Jerry Fodor (Putnam, 1960; Fodor, 1968). In their view, a mental state is constituted not by a neural state, but by the functional role it plays. Its functional role consists in its causal relations to other mental states and to sensory inputs and behavioral outputs. For example, according to functionalists pain is caused by bodily injury to produce the awareness that something is wrong with the body and the desire to ameliorate that condition, to produce escape attempts, wincing, moaning, etc. All these causal relations constitute the pain. Obviously, a mental state is conceived of as a causally effective entity in the body. Since members of different species have distinct biological structures, it is argued that a mental state may be realized by different types of physical state. This is the so-called thesis of multiple realizability from which they conclude that the identity theory sketched above must be false. Some functionalists even compare minds with computer programs that may run on different types of machines. It has been convincingly demonstrated, however, that this computational view is untenable. Minds are not analogs of computer programs and mental acts are not computations (Searle, 1980, 1992). For details on functionalism, see (Beakley and Ludlow, 2006; Goldman, 1993; Rosenthal, 1991).

Emergentism (psychophysical supervenience)

According to this theory, mental states and processes exist and at least some of them, e.g., phenomenal consciousness, are not reducible to physical states and processes, although they are dependent on the physical and covary with its alterations. Specifically, they are systemic properties and are caused not by a single body part such as brain, liver, or any other substructure, but by the interaction of all parts of the body. However, they are causally inert.

They only *supervene* on the physical. In line with what has been said about emergent phenomena on page 119, *supervenience* means the following type of dependence:

A class of properties $\{Q_1, \ldots, Q_n\} = B$, say B-properties, depend on another class of properties $\{P_1, \ldots, P_m\} = A$, say A-properties, if it is true that whenever an individual has A-properties, then she also has B-properties. Thus, B-properties are determined by A-properties. If A-properties vary, B-properties will also vary. That is, supervenience is a dependence relation between two classes of properties. This intuitive notion is made precise by the following definition.

Definition 176 (Supervenience). *For all objects x and y, for all possible worlds w_1 and w_2, and for all classes $A = \{P_1, \ldots, P_m\}$ and $B = \{Q_1, \ldots, Q_n\}$ of $m, n \geq 1$ properties: The properties B supervene on the properties A iff whenever x in w_1 and y in w_2 possess the properties A, then x in w_1 and y in w_2 possess the properties B.*

Concisely, a property Q supervenes on, or *emerges* from, the property P iff P underlies Q. On the basis of the definition above, the psychophysical supervenience thesis means that the mental supervenes on the physical. That means that two individuals have the same mental properties if they have the same physical properties. Otherwise put, physical duplicates are also mental duplicates. Since the supervenience of mental on the physical is brought about by the interaction of all body *parts,* it is referred to as *mereological* supervenience. Our mind-body conception sketched on pages 131–142 is such an emergentist theory of mereological supervenience. It falls under non-reductive physicalism because it doesn't reduce the mental to the physical. For details on emergence and supervenience, see (Broad, 1925; Morgan, 1923; Davidson, 1970; Kim, 2006; Stephan, 2007).

That something, B, is reducible to something else, A, means that B is nothing more than A. For example, the claim that the mind is reducible to the body says that the mind is nothing more, or other, than the body. This amounts to the theory of psychoneural identity mentioned above. Our emergentist theory, however, does not reduce the mind to the body. It concedes that the mind has properties that the body lacks, although it is causally dependent on the body (see pp. 131–142).

19.3.2 Mental States

In the ontology of mental diseases with which we shall concern ourselves in the next section, the central question is whether there are minds and mental states to become afflicted with diseases at all. To prepare our discussion, on page 132 we distinguished between subjective and objective mental states, where mental states proper are the subjective states, as well as gave a brief sketch of the main theories of mind and mental states in preceding sections.

We saw that each of them either affirms or denies the existence of mind and tries, respectively, to explain the supposedly existent mind or to replace the supposedly non-existent mind with another entity, e.g., the brain. But such an affirmation or denial is only an ontological stance. It is not an ontological proof or disproof whether mind and mental states exist.

To prove, substantiate, or disprove the ontological assertion that a particular mental state such as *emotion* exists, one first needs an idea of that state in order to be able to distinguish it from other entities, e.g., bricks. The idea may be a more or less simple concept such as "x is an emotion if and only if it is such and such ...", or it may be a more or less complex theory such as a detailed theory of emotions. The former approach may be referred to as a definitional approach, the latter as a theoretical approach. We undertook, on pages 139–142, a theoretical approach of the emergentist type to suggest that mental states be construed holistically. That is, a mental state is a state of the whole organism and not of any of its constituent parts, e.g., brain. As we stated previously on page 142, mind is not just in the head. That someone hallucinates, is pleased, or is sad, is an attitude ascribed to a person rather than to her liver or brain. Thus, there is no dividing line between mind and body as a whole. Mental states are systemic properties of the organism, body, individual, person, or whatever name you may use to refer to a human being. In what follows, we shall try to utilize this conception in the ontology of mental diseases.

19.3.3 The Ontology of Mental Diseases

Are there mental diseases? This question may sound odd because psychiatry as a medical discipline claims to be concerned with patients suffering from just such diseases. Accordingly, psychiatric text- and handbooks present hundreds of mental diseases such as schizophrenia, cyclothymia, depression, and others. Many clinical institutions are psychiatric institutions devoted either to the management of mentally ill patients or to mental health research.

However, not everybody agrees on the claim that mental diseases exist. For example, the prominent antipsychiatrist Thomas Szasz maintains that the idea of mental disease is a myth. Psychiatry is a pseudo-scientific social control system that interprets problems in living as mental diseases to medicalize everyday life (Szasz, 1984, 2007, 2008). Medicalization of conflict as disease and psychiatric coercion as treatment is medicalized terrorism (Szasz, 2009a). In a similar vein, the labeling theory considers the psychiatric diagnosis of a mental disease as a label that a group attaches to an individual whose behavior violates social norms. Prior to the labeling, the deviant individual does not have any mental disorder. The role she assumes is imposed on her through labeling and the subsequent treatment by societal agents and persons (Scheff, 1966). This sociological theory had its apogee in the 1970s. Its significance has continuously decreased since (Scheff, 1999, x).

The critiques of the foundations of psychiatry mentioned above have given rise to a debate over whether mental diseases 'really' exist or are merely fictitious (Szasz, 2009b; Ghaemi, 2007; Reznek, 1991). To decide this question first requires a *concept of mental disease* in order to know what the subject of the ontological debate and analysis is at all. Regrettably, there is as yet no such concept in medicine. For this reason, the whole debate on the ontology of mental diseases cannot be taken seriously. One of the main obstructions to progress in the discussion is the term "mental disease" itself, also called "mental illness". It is inherently ambiguous in that it does not tell us to what the term "mental" refers. At least the following two interpretations are possible:

1. In the term "mental disease", the adjective "mental" means that the *mind* is afflicted by a disease. So, a mental disease is a *disease of the mind*.
2. It means that the patient is afflicted by a disease or disorder that causes disordered *mental states*.

According to the first interpretation, a patient who is diagnosed with a mental disease such as schizophrenia, is someone whose mind has a disease. This position can only be held by dualists, and the concept of mental disease that they might put forward would be a mentalistic one like the theory of psychoanalysis. In a conceptual system of this type, one can without fear of any argument maintain the existence of anything and everything, as it is impossible to create an intersubjective methodology that would enable the critics to refute a mentalistic hypothesis. Thus, every imaginable disease entity can be invented in the realm of a mentalistic concept of mental disease. Therefore, ontological analyses of mentalistic nosologies are fruitless. For instance, when a psychiatrist claims that "there is a mental disease called *ego anachoresis*" that is characterized by the retiring of ego from the world into itself (Winkler, 1954), it is impossible to refute her existence claim because (i) as outlined on page 396, indefinite existence claims are not falsifiable; and (ii) thanks to her mentalistic frame of reference, the proponent is always capable of verifying her claim by presenting an individual whose mind, in the proponent's language, displays ego anachoresis. We have seen previously that the validity of existence claims is relative to languages (p. 693 f.).

The second interpretation above conforms to the public knowledge about the human organism and suffering human beings gathered during the long history of medicine, as well as to the general concept of disease analyzed on pages 151–183. There are many diseases with mental manifestations such as brain tumors and other brain-based diseases, endocrinological and metabolic disorders, hepatic diseases and others. Thus, in line with the second interpretation above, we consider a mental disease emergentistically, i.e., as a disease of this type upon which *disordered mental states* in terms of mental symptoms and signs *supervene*. Otherwise put, a mental disease represents a supervenient aspect of a disease in the usual sense, which has been dismissively labeled the "medical model" or "biomedical model". Since such a disease is traditionally understood as a bodily malady, we avoid ontological difficulties about whether there are mental diseases or not because we can always interpret them trope-theoretically as bundles of tropes. For example, if someone claims that there is a mental disease called *depression* whose bodily features consist in serotonin and norepinephrine deficiency in the brain, then it should not be difficult for her to convince us that this mental disease indeed exists. To this end, she only needs to present an individual with depression who has serotonin and norepinephrine deficiency.

However, while our emergentist interpretation of mental diseases as supervenient features or processes resolves the ontological problem associated with them, it does not maintain or imply that mental diseases are brain diseases. As pointed out previously, we consider mental states as systemic properties of the whole individual. In consequence, a mental disease with disordered mental states cannot be attributed to a proper part of the individual, e.g., her brain.[140]

Suppose there is a patient x presenting with a human condition H, such as 'schizophrenia' or 'myocardial infarction', that consists of a number of features $\{F_1, \ldots, F_n\}$. Whether this patient is categorized as having a somatic disease or as having a mental disease, D, means, according to our *nosological categorization postulate* outlined on page 429, that (i) there is a particular theory T of disease D such that (ii) the structure $\langle \{x\}, H \rangle$ consisting of the patient x and her condition H can be extended, by adding T-theoretical components of the nosological predicate D, to become a model for theory T.

The prototype resemblance theory of disease presented previously does not distinguish between somatic and mental diseases. It advertises for only one category of diseases encompassing all types of diseases. There is no objection, however, to refer to those diseases as mental which primarily generate disordered mental states. A mental disease is established in the same fashion as all other diseases, i.e., with reference to a prototype disease and in the spirit of our prototype resemblance theory of disease. Viewed from the historical perspective, psychiatry as the discipline concerned with mental diseases began in exactly this way with the work of the French physician Philippe Pinel (1745–1826). When he was the physician of the infirmaries at the Bicêtre Hospital near Paris 1793 to 1795, he *declared* that instead of being criminals, the myriads of men who were imprisoned there were *mentally ill* (Pinel, 1798, 1801).

---

[140] The well-known slogan "mental diseases are brain diseases" is usually attributed to Wilhelm Griesinger (1817–1868), a prominent German neurologist and psychiatrist of the nineteenth century. Although the quoted wording is not to be found in his writings, Griesinger was indeed of this opinion, which he expressed in several places in his early work *Pathology and Therapy of Mental Diseases* (Griesinger, 1845). For example, "Since insanity is a disease, namely a brain disease, there cannot exist another, more adequate method of studying it than the medical one" (ibid., 8).

In closing this section, we may emphasize once again that the basic difficulty of the ontology of mental diseases lies in the deficiency of the language of psychiatry. It is still an unscientific language and very much in need of improvement. Nosological predicates in psychiatry denoting clinical-psychiatric entities, i.e., individual mental diseases, are seldom, or seldom adequately, defined. As a result, every psychiatrist has more or less a private conceptual system, making reasonable research and communication impossible. The same diagnosis applies to psychosomatics the ontology of which is analyzed below.

19.3.4 The Ontology of Psychosomatic Diseases

Today, the adjective "psychosomatic" refers to the doctrine of mind-body causation, propounding that there are bodily effects caused by the psyche. Upon this postulate of psychosomatic causation rests the discipline of *psychosomatic medicine,* or psychosomatics for short, that is concerned with psychosomatic diseases or disorders, nowadays called *psychophysiological disorders.* This category of disorders encompasses health conditions such as non-allergic asthma bronchiale, anorexia nervosa, colitis ulcerosa, and others which are supposed to be caused by psychic, i.e., mental, factors and disturbances.

Do psychosomatic disorders 'really' exist? No doubt, there are individuals suffering from such clinical disorders as listed above. Our ontological question thus reduces to an etiological and epistemological one: Is the postulate of psychosomatic causation true, i.e., are the so-called psychosomatic disorders 'really' *psycho*-somatic, and as such, caused by psychic factors? This question can be answered in the affirmative in a dualistic-interactionistic system only. For only such a system allows for the existence of an independent mind capable of causally acting upon the body. In our emergentist view, however, the term "psychosomatic" is a misnomer. It is due to *the-barometer-causes-storm fallacy*, discussed on pages 225 and 253, that is based on the mistaking of spurious causes for genuine causes. What is traditionally categorized as "psychosomatic", is in fact *sociosomatic* and requires a sociological approach rather than an approach concerning the psychology of the individual. To help us understand why, let us look briefly at the history of the concept.

According to detailed medical-historical analyses by Steinberg (2004, 2005, 2007), the hyphenated adjective "psycho-somatic" was coined in the early nineteenth century by the German physician Johann Christian August Heinroth (1818, Vol. 2, 49). This was prior to Rudolf Virchow's theory of cellular pathology, which appeared in 1858 to significantly contribute to the association of clinical medicine with natural sciences. As of 1811, Heinroth (1773–1843) held the then newly founded chair of "psychic therapy" at the University of Leipzig in Germany, and was the first academic psychiatrist in Europe. In his extremely theocentric view, the immaterial soul has primacy over, and interacts with, the body as an instrument. Disordered thoughts and emotions due to sin and guilt have negative effects on both soul and body, and cause mental as well as bodily diseases and disorders (Heinroth, 1818, 1823).

Heinroth's dualistic-interactionistic doctrine of psychogenesis was a stopgap. Lacking adequate biomedical knowledge as a basis for judgment, he explained observable diseases and disorders by unobservable mental states and processes. By the end of the century, Sigmund Freud and his colleague Josef Breuer used the same postulate to explain hysterical paralysis, which they interpreted as a *conversion* disorder. The paralysis was caused, they argued, by a mental process highly charged with affect whose path to consciousness was blocked such that it would divert along the wrong paths and flow into the somatic sphere (Freud and Breuer, 1895). Yet they did not explain how the conversion of the mental into the physical occurred. Their reasoning is reminiscent, and an analog, of Heinrothean conversion of sin and guilt into disease. On their speculative assumption, Freud developed his theory of psychoanalysis to explain everything by means of the Oedipus complex and its ancillaries. Some of his followers, primarily Franz Alexander (1891–1946), similarly applied psychoanalysis to internistic diseases and disorders (Alexander, 1934, 1939, 1950), and founded in 1939 the journal *Psychosomatic Medicine*. Psychosomatic societies were established worldwide to spread the dualistic-interactionistic doctrine of psychogenesis as an etiologic presumption. At almost every medical school today, there are psychosomatic departments that teach medical students this same principle. However, in the long run, the natural course of inquiries, evidence, and reasoning demonstrate that a speculative, unscientific stopgap cannot serve as a useful scientific principle to compete with empirically supported ideas. A good example in favor of this thesis is the recategorization of peptic ulcer diseases that we considered in Section 11.2.4 on page 490. From the commencement of psychosomatics onwards, these diseases were viewed and treated as psychosomatic diseases, and subjected to thousands of bombastic psychodynamic theories about their genesis and therapy. That remained the case until Helicobacter pylori was discovered as the culprit in the early 1980s. The same ulcers are nowadays viewed as infectious diseases and successfully treated by antibiotics (Warren and Marshall, 1983; Marshall 2002a).

This is not to say that behind every psychosomatic disorder there is a bodily cause, a bacterium, a toxic substance, and the like such that in the not-too-distant future every such disorder would turn out a somatic disorder. Our claim is only that the idea of psychosomatics has been a mistake since its inception by Heinroth. The pathogenic forces come not from the psyche, but rather from the social structure and values of the group and community in which an individual interacts with others, as well as from the mode of their interaction. What psychosomatics has been unable to accomplish until now, could be better managed by *sociosomatics* (see page 143).

In sociosomatics as an intersubjective, empirical science of health-relevant interaction between individuals and groups, there would be no need for speculative theories of mind-body interaction and the obscure psychogenesis of diseases. Based on a theory of sociogenesis, ineffective psychotherapies could be replaced with interaction modification, moral criticism, and ethics in order to reshape the individual's preference behavior. For example, it is more sensible and efficacious to analyze and prevent a phenomenon such as obesity by inquiring into, and dealing with, the behavioral impact of the food industry and media than by recourse to, and therapy of, the Oedipus complex.

19.4 Biomedical Ontology Engineering

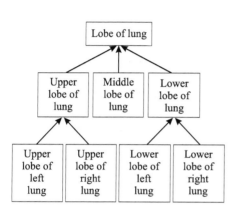

Fig. 85. Part of the FMA ontology of anatomy of the lung. FMA is the "Foundational Model of Anatomy". The arrows represent the taxonomic relation *is_a*. See (Rosse and Mejino, 2003)

As mentioned on page 698, a recent discipline in applied ontology is the so-called ontology engineering. It is referred to in biomedical sciences as biomedical ontology engineering or biomedical ontology (Jansen and Smith, 2008). Biomedical ontologists and ontology engineers analyze nomenclatures such as Nomina Anatomica, partial nomenclatures such as the terminology of mouse genomics, thesauri such as SNOMED, coding systems such as ICD, and the semantic relations between the terms of such vocabularies. Through their analysis they produce a list, semantic network, database, or computer program, and refer to it as *an* ontology. For example, after having analyzed ICD, SNOMED, or a partial nomenclature, e.g., the nomenclature of the respiratory system, their results are presented, respectively, as "ICD ontology", "SNOMED ontology", and "the ontology of respiratory system" (see Figures 85–86).

The odd phrase "ontology engineering" is due to the ambiguation of the term "ontology" in the information sciences in the 1990s. While the term "ontology" initially meant, and in philosophy still means, the theory of being, in informatics and natural sciences it is nowadays understood as a *system of concepts* that are used in a domain such as anatomy, physiology, or orthopedics. Extensive investigations into such systems are undertaken under the label "biomedical ontology engineering", although the whole endeavor merely recapitulates the received conceptual and semantic analysis. For example, according to a most widely quoted source, (i) "A specification of a representational vocabulary for a shared domain of discourse – definitions of classes, relations, functions, and other objects – is called *an* ontology" and (ii) "An *ontology* is an explicit specification of a conceptualization" (Gruber, 1993,

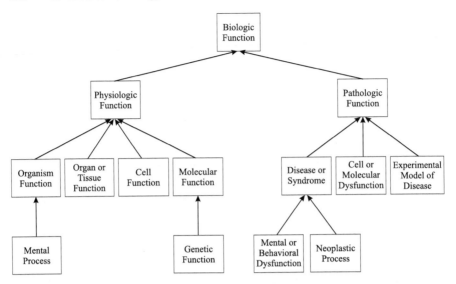

Fig. 86. Part of the semantic network of the UMLS ontology. The arrows represent the taxonomic relation *is_a*. UMLS is the "Unified Medical Language System". See http://www.nlm.nih.gov/research/umls/. Last accessed December 2, 2010

199). We are thus currently witnessing a semantic branching of the phrase "ontology" from its original meaning to also include something like "terminology" or "conceptology". But be aware that it would be more adequate to consider either of these two research fields as a branch of syntax and semantics, or more generally, linguistics. The so-called biomedical ontology, then, would present itself as a medical-linguistic branch concerned with medical language and medical-linguistic structures rather than with medical ontology. Biomedical ontology engineers do not inquire into the question of what exists at all in a specific domain, or whether the referents of the concepts they are dealing with exist. They are convinced, or presuppose, a priori that such is the case. These supposed existents include, for example, not only atoms, molecules, bones, muscles, and brains, but also biomedical holes, boundaries, sites, features, biological functions, regulatory and pathogenetic processes, medical procedures, bodily and mental diseases, genes, diseases thereof, gene products, and so forth. Genuine ontological questions such as "do diseases, or genes, exist or are they human inventions?" are not addressed. Interestingly, the results of their research, so-called ontologies, are provided as portable databases internationally accessible through the Internet. Databases originating with different research groups in distinct places are accessed remotely and are matched, merged, modified, pruned, integrated, used, reused, and so on. Thus, biomedical ontologies themselves are handled as tangible objects and unquestioned facts paving the way for the autoevolution of artificial species of hypostatized entities. For instance, see (Burger et al., 2008; Pisanelli, 2007).[141]

Summarizing, there is currently an inflationary use of the label "ontology" to the effect that the term is being reified and materialized. Vocabularies and thesauri are put forward in terms of listings and dictionaries, semantic networks, diagrams, computer programs, representations of interconceptual relations, and mereological relationships, which biomedical ontology engineers refer to as ontologies. What has been called a nomenclature such as Nomina Anatomica, a coding system such as ICD, a thesaurus such as SNOMED in the past, is nowadays said to be an ontology that represents *the reality* in the world out there (Grenon et al., 2008; Smith, 2004, 2008). As an avowed ontological realist, Barry Smith even defends the thesis that "ontologies [...] should be understood as having as their subject matter, not concepts, but rather the universals and particulars which exist in reality and are captured in scientific laws" (Smith, 2004, 73). By so doing, the difference between a conceptual system that always and unavoidably is an abstract human construct, on the one hand, and a real system, on the other, is naïve-realistically blurred. This attitude may be confusing and detrimental in areas where the ontological question of whether a particular entity exists, is of paramount importance, e.g., in nosology and metanosology concerned with diseases and the problems of their existence or non-existence. There are even scholars who by "comparing mouse and man" (Schofield et al., 2008, 125) analyze the genetics of a mouse to suggest a *disease ontology* of human diseases (ibid., 119).

To judge the critical comments above, it is worth noting that according to our approach presented in Section 19.1.1 on page 712, applied ontology is best accomplished by investigating the ontological commitments of some item of knowledge, X, to identify that part of the world knowledge X talks about. Using the jargon of biomedical ontology engineers, let us call "that part of the world knowledge X talks about" X's *ontology*°. The latter word is tagged in order to clearly distinguish between:

a. ontology as philosophy within a particular language $\mathcal{L}$ and
b. ontology° as a world sector outside a language $\mathcal{L}$.

As outlined on page 715, the ontology° of a particular item of knowledge is in fact a model for that knowledge and consists of a generalized relational structure $\langle \Omega_1, \ldots, \Omega_m; R_1, \ldots, R_n; a_1, \ldots, a_p \rangle$ such that $\Omega_1, \ldots, \Omega_m$ are $m \geq 1$ categories of objects; $R_1, \ldots, R_n$ are $n \geq 1$ subsets, relations, or functions over these categories; and $a_1, \ldots, a_p$ are $p \geq 0$ particular individual objects

---

[141] To this prolific undertaking has even been devoted a recent international journal, *Applied Ontology*, to investigate the "ontology of time, events and processes; ontology of space and geography; ontology of physics and physical objects; ontology of biomedicine; ontology of mental entities; ontology of agents and actions; ontology of organizations and social reality; ontology of the information society; ontology of business and e-commerce; ontology of law; ontology of history, culture and evolution" (Guarino and Musen, 2009).

originating from these categories. But in contrast to the analysis of such models as world sectors, a *vocabulary* such as {mouse, man, AIDS} talks about the world just as little as the vocabulary {cacochymia, drapetomania, Pegasus} does. Both of them are void of ontological commitments because a vocabulary does not consist of sentences *that talk about any world sector* and that make any assertion thereby. Hence, it lacks any model. It is therefore inappropriate to associate ontologies° with proliferating vocabularies and databases such as ICD, SNOMED, SNOMED-CT®, ULMS, OpenCyc, SUMO, FMA, DOLCE, DOLCE+, GO, LinkBase®, and so forth. Otherwise, it can be argued that there are no boundaries between such ontologies° and fictional entities. See Section 19.6 below.

Sentences have a totally different ontological relevance. First, regarding scientific theories, the method of set-theoretical reconstruction discussed on page 403 provides an ideal extensional tool to make explicit the ontology° of a given theory by identifying those relational structures which are its *models*. Let there be a theory that has been axiomatized by a set-theoretical structure $\langle \Omega_1, \ldots, \Omega_m; R_1, \ldots, R_n \rangle$, then this structure is just the ontology° of that theory. For example, the ternary structure ⟨living organisms, harmful agents, antibodies against these agents⟩ is the ontology° of the theory of *active immunity structure* axiomatized in Definition 129 on page 422.

Second, note that not only theories, but every item of knowledge, i.e., any sentence, is set-theoretically axiomatizable. In this way, one can easily identify its ontology°. For instance, the ontology° of the philosophically as well as medically insignificant statement "Elroy Fox is a diabetic" may in the following way be revealed as the sector of the world ⟨a set of diabetics, Elroy Fox⟩:

Definition 177. ξ *is an Elroy Fox' diabetes structure iff there are D and x such that:*

1. $\xi = \langle D, x \rangle$,
2. *D is a set of diabetics,*
3. $x = $ *Elroy Fox,*
4. $x \in D$.

By virtue of axioms 2–4, the structure $\langle D, x \rangle$ is exactly the sector of the world ⟨a set of diabetics, Elroy Fox⟩. Thus, the latter structure is the ontology°, or a model, for the statement "Elroy Fox is a diabetic". Otherwise put, the truth of the statement "Elroy Fox is a diabetic" requires the *existence* of the particular sector of the world ⟨a set of diabetics, Elroy Fox⟩.

19.5 Formal Medical Ontology

In line with what has been said about formal ontology on page 698, formal ontology in medicine is a recent, non-empirical research field that analyzes formal properties of medical objects and formal relations between them to construct general axiomatic theories about them. For example, every object is a part of itself. That is, $\forall x \big(is\_a\_part\_of(x, x) \big)$. Thus, the binary relation $is\_a\_part\_of$ expressing parthood is a reflexive relation. That means that every medical object stands in this relation to itself. As trivial as such formal knowledge may seem, it is instrumental in medical knowledge-based decision support systems because computers executing such programs do not know that, and need it in order to draw useful conclusions when in a reasoning process the question arises whether, for instance, the hypophysis of a patient is part of the hypophysis of this patient or not. *Formal medical ontology* conducts formal, *protomedical* research of this type in medicine to provide axiomatic theories of medical entities. A minor, meaningful part of what biomedical ontology engineers do, is in fact formal medical ontology. By formalizing ontologically relevant parts of medical knowledge, they serve medical informatics, expert systems research, and related areas and facilities. Examples are medical applications of (i) ordinary taxonomy, (ii) mereology, and (iii) mereotopology. Ordinary taxonomy was outlined on page 60. The latter two areas will be briefly considered in the following two sections:

    19.5.1   Mereology and Mereotopology
    19.5.2   Fuzzy Formal Ontology.

For details, see (Bittner and Donnelly, 2007; Hovda, 2009; Koslicki, 2008; Schulz and Hahn, 2005):

19.5.1 Mereology and Mereotopology

Mereology was briefly introduced on pages 591–592. It is a formal theory of parthood relations such as $is\_a\_part\_of$ and $is\_a\_proper\_part\_of$ to enable part-whole as well as spatial reasoning, e.g., in anatomy, imaging disciplines, and surgery. For instance, since parthood is a transitive relation, we can infer from the statements "lens $is\_a\_proper\_part\_of$ eye" and "eye $is\_a\_proper\_part\_of$ visual system" the statement that "lens $is\_a\_proper\_part\_of$ visual system". See the mereological axioms, definitions, and theorems in Tables 15–16 on page 591 f. A combination of taxonomy and mereology is illustrated in Figure 87.

Mereotopology is an extension of mereology by adding some topological concepts dealing with spatial objects and relations such as boundaries, surfaces, interiors, neighborhood, connection, and others. As a simple example, consider the notion of an *interior part*, for instance, an interior part of an organ. When an object x is_a_part_of another object y, written Pxy, such that it does not touch y's boundaries, then it *is_an_interior_part_of* y, written $IPxy$. A few axioms, definitions, and theorems listed in Table 26 may illustrate how such mereotopological concepts are formally characterized and how they relate to others. In the table, the following predicates are used, the first one of which is a primitive and defines our second topological predicate E, i.e., "encloses". They read:

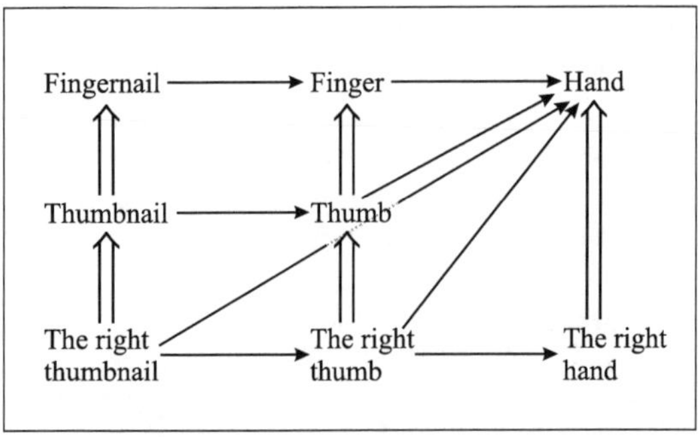

Fig. 87. A combination of the taxonomic relation *is_a* (⇑) and partonomic relation *is_a_part_of* (→). Adapted from (Zaiß et al., 2005, 64)

$$Cxy \equiv x \text{ is\_connected\_to } y$$
$$Exy \equiv x \text{ encloses } y$$

e.g., the retina is connected to the optic nerve, the pericardium encloses the myocardium.

The remaining predicates are mereological ones. We take the predicates P, PP, and O from Table 15 on page 591:

$$
\begin{aligned}
Pxy\ &\equiv\ x \text{ is\_a\_part\_of } y \\
PPxy\ &\equiv\ x \text{ is\_a\_proper\_part\_of } y \\
Oxy\ &\equiv\ x \text{ overlaps } y \\
IPxy\ &\equiv\ x \text{ is\_an\_interior\_part\_of } y
\end{aligned}
$$

For the sake of readability, the quantifiers in Table 26 are omitted. All sentences are tacitly universally quantified, i.e., universal closures.

Table 26: Some mereotopological axioms, definitions and theorems

Axioms:

1. Cxx — Connection is reflexive,
2. $Cxy \rightarrow Cyx$ — connection is symmetric,

Definitions:

3. $Exy \leftrightarrow (Czx \rightarrow Czy)$ — x encloses y iff whenever something connects to it, then it also connects to y,

4. $IPxy \leftrightarrow \big(Pxy \wedge (Czx \rightarrow Ozy)\big)$ — x is an interior part of y iff it is a part of y and everything that connects to it, overlaps y,

Axioms:

5. $(Exy \leftrightarrow Ezy) \leftrightarrow x = z$ — two objects are identical iff whenever one of them encloses a third object, the other one encloses it too,

6. Exx — enclosure is reflexive,
7. $Exy \wedge Eyz \rightarrow Exz$ — enclosure is transitive,

Theorems:

8. $Exy \wedge Eyx \rightarrow x = y$ — enclosure is antisymmetric,

Table 26: Some mereotopological axioms, definitions and theorems

9. $Pxy \rightarrow Eyx$	an object encloses its parts,
10. $Oxy \rightarrow Cxy$	two overlapping objects are connected,
11. $IPxy \rightarrow Pxy$	IP is a particular type of parthood,
12. $IPxy \wedge Pyz \rightarrow IPxz$	left monotonicity.
13. $Pxy \wedge IPyz \rightarrow IPxz$	right monotonicity.[142]

Sentence 3 defines enclosure by connection. Sentence 4 defines interior parthood by parthood, connection, and overlap. The latter was defined in Table 15 on page 591. Theorems 9–10 are bridges between mereology and topology ("mereotopology").

As pointed out above, the goal of such axiomatizations and studies is, first, to implicitly or explicitly define the respective concepts, and second, to provide the necessary formal-ontological knowledge for use in medical decision-support systems. For details on mereotopology, see (Simons, 2000b; Casati and Varzi, 1999; Cohn and Varzi, 2003).

19.5.2 Fuzzy Formal Ontology

The mereology and mereotopology discussed up to this point must be qualified as *classical, ordinary,* or *crisp* because their underlying logic is the classical predicate logic and set theory. In spite of the obvious vagueness of the entire world surrounding us, formal ontologists still adhere to this classical approach. Medical entities, however, are vague and for this reason, coping with them requires a fuzzy approach. We saw, for example, that we do not know when a person begins and when she ends; where exactly the boundaries lie between two or more cells in a tissue, or between a cell and the extracellular space; how to draw a sharp demarcation line between two different diseases in an individual; when exactly a pathogenetic process in the organism begins; how long exactly the incubation period of an infectious disease is; and so on. Consequently, the crisp mereology and mereotopology may not be very relevant in medicine because the parts of vague entities are vague, as are the relations between them. To use the example above once again, (i) if personhood begins *discretely* at a particular time *t*, say on the 91st day of gestation, then according to Definitions 5–6 in Table 15 on page 591, the embryo preceding *t* cannot be a part of the person. Definition 6 implies that if they are discrete from one another, then they do not overlap. In this case it follows from Definition 5 that they do not have a common part, and thus, the embryo before *t* is not a part

---

[142] Mereotopology comes from the philosophy of the British mathematician Alfred North Whitehead (1861–1947), especially from his work *Process and Reality* (1929) in which he enriched mereology with some topological notions such as *connection* and *contiguity* (Clarke, 1981, 1985; Simons, 2000b; Cohn and Varzi, 2003).

of the person. This, however, is counterintuitive. Where does the person come from if not from the early embryo? Conversely, (ii) if personhood emerges *continuously* during a period of time and t is a point of this period, then personhood *vaguely overlaps* the embryo preceding t. Their overlapping part is a vague region such that its vagueness retrogradely increases because the region has no *earliest* point. A similar example concerns intracerebral bleedings, as displayed by imaging techniques like X-ray, magnetic resonance imaging, or positron emission tomography, since they have no exact boundaries. In this case, the bleeding structure in the brain also constitutes a vague region to the effect that it cannot always be determined whether an area in the penumbral surrounding is or is not a part of that region. Thus, in medicine and other fields as well, the crisp mereological primitive "is_a_part_of" should be replaced with the more general, fuzzy term "is_a_vague_part_of". This vagueness may also be mapped to $[0, 1]$ to yield degrees of parthood. What we would obtain in this way, is a concept of fuzzy parthood that could be supplemented with additional fuzzy-mereological concepts to construct a *fuzzy mereology*. The analogous fuzzifying of topological notions such as those used above, then, would pave the way toward fuzzy mereotopology. A full exposition is beyond our present scope, but in the following two sections:

▶ Fuzzy subsethood
▶ Fuzzy mereology

the first steps are taken toward fuzzy mereotopology in order to stimulate further research (Sadegh-Zadeh, Forthcoming).

Fuzzy subsethood

In preparation for our discussion of fuzzy mereology in the next section, we will first introduce the basic relation of *fuzzy subsethood* that will be used as an auxiliary. Initially, such a concept was presented by Lotfi Zadeh (1965a, 340). It says that a fuzzy set A is a subset of a fuzzy set B if and only if the membership degree of every object x_i in set A is less than or equals its membership degree in set B. That is:

$$A \subseteq B \text{ iff } \mu_A(x_i) \leq \mu_B(x_i) \tag{182}$$

for all x_i in the universe of discourse Ω. For example, if in the universe of discourse $\Omega = \{x_1, x_2, x_3, x_4, x_5\}$ we have the following two fuzzy sets:

$A = \{(x_1, 0.3), (x_2, 0.6), (x_3, 0.5), (x_4, 0), (x_5, 0)\}$,
$B = \{(x_1, 0.4), (x_2, 0.6), (x_3, 0.8), (x_4, 0), (x_5, 1)\}$,

then $A \subseteq B$. Surprisingly, this old concept of containment is still in use in fuzzy research and practice. However, Bart Kosko showed that it is a *crisp* concept and therefore deviates from the intentions of fuzzy set theory and logic

(Kosko, 1992, 278). It is crisp because it allows only for definite subsethood or definite non-subsethood between two fuzzy sets. All membership degrees in a fuzzy set B must dominate those in a fuzzy set A in order for A to be a subset of B. If 999 membership degrees in a set B of length 1000 dominate those in a set A, while only a single membership degree, the 1000th one in set B, falls short of the corresponding degree in set A, then the subsethood relation $A \subseteq B$ does not hold, although set A is actually a subset of B in 999 instances. The 1000th instance in B violates Zadeh's definition above and upsets the inclusion of A in B. So, the degree of subsethood between two fuzzy sets, A and B, is either 1 or 0. In its original formulation, then, there is no fuzziness of subsethood. To avoid such a bivalent relation, Kosko makes an alternative proposal, which we will briefly sketch below in order to use it in the next section.

Consider now what will happen if the membership degrees of objects in set A steadily increase so that more and more of them exceed the corresponding membership degree in set B. In such a case one will gradually approach a point where set A gains dominance, i.e., supersethood, over B. By quantifying this *gradual growth* of A's dominance over B we obtain a degree of *supersethood*. So, we shall first introduce a notion of fuzzy supersethood and derive subsethood by the formula $1 - supersethood$. To this end, we measure the dominance that set A gradually acquires, or fails to acquire, over set B by (i) determining the actual overhang of each individual membership degree in set A:

$$max\big(0, \mu_A(x_i) - \mu_B(x_i)\big)$$

and (ii) summing up all of them:

$$\sum max\big(0, \mu_A(x_i) - \mu_B(x_i)\big)$$

for all members x_i, and (iii) normalizing the result by dividing it through the count of set A:

$$\frac{\sum max\big(0, \mu_A(x_i) - \mu_B(x_i)\big)}{c(A)}. \tag{183}$$

(For the notion of fuzzy set *count c*, see Definition 32 on page 172.) The component 0 in the formula (183) guarantees that only overhangs in set A are gathered and used to yield a measure of dominance of set A over set B. The normalized measure (183) is just the degree of *supersethood* of set A over set B, and lies between 0 and 1 inclusive. If we symbolize the phrase "degree of supersethood of A over B" by "$supersethood(A, B)$", we may define this function, *supersethood*, in the following way:

Definition 178 (Fuzzy supersethood).

$$supersethood(A, B) = \frac{\sum max\big(0, \mu_A(x_i) - \mu_B(x_i)\big)}{c(A)}.$$

For example, if in the universe of discourse $\Omega = \{x_1, x_2, x_3, x_4, x_5\}$ our fuzzy sets are:

$$A = \{(x_1, 0.3), (x_2, 0.6), (x_3, 0.5), (x_4, 0), (x_5, 0)\},$$
$$B = \{(x_1, 0.4), (x_2, 0.6), (x_3, 0.8), (x_4, 0), (x_5, 1)\},$$
$$C = \{(x_1, 1), (x_2, 1), (x_3, 1), (x_4, 1), (x_5, 1)\},$$
$$D = \{(x_1, 1), (x_2, 1), (x_3, 0), (x_4, 1), (x_5, 0)\},$$
$$\varnothing = \{(x_1, 0), (x_2, 0), (x_3, 0), (x_4, 0), (x_5, 0)\},$$

then we have:

$$supersethood(A, A) = \frac{(0 + 0 + 0 + 0 + 0)}{1.4} = 0$$

$$supersethood(A, B) = \frac{(0 + 0 + 0 + 0 + 0)}{1.4} = 0$$

$$supersethood(B, A) = \frac{(0.1 + 0 + 0.3 + 0 + 1)}{2.8} = 0.5$$

$$supersethood(C, D) = \frac{(0 + 0 + 1 + 0 + 1)}{5} = 0.4$$

$$supersethood(D, C) = \frac{(0 + 0 + 0 + 0 + 0)}{5} = 0$$

$$supersethood(A, \varnothing) = \frac{(0.3 + 0.6 + 0.5 + 0 + 0)}{1.4} = 1$$

$$supersethood(\varnothing, A) = \frac{(0 + \cdots + 0)}{0} = 0.$$

Now, fuzzy *subsethood* is defined as a dual of the fuzzy supersethood, and is written $subsethood(A, B) = r$, to say that to the extent r fuzzy set A is a subset of fuzzy set B:

Definition 179 (Fuzzy subsethood).

$$subsethood(A, B) = 1 - supersethood(A, B).$$

Regarding the seven fuzzy sets above we have:

$subsethood(A, A) = 1 - 0 = 1$
$subsethood(A, B) = 1 - 0 = 1$
$subsethood(B, A) = 1 - 0.5 = 0.5$
$subsethood(C, D) = 1 - 0.4 = 0.6$
$subsethood(D, C) = 1 - 0 = 1$
$subsethood(A, \varnothing) = 1 - 1 = 0$
$subsethood(\varnothing, A) = 1 - 0 = 1.$

This concept of fuzzy subsethood is powerful enough to include both Zadeh's initial concept as well as the classical, crisp subsethood relation "$\subseteq$" between classical sets. See, for example, the latter three subsethood degrees. They show that:

If $X \subseteq Y$ in classical sense, then $subsethood(X, Y) = 1$,

if $X \subseteq Y$ in Zadeh's sense, then $subsethood(X, Y) = 1$.

The above procedure of determining the degree of $subsethood(A, B)$ indirectly by first determining the degree of $supersethood(A, B)$ is obviously a roundabout way. Fortunately, Bart Kosko proved a theorem called the *Subsethood Theorem* that enables a straightforward calculation thus (Kosko, 1992, 287):

Theorem 6 (Subsethood Theorem).

$$subsethood(A, B) = \frac{c(A \cap B)}{c(A)}.$$

By applying this theorem to the first two examples above, we will show that this relationship may be used instead of Definition 179:

$A = \{(x_1, 0.3), (x_2, 0.6), (x_3, 0.5), (x_4, 0), (x_5, 0)\},$

$B = \{(x_1, 0.4), (x_2, 0.6), (x_3, 0.8), (x_4, 0), (x_5, 1)\},$

$A \cap B = B \cap A = \{(x_1, 0.3), (x_2, 0.6), (x_3, 0.5), (x_4, 0), (x_5, 0)\}$

$c(A \cap B) = c(B \cap A) = 1.4$

$c(A) = 1$

$c(B) = 2.8$

$$subsethood(A, B) = \frac{c(A \cap B)}{c(A)} = \frac{1.4}{1.4} = 1$$

$$subsethood(B, A) = \frac{c(B \cap A)}{c(B)} = \frac{1.4}{2.8} = 0.5.$$

Thus, fuzzy $subsethood(A, B)$ is a binary function such that given a universe of discourse Ω, it maps the binary Cartesian product of Ω's fuzzy powerset, i.e., $F(2^\Omega) \times F(2^\Omega)$, to the unit interval. That is, $subsethood: F(2^\Omega) \times F(2^\Omega) \mapsto [0, 1]$.

Fuzzy mereology

With the concept of fuzzy subsethood in hand, we shall briefly outline a tentative fuzzy-logical approach to mereology by introducing some of its basic concepts: *fuzzy parthood*, *fuzzy proper parthood*, *fuzzy overlap*, and *fuzzy discreteness*. We shall also demonstrate some fuzzy-mereological theorems to show that they preserve classical-mereological relationships.

The classical, crisp mereology and mereotopology that we studied previously, are tacitly based on what we may call the *definiteness postulate* according to which parts as well as wholes are clear-cut objects with a definite constitution and sharp boundaries. This definiteness allows categorical judgments about whether an object x is part of another object y or not, overlaps it or not, and so on. An example is "the right thumb is a part of the right hand". Both the right thumb as well as the right hand are required to be definite entities. However, it is often the case that neither an object y as *the whole* nor an object x as its *part* can be delimited by clear-cut, declarative statements. For instance, in an injured tissue it is often impossible to say whether at the margin of a wound, y, a particular bunch of cells, x, is or is not a part of the wound. It is only to a particular extent a part thereof because the wound does not have a clear-cut boundary. The definiteness postulate above precludes even the possibility of such vague objects.

Otherwise put, the relations of parthood, connection, overlap, and others dealt with in classical mereology and mereotopology are Aristotelean, crisp relations that hold between clear-cut entities. Questions of the type "is x a part of y?", "is x connected to y?" and similar ones can only be answered either Yes or No by categorical statements of the type "x is a part of y", "a is not a part of b", and so on. It is impossible to state, for instance, that "x is barely a part of y" or "x is strongly connected to y". For practical considerations, then, we must abandon the definiteness postulate of classical mereology and mereotopology in favor of a fuzzy approach.

Our approach begins with the introduction of a concept of *fuzzy parthood* that does not presuppose the definiteness postulate. Through fuzzy parthood we access the entire corpus of fuzzy logic, thereby rendering fuzzy mereology useful in all practical domains whose objects and relations are vague, e.g., medical practice and research. We shall conceive fuzzy parthood as a binary function of the form "object x is a part of object y to the extent z", or:

The degree of parthood of x in y is z

symbolized by:

$$parthood(x, y) = z$$

where z is a real number in the unit interval $[0, 1]$. The relata x and y, i.e., the *part* and the *whole,* will be represented as fuzzy sets. For example, the clear-cut *right_hand* above may in a particular context be the fuzzy set displayed in (184) below. For the sake of readability, the following abbreviations will be used:

r	≡	right
r_t	≡	right thumb
r_f	≡	right forefinger
r_m	≡	right middle finger
r_r	≡	right ring finger
r_s	≡	right small finger.

For our purposes, the human right hand will be represented as an anatomically incomplete hand consisting of fingers only. However, larger sets can be made to represent the right hand as complete as 'it is in reality' consisting of muscles, bones, fingers, etc., by continuing the fuzzy set accordingly:

$$r\_hand = \{(r\_t, 1), (r\_f, 1), (r\_m, 1), (r\_r, 1), (r\_s, 1)\}. \tag{184}$$

This right hand is obviously a hand in anatomy atlases and contains each of the five fingers to the extent 1. However, consider the right hand of my neighbor Oliver who worked in a sawmill until recently:

$$Oliver's\ r\_hand = \{(r\_t, 0), (r\_f, 0.3), (r\_m, 0.5), (r\_r, 0.8), (r\_s, 1)\}.$$

Now, if you ask "is the right thumb a part of the right hand?", the answer will be "yes, insofar as you mean the right hand in anatomy atlases as listed in (184) above. But if you mean Oliver's right hand, no". More precisely, in anatomy atlases the right thumb is a part of the right hand to the extent 1. But regarding Oliver's right hand, which has no thumb, it is a part thereof to the extent 0. Likewise, in anatomy atlases the right forefinger is a part of the right hand to the extent 1. But regarding Oliver's right hand, it is a part thereof only to the extent 0.3, and so on.

The intuitive consideration above is based on our understanding that (i) parts and wholes are vague objects and are therefore best represented as fuzzy sets; (ii) parthood is a matter of degree; and (iii) this degree will be determined by defining *fuzzy parthood* by the degree of the *fuzzy subsethood* of the part in the whole. To this end, we must realize that the relation of fuzzy subsethood holds only between fuzzy sets of equal length because they must be fuzzy sets in the same universe of discourse $\Omega = \{x_1, \ldots, x_n\}$. Two fuzzy sets which are either of unequal length or do not stem from the same universe of discourse cannot be compared with one another. So, we face a problem:

Since a part is usually 'smaller' than the whole, the fuzzy set representing a part will be shorter than the fuzzy set that represents the whole. Consider, for example, a question of the form "is the right forefinger a part of the right hand?" that is based on data of the following type:

$$\begin{aligned} \{(r\_f, 1)\} &= \text{a right forefinger} \\ \{(r\_t, 1), (r\_f, 1), (r\_m, 1), (r\_r, 1), (r\_s, 1)\} &= \text{a right hand} \end{aligned} \tag{185}$$

such that the question reads:

Is $\{(r\_f, 1)\}$ *a part of* $\{(r\_t, 1), (r\_f, 1), (r\_m, 1), (r\_r, 1), (r\_s, 1)\}$?

In order to answer such a question regarding base entities of different size, we introduce the following method of representing mereological entities as fuzzy sets of equal length. We will divide a fuzzy set such as the right hand (185) above into two segments:

$$\{head \,|\, body\}$$

such that it starts with a head separated by a stroke "|" from the body that succeeds it. For example, the right hand in (185) above may be restructured in the following or in any other way:

$$\{(r\_t, 1)\} \,|\, \{(r\_f, 1), (r\_m, 1), (r\_r, 1), (r\_s, 1)\}.$$

What the head of such a restructured fuzzy set contains, depends on the *subject* x of the mereological question "is x a part of y?". For instance, if it is asked "is a *right forefinger* a part of the *right hand*", the subject of the question, referred to as the query subject, is a right forefinger:

$$\{(r\_f, 1)\}$$

and thus its object y, referred to as the query object, is the restructured fuzzy set:

$$\{(r\_f, 1)\} \,|\, \{(r\_t, 1), (r\_m, 1), (r\_r, 1), (r\_s, 1)\}$$

whose segment $(r\_f, 1)$ is taken to be its head and the remainder of the set to be its body. By so doing we need not examine the entirety of a *whole* to determine whether the query subject $\{(r\_f, 1)\}$ is a part thereof or not. We look only at the *head* of the restructured fuzzy set to examine whether, and to what extent, the *query subject* matches it. In our present example, the query subject, i.e., $(r\_f, 1)$, and the head of the restructured fuzzy set match completely. So, the answer to the query is "a right forefinger is a part of the right hand to the extent 1". This extent, 1, we obtain by determining the degree of fuzzy subsethood of the query subject, i.e., $(r\_f, 1)$, *in the head* of the restructured fuzzy set that represents the right hand. Asking the same question of the following restructured fuzzy set:

$$\{(r\_f, 0.3)\} \,|\, \{(r\_t, 0), (r\_m, 0.5), (r\_r, 0.8), (r\_s, 1)\} = \text{Oliver's right hand}$$

the answer is "a right forefinger is a part of Oliver's right hand only to the extent 0.3". We obtain this extent, 0.3, in the same fashion as above by determining the degree of fuzzy subsethood of the query subject $\{(r\_f, 1)\}$ in the head of the restructured fuzzy set that represents Oliver's right hand. It is of course possible that when inquiring into whether an entity x is a part of an entity y, the entity x is not elementary such as "a right forefinger". It may also be a compound such as "a right forefinger and a right middle finger" to ask whether "a right forefinger and a right middle finger are a part of the right hand". In this case, our query subject and restructured fuzzy sets are:

$$\{(r\_f, 1), (r\_m, 1)\} \qquad = \text{a right forefinger and a right middle finger,}$$
$$\{(r\_f, 1), (r\_m, 1)\} \,|\, \{(r\_t, 1), (r\_r, 1), (r\_s, 1)\} = \text{a right hand in anato-}$$
$$\text{my atlases,}$$
$$\{(r\_f, 0.3), (r\_m, 0.5)\} \,|\, \{(r\_t, 0), (r\_r, 0.8), (r\_s, 1)\} = \text{Oliver's right hand.}$$

Regarding the fuzzy parthood of the compound query subject $\{(r\_f, 1), (r\_m, 1)\}$ in each of the two right hands above we obtain the following results:

- $\{(r\_f, 1), (r\_m, 1)\}$ is a part of the right hand in anatomy atlases to the extent 1,
- $\{(r\_f, 1), (r\_m, 1)\}$ is a part of Oliver's right hand to the extent 0.4.

It is worth noting that a restructured fuzzy set, represented as $\{head \mid body\}$, may either have an empty head or an empty body:

$$\{\varnothing \mid body\}$$
$$\{head \mid \varnothing\}$$

depending on the extent of overlap between the query subject and the query object. In any event, it can easily be determined whether and to what extent the query subject is a fuzzy subset of the head of the query object. This is exactly our concept of fuzzy parthood introduced in the Definition 180 below. To this end, we denote the head of a restructured fuzzy set A by $head(A)$. For example, if A is Oliver's restructured right hand $\{(r\_f, 0.3), (r\_m, 0.5)\} \mid \{(r\_t, 0), (r\_r, 0.8), (r\_s, 1)\}$, then we have $head(A) = \{(r\_f, 0.3), (r\_m, 0.5)\}$.

We must now establish how to decide the *length* of a fuzzy set in a mereological discourse. For example, it does not make sense to ask whether a hand is a part of the forefinger because a hand, represented as a fuzzy set, is longer than a forefinger as a fuzzy set. So, a comparison will not be feasible. We may prevent such cases using the following three auxiliary notions:

First, two universes of discourse, Ω_1 and Ω_2, are said to be related if one of them is a subset of the other one, i.e., if either $\Omega_1 \subseteq \Omega_2$ or $\Omega_2 \subseteq \Omega_1$. Otherwise, they are unrelated. For example, {thumb, forefinger, middle_finger} and {thumb, middle_finger} are related, while {thumb, forefinger, middle_finger} and {eye, ear} or {ring_finger, small_finger} are unrelated.

Second, two fuzzy sets A and B are said to be *co-local* if their universes of discourse, Ω_A and Ω_B, are related, i.e., (i) A is a fuzzy set in Ω_A; (ii) B is a fuzzy set in Ω_B; and (iii) Ω_A and Ω_B are related. For example, $\{(r\_t, 1), (r\_f, 1), (r\_m, 1)\}$ and $\{(r\_t, 0), (r\_f, 0.3)\}$ are co-local, while $\{(r\_t, 1), (r\_f, 1), (r\_m, 1)\}$ and $\{(eye, 1), (ear, 0.7)\}$ are not co-local.

Third, two fuzzy sets A and B are of equal length if they have the same number of members. For instance, $\{(r\_t, 1), (r\_f, 1), (r\_m, 1)\}$ and $\{(r\_t, 0), (r\_f, 0.3), (r\_m, 0.5)\}$ are of equal length, while $\{(r\_t, 1), (r\_f, 1), (r\_m, 1)\}$ is longer than $\{(r\_t, 0), (r\_f, 0.3)\}$. The phrase "the length of the fuzzy set A" is written "$length(A)$".

Definition 180 (Fuzzy parthood). *If X and Y are co-local fuzzy sets, then:*

$$parthood(X, Y) = \begin{cases} 0 & \text{if } head(Y) = \varnothing \text{ or} \\ & lenght(X) > lenght(Y) \\ subsethood(X, head(Y)) & otherwise. \end{cases}$$

As an example, we will now calculate the degree of parthood of the fuzzy set:

$$A = \{(a, 1), (b, 0.4), (c, 0.6)\}$$

in following fuzzy structures :

$$
\begin{aligned}
A &= \{(a, 1), (b, 0.4), (c, 0.6)\} \\
  &= \{(a, 1), (b, 0.4), (c, 0.6)\} \mid \varnothing \\
B &= \{(x, 0.9), (a, 0.6), (y, 1), (b, 0.2), (z, 0.5), (c, 1)\} \\
  &= \{(a, 0.6), (b, 0.2), (c, 1)\} \mid \{(x, 0.9), (y, 1), (z, 0.5)\} \\
C &= \{(x, 1), (a, 1), (y, 0), (b, 0.4), (z, 1), (c, 0.6)\} \\
  &= \{(a, 1), (b, 0.4), (c, 0.6)\} \mid \{(x, 1), (y, 0), (z, 1)\} \\
D &= \{(x, 1), (a, 0), (y, 0), (b, 0), (z, 1), (c, 0)\} \\
  &= \{(a, 0), (b, 0), (c, 0)\} \mid \{(x, 1), (y, 0), (z, 1)\} \\
  &= \varnothing \mid \{(x, 1), (y, 0), (z, 1)\} \\
E &= \{(a, 0), (b, 0), (c, 0)\} \\
  &= \{(a, 0), (b, 0), (c, 0)\} \mid \varnothing \\
  &= \varnothing \mid \varnothing \\
F &= \{(a, 1), (b, 0.4), (c, 0.6)\} \\
  &= \{(a, 1), (b, 0.4), (c, 0.6)\} \mid \varnothing
\end{aligned}
$$

By employing the Subsethood Theorem, i.e., Theorem 6 on page 745, we obtain the following degrees of parthood:

$$
\begin{aligned}
parthood(A, A) &= 1 \\
parthood(A, B) &= subsethood(A, head(B)) \\
&= \frac{0.6. + 0.2 + 0.6}{1 + 0.4 + 0.6} = \frac{1.4}{2} \\
&= 0.7 \\
parthood(A, C) &= 1 \\
parthood(A, D) &= 0 \\
parthood(A, E) &= parthood(A, \varnothing) = 0 \\
parthood(A, F) &= parthood(A, A) = 1.
\end{aligned}
$$

Since fuzzy parthood is defined by fuzzy subsethood, its degree lies in the unit interval $[0, 1]$. The last examples show that an object is a part of itself to the extent 1 and a part of the empty object $\varnothing$ to the extent 0.

Something may be partially or completely a part of something else. The question arises whether it is a proper part thereof. We define the degree of *fuzzy proper parthood* of an object A in another object B, written *p-parthood*(A, B), by the notion of fuzzy parthood thus:

Definition 181 (Fuzzy proper parthood). *If X and Y are co-local fuzzy sets with $length(X) \leq length(Y)$, then:*

$$p\text{-}parthood(X,Y) = \begin{cases} 0 & \text{if } head(Y) = \varnothing \text{ or } X = Y \\ parthood(X,Y) & \text{otherwise.} \end{cases}$$

For instance, the degree of proper parthood of the above example fuzzy set $A = \{(a,1),(b,0.4),(c,0.6)\}$ in fuzzy sets A-F are:

$p\text{-}parthood(A,A) = 0$

$p\text{-}parthood(A,B) = 0.7$

$p\text{-}parthood(A,C) = 0$

$p\text{-}parthood(A,D) = 0$

$p\text{-}parthood(A,E) = p\text{-}parthood(A,\varnothing) = 0$

$p\text{-}parthood(A,F) = p\text{-}parthood(A,A) = 0.$

Without fuzzifying the entities we may give some intuitive examples to show that our fuzzy approach preserves the classical relations of parthood and proper parthood:

$parthood(r\_thumb, r\_thumb)$	$= 1$	$p\text{-}parthood(r\_thumb, r\_thumb) = 0$	
$parthood(r\_thumb, r\_hand)$	$= 1$	$p\text{-}parthood(r\_thumb, r\_hand) = 1$	
$parthood(r\_thumb, r\_kidney)$	$= 0$	$p\text{-}parthood(r\_thumb, r\_kidney) = 0$	
$parthood(r\_thumb, \varnothing)$	$= 0$	$p\text{-}parthood(r\_thumb, \varnothing) = 0$	
$parthood(\varnothing, r\_hand)$	$= 1$	$p\text{-}parthood(\varnothing, r\_hand) = 1$	
$parthood(\varnothing, r\_thumb)$	$= 1$	$p\text{-}parthood(\varnothing, r\_thumb) = 1.$	

Parthood and proper parthood are binary functions which map the fuzzy powerset of the Cartesian product of two categories of entities, Ω_1 and Ω_2, to the unit interval $[0,1]$. That is:

$parthood \colon F(2^{\Omega_1}) \times F(2^{\Omega_2}) \mapsto [0,1]$

$p\text{-}parthood \colon F(2^{\Omega_1}) \times F(2^{\Omega_2}) \mapsto [0,1].$

We may now move on in our discussion to the fuzzy-mereological concepts of *fuzzy overlap* and *fuzzy discreteness*. They have the following syntax:

$overlap(X,Y) = r$	$\equiv$	X overlaps Y to the extent r,
$discrete(X,Y) = r$	$\equiv$	X is discrete from Y to the extent r.

To apply these concepts, we need the following, auxiliary notion of the *degree of intersection* of two fuzzy sets. Its syntax is:

$intersection(X,Y) = r \qquad \equiv \qquad$ the degree of intersection of X and Y is r.

Definition 182 (Degree of fuzzy intersection). *If X and Y are two fuzzy sets in the universe of discourse Ω, then:*

$$intersection(X, Y) = \frac{c(X \cap Y)}{c(X \cup Y)}.$$

For example, if our entities are the following fuzzy sets in the universe $\Omega = \{x, y, z\}$:

$A = \{(x, 0.3), (y, 0.8), (z, 0.4)\},$
$B = \{(x, 1), (y, 0.5), (z, 0.3)\},$

then we have: $intersection(A, B) = \frac{(0.3 + 0.5 + 0.3)}{(1 + 0.8 + 0.4)} = \frac{1.1}{2.2} = 0.5.$

Definition 183 (Degree of fuzzy overlap). *If X and Y are co-local fuzzy sets, then:*

$$overlap(X, Y) = \begin{cases} intersection(X, head(Y)) & \text{if } lenght(X) \leq lenght(Y) \\ intersection(head(X), Y) & otherwise. \end{cases}$$

For instance, the two co-local fuzzy sets A and B mentioned above overlap to the extent 0.5. A more instructive example may be:

$\{(r\_f, 1), (r\_m, 1)\}$ = a right forefinger and a right middle finger,
$\{(r\_f, 0.3), (r\_m, 0.5)\} \mid \{(r\_t, 0), (r\_r, 0.8), (r\_s, 1)\}$ = Oliver's right hand.

These two fuzzy sets of unequal length, referred to as C and D, respectively, overlap to the following extent:

$$overlap(C, D) = \frac{(0.3 + 0.5)}{1 + 1} = 0.4$$

where $head(D) = \{(r\_f, 0.3), (r\_m, 0.5)\}$ because $D = \{(r\_f, 0.3), (r\_m, 0.5)\} \mid \{(r\_t, 0), (r\_r, 0.8), (r\_s, 1)\}$.

Definition 184 (Degree of fuzzy discreteness). *If X and Y are co-local fuzzy sets, then $discrete(X, Y) = 1 - overlap(X, Y)$.*

For instance, the last two fuzzy sets C and D mentioned above are discrete from one another to the extent $1 - 0.4 = 0.6$. But the same set C is totally discrete from the following fuzzy set:

$E = \{(r\_f, 0), (r\_m, 0)\}.$

That is, $discrete(C, E) = 1$ because $overlap(C, E) = 0$ and $1 - 0 = 1$.

So far we looked at the following concepts: degrees of parthood, proper parthood, intersection, overlap, and discreteness. All of them were defined by means of purely fuzzy set-theoretical notions. Thus, none of them is a primitive. Table 27 displays some corollaries of the definitions above. They express important fuzzy-mereological relationships and show that classical-mereological relationships are only limiting cases thereof, i.e., bivalent instances of them with limiting values 0 and 1. For example, the first corollary corresponds to the axiom of reflexivity of classical parthood, and the second one corresponds to its axiom of symmetry.

Table 27. Some fuzzy-mereological theorems

1. $parthood(A, A) = 1$
2. $parthood(A, B) = parthood(B, A) = 1 \rightarrow A = B$
3. $parthood(A, B) > 0 \land parthood(B, C) > 0 \rightarrow parthood(A, C) > 0$
4. $parthood(A, B) > 0 \rightarrow overlap(A, B) > 0$
5. $parthood(A, B) > 0 \rightarrow parthood(A, B) = overlap(A, B)$
6. $A \neq B \rightarrow p\text{-}parthood(A, B) = parthood(A, B)$
7. $p\text{-}parthood(A, A) = 0$
8. $p\text{-}parthood(A, B) = r \land r > 0 \rightarrow parthood(A, B) = r$
9. $p\text{-}parthood(A, B) > 0 \rightarrow p\text{-}parthood(A, B) = parthood(A, B)$
10. $p\text{-}parthood(A, B) > 0 \land p\text{-}parthood(B, C) > 0 \rightarrow p\text{-}parthood(A, C) > 0$
11. $overlap(A, A) = 1$
12. $overlap(A, B) = overlap(B, A)$
13. $overlap(A, B) > 0 \land parthood(B, C) > 0 \rightarrow overlap(A, C) > 0$
14. $overlap(A, B) > 0 \rightarrow \exists C (parthood(C, A) > 0 \land parthood(C, B) > 0)$
15. $discrete(A, B) = 1 \rightarrow overlap(A, B) = 0$

19.6 Medical Ontology *de re* and *de dicto*

On page 707 we distinguished between existence *de re* and existence *de dicto* in order to appraise and characterize the mode of existence of fictional entities. This was made possible by introducing the modal operator $\mathcal{A}_S$ that reads "it is asserted in story S that". The "story S" is to be understood in a more general sense as a variable denoting any narrative, i.e., linguistic, context and narrated source to which one may refer. For example, we refer to clonal selection theory of immunity when we say:

It is asserted in *the clonal selection theory of immunity* that ...   (186)

there are antigens, antibodies, and lymphocytes such that an antigen selects from among a variety of lymphocytes those which are capable of expressing complementary, antigen-specific receptors ... etc. Thus, (186) says:

$\mathcal{A}_{the\ clonal\ selection\ theory\ of\ immunity}$ $\cdots$

In the subscript of this operator, the clonal selection theory of immunity is the story S. Therefore, from now on the operator $\mathcal{A}_S$ may read more generally "it is asserted in the context S that" where "context S" stands for any quotable source, e.g., story, theory, sentence, conversation, sermon, decree, myth, and the like.

We saw in preceding sections that the question of whether something, e.g., schizophrenia, does or does not exist, is controversial in medicine. A method of reasoning that differentiates between *de re* and *de dicto* ontology may be used to settle such ontological debates in the following way:

Consider, for example, that in response to Thomas Szasz' antipsychiatric reproaches referred to on page 730, an orthodox psychiatrist might retort that certainly there are mental disorders. She is therefore recommended to clearly state what she means by her claim "there are mental disorders". Which one of the following claims does she intend to make, the de re or the de dicto one?

de re: $\exists x \mathcal{A}_S(x$ is a mental disorder$)$
de dicto: $\mathcal{A}_S \exists x(x$ is a mental disorder$)$.

Here, context S could be further specified, for example, as a work by Sigmund Freud or the "Diagnostic and Statistical Manual of Mental Disorders, Fourth Edition", DSM-IV for short:

de re: $\exists x \mathcal{A}_{DSM\text{-}IV}(x$ is a mental disorder$)$
de dicto: $\mathcal{A}_{DSM\text{-}IV} \exists x(x$ is a mental disorder$)$.

In the first, de re case she would have to explicitly specify what the entity x is that she contends to exist while reporting in addition that DSM-IV declares that existent x to be a mental disorder. Since the existence claim "$\exists x$" and the predication step "x is a mental disorder" are detached from one another, they are obviously two different acts of asserting and must therefore be justified independently. In the second, de dicto case she would merely be reporting on an existence claim made in a story S, i.e., DSM-IV in the present example, for which she is not responsible and that she may not share. What will be gained in both cases is the clarity of the ontological discourse, on the one hand; and the following epistemologically significant result, on the other.

Obviously, the de dicto ontological statement above is an analog of the ontology of fictional entities discussed in Section 18.3.2 on page 706. It mimics reports of the form "According to Arthur Conan Doyle's story *A Study in Scarlet* there is a detective called Sherlock Holmes whose place of residence is 221B Baker Street in London". To prove that a medical entity, be it a disease, a gene, or something else, is not an invented artifact like a fictional character, one must scrutinize the conceptual framework of the dispute, including its logic, and the epistemological status of the context S with respect to which an existence claim is made. What is particularly important is that in each case the ontological discourse turns out to be a context-relative, conceptual, logical, and epistemological inquiry.

Biomedical ontology engineering, discussed in Section 19.4 on page 735, may also be categorized as a *de dicto* ontology if it is an ontological endeavor at all. The reason of this skepticism is that biomedical ontology engineers confine themselves to the analysis of biomedical vocabularies and make their ontological claims on the basis of such a vocabulary V, e.g., SNOMED. Thus, their claims are reconstructible in the following fashion:

de dicto: $\mathcal{A}_{vocabulary\text{-}V} \exists x(x \ is \ P).$

What they declare as existent and as the ontology° of a discipline such as anatomy or genetics, is based merely on the fact that the names of the entities they are talking about, are written in the vocabulary V. Had the vocabulary V contained other names, e.g., "dyscrasia", "drapetomania" and "Pegasus", then they would of course advocate the existence of these dubious entities and would analyze their fictitious ontologies°.

With the existence predicates in Definitions 172–173 on page 692 and the discussion above, we demonstrated that the ontological analysis and adjudication of a medical existence claim such as "mental disorders exist" as well as its denial, is inextricably intertwined with the underlying language, conceptual system, knowledge, and logic. It is impossible to conduct ontology in a vacuum. Our ontological beliefs are relative to the respective contexts and logics, say theories, that we endorse or use, or to which we refer. On this account, the naive-ontological realism held by biomedical ontologists and others represents a kind of dogmatism. When the context and logic that serve as the frame of reference of an ontological discourse die out such as, for example, the Hippocratic medicine, the entities claimed with respect to that frame will also disappear. Examples are obsolete diseases such as cacochymia and leucophlegmatia. "If I ask about the world, you can offer to tell me how it is under one or more frames of reference; but if I insist that you tell me how it is apart from all frames, what can you say?" (Goodman, 1975, 58).

19.7 Summary

We briefly discussed some basic notions of ontology. We also showed that existence may arguably be conceived as a predicate. Without this legitimate option, nobody could talk of the *category of existent entities* and that of non-existens. In addition, we introduced a concept of fuzzy existence, referred to as the Heraclitean operator, that renders the transition between being and nothingness continuous. Both approaches advance a thesis of ontological relativity with respect to the language and logic used. We showed that the analysis of the ontological commitments of medical knowledge represents an ideal method of medical-ontological research. We also discussed the ontology of nosology in general, and of mental and psychosomatic disorders in particular. We argued that nosological nominalism and tropism may be defendable, on the one hand; and compatible with social constructivism, on the other. We advanced an emergentist theory of mind according to which the psychogenesis of mental and psychosomatic disorders cannot exist. Their sociogenesis was advocated instead. The so-called biomedical ontology engineering was demonstrated to deal primarily with medical vocabularies and thesauri, but not with medical ontology. It is thus a *de dicto* ontology, and as such, a medical-linguistic enterprise. Our dichotomy of ontology into *de re* versus *de dicto* ontology was applied to diseases to show how the ontology of nosology may benefit from this distinction. We in addition outlined a fuzzy approach to formal ontology by taking the first steps toward fuzzy mereology.

On Medical Truth

20.0 Introduction

Since the advent of the natural sciences, natural scientists have spread the idea that the pursuit of truth about the facts of the world is the main drive of scientific research. The aim, they say, is to acquire knowledge and to provide explanations and predictions of phenomena and events. Surprisingly, even in our contemporary world in which scientific research is strongly involved in seeking solutions to the practical problems pertaining to the pursuit of food, water, energy, health, labor, peace, war, nuclear weapons, and the like, *the pursuit-of-truth postulate* nevertheless enjoys vigorous advocacy, especially in philosophy (see Goldman, 2003). In this chapter, the role that truth actually plays in medicine will be examined. Our discussion of this issue divides into the following four sections:

    20.1 Truth in Medical Sciences
    20.2 Truth in Clinical Practice
    20.3 Misdiagnoses
    20.4 Truth Made in Medicine.

20.1 Truth in Medical Sciences

Like other branches of scientific research, medical research is usually considered a pursuit-of-truth endeavor whose aim is the explanation and prediction of events, for example, the explanation of morbidity and the prediction of treatment effects. Supposedly, medical research records all the truths in its domain by gaining knowledge about cells, genes, genetic diseases, clonal selection theory, AIDS, and so on in order to achieve its aim. But how is one to know whether an entry in this record of truths, e.g., the clonal selection theory of immunity, is true? The answer is simple: A theory of truth is needed that (i) defines the term "true", tells us how the term functions in the language

K. Sadegh-Zadeh, *Handbook of Analytic Philosophy of Medicine*,
Philosophy and Medicine 113, DOI 10.1007/978-94-007-2260-6_20,
© Springer Science+Business Media B.V. 2012

of medicine, and what the properties of truth are; and (ii) informs us how to find out whether an item of medical knowledge under discussion satisfies that theory. These two criteria may be referred to as *truth theory* and *truth determination,* respectively. As discussed in Section 11.1.1 on page 460, however, there are a variety of conflicting truth theories and no method of truth determination. Only one of these theories of truth is relevant in the present context, i.e., the semantic theory of truth. To ascertain whether in the light of this theory the pursuit-of-truth postulate holds in medicine, we must recall that for reasons outlined in several places in previous chapters there are scarcely any truths in medical sciences. This lack of truth is mainly due to the circumstance that a major part of medical knowledge either consists of unverifiable hypotheses or deontic rules. When truth is principally unattainable, it cannot be pursued.

That there is so little truth in medical sciences should not be surprising or disappointing. The deeply entrenched belief in the truth of scientific knowledge originates from Greek antiquity. However, by thorough analyses of language and truth, we have since learned that truth is not a property that every empirical sentence could possess because it also depends on the syntax of the sentence. As pointed out in Section 9.3, there are truth-repelling syntaxes such as the combination of $\forall$ and $\exists$ in a statement of the form $\forall x \exists y \alpha$, e.g., $\forall x \exists y (Px \rightarrow Qyx)$. Examples are the well-known slogans "everybody loves someone"; "every cell stems from another cell"; and "every event has a cause". Moreover, truth cannot be separated from human intentionality and worldmaking. It is formed and created rather than discovered.

20.2 Truth in Clinical Practice

In diagnostic-therapeutic decision-making, the physician needs and uses information on the present and past state of the patient. Apart from the physician's own observations, the sources of most of the data she uses are the patient's reports, the reports of the patient's family members, and the reports of other physicians as well as reports from laboratories, the physician's assistants, and others. The physician seldom knows which data are true and which data are false. They are mostly *uncertain.* She groups them according to the extent of their certainty, i.e., credibility, probability, or plausibility. The only option she has in this situation is to epistemically trust the testifiers from whom she receives the data as testimonies. Even the testifiers themselves do not know whether the data that they gather from tests, apparatuses, or measurements are true. Both their and the physician's uncertain observations require all of them to epistemically trust each other. In addition, they must also trust other persons involved such as engineers and mathematicians who have constructed the methods and apparatuses they use to take, for example, ECGs, EEGs, ultrasonic or other images such as CT, MRT, PET, and SPECT. The same requirement of epistemic trust obtains with regard to the medical knowledge that the doctor explicitly uses to attain a diagnosis, prognosis, or therapeutic judgment, knowledge which we showed in the preceding section cannot be true. Thus, not epistemic truth of knowledge, but epistemic trust in testifiers is a fundamental characteristic of clinical decision-making. There can be no doubt that from a context of this type where the truth values of the premises are unknown, merely conjectural diagnoses and prognoses can arise. However, even without possessing the truth value *true,* diagnoses and prognoses create facts, and thus *truth,* because they are performatives. This we have stressed in several places in previous chapters.

20.3 Misdiagnoses

An issue central to medical truth is the problem of misdiagnosis. Although it could be used as a point of departure for the philosophy of medicine, neither in medicine nor in the philosophy of medicine has it received the attention it deserves. It is neglected primarily because the term "misdiagnosis" is ill-defined and gives the impression of triviality. It is usually taken to mean: "A misdiagnosis is a diagnosis that turns out wrong". This customary view may be reconstructed as a conditional definition of the following form:

If α is a diagnosis, then α is a misdiagnosis iff α is wrong.   (187)

Being "wrong" includes the plain falsehood, incompleteness, and overcompleteness of a diagnosis. For example, if a patient has diabetes and hepatitis, then a diagnosis of her state is (i) false when it ignores both diseases and says, e.g., that the patient has gastritis; (ii) it is incomplete when it ignores one of the two diseases and only says, e.g., that she has diabetes; and (iii) it is overcomplete when it adds, superfluously, a third disease that the patient does not have and says, e.g., that the patient has diabetes, hepatitis, and gastritis.

The provisional reconstruction of the received view in (187) above shows that in order for something to be a misdiagnosis, it must first be a diagnosis. The concept of diagnosis was defined in Sections 8.2.6–8.2.8. Taking that concept into account, a misdiagnosis may be a wrong categorical diagnosis or a wrong conjectural diagnosis. For example,

- the *categorical* diagnosis "Elroy Fox has diabetes and he does not have hepatitis" is a misdiagnosis if the patient does in fact have hepatitis. Likewise, the categorical fuzzy diagnosis "the extent to which Elroy Fox has acute leukemia is 0.6" is a misdiagnosis if the patient does not have leukemia, i.e., the extent to which he has leukemia is 0.
- the *conjectural* diagnosis "the probability that Elroy Fox has acute appendicitis, is 0.6" is a misdiagnosis if the patient definitely has acute appendicitis. In this case, the probability that he has the disease is $1 \neq 0.6$ falsifying the conjectural diagnosis. This is interesting as well as disturbing because *all* probabilistic diagnoses with $0 < p < 1$ will turn out misdiagnoses as soon as true alternative diagnoses become known.

In line with (187) above, a diagnosis α can be considered a misdiagnosis only if there is a true statement β, e.g., a finding, that shows that α is incomplete, overcomplete, or false. Such a statement β falsifies a wrong diagnosis and is therefore referred to here as a falsifying evidence. The falsifying evidence is almost always itself an *alternative diagnosis* that replaces the misdiagnosis.

Where does an alternative diagnosis come from? It may be the result of new data about the patient gathered by additional examination or by autopsy, of new medical knowledge, or of a new method of diagnostic inquiry and reasoning. In order that a statement can be considered an alternative diagnosis, it must have some conceptual basis in common with the diagnosis which it is replacing. To this end, the knowledge base from which it emerges must be commensurable with the knowledge base from which the misdiagnosis emerged. For example, a Hippocratic diagnosis such as "the patient has cacochymia" cannot be falsified by a modern, hematological diagnosis such as "the patient has leukemia" because modern hematological knowledge has nothing in common with Hippocratic medicine. Otherwise put, they have different ontologies and are talking about two different worlds. Thus, in order to replace a diagnosis α about a patient x with an alternative diagnosis:

1. there must exist a knowledge base KB, a diagnostic method M, a patient data set D, and a sentence β about the patient x such that β is a diagnosis about x relative to D and $KB \cup M$ as its frame of reference. That is, $diagnosis(x, D, KB \cup M) = \{\beta\}$. See Sections 8.2.6 and 8.2.10;
2. the knowledge base KB must be commensurable with the knowledge base KB' by use of which the initial diagnosis α has been obtained. That is, if $\{\alpha\} = diagnosis(x, D', KB' \cup M')$, then KB and KB' must be commensurable;
3. the diagnosis α, as compared to β, must be false, incomplete, or overcomplete.

For instance, suppose that the patient Elroy Fox undergoes surgery because of the diagnosis "Elroy Fox has acute appendicitis". However, the histological examination of his removed appendix shows that it is not inflammated. This new data in conjunction with clinical-pathological knowledge yields the alternative diagnosis "Elroy Fox does not have acute appendicitis". This statement is now considered true and falsifies the initial diagnosis. Note that if the initial diagnosis were a probabilistic one, e.g., $p(\alpha) = 0.6$, it would be impossible to falsify it by a new probabilistic diagnosis of the form $p(\beta) = r$ whenever $0 < r < 1$. That means that for a diagnosis to turn out a misdiagnosis, a *true categorical statement* is required that falsifies it. A conjectural diagnosis can never falsify another diagnosis because a conjectural diagnosis does not have the truth value *true*. Therefore, it can only serve as a competing diagnosis.

It was pointed out above that a frame of reference from which an alternative diagnosis emerges, must have common conceptual ground with the frame of reference that produced the falsified diagnosis. Diagnoses originating from disjoint conceptual systems cannot falsify each other. For example, a student of contemporary Western medicine cannot reasonably argue that Hippocratic diagnoses were all false or the diagnoses made on the basis of the traditional Chinese medicine are wrong. It is worth noting that our contemporary medicine is a *multiparadigmatic discipline* which comprises many different theories, e.g., cell theory, theory of infectious diseases, theory of autoimmune diseases, theory of genetic diseases, psychosomatics, etc. As a result, it contains sub-areas which are conceptually incommensurable, for example, infectiology and psychoanalysis. Thus, a diagnosis which says that the patient has peptic ulcer disease caused by helicobacter pylori will be unable to falsify the psychoanalytic diagnosis that she has a psychosomatic disease, and vice versa. Both diagnoses may exist simultaneously with advocates in two different professional communities. That means that like diagnoses, misdiagnoses are also relative to frames of reference. A statement that is considered a misdiagnosis from a particular point of view, need not be a misdiagnosis from another point of view.

Up to now, we considered the truth of the falsifying evidence a prerequisite. This leads to several problems. First, we know how difficult it is to obtain true statements about the patient's health condition. Second, the very concept of truth is problematic. Third, since the class of alternative diagnoses itself is a class of diagnoses, we may legitimately ask how many of these new diagnoses may turn out wrong in the future. For example, a diagnosis α made by the pathologist is often considered a falsifying diagnosis against the clinician's diagnosis β if they differ from one another. However, it may be that the pathologist's diagnosis will itself be falsified by an alternative diagnosis made by a clinical chemist. That means that not only the truth value of a diagnosis, but also the truth value of a falsifying alternative diagnosis is always something provisional. The ultimate truth of a diagnosis is never known definitely. A sensible concept of diagnosis, therefore, should not require that a diagnosis be a true statement about the patient.

The considerations above demonstrate that the ordinary concept of misdiagnosis reconstructed in (187) above is too simplistic. An acceptable concept of misdiagnosis has to take into account all of the relativities that we briefly mentioned in our discussion.

20.4 Truth Made in Medicine

According to the non-statement view of theories discussed previously, a medical theory is an artifactual, conceptual structure by means of which one may inquire into whether some particular objects belong to its application domain. For example, with reference to our miniature theory of active immunity sketched in Definition 129 on page 422, someone may ask whether human beings could be successfully vaccinated against myocardial infarction. Such a question should of course have some rationale behind it in order not to be odd and unanswerable. The rationale behind the present question is that coronary heart disease, as a cause of myocardial infarction, is likely to be caused by Chlamydophila pneumoniae. This hypothesis was dealt with in Section 6.5.3. Should it be possible to prevent or reduce the incidence of coronary heart disease in the population of those who are vaccinated against Chlamydophila pneumoniae, then this would mean that we have succeeded in rendering the following structure a model for our theory: ⟨set of human beings, Chlamydophila pneumoniae infection, antibodies against Chlamydophila pneumoniae⟩. Such an active immunity structure, then, would provide a basic immunity against coronary heart disease and myocardial infarction.

Through such a process of interrogation and exploration based on theories, we may design research programs that produce medical knowledge. Note that not a theory itself, but the knowledge acquired thereby is subject to epistemic qualifications such as true, false, believable, quite true, very true, probable, plausible, etc. Like theories, medical nomenclatures, thesauri, taxonomies, and terminologies are also artifactual systems constructed by medical communities and added to the language of medicine as a natural language. Medical and biomedical knowledge about any subject, e.g., organisms, cells, genes, diseases and therapies, is gained on the basis of such artifactual structures and systems.

Diagnoses, prognoses, and therapeutic and preventive decisions as the ultimate products of medicine are obtained by employing medical language and knowledge. They are thus made on the basis of artifactual-medical structures and systems. We can therefore conclude that when anything said about a patient, malady, or therapy is true in a particular health care system such as Western medicine or traditional Chinese medicine, then this truth is made in that system itself. The history of medicine demonstrates that another health care system may make other truths. Medical truths are system-relative.

20.5 Summary

Medical knowledge does not contain much truth because it mainly consists of hypotheses and deontic rules. The truth values of the former are unknown. The latter have no truth values. Likewise, in clinical practice true diagnoses and prognoses are not always attainable because (i) medical knowledge is inevitably vague, uncertain, and unreliable; (ii) this also holds true for most parts of patient data; (iii) physicians are not trained in viable and efficient methodology of clinical reasoning; and (iv) neither clinical decision support systems nor the automation of clinical decision-making will be able to compensate for the first two shortcomings. So, misdiagnoses will remain unavoidable forever, although their frequency may be reduced by improving the techniques of clinical judgment. Since medical theories are artifactual structures and medical languages are artifactual systems, the truth of the diagnoses and prognoses based upon them is made in medicine (Sadegh-Zadeh, 1981c).

On the Nature of Medicine

21.0 Introduction

The quality of medical practice, research, and education depends considerably on the image medical professionals, researchers, and teachers have of their discipline because that image determines the modes of their professional, scientific, and educational conduct. This image refers to what they usually term 'the nature of medicine'. Accordingly, the nature of medicine is often a central theme in metamedical discussions concerned with the question "what is medicine?". Is it a natural science? Is it an applied science? Is it an A or a B or a C? The preceding chapters revealed many new and interesting features of medicine, casting a new light on that question.

We outlined on pages 103–105 that due to the polysemy of the particles "what" and "is", a what-is-X question such as "what is medicine?" is usually misunderstood. It gives the impression that an answer to it in the form of "X is_a P", e.g., "medicine is_a practical science", provides a definition of X as if X were nothing else than P. However, the particle "is_a" in an answer of the form "medicine is_a practical science" is a descriptive, taxonomic subsumption predicate and merely characterizes X as having the feature P among its features such as "melanoma is a skin disease" or "Einstein is_a physicist".

Every object has a practically infinite number of features, and thus, it *is_a* member of a practically infinite number of categories. For instance, Einstein is a human being; he is a violinist; he is a Nobel Prize laureate; he is born in Ulm, Germany; he is married; he is a believer; he has a mistress; and so on. That is, Einstein is a member of the categories A, B, C, D, etc. That means that an answer to a what-is-X question never defines X. It only describes X, rightly or wrongly, adequately or inadequately.

What has just been said also holds for medicine. Depending on what feature A, B, C, D, ... of medicine one is highlighting, one will assert that "medicine is an A" or "medicine is a B" or "medicine is a C", and so on such as, for example,

K. Sadegh-Zadeh, *Handbook of Analytic Philosophy of Medicine*,
Philosophy and Medicine 113, DOI 10.1007/978-94-007-2260-6_21,
© Springer Science+Business Media B.V. 2012

medicine is a healing profession,
medicine is a biological science,
medicine is an art,
medicine is a moral enterprise,
medicine is a service business,
medicine is a social science,

etc. The proponents of such judgments are often in a permanent state of feud with one another because each of them believes that only she is right and the other ones err, although all of them are right. The odd belief that medicine may belong to only one class also brought with it the debate about the popular either-or question whether medicine is a science or an art. The question ignores that science and art are not mutually exclusive. Medicine might indeed be a science as well as an art. Most importantly, in order that the question "is *medicine* a *science* or an *art?*" can be taken seriously, the questioner ought to clearly specify what the three italicized terms mean. The latter term is one of the extremely vague elements of our languages. Every human activity, including medicine, can be interpreted as an art. Such categorizations are uninformative. Regarding the term "science", there is as yet no acceptable concept of it to examine whether medicine is or is not a science. The third term, "medicine", similarly needs a clear concept. In the present chapter, we will inquire into such issues to understand what scientific, non-scientific, and extra-scientific features medicine may have. Our discussion consists of the following seven sections:

21.1 The Subject and Goal of Medicine
21.2 Is Medicine a Natural Science?
21.3 Is Medicine an Applied Science?
21.4 Does Medicine Belong to the Humanities?
21.5 Is Medicine a Practical Science?
21.6 Medicine is Practiced Morality as well as Ethics
21.7 Quo Vadis Medicina?

21.1 The Subject and Goal of Medicine

The first step in inquiring into the nature of medicine is to clarify its subject and goal. As pointed out above, however, in the effort to be clear about its subject and goal one must be aware of the ambiguity of the term "medicine" itself. Many different activities fall under the purview of this term, making it difficult to form a judgment covering all of them. Examples are pediatrics, orthopedic surgery, bone research, muscle physiology, physiotherapy, cosmetic surgery, hygiene, water pollution research, cell research, blood research, virology, genetics, DNA research, protein research, psychiatry, dream analysis, social psychiatry, and so on. Since many of these activities can also be conducted outside medicine, e.g., in biology and mineralogy, the question arises as to what kind of activity inherently does or does not belong to medicine. We shall not attempt to explicate the term "medicine" and delimit its scope here. However, we may recall what was emphasized several times in our earlier discussions:

Medicine is characterized by its subject and goal. Its subject is the *Homo patiens*. Its goal is to promote, protect, and restore health through the prevention of maladies in individuals and communities, curing sick people, and caring for sick people. To this end, medicine involves the investigation of the nature, genesis, diagnostics, therapy, and prevention of maladies. It has become common to distinguish between clinical medicine and non-clinical medicine in the following fashion:

- Clinical medicine deals with patients and patient-related issues. It encompasses diverse sub-fields from surgery to internal medicine to psychiatry to obstetrics to reconstructive orthopedics. They are concerned with diagnosing and treating patients' maladies. Their task is both *clinical practice* and *clinical research*.
- Non-clinical or preclinical medicine does not deal with patients. It investigates the structures and functions of the body and body parts, and comprises many different disciplines such as anatomy, histology, cytology, physiology, neurophysiology, biochemistry, biophysics, and so on. Non-clinical medicine is concerned exclusively with research.

In the landscape sketched above, it is difficult to determine where *medicine* begins and where it ends. For our purposes, then, we will understand by "medicine" primarily the core of medicine consisting of clinical practice and research, or *clinical medicine* for short. Issues in the periphery, not directly related to this core, i.e., non-clinical medicine, can be undertaken equally well in zoology, botany, chemistry, physics, etc. The disciplines concerned with these issues have come to be known as medical biosciences, biomedical sciences, or *biomedicine* for short. Biomedicine is by no means identical with medicine. Biomedical sciences are auxiliaries and do not necessarily belong to medicine proper. We will therefore clearly distinguish between these two areas in our discussion of the nature of medicine below. For, as we shall see, regarding their 'nature' they significantly differ from one another.

When someone argues that "medicine is a *P*", for example, "medicine is concerned with Homo patiens", it is important to know whether she uses the particle "is" (i) in a *descriptive* sense to say that real-world medicine has the property of being a *P;* or rather (ii) in a *prescriptive* sense to require that medicine has to be a *P*. A description can easily be falsified when it is wrong. However, many stubborn conflicts and fruitless debates arise from pseudo-descriptive utterances that are implicitly intended to be prescriptive. In the present chapter, we shall be explicit about our judgments on the nature of medicine when we argue that "medicine is such and such". For instance, what was stated above about the subject and goal of medicine was meant in the prescriptive sense to say that "medicine has to concern itself with Homo patiens ... and so on". It does not have to concern itself with cells, proteins, DNA, and the like for their own sake.

21.2 Is Medicine a Natural Science?

Disciplines such as physics, chemistry, biology, and geology are referred to as *natural sciences* because they are concerned with nature, i.e., with natural phenomena, objects, and processes. The class of entities with which biomedical disciplines such as anatomy, physiology, and biochemistry are concerned also include natural entities such as organisms, cells, genes, and DNA. Hence, biomedicine may also be viewed as natural science. As we emphasized in the preceding section, however, biomedicine is not identical with medicine. Medicine proper is clinical medicine, the rest is zoology, botany, physics, and chemistry. By overlooking this fact one may erroneously judge that medicine is_a natural science ("is_a" in what sense: descriptive or prescriptive?).

From the descriptive point of view, the characterization of *medicine* as natural science is wrong for the following simple reason. The knowledge gained by natural-scientific investigations consists of declarative sentences, specifically, of constatives, that describe nature, such as "most cells have a nucleus". It does not contain deontic sentences of the form "you ought to tell the truth" and the like. However, we saw previously that clinical-medical knowledge almost exclusively consists of deontic sentences, for example, "if you observe symptoms $A_1, \ldots, A_m$ in the patient, then you ought to do $B_1, \ldots, B_n$". Natural sciences merely describe how things are. Clinical-medical knowledge prescribes how the physician *ought to act*. Thus, clinical medicine is not a natural science (see Chapter 15).

Interpreted in a prescriptive sense, it would be meaningless to require that "medicine has to be a natural science". As shown in Chapter 14, maladies are not natural entities independent of human mind, intentions, and values. They are deontic constructs. On this account, the investigation into maladies and their etiology, diagnostics, and therapy is investigation into deontic constructs, and as such, cannot be natural-scientific research. More importantly, we shall see below that clinical-medical research inquires into the efficacy of diagnostic and therapeutic rules of action and evaluates them. They are deontic rules and represent complex human action rules to be followed in clinical settings by physicians and other care providers. The search for, and the evaluation of, human action rules is not natural-scientific research because action rules are not natural entities to be found 'in the world out there' (see Chapter 15). To be clear, even though medicine has natural-scientific sub-disciplines, i.e., biomedicine, clinical medicine as its core is not a natural science.

21.3 Is Medicine an Applied Science?

The commonly used term "applied science" is ambiguous. On the one hand, a scientific discipline such as archeology or mineralogy in which knowledge and methods from other disciplines are applied, is called an *applied science* or discipline. On the other hand, an applied science is understood as the application of some basic science, such as physics or chemistry, to solve practical problems. For example, an engineering science is considered an applied science in this sense. However, the latter meaning of the term is inappropriate. It is better captured by the concept of "practical science" that will be discussed below.

We often encounter the view which says that medicine is an applied science. Specifically, we are told that medicine is an *applied natural science* because natural-scientific knowledge and methods are applied to solve medical problems. For example, cardiological diagnostics and therapy employ chemical and physical knowledge to collect and interpret patient data. Nevertheless, medicine cannot be considered an applied natural science for the following reasons:

First, the knowledge and methods applied in medicine come not only from the natural sciences, but also from a wide variety of other disciplines, e.g., mathematics, psychology, sociology, history, engineering sciences, and others. Does the use of knowledge from such sources justify viewing medicine as applied mathematics, applied psychology, applied sociology, applied history, applied engineering, and so on? If it does not, what is it that justifies viewing medicine as applied *natural science?* Even the natural sciences themselves, e.g., physics and chemistry, extensively apply mathematics. Does this justify viewing physics and chemistry as applied mathematics? If it does, would the transitivity of the application relation:

A is applied *B* and *B* is applied *C,* therefore, *A* is applied *C*

not justify the strange view that medicine is applied mathematics? The idea of viewing some particular science as an applied science is based on the understanding that applied sciences are those fields in which some basic or foundational sciences are applied. Specifically, some logical empiricists have claimed that every empirical science can be reduced to physics, a doctrine known as physicalism. This doctrine, however, is false (see footnote 138 on page 724).

Second, supposing that a particular science were an applied natural science, we must then ask what this science is doing in *applying* natural-scientific knowledge or methods? It is of course not the mere application for its own sake. Nor is the research task of the discipline exhausted by the application of natural-scientific knowledge or methods. Generally there is something else to achieve thereby, for example, solving particular problems such as how to accurately diagnose myocardial infarction, AIDS, or any other disease. *Such* problems, however, are genuinely practical ones. The pursuit of solutions for practical problems in a discipline *A* such as cardiology by means of auxiliary knowledge from another discipline B such as physics does not render A an applied B. Discipline A still remains, as we shall see below, a practical discipline sui generis which, among other things, *also* uses knowledge from discipline B.

Third, as we have already mentioned and as will be shown below, clinical-medical research establishes diagnostic and therapeutic rules of action and evaluates them by comparative inquiries into their efficacy. As *deontic rules,* they cannot be the subject of natural sciences. The act of establishing or evaluating an action rule takes place in a system of human values that is something social and cultural, but not physical, chemical, or biological. It may supervene on the physical, chemical, and biological, but there is no identity between them.

21.4 Does Medicine Belong to the Humanities?

The humanities are concerned with the study of man's intellect, spirituality, works, culture, and history. Examples are language studies, literature, history, philosophy, and theology. There are scholars who argue that medicine belongs to the humanities. Edmund Pellegrino, for instance, says: "But medicine is equally well one of the humanities because its concerns are for all dimensions of the life of man which in any way impinge on his well-being" (Pellegrino, 2008, 326). Note, however, that along the same line of argumentation one could also maintain that medicine is chemistry, physics, psychology, mathematics, ornithology, ethnology, theology, and the like. It is obvious that we do not gain anything reasonable by such arbitrariness in dealing with the subsumption relation *"is_a"* to categorize medicine according to our liking.

21.5 Is Medicine a Practical Science?

The answer to this question is a plain Yes. But it requires an explanation of its philosophical consequences. To this end, we shall distinguish between theoretical and practical sciences and shall demonstrate that medicine is an instance of both types of science. Our discussion divides into the following four parts:

21.5.1 Practical *vs.* Theoretical Sciences
21.5.2 Means-End Research
21.5.3 Clinical Research is a Practical Science
21.5.4 Relationships Between Biomedicine and Clinical Medicine.

21.5.1 Practical *vs.* Theoretical Sciences

Traditionally, scientific fields are divided into two categories, *theoretical* sciences and *practical* sciences. It is said, for example, that physics, chemistry, biology, genetics, and similar disciplines are theoretical sciences, whereas pedagogy, surgery, gynecology, and pediatrics are practical disciplines. But there are two problems associated with this dichotomy. First, as pointed out on page 450, the contrasting pair "theoretical" and "practical" is ambiguous because the adjective "theoretical" in this pair has nothing to do with theories and theoretical terms as discussed in Section 9.4. Second, most people, including scientists, believe that a practical science is so called because practical scientists practice something, e.g., clinicians treat patients, whereas a theoretical science such as physics and chemistry is void of any practice. But this belief is wrong. First, theoretical scientists practice scientific research. And second, the practicality of a practical science does not refer to any kind of practice in that science. In line with our definition of the terms "theoretical knowledge" and "practical knowledge" on page 450 ff., a theoretical science is one that produces theoretical knowledge, whereas a practical science produces practical knowledge. This production of practical knowledge is accomplished by *means-end research* in order to find out optimal means of achieving an end.

21.5.2 Means-End Research

An end, or goal, is a condition that some agent may desire and intend to achieve. For instance, a physician's goal may be to achieve a correct diagnosis of a patient's token disease who is suffering from upper abdominal pain. The patient's recovery, which both she and her physician desire, is also a goal. A means is not a tool, but a method, i.e., a more or less complex mode of action the performance of which may help someone achieve some goal. For instance, gastroscopy is a means of inspecting the cavity and mucous membrane of the stomach. Aspirin use is a means to reduce the risk of, and to prevent, myocardial infarction.

There may be no or a number of $n \geq 1$ means by each of which a goal may be attained. In the latter case, the means are said to be associated with the goals, or to point to them. For instance, gastroscopy is associated with the visualization of the cavity and mucous membrane of the stomach. Aspirin use is associated with reductions in the risk, and prevention, of myocardial infarction. Such an association between a means and an end has come to be termed a *means-end relation*. Means-end relations are *interventional-causal* relations between actions and goals. That is, a means includes at least one action to bring about the associated end.

The set of distinct means that point to the same goal defines the *equifinality* set. And the set of distinct goals associated with a given means constitutes the *multifinality* set. For instance, the set of different diagnostic measures which enable the diagnosis of Helicobacter gastritis yields an equifinality set, while the set of different goals that are attainable by aspirin use is a multifinality set, e.g., {alleviation of fever, pain relief, thrombosis prevention, reduction in the risk of myocardial infarction, ... etc. ... }. With respect to the effectiveness of their means, there are three types of means-end relations:

1. those with sufficient means,
2. those with weakly sufficient means, and
3. those with necessary means.

A sufficient means is one that is always effective; a weakly sufficient means is one that is only sometimes, but not always, effective; and a necessary means is one without which the goal cannot be achieved. Thus, means-end relations of the type 1 and 3 are deterministic interventional-causal relations between means and ends, while those of the type 2 are probabilistic interventional-causal relations sketched in the following schemes in turn:

- $C \,\&\, A \rightarrow G$ reads: if under circumstances C action A is conducted, then goal G will be attained;
- $p(G \,|\, C \cap A) = r$ the probability of attaining goal G by conducting action A under circumstances C, is r.

Means-end research is the investigation into such means-end relationships in order to find or construct novel means of achieving a particular goal as well as to enhance their efficacy. A practical science is a *means-end research* field. Thus, it constitutes a *science of practicing* or science of praxis. Specifically, it inquires into purposeful human actions, their consequences, efficiency, and planning. A good example is clinical research as will be shown in the next section.

21.5.3 Clinical Research is a Practical Science

On page 765 we distinguished between clinical medicine and biomedicine. Clinical medicine, referred to as the core of medicine, comprises clinical disciplines such as internal medicine, pediatrics, surgery, and others. Biomedicine includes the so-called medical biosciences such as anatomy, physiology, biochemistry, medical physics, and similar ones. They are auxiliaries to clinical medicine. We saw that they are best characterized as interventional-causal research fields insofar as they conduct experimental research.

Clinical medicine, however, is something different. To explain, we need an additional differentiation. Clinical medicine unites two not sharply separable endeavors, i.e., clinical research and clinical practice. We shall here be concerned with *clinical research* only. By systematically inquiring into all clinical issues from suffering to disease to diagnostics to therapy and prevention, clinical research serves clinical practice to enhance its knowledge-base, efficiency, and quality. To put it concisely, clinical research is a science, not a practice, of optimal clinical decision-making. Because of the epistemological and metaphysical significance of this understanding, we will now carefully demonstrate that clinical research represents a *practical science* par excellence. Our analyses will enable us to uncover how this peculiar practicality turns clinical medicine into both practiced morality and ethics.[143]

One will easily discern what type of science clinical research is, by considering the type of studies it undertakes and the type of knowledge it acquires thereby. To begin with the former point, clinical research may be categorized as a practical science for the following three reasons: (i) the central subject of its investigations is the *goal-driven praxis*, i.e., goal-driven doing and acting, of physicians and other health personnel in diagnostic, therapeutic, and preventive contexts who are concerned with:

- the *construction* of methods of diagnostics, treatment, and prevention of a new malady, or
- the *improvement* of available methods of diagnostics, treatment, and prevention of a known malady;

(ii) its primary aim is to analyze *means-end relationships* in diagnostics, treatment, and prevention to find out the optimal strategies of clinical decision-making that enable more accurate diagnoses and more efficacious treatments and prevention than currently possible; and (iii) to establish clinical action rules that guide the goal-driven doing and acting of physicians and other health personnel. To accomplish these tasks requires (a) structured research group activities that take place in special, more or less complex social environments, e.g., in long-term departmental, national, or international collaborative studies of the diagnostics, treatment, and prevention of a malady such as myocardial infarction, AIDS, or leukemia; and (b) practical reasoning in contrast to the theoretical reasoning of theoretical sciences, i.e., logic. See Section 22.3 on page 799.

To illustrate the ideas above, we shall extend the notion of a conditional action, introduced in Definition 151.4 on page 563, to obtain the notion of a conditional, goal-driven action. If C denotes some circumstances under which a goal G is pursued, then the statement:

If condition C obtains and goal G is pursued, then action A is performed,

describes a *conditional, goal-driven action*. It may conveniently be formalized as follows:

$$C \,\&\, G \rightarrow A. \tag{188}$$

A simple example is: If a patient complains of upper abdominal pain (condition C) and the physician wants to explore whether she has gastritis (desired

---

[143] The inspiration for my view of medicine as a practical science came from Wolfgang Wieland (1975, 1986). Likewise, the inspiration for my view of medicine as a moral enterprise came from Edmund Pellegrino and David Thomasma (1981) and Thomasma and Pellegrino (1981). In both cases, however, our reasoning, methods, and results are very different from one another.

goal G), then she performs gastroscopy (action A). Clinical-medical research consists in inquiring into conditional, goal-driven actions of the type (188) to analyze their effects, side-effects, efficacy, benefits, harms, and costs in order to identify what action is optimal under circumstances C to attain the desired goal G. For instance, when:

condition C $\equiv$ the patient complains of upper abdominal pain,
desired goal G $\equiv$ explore whether the patient has gastritis or peptic ulcer disease,
possible actions $\equiv$ {gastroscopy, computed tomography, ^{13}C-urea breath test, ELISA} $= \{A_1, A_2, A_3, A_4\}$,

then by testing each of these possible four actions $A_1, \ldots, A_4$ in a sample of patients and comparing the results we may eventually obtain a statement of the form:

IF a patient complains of upper abdominal pain AND you want to explore whether she has gastritis or peptic ulcer disease, THEN the optimal action is gastroscopy.

That is:

A patient complains of upper abdominal pain $\wedge$ you want to explore whether she has gastritis or peptic ulcer disease $\rightarrow$ the optimal action is gastroscopy.

This is, according to Exportation and Importation Rules of deduction in Table 36 on page 895, classical-logically equivalent to:

A patient complains of upper abdominal pain $\rightarrow$ (you want to explore whether she has gastritis or peptic ulcer disease $\rightarrow$ the   (189) optimal action is gastroscopy).

That means in a generalized form:

Condition C obtains $\rightarrow$ (goal G is desired $\rightarrow$ the optimal action is A),

or equivalently:

$$C \rightarrow (G \rightarrow is\_optimal(A)), \qquad (190)$$

where action A in the present example is one of the four alternative actions $\{A_1, A_2, A_3, A_4\}$ mentioned above, e.g., gastroscopy. Note that (190) is an empirical proposition, i.e., a declarative *statement* that reports on the result of a comparative action research. The emphasis is important. We shall see below that on the basis of propositional knowledge of the type (190) clinical action rules are advanced as *imperatives*.

Generalizing the above observation, a clinical research program may be reconstructed as a branching project such that under more or less complex circumstances of the type $C \equiv C_1 \& \ldots \& C_h$ with $h \geq 1$, many possible goals $G_1, \ldots, G_n$ may come into consideration each of which is attainable by performing any of the alternative actions $A_{i_1}, A_{i_2}, \ldots, A_{i_m}$ with $i, m \geq 1$:

$$
C \rightarrow \begin{cases} G_1 \rightarrow \text{ possible actions are } A_{1_1}, A_{1_2}, \ldots, A_{1_k} \\ \vdots \\ G_n \rightarrow \text{ possible actions are } A_{n_1}, A_{n_2}, \ldots, A_{n_p} \end{cases} \tag{191}
$$

with $i, k, n, p \geq 1$. For instance, there are patients complaining of upper abdominal pain. This is the condition, or circumstance, C. But their suffering may be due to many different causes. How are we to track down which of these possible causes is, or has been, effective in a particular patient such as Elroy Fox who is complaining of upper abdominal pain? To this end, we need to know the optimal *methods* of diagnostics to be used in such a situation. The knowledge required for making this diagnostic decision is acquired in *prior clinical research*. Specifically, the clinical research under discussion concerns itself with clinical circumstances of the type:

- the patient complains of upper abdominal pain $\equiv C$

where many different goals come into consideration, e.g., the goals to examine whether the patient has:

- gastritis or peptic ulcer disease $\equiv G_1$
- stomach carcinoma $\equiv G_2$
- gallstones $\equiv G_3$
- gallbladder inflammation $\equiv G_4$
- acute pancreatitis $\equiv G_5$
- liver cirrhosis $\equiv G_6$
- and so on,

while according to (191) each of these goals is attainable by a number $m \geq 1$ of alternative diagnostic actions $A_{i_1}, A_{i_2}, \ldots, A_{i_m}$ with $1 \leq i \leq 6$. The aim of clinical *research* is to identify which one of these alternative actions is the optimal one to attain the corresponding goal G_i. The alternative actions are performed in different samples of patients, and their effects are evaluated according to particular, agreed-upon criteria. Depending on their respective values, the actions are ranked in the order of their preferability such that eventually we obtain a highest-ranked assertion of the type $C \rightarrow \big(G_i \rightarrow is\_optimal(A_{i_j})\big)$ with $i, j \geq 1$. The statements (189–190) above are just such assertions without indices. On the basis of such final, empirical assertions a *conditional imperative* of the following form is advanced by research groups, medical communities, or even health authorities:

$$
C \rightarrow (G \rightarrow do\ A). \tag{192}
$$

An example is:

> IF a patient complains of upper abdominal pain, THEN (IF you
> want to explore whether she has gastritis or peptic ulcer disease,   (193)
> THEN do gastroscopy).

Recall that (189–190) are empirical statements and assert "what is the case". Thus, they have a truth value. By contrast, (193) is not a statement and does not assert anything. It is an imperative, specifically a *conditional action rule* of the form (192) that commands: "Under circumstances C, if goal G is desired, do $A!$". Therefore, it is not true or false, but more or less efficacious. That is, it has an *efficacy value*. Let there be two competing conditional action rules of the form:

$$C \rightarrow (G \rightarrow do\ A),$$
$$C \rightarrow (G \rightarrow do\ B),$$

each of which recommends, under the same circumstances C, a different action to attain the same goal G, then they can be compared with each other with respect to their efficacy values so as to execute the one with the higher efficacy. That means that we choose a conditional action rule because of its efficacy value and not its truth value. This is so simply because it has no truth value. The efficacy of a conditional action rule can be defined as follows:[144]

Regarding a conditional action rule $C \rightarrow (G \rightarrow do\ A)$, it may be asked in how many situations of the type C the goal G is attained by performing action A. And in how many situations of the same type C the same goal G is attained without doing anything? The difference between the two we call the efficacy value or *degree of efficacy* of the action rule $C \rightarrow (G \rightarrow do\ A)$. This idea may be conceptualized as follows by using the notion of probabilistic relevance introduced in Definition 65 on page 239.

The probability that under circumstances C the goal event G occurs if action A is performed, is expressed by sentence 1 below. The probability that under circumstances of the same type C a goal event of the same type G occurs if *no* action is performed at all, is expressed by sentence 2 below. The arithmetical difference $r_1 - r_2$ between both probabilities yields the degree of probabilistic relevance of action A to attaining goal G under circumstances of the type C. This degree of probabilistic relevance, expressed in sentence 3, we refer to in sentence 4 as the *degree of efficacy* of the conditional action rule $C \rightarrow (G \rightarrow do\ A)$, written $\mathit{eff}\big(C \rightarrow (G \rightarrow do\ A)\big)$:

1. $p(G\,|\,C \cap A) = r_1$
2. $p(G\,|\,C) = r_2$

---

[144] The inspiration for my ideas on the efficacy of what I have termed *conditional action rules* (Sadegh-Zadeh, 1978b) came from Mario Bunge's pragmatics (Bunge, 1967, 121–150). Bunge, however, uses another framework and approach that cannot be discussed here.

3. $probabilistic\_relevance\_of(A\ to\ G\ under\ C) = r_1 - r_2$
4. $eff\big(C \rightarrow (G \rightarrow do\ A)\big) = probabilistic\_relevance\_of(A\ to\ G\ under\ C)$
   $= r_1 - r_2.$

The degree of efficacy of a conditional action rule is a real number in the interval $[-1, 1]$, i.e., positive, negative, or zero. Only in the first case is action A efficacious. In the second case it has a negative effect. And in the third case it is useless. Two or more different, equifinal action rules of the type:

$$C \rightarrow (G \rightarrow do\ A_1), \qquad\qquad (194)$$
$$C \rightarrow (G \rightarrow do\ A_2),$$
$$C \rightarrow (G \rightarrow do\ A_3),$$

and so on,

which under circumstances of the same type recommend different actions to attain the same goal, may be compared in terms of their efficacy values so as to determine the most efficacious, the best, one. By so doing, clinical research enhances the efficacy and quality of clinical practice. See also Sections 8.5.2 and 22.3.2 on page 801.

More generally, a conditional action rule $C \rightarrow (G \rightarrow do\ A)$ may recommend an action A that consists in several alternative options, i.e., $A \equiv A_1 \vee A_2 \vee \ldots \vee A_q$ with $q \geq 1$, such that the physician is encouraged to choose among the alternatives $A_1, A_2, \ldots, A_q$ depending on which one of them is most appropriate in an individual situation. Thus, a single conditional clinical action rule advanced by clinical research assumes the following general structure:

$$C \rightarrow (G \rightarrow do\ A_1 \vee A_2 \vee \ldots \vee A_q) \qquad\qquad (195)$$

which says: Under circumstances C do any of the actions $A_1 \vee A_2 \vee \ldots \vee A_q$ if goal G is desired. A quick look at our previous reconstruction (116) of *practical knowledge* on page 454 will demonstrate that the present conditional action rule (195) is exactly the basic form of that type of practical knowledge whose sentential constituents were represented as follows:

$$If\ \alpha_1 \wedge \ldots \wedge \alpha_k\ then\ \Big(if\ \beta_1 \wedge \ldots \wedge \beta_m,\ then$$
$$do\ \big((\gamma_1 \wedge \ldots \wedge \gamma_n)_1 \vee \ldots \vee (\delta_1 \wedge \ldots \wedge \delta_p)_q\big)\Big)$$

with $k, m, n, p, q \geq 1$ such that:

- $\alpha_1 \wedge \ldots \wedge \alpha_k$ are $k \geq 1$ statements describing the condition C,
- $\beta_1 \wedge \ldots \wedge \beta_m$ are $m \geq 1$ statements describing the goal G pursued,
- $(\gamma_1 \wedge \ldots \wedge \gamma_n)_1 \vee \ldots \vee (\delta_1 \wedge \ldots \wedge \delta_p)_q$ are statements describing the recommended, alternative actions $A_1 \vee A_2 \vee \ldots \vee A_q$ with $(\gamma_1 \wedge \ldots \wedge \gamma_j)_i = A_i$ and $q \geq 1$.

Medicine is a practical science as it seeks and acquires practical knowledge of the form above through clinical research. That medicine turns out a practical science, has two interesting consequences that can easily be recognized on the basis of our reconstructions. Concisely put, it makes medicine practiced morality and ethics as well as an engineering science. We shall discuss these issues in Sections 21.6 and 21.7.1 below.

21.5.4 Relationships Between Biomedicine and Clinical Medicine

We saw that the subject of inquiry in clinical research primarily includes intentional, goal-driven human actions, action rules, and their efficacy. Intentions, goals, actions, action rules, and rule efficacies are not natural objects, phenomena, or processes. Rather, they are man-made, cultural artifacts, and human values. Hence, the categorization of clinical research as a natural science or as an applied natural science is incorrect.

A considerable amount of discourse in clinical research is concerned with analyzing, criticizing, reconstructing, and constructing different types of intentions, goals, and actions of health care professionals such as, for example, assistance in dying, xenotrasplantation, stem cell research and technology, therapeutic cloning, and others. In dealing with these and similar subjects, value systems and considerations are indispensable. The reasoning proceeds not causalistically, but consequentialistically and teleologically by asking the following question: *What are the consequences of our conduct in this or that way and what is good for patients as human beings?* The same holds true for the relationships between the theoretical knowledge of biomedicine and the practical knowledge of clinical medicine. It is important to note that the theoretical knowledge provided by biomedicine does not imply any clinical-conditional action rule. For example, when the following item of knowledge:

> Streptomycin inhibits the growth of strains of tubercle bacilli   (196)

is put forward by bacteriology as an experimental science, we cannot logically infer from this statement (196) a clinical-conditional action rule of the type:

> If a patient suffers from lung tuberculosis, then (if you want to cure her, then administer streptomycin!).   (197)

The reason is that there is no logic that allows for an inference from (196) to (197). Before streptomycin is tested on human subjects, we cannot know whether it will cure or kill. Empirical knowledge acquired by experimentation with micro-organisms does not imply *what we should do* in the human sphere. But it is capable of guiding our imaginations and value decisions. So, before we are able to advance the conditional action rule (197) for use in clinical practice, specific clinical research is needed to find out whether the following assertion of an optimal action can be justified:

If a patient suffers from lung tuberculosis, then (if you want to cure her, then the optimal action is administration of strepto-   (198) mycin).

Only on the basis of such investigations and results can a conditional action rule of the form (197) be advanced, even though behind the transition from (198) to (197) lies no system of pure logic, but of *practical reasoning* discussed in Section 22.3 below. It establishes value axioms of the type "An action A is to be preferred to an action B if it is better than B" based on the axiom "An action rule is to be preferred to another one if it is more efficacious than the latter". Thus, the advancement of the conditional imperative (197) is a practical value decision based on the medical-moral axioms of beneficence and non-maleficence (Sadegh-Zadeh, 1978b).

21.6 Medicine is Practiced Morality as well as Ethics

So far we have represented clinical action rules as conditional imperatives of the form $C \to (G \to do\ A_1 \vee A_2 \vee \ldots \vee A_q)$ with $q \geq 1$. We will now go one step further to recognize that they are in fact conditional ought-do-do rules, i.e., conditional obligations, of the structure $C \to \big(G \to OB(A_1 \vee A_2 \vee \ldots \vee A_q)\big)$ where the predicate "OB" is the obligation operator "it is obligatory that" and replaces the imperative "do!". Thus, the social origin and authority of clinical action rules will be shown in the following two sections:

    21.6.1   Clinical Practice is Practiced Morality
    21.6.2   Clinical Research is Normative Ethics.

21.6.1 Clinical Practice is Practiced Morality

Malpractice suits demonstrate that there are clinical actions which violate the standards of clinical practice and thereby give rise to litigation. We discussed this issue on page 579. In the example given there, the failure of the physician to perform at least one of the following two alternative diagnostic actions prevented her from diagnosing the patient's lethal myocardial infarction:

    a. record an ECG in the patient, or
    b. determine the concentration of heart-relevant enzymes in her blood.

The physician's omission was interpreted as clinical malpractice. That a particular type of physician conduct counts as a violation of some standards of practice and thereby gives rise to a malpractice suit, is proof that those standards of practice are obligatory goals and are thus based on deontic rules. More specifically, they are clinical ought-to-do rules of the form:

$$C \to \big(G \to OB(A_1 \vee A_2 \vee \ldots \vee A_q)\big)$$

whose micro-logical structure was outlined in (134) on page 579. As conditional obligations, they regulate physician conduct in the diagnostics, therapy, and prevention of maladies. If every physician were allowed to act according to what she deems right, there would be no offence, and hence, no malpractice suits. In Chapter 15 we concluded from this fact that clinical practice is a deontic domain. A deontic domain is either a legal or a moral domain. Clinical ought-to-do rules, as clinical standards, are not prescribed by legal authorities. They are advanced by medicine itself. So we may conclude that they are domain-specific moral rules. That is, the modal operator "it is obligatory that" contained in a conditional clinical action rule such as the following one is to be interpreted as expressing a moral obligation:

- If a patient complains of acute chest pain that radiates to her left arm, then
- if you want to know whether she has myocardial infarction, then
- *it is obligatory that* you record an ECG or determine the concentration of heart-relevant enzymes in her blood.

The obligation prescribes what type of clinical *actions* are right and good under certain clinical circumstances. In a nutshell, clinical practice as a historical institution – and not as a praxis of individual physicians – is *practiced morality* because it executes such rules. Its moral norms are codified into clinical ought-to-do rules like above usually called clinical knowledge, specifically diagnostic-therapeutic knowledge. See Section 10.7. Clinical knowledge at a particular time represents the practical-moral corpus of medicine at that time (Sadegh-Zadeh, 1983, 14).

21.6.2 Clinical Research is Normative Ethics

Recall that the conditional clinical ought-to-do rules referred to above are exactly the clinical indication and contra-indication rules that we studied in indication structures and contra-indication structures in Sections 8.2.3 and 8.2.4. By advancing such action rules as *clinical knowledge* for use in clinical decision-making, clinical research and the medical community regulate physicians' conduct in that physicians are bound to obey those rules. In medical education the rules are taught as medical knowledge. And they are disseminated as knowledge in textbooks and other medical literature. Since the totality of this practical-medical knowledge provides a practical-moral corpus for physician conduct in clinical practice, the pursuit thereof in medicine and the continuing effort to improve and justify it by practical-medical research and practical-medical reasoning are *normative ethics*. The characteristics and quality of the moral corpus reflect the nature and quality of that normative ethics.

Our view of clinical research as normative ethics is based on the following observation. Conditional clinical obligations regulate, as indication and contra-indication rules, the physician's clinical decision-making and are thus her local, i.e., domain-specific, rules of conduct. The search for such rules by clinical investigations and practical reasoning constitutes an ethical inquiry because their subject consists of *rules* of morally relevant conduct. The ethical reasoning we are supposing is comparative reasoning in that the clinical efficacies of at least two different rules of the following form:

$$eff\left(C \rightarrow \left(G \rightarrow OB(A_1 \vee A_2 \vee \ldots \vee A_p)\right)\right)$$
$$eff\left(C \rightarrow \left(G \rightarrow OB(B_1 \vee B_2 \vee \ldots \vee B_q)\right)\right) \qquad \text{with } p, q \geq 1$$

each of which prescribes particular actions, are compared so as to prefer and advance the one with the higher efficacy. For example, comparative clinical research may result in the decision to give the following rule preference over all other, competing rules: "If a patient complains of upper abdominal pain, then, if you want to know whether she has gastritis or peptic ulcer disease, then it is obligatory that gastroscopy is performed and a biopsy is taken". The comparative character of clinical research as ethics may evolve in the future by employing the methodology of fuzzy deontics that we proposed in Section 16.5.5, and advancing clinical indication and contra-indication rules in terms of what we called comparative conditional norms on page 662. It will then be justified to view clinical research as comparative-normative ethics (Sadegh-Zadeh, 1983, 13).

21.7 Quo Vadis Medicina?

There are numerous moralities on earth. The morality of Germans is different from that of Tutsi. Correspondingly, there are a large number of ethics concerned with these distinct moralities. For instance, the normative Catholic ethics deviates from Tutsi normative ethics. Thus, there is not one ethics on earth, but many. The same holds true for medicine interpreted as ethics. Medicine as ethics changes through time. Convincing evidence for this is the impact on medicine that biosciences and technology have developed since the 1950s. Artificial insemination and designing babies, genetic manipulation of the embryo, termination of life and physician-assisted suicide, transplantation of organs and tissues, nanomedicine, and many other innovations demonstrate that medicine is continuously redefining man, life, death, and health care through changes to its moral corpus. The emergence of bioethics in the 1960s was a reaction to this increasing moral and ethical hegemony of medicine in life and death matters (Jonsen, 1998; Jecker et al., 2007).[145]

---

[145] Whoever has difficulty understanding medicine as ethics, may distinguish between implicit and explicit ethics and reinterpret clinical research as an implicit ethics that does not explicitly regard itself as ethics because clinical researchers do not sufficiently reflect about what ethics might be.

Although bioethics, including medical ethics, has since been very successful, it is highly unlikely that it will take precedence over medicine as an implicit
ethics of human life before and after birth. The reasons for this skepticism are
briefly outlined in the following two sections:

21.7.1 Medicine as an Engineering Science
21.7.2 Medicine Toward Anthropotechnology and Posthumanism.

21.7.1 Medicine as an Engineering Science

The picture painted of medicine as a deontic, rule-based healing profession
represents the institution of medicine up to this point in time. But states of
affairs are in rapid transition, and medicine is increasingly assuming the role
of an engineering science. In the next five sections, the nature of engineering
sciences will be analyzed so as to recognize and examine how medicine is going
to engineer its knowledge and modes of action:

▶ What is an engineering science?
▶ The engineering of medical knowledge
▶ The engineering of therapeutica
▶ Clinical decision-engineering
▶ Health engineering.

What is an engineering science?

We must first distinguish between engineering as practice, on the one hand;
and engineering research or science, on the other. Engineering practice is the
design of a material or device, by means of which a specified goal may be
attained, using engineering knowledge. Such knowledge is provided by engineering sciences. An engineering science is a research field that investigates
methods of designing materials and devices by means of which specified goals
may be attained more efficiently than by alternative actions. Otherwise put,
an engineering science inquires into efficient means-end relations whose means
are materials or devices. Thus, it is *means efficiency research*. The efficiency
knowledge that it produces has the structure of practical knowledge sketched
in (195) on page 775. On this account, engineering sciences are practical sciences. The actions that they recommend for achieving goals under certain
circumstances, are *applications* of materials or devices.

In preceding sections and on page 768, we categorized medicine as a practical science because, by means of clinical and biomedical research, it inquires
into means-end relations to advance efficient *clinical-practical knowledge*. The
alternative actions $A_1 \vee \ldots \vee A_q$ prescribed in an item of clinical-practical
knowledge $C \rightarrow (G \rightarrow OB(A_1 \vee \ldots \vee A_q))$ are *invented*, and in most cases
novel, types of action such as particular diagnostic or therapeutic methods,
e.g., the diagnostics of Alzheimer's disease, AIDS, or any other malady. In

contrast to theoretical sciences, a practical science such as clinical research not only investigates the efficacy of *modes of praxis*. It even invents goals, e.g., therapeutic use of stem cells, as well as appropriate action modes to achieve those goals, and is for that matter, in addition, a poietic science in the Aristotelean sense. The Greek term "poiesis" means *creating, making,* and *producing* (see page 112). Examples of poietic acts in medicine are the invention and design of diagnostic, therapeutic, and preventive measures. Such measures employ more or less sophisticated algorithms and devices, including machines, or are accomplishments of such devices that work automatically and without human assistance. Consider, for instance, the human-machine complex in an intensive care unit, cardiologic-diagnostic laboratory, or neurosurgical operating theater. The measures as well as the devices are created, designed, and engineered. For instance, insulin is synthesized by genetically engineered bacteria and is injected by an insulin pump as a fuzzy controller. It is only this poietic aspect of medicine that justifies viewing it as an *art*. But why call this type of creativity an art and not a productive or *engineering science?* Medical poiesis is strongly represented by *biomedical engineering,* including medical biotechnology, that has become a major and influential source of both research and technology in medicine. Without it no health care would be possible today. It is therefore no exaggeration to say that by virtue of biomedical engineering health care is becoming, or has already become, health engineering science and health engineering practice. That means, in the light of our observations above, that the moral acts that clinical research as normative ethics prescribes, are health engineering acts.

Medicine is well on the way to designing and engineering all of its relevant subject areas, from knowledge to remedies to devices to clinical decision-making. This transformation to an engineering science and practice, or technology, is caused by pervasive economization of our life affairs to the effect that medical services and health care have been increasingly commodified. The emergence of information technologies and the Internet in the end of the twentieth century has only accelerated this process.

The engineering of medical knowledge

A cursory glance at the current philosophy of science journals shows that philosophers of science to this day take delight in theorizing about the truth, truthlikeness, or probability of the entities that science in general and experimental sciences in particular present as *knowledge*. However, from another perspective, the concepts and theories of truth, truthlikeness, and probability are unsuitable for analyzing and evaluating experimental knowledge. The reason is that this type of knowledge is increasingly being engineered as a commodity in epistemic factories. A commodity, be it an automobile or experimental-scientific knowledge, is not true, truthlike, or false, but more or less profitable for its producer and more or less valuable to its users. We will explain this perspective below, taking the medical-experimental sciences as our examples.

In Chapter 12, we reconstructed scientific experiments as epistemic machines that engineer knowledge, and an experimental research laboratory as an epistemic factory housing such machines. As the main sources of knowledge in medicine, biomedical and clinical research laboratories are such factories equipped with different types of devices and networked with other laboratories via intranets and the Internet. Their product, i.e., medical-experimental knowledge, plays the role of a blueprint for the production of commodities such as vaccines, antibodies, receptor blockers, pacemakers, stem cells, in vitro embryos, and so on. As a blueprint, it has become a commodity itself, even a basic commodity that is considered worth having at any price. To ascertain the validity and consequences of this image, one must look beyond the momentary state of a particular research program, e.g., a series of experiments on DNA, tubercle bacilli, stem cells, or a single publication on a particular topic. One needs instead survey its entire history, from its inception until its productive end, in order to see its final product or products materialize step by step. Consider, for example, the following:

- genetic engineering, gene chips, and gene-diagnostic devices arising from decades-long DNA research,
- cervical cancer vaccine arising from 30 years of research on human papilloma virus.

Let X be the subject of a particular research project such as the human papilloma virus. Over the course of the project, a number of publications on this subject X are produced by the research team, or by generations of such teams; and the successful conclusion of the project yields a final commodity Y, e.g., cervical cancer vaccine. Now, the message of our epistemic engineering thesis is twofold. It says, first, that the content of publications on the subject X is engineered in epistemic factories, and second, that these publications are not knowledge about X, but a successively evolving blueprint for the production of the final commodity Y. More specifically, the central sentences in an item of experimental knowledge are *interventional-causal*, or *operational*, *sentences* talking about what occurs when a particular material is subjected to specific operations, say actions, methods, or techniques. They are either deterministic sentences of the structure:

> If M is some material, then, if it is subjected to action A, then R will result, $\qquad(199)$

or probabilistic sentences of the form:

> If M is some material, then the probability that R will result on the condition that M is subjected to action A, is r. $\qquad(200)$

Here, M is any material of arbitrary complexity, e.g., a bunch of human papilloma viruses, stem cells, other types of cells or molecules, an organ or organism, etc.; while action $A = \{A_1, \ldots, A_m\}$ is composed of $m \geq 1$ operations;

and the result $R = \{R_1, \ldots, R_n\}$ consists of $n \geq 1$ components, all of which yields the following structure:

$$M \rightarrow (A \rightarrow R)$$
$$M \rightarrow p(R \mid A) = r \qquad \text{or} \quad p(R \mid M \cap A) = r.$$

Both sentences are conditional operational sentences and formalize sentences (199–200) above. See also the concept of operational definition on page 91. The material M is what is analyzed in an experiment; R is the experimental result; and the operation A is the entirety of experimental methods, techniques, and devices applied to M to yield R. To illustrate, we will return to an example used in our discussion of epistemic machines in Section 12.2 on page 535:

> Let M be a set of some epileptic hippocampal neurons, then the probability that their spikes are reduced if they are treated with GABA (Gamma Amino Butyric Acid), is 0.8.

That means:

> M is a set of epileptic hippocampal neurons $\rightarrow p$(their_spikes_is_reduced | GABA_is_administered) = 0.8

or equivalently:

> p(their_spikes_is_reduced | M is a set of epileptic hippocampal neurons $\cap$ GABA_is_administered) = 0.8.

Action A in conditional-operational sentences of this type is always a machine-aided action or conducted by machines. It demonstrates the central role technology plays in medical-experimental knowledge. It also demonstrates the production of R by the technological transformation of the material M. In other words, experimental findings of the type above ensure the technological producibility of the component R from material M. Thus, they are technological production rules, i.e., *methods of engineering of something*. This explains, first, why experimental researchers patent their findings; and second, why medical-experimental research is mostly carried out in industrial laboratories where the commodities are directly manufactured. Examples are pharmaceutical factories and biotech companies. Even research projects at medical schools today are funded by the production industry, a relationship that has come to be termed research transfer, cooperation, or sponsoring. In this context, the following philosophical question arises: Does medical-experimental *knowledge* contribute to the engineering of health commodities, or is it a gratuitous by-product of the engineering history of these commodities?

The engineering of therapeutica

Any intervening action that aims to ameliorate the health condition of a patient we call therapy. Correspondingly, we introduced the term "therapeuticum" on page 366 as a general label to denote any substance, device, or procedure, including surgical techniques, that is a constituent of an efficacious therapy. Drugs and prosthetics are typical examples. Nowadays all therapeutica are engineered. For example, drugs and vaccines are products of chemical, biotechnological, and pharmaceutical engineering. The production of devices such as insulin pumps, pacemakers, defibrillators, and neurochips would be impossible without highly sophisticated engineering theory and practice behind them. As pointed out above, biomedical engineering has become a major and influential source of research as well as technology in medicine, without which no health care would be possible today. There would exist no invasive diagnostics and therapy, no surgery, emergency medicine, intensive care units, prevention, and so on.

Clinical decision-engineering

In the past, clinical judgment was considered the expert task of the physician. But the advent of computer technology and artificial intelligence changed this situation. In the 1960s, a new discipline emerged that has come to be termed medical informatics, including clinical informatics. The latter is in the process of taking over clinical judgment. This development is closely associated with the publication of a short article in Science in 1959 by the engineer Robert Steven Ledley and the physician Lee B. Lusted about the reasoning foundations of medical diagnosis (Ledley and Lusted, 1959). These two pioneers explained how the "digital electronic computer" could assist physicians and medical students in learning methods of clinical reasoning. "But to use the computer thus we must understand how the physician makes a medical diagnosis", they said (ibid, 9). To this end, they started with an elementary application of sentential logic, Bayes's Theorem, and some decision-theoretic concepts. They thereby paved the way for a probabilization of clinical judgment and founded a new discipline termed *medical decision-making* (Lusted, 1968).

During about twenty years of clinical probabilism that followed (Sadegh-Zadeh, 1980b), a new field of clinical computing developed that contributed to an intense application of information sciences to clinical reasoning. As a result, special computer programs emerged that have come to be termed 'computer-aided medical decision support systems', 'medical expert systems', 'medical knowledge-based systems', and the like. Initially, they were mostly based on one-sided probabilistic approaches and Bayes's Theorem. However, a variety of additional approaches have been introduced since about 1975, especially the application of fuzzy logic and neuro-fuzzy methodology.[146] Under the umbrella name "artificial intelligence in medicine", AIIM for short, the software products of this new research and technology are more and more invading clinical decision-making and patient management. A new subdiscipline

---

[146] Neuro-fuzzy methodology is a combination of neurocomputing with fuzzy-logical methodology. See, for example (Fullér, 2000; Teodorescu et al., 1999).

of medical informatics has come into being that is exclusively concerned with AIIM. As pointed out on page 323, this subdiscipline is increasingly becoming an engineering science of clinical practice. The whole process of clinical decision-making is being computerized and based on knowledge-based systems and the World Wide Web, from history-taking to the interpretation of recordings and patient data to the making of diagnostic-therapeutic decisions to follow-ups. Since the programs are engineered, their WWW-integrated use in individual clinical settings must be viewed as *clinical decision-engineering*. That is, clinical judgment is more and more being engineered today. Future generations of physicians will probably constitute only dependent parts within a global health care machine and will play mere auxiliary roles as some sort of mobile peripherals for gathering patient data requested by the machine to engineer clinical decisions (Sadegh-Zadeh, 2001b, IX).

Health engineering

Medical knowledge, therapeutica, and clinical decisions are the main constituents of health care. Now that all of them are being engineered, what has traditionally been called health care is increasingly becoming health engineering.

21.7.2 Medicine Toward Anthropotechnology and Posthumanism

We tried above to sketch the way that contemporary medicine has taken toward technology. The beginning of this transition of health care to health engineering cannot be placed exactly. The obvious transition, however, indicates that a new mode of medical worldmaking is emerging behind which lies a new concept of man. The concept seems to consist in the view of the human being as a modular system consisting of exchangeable modules, from organ systems to organs to tissues to cells to molecules to atoms. This type of medical anthropology is a product of the field of medicine that followed the German pathologist Rudolf Virchow's cellular pathology propounded in 1855. Only because of such a *modular anthropology* is it possible to transplant body parts, organs, tissues, and cells; to implant pacemakers and chips; to conduct in vitro fertilization and genetic interventions; to screen embryos for the sake of designing babies; to pursue human enhancement by chemistry and nanotechnology; and to exchange or insert many other modules in the future. There is no doubt that this new medicine as technology will develop a remarkable evolutionary impact on man. A new man is being made by medicine. That this anthropotechnology is only a part of the imminent Grand Biotechnology need not be stressed. Inspired by the belief that science and technology can be used to transcend the natural limitations of human body and mind, medical anthropotechnology is on the best way even to transcend the Homo sapiens and to contribute, in collaboration with other technological branches, to posthumanism that is characterized by the supremacy of machine over man.

We have interpreted this trans-Darwinian evolution as a Darwin-Lamarckian autoevolution of life on earth (Sadegh-Zadeh, 2000d, 113).

21.7.3 Summary

Like any other entity, medicine has numerous properties. Characterizing it by limiting its 'nature' to only one of these properties, is prone to dogmatism. In our analysis of this issue we found that clinical research is a practical science, while biomedical-experimental disciplines represent theoretical sciences. By virtue of its practicality, clinical *research* belongs to the discipline of normative ethics, for it seeks and establishes deontic-clinical rules of action usually called clinical-practical knowledge. The execution of these deontic rules in clinical *practice* turns this practice into a moral activity. *The good old medicine* characterized as practiced morality and normative ethics is currently in transition to an engineering discipline. Medical knowledge, therapeutica, clinical decisions, organs, tissues, cells, genes, molecules, and even health are being engineered today to the effect that medicine is on the way toward anthropotechnology as a branch of biotechnology.

Part VII

Epilog

Science, Medicine, and Rationality

22.0 Introduction

In preceding chapters, we tacitly presumed that medicine is a science, adding in the last chapter the view that it is (i) a practical science and (ii) in transition to an engineering science. What was left out until now is to determine what it means to say that medicine is a science. What is science? In order for judgments (i) and (ii) above to be testable, this basic question requires some clarity. Before we proceed to our logic précis, in the present part of our analytic philosophy of medicine we shall try to shed some light:

    22.1 On the Concept of Science
    22.2 On the Scientific Status of Medicine
    22.3 On Rationality in Medicine

as rationality is usually considered a feature of science.[147]

22.1 On the Concept of Science

We deliberately avoided starting this book with a definition of science because in the wrong place such a definition would either be superficial or unintelligible. It might come as a surprise that there is as yet no agreement on what science is. Although attempts to characterize or even to define it have a long history, going all the way back to Aristotle, it was not until the British

---

[147] In English-speaking countries, one distinguishes between science and humanities equating science with natural science. Our terminology follows the German usage of the word "science" that is more adequate. In Germany, *science* is not identified with *natural science*. Rather, *science* is the general category of all sciences. We thus distinguish between natural sciences, humanities, mathematical sciences, medicine, and many other types of sciences. All of them constitute the class *science* (in the singular) or the class of *sciences* (in the plural).

K. Sadegh-Zadeh, *Handbook of Analytic Philosophy of Medicine*,
Philosophy and Medicine 113, DOI 10.1007/978-94-007-2260-6_22,
© Springer Science+Business Media B.V. 2012

empiricism of the seventeenth and eighteenth centuries that definite criteria were suggested for differentiating science from non-science and pseudoscience. We saw previously that the first criteria put forward by British empiricists comprised observation, experimentation, and induction. These, however, are too narrow and preclude all non-experimental sciences, e.g., mathematics, economics, logic, and others. We also saw in Section 11.5.1 that still more explicit criteria such as verifiability and confirmability as well as the falsifiability of statements, hypotheses, and theories were suggested by logical empiricists and critical rationalists in the twentieth century. As pointed out, however, these criteria are not satisfiable and, in addition, too simplistic. Not every verifiable or falsifiable statement is scientific. For example, the verifiable statement "this sentence consists of six words" is none. Science is too complex a phenomenon to be characterized by a single, simple demarcation criterion. A multicriterial concept of science will be necessary to capture its degree of complexity. We proposed such a concept in terms of an eleven-place predicate a couple of years ago (Sadegh-Zadeh, 1970c). A slightly similar concept was also suggested by Mario Bunge (1983, 197 ff.). On the basis of these two proposals, an amended notion of science will be sketched in the following four sections:

22.1.1 Research Institutions

Note at the outset that the question "what is science?" is to be understood as a what-is-X question in the *quid mode* discussed on page 104. In answering the question, some measures of precaution should be taken into account. The most important one is that science as a complex phenomenon cannot be adequately conceptualized as a one-dimensional entity, i.e., it cannot be adequately defined solely by its subject matter, its method, the quality of knowledge it provides, or something like that. The explication of the concept of science that we are here undertaking, provides a 10-dimensional construct. We will first briefly outline its ten dimensions:

1. **Community, C:** A group of human beings with a joint intention who regularly interact with each other is called a community. When dealing with social and communitarian epistemology, we pointed out that scientific knowledge comes from scientific communities and not from individual scientists. The productive units of science are thus scientific *communities*. In our concept below, a scientific community will be represented by the symbol "C".

2. **Society, S:** A scientific community, C, is a subset of a larger human *society*, denoted by the variable "S". For instance, physiologists in China

are a part of the Chinese society, while German mathematicians constitute a subgroup of the German society. Of course, Chinese physiologists as well as German mathematicians are also communities in a larger human society, say world population. The society, represented by one or more states, hosts such communities and regulates, supports, or hinders their work. There is an intense interaction between society and scientific communities to the effect that society impacts on science and vice versa.

3. **Domain, _D:_** Every scientific discipline is concerned with particular objects, relations, phenomena, or processes, entities for short. For example, bacteriology is concerned with bacteria, and linguistics is concerned with languages. The set of entities with which a scientific community is concerned, is referred to as the _domain_ of its concern or discourse, symbolized by _"D"_.

4. **Problems, _P:_** In dealing with a domain _D,_ a scientific community _C_ is interested in solving particular puzzles or problems. For instance, in analyzing the brain tissues of patients with Alzheimer's disease, a pathologist's problem may be whether there are any intracellular pathogens in these tissues which play a causative role. The set of $m \geq 1$ problems, {problem 1, problem 2, ..., problem m}, that a scientific community _C_ is analyzing, may be denoted _"P"_.

5. **Goals, _G:_** In analyzing some particular problems, _P,_ a scientific community pursues some goals. For example, they want to causally explain the genesis of Alzheimer's disease, or they want to analyze the molecular structure of HIV in order to construct a vaccine. The set of $n \geq 1$ goals, {goal 1, goal 2, ..., goal n}, that a scientific community pursues in dealing with some problems, is symbolized by _"G"_.

6. **Axiomatic basis, _A:_** In conducting particular research, a scientific community _C_ shares some basic metaphysical axioms and postulates which are not a part of the research project itself, but are supposed to be indisputably relevant to the project and valid. For example, in the above-mentioned research concerned with the etiology of Alzheimer's disease, the so-called 'Principle of Causality' is supposed to be true which says that "every event has a cause". One may of course ask the etiologist "how do you know that? Have you ever examined _all_ of the events in the universe to know that each one of them has a cause? Maybe there are some events in the world without any causes, spontaneous events so to speak, e.g., Alzheimer's disease". She will never be able to prove that her 'Principle of Causality' is true simply because it is an unbounded universal statement. Thus, it represents a protoscientific postulate. Another example is the same etiologist's ontological realism according to which she contends "the entities that I am investigating in my research exist independently of the human mind". She will not be able to prove this postulate either. The set of all protoscientific beliefs of this type that a scientific community _C_ holds, is referred

to as the *axiomatic basis* of the research, denoted "*A*". For example, $A = \{$Every event has a cause; Entities investigated in this research exist independently of the human mind; There are objective natural laws$\}$. The axiomatic basis, A, is a pool of dogmas like in ideology and religion. The Greek term δόγμα (dogma) means "belief, opinion, doctrine, assumption".

7. **Conceptual basis, *CB*:** The scientific analysis of a problem is never conducted in a conceptual-epistemic vacuum. Rather, it always takes place on the basis of some antecedently available conceptual frameworks and knowledge consisting of any pool of concepts, descriptions, hypotheses, and theories. For example, when inquiring into the physiology of human vision, a physiologist uses some particular, already existing medical-physiological vocabulary, anatomical knowledge about the eye, some theories from other disciplines such as laws of geometric optics, laws of physical optics, etc. The entirety of such antecedently existing conceptual systems used by a scientific community in dealing with a research domain D constitutes the *conceptual basis* of this research, symbolized by "*CB*".

8. **Methodological basis, *M*:** Like the preceding item, scientific research is not conducted in a methodological vacuum. In inquiring into a domain D to solve some particular problems, P, a scientific community employs some specific methods such as, e.g., examination under a microscope, or statistical analysis of experimental data obtained by conducting a series of controlled clinical trials. A method may consist in using some concrete devices and machines, in employing some abstract mathematical or logical theories and algorithms, or in similar procedures. The set of such concrete and abstract methods applied in scientific research constitutes its *methodological basis,* denoted "*M*".

9. **Deontic basis, *DB*:** Medical research is a good example to demonstrate that scientific research also has a *deontic basis,* denoted "*DB*". It comprises some moral and legal rules that regulate the research by prescribing what types of action are permitted, forbidden, or obligatory. Examples are medical-ethical principles in clinical research as well as patients' rights. See also Section 15.2.

10. **Research product, *RP*:** The yield of a scientific inquiry, which is usually made publicly available by publishing it in journals, books or other media, is generally viewed as knowledge. It may consist of any surveys, reports, hypotheses, theories, or some other product. We shall therefore refer to it as the *research product* of the inquiry, symbolized by "*RP*".

The ten components above constitute a 10-dimensional structure of the following form that will be referred to as a *research institution,* denoted "$\mathcal{RI}$":

$$\mathcal{RI} = \langle C, S, D, P, G, A, CB, M, DB, RP \rangle.$$

Our explication of the concept of science will follow the order in which we introduce the following terms, where "A ⇐ B" means that B is dependent on A:

- Research frame ⇐ research institution ⇐ scientific research institution ⇐ scientific research field ⇐ science.

We start by introducing the basic, auxiliary predicate "is a research frame" with the following set-theoretical definition:

Definition 185 (Research frame). ξ *is a* research frame *iff there are D, P, G, A, CB, M, DB such that:*

1. $\xi = \langle D, P, G, A, CB, M, DB \rangle$,
2. *D, the domain, is a set of any entities (objects, relations, processes, phenomena, etc.), e.g., a collection of patients with Alzheimer's disease,*
3. *P is a set of $k \geq 1$ problems over D, e.g., {What causes Alzheimer's?, Is it an infectious disease?, Is it an autoimmune disease?, ... etc. ...},*
4. *G is a set of $m \geq 1$ goals,*
5. *A is a set of $n \geq 1$ axioms, referred to as the axiomatic basis of the research frame,*
6. *CB is a set of $p \geq 1$ available conceptual systems, referred to as the conceptual and epistemic basis of the research frame, e.g., {neuroanatomy, neuropathology, immunology, microbiology, biochemistry, ... etc. ...},*
7. *M is a set of $q \geq 1$ methods, called the methodological basis of the research frame,*
8. *DB is a set of $s \geq 0$ deontic rules regulating the handling of the domain D, of the problems P, and the pursuit of the goals G, called the deontic basis of the research frame,*
9. *On the basis of A, CB and DB, methods M are applied to D to solve the problems P and to attain the goals G.*

A group of persons may work on such a research frame $\langle D, P, G, A, CB, M, DB \rangle$ to solve the problems, P, of the frame and to put forward some research products. The new structure that ensues, we will call a *research institution*, denoted "$\mathcal{RI}$". It is introduced by a second set-theoretical definition as follows:

Definition 186 (Research institution). $\mathcal{RI}$ *is a* research institution *iff there are C, S, D, P, G, A, CB, M, DB, RP such that:*

1. $\mathcal{RI} = \langle C, S, D, P, G, A, CB, M, DB, RP \rangle$,
2. *C is a coherent group of human beings called a research community,*
3. *S is a human society with C being a subset thereof,*
4. *$\langle D, P, G, A, CB, M, DB \rangle$ is a research frame,*
5. *RP is a set of research products, e.g., knowledge,*
6. *The community C works on the research frame $\langle D, P, G, A, CB, M, DB \rangle$ and outputs the research product RP.*

For instance, consider the following groups:

- a community C_1 of researchers consisting of a neurologist x_1 and her assistant x_2, i.e., $C_1 = \{x_1, x_2\}$;
- a community C_2 of researchers consisting of a group of seven neurologists, pathologists, and statisticians $\{y_1, \ldots, y_7\}$;
- a community C_3 of researchers consisting of a group of 245 multidisciplinary scholars $\{z_1, \ldots, z_{245}\}$ who are working on a multi-center research project to investigate the causes of Alzheimer's disease;
- a community C_4 of researchers consisting of a group of 30,000 physicists and mathematicians distributed over the world who are associated with CERN (see page 535) to analyze some nuclear phenomena and put forward some RPs, e.g., a number of journal articles, books, DVDs, etc.

Each of these communities constitutes a research institution if we complete their structure $\langle C, S, D, P, G, A, CB, M, DB, RP \rangle$. There are scores of such research institutions in the world. Among them are not only disciplines such as mathematics, nuclear physics, ethnology, and immunology, but also astrology, homeopathy, anthroposophic medicine, bioharmonics, and osteopathy. Consider astrology as an example. Some people concern themselves, by means of some specific methods, with the constellation of celestial bodies and correlate them with human affairs to put forward a jumble of assertions about everything under the sun and stars. What they do is perfectly reconstructible as a research institution according to Definition 186 above. Yet, is it a science? It becomes apparent that not every type of research institution can be reasonably categorized as a science. Only a particular type of research institution deserves that name. We shall try to identify this type in what follows.

22.1.2 Scientific Research Fields

We shall first introduce the notion of a *scientific* research institution, denoted $\mathcal{SRI}$, by means of a set-theoretical definition. An $\mathcal{SRI}$ is a particular subcategory of research institutions. Note, however, that the new adjective "scientific" in our compound term "scientific research institution" is a basic term and does not presuppose a concept of science that we are pursuing. On the contrary, the latter will be introduced by the former. The procedure is thus void of any circularity. That is, we define the term "science" by the term "scientific", but not conversely.

Definition 187 (Scientific research institution). *$\mathcal{SRI}$ is a scientific research institution iff there are C, S, D, P, G, A, CB, M, DB, RP such that:*

1. *$\mathcal{SRI} = \langle C, S, D, P, G, A, CB, M, DB, RP \rangle$,*
2. *$\langle C, S, D, P, G, A, CB, M, DB, RP \rangle$ is a research institution,*
3. *Members of the community C have enjoyed a specialized training about the domain of discourse D, the conceptual basis CB, and the methodological basis M,*

4. They communicate with each other and learn from one another,

5. In dealing with the domain of discourse D and the problems P, the community C uses a transparent and well-structured language,[148]

6. A does not contain metaphoric, falsified, or cryptic axioms (such as "the stars don't lie" or "like cures like"),

7. M comprises reliable methods of inquiry including at least one public system of logic that is used in producing RP,

8. The research product RP is reliable,

9. The research frame $\langle D, P, G, A, CB, M, DB \rangle$ of the institution stands in a tradition of other research frames and research products $RP_1, RP_2, \ldots$ produced by other scientific research institutions.

The latter clause ensures that a scientific research institution is an element of a long-term scientific *research program* in the sense of Imre Lakatos (1978). It is not a nine-days wonder. In characterizing scientific methods and products, we deliberately used the humble term "reliable" in order to avoid controversies about their detailed epistemological qualities and about how these qualities are guaranteed. This is not the right place to develop the issue. We are here giving only a formal sketch of how to come to grips with the notoriously intractable concept of science. A complete explication of our concept will require us to be more precise about what we have here labeled "reliable".

A scientific research institution may be local, regional, national, or global. The overarching institution regarding a particular domain constitutes a scientific field:

Definition 188 (Scientific field). *If $\langle C, S, D, P, G, A, CB, M, DB, RP \rangle$ is a scientific research institution, then it is a scientific research field, or a scientific field for short, iff its research community C is the union of all scientific research communities concerned with the domain D.*

For example, all scientific research institutions in the world concerned with Alzheimer's disease constitute a scientific field called *Alzheimer research*. All scientific research institutions concerned with the biological functions of the human body and its parts yield a scientific field traditionally called *human physiology*. And so on.

22.1.3 Science in General

On the basis of our discussions in the preceding two sections, we will now suggest a general concept of science, which we shall further differentiate in the next section.

---

[148] We do not require a 'precise' language because in this case only mathematical sciences and logic would turn out scientific research institutions. The languages of all other branches are irremediably imprecise because they are derivatives of natural language. But we have seen in previous chapters that this unavoidable vagueness of scientific languages is not a disadvantage. See, for example, Section 16.5.1.

Definition 189 (Science_in_general). *An object is a science iff it is a scientific field.*[149]

That means that science (in the singular) is the class of all scientific fields as defined in Definition 188. Its members are the individual sciences (in the plural), i.e., individual scientific fields. Thus, a scientific field *is_a* science. Astrology and homeopathy do not turn out sciences because they do not satisfy clauses 5–8 of Definition 187. Bacteriology and English studies, however, satisfy the criteria and thus turn out sciences.

Nevertheless, the resulting concept of science in our Definition 189 is not a clear-cut category. When a discipline is inhomogeneous or in the process of degenerating, it may be impossible to discern whether it is a science or not. Consider psychiatry as an example. Although it has areas that unquestionably count as scientific fields, e.g., biological psychiatry and psychopharmacotherapy, it also has subdisciplines that turn out unscientific. Psychopathology is an example because its ill-structured and opaque language violates clause 5 of Definition 187. This and similar findings make it difficult to judge whether psychiatry as a whole is definitely a science (Sadegh-Zadeh, 1970c).

The vagueness of our general concept of science is mainly due to the complexity of its referent, which we reconstructed as entities of the structure $\langle C, S, D, P, G, A, CB, M, DB, RP \rangle$. In the spirit of tradition, we treated this concept – like the other ones we dealt with – as if it were a *classical concept* definable by some necessary and sufficient conditions as discussed on pages 161 and 230. This traditional approach may be the reason why the concept of science has been so notoriously intractable. A classical concept cannot capture a complex, irreducible category (see Section 6.3.1).

An alternative is to treat the concept of science as a *non-classical* concept, which we discussed on page 162. In this case it may be explicated as a fuzzy category with grades of membership for individual sciences, thus enabling us to state, for example, "to the extent 1 physics is a science"; "psychiatry is a science to the extent 0.5"; and "astrology is a science to the extent 0". There are many ways to introduce such a fuzzy concept of science. One such possibility, for example, is to require a number of n ideal properties, say $n = 100$, of which a research institution may present m properties. The quotient $\frac{m}{n}$, then, would be the degree to which it is a science. Since $\frac{m}{n}$ is a real number in the unit interval $[0, 1]$, this method yields a membership function $\mu_{science}$ that makes it possible to represent the above statements as follows: $\mu_{science}(\text{physics}) = 1$; $\mu_{science}(\text{psychiatry}) = 0.5$ and $\mu_{science}(\text{astrology}) = 0$.

Another possibility is the prototype resemblance method of concept formation introduced on pages 174–183. Using this method, one would first have to decide which research institution or institutions could serve as prototype

---

[149] Note that Definition 189 is a convenient abbreviation of the following set-theoretical definition: ξ is a *science* iff there are C, S, D, P, G, A, M, CB, DB, RP such that (i) $\xi = \langle C, S, D, P, G, A, CB, M, DB, RP \rangle$ and (ii) $\langle C, S, D, P, G, A, CB, M, DB, RP \rangle$ is a scientific field.

members of the envisaged category *science*. With $n \geq 1$ such prototypes, say physics and history, we could recursively delineate the category *science* by definitions of the following type or similar ones (see also Definitions 37 and 39 on pages 176 and 178, respectively):

Definition 190 (Science_in_general as a prototype resemblance category: 1).

1. *Physics as well as history is a* science, *referred to as a* prototype science,
2. *a research institution is a* science *if the minimum degree of its similarity to prototype sciences exceeds 0.5 (or any other number $r \in (0, 1]$ to be fixed).*

Definition 191 (Science_in_general as a prototype resemblance category: 2).

1. *Physics as well as history is a* science *to the extent 1, referred to as a* prototype science,
2. *a research institution is a* science *to the extent r iff r is the minimum degree of its similarity to prototype sciences and $r > 0.5$ (or any other number $r \in (0, 1]$ to be fixed).*

The emerging category of sciences, then, would be n-focal depending on the number n of prototype sciences chosen in clause 1 to the effect that a soft science such as ethnology would not need to be compared with physics to be excluded as a science, but with history. Despite the disparity between physics and ethnology, the latter would turn out a science nonetheless because it is sufficiently similar to the soft prototype science history. Here two problems arise:

First, it might be a difficult task to construct an appropriate similarity relation between research institutions.[150] Second, it is questionable whether statements such as "economics is a science to the extent 0.7" and "psychiatry is a science to the extent 0.51" are useful utterances at all. Do they have any practical consequences and value? This reminds us that although a fuzzy approach to the concept of science may be intellectually interesting, it will remain practically sterile if it does not advise us how to act. An additional problem is the limiting degree of similarity to a prototype science. Tentatively, we chose the limiting degree 0.5. But what instances should decide this minimum degree of similarity? Taking these problems into account, which we cannot resolve here, we must be content with a classical concept of science like in Definition 189 above even though it is basically impossible to make it precise.

However, an important aspect of the concept of science discussed thus far should not be overlooked. Since it also includes among its ten dimensions the

---

[150] Tentatively, take 100 criteria and examine to what extent $r \in [0, 1]$ they are satisfied by a prototype science. Call the score the SCI index of that prototype. Now, examine a candidate research institution in the same fashion. The result is the SCI index of that institution. Calculate the similarity between both SCIs using the Similarity Theorem given on page 173. Go to Definitions 190 and 191.

scientific community and the society hosting that community, it is a pragmatic concept that is not confined to identifying science with a body of knowledge, as it is traditionally. It shows that science is not merely a cognitive, but also a social, and consequently a political, moral and economic, institution. However, it is still incomplete in an essential respect. This is the subject of our discussion in the next section.

22.1.4 Types of Science

Philosophers of science concerned with this concept have been inclined to identify science with empirical and mathematical sciences. The research products of these sciences are empirical or formal descriptions, hypotheses, theories, and theoretical frameworks, i.e., what has traditionally come to be termed *knowledge* consisting of declarative sentences of the form "the earth revolves around the sun"; "AIDS is caused by HIV"; "$2 + 2 = 4$"; and the like. Let us call them declarative or descriptive sciences. There are other, non-descriptive types of science, however, whose research products are not descriptions, e.g., diagnostic-therapeutic research in medicine, normative ethics, and law. None of these sciences is covered by traditional concepts of science.

Because of the above-mentioned diversity of scientific research products, it was not possible to specify the term "research product" in our definitions above to the effect that the resulting concept of science in Definition 189 is too general and does not discriminate between descriptive and non-descriptive sciences. Distinct types of science will now be identified by further differentiating the Definition 189. To this end, we first consider three different categories of research products that characterize distinct species of science. The research product of a scientific field may be:

1. **theoretical knowledge.** It consists of declarative-descriptive sentences as demonstrated above, e.g., quantum theory, theory of cellular pathology, theory of evolution, theory of autoimmune diseases, "AIDS is caused by HIV", etc.;
2. **practical knowledge.** It consists of imperatives of the form $X \rightarrow (Y \rightarrow do\ Z)$ which say: Under circumstances X, if goal is Y, do $Z!$ See Sections 10.6, 21.5.3, and below;
3. **deontic rules.** Examples are medical-ethical principles and laws.

While research products of the type 1 are descriptive, those of the types 2–3 are prescriptive. Scientific activities that provide products of the type 1 are usually the so-called theoretical sciences. A scientific field whose products are imperatives of the type 2, such as diagnostic-therapeutic research, was referred to in Section 21.5.3 as a practical science. Those fields of research whose products are deontic rules like in 3 above, are deontic or normative sciences. We thus arrive at a tripartite concept of science that categorizes sciences according to the syntax of their products:

Definition 192 (Types of science). *A scientific field is:*

1. *a* theoretical science *iff its research products, RP, consist of theoretical knowledge,*
2. *a* practical science *iff its research products, RP, consist of practical knowledge,*
3. *a* deontic science *('deontology') iff its research products, RP, are deontic rules.*

Examples of theoretical sciences are natural sciences, mathematics, biomedical sciences, sociology, history, and linguistics. Practical sciences are, e.g., clinical research, engineering sciences, and pedagogy. Examples of deontic sciences are normative ethics, diagnostic-therapeutic research, and law. The advantage of our approach above is that it provides precise, syntactic criteria of categorization and thereby prevents philosophical controversies.

22.2 On the Scientific Status of Medicine

Medicine embraces more than a hundred different research fields from cytology to medical physics to internal medicine to psychiatry to medical ethics. Many of these fields are themselves heterogeneous and consist of several subfields. For example, internal medicine unites clinical endocrinology, gastroenterology, cardiology, rheumatology, nephrology, oncology, and many other subfields. Psychiatry unites biological psychiatry, psychopathology, psychotherapy, child and adolescent psychiatry, etc. For different reasons, not all of such subfields have the same degree of scientificity. As a result, it is impossible and thus not recommendable to judge the scientific status of medicine all at once. What is more interesting is that medicine constitutes an heterogeneous scientific field in another respect:

> **Medicine unites all three types of science** distinguished in
> Definition 192 above: It is a theoretical science, a practical science,   (201)
> and a deontic science at the same time.

For example, while biomedical research fields such as cytology, medical physics, and physiology are theoretical sciences, clinical research fields in all clinical disciplines from pediatrics to psychiatry are practical sciences. Medical ethics, when it acts as normative ethics by putting forward moral principles for use in research and practice, is a deontic science. In Section 21.6 on page 777, we also categorized diagnostic-therapeutic research as a deontic discipline because it advances clinical ought-to-do rules for use in clinical decision-making.

22.3 On Rationality in Medicine

We avoided the term "rationality" until now because it is exceedingly ambiguous. Only one of its many meanings will be of interest here, however.

Specifically, we will ask the question whether medicine and health care are rational undertakings and how rational medical decisions are. We need to examine these questions with regard both to medical research and medical practice. In these two areas, two different types of rationality are primarily operative: theoretical rationality and practical rationality. In the present section, we shall therefore briefly discuss the following issues:

22.3.1   Theoretical and Practical Rationality
22.3.2   Rationality in Medical Sciences
22.3.3   Rationality in Clinical Practice
22.3.3   The Relativity of Rationality.

22.3.1 Theoretical and Practical Rationality

Rationality is the ability to reason and has at least two dimensions, theoretical rationality and practical rationality. Theoretical rationality is the ability to perform *theoretical reasoning,* while practical rationality is the ability to perform *practical reasoning*. What is usually called *moral reasoning* is partly theoretical and partly practical reasoning. So, we need not consider it separately.

Suppose Mr. Elroy Fox has an acute fever and cough. He decides to consult Dr. Smith, who takes a brief patient history and finds no additional complaints or symptoms. He thus assumes on the basis of his background knowledge that the patient may have bronchitis. He examines the patient's chest, and during auscultation hears massively altered breath sounds and rales. So he changes his belief and hypothesizes that Mr. Elroy Fox might have pneumonia. To support or falsify this diagnostic hypothesis, he conducts chest radiography and observes wide opaque areas in both lungs. On the basis of this new evidence and his medical knowledge, he now strongly believes that the patient has acute pneumonia. Dr. Smith's reasoning in this case is *theoretical* because it is concerned with states of affairs in order to gather evidence for deciding *what to believe*. It thus leads to beliefs or belief changes regarding "what was, is, or will be the case".

After having formed a belief about Mr. Elroy Fox's state of health, Dr. Smith now thinks about how to treat the patient. He deems immediate antibiotic therapy indispensable for addressing the cause of the patient's complaints and symptoms. The most efficacious antibiotic that he could administer by injection is a penicillin derivative. But the patient has a history of penicillin allergy. Dr. Smith therefore decides to use erythromycin. His reasoning to reach this decision is *practical* because it is concerned with deciding *what to do*. It leads to intentions, plans, and actions. In contrast to theoretical reasoning, which examines descriptive questions, practical reasoning examines a normative question by asking which among a set of alternative actions would be best to do. Otherwise put, practical reasoning asks what one ought to do. It is not concerned with beliefs, but rather with values.

There are a large number of methods from logic to decision theory to game theory to ethics that assist theoretical and practical reasoning in science and everyday life. But none of them is applicable in every situation. Their respective presuppositions must be fulfilled. We will briefly examine how medicine can benefit from them.

22.3.2 Rationality in Medical Sciences

Above, medical sciences were divided into three types: (i) theoretical sciences that produce theoretical knowledge by theoretical reasoning; (ii) practical sciences that produce practical knowledge by practical reasoning; and (iii) deontic sciences that produce ought-to-do rules of action. Since reasoning in the latter fields is either theoretical or practical, they will not be considered separately. We shall consider the first two in turn. What is important to note at the outset is the distinction between reasoning and rhetoric. Rhetoric is not reasoning. It is an artful use of the language.

Theoretical reasoning in medical sciences

According to the classical concept of knowledge presented in Definition 116 on page 385, belief is a main component of theoretical knowledge. It is therefore commonly supposed that theoretical reasoning is needed to justify knowledge in general and theoretical-scientific knowledge in particular. We may take the subject of theoretical reasoning to be sentences, as scientific knowledge is communicated using sentences.

It is traditionally assumed that scientific sentences are justified deductively or inductively, so we will look at these two possibilities in turn. (i) Medical-scientific knowledge consists of universal hypotheses of a deterministic, statistical, or fuzzy type. They do not deductively follow from empirical evidence because empirical evidence, consisting of the so-called scientific data and descriptions of facts, is represented by singular sentences. No universal sentence is implied by singular sentences. Medical-empirical knowledge is therefore not deductively justifiable by experience. (ii) As regards its inductive justification, we shall see in Section 29.2 that there is as yet no inductive logic of justification. We know already that confirmation also does not work (see Section 11.1.2). The *comparative support* of empirical-medical knowledge either by means of likelihood tests or statistical significance tests, discussed on pages 477 and 480, remains the gold standard for inductive support. If according to Definition 143 on page 478, a hypothesis is empirically *better supported* than the alternative hypothesis, then it is rational to believe in it *more than* in the latter. It is thus possible to rationally ground theoretical-medical knowledge on experience and to advocate a moderate fuzzy-logical empiricism (Sadegh-Zadeh, Forthcoming).

Practical reasoning in medical sciences

Medical sciences do not only produce theoretical knowledge. Practical-medical sciences in terms of clinical research in clinical disciplines produce, in addition, practical knowledge. As discussed in previous sections, practical-medical knowledge consists either of imperatives or ought-to-do rules. Both of these types of *practical* sentences, e.g., the imperative:

> IF a patient complains of upper abdominal pain, THEN (IF you want to explore whether she has gastritis or peptic ulcer disease,   (202) THEN *do* gastroscopy)

are obtained on the basis of *declarative*, i.e., theoretical, sentences of the following type:

> IF a patient complains of upper abdominal pain, THEN (IF you want to explore whether she has gastritis or peptic ulcer disease,   (203) THEN the optimal action is gastroscopy).

As outlined by demonstrating a set of equifinal rules in (194) on page 775, an action such as gastroscopy recommended in (202) has been found in previous research to be the optimal action based on a comparison to alternative actions. It is obvious that there are no logical relationships between such a descriptive result (203) and the prescriptive rule (202). But if there are no such relationships, why do the researchers investigating upper abdominal pain not recommend any other prescriptive rule than rule (202)? What is the rationale behind their transition from theoretical sentence (203) to practical sentence (202)? Otherwise put, why and by virtue of which logic or canon of reasoning does the research team or the scientific-medical community choose to recommend the action rule (202) on the basis of the empirical finding (203)?

It is commonly assumed that an action rule such as (202) above is recommended because this decision is *the best one* according to the preferences of the clinical researchers as decision-makers. Their preferences in the present example consist in achieving their goal, i.e., the greatest number of accurate diagnoses, at the lowest cost in terms of side-effects such as pain, damage, and death as well as money in relation to the value of their goal. In the theory of rational choice, a decision to act in a way – to choose rule (202) instead of a competing one – that maximizes the benefits and minimizes the costs, is called a rational decision. Research based on this type of practical reasoning may therefore be viewed as rational research *relative to this type of reasoning*. The recommendation of a particular therapeutic action rule such as:

> IF a patient has peptic ulcer disease and is Helicobacter pylori positive, THEN (IF you want to cure her disease, THEN administer antibiotics XYZ for 1 week)   (204)

on the basis of a controlled clinical trial follows the same principle of practical reasoning. There are of course also other issues of practical rationality in medical sciences such as:

- the question of whether the decision of a scientific community to investigate a particular subject, say xenotransplantation, is a practically-rational one, or more practically-rational than the decision to spend the required resources on animal protection or 'bread for the world';
- likewise, the decision of an individual medical scientist to devote herself, say, to HIV research instead of stem cell research or history of medieval medicine may be analyzed with respect to its practical rationality.

In either case, practical reasoning will be at work because the subject of inquiry is to find out what to do or prefer to do. Again, the question can only be answered by taking into account the goal or goals that the research community or the individual scientist pursues. The rationality of an action as a means to attain an end is relative to the *end* because it can only be judged by considering the comparative optimality of the respective means-end relation. The basic question of practical rationality is, therefore, which ends are worth pursuing at all so that one could choose among them. This is an explicitly ethical question and shows that practical reasoning is basically ethics.

22.3.3 Rationality in Clinical Practice

We saw throughout our analyses that the diagnostic-therapeutic decision-making in clinical practice represents a *process* of reasoning in which theoretical and practical reasoning cannot be sharply separated from one another. Each step in diagnostic reasoning as theoretical reasoning is intertwined with practical reasoning about *what to do next* differential-diagnostically to test a diagnostic hypothesis, *what to do* therapeutically now, etc. While the theoretical component of such reasoning requires logical augmentation and application of methodological frameworks such as the Bayesian logic discussed on page 988, its practical component by and large consists in the use of practical-clinical knowledge, i.e., clinical imperatives and ought-to-do rules, and procedural frameworks such as branching clinical questionnaires discussed in Section 8.1.2 on page 283. An ideal physician who has the capability of multi-logical reasoning, would have no problems accomplishing these tasks. But it is well-known that one can scarcely find such capabilities in real-world clinical practice. For this reason, rationality in clinical practice is hard to come by. Clinical rationality is also hindered by the fact that the clinical encounter and patient management are game-theoretical settings (Osborne, 2004). As a player in this game the physician, as well as the patient, acts in anticipation of other player's behavior to the effect that the outcome of their interaction depends on what the parties jointly do. When the physician does not *know* in advance, as is always the case, what the patient will do and how she, as a bio-psycho-social system, will react to the physician's actions, the physician's reasoning will only be based on guesses that impede rational decision-making.

The Relativity of Rationality

As pointed out above, neither in medical research nor in medical practice are theoretical and practical reasoning operative in isolation from one another. The decision about *what to do* in a particular setting is often dependent on the judgment about *what to believe* in this setting and vice versa. One may therefore consider them together in terms of global rationality, or *rationality* for short.

It is important to note that what appears rational to someone, need not appear equally rational, or rational at all, to someone else. This is so because what is commonly called rationality is in fact relative to a number of parameters that vary across individuals and circumstances. Specifically, (i) theoretical rationality is relative to the system of logic followed in reasoning. For example, what appears rational relative to Zande Logic (da Costa et al., 1998; Jennings, 1989; Triplett, 1988), is just absurd relative to our Western systems of logic. Here is another example: Given some evidence, paraconsistent logic is able to draw more conclusions therefrom than classical logic does; and fuzzy logic is able to draw even more conclusions than paraconsistent logic does. That is, on the basis of some given evidence, fuzzy logic supports more beliefs than paraconsistent logic does; and the latter supports more beliefs than classical logic does. Thus, behaving rationally is much easier by following fuzzy logic than paraconsistent logic or classical logic, and much easier by following paraconsistent logic than classical logic. Otherwise put, the set of rational beliefs and actions relative to classical logic is a subset of those relative to paraconsistent logic; and the latter set of rational beliefs and actions is a subset of those relative to fuzzy logic. (ii) Practical rationality is in addition relative to the decision-maker's methodology of practice as well as goals and values.

Because of the philosophical significance of the term "relative", we should clarify its meaning. Conspicuously, it is an antonym of the term "absolute". For example, that according to Einstein's general theory of relativity time is something relative means that there is no absolute time, i.e., something that can unconditionally be called "x is a time duration of the length such and such", e.g., 1 hour, because time duration is dependent on some factors, specifically on the motion and speed of the observer. Likewise, that according to our conception rationality is something relative, means that there is no absolute rationality, i.e., a property to be attributed to a belief or decision alone in isolation from everything else. For example, let α be a sentence that describes a diagnostic belief or a therapeutic decision. It is inappropriate to say, using the *unary* predicate "is rational", that α *is rational*. Rather, it is more appropriate to conceive rationality as a many-place *relation* that we may conceptualize by the following *many-place* predicate:

- A belief or decision α is rational with respect to the circumstances C, goals G, values V, logic L, methods M, and conceptual system CS iff
  . . .

symbolized by:

- $R(\alpha, C, G, V, L, M, CS)$.

This seven-place predicate says that a belief or decision α is rational with respect to six different factors. They are:

1. $C \equiv$ the circumstances under which the belief α is formed or the decision α to act is made. C is in fact a set of premises or data that describe the circumstances. Different circumstances justify different beliefs and actions. There may be many possible circumstances $C_1, C_2, C_3, \ldots$ and so on one of which will actually be present when forming a belief or decision-making, symbolized by "C" above.

2. $G \equiv$ a set of goals that one pursues in forming the belief or making the decision α to act. There may be many different possible goal sets $G_1, G_2, G_3, \ldots$ and so on one of which will actually be pursued, symbolized by "G" above.

3. $V \equiv$ a set of values in the light of which goals G are evaluated. There may be many different sets of competing values $V_1, V_2, V_3, \ldots$ and so on to one of which an agent subscribes, symbolized by "V" above. Under the same circumstances C and in pursuing the same goals G, two agents' beliefs and decisions will usually differ from one another if they do not share the same system of values;

4. $L \equiv$ a logic that is used in reasoning. There are indeed a number of different logics $L_1, L_2, L_3, \ldots$ and so on each of which, symbolized by "L" above, may be used in the reasoning process;

5. $M \equiv$ a set of methods that supplement the logic L in reasoning, e.g., likelihood tests, statistical significance tests, or any decision theory assisting in making the decision α. There are indeed a number of different methods of judgment and decision-making $M_1, M_2, M_3, \ldots$ and so on each of which, symbolized by "M" above, a reasoner or decision-maker may apply to get the belief or decision α;

6. $CS \equiv$ a conceptual system consisting of any knowledge-base or conceptual framework used in interpreting C, evaluating G, applying M, and forming the belief or making the decision α. There are indeed a large number of different conceptual systems $CS_1, CS_2, CS_3, \ldots$ and so on each of which, symbolized by "CS" above, may be used.

One and the same belief or action α may appear differently rational if in belief forming and decision-making we replace any of the variable factors C, G, V, L, M, CS with another, competing one. Rationality, R, in $R(\alpha, C, G, V, L, M, CS)$ is not meaningfully attributable to the belief or action α alone because it is an attribute of the entire structure $\langle \alpha, C, G, V, L, M, CS \rangle$. By changing any of the seven variables of the structure, say from $\langle \alpha, C, G, V, L, M, CS \rangle$ to $\langle \alpha, C', G, V, L, M, CS \rangle$ or $\langle \alpha, C', G, V, L', M, CS \rangle$ where $C \neq C'$ and $L \neq L'$, the rationality of the belief or action α may vary. A belief or action α that appears rational in the structure $\langle \alpha, C, G, V, L, M, CS \rangle$, may not appear so in another structure such as $\langle \alpha, C', G, V, L, M, CS \rangle$ or $\langle \alpha, C', G, V, L', M, CS \rangle$ or $\langle \alpha, C', G', V', L', M', CS' \rangle$. For example, everything else being equal, when $C \equiv$ "the patient has acute pneumonia" the administration of antibiotics to the patient may be rational, whereas it is not rational when $C \equiv$ "the patient has depression". We therefore consider rationality something relative.

The considerations above elucidate what the *relativity* of an attribute such as "is rational" actually means. It means simply that the rationality of a belief or action x is a *relation* such that it needs to be represented by a relational, i.e., many-place, predicate R with the correct syntax $R(x, y_1, \ldots, y_n)$ where $n \geq 1$. Hence, it is not a one-place property of the type "x is rational". As a result, we are not allowed to say that Rx, e.g., "this therapeutic action is rational" and "the other one is not rational". This is the plain solution to the mystery surrounding the term *"relativity"*.

It is not our aim here to define the seven-place predicate of rationality above. Such a task requires the construction of a theory of rationality. We have merely tried to argue that in medicine rationality in the colloquial sense cannot be viewed as the decisive criterion for preferring a particular diagnostic belief over another one, a particular therapeutic decision over another one, a particular theory over another one, a system of medicine as a whole over another one, and so on because rationality is not an elementary attribute of a unary entity x, but a complex attribute of a multidimensional structure $\langle x, y_1, \ldots, y_n \rangle$ and may therefore be viewed from different dimensions of the structure, i.e., from many different perspectives. Since this perspectivity of judgments is of paramount epistemological and metaphysical importance, it will be the subject of our discussion in the next, penultimate chapter, which completes our medical-philosophical considerations.

22.4 Summary

A ten-place concept of science was proposed which shows that science is not a semantic process of searching for truth, but a pragmatic process in which a scientific community in interaction with a larger society produces some research products usually called knowledge. Some syntactic criteria of research products were put forward which enable a differentiation between three types of science, theoretical science, practical science, and deontic science. Medicine encompasses all three types of science. To each type of science belongs a specific mode of reasoning. Thus, medical reasoning is either theoretical or practical reasoning because deontic reasoning itself is either theoretical or practical. This does not imply that medical reasoning is rational. Rationality is a much more complex, relational attribute and may be judged differently depending on the perspective.

Perspectivism

The relativistic concept of rationality above is consonant with our relativism throughout the preceding chapters. In the following two sections:

we shall demonstrate that (i) relativism enables a viable theory of knowledge and action that may be termed *perspectivism*; and (ii) perspectivism may be conceived as a modal theory that has both *de re* and *de dicto* aspects with significant metaphysical consequences. The basic idea of perspectivism, which we shall further elaborate here, comes from the German philosophers Leibniz, Kant, and Nietzsche (Kaulbach, 1990; Hales and Welshon, 2000; Baghramian, 2004; Giere, 2006; Ibbeken, 2008; DeRose, 2009).

23.1 Relativism, Contextualism, Perspectivism

The universal relativism that we hold must not be confused with the folk understanding "anything goes". For example, when we say that diagnosis, prognosis, therapy, and prevention are relative, or that rationality in general and the rationality of medical judgments and decisions in particular are relative, we do not maintain that there is no common ground and everybody is allowed to do or to believe what she wants. Our relativism emerges from, and reflects, the recognition that in human languages, most predicates and all functions represent n-ary relations with $n > 1$, and thus, concern objects and states of affairs *in relation to, i.e. relative to, one another* and ought to be treated accordingly. It is a methodological approach to representing complex entities and realities as multidimensional, *relational structures* of the form $\langle x, y_1, \ldots, y_n \rangle$, e.g., the concepts of science, rationality, diagnosis, and diagnostic structure discussed earlier (for the notion of a relational structure, see pages 72 and 878):

K. Sadegh-Zadeh, *Handbook of Analytic Philosophy of Medicine*,
Philosophy and Medicine 113, DOI 10.1007/978-94-007-2260-6_23,
© Springer Science+Business Media B.V. 2012

- $\langle C, S, D, P, G, A, M, CB, DB, RP \rangle$ (science: Definition 188, p. 795)
- $R(\alpha, C, G, V, L, M, CS)$ (rationality: p. 805)
- $diagnosis^*(\Delta, p, D, KB \cup M)$ (diagnosis*: Definition 103, p. 322)
- $\langle p, d, t_1, \mathfrak{D}, \mathfrak{A}, D_1, A_1, f, OB, t_2, D_2, D, \Delta, PO, nv, T(nv), cr, dg \rangle$
    (diagnostic structure: Definition 101 , p. 321)

All these structures are of the general form:

$$\langle x, y_1, \ldots, y_n \rangle \tag{205}$$

such that an object x is viewed, or judged, on the basis of an n-dimensional substructure $\langle y_1, \ldots, y_n \rangle$, with $n \geq 1$, that we therefore term a *perspective*. We say that object x is viewed, or judged, from the perspective $\langle y_1, \ldots, y_n \rangle$. For example, the many-place concept of diagnosis* above shows that a set of statements, Δ, such as:

$$\{\text{Elroy Fox has myocardial infarction, he has no hepatitis}\} \tag{206}$$

is considered a diagnosis from the perspective $\langle p, D, KB \cup M \rangle$ that is constituted by the patient p; a particular set of patient data, D; and some knowledge base and method of reasoning, $KB \cup M$. Viewed from another perspective, say $\langle p, D', KB' \cup M' \rangle$ that is different from the first perspective $\langle p, D, KB \cup M \rangle$ because of $D \neq D'$ and $KB \cup M \neq KB' \cup M'$, the statement 206 may not turn out a diagnosis (see below).

As we saw in preceding chapters, 'when looking at the world' the beholder always stands in, and is a component of, such a structure as 205. The awareness of such multidimensional, perspectival structures $\langle x, y_1, \ldots, y_n \rangle$ in both everyday life and science is methodologically and epistemologically illuminating and instrumental. At this juncture, some equally important metaphysical consequences will be noted that may help reduce the epistemic hubris that is prevalent in natural-scientifically oriented disciplines like biomedicine. They will remind us that one views the objects of one's concern, say the world, always from a particular perspective such that by changing one's perspective one's views about the object will change.

For instance, you will see a cell differently depending on whether you use an optical microscope, a transmission electron microscope, a scanning electron microscope, or another device. The particularity of a perspective $\langle y_1, \ldots, y_n \rangle$ used in a structure $\langle x, y_1, \ldots, y_n \rangle$ means that the perspective is only one of the many alternatives from which the object x may be viewed because each of the n dimensions $y_1, \ldots, y_n$ of the perspective $\langle y_1, \ldots, y_n \rangle$ is exchangeable by any other variety of the same type, e.g., the dimension y_1 by y_1', or by y_1'', or by y_1''', and so on where $y_1 \neq y_1' \neq y_1'' \neq y_1'''$. For example, regarding the concept of rationality sketched above, i.e., $R(\alpha, C, G, V, L, M, CS)$, one can judge the rationality of a diagnostic belief or therapeutic action α not only under circumstances C, but also under completely different circumstances C', or C'', or C''' where $C \neq C' \neq C'' \neq C'''$. The same holds for the remaining dimensions of the structure. Each constellation of the variable dimensions yields a particular perspective. Given an n-dimensional perspective $\langle y_1, \ldots, y_n \rangle$ in a judgmental structure $\langle x, y_1, \ldots, y_n \rangle$ such that $m_i \geq 1$ is the number of the varieties of the dimension y_i, then there are $m_1 \times m_2 \times \cdots \times m_n$ different perspectives from which object x may be viewed. Each of them will of course show the object x in a different shape and manner due to differences between the angles of inquiry, i.e., the German "Blickwinkel".

As a result, one's knowledge of the world is perspective-dependent or perspective-relative, a perspective being a point of view in the above sense, i.e., where one stands to look at some particular object. It may be an opinion or theory, a look through an optical microscope, telescope, PET machine or something else. And there are so many perspectives that one can take! Distinct languages that one may use are distinct perspectives; distinct logics are distinct perspectives; distinct theories are distinct perspectives; distinct devices, techniques, and methodologies are distinct perspectives; distinct knowledge-bases are distinct perspectives; distinct value systems are distinct perspectives; distinct people whom one admires, loves, or hates engender different perspectives; and so on. None of them gives you "the true picture" of the object because no perspective can be identified as "the right one" to produce "the true picture of the object". We hold in our hands only different perspectival pictures of the represented object, which were taken from distinct perspectives, and in describing the object we never describe the "object-in-itself". We describe *the picture* we have taken of it from our perspective. We never judge whether a picture is true or not by comparing it with the depicted object in-itself to determine the degree of correspondence between them. We only compare a perspectival picture of the object with another perspectival picture thereof. For every perception and observation that we make about the object, and any theorizing we conduct about it, generates a new perspectival picture of the object to the effect that the object is accessible to us through its perspectival pictures only. What it is "in itself" remains inaccessible forever.

Is it conceivable, then, that there is no such ontic state as "being in-itself"? That the object is created by the perspectives, and does not exist at all independently of them? This possibility is in line with the ontological relativity advanced in Chapter 18. But a precise answer to the question will be given in the next section.

It is obvious that perspectivism is at variance with realism, objectivism, and absolutism because it excludes the possibility of objective knowledge. It is closely related with *contextualism* touched upon in previous chapters. In contrast to traditional epistemology, which is an absolutist view, contextualism is relativistic according to which the context determines meaning, truth, and relevance. That is, the meaning of expressions and the semantic-pragmatic features of statements such as their truth values, credibility, plausibility, and probability are subject to circumstantial variation in that they fluctuate across contexts of utterance and frames of reference. Examples par excellence are indexicals such as "I", "here", and "now", discussed on page 135. Another, less salient example encountered on page 337 is the notion of "diagnosis". We saw that it is a context-sensitive expression in that it applies to one and the same object in different contexts differently. While a statement such as "Mr. El-roy Fox has Hashimoto's thyroiditis" is a *diagnosis* in our current Western medicine, it is *none* in the Hippocratic humoral pathology or in traditional Chinese medicine, TCM, simply because the latter two systems of medicine do not include a concept of Hashimoto's thyroiditis. For another example, see the contextuality of causes on page 245. That is, diagnoses and etiologies are context-relative.

These examples strengthen the view that even what is called knowledge, is knowledge in a particular context and may lose this attribute in another circumstance and context. They thus corroborate the idea of *contextuality of knowledge* that we had already expressed on page 518. Contextualism not only supports perspectivism because a context, as a frame of reference, is arguably a perspective, but it may also benefit from our following analysis of perspectivism reconstructed as a modal epistemology.

23.2 Perspectivism *de re* and Perspectivism *de dicto*

To answer the ontological question above of whether the object of a perspec-tival inquiry is created by the perspective or exists independently, we shall ground perspectivism on a binary modal operator that renders it amenable to logical-ontological analyses. To introduce the operator, consider first the following sentence:

> Viewed from the perspective of cellular pathology, all diseases result from changes that occur in cells. (207)

This sentence may be construed as a tripartite compound consisting of (i) the two-place operator "Viewed from the perspective ..." that bears the follow-ing two operands: (ii) the name "cellular pathology", and (iii) the sentence "all diseases result from changes that occur in cells". Rewritten in a more structured, operator-operand syntax, it says:

> Viewed_from_the_perspective(cellular pathology, all diseases re-sult from changes that occur in cells).

The operator, being a binary predicate of a many-sorted language of higher order, is prefixed to its operands within parentheses. The first operand, the Virchowian cellular pathology, represents the perspective; and the second operand, "all diseases result from changes that occur in cells", is a sentence describing a view from that perspective. Thus, the statement (207) has the following syntax:

$$VfP(X, \varphi) \tag{208}$$

where:

VfP	is:	the operator "Viewed_from_the_perspective ..." referred to as the *perspective operator;*
X		is a place-holder for any perspective *A, B, C, ...*, e.g., "cellular pathology" in the present example; and
φ		is a sentence variable representing any sentence $\alpha, \beta, \gamma, ...$ of arbitrary complexity, e.g., "all diseases result from changes that occur in cells" in the present example.

A statement of the form (208) will be referred to as a *perspectival statement,* assertion, or report. For instance, the perspectival statement (207) says that:

$$VfP(A, \alpha) \tag{209}$$

with $A \equiv$ "cellular pathology", and $\alpha \equiv$ "all diseases result from changes that occur in cells". A pathologist taking a perspective other than cellular pathology will certainly maintain something different. A molecular pathologist, for example, may maintain that viewed from the perspective of molecular pathology, all diseases result from changes that occur in molecules. That is:

VfP(molecular pathology, all diseases result from changes that occur in molecules)

or formally:

$$VfP(B, \beta) \tag{210}$$

where $B \equiv$ "molecular pathology", and $\beta \equiv$ "all diseases result from changes that occur in molecules". Obviously, diseases viewed from two different perspectives are represented, or explained, differently.

That "*VfP*" is an intensional, i.e., modal, operator is plainly revealed by the following test. Suppose that both the perspectival statement (209) and the statement β are true. If we now substitute this true statement β for the true statement α in (209), we obtain a false perspectival statement, i.e., $VfP(A, \beta)$, which says that "viewed from the perspective of cellular pathology, all diseases result from changes that occur in molecules". Since the substitution of *truth* for *truth* yields *falsehood,* the operator *VfP* cannot be an extensional one. It must be considered a modal operator, as the *content* of the second operand in a perspectival statement apparently plays an essential role. Otherwise put, *VfP* operates on the intension of its operands and not on their extension. See the definition of the term "modal operator" on page 912.

To simplify our analyses, the binary perspective operator *VfP* will be transformed into a pseudo-unary one by attaching the perspective name as a subscript to it and writing, in general:

$$VfP_X(\varphi) \qquad \text{instead of:} \quad VfP(X, \varphi)$$

such as, for example:

$$VfP_A(\alpha) \qquad \text{instead of:} \qquad VfP(A,\alpha)$$
$$VfP_B(\beta) \qquad \text{instead of:} \qquad VfP(B,\beta)$$
$$VfP_C(\gamma) \qquad \text{instead of:} \qquad VfP(C,\gamma)$$

and so on where A, B, and C are particular, specified perspectives; and α, β, and γ represent statements of arbitrary complexity as in the following example about HIV infection and in subsequent examples (211–214):

- VfP_{aids_theory}(the hallmark of symptomatic HIV infection is immunodeficiency caused by continuing viral replication. The virus can infect all cells expressing the T4 antigen, which HIV uses to attach to the cell. Chemokine receptors are important for virus import, and individuals with CCR5 deletions are less likely to become infected...) (Tierney et al., 2004, 1266).

- $VfP_{cellular\_pathology}$(all diseases result from changes that occur in cells) (211)

- $VfP_{molecular\_pathology}$(all diseases result from changes that occur in molecules) (212)

- $VfP_{autoimmune\_pathology}$(all diseases are autoimmune processes) (213)

- $VfP_{humoral\_pathology}$(all diseases result from dyscrasia of the four humors *blood, phlegm, yellow bile,* and *black bile*) (214)

Now, to answer the afore-mentioned ontological question of whether the object of a perspectival view really exists or is a creation of the perspective, we will introduce a distinction between perspectivism *de re* and perspectivism *de dicto* like in the other modalities studied in Chapter 27 in Part VIII, i.e., alethic, deontic, epistemic, temporal, and asserted truth modalities (the latter was discussed on page 707). To this end, consider the following two statements first:

- $VfP_{cellular\_pathology}$(for all x, if x is a disease, then x results from changes that occur in cells) (215)

- For all x, if x is a disease, then $VfP_{cellular\_pathology}$(x results from changes that occur in cells). (216)

The first statement is the same as (211) above. The reformulation in (215) brings the universal quantifier "for all x" explicitly to light that was implicit in (211). It shows that the persepctive operator $VfP_{cellular\_pathology}$ precedes the universal quantifier that is included in its scope to the effect that the operator $VfP_{cellular\_pathology}$ applies to the whole sentence following it. Thus, (215) is a perspectival statement *de dicto*. By contrast, (216) is a perspectival statement *de re* because it talks about disease as something extra-perspectival referred to by the prefixed, universal antecedent "For all x, if x is a disease" that precedes the perspective operator $VfP_{cellular\_pathology}$. The distinction becomes salient by formalizing the two statements (for the definition of *de re* and *de dicto,* see also page 925):

de dicto: $VfP_{cellular\_pathology}\big(\forall x(Dx \rightarrow Cx)\big)$ (217)

de re: $\forall x\big(Dx \rightarrow VfP_{cellular\_pathology}(Cx)\big),$ (218)

or more generally:

de dicto: $VfP_A\big(\forall x(\alpha \rightarrow \beta)\big)$

de re: $\forall x\big(\alpha \rightarrow VfP_A(\beta)\big).$

Note the order of the two operators, VfP and $\forall x$, in each of these two sentences. We have finally arrived at the solution to our ontological problem above. It is simply this. Only a *de dicto* perspectival statement of the form:

$VfP_X\big(\exists x\varphi\big)$

whose perspective operator includes an existential quantifier $\exists x$ in its scope, can be said to postulate the very existence of the object x intra-perspectivally. In this case, the existence of the objects x depends on the perspective. An example is the perspectival *de dicto* statement:

- $VfP_{cellular\_pathology}$(there is an x such that x is a disease and results from changes that occur in cells).

In this example, it is intra-perspectivally postulated that there is something that is a disease and results from changes which occur in cells. Maybe it doesn't exist and is merely invented by the perspective? Such skeptical questions cannot arise with respect to a perspectival statement *de re:*

- There is an x such that x is a disease and $VfP_{cellular\_pathology}$(x results from changes that occur in cells).

Rewritten formally, it looks:

$\exists x\alpha \wedge VfP_A(\beta)$

and is extra-perspectivally preceded by an independent existence postulate. Note that the perspective operator is somewhat similar to the binary assertion operator $\mathcal{A}(S, \varphi)$ used on pages 707 and 753 when discussing the ontological state of fictional objects. But the two operators are neither identical nor synonymous. Both are promising conceptual tools and may be of valuable service in dealing with epistemological and metaphysical problems of medicine and other sciences, e.g., in resolving the conflict between psychiatry and antipsychiatry on whether "there really are" mental diseases or not. The problem of theoretical terms dealt with on page 409, can be tackled anew with the aid of perspectivism de re and de dicto to find novel solutions. However, we will refrain from making this book bigger than it has turned out, and leave the inquiry to the reader. As a point of departure, you may use the question from which perspective X it can be asserted that there are cells, and whether "cell" is a theoretical term of that perspective; or from which perspective X it can be asserted that there are mental diseases, and whether "mental disease" is a theoretical term of that perspective; and so on. You may then go on to examine whether any of the following relationships hold:

- $VfP(X, \varphi) \leftrightarrow \neg VfP(X, \neg \varphi)$
- $VfP(X, \neg \varphi) \leftrightarrow \neg VfP(X, \varphi)$
- $VfP(X, \varphi) \wedge VfP(X, \psi) \rightarrow VfP(X, \varphi \wedge \psi)$
- $VfP(X, \varphi) \vee VfP(X, \psi) \rightarrow VfP(X, \varphi \vee \psi)$
- and search for additional ones.

The Doubter

In the heyday of philosophy of science in the last century, special philosophies of science such as philosophy of physics, philosophy of biology, philosophy of mathematics, and others branched from the general philosophy of science. Philosophy of medicine, which has existed since Hippocrates and Galen as casual philosophizing about medical issues, also emerged as a field of scholarly research in the 1920s. It counted, and continues to count, as one of the special philosophies of science. We should be aware, however, that philosophy of medicine is, strictly speaking, neither a philosophy of science nor philosophy of a science. It is in fact philosophia universalis and not confined to medicine as a science or merely to scientific problems and issues in medicine. Beside genuinely metatheoretical concerns such as medical epistemology and medical concept formation, it also inquires into object-theoretical issues such as organism, life, death, suffering, disease, diagnostic-therapeutic methodology, caring and curing, personhood, mind, anthropology, human values, deontics, and so on. In this capacity, it convincingly demonstrates that medicine could serve as a highly fertile ground both for philosophy in general and philosophy of science in particular.

When I started working on philosophy of medicine in 1970, this field of research was not well known. Only a few scholars in the USA, Germany, and some other Western European countries concerned themselves with medical-philosophical problems. "In the 1960s and early 1970s, the number of persons who credited the importance of the philosophy of medicine and bioethics could have easily assembled in a small room. Of these, few had an appreciation of the breadth of philosophical issues at stake in medicine and the biomedical sciences" (Engelhardt, 2000, 1). Three publication series changed the situation and considerably contributed to a philosophy of medicine movement in the last thirty-five years: the present book series *Philosophy and Medicine* (USA); *The Journal of Medicine and Philosophy* (USA); and *Metamedicine* (Germany), now known as *Theoretical Medicine and Bioethics* (USA). Medical students in many countries today have the opportunity of attending classes, courses, and seminars teaching philosophy of medicine or at least

K. Sadegh-Zadeh, *Handbook of Analytic Philosophy of Medicine*,
Philosophy and Medicine 113, DOI 10.1007/978-94-007-2260-6_24,
© Springer Science+Business Media B.V. 2012

some medical-philosophical subjects. But there is as yet no internationally uniform catalog of subjects to be taught in the curriculum. A cursory glance at the course catalogs of universities shows that there is no general agreement on what does, and what does not, belong to philosophy of medicine. Rather, the teachers are allowed to freely choose the themes they want, or are able, to teach. Themes from bioethics, medical ethics, history of medicine, and humanities predominate. There are as yet no agreed-upon, explicit methods of medical-philosophical inquiry, and trained teachers are also widely lacking. So, it comes as no surprisee that most of the subjects taught are not genuinely medical-philosophical issues.

We can only hope that the unfruitful state of affairs sketched above will improve in the near future to bring about a scientific philosophy of medicine that can be taken seriously and is useful to students, physicians, medicine, and patients. The present book attempts to bring us a bit closer to this desirable state. It treats central themes of the philosophy of medicine by means of an explicit, transparent, and learnable method, i.e., logical and conceptual analysis. Should it be able to gain a few sympathizers for analytic philosophy of medicine, that would reward me more than I merit. In order for you to estimate how many cycles during the long period of thinking and re-thinking on its subject I have taken through what you now hold in your hands, I would like to conclude with citing the German writer Bertolt Brecht's (1898–1956) poem *The Doubter*, written in 1937 (Willett and Manheim, 1987, 270), and then referring you to the opening Section 0.1 of the book in its Introduction:

```
Whenever we seemed
To have found the answer to a question
One of us untied the string of the old rolled-up
Chinese scroll on the wall, so that it fell down and
Revealed to us the man on the bench who
Doubted so much.

I, he said to us,
Am the doubter. I am doubtful whether
The work was well done that devoured your days.
Whether what you said would still have value for anyone
If it were less well said.
Whether you said it well but perhaps
Were not sure of the truth of what you said.
Whether it is not ambiguous; each possible misunderstanding
Is your responsibility. Or it can be unambiguous
And take the contradictions out of things;
Is it too unambiguous?
If so, what you say is useless. Your thing has no life in it.
Are you truly in the stream of happenings? Agreeable to
All that develops? Are you developing? Who are you? To whom
```

Do you speak? To whom is what you say useful?
And, by the way:
Is it sobering? Can it be read in the morning?
Is it also linked to what is already there?
Have the sentences spoken before you
Been made use of or at least refuted?
Is everything verifiable? By experience? By which one?
But above all
Always above all else: how does one act
If one believes what you say? Above all: how does one act?

Reflectively, curiously, we studied the doubting
Blue man on the scroll, looked at each other and
Made a fresh start.

***

Part VIII

Logical Fundamentals

Classical Sets

25.0 Introduction

Medicine counts as a scientific discipline. It is commonly said that in a scientific discipline knowledge and action are justified by reasoning. In the present book we are concerned, among many other things, with medical knowledge and action, and thus, with the nature, methods, and problems of reasoning in medical practice and research. To this end, we shall need theories and techniques of reasoning, i.e., *logic,* to analyze whether any logic is used, or may be instrumental, in medical reasoning. Since it would be unfair to leave the reader in the dark about what we understand by the term "logic", we have explained it in the present, final Part VIII by introducing some useful fruits of the science of logic, deductive and inductive ones, so that we may apply them in other parts of the book. The terms "deductive" and "inductive" will be explained later.

Logic provides, among other services, tools for facilitating the reasoning by formalizing it. To properly assess the instrumental value of formalizing reasoning processes by logic, consider the following example. Suppose you are making a diagnosis in a patient who is having heart problems. Your suspicion is that she has coronary heart disease. To test this diagnostic hypothesis, you measure the areas of a couple of wavelets in her electrocardiogram, ECG. While so doing, you need to calculate *the sum of 2a and 3b squared.* You may of course use the following binomial rule:

> The sum of two numbers squared equals the sum of the first
> number squared and the second number squared and the double (219)
> of the first number times the second number.

However, this informal exposition of the rule is confusing. Why not use its transparent, formal version:

$$(x + y)^2 = x^2 + y^2 + 2xy \qquad (220)$$

K. Sadegh-Zadeh, *Handbook of Analytic Philosophy of Medicine,*
Philosophy and Medicine 113, DOI 10.1007/978-94-007-2260-6_25,
© Springer Science+Business Media B.V. 2012

to resolve your ECG query in the following simple fashion?

$$(2a + 3b)^2 = 4a^2 + 9b^2 + 12ab.$$

Likewise, try to determine whether the Catholic, the Protestant, or the Utilitarian moral system implies that therapeutic cloning and designer babies are permissible. If it turns out impossible to answer this question intuitively, what may account for *that* impossibility and how could we overcome it? Again, logic provides tools for facilitating the reasoning by formalizing it, similar to the facilitation of the calculation above by formalizing the binomial rule (219) in (220). Therefore, for the purposes of this book, we shall need some knowledge of logic to reason about medical matters since they are too complex for intuitive analysis, discussion, and judgment.

We should be aware at the outset that the term "logic" plays two different roles, a generic one and a specific one. As a generic term, it refers to *the science of logic* that is concerned with formal languages and methods of reasoning. From this broad area emerge a wide variety of individual theories each of which, in particular, is also called *a* logic, such as predicate logic, epistemic logic, tense logic, paraconsistent logic, and so on. Thus, there is not only one single logic, 'the logic that everyone of us ought to accept and obey' so to speak. There are in fact infinitely many different and competing logics. In the following, we shall consider several exemplars of such individual logics. In doing so, our aim is to assemble some powerful methods of analyzing medical language, knowledge, reasoning, action, morality, metaphysics, and in addition to examine whether there is a specific *logic of medicine*.

We shall start with an elementary introduction to the essentials of *classical logic* that is usually viewed as 'the logic' itself. The introduction will be preceded by a few basic notions of *classical set theory* for two reasons. First, we shall use them as technical means throughout. Second, they are indispensable for an adequate understanding and appraisal of the novelties, peculiarities, and strengths of *fuzzy logic*, which constitutes one of the main tools of our analytic philosophy of medicine and will be sketched later in Chapter 30. Thus, our logical fundamentals include the following six chapters:

25 Classical Sets
26 Classical Logic
27 Modal Extensions of Classical Logic
28 Non-Classical Logics
29 Probability Logic
30 Fuzzy Logic.

To repeat what has been said in the Preface, the following may at first glance look hieroglyphic. But everything said on these pages is absolutely self-contained, on the one hand; and indispensable for understanding the preceding seven parts of the book, on the other. The only recommendation is to proceed step by step and not to skip anything.

Among the philosophically most important issues in medicine are suffering, maladies, disease, diagnosis, therapy, and the ethics of clinical decision-making. Now, suppose you are interested in the philosophy of these subjects. You wonder whether a disease, such as *diabetes mellitus* that a doctor refers to in a diagnosis like "the patient Elroy Fox has diabetes mellitus", is a natural kind rather than an artificial cluster of complaints, symptoms, and signs constructed by human society on the basis of human values. To answer your question, you need to know what you understand by the terms "natural kind" and "artificial cluster". What is a *natural kind?* What is an *artificial cluster?* And how are we to gauge whether patients such as Elroy Fox, whom we classify as diabetics, are members of a natural kind like elephants in a zoo are members of the natural kind of elephants, or of an artificial cluster? Let us try to examine whether the theory of classes that has come to be known as *set theory,* may be of any assistance in our philosophizing on such issues and on suffering, maladies, disease, diagnosis, therapy, and clinical decision-making in general.

There are two principal ways of talking about the objects one is considering. On the one hand, one may consider the *properties* an object has, and the *relations* in which it stands. Properties and relations are called *attributes.* For example, the statement "Elroy Fox has diabetes" ascribes to the patient Elroy Fox the attribute *diabetes.* This disease state is in fact an attribute, although a very complex one consisting of problems, complaints, symptoms, signs, and findings *A, B, C, D,* etc. On the other hand, one may consider a list on which the object stands, i.e., the *class* or *set* to which it belongs, e.g., "Elroy Fox is a diabetic". That is, he belongs to the set of diabetic people. These two approaches are referred to as the *intensional* and the *extensional* approach, respectively. The adjectives "intensional" and "extensional" derive from the following terminology.

We distinguish between the *intension* and the *extension* of a linguistic entity: (i) The extension of a proper name such as "Elroy Fox" or "the Eiffel Tower" is the *individual object* to which it refers. For example, the neurophysiologist Dr. Elroy Fox is the extension of the word "Elroy Fox". The intension of a proper name consists of the *attributes* of the individual object it denotes. (ii) The extension of a predicate is the *set* of all objects it applies to. For instance, the extension of the predicate "has diabetes" is the set of all diabetics. The intension of a predicate is the attribute it denotes. For example, the intension of the predicate "has diabetes" is a compound attribute composed of a couple of subattributes such as hyperglycemia, glucosuria, etc. From now on, we shall use the following four terms as synonyms: "attribute", "property", "feature", and "quality". In addition to proper names and predicates, we also need to consider the statements. (iii) The extension of a statement is its truth value. For instance, the extension of "The Eiffel Tower is in Paris" is the truth value *true.* The intension of a statement is the state of affairs it describes. For example, "Elroy Fox has diabetes" denotes the state of affairs that consists in a particular health condition of Mr. Elroy Fox.

In our discussions and analyses we shall prefer the extensional approach because it enables us to apply to the subjects of our concern the reasoning methods of set theories and logics. The technical term "set" renders precise what is meant by the colloquial term "class". Sets are formally constructed entities to study the formal and logical laws of classes, and to thereby enable class calculations in analogy to $5+7 = 12$. We distinguish between ordinary or *classical sets,* on the one hand; and *fuzzy sets,* on the other. Since in the present chapter we are only concerned with classical sets, we omit the qualifying adjective "classical". Our study is divided into the following sections:[151]

25.1 Sets
25.2 Operations on Sets
25.3 Relations
25.4 Functions.

The aim of our introduction to these basic notions is confined to assembling some elementary, formal tools of inquiry that are used in our analytic philosophy of medicine in Parts I–VII. We do not intend to go into details. So, our presentation will necessarily appear something superficial from the perspective of the expert.[152]

25.1 Sets

A set is any collection of distinct objects called its elements or members. An example is the collection of *the three wise men.* If a set comprises the elements $a_1, \ldots, a_n$ with $n \geq 1$, it is conveniently represented by listing them, separated by commas, between two braces { } such that the set is written simply $\{a_1, \ldots, a_n\}$. For instance, the set of the three wise men is {Balthasar, Caspar, Melchior}. In the names of the objects $a_1, \ldots, a_n$ used above, the subscripts 1 through n with $n \geq 1$ are positive integers to conveniently form different names from a single variable "a". The symbol "$\geq$" means "equals or is greater than".

A set may be finite or infinite. In the former case, the elements of the set are countable in a finite period of time. For example, {Balthasar, Caspar, Melchior} is a finite set. Otherwise, the set is said to be infinite, e.g., the set of positive integers 1, 2, 3, etc. An infinite set cannot be represented by listing its elements within two braces { }. Rather, it is formed by indicating some

---

[151] The study of classical sets and their properties is the task of classical set theory. This theory serves as the foundation of contemporary mathematics and is closely associated with classical logic. It was founded by the German mathematician Georg Cantor (1845–1918) (Dauben, 1990). However, it is seriously challenged by fuzzy set theory, which we shall study in Chapter 30 on page 993.

[152] In what follows, we shall use the terminology of naive set theory. Axiomatic set theory is too remote from our purposes.

condition C that its elements satisfy. To this end, we use the set construction operator $\{x \mid \ldots\}$ that reads "the set of all objects x such that...", and write $\{x \mid x \text{ satisfies condition } C\}$ to mean "the set of all objects x such that x satisfies condition C". For instance, "the set of all numbers which are greater than 9" is written $\{x \mid x > 9\}$ and "the set of all human beings" is written $\{x \mid x \text{ is a human being}\}$. Of course, we may also represent a finite set in the same, general fashion by indicating a property that its elements posses. Here are some examples:

$\{x \mid x \text{ is a coin in your purse right now}\}$,
$\{x \mid x \text{ is a Gothic cathedral in London}\}$,
$\{x \mid x \text{ is a resident of New York City and has diabetes mellitus}\}$.

We say that a set contains its members or that the members belong to the set. For example, the set of the three wise men, i.e., {Balthasar, Caspar, Melchior}, contains Balthasar, Caspar, and Melchior.

We refer to sets by their names, e.g., "the set of the three wise men". For notational convenience, however, we shorten such set names in that we represent them by Roman upper-case letters A, B, C, ... To prevent confusion with their members, the latter ones are represented by lower-case letters a, b, c, ... The 3-dot ellipsis "..." is used to shorten a sequence of objects that we cannot or do not want to write down. For example, we abridge a set such as $\{1, 2, 3, 4, 5, 6, 7, 8, 9, 10\}$ by writing $\{1, 2, \ldots, 10\}$. If A is a set, we write:

$$x \in A$$

to say that x *is an element of A*, or x *is a member of A*, or x *is in A*. And we write $x \notin A$ to indicate that x is *not* an element of A, or x is *not* a member of A, or x is *not* in A. For instance, we have Caspar $\in$ {Balthasar, Caspar, Melchior} and $5 \notin$ {Balthasar, Caspar, Melchior}.

The symbol "$\in$", a styled εlementhood, is the basic concept of classical set theory and designates the elementhood or *membership relation* between an object x and a set A such that $x \in A$ when x is a member of A. If A is a set and we want to say that both $x \in A$ and $y \in A$, we write conveniently $x, y \in A$. We have, for example:

- Caspar, Balthasar $\in$ {Balthasar, Caspar, Melchior},
- AIDS, measles, cholera $\in \{x \mid x \text{ is an infectious disease}\}$.

A set such as $\{a\}$ or {Einstein} with only one member is called a *singleton*. A singleton $\{x\}$ must be distinguished from its only member x because $\{x\} \neq x$. The inequality sign "$\neq$" is the negation of "$=$" and simply means "does not equal". A set with no members is the null or *empty set* and is written $\{\ \}$ or $\varnothing$. There is no $x \in \varnothing$. For example, there is currently no human being on earth older than 500 years. So, we have that $\{x \mid x \text{ is a human being older than 500 years}\} = \varnothing$. That is, the set that consists of 500-year-old people is empty. A set may also have other sets as its members such as, for instance, $B = \{3, \{a, b\}\}$. Here, we have $3, \{a, b\} \in B$.

An ordinary or classical set A as sketched above has the following, characteristic property: The membership relation '$\in$' is an all-or-nothing attribute. That means that an object x is either definitely a member of the set, $x \in A$; or it is definitely not a member of that set, $x \notin A$. There is no intermediate option between membership and non-membership. Otherwise put, there exist no borderline cases, no quasi, partial or semi-members so to speak. This brings with it that a classical set such as the set of odd numbers between 0 and 10, i.e., $\{1, 3, 5, 7, 9\}$, has a sharp boundary dividing the entire world into members of the set, on the one hand; and non-members of the set, on the other. Something like the number 16 is

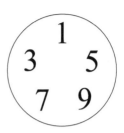

Fig. 88. The set of odd numbers between 0 and 10 with its sharp boundary, represented by a Venn diagram. Classical sets are usually represented by such Venn diagrams named after the British logician John Venn (1834–1923) who introduced them in 1880

either within or outside that boundary. Classical sets are therefore also called *crisp sets*. As we shall see later, fuzzy sets behave differently than crisp sets (Figure 88).

25.2 Operations on Sets

We stated already that sets are formal constructs to enable class calculations. The calculations are formal operations performed on sets. In this section, the following five basic set operations that we shall need thoroughout are outlined:

    25.2.1   Intersection
    25.2.2   Union
    25.2.3   Subset
    25.2.4   Complement
    25.2.5   Powerset.

We shall in addition present some basic laws of set theory in Section 25.2.6 below. In definitions and other contexts, the phrase "iff" will serve as a convenient shorthand for "if and only if" throughout.

25.2.1 Intersection

The *intersection* of two sets A and B, written $A \cap B$, is the set of all objects that are elements of both A and B. That is:

Definition 193 (Intersection). $A \cap B = \{x \mid x \in A \text{ and } x \in B\}$.

The formally correct version of the definition would be this: $A \cap B = C$ *iff* $C = \{x \mid x \in A \text{ and } x \in B\}$. But we shall simplify the formal presentation of our definitions to keep them readable. For a justification of this practice, see methods of definition in Section 5.3 on page 85.

As an example, we consider two minor sets. One of them, X, consists of the females Amy, Beth, and Carla. The other one, Y, contains the physicians Beth, Carla, Dirk, and Elroy. Thus, we have:

females:	$X = \{$Amy, Beth, Carla$\}$	abbreviated to $\{a, b, c\}$
physicians:	$Y = \{$Beth, Carla, Dirk, Elroy$\}$	abbreviated to $\{b, c, d, e\}$.

We now determine, based on Definition 193 above, the set of those persons who are both female *and* physician, that is, the set of female physicians:

$$X \cap Y = \{a, b, c\} \cap \{b, c, d, e\} = \{b, c\}.$$

This calculation may also be graphically illustrated by a Venn diagram (Figure 89).

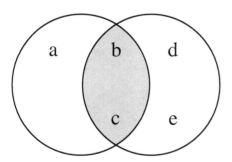

Fig. 89. The intersection of two sets, i.e., the shaded region of this Venn diagram, contains those members which belong to both sets

Two sets A and B are said to be *disjoint* if they have no members in common, that is, if their intersection is empty: $A \cap B = \varnothing$. For instance, $\{a, b\}$ and $\{c, d\}$ are disjoint since we have $\{a, b\} \cap \{c, d\} = \varnothing$. Note that due to Definition 193, set intersection reflects the standard, classical meaning of the connective "and".

25.2.2 Union

The *union* of two sets A and B, written $A \cup B$, is the set of all objects that are either elements of A or B. That is:

Definition 194 (Union). $A \cup B = \{x \mid x \in A \text{ or } x \in B\}$.

Using the example sets X and Y above, we now determine the set of those persons who are female *or* physician, that is, the union $X \cup Y$:

$$X \cup Y = \{a, b, c\} \cup \{b, c, d, e\} = \{a, b, c, d, e\}.$$

Note that due to Definition 194, set union reflects the standard, classical meaning of the connective "or". See Figure 90.

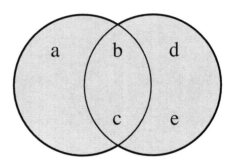

Fig. 90. The union of two sets, i.e., the shaded regions of this Venn diagram, contains all members of both sets

25.2.3 Subset

A set A is a *subset* of a set B, written $A \subseteq B$, iff every member of A is also a member of B. It is also said that B is a superset of A, written $B \supseteq A$.

Definition 195 (Subsethood). $A \subseteq B$ *iff* (*if* $x \in A$, *then* $x \in B$).

For example, we may easily observe that $\{a, b\} \subseteq \{a, b, Einstein, Freud\}$. See Figure 91. Two particular, 'extreme' subsets of any set A are the set A itself and the empty set $\varnothing$. That means that the following relationships hold: $A \subseteq A$ and $\varnothing \subseteq A$. Note that due to Definition 195, subsethood reflects the standard, classical meaning of the connective "if-then".

Two sets A and B are *equal*, written $A = B$, if and only if each member of A is also a member of B and each member of B is also a member of A. This is the case exactly if and only if both $A \subseteq B$ and $B \subseteq A$. For instance, regarding a set with members a, b, c we have $\{a, b, c\} = \{b, c, a\} = \{c, a, b\}$. If two sets A and B are not equal, we write $A \neq B$. For example, $\{a, b\} \neq \{a, b, c\}$. From these considerations it follows that:

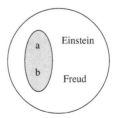

Fig. 91. The encircled region within the larger circle is a subset of the whole. That is, we have $\{a, b\}$ is a subset of $\{a, b, Einstein, Freud\}$

- there is no particular order of the members of an ordinary set,
- there are no redundant occurrences of members in a set.

The latter statement means that a set does not contain a member more than once. Thus, an entity such as $\{a, b, a, d, d\}$ is not a set. It is a *bag*, also called a multiset. A bag is usually written in square brackets $[\,]$ such as $[a, b, a, d, d]$.

The subsethood $A \subseteq B$ between a set A and a set B does not exclude that also $B \subseteq A$ to the effect that $A = B$. But if a set A is a subset of a set B, i.e., $A \subseteq B$, it is said to be a *proper subset* of B if $A \neq B$. In this case, B has at least one member that is not contained in A. Proper subsethood is written $A \subset B$. For example, we have $\{a, b\} \subset \{a, b, c\}$.

25.2.4 Complement

If a set is a subset of another set, then this latter, underlying set will be referred to as the *base set* or the *universe of discourse*, or *universe* for short. It will be denoted by Greek Omega Ω throughout. Given a subset A of a base set Ω, the set of all remaining members of Ω that do not belong to A is called *Not A* or the *complement* of A in Ω, written $\overline{A}$.

Definition 196 (Complement). *In a base set Ω with $A \subseteq \Omega$, we have $\overline{A} = \{x \in \Omega \mid x \notin A\}$.*

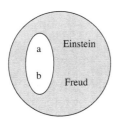

Fig. 92. The complement of a set in a base set $\{a, b, Einstein, Freud\}$. The shaded set is the complement of the set $\{a, b\}$ and conversely

For example, in our base set $\Omega = \{a, b, Einstein, Freud\}$ with its subset $\{a, b\}$ shown in Figure 92, the complement of this set $\{a, b\}$ is $\overline{\{a, b\}} = \{Einstein, Freud\}$. Note that according to Definition 196, the complement reflects the standard, classical meaning of the negation "not".

Analogously, the *relative complement* of a set A in a set B, written $B \setminus A$ and referred to as the *set difference* of B and A, is the set of all members of B which do not belong to A. We shall write $B - A$ instead of $B \setminus A$. Thus, we have $B - A = \{x \in B \mid x \notin A\}$. For instance, $\{a, b, c\} - \{b\} = \{a, c\}$.

25.2.5 Powerset

A set whose members are themselves sets is usually called a *family of sets*, or set family for short. For instance, a school with its classes as sets of pupils is such a set family. A particular set family is the so-called *powerset* of a set. The powerset of a set Ω, written *powerset*(Ω) or 2^{Ω}, is the set of *all* subsets of Ω.

Definition 197 (Powerset). $powerset(\Omega) = \{A \mid A \subseteq \Omega\}$.

For example, if our base set is $\{a, b\}$, then we have the following powerset:

$$powerset(\{a, b\}) = \{\{a\}, \{b\}, \{a, b\}, \varnothing\}.$$

The name "powerset" is due to the fact that if a set Ω has $n \geq 0$ members, its powerset contains 2^n members. For instance, our set $\{a, b\}$ above with 2 members has a powerset of $2^2 = 4$ members. A set of 3 members has a powerset of $2^3 = 8$ members, ... , and a set of 15 members has a powerset of $2^{15} = 32,768$ members. Therefore, the standard symbol for the powerset of a set Ω is 2^Ω. From now on, we shall use this exponential notation, 2^Ω.

25.2.6 Two Basic Laws

The basic notions of classical set theory sketched above imply a number of relationships between sets known as set-theoretical principles or laws. These principles form the foundations of Boolean algebra that is an important part of theories in logic and computer science. A few of them which we shall use may serve as examples. For details, see (Givant and Halmos, 2009):[153]

$A \cap B = B \cap A$	Commutative Law
$A \cup B = B \cup A$	Commutative Law
$A \cap (B \cap C) = (A \cap B) \cap C$	Associative Law
$A \cup (B \cup C) = (A \cup B) \cup C$	Associative Law
$A \cap (B \cup C) = (A \cap B) \cup (A \cap C)$	Distributive Law
$A \cup (B \cap C) = (A \cup B) \cap (A \cup C)$	Distributive Law
$\overline{(A \cap B)} = \overline{A} \cup \overline{B}$	De Morgan's Law
$\overline{(A \cup B)} = \overline{A} \cap \overline{B}$	De Morgan's Law
$\overline{\overline{A}} = A$	Involution Law

As we shall see in Chapter 30 below, fuzzy set theory is a non-classical set theory. As such, it is at variance with classical set theory and falsifies two of its basic laws indicating that classical set theory cannot be the ultimate measure. To understand this conflict and to be able to decide which one of these set theories is preferable, requires some knowledge of the two laws mentioned. They parallel the following two, well-known classical-logical laws of

---

[153] George Boole (1815–1864) was a British mathematician and logician. He contributed significantly to the emergence of what has come to be termed symbolic, formal, modern, or mathematical logic. See (Boole, 1847, 1848, 1854). *Boolean algebra* or *Boolean logic* is a calculus of the truth values *true* and *false,* and of the connectives "not", "or", and "and" (i.e., complement, union, intersection) by means of the binary set $\{0, 1\}$. See (Brown, 2003; Givant and Halmos, 2009).

our ordinary logic, mathematics, and common sense, i.e., the Law or Principle of Non-Contradiction and the Law or Principle of Excluded Middle. If Ω is any base set and A is a subset of it with the complement $\overline{A}$, then we have:

$$A \cap \overline{A} = \varnothing \qquad \text{Principle of Non-Contradiction} \qquad (221)$$

$$A \cup \overline{A} = \Omega \qquad \text{Principle of Excluded Middle} \qquad (222)$$

The Principle of Non-Contradiction, also called the Principle of Contradiction, says that a set and its complement are disjoint. They have nothing in common. This law parallels a well-known law of classical logic according to which the conjunction of a statement and its negation such as "Mr. Elroy Fox is a diabetic and he is not a diabetic" is contradictory and for that reason never true.

The Principle of Excluded Middle says that in a base set Ω, the union of a set A and its complement $\overline{A}$ exhausts Ω. "There is nothing between them". For instance, "Mr. Elroy Fox is a diabetic or he is not a diabetic". A third option does not exist. Also this law has an analog in logic (see Table 36 on page 895).

Let Ω be the base set $\{1, 3, 5, 7, 9\}$ with the subset $A = \{1, 3, 5\}$. The complement of A is $\overline{A} = \{7, 9\}$. The two laws above are easily confirmed: $\{1, 3, 5\} \cap \{7, 9\} = \varnothing$, whereas $\{1, 3, 5\} \cup \{7, 9\} = \Omega$. But we shall be surprised to see in Chapter 30 that these time-honored laws are not valid in fuzzy set theory. See also Sections 6.3.4 and 17.1.

25.3 Relations

Relations play a ubiquitous role in medicine and other branches of science. Most objects, structures, and processes are described in terms of *relations*. For example, in the statement "AIDS is caused by HIV" the phrase "is caused by" represents the relation of causation between two events, HIV infection and AIDS. Many relations are *functions* in the mathematical sense of this term. Thus, the notions of relation and function will be two indispensable tools of our inquiry. They are explained in this section and the next. We start by introducing the notion of a relation in the following three subsections:

   25.3.1 Ordered Tuples
   25.3.2 Cartesian Products
   25.3.3 n-ary Relations.

25.3.1 Ordered Tuples

A *pair*, dyad, or 2-tuple is a set with two members such as $\{x, y\}$. A *triple*, triplet, triad, or 3-tuple is a set with three members such as $\{x, y, z\}$. A *quadruple*, quadruplet, tetrad, or 4-tuple is a set with four members such as $\{w, x, y, z\}$. And generally, an n-tuple $\{x_1, \ldots, x_n\}$ is a set with $n \geq 1$ members $x_1, \ldots, x_n$.

If the ordering of the members in a pair $\{x, y\}$ is significant such that $\{x, y\} \neq \{y, x\}$, the pair is said to be an *ordered pair* and written $\langle x, y \rangle$ or (x, y) to distinguish it from an unordered pair $\{x, y\}$. For instance, the request "please indicate a pair of numbers such that the first number is *greater than* the second one" is satisfied by $\{9, 5\}$, but not by the reverse pair $\{5, 9\}$, although both sets contain the same objects. This observation demonstrates that the former set, $\{9, 5\}$, with its first member being *greater than* its second member, is an ordered pair. So, it is better written $\langle 9, 5 \rangle$ to distinguish it from $\{9, 5\}$ at the first glance. Generally, for an ordered pair $\langle x, y \rangle$ it is true that $(x, y) = (x', y')$ if and only if $x = x'$ and $y = y'$. Thus, $\langle x, y \rangle \neq \langle y, x \rangle$.

An ordered pair of the form $\langle \langle x_1, x_2 \rangle, x_3 \rangle$ whose first member is a pair, is written $\langle x_1, x_2, x_3 \rangle$ and referred to as an ordered triple. An ordered pair of the form $\langle \langle x_1, x_2, x_3 \rangle, x_4 \rangle$ whose first member is an ordered triple, is written $\langle x_1, x_2, x_3, x_4 \rangle$ and referred to as an ordered quadruple. In general, an ordered pair of the form $\langle \langle x_1, \ldots, x_{n-1} \rangle, x_n \rangle$ whose first member is an ordered $(n\text{-}1)$-tuple $\langle x_1, \ldots, x_{n-1} \rangle$ with $n > 1$ is written $\langle x_1, \ldots, x_n \rangle$ and referred to as an ordered n-tuple. Thus, the notion of an ordered pair is the basic term defining all n-tuples. An ordered n-tuple $\langle x_1, \ldots, x_n \rangle$ with $n > 1$ may simply be defined as an ordered pair $\langle a, b \rangle$ of the form $\langle \langle x_1, \ldots, x_{n-1} \rangle, x_n \rangle$ such that $a = \langle x_1, \ldots, x_{n-1} \rangle$ and $b = x_n$.

An ordered n-tuple has an ordering in it such that the tuple is destroyed by changing that ordering. Consider as an example any sentence we write down. It does have an ordering of its words. In the latter sentence, for instance, the word "It" is the first word, the word "does" is the second word, the word "have" is the third word, and so on. The entire sentence forms the ordered 8-tuple $\langle It, does, have, an, ordering, of, its, words \rangle$ that cannot be altered without doing damage to the meaning of the sentence.

Two ordered n-tuples $\langle x_1, x_2, \ldots, x_n \rangle$ and $\langle y_1, y_2, \ldots, y_n \rangle$ are said to be equal, $\langle x_1, x_2, \ldots, x_n \rangle = \langle y_1, y_2, \ldots, y_n \rangle$, if and only if $x_1 = y_1$ and $x_2 = y_2$ and $\ldots$ and $x_n = y_n$. In short, if and only if $x_i = y_i$ for $1 \leq i \leq n$. The symbol "$\leq$" means "less than or equal to". For example, we have $\langle 2, 6, 7, 9 \rangle = \langle 2, 6, 7, 9 \rangle$, whereas $\langle a, b, c \rangle \neq \langle a, c, b \rangle$. From the considerations above it follows that in contradistinction to an unordered set,

- there is an ordering of members of an ordered n-tuple,
- there may be redundant occurrences of members in an ordered n-tuple.

For instance, $\langle 8, 4, 4 \rangle$ is a correctly formed ordered triple which in a particular context may stand for the information that 8 minus 4 equals 4. Despite their peculiarities mentioned, ordered tuples are also called ordered sets because they are definable in terms of sets. Summarizing, we have:

sets: $\qquad\qquad \{a, b, c\} = \{a, c, b\} = \{c, a, b\} \neq \{c, a\}$

ordered tuples: $\quad \langle a, b, c \rangle = \langle a, b, c \rangle \neq \langle a, c, b \rangle \neq \langle c, a, b \rangle.$

25.3.2 Cartesian Products

The concept of *relation* embraces any kind of connection and association of objects. Here it will be defined by means of the notion of a *Cartesian product*.

When we talk about the family relationship between two individuals by saying, for example, that "Anna Freud is a daughter of Sigmund Freud", then the object of our concern is the ordered pair $\langle \text{Anna, Sigmund} \rangle$ whose first member is a daughter of its second member. Each member of such an ordered pair comes from a particular set. In the present example, the first member comes from the set of females, and the second member comes from the set of parents. Let A and B be any sets. Then $A \times B$ is referred to as their *cross product* or *Cartesian product*, named after the French mathematician and philosopher René Descartes (Renatus Cartesius: 1596–1650). The Cartesian product $A \times B$ is the set of all ordered pairs $\langle x, y \rangle$ such that the first member x of a pair comes from A and its second member y comes from B.

Definition 198 (Cartesian product). $A \times B = \{\langle x, y \rangle \mid x \in A \text{ and } y \in B\}$.

For example, if $A = \{a, b\}$ and $B = \{1, 2\}$, then we have:

$$A \times B = \{\langle a, 1 \rangle, \langle a, 2 \rangle, \langle b, 1 \rangle, \langle b, 2 \rangle\}.$$

In a Cartesian product $A \times B$, the sets A and B are referred to as its components. $A \times B$ with two components is said to be a two-place or a *binary* Cartesian product. A binary relation or simply a *relation* R from a set A to, or into, a set B is a subset of the binary Cartesian product $A \times B$, i.e., a set of ordered pairs. For example, if A_1 is the set of females and A_2 is the set of parents, then the relation of being *a daughter of* someone is a subset of $A_1 \times A_2$:

$A_1 = \{x \mid x \text{ is a female}\}$

$A_2 = \{y \mid y \text{ is a parent}\}$

$A_1 \times A_2 = \{\langle x, y \rangle \mid x \in A_1 \text{ and } y \in A_2\}$

$R = \{\langle x, y \rangle \mid x \text{ is a daughter of } y\}$

$R \subseteq A_1 \times A_2$.

In this example, set $A_1 \times A_2$ is the set of all ordered pairs of the form $\langle x, y \rangle$ where x is any female and y is any parent. It is obvious that the relation of daughterhood, R, is a subset of $A_1 \times A_2$ because it comprises alls pairs $\langle x, y \rangle \in A_1 \times A_2$ such that x is a daughter of y. Therefore, we write $\langle a, b \rangle \in R$ to say that a and b stand in the relation R. For instance, $\langle Anna, Sigmund \rangle \in$ *Daughter_of*. Since a Cartesian product as well as its components are sets, it is worth noting that any of these components may itself be a Cartesian product. So, by recursions of the form:

$(A \times B) \times C$ abbreviated to: $A \times B \times C$

$(A \times B \times C) \times D$ $A \times B \times C \times D$

$\vdots$

$(A_1 \times \cdots \times A_{n-1}) \times A_n$ $A_1 \times \cdots \times A_n$

we obtain the general concept of a many-place, n-place, or n-ary Cartesian product in the following way:

$$A_1 \times \cdots \times A_n = \{\langle x_1, \ldots, x_n \rangle \mid x_i \in A_i\} \quad \text{for } 1 \leq i \leq n.$$

Here, $A_1, \ldots, A_n$ with $n > 1$ are any sets, and the number n is referred to as the *arity* of the Cartesian product. For instance, when there are three sets:

$A = \{a, b\}$

$B = \{c\}$

$C = \{1, 2\}$

then we have the three-place or *ternary* Cartesian product:

$$A \times B \times C = \{\langle a, c, 1 \rangle, \langle a, c, 2 \rangle, \langle b, c, 1 \rangle, \langle b, c, 2 \rangle\}.$$

In an n-ary Cartesian product $A_1 \times \cdots \times A_n$, all components $A_1, A_2, A_3, \ldots$ may also be the same set A such that in this case we have the n-ary Cartesian product $A \times \cdots \times A$ for which the shorthand A^n is used. For example, if $A = \{a, b\}$, then we have the following binary, ternary, and quaternary Cartesian products:

$$\begin{aligned}
A \times A &= A^2 &&= \{\langle a, a \rangle, \langle a, b \rangle, \langle b, a \rangle, \langle b, b \rangle\} \\
A \times A \times A &= A^3 &&= \{\langle a, a, a \rangle, \langle a, a, b \rangle, \ldots, \langle b, b, b \rangle\} \\
A \times A \times A \times A &= A^4 &&= \{\langle a, a, a, a \rangle, \langle a, a, a, b \rangle, \ldots, \langle b, b, b, b \rangle\}
\end{aligned}$$

and so on.

25.3.3 n-ary Relations

Based on the above concept of Cartesian product we have arrived at, we are now able to define what a relation in general is. A many-place, n-place or n-ary *relation* on some particular sets $A_1, \ldots, A_n$ with $n > 1$ is a subset of their Cartesian product $A_1 \times \cdots \times A_n$. For instance, when we say that:

4 is less than 8

3 is less than 5

then we are stating that there is a binary Cartesian product $A \times B$ and a set of ordered pairs $\{\langle x, y \rangle \mid x \text{ is less than } y\}$, which we may call "$<$", such that:

$$< \subseteq A \times B$$

and:

$$\langle 4, 8 \rangle \in <$$
$$\langle 3, 5 \rangle \in < .$$

The same is true of Anna Freud's and Jesus Christ's fathers when we state that the father of Anna is Sigmund and the father of Jesus is Joseph. In this case, we are maintaining that there is a set, i.e., *Father_of* $=$ $\{\langle x, y \rangle \mid \textit{the father of } x \textit{ is } y\}$, such that:

$$\langle Anna, Sigmund \rangle \in Father\_of$$
$$\langle Jesus, Joseph \rangle \in Father\_of.$$

Obviously, the two binary relations of being *less than* something and being the *father of* someone are also sets containing ordered pairs as their members. Thus, we may define:

Definition 199 (Relation).
  a. R is a relation *on*, or *over*, sets $A_1, \ldots, A_n$ iff $R \subseteq A_1 \times \cdots \times A_n$.
  b. R is an n-ary relation *iff there are sets* $A_1, \ldots, A_n$ *such that R is a relation on these sets. R is binary if $n = 2$, ternary if $n = 3$, quaternary if $n = 4$, and so on.*
  c. *In order to have an homogeneous terminology, an ordinary set A may also be referred to as an n-place relation with $n = 1$, i.e., as a unary one.*

The objects $x_1, \ldots, x_n$ of an n-tuple $\langle x_1, \ldots, x_n \rangle$ that stand in the relation R, are called the *relata* of the relation. For instance, Anna Freud and Sigmund Freud are the relata of the relation "the father of Anna is Sigmund". If R is an n-ary relation such as $<$ or *Father_of* having the n-tuple $\langle x_1, \ldots, x_n \rangle$ among its members, there are three options to express that "the objects $x_1, \ldots, x_n$ stand in the relation R":

postfix notation:	$\langle x_1, \ldots, x_n \rangle \in R$	or:	$(x_1, \ldots, x_n) \in R$
prefix notation:	$R \ni \langle x_1, \ldots, x_n \rangle$	or:	$R(x_1, \ldots, x_n)$
infix notation:			$x_1 \ldots x_{n-1} R x_n.$

For example:

4 *is less than* 8	(infix)
$4 < 8$	(infix)
$(4, 8) \in <$	(postfix)
$< \ni (4, 8)$	(prefix)
Romeo *loves* Juliet	(infix)
Elroy Fox *gives* Amy the book	(infix).

The infix mode is used in natural languages. We shall in general use the prefix notation $R(x_1, \ldots, x_n)$ to say that the predicate "R" applies to the ordered tuple $(x_1, \ldots, x_n)$. For instance, we shall write *Father_of* (*Anna, Sigmund*) to indicate that *Father_of* of Anna is Sigmund. As these examples demonstrate, the name of a relation is written with an initial capital letter.

25.4 Functions

The term "function" is ambiguous. In everyday life, biology, and other empirical sciences it means the role that an organ, instrument, person, or institution plays in a particular system. It is said, for instance, that "the function of the heart is to pump blood through the body". In addition to this imprecise teleological meaning, the term "function" has also another, precise, mathematical meaning. In will be used here in this latter, non-teleological sense throughout. A few types of functions are introduced in the following four sections:

    25.4.1 Functions are Single-Valued Relations
    25.4.2 Composition of Functions
    25.4.3 Restriction of a Function
    25.4.4 Point and Set Functions.

25.4.1 Functions are Single-Valued Relations

Functions are a particular type of relation. They make life easier by bringing order into our thoughts, morals, and life affairs. Concisely, a function is a natural or an artificially constructed relation between two sets such that an object from the first set is associated with *one and only one* object in the second set. Consider a simple example. The tax law "everybody has to pay 10% income tax" institutes a function, call it *tax rate*, that associates the set of incomes with the set of tax liabilities such that tax_rate(income) = 10% of income = tax liability. For instance, if someone's income is \$12,530, then she must pay \$1,253 tax because tax_rate(12,530) = 1,253. We will explain:

A relation R from a set $A = A_1 \times \cdots \times A_{n-1}$ to a set B associates some or all members of A with some or all members of B. Those members of set A which are associated with any members of set B, are called the *domain* of the relation and written *domain*(R). Those members of set B with which members of *domain*(R) are associated, are referred to as the codomain or *range* of the relation, and written *range*(R). That is:

$$domain(R) = \{x \mid x \in A \text{ and there exists } y \in B \text{ such that } \langle x, y \rangle \in R\},$$
$$range(R) = \{y \mid y \in B \text{ and there exists } x \in A \text{ such that } \langle x, y \rangle \in R\}.$$

For instance, let R be the relation of being a daughter of someone, "x is a daughter of y". It associates members of the set of females, A, with members of the set of parents, B. The domain of the relation, i.e.:

$domain(Is\_a\_daughter\_of)$

is the set of daughters. Conversely, the range of the relation, i.e.:

$range(Is\_a\_daughter\_of)$

is the set of all parents who have a daughter. Since everybody has two parents, the relation *daughterhood* obviously associates a member of its domain with $n > 1$ members of its range. For example, Anna Freud (1895–1982) is a daughter of Sigmund Freud and a daughter of his wife Martha:

$Is\_a\_daughter\_of(Anna, Sigmund)$

$Is\_a\_daughter\_of(Anna, Martha)$.

There are two members of the $range(Is\_a\_daughter\_of)$ with whom Anna is associated, with Sigmund and Martha. But Sigmund Freud and his wife Martha have also two additional daughters. One of them is Mathilde (1887–1978). So, we have:

$Is\_a\_daughter\_of(Mathilde, Sigmund)$

$Is\_a\_daughter\_of(Mathilde, Martha)$.

These examples show that the relation of being a daughter of someone is apparently a *many-to-many* one, that is, a relation that associates many members of its domain with many members of its range. Thus it is *not* a function.

As was stated above, a function is a relation R from a set A to a set B which uniquely associates members of A with members of B. The term "uniquely" means that a member of its $domain(R)$ is associated with exactly one member of its $range(R)$. Thus, a function is a *many-to-one* relation, including one-to-one. For instance, the relation of fatherhood is a function such that we have "Father of Anna is Sigmund" and "Father of Mathilde is Sigmund". There is no second male who is their father. We shall elaborate on this basic idea in what follows (Figure 93).

We have already pointed out that any ordered n-tuple $\langle a_1, \ldots, a_n \rangle$ may be viewed as an ordered pair $\langle x, y \rangle$ of the form $\langle \langle a_1, \ldots, a_{n-1} \rangle, a_n \rangle$ such that $x = \langle a_1, \ldots, a_{n-1} \rangle$, and $y = a_n$. Thus, for simplicity's sake we may confine our discussion to the general case of ordered pairs, $\langle x, y \rangle$, whose first member x is a single object or any tuple.

Let R be any relation on sets A and B such that for $x \in A$ and $y \in B$ we have $R(x, y)$. The relation R may be conceived of as a rule that assigns to object $x \in A$ another object $y \in B$ to yield the ordered pair $\langle x, y \rangle$ such that $R(x, y)$. For example, the relation *Divides* assigns to the number 4 the number 8 such that $Divides(4, 8)$. And the relation *Father_of* assigns to Jesus the individual Joseph such that $Father\_of(Jesus, Joseph)$. See Figure 94.

If R is any relation on sets A and B such that $R(x, y)$, the object $y \in B$ in its range is said to be the image or the value of the relation for, or at, the

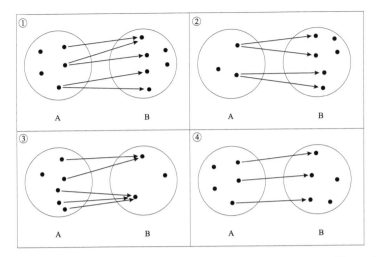

Fig. 93. Four types of relations illustrated by sagittal diagrams. Example 1 is a many-to-many relation. A one-to-many relation we find in 2. The many-to-one relation in 3 represents a function. Another function is the one-to-one relation in 4

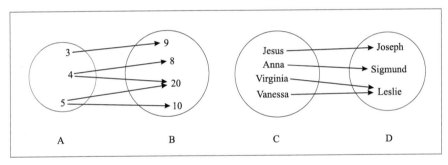

Fig. 94. In the left sagittal diagram, the relation *Divides* assigns to numbers in set *A* other numbers in set *B*. Some numbers from *A* are associated with more than one number in *B*. For instance, 4 divides 8 and 20. The relation is one-to-many. The graph on the right-hand side shows who the father of a person is. In contradistinction to the former relation, this one assigns to a member of set *C* exactly one member of set *D* as her father. This relation is one-to-one or sometimes many-to-one. It is thus a *function*. See body text

point $x \in A$ of its domain. For instance, in *Divides*$(4, 8)$ in Figure 94 the value of the relation *Divides* at the point 4 is 8. The value of the relation *Father_of* at the point Jesus is Joseph.

A relation R may be single-valued in that whenever $R(x, y)$, then the value y at the point x is unique. There exists no other object $z \neq y$ such that "$R(x, z)$" also holds. For example, the relation *Father_of* is single-valued. It always assigns to an individual a unique person as her father. Such a single-valued relation is called a *function*. By contrast, the relation *Divides* is not single-valued and thus no function because it assigns to a number such as 4 many numbers each of which 4 divides, e.g., 8, 12, 16, etc.

Definition 200 (Single-valued relation). *If R is a relation on sets A and B, then R is single-valued iff for all $x \in A$ and for all $y, z \in B$ it is the case that if $R(x, y)$ and $R(x, z)$, then $y = z$.*

Definition 201 (Function).

    a. *A single-valued relation is called a* function.
    b. *If a relation F is a function, we symbolize it by a lower-case letter, f, to distinguish it from non-functional relations, and write $f(x) = y$ instead of $F(x, y)$. That is:*
    c. $f(x) = y$ *iff there is a single-valued relation F such that $F(x, y)$.*

The expression "$f(x)$" in the last definition reads "f of x", or "f applied to x", or "f at x". The definition shows that (i) we shall write functions as equations because their values are unique; and (ii) we shall symbolize them by lower-case letters to easily distinguish them from relations that are not single-valued. Functions are usually denoted by symbols like "f", "g", "h", etc. We have, for example:

$father(Jesus) = Joseph$

$log(2, 32) = 5$ (from $2^5 = 32$)

$plus(1, 5) = 6$

$minus(8, 4) = 4.$

The above examples were presented in prefix notation. The familiar infix notation for the latter two mathematical functions is:

$1 + 5 = 6$

$8 - 4 = 4$

which in prefix notation, as above, mean:

$+(1, 5) = 6$

$-(8, 4) = 4.$

The latter two reconstructions demonstrate that formal signs such as "+" and "−" are indeed such function symbols as "f" above. The same applies to *log* as a shorthand for "logarithm".

    Let f be a function from a set A to a set B, for example, the function *father* from the set of offspring to the set of males such that $f(x) = y$ for $x \in A$ and $y \in B$. In a functional relation of the form $f(x) = y$ we distinguish (i) function, f; (ii) *argument* of the function, x; and (iii) *value* of the function at the argument x, i.e., y. Note that this value y is just $f(x)$. For instance, due to *father(Jesus)* = *Joseph* we may state that Joseph is the value of the function *father* at the argument *Jesus*.

In a functional relation $f(x) = y$, we say also that the object $y \in B$ is the image of $x \in A$ under f, and that the object $x \in A$ is the preimage of y under f. The function f *maps* the argument or preimage x to the value or image y. The set of all arguments of the function f, i.e., set A, is referred to as the domain of f, or *domain(f)* for short; and the set of its values, i.e., set B, is the codomain or range of f, or *range(f)* for short. We also say that the function f maps *domain(f)* to *range(f)*, or that f is a *mapping* from set A to set B. Thus, a mapping is a triple $\langle A, B, f \rangle$ such that A and B are non-empty sets, and f is a function from A to B. The triple is usually written in the following suggestive form:

$$f : A \mapsto B \tag{223}$$

that reads "f maps A to B". For example, we have the mappings:

father : *humans* $\mapsto$ *humans*

weight : *objects* $\mapsto$ *real numbers*.[154]

If the domain of a function f is an n-ary Cartesian product $A_1 \times \cdots \times A_n$ with $n \geq 1$ such that:

$$f : A_1 \times \cdots \times A_n \mapsto B$$

with $f(x_1, \ldots, x_n) = y$, then f is an n-ary function and we say that it has n arguments $x_1, \ldots, x_n$. An n-ary function is called *unary* or one-place if $n = 1$; *binary* or two-place if $n = 2$; *ternary* or three-place if $n = 3$; *quaternary* or four-place if $n = 4$; and so on. For instance, 'father' is a unary function and has only one argument; 'plus' and 'minus' are binary functions and have two arguments:

father(Jesus) = *Joseph*	$\equiv$	$f(x) = y$	unary
$1 + 5 = 6$	$\equiv$	$+(1, 5) = 6$	binary
$8 - 4 = 4$	$\equiv$	$-(8, 4) = 4$	binary.

Note that an n-ary function is a single-valued $(n+1)$-ary relation. A function is called an *operator* if it acts on another function to produce a new function. It is more and more becoming customary, however, to view any function as an operator. More specifically, an operator on a set A is a function that takes values in the same set A. A unary operator on A is a function f from A to A. For example, the human fatherhood function *father* above is a unary operation on the set of human beings. A binary operation on a set A is a function f from $A \times A$ to A. Examples are the arithmetical operations of addition and subtraction above, and multiplication and division. And generally, an n-ary operation on a set A is a function f form $A_1 \times \cdots \times A_n$ to A.

---

[154] See footnote 12 on page 74.

25.4.2 Composition of Functions

The value $f(x)$ of a function f may serve as the argument of another function g to yield the value $g\big(f(x)\big)$. For instance, the familiar expression $(1+5)^2 = 36$ says that $squared\big(plus(1,5)\big) = 36$. In this expression, the squaring function *squared*, or *square_of*, is applied to the value $plus(1,5)$ of the function *plus* at the arguments 1 and 5:

$$plus(1,5) = +(1,5) = 1 + 5 = 6$$
$$squared\big(plus(1,5)\big) = squared(1+5) = squared(6) = 6^2 = 36.$$

The nesting of two or more functions in this fashion to construct a new one is referred to as their *composition*. The function composition is simply the application of a function g to the values of another function f. This yields a third function $g \circ f$. We will explain (see Figure 95).

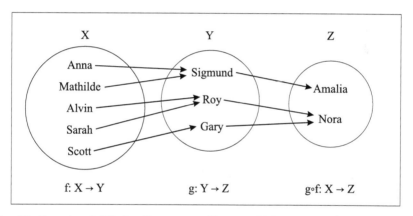

Fig. 95. Function f ("father") maps set X to set Y. Function g ("mother") maps set Y to set Z. They jointly yield a new function $g \circ f$ ("paternal grandmother"), i.e., their composition, that maps X to Z

Even in our day-to-day communications we compose of available functions new ones when we say, for example, that Amalia Freud is Anna Freud's *grandmother*. The term "grandmother" emerges from the composition of two functions. To illustrate, we will first differentiate between the two familiar, paternal and maternal, grandmothers. Let *"p-grandmother"* denote the paternal grandmother, i.e., the mother of one's father, whereas the maternal grandmother may be termed *"m-grandmother"*. Suppose now that there are three individuals, e.g., Anna, Sigmund, and Amalia Freud, such that:

1. $father(Anna) = Sigmund$
2. $mother(Sigmund) = Amalia$.

By equation 1, we may in equation 2 substitute the value *father(Anna)* for the argument *Sigmund* to obtain:

3. $mother(father(Anna)) = Amalia.$

One can then introduce a new function termed "*p-grandmother(x)*" and define it as follows:

$$p\text{-}grandmother(x) = mother(father(x)).$$

By this definition, we obtain from equation 3 the information that:

$$p\text{-}grandmother(Anna) = Amalia.$$

In this example, the function *p-grandmother* is a perfect composition of the two unary functions *mother* and *father*. It emerges in the following way. Let *f* and *g* be two functions as above such that *range(f)* houses in *domain(g)*:

$$f : A \mapsto B$$
$$g : C \mapsto D \qquad \text{with } B \subseteq C.$$

The composition of *g* and *f*, written $g \circ f$, is a new function that is defined by:

$$(g \circ f)(x) = g(f(x))$$

to the effect that:

$$g \circ f : A \mapsto D.$$

The composition $g \circ f$ thus maps set *A* to set *D*, i.e., *domain(f)* to *range(g)*. When $g \circ f$ is given a proper name, say *h*, then we have $h : A \mapsto D$ such that $h(x) = g(f(x))$. That means that first the function *f* is applied to $x \in A$, and then the function *g* is applied to the resulting value $f(x)$ to return an output such as $y \in D$. For example, if we have:

$$f(x) \equiv father(x)$$
$$g(x) \equiv mother(x)$$
$$p\text{-}grandmother(x) \equiv (g \circ f)(x),$$

then:

$$f(Anna) = Sigmund$$
$$g(Sigmund) = Amalia$$
$$p\text{-}grandmother(Anna) = (g \circ f)(Anna) = g(f(Anna)) = Amalia.$$

By generalizing the method above, we can compose of $n > 1$ functions $f_1, f_2, \ldots, f_n$ the new function $f_n \circ f_{n-1} \circ \cdots \circ f_1$ such that:

$$(f_n \circ f_{n-1} \circ \cdots \circ f_1)(x) = f_n\left(f_{n-1}\left(\cdots (f_1(x)) \cdots\right)\right).$$

25.4.3 Restriction of a Function

Informally, a restriction of a function is the result of trimming its domain. If f is a function from domain A' to range B, and A is a subset of A', then the *restriction* of f to A, written $f|_A$, is that part of f that maps only the smaller set A to B. That is, when:

$$f : A' \mapsto B$$

and $A \subseteq A'$ and:

$$f|_A : A \mapsto B$$

then the function $f|_A$ is a restriction of f to $A \subseteq A'$. For example, the function "paternal grandmother" is a restriction of the function "grandmother" to the set of fathers; and the function "maternal grandmother" is a restriction of the same function "grandmother" to the set of mothers:

$$grandmother : parents \mapsto females$$
$$p\text{-}grandmother : fathers \mapsto females \qquad where : \quad fathers \subseteq parents$$
$$m\text{-}grandmother : mothers \mapsto females \quad where : \quad mothers \subseteq parents.$$

Thus we have:

$$p\text{-}grandmother \equiv grandmother|_{fathers}$$
$$m\text{-}grandmother \equiv grandmother|_{mothers}.$$

Conversely, if g is a function such that $g : A \mapsto B$, and another function $f : A' \mapsto B$ has a larger set A' as its $domain(f)$ such that $A \subseteq A'$, then f is said to be an extension of g to A'. For instance, the function $grandmother$ above is an extension of both $p\text{-}grandmother$ and $m\text{-}grandmother$ to the set of parents. In general, if $f|_A$ is a restriction of a function f to A, then f is an extension of $f|_A$ to A' when $A \subseteq A'$.

25.4.4 Point and Set Functions

A final distinction we have to make is between point functions and set functions: If f is a function such that $f : A \mapsto B$, then (i) it is a *point function* if its arguments, being elements of its domain A, are single objects. Examples are the functions *square of* a number and *father of* a human being. The former one maps single numbers such as 4 to their squares: $square(4) = 16$. The latter one maps individual human beings to males: $father(Jesus) = Joseph$. By contrast, (ii) f is a *set function* if its arguments, i.e., elements of A, are sets. An example is the *probability* discussed in Section 29.1.1 on page 973.

To distinguish from the function types above are point-valued and set-valued functions. If f is a function such that $f : A \mapsto B$, then (i) it is *point-valued* if its values, being elements of its range B, are single objects. An example is the quantitative function *the_blood_sugar_of* in a statement of the form "the blood_sugar_of Elroy Fox is 215 mg%". The number 215 is a point in the range of the function. By contrast, (ii) f is *set-valued* if it has sets as its values, i.e., when elements of its range B are sets. For example, *square_root_of* and *full_siblings_of* are such set-valued functions. The former one assigns to a number the set of its square roots, e.g., *square_root_of*$(16) =$ $\{+4, -4\}$, while the latter one returns for every human being x a possibly empty set $\{y_1, \ldots, y_n\}$ of other human beings as her full siblings. For example, *full_siblings_of*(Michael_Jackson) $=$ {Rebbie, Jackie, Tito, Jermaine, ... etc.}, whereas *full_siblings_of*(Jesus) $= \varnothing$.

25.5 Summary

Some basic notions of classical set theory have been briefly introduced. Specifically, the concept of classical set has been outlined and the main operations on classical sets, such as intersection, union, complement, subset, and power-set, have been explained. By means of these tools a sketch has been given of the concept of Cartesian product to serve as a basis for the introduction of the concepts of relation and function. Also the composition and restriction of functions have been very briefly described. Finally, a distinction has been made between point functions and set functions, as well as between point-valued functions and set-valued functions. These formal devices will be instrumental in our discussions throughout.

Classical Logic

26.0 Introduction

In doing analytic philosophy of medicine, we shall need some acquaintance with logic. However, like many other terms in our natural languages, the terms "logic" and "logical" are ambiguous. We will therefore provide a brief introduction to the meaning of these notions in what follows. Unless stated otherwise, the term "logic" will refer to deductive logic, the precise meaning of which is discussed below.

Western deductive logic originated in Greek antiquity. It found its first expression in the works of the great philosopher Aristotle (384–322 BC) which have come to be known as the *Organon*, i.e., 'instrument'. Aristotle's logic, also known as *syllogistics,* was unsystematically concerned with patterns of reasoning and argumentation. It remained in this fragmentary state relatively unchanged and unchallenged until the second half of the nineteenth century. At that time, logic underwent a period of reform and modernization, due in large part to the German mathematician Gottlob Frege (1848–1925) (Frege, 1879; van Heijenoort, 1971), and became more and more a mathematical endeavor of studying the structure and peculiarities of artificial, formal languages. In this new form, logic gave rise in the twentieth century to disciplines such as theoretical informatics and programming languages, and transformed our lives through computation, information processing, and the Internet.[155]

---

[155] The reason why for over two millennia Aristotle's syllogistic logic persisted in its rudimentary state lies in his conception of logic as a mere ad hoc gathering of a certain type of reasoning schemas known as *syllogisms*. He and his followers spent much time finding such schemas and assembled some twenty syllogisms. Well-known examples are arguments of the form "All men are mortal. Socrates is a man. So, Socrates is mortal" and "Every A is B. Every B is C. So, every A is C". However, they didn't ask what it is that makes such schemas valid patterns of reasoning. The watershed between their naive approach and modern, symbolic, or formal logic lies in 1847 when the British mathematician George Boole published his books mentioned in footnote 153 on page 830 (Boole, 1847, 1848, 1854).

K. Sadegh-Zadeh, *Handbook of Analytic Philosophy of Medicine,*
Philosophy and Medicine 113, DOI 10.1007/978-94-007-2260-6_26,
© Springer Science+Business Media B.V. 2012

A formal language consists, in effect, of a particular alphabet and some rules of forming, and transforming, strings over this alphabet. There are several types of formal languages analyzed in logic. Depending on their structure, they are called first-order languages, second-order languages, and so on. Today a logic is considered a theory of such a language and is, correspondingly, referred to as a first-order logic, second-order logic, and so on. In this chapter, we shall outline a *first-order logic* as a paragon of deductive logic. Its full name is: Classical, first-order predicate logic with identity. What all these expressions mean exactly, will become clear below. Our approach will be an elementary one because our précis of logic is not intended to be a textbook. Similar to our discussion of classical set theory in the preceding chapter, it tries to assemble, as briefly as possible, formal tools for use in our medical-philosophical inquiries in Parts I–VII. For special literature, see (Shoenfield, 2001; Barwise, 1977; Hermes, 1995; Church, 1956; Kleene, 1952).

The logic we shall study first is termed *classical logic* because the idea to create such an instrument, or 'organon', is rooted in Greek antiquity. Owing to its origin, it is based on three time-honored Aristotelean doctrines sketched on page 874. For these and several other reasons that we shall discuss later in this chapter, it is also called a logic of the Aristotelean style, or an *Aristotelean logic* for short.

As the traditional method of reasoning and proof, classical logic underlies mathematics and all other sciences, including medicine. We shall see later in Chapter 30 that what is currently being eradicated by the so-called *fuzzy logic*, is exactly this Aristotelean style of scientific reasoning. This eradication will completely change medicine, other sciences, technology, and culture. For this reason, a relatively complete, albeit small, picture of classical logic will be presented in this chapter to evaluate its replacement with fuzzy logic. Our exposition consists of the following two parts:

26.1 Basic Concepts
26.2 Classical First-Order Predicate Logic with Identity.

We shall first introduce a few basic, intuitive concepts to aid in understanding the otherwise highly abstract apparatus of logic.

What is known as 'sentential logic' today is due to his studies (see body text and Section 26.1.2). The next, truly innovative step that is generally acknowledged as the beginning of modern logic proper was taken by the inventor of the *predicate logic,* the German mathematician Gottlob Frege. His works (1879, 1884, 1893) inspired the British mathematician and philosopher Bertrand Russell (1872–1970) to write, in collaboration with his teacher Alfred North Whitehead, the monumental logic work *Principia Mathematica* (Whitehead and Russell, 1910). Today it counts as the international start of the rapid development of modern logic. For a detailed history of logic, see (Bochenski, 1961; Kneale and Kneale, 1968).

26.1 Basic Concepts

The first basic concept is of course the classical concept of *logical reasoning* itself. For classical logic is concerned, among other things, with the study of rules and techniques that enable such reasoning. We shall also touch on some additional key notions that will be used throughout. Our discussion of these is divided into the following five sections:

26.1.1 Reasoning, Argumentation, and Proof
26.1.2 The Classical Concept of Inference
26.1.3 Object Language and Metalanguage
26.1.4 Syntax, Semantics, and Pragmatics
26.1.5 Material and Formal Truth.

26.1.1 Reasoning, Argumentation, and Proof

We all reason. We do so in our daily lives as well as in science, politics, theology, and elsewhere. The physician who seeks a diagnosis for her patient, the student who comes too late to class, and the man or woman who wants to divorce, all of them answer a why-question by providing reasons. How are we to know whether their reasoning is acceptable? Consider the following examples:

- How does a produce vendor justify her claim that the tomato she is selling a customer is ripe?
- How does a physician convince a patient that she has acute hepatitis and ought to consent to a particular treatment?
- How does a medical ethicist convince politicians that therapeutic cloning should be legalized?
- How does a pharmacologist support her assertion that her new drug cures AIDS?
- How does a mathematician prove that 2 + 2 equals 4 and not 5?

What these examples demonstrate, is that we often have to convince people of the credibility and acceptability of a particular statement that we make, such as "this tomato is ripe", "you have acute hepatitis", "therapeutic cloning is necessary", "this drug cures AIDS", and "2 + 2 = 4". For our efforts at persuasion to succeed, we use a technique called reasoning or argumentation, to put forward an argument or proof. An *argument* or *proof* is a finite sequence of one or more sentences called *premises* followed by a word such as:

so, therefore, for this reason, it follows that, consequently

followed by a single sentence called the consequence or *conclusion*. A simple, typical example that might have been used by the produce vendor above is this:

Example 1.

All red tomatoes are ripe,	Premise
This is a red tomato,	Premise
So:	Reasoning step
This tomato is ripe	Conclusion.

In non-logical contexts, an argument is not always delivered in this order. Sometimes the conclusion comes first and phrases such as "because", "since", "for", or "as" are used to indicate that an argument is being given. For example, "this is a ripe tomato because it is red, and red tomatoes are ripe" is a usual form of the structured argument above.

The premises of an argument may be arbitrarily simple or complex. When the argument is correct, its premises constitute the *reason* or *reasons* for its conclusion. They *justify* the conclusion. They *support* it. They *prove* it. The argument as a whole is a *proof* of its conclusion. All of these verbal qualifications are equivalent. A correct argument is also called valid. We need to distinguish between valid and invalid arguments so as to put forward valid ones only. Their premises prove what we assert in their conclusions. For instance, Example 1 above is a valid argument, whereas the following four example arguments are fallacious and thus invalid:

Example 2.

All ripe tomatoes are red,
This is a red tomato,
 So:
This tomato is ripe.

Example 3.

All viral diseases are infectious diseases,
AIDS is an infectious disease,
 So:
AIDS is a viral disease.

Example 4.

Whoever has acute hepatitis has hyperbilirubinemia,
If someone has hyperbilirubinemia, then she has jaundice,
 So:
If someone has jaundice, then she has acute hepatitis.

Example 5.

All viral diseases are infectious diseases,
Myocardial infarction is not a viral disease,
 So:
Myocardial infarction is not an infectious disease.[156]

---

[156] "Hyperbilirubinemia" means *elevated level of bilirubin in the blood. Myocardium* is the heart muscle.

Why are these arguments invalid and what features characterize a valid argument? Whether an argument is valid or invalid, does not depend on the truth or falsehood of its premises or conclusion. An argument that has true premises and a true conclusion may be invalid nonetheless. For instance, in Example 3 above everything is true, whereas the argument is fallacious. Likewise, Examples 2 and 5 are invalid arguments, but not because their premises or conclusions were false. Conversely, the following argument is a valid one despite its evidently false premise and conclusion:

Example 6.
AIDS is a gastric tuberculosis,
　So:
Whoever has AIDS has gastric tuberculosis.

The validity or invalidity of an argument is neither a property of its premises nor a property of its conclusion. Rather, it consists in a particular *relation* between its premises and conclusion whether they be true or false. We will now elucidate the nature of this relation.[157]

26.1.2 The Classical Concept of Inference

The drawing of a conclusion from some premises is also called an inference. The four notions mentioned thus far are synonymous, i.e., reasoning, argument, proof, and inference. Henceforth we shall use the latter one only. All four notions are to be understood with the qualification "deductive". Since we shall be interested in deductive inferences only, the qualifying adjective "deductive" will be omitted. We also distinguish between valid and invalid inferences, but are interested in valid inferences only. Therefore, the qualifying adjective "valid" is also omitted.

A concept of inference that defines what is to be understood under the term "inference", is the basic concept of a logic. Aristotle's syllogistic logic made no progress for over two millennia because it lacked a concept of inference. Consequently, it was unable to bring about a general and fruitful method of doing logic and eventually ceased in the nineteenth century. Modern, symbolic, or formal logic as a theory of inference developed in close connection with the emergence of the concept of inference in the nineteenth century, and replaced Aristotle's rudimentary, syllogistic logic. A concept of inference appeared for

---

[157] After a suggestion by the U.S.-American philosopher and semioticist Charles Sanders Peirce (1839–1914), an inference of the type 2 and 3 is called *abduction*: From "(If A, then B) and B" infer A. Many attempts are being made in information sciences to construct a logic of abduction called "abductive reasoning" and "abductive inference" (Josephson and Josephson, 1996; Walton, 2005). Although the outcome of this research may be viewed as a useful conceptual framework, it does not deserve the name "logic" or "reasoning" because all abductive inferences lack any trace of validity.

the first time in Bernard Bolzano's *Theory of Science* in 1837 (Bolzano, 1837, § 154):[158]

"Propositions M, N, O, ... follow from propositions A, B, C, D, ... with respect to the constituents i, j, ... if every set of ideas whose substitution for i, j, ... renders all of A, B, C, D, ... true also makes M, N, O, ... true".

This concept is immature and tainted with psychologism. Nevertheless, it already betrays the spirit of the classical concept of inference that would emerge in the twentieth century: The premises of a valid inference entail its conclusion. This means that whenever its premises are true, its conclusion is true. Like Example 1 in the preceding section, the following three arguments demonstrate this entailment relation. The arguments are presented in the standard form without using colloquial phrases such as "so". Instead of such phrases, the line between premises and conclusion indicates the reasoning step, i.e., the drawing of the conclusion from the premises:

Example 7.
All viral diseases are infectious diseases,
AIDS is a viral disease,

AIDS is an infectious disease.

Example 8.
$x + y = y + x$

$35 + 2 = 2 + 35.$

Example 9.
Amy has higher blood pressure than Beth,
Beth has higher blood pressure than Carla,

Amy has higher blood pressure than Carla.

Each of the inferences above is valid, for its conclusion is true whenever its premises are true. Otherwise put, it is impossible that if the premises are true, the conclusion is false. In a valid inference it is said that:

- the conclusion *follows from* the premises,

---

[158] Bernardus Placidus Johann Nepomuk Bolzano (1781–1848) was a Czech philosopher, mathematician, and theologian. He joined the theology department at the university of Prague and was ordained a Catholic priest in 1804. Despite his dedication to the Church, he did not give up his mathematical and logical interests. He did some foundational work on differential calculus, real numbers, and real functions. Due to his politically liberal views and his lecture on *"propaganda for freethinking"*, he was suspended from his professorship in 1819, forbidden to publish, and put under police surveillance. For his detailed biography, see (van Rootselaar, 1970).

- the conclusion *is a consequence of* the premises,
- the premises *imply* the conclusion.

Depending on context and convenience, we shall use these three wordings interchangeably. Correspondingly, we shall refer to the relation between premises and conclusion as a:

consequence relation,
relation of implication.

We thus obtain the preliminary version of the *classical concept of inference:* A set $\{\alpha_1, \ldots, \alpha_n\}$ of $n \geq 1$ sentences imply a sentence β if and only if, whenever the sentences $\alpha_1, \ldots, \alpha_n$ are true, β is true. In order to bring out the relational character of this concept, we shall henceforth symbolize the sentence "$\{\alpha_1, \ldots, \alpha_n\}$ *implies* β" by "$\{\alpha_1, \ldots, \alpha_n\} \vDash \beta$". That is, the symbol "$\vDash$" reads "implies".

Definition 202 (Inference,implication). $\{\alpha_1, \ldots, \alpha_n\} \vDash \beta$ *iff* (*if* $\{\alpha_1, \ldots, \alpha_n\}$ *are true, then β is true*).

In all of our examples above we have presented inferences in the following vertical form:

α_1

α_2

$\vdots$

α_n

———

β

such that any a_i with $1 \leq i \leq n$ as well as β were single statements. The straight line between premises and conclusion illustrates the implication relation $\vDash$ between them. The conditional in the definiens of Definition 202, i.e., "*if* $\{\alpha_1, \ldots, \alpha_n\}$ are true, *then* β is true", shows that the relation $\vDash$ consists in the propagation of truth from premises to conclusion. Thus, the characteristic of the implication relation $\vDash$ is that it is truth propagating and thus *truth preserving*. Since the validity of an inference depends only on this *relation* between premises and conclusion and is independent of their actual truth and falsehood, one can both conduct and analyze an inference even though one is ignorant of the truth and falsehood of its premises and conclusion. The independence of the implication relation $\vDash$ from the actual truth and falsehood of the premises and conclusion amounts to the important fact that an inference is not content dependent. For example, it is irrelevant what the variable X in the following inference means (for the notion of a variable, see footnote 10 on page 58):

Example 10.

Amy has higher X than Beth,
Beth has higher X than Carla,

Amy has higher X than Carla.

According to Definition 202, this is a valid inference, although the variable X has no definite meaning. It may be interpreted by anything. In Example 9 above it has been interpreted by "blood pressure". If it is interpreted by something else, e.g., "salary" or "white blood cell count", a valid inference emerges anew. This finding reveals that the validity of an inference does not depend on the specific content of the argument. It depends solely on its structural features, say inner *form*. To better understand this essential feature we shall shed some more light on it in what follows.

In the above discussion, we have often talked about true and false sentences and statements. But we clearly discriminated between *statements* and *sentences* in previous sections and showed that the genuine bearers of the truth values *true* and *false* are a subclass of declarative statements called constatives such as "The Eiffel Tower is in Paris" or "All humans are mortal". See (5) on page 22.

26.1.3 Object Language and Metalanguage

It is trivial to state that tables, chairs, and the human disease AIDS are some things in the world outside of mere language, whereas the *words* "tables", "chairs", and "AIDS" denoting them reside solely in the language. A word, on the one hand; and what it refers to, on the other, are obviously two different things and must therefore be clearly distinguished. However, by means of language we not only talk about the world outside it. We also talk about the world inside, i.e., about language itself. We say, for example, that the word "AIDS" is an acronym. By using language to talk about language itself, different layers of language emerge which must be carefully distinguished from one another to prevent confusion and paradoxes.

Metalanguage is the language that is used to describe or analyze another language as its object, called *object language*. For example, when speaking in English about the meaning of the German word "Sprache", English is our metalanguage and German is our object language. Object language and metalanguage need not be two different languages, however. One and the same language may at the same time serve as both metalanguage and the object language of itself. For instance, the English statement:

Elroy Fox is ill   (224)

is the *object statement* of the following English *meta-statement:* "The statement (224) consists of four words". Finally, a *metalinguistic term* is a term of metalanguage that refers to something in the object language. For example, the term "acronym" that we have used above is a metalinguistic term. It classifies particular elements of language such as "AIDS" and "WHO" as *acronyms.*

Likewise, the concept of inference we have introduced in the last section, is a metalinguistic concept. When we say, for example, that "Elroy Fox is ill" implies "Elroy Fox is ill or Elroy Fox is healthy", the metalinguistic term *"implies"* in our claim denotes a particular linguistic relation between statements, i.e., between the premise and the conclusion of our argument:

$$\text{"Elroy Fox is ill"} \vDash \text{"Elroy Fox is ill or Elroy Fox is healthy"}. \qquad (225)$$

It does not denote any fact outside of language. It would therefore be incorrect to assert that "this fact follows from that fact". It is not facts, but only statements that follow from one another simply because the term "implies" is defined for statements and not for facts.

What we need to be aware of is that words and sentences are *used* in object language to make statements, whereas in metalanguage they are merely *mentioned* to make meta-statements about them. For instance, in the object-statement "AIDS is a viral disease" the term "AIDS" is used to refer to a particular disease. However, in the meta-statement "the word 'AIDS' is an acronym" it is not used. It is only mentioned in that it is put in quotation marks to give a metalinguistic name to it and to talk about it by using this name. One should be very careful not to confuse the *using* of linguistic phrases with the *mentioning* of them.

Only when in a particular context there is no fear of mistake, an object-linguistic sign may serve as its own metalinguistic name, i.e., it may be used *autonymously.* For example, rewriting the inference (225) above autonymously, we obtain the meta-statement: Elroy Fox is ill $\vDash$ Elroy Fox is ill or Elroy Fox is healthy. From now on we shall sometimes use words and sentences autonymously.

26.1.4 Syntax, Semantics, and Pragmatics

As was pointed out above, the implication relation $\vDash$ depends solely on the inner *form* and not on the content of an argument. The details of this point are important and therefore briefly explained in this section. To this end, we distinguish between syntax, semantics, and pragmatics. Roughly, we may say that they are concerned, respectively, with the structure of language, with meaning, and with the use and effects of language. We shall consider them in reverse order.[159]

---

[159] Syntactics, semantics, and pragmatics have been clearly introduced as subfields of *semiotics* by Charles William Morris (1901–1979) (Morris, 1938). Semiotics, from the ancient Greek word σημεῖον (semeion) meaning "sign", is the study of the nature and function of signs including the systems and processes under-

Pragmatics, from the Greek term πράγμα (pragma) meaning "action", explores the relations between language and its users. Its focus of interest is people's use of language and the role that language and its elements play in the context of society and human life in general. Phenomena that have come to be termed the *meaning* of expressions and the *truth* of statements, are considered issues of communication and social behavior, i.e., as pragmatic phenomena. For instance, the word "disease" is usually thought to signify something in 'the world out there', say the category of attributes such as diabetes, myocardial infarction, and the like. A pragmatic perspective, however, reveals it to be the product of a complex social practice in human communities (see Sections 6.3.1 and 14.4).

Semantics leaves out the users of language. It studies issues such as 'meaning' and 'truth' as mere relations between elements of language and what they refer to. These elements may be words or structures of higher order such as simple sentences, compound sentences, theories, etc. For example, the term "true" in a sentence like "the following statement is true":

AIDS is a viral disease   (226)

refers to the statement (226) above to characterize it as true. In this capacity, "true" is a semantic term of metalanguage ascribing a relational property to an object-linguistic statement.

The syntactics or *syntax* ignores, in addition, also the content of words and statements. It considers the signs of a language as blank geometric objects only and disregards both their meaning and their users. The syntax of a language is in principle its grammar consisting of a set of rules that specify its formal structure. The rules provide a set of basic signs such as $\langle A, B, C, \ldots \rangle$, called the alphabet of the language, and fix what is an expression over this alphabet, what is a sentence, how expressions and sentences may be formed and transformed in this language, etc. For example, according to English syntax, the string (226) above is a sentence, whereas "viral a AIDS disease is" is none.

With the above in hand, we are now in a position to ascertain the status of the classical concept of inference presented in Definition 202. The notion of implication introduced by that definition, ⊨, is a semantic concept of metalanguage, i.e., a *semantic-metalinguistic* concept, because it denotes a *truth* preserving relation between premises and conclusion formulated in object-language. The revolutionary achievement of modern, symbolic, or formal logic that we shall study below has been to show that this semantic concept of

---

lying signification, expression, representation, and communication. Semiotics as *medical* symptomatology ('symptoms as signs of diseases') has existed since Hippocrates. As a linguistic and philosophical issue, however, it is largely the creation of the Swiss linguist Ferdinand de Saussure (1857–1913) and the U.S.-American philosophers Charles Sanders Peirce (1839–1914) and C.W. Morris (Saussure, 1916; Peirce, 1931; Morris, 1938; Danesi, 1994).

inference can equivalently be replaced with a *syntactic* one disregarding controversial issues of meaning and truth. To proceed to the theory and practice of this groundbreaking idea, we need only to take one final step.[160]

26.1.5 Material and Formal Truth

Issues of meaning and truth are controversial in human societies. In light of this, it might be practically impossible in many cases to attain agreement over whether some particular premises imply a particular conclusion were the measure of inference solely the semantic concept of inference introduced in Definition 202 above. Fortunately, however, this semantic concept can be replaced with a syntactic one that does not need to consider the content of the statements at all. To understand how such a replacement of semantics with syntax is possible, we need to distinguish between *material* and *formal* truth.

In the present context, our considerations are confined to the realm of everyday language and to common sense. For example, when the patient Elroy Fox is ill and we therefore state that "Elroy Fox is ill", this sentence is true because it expresses a fact. Its truth is factual or, as we shall say, *material* truth. Now, let us substitute in our sentence the term "a car" for the word "ill" to see what will ensue. Clearly, we get the false statement "Elroy Fox is a car". Obviously, by changing a single component of our statement "Elroy Fox is ill", we change its truth value from *true* to *false*. This is because the constituent parts of our sentence are relevant to its truth. Interestingly, however, there are true sentences of another type whose constituent parts are irrelevant to their truth. For instance, consider the following sentence:

Elroy Fox is ill or Elroy Fox is not ill.   (227)

According to the common-sense understanding of the particle "or", this sentence is true because at least one of its double constituent sentences preceding or succeeding "or", is true. In this case, however, the truth of the compound sentence is independent of whether Elroy Fox is actually ill or not. Facts are immaterial to this type of truth since the truth of the sentence as a whole is independent of the truth of its constituent sentences. If we substitute for its true constituent sentence "Elroy Fox is ill" any other sentence, e.g., the false sentence "Elroy Fox is a car", the original truth of sentence 227 above will not change, and we shall obtain a true sentence anew: "Elroy Fox is a car or Elroy Fox is not a car". This is because both sentences have a syntax of the following form:

α or not-α

---

[160] Any system of logic that abstracts the syntactic *form* of statements away from their semantic content in order to establish content-independent principles, is said to be a *formal* or symbolic one. Modern logic is a formal logic.

where α represents any sentence. Every sentence of this *form* is true, for example:

- AIDS is a viral disease or AIDS is not a viral disease,
- $2 + 2 = 5$ or $2 + 2 \neq 5$,
- Elroy Fox has diabetes or Elroy Fox does not have diabetes.

Since the truth of sentences of this type is independent of the content of their constituent sentences and depends soley on their form, their truth is said to be of formal origin or a *formal truth*. Modern, symbolic, or formal logic emerged in the second half of the nineteenth century as a study of formal truth. It was found that there are a few particular signs which in compound statements are essential to their truth. In the above examples, it is a specific combination of the particles "or" and "not" in the form of "α or not-α". By changing this form the truth of the statement will be destroyed. For example, in contrast to (227) above the statement "Elroy Fox is ill and Elroy Fox is not ill" is not true because it contains the particle "and" instead of "or".

We shall see below that the semantic relation of inference, $\vDash$, as introduced in Definition 202 above, is grounded in formal truth. Specifically, it will turn out that a set of sentences $\{\alpha_1, \ldots, \alpha_n\}$ implies a sentence β if the *if-then* statement:

If α_1 and ... and α_n, then β

consisting of $\{\alpha_1, \ldots, \alpha_n\}$ as its antecedent and β as its consequent is a formal truth, as is the case in the following example:

If Elroy Fox has pneumonia and fever, then Elroy Fox has fever.

Thus, inference, $\vDash$, can be both practiced and analyzed syntactically. After the next section, we shall turn to a particular system of logic concerned with just this task.

26.1.6 Summary

We have distinguished between object language and metalanguage and have briefly introduced the notions of syntax, semantics, and pragmatics. We have also given a sketch of the notions of reasoning, argumentation and proof, and of the classical concept of deductive inference. This concept is a semantic one and signifies a relation of formal truth between the premises and the conclusion of an argument. It will be replaced with a syntactic one in the next section to formalize inference. The intended syntactic concept of inference and the methods of how to manage it constitute the formal logic we shall introduce.

26.2 Classical First-Order Predicate Logic with Identity

Natural languages such as English, German, or Chinese are complicated, highly unkempt, and vague. These features make it impossible in non-trivial cases to decide whether some particular natural language statements imply another statement. For example, try to determine whether it follows from the Bible that human cloning is morally bad and should therefore be forbidden. It is absolutely impossible to accomplish this and similar tasks by means of natural language. A logic provides simple methods for resolving just such inference problems, however complex they may be. To this end, it constructs an artificial, formal language into which natural language statements can be translated to examine what they imply. As discussed earlier, a logic is in effect a theory of such a formal language. In this section, we shall briefly introduce a logic termed *classical first-order predicate logic with identity,* or first-order predicate logic for short. The formal language of which it is a theory is a first-order language that we shall therefore refer to as $\mathcal{L}_1$, i.e., 'language of the first order'. This will be explained later on page 873. Our natural language statements can be translated into $\mathcal{L}_1$ to conduct logical inferences.

To study its logic, we need to present the language $\mathcal{L}_1$ first. To this end, we shall fix its *syntax* and explain its semantics. Once we have laid out the language, we can inquire into its logic, the presentation of which consists of the following four parts:

26.2.1 The Syntax of the Language $\mathcal{L}_1$
26.2.2 The Semantics of the Language $\mathcal{L}_1$
26.2.3 A Predicate-Logical Calculus
26.2.4 Metalogic.

26.2.1 The Syntax of the Language $\mathcal{L}_1$

The formal language $\mathcal{L}_1$ is the object language we want to construct. In this language, inferences are conducted syntactically. To utilize the construct as a *logic,* natural language statements such as "Elroy Fox is ill", "AIDS is a viral disease", "All men are mortal", and others are easily translated into $\mathcal{L}_1$ to enable the drawing of conclusions from them. The effect of the procedure is comparable to what we did at the beginning of Part VIII, on page 821, when we translated the natural language sentence:

> The sum of two numbers squared equals the sum of the first number squared and the second number squared and the double of the first number times the second number.

into the algebraic sentence:

$$(x + y)^2 = x^2 + y^2 + 2xy$$

to perform a calculation. The language $\mathcal{L}_1$ is constructed step by step in the following eight sections:

- ▶ Some elementary notions
- ▶ The alphabet of $\mathcal{L}_1$
- ▶ Terms in $\mathcal{L}_1$
- ▶ Formulas in $\mathcal{L}_1$
- ▶ Syntax simplified
- ▶ Bound and free individual variables
- ▶ Substitution
- ▶ The name of the logic.

Some elementary notions

We shall use some simple examples to intuitively familiarize ourselves with the syntax of $\mathcal{L}_1$. This language is a very economical one and consists of only a few types of signs. Among the important ones are *individual symbols,* predicate symbols or *predicates,* and *function symbols.* They will be briefly explained in the following three paragraphs first. Note that the syntax of $\mathcal{L}_1$ has nothing in common with the grammar of natural language. But natural language sentences are translatable into $\mathcal{L}_1$. We shall give many examples.

Individual symbols

In natural language statements such as "Elroy Fox is a diabetic" or "7 is greater than 3", individual objects are denoted by proper names such as "Elroy Fox", "7", and "3". We call them *individual constants* because they denote particular individuals such as Elroy Fox, 7, and 3, respectively, and have constant meanings. There are also a second type of individual symbols in a natural language which range over all particular individual objects. That is, they do not denote determinate individuals. For example, when we say that "someone is a diabetic" or "when a number is greater than another one, then ...", we do mean individual objects, although do not mean particular ones. We mean any human being x who is a diabetic and any number y that is greater than any other number z. Such an x, $y,$ and z may be Elroy Fox, the Eiffel Tower, 7, or some other individual object. Individual symbols of this type obviously represent variable objects and are therefore called *individual variables*. Individual constants *and* individual variables constitute the set of individual symbols.

Predicates

If from an elementary statement such as "Elroy Fox is a diabetic" or "7 is greater than 3" we remove all individual symbols, the remainder is called a predicate symbol, or a *predicate* for short. For example, "is a diabetic" and "is greater than" in the afore-mentioned examples are predicates. The number of individual symbols that a predicate requires to form a statement, is referred to as its *arity*. The predicate "is a diabetic" is a unary or one-place predicate because it needs only one individual symbol such as "Elroy Fox" to form the statement "Elroy Fox is a diabetic". Accordingly, the predicate "is greater than" is a binary or two-place predicate. It needs two individual symbols such as "7" and "3" to form the statement "7 is greater than 3". In general, a predicate is n-ary with $n \geq 1$.

Viewed from the extensional perspective, a one-place predicate denotes a set or class. For instance, "is a diabetic" denotes the class of all diabetics. An n-place predicate denotes an n-place relation if $n > 1$. An example is the binary predicate "is greater than". It denotes the Cartesian product $A \times B$ of two sets A and B such that each $x \in A$ is greater than $y \in B$, i.e., $\langle x, y \rangle \in$ *Greater_than*. Viewed from the intensional perspective, a one-place predicate denotes a property, i.e. a one-place attribute. For instance, "is a diabetic" denotes the property of being a diabetic. An n-place predicate denotes an n-place attribute that characterizes an n-tuple $\langle x_1, \ldots, x_n \rangle$, i.e., a relation. For example, the binary predicate "is greater than" denotes the property of being greater than something. We shall always choose the extensional approach. (For the terms *extensional* and *intensional*, see page 823.)

Function symbols

A function symbol denotes a function in the formal, mathematical sense of this term as it has been defined in Section 25.4. For example, the phrase "the father of" in a statement such as "the father of Jesus is Joseph", i.e., $father(Jesus) = Joseph$, is a function symbol. A function symbol has the arity of the function it denotes. The function symbol "the_father_of", or "father" for short, is unary because it takes only one argument. The function symbol "the_sum_of" or "sum" for short, i.e., $+$, is binary: $sum(x, y)$, because it takes two arguments. For instance, $sum(3, 5) = 8$, or $+(3, 5) = 8$, or $3 + 5 = 8$. In general, a function symbol is n-ary with $n \geq 1$.

In order to talk about sentences, we shall use variables that refer to them. They are lower-case letters α, β, γ, $\ldots$, α_1, α_2, α_3, $\ldots$ from the beginning of the Greek alphabet. We shall say, for example, let α be the sentence "Elroy Fox is a diabetic".

The alphabet of $\mathcal{L}_1$

The alphabet of the language we are constructing consists of three types of signs: logical signs, material or descriptive signs, and auxiliary signs. They are specified below.

LOGICAL SIGNS:

Sign:	Reads:	Name:
$\neg$	*not; it is not the case that...*	negation sign

$\vee$	or; either ... or ...	disjunction sign (the inclusive "or")
$\exists$	there exists a / an	existential quantifier, particularizer
	there is a / an; some	
$=$	equals, is identical with	equality sign, identity sign.

DESCRIPTIVE SIGNS:

- Finitely many individual constants: $a, b, c, \ldots, a_1, a_2, a_3, \ldots$ They are symbolized by lower-case letters toward the beginning of the Roman alphabet and denote particular individuals such as Elroy Fox, Einstein, 7, Paris.
- countably many individual variables: $x, y, z, \ldots, x_1, x_2, x_3, \ldots$ They are symbolized by lower-case letters toward the end of the Roman alphabet and range over domains of individual objects. They do not denote particular objects. They are placeholders of arbitrary individual objects such as in the sentences "x is a diabetic" and "x is greater than y".
- finitely many m-place predicates with $m \geq 1$: $P, Q, R, \ldots, P_1, P_2, P_3, \ldots$ They are constants and are symbolized by Roman upper-case letters. From the extensional perspective, they denote particular sets of individual objects or relations between individual objects such as "is a diabetic" and "is greater than".
- finitely many n-place function symbols with $n \geq 1$: $f, g, h, \ldots, f_1, f_2, f_3,$ $\ldots$ They will be symbolized by Roman lower-case letters f, g, $h, \ldots$ They are constants and denote n-place functions in the formal, mathematical sense of this term. Natural language examples are the unary function symbol "the_father_of" and the binary summation symbol "+".
- countably many Greek lower-case letters $\alpha, \beta, \gamma, \ldots, \alpha_1, \alpha_2, \alpha_3, \ldots$ from the beginning of the Greek alphabet. They serve as variables for sentences and are referred to as formula variables.

AUXILIARY SIGNS:

- Left bracket "("; right bracket ")"; and comma ",".

All words and sentences of the language $\mathcal{L}_1$ will be formed over the alphabet introduced above that is summarized in Table 28.

Table 28. The alphabet of the language of the first-order predicate logic, $\mathcal{L}_1$

1. Logical signs	$\neg, \vee, \exists, =$
2. Individual constants	$a, b, c, \ldots, a_1, a_2, a_3, \ldots$
3. Individual variables	$x, y, z, \ldots, x_1, x_2, x_3, \ldots$
4. m-ary predicates with $m \geq 1$	$P, Q, R, \ldots, P_1, P_2, P_3, \ldots$
5. n-ary function symbols with $n \geq 1$	$f, g, h, \ldots, f_1, f_2, f_3, \ldots$
6. Formula variables	$\alpha, \beta, \gamma, \ldots, \alpha_1, \alpha_2, \alpha_3, \ldots$
7. Auxiliary signs	$(,)$

Terms in $\mathcal{L}_1$

Finite sequences of signs of the alphabet introduced above yield strings of signs. There are only two types of meaningful strings in $\mathcal{L}_1$. They are called *terms* and *formulas*. We shall define them in this section and the next.

Definition 203 (Strings in $\mathcal{L}_1$).

1. *Every sign of the alphabet of $\mathcal{L}_1$ is a* string *over this alphabet.*
2. *If s_1 and s_2 are strings, their concatenation $s_1 s_2$ is a* string.

Note that in the definition above, s_1 and s_2 are metavariables that denote variable, not particular, signs of object language $\mathcal{L}_1$. Metavariables will often be used in our discussions below as metalinguistic tools. According to Definition 203, the following phrases are strings: $a, b, faaba, x, Px, P(x), \neg aP\neg f$, $Pxx)x\exists$. The question of whether or not they are meaningful, is not relevant. Note, however, that the following phrases are not strings over the alphabet of $\mathcal{L}_1$ simply because they contain inadmissible signs: $x\circ, \neg P + f\&$.

Definition 204 (Terms in $\mathcal{L}_1$).

i) *An individual constant and an individual variable is a term.*
ii) *If f is an n-ary function symbol and $t_1, \ldots, t_n$ are $n \geq 1$ terms, then* $f(t_1, \ldots, t_n)$ *is a term.*
iii) *A term of the form:*
   - *$a, b, c, \ldots, x, y, z, \ldots$ introduced in (i) is called an* atomic term,
   - *$f(t_1, \ldots, t_n)$ introduced in (ii) is referred to as a* compound term.

As this definition shows, t is a metavariable to refer to terms of the object language $\mathcal{L}_1$. A term of the form $f(t_1, \ldots, t_n)$ may be read "f of $t_1, \ldots, t_n$". Here are some examples:

The following strings are atomic terms: a, b, c, d, x, y. Let f be a unary, and g and h two binary function symbols. The following strings are compound terms: $f(a), f(y), g(a, x), g(b, b), g(f(b), c), h(g(b, c), d)$. This may be illustrated by some natural language examples. The metalinguistic sign "$\equiv$" that we shall frequently use as a shorthand, means "is the same as":

Semiformal:	**In $\mathcal{L}_1$:**	**Natural language:**
father(*Jesus*)	$\equiv f(a)$	Joseph
father(*father*(*Jesus*))	$\equiv f(f(a))$	paternal grandfather, Jacob
father(*father*(*father*(*Jesus*)))	$\equiv f(f(f(a)))$	paternal great grandfather, Matthan
father(*mother*(*Jesus*))	$\equiv f(g(a))$	maternal grandfather, Joachim
$+(5, 3)$	$\equiv g(b, c)$	The sum of 5 and 3
$-(+(5, 3), 4)$	$\equiv h(g(b, c))$	The difference of (sum of 5 and 3) and 4.

Formulas in $\mathcal{L}_1$

What we will here briefly call a "formula", usually termed "well-formed formula", is meant to capture natural language sentences and statements. However, we shall avoid these expressions to prevent associations with natural language and its imprecise syntax. The following recursive Definition 205 determines the set of all formulas in $\mathcal{L}_1$. The Greek lower-case letters $\alpha, \beta, \gamma, \ldots, \alpha_1, \alpha_2, \alpha_3, \ldots$ that we shall use, are formula variables and belong to the alphabet of $\mathcal{L}_1$, as displayed in Table 28 on page 860. They represent any $\mathcal{L}_1$ formulas. Note that they are not metalinguistic symbols. We use them autonymously only to avoid troublesome quotation marks such as "α", "β", and so on.

Definition 205 (Formulas in $\mathcal{L}_1$).

1. *If t_1 and t_2 are terms, then $t_1 = t_2$ is a formula.*
2. *If P is an n-place predicate and $t_1, \ldots, t_n$ are terms, then $P(t_1, \ldots, t_n)$ is a formula.*
3. *If α is a formula, then $\neg \alpha$ is a formula.*
4. *If α and β are formulas, then $(\alpha \vee \beta)$ is a formula.*
5. *If x is an individual variable and α is a formula, then $\exists x \alpha$ is a formula.*
6. *A formula of the form:*
   - *$t_1 = t_2$ introduced in (1) is called an equality or identity,*
   - *$P(t_1, \ldots, t_n)$ introduced in (2) is referred to as a predication,*
   - *Equalities and predications are called atomic formulas,*
   - *$\neg \alpha$ introduced in (3) is termed a negation,*
   - *$(\alpha \vee \beta)$ introduced in (4) is called a disjunction,*
   - *$\exists x \alpha$ introduced in (5) is referred to as an existential quantification or particularization.*

Formulas read in the following way:

Formula:	**Reads:**
$t_1 = t_2$	t_1 equals t_2 (or: t_1 is identical with t_2)
$P(t_1, \ldots, t_n)$	$t_1, \ldots, t_n$ are P
$\neg \alpha$	not α; it is not the case that α
$(\alpha \vee \beta)$	α or β
$\exists x \alpha$	There is an x, α
	There exists an x, α
	There is an x such that α
	There exists an x such that α
	There are (exist) some x such that α
	For some x, α.

Here are a few examples. Atomic formulas are presented first, followed by compound formulas. Let f be a unary function symbol and g a binary one. The following strings are equalities, and thus atomic formulas:

$a = a$

$a = x$

$f(a) = y$

$f(y) = g(a, b).$

Note that the well-known inequality sign "$\neq$" is defined by the equality sign and negation as follows:

$t_1 \neq t_2$ iff $\neg (t_1 = t_2).$

Let P be a unary predicate and Q a binary one. The following strings are predications, and thus atomic formulas:

$P(a)$

$Q(a, b)$

$P\big(f(a)\big)$

$Q\big(a, f(a)\big).$

The following natural language examples may illustrate:

Natural language:	Semiformal atomic formulas:	In $\mathcal{L}_1$:
4 equals 4	4 = 4	$a = a$
4 equals 16	4 = 16	$a = b$
4 squared is 16, $4^2 = 16$	squared(4) = 16	$f(a) = b$
4 squared is $4 \cdot 4$	squared(4) = $\times(4, 4)$	$f(a) = g(a, a)$
Elroy Fox is a diabetic	Is_a_diabetic(Elroy_Fox)	$P(a_1)$
Dr. Osler examines Elroy Fox	Examines(Dr._Osler, Elroy_Fox)	$Q(a_2, a_1)$
Jesus loves his mother	Loves(Jesus, mother(Jesus))	$R\big(a_3, h(a_3)\big)$
The mother of Jesus is dead	Is_dead(mother(Jesus))	$S\big(h(a_3)\big)$

Atomic formulas are atomic in the sense that they cannot be broken into smaller formulas. But they are also not powerful enough to express more complex states of affairs. In Definition 205.3–5 they have been supplemented by compound formulas. We shall present some examples below. From now on we shall suppose that all $\mathcal{L}_1$ terms and formulas are formed correctly. That is, we shall assume that we need not ensure whether in a formula such as $Q(a, b)$ the predicate Q is actually a binary one and is allowed to bear two individual signs. Likewise, we assume that all $\mathcal{L}_1$ formulas are meaningful and none of them has a damaged syntax such as "examines Elroy Fox". Here are a few examples:

These strings are formulas:	These strings are not formulas:
$P(a)$	$P(a))$
$\neg P(a)$	$\neg P(\neg a)$
$\big(P(a) \vee \neg P(a)\big)$	$\big(P(a)\neg \vee \neg P(a)\big)$
$\exists x P(a)$	$\exists x, P(a)$

$$\neg\exists x\neg P(a)$$
$$\bigl(\neg\exists x\neg P(a)\vee Q(x,y)\bigr)$$
$$\Bigl(\bigl(\neg P(a)\vee\neg\neg Q(x,y)\bigr)\vee R(a,b,z)\Bigr)$$

$$\neg\exists x\vee P(a)$$
$$\bigl(\neg\exists x\neg P(a)\neg Q(x,y)\bigr)$$
$$\Bigl(\bigl(\neg P(a)\vee\neg Q\neg(x,y)\bigr)\vee R(a,b,z)\Bigr)$$

This may be illustrated by a few natural language examples. In these examples, the predicate constant P stands for the one-place predicate "is a diabetic", and the predicate constants Q and R stand, respectively, for the two-place predicates "examines" and "loves". The individuals Elroy Fox, Dr. Osler, Kaspar Hauser, and Jesus are represented by the individual constants "a", "b", "c", and "d", respectively:

Natural language sentences:	Written in $\mathcal{L}_1$:
Elroy Fox is a diabetic or Dr. Osler examines him	$\bigl(P(a)\vee Q(b,a)\bigr)$
x is a diabetic	$P(x)$
There is someone who is a diabetic,	$\exists x\,P(x)$
There are diabetics	$\exists x\,P(x)$
There is someone whom Dr. Osler examines	$\exists x\,Q(b,x)$
There is nobody who examines Kaspar Hauser	$\neg\exists x\,Q(x,c)$
There is someone whom Jesus loves	$\exists x\,R(d,x)$
There exists nobody whom Jesus does not love	$\neg\exists x\neg R(d,x)$
Elroy Fox is a diabetic or he is not a diabetic	$\bigl(P(a)\vee\neg P(a)\bigr)$
There are diabetics or there are none	$\bigl(\exists x\,P(x)\vee\neg\exists x\,P(x)\bigr)$

From Definition 205.4 it follows that if α,β,γ, and δ are formulas, then the string $\Bigl(\bigl((\alpha\vee\neg\beta)\vee\gamma\bigr)\vee\neg\delta\Bigr)$ is a formula. We are thus able to build formulas of arbitrary complexity. However, some types of natural language statements cannot be translated into the language $\mathcal{L}_1$ yet. Among them are compound statements composed of elementary ones by using particles such as "and", "if-then", and others. In order to be able to also translate them into $\mathcal{L}_1$, we must extend the alphabet of $\mathcal{L}_1$ by introducing some additional logical signs. They will be defined by the available ones, i.e., by $\neg,\vee$, and $\exists$. That means that the new signs we shall introduce are in principle dispensable and could be represented by a combination of $\neg,\vee$, and $\exists$. Thus, they are mere shorthands for longer strings. We will first describe how they read:

DERIVED LOGICAL SIGNS ADDED TO THE ALPHABET OF $\mathcal{L}_1$:

Sign:	Reads:	Name:
$\wedge$	and; as well as	conjunction sign
$\rightarrow$	if..., then ...; when; whenever; avoid: "implies", "implication"	conditional sign
$\leftrightarrow$	... if and only if ...	biconditional sign
$\forall$	all; for all; every; each	universal quantifier, generalizer.

To simplify the definitions, we use our metalinguistic sign of identity, i.e., $\equiv$. A string of the form $\alpha\equiv\beta$ reads "α is the same as β" or "α stands for β".

Definition 206 (Conjunction, conditional, biconditional, universal quantifier).

1. $(\alpha \wedge \beta) \equiv \neg(\neg\alpha \vee \neg\beta)$
2. $(\alpha \rightarrow \beta) \equiv (\neg\alpha \vee \beta)$
3. $(\alpha \leftrightarrow \beta) \equiv (\alpha \rightarrow \beta) \wedge (\beta \rightarrow \alpha)$
4. $\forall x\alpha \equiv \neg\exists x\neg\alpha$
5. *A formula of the form:*
   - $(\alpha \wedge \beta)$ *introduced in (1) is termed a* conjunction,
   - $(\alpha \rightarrow \beta)$ *introduced in (2) is called a* conditional, *and sometimes also incorrectly* "implication" *(see also page 898),*
   - $(\alpha \leftrightarrow \beta)$ *introduced in (3) is referred to as a* biconditional,
   - $\forall x\alpha$ *introduced in (4) is called a* universal quantification *or a* generalization.

The new formulas read as follows:

Formula:	Reads:
$(\alpha \wedge \beta)$	α and β
$(\alpha \rightarrow \beta)$	If α, then β; when α, β; β provided that α
$(\alpha \leftrightarrow \beta)$	α if and only if β
$\forall x\alpha$	For all x, α; For every x, α.

In a conditional $(\alpha \rightarrow \beta)$, the formula α is referred to as the *antecedent,* and β is referred to as the *consequent.* A few examples may illustrate the new formulas.

These strings are formulas:	These strings are not formulas:
$(P(a) \wedge \neg P(a))$	$(P(a) \wedge \neg P(a)$
$(P(a) \rightarrow P(b))$	$(a \rightarrow b)$
$(P(a) \rightarrow \neg P(b))$	$(P(a) \rightarrow, \neg P(b))$
$(\neg P(a) \leftrightarrow \neg\neg P(b))$	$(P\neg(a) \leftrightarrow \neg\neg P(b))$
$\forall x P(a)$	$\forall xx P(a)$
$\forall x(P(x) \rightarrow Q(x, x))$	$\forall\neg x(P(x) \rightarrow Q(x, x))$
$\neg\forall x\neg\exists y Q(x, y)$	$\neg\forall(x\neg\exists y Q(x, y)$
$\left(\forall x(P(x) \leftrightarrow \neg\exists x\neg P(x))\right)$	$\left(\forall x(P(x) \leftrightarrow: \neg\exists x\neg P(x))\right)$
$\left(\forall x(P(x) \leftrightarrow \neg\exists y\neg P(y)) \wedge Q(x, z)\right)$	$\left(\forall x(P(x) \leftrightarrow \neg\exists y\neg P(y)) \wedge Q(x\neg z)\right)$

For instance, the latter formula reads: (For all $x(x$ is P if and only if there is no y such that y is not P) and x and z are Q). Let $\alpha, \beta, \gamma, \ldots, \alpha_1, \alpha_2, \ldots$ be any formulas. The following strings are formulas:

$$\left((\alpha \wedge \beta) \rightarrow \exists x\forall y(Q(x, y) \vee \neg\beta)\right)$$

$$\left((\neg\neg Q(x, y) \leftrightarrow \neg(\alpha \vee \neg\beta)) \wedge \gamma\right)$$

Here are some natural language examples. They contain, in addition to the predicate constants P and Q that we have already used above, the following two predicate constants: H stands for the one-place predicate "is happy", and L stands for the two-place predicate "loves":

Elroy Fox is a diabetic and Dr. Osler examines him $\equiv$ $\big(P(a) \wedge Q(b,a)\big)$
If Elroy Fox is not a diabetic, then he is happy $\equiv$ $\big(\neg P(a) \to H(a)\big)$
Dr. Osler examines Elroy Fox if and only if he is a diabetic $\equiv$ $\big(Q(b,a) \leftrightarrow P(a)\big)$
Everyone loves someone $\equiv$ $\forall x \exists y L(x,y)$
Everyone is loved by someone $\equiv$ $\forall x \exists y L(y,x)$
Everyone who is loved by someone is happy $\equiv$ $\Big(\forall x\big(\exists y L(y,x) \to H(x)\big)\Big)$

In closing this section, all logical signs of $\mathcal{L}_1$ are summarized:

$\neg, \vee, \wedge, \to, \leftrightarrow$ are called *sentential connectives* or sentential operators. They operate on formulas to produce new formulas.

$\exists, \forall$ are called *quantifiers*. They operate on individual variables $x,\ y,\ z, \ldots$

Syntax simplified

We have seen in the example formulas above, e.g., $\Big(\forall x\big(\exists y L(y,x) \to H(x)\big)\Big)$, that brackets and commas as auxiliary signs may reduce the readability of expressions. To address this, four rules of parsimony are given below, according to which auxiliary signs may be omitted.

RULES OF PARSIMONY:

1. Spare outer brackets:

$\alpha \vee \beta \quad \equiv \quad (\alpha \vee \beta)$

$\alpha \wedge \beta \quad \equiv \quad (\alpha \wedge \beta)$

$\alpha \to \beta \quad \equiv \quad (\alpha \to \beta)$

$\alpha \leftrightarrow \beta \quad \equiv \quad (\alpha \leftrightarrow \beta)$

2. Spare left brackets:

$\alpha_1 \vee \ldots \vee \alpha_n \quad \equiv \quad \big(\ldots((\alpha_1 \vee \alpha_2) \vee \alpha_3) \vee \ldots\big) \vee \alpha_n$ with $n \geq 1$

$\alpha_1 \wedge \ldots \wedge \alpha_n \quad \equiv \quad \big(\ldots((\alpha_1 \wedge \alpha_2) \wedge \alpha_3) \wedge \ldots\big) \wedge \alpha_n$ with $n \geq 1$.

The two rules above concern only uniform disjunctions and conjunctions. To prevent confusions, these rules do not apply to formulas that are not similarly uniform, e.g., $(\alpha \vee \beta) \wedge \gamma$, on the grounds that $(\alpha \vee \beta) \wedge \gamma$ and $\alpha \vee (\beta \wedge \gamma)$ are two different formulas. To confirm, consider the following example:

$(\alpha \vee \beta) \wedge \gamma \quad \equiv \quad$ Elroy Fox is ill or he is healthy, and he is happy;

$\alpha \vee (\beta \wedge \gamma) \quad \equiv \quad$ Elroy Fox is ill, or he is healthy and happy.

3. Spare term brackets and commas in terms and predications:

$$ft_1 \ldots t_n \quad \equiv \quad f(t_1, \ldots, t_n) \qquad \text{with } n \geq 1$$
$$Pt_1 \ldots t_n \quad \equiv \quad P(t_1, \ldots, t_n) \qquad \text{with } n \geq 1.$$

4. Binding strength:

$\neg, \exists, \forall$ dominate, i.e., bind stronger than $\vee, \wedge$

$\vee, \wedge$ dominate $\rightarrow, \leftrightarrow$

What is meant by "A binds stronger than B" is that the sign A seizes a string on which it operates, rather than does the competing sign B. The following examples may illustrate:

$$\alpha \wedge \beta \rightarrow \gamma \quad \text{is:} \quad (\alpha \wedge \beta) \rightarrow \gamma \quad \text{but not} \quad \alpha \wedge (\beta \rightarrow \gamma)$$
$$\alpha \leftrightarrow \beta \vee \gamma \quad \text{is:} \quad \alpha \leftrightarrow (\beta \vee \gamma) \quad \text{but not} \quad (\alpha \leftrightarrow \beta) \vee \gamma$$
$$\exists x Px \wedge Qy \quad \text{is:} \quad (\exists x Px \wedge Qy) \quad \text{but not} \quad \exists x (Px \wedge Qy).$$

Using the syntactic agreements above we may now write and read the formula $\Big(\forall x \big(\exists y L(y, x) \rightarrow H(x)\big)\Big)$ cited previously in the following simplified way:

$$\forall x (\exists y Lyx \rightarrow Hx) \quad \equiv \quad \text{For all } x, \text{ if there is a } y \text{ such that } y \text{ loves } x, \text{ then}$$
$$x \text{ is happy. } (\equiv \text{ Whoever is loved is happy.})$$

Bound and free individual variables

In the formula $\forall x (\exists y Lyx \rightarrow Hx)$ just used, the individual variable x physically occurs three times. We say that there are three *occurrences* of the individual variable x in $\forall x (\exists y Lyx \rightarrow Hx)$. And there are two occurrences of the individual variable y in the formula. An occurrence of an individual variable in a formula may or may not be controlled by a quantifier. What that means and causes, is explained in this section. In conducting inferences, the question of whether or not an occurrence of an individual variable in a formula is quantifier controlled, will play a central role. We must therefore clearly define this notion.

In $\mathcal{L}_1$, there are no variables other than individual variables. For convenience, we shall therefore talk simply of 'variables' throughout instead of 'individual variables'. A distinction will be made between *bound* and *free* variables in a formula. The precise definition of these two notions, presented at the end of this section, is a demanding one. For this reason, we will here prefer less complex definitions to keep them readable, although they may appear less precise. The auxiliary notion of "the scope of a quantifier" will be introduced first.

Definition 207 (The scope of a quantifier). *If Qv is a string occurring in a formula with Q being any quantifier and v any individual variable, e.g., $\exists x$ in $\exists x Px$, then the* scope *of the quantifier Q in the formula is Qv together with the smallest formula immediately succeeding it.*

For instance, in the formula $\exists x(Px \wedge Qx)$ the scope of the quantifier $\exists$ is the entire formula, whereas the scope of $\exists$ in $\exists x Px \wedge Qx$ is only $\exists x Px$. The scope of the quantifier $\forall$ in the formula $\forall x Px \rightarrow \exists y Qxy$ is $\forall x Px$. The scope of $\forall$ in the formula $\forall x(Px \rightarrow \exists y Qxy)$ is the entire formula, while the scope of $\exists$ therein is $\exists y Qxy$.

Definition 208 (Bound and free occurrences of individual variables).

  a. *An occurrence of an individual variable in a formula is* bound *iff this occurrence is within the scope of a quantifier using it.*
  b. *An occurrence of an individual variable in a formula is* free *iff it is not bound.*

To illustrate, consider the formula $\exists x(Px \wedge Qxy)$. Each occurrence of the variable x in this formula is bound, whereas the occurrence of y is free. In the formula $\exists x Px \wedge Qxx$, the occurrences of x in $\exists x Px$ are bound and in Qxx are free. In the formula $\forall x Px \rightarrow \exists y Qxy$, the occurrences of the variable x in $\forall x Px$ are bound, and its occurrence in $\exists y Qxy$ is free. However, in the formula $\forall x(Px \rightarrow \exists y Qxy)$, every occurrence of the variable x is bound. Note, therefore, that it is the *occurrences* of variables that are said to be bound or free. One and the same variable may occur both bound and free in the same formula as does x, for example, in $\exists x Px \wedge Qxx$. Thus, we have:

Formula:	**Bound occurrences:**	**Free occurrences:**
$\exists x Px \wedge Qxx$	x in $\exists x Px$	x in Qxx
$\exists x(Px \wedge Qxy)$	x in the entire formula	y in Qxy
$\exists y(Py \wedge Qyz)$	y in the entire formula	z in the entire formula
$\forall x Px \rightarrow \exists y Qyy$	x in $\forall x Px$, y in $\exists y Qyy$	
$\forall x(Px \rightarrow \exists y Qxy)$	x in the entire formula, y in $\exists y Qxy$	
$\forall x(Px \rightarrow \neg \exists y Rxyz)$	x in the entire formula, y in $\neg \exists y Rxyz$	z in $\neg \exists y Rxyz$

Definition 209 (Free individual variables and closed formulas).

  a. *A variable in a formula is a* free variable *iff at least one of its occurrences in the formula is free.*
  b. *A formula is said to be* variable-free *or* closed *iff it doesn't contain free variables;* open, *otherwise.*
  c. *A closed formula in $\mathcal{L}_1$ is referred to as a* sentence.

For instance, $\exists x Px \wedge Qxx$ is an open formula, whereas $\exists x(Px \wedge Qxx)$ is closed and thus a sentence. When a natural language statement is correctly translated into $\mathcal{L}_1$, the emerging string should be a closed formula, i.e., a sentence according to Definition 209.c above. We shall see below that non-sentences are not suitable objects for logical inferences. Note that if a variable x occurring in a formula α lies within the scope of a quantifier $\mathcal{Q}$ such that it is *bound* in $\mathcal{Q}x\alpha$, then the quantifier $\mathcal{Q}$ is said to *bind* the variable x.

By means of the above terminology, we now introduce an important notion that we shall use frequently in later chapters: The *universal closure* of a formula is a sentence obtained by binding all free variables of the formula with universal quantifiers *prefixed* to the formula. For example, the universal closure of the open formula Px is $\forall x Px$; and of the formula $Px \wedge Qxy$ is $\forall x \forall y (Px \wedge Qxy)$. The formula $\forall x \forall y \exists z (Px \rightarrow Qxy \vee Rxyz)$ is the universal closure of $\exists z (Px \rightarrow Qxy \vee Rxyz)$. The following definition gives a concise formulation of the concept by using a notion from the subsequent Definition 211.

Definition 210 (Universal closure). *If $\mathcal{F}(\alpha) = \{x_1, \ldots, x_n\}$, then β is the universal closure of α iff $\beta \equiv \forall x_1 \ldots \forall x_n \alpha$.*

In closing this section, we present a precise, direct definition of the notions of a free variable and bound variable without recourse to the less precise notion of a quantifier's scope. Some readers may want to skip the following recursive definition. The symbols "$\mathcal{V}$" and "$\mathcal{F}$" denote metalinguistic functions. They are set-valued functions as defined in Section 25.4.4 on page 843.

Definition 211 (The set of free individual variables of a formula).

1. *The set of* variables in a term t, *written $\mathcal{V}(t)$:*
   1.1. $\mathcal{V}(a) = \varnothing$
   1.2. $\mathcal{V}(x) = \{x\}$
   1.3. $\mathcal{V}(ft_1 \ldots ft_n) = \mathcal{V}(t_1) \cup \ldots \cup \mathcal{V}(t_n)$.

2. *The set of* variables in a formula α, *written $\mathcal{V}(\alpha)$:*
   2.1. $\mathcal{V}(t_1 = t_2) = \mathcal{V}(t_1) \cup \mathcal{V}(t_2)$
   2.2. $\mathcal{V}(Pt_1 \ldots t_n) = \mathcal{V}(t_1) \cup \ldots \cup \mathcal{V}(t_n)$
   2.3. $\mathcal{V}(\neg \alpha) = \mathcal{V}(\alpha)$
   2.4. $\mathcal{V}(\alpha \vee \beta) = \mathcal{V}(\alpha) \cup \mathcal{V}(\beta)$
   2.5. $\mathcal{V}(\exists x \alpha) = \{x\} \cup \mathcal{V}(\alpha)$.

3. *The set of* free variables in a formula α, *written $\mathcal{F}(\alpha)$:*
   3.1. $\mathcal{F}(t_1 = t_2) = \mathcal{V}(t_1 = t_2) = \mathcal{V}(t_1) \cup \mathcal{V}(t_2)$
   3.2. $\mathcal{F}(Pt_1 \ldots t_n) = \mathcal{V}(Pt_1 \ldots t_n) = \mathcal{V}(t_1) \cup \ldots \cup \mathcal{V}(t_n)$
   3.3. $\mathcal{F}(\neg \alpha) = \mathcal{F}(\alpha)$
   3.4. $\mathcal{F}(\alpha \vee \beta) = \mathcal{F}(\alpha) \cup \mathcal{F}(\beta)$
   3.5. $\mathcal{F}(\exists x \alpha) = \mathcal{F}(\alpha) - \{x\}$.

4. *A variable x is* free *in a formula α iff $x \in \mathcal{F}(\alpha)$.*
5. *A formula α is* closed *iff $\mathcal{F}(\alpha) = \varnothing$.*

For example, the variables of the term $f(y, z, a)$ are $\{y, z\}$, i.e., $\mathcal{V}(f(y, z, a)) = \{y, z\}$. The formulas Pxy and $\forall x \exists y Pxy$ have the same variables, i.e., $\{x, y\}$. They are free in the first and bound in the second formula. The variable z is free in $\forall x (Pxz \rightarrow \exists y Qxy)$, whereas the formula $\forall x \forall z (Pxz \rightarrow \exists y Qxy)$ is closed, i.e., it has no free variables. For simplicity's sake, Definition 211 does not explicitly consider conjunctions, conditionals, biconditionals, and universal generalizations because these formulas have been defined, as shorthands, by negations, conjunctions, and existential quantifications (see Definition 206 on page 865 above).

Substitution

Logical inferences are conducted by syntactically transforming sentences into other sentences. In the process of transformation, referred to as "drawing a conclusion", very often a particular syntactic operation is required that replaces in a formula an *individual variable* with a new term to produce a new formula. The operation is called "substitution of a term for an individual variable", or *substitution* for short. The substitution is carried out by replacing each *free occurrence* of the variable by an occurrence of the new term. For example, to replace in the formula "x is a diabetic" a free occurrence of the variable x with the term "Elroy Fox" means "Elroy Fox is a diabetic". Analogously, by substituting an occurrence of the individual constant b for each free occurrence of the variable x in the formula $Px \rightarrow Qx$ we obtain the formula $Pb \rightarrow Qb$.

In this section, the concept of substitution sketched above will be precisely introduced in two steps. Since substitution regulates a central inferential operation, it is important that we have a clear understanding of it. As a first step, we shall define how variables are substituted in *terms*. On this basis, a second notion of substitution will be defined for *formulas*. To begin, the metalinguistic term $\hat{s}(t_\circ, x, t)$ that we shall first define, reads:

- "the result of substituting in term $t_\circ$ the term t for the variable x", or
- "the result of replacing in term $t_\circ$ the variable x with the term t".

We shall use the smooth, second wording. Note that $t_\circ$ is an antecedently available term in which an individual variable, x, is replaced with a new term. For example, $\hat{s}(x, x, b) = b$. That is, "the result of replacing in term x the variable x with the term b is b". The substitution sign $\hat{s}$ is a ternary metalinguistic operator, called *substitution operator,* such that it produces new terms from other terms. It will be introduced by means of a *definition by cases* for atomic terms first, followed by a separate definition for compound terms.[161]

Definition 212 (Substitution in atomic terms).

$$\hat{s}(y, x, t) = \begin{cases} t & \textit{if } x \equiv y \\ y & \textit{otherwise, i.e., if } x \not\equiv y. \end{cases}$$

---

[161] For the notion of *definition by cases,* see page 94. The two definitions, 212–213, are representable by a single recursive definition by cases. For the sake of readability, we have split it up into two separate definitions. In the present context, the unified definition might appear too complicated. It will be presented as an example at the end of Section 5.3.5, i.e. Definition 23 on page 99.

That means that in an atomic term y an individual variable x can be replaced with a term t only if x and y are identical. Otherwise put, (i) an individual variable is replaceable by any term only if it is present at all; and (ii) *individual constants are not replaceable*. This may be illustrated by a few examples:

Substitution:	Reads:
$\hat{s}(x, x, a) = a$	the result of replacing in x the variable x with a is a.
$\hat{s}(y, y, b) = b$	the result of replacing in y the variable y with b is b.
$\hat{s}(x, x, y) = y$	the result of replacing in x the variable x with y is y.
$\hat{s}(a, x, b) = a$	the result of replacing in a the variable x with b is a.
$\hat{s}(x, y, a) = x$	the result of replacing in x the variable y with a is x (because there is no y in x to be replaced with a).
$\hat{s}(y, y, f(x)) = f(x)$	the result of replacing in y the variable y with $f(x)$ is $f(x)$.
$\hat{s}(y, y, g(a, y)) = g(a, y)$	the result of replacing in y the variable y with $g(a, y)$ is $g(a, y)$.

The following definition concerns substitution in compound terms such as $g(x, y), h(y, a, z)$, etc. As the definition shows, in such a term each of its constituent terms has first to be treated individually according to Definition 212 above.

Definition 213 (Substitution in compound terms).

$$\hat{s}(ft_1 \ldots t_n, x, t) = f\hat{s}(t_1, x, t) \ldots \hat{s}(t_n, x, t).$$

The definition says that by replacing in a compound term $ft_1 \ldots t_n$ a variable x with a new term t, we obtain the value $f\hat{s}(t_1, x, t) \ldots \hat{s}(t_n, x, t)$, *after* the new term t has been successively substituted for the variable x in each of the constituent terms $t_1, \ldots, t_n$. For instance, let g be a binary and h be a ternary function of the form gt_1t_2 and $ht_1t_2t_3$. Consider now the compound term $h(y, a, g(x, y))$. This is, written without brackets, the term $hyagxy$. In this compound term, the variable y is to be replaced with the term z. What is the result $\hat{s}(hyagxy, y, z)$? We will compute the result of the substitution according to Definition 213:

$$\hat{s}(hyagxy, y, z) = h\hat{s}(y, y, z)\hat{s}(a, y, z)\hat{s}(gxy, y, z)$$
$$= h\hat{s}(y, y, z)\hat{s}(a, y, z)g\hat{s}(x, y, z)\hat{s}(y, y, z)$$
$$= hzagxz.$$

The concept of substitution for formulas that we are pursuing, will now be introduced with the aid of the substitution operator $\hat{s}$ for terms. Before doing so, a simple example may explain the procedure.

Obviously, the formula Px yields by replacing its free variable x with the term b the formula Pb. This process of term substitution in formulas is captured by a quaternary metalinguistic *predicate* usually written $Subst(\alpha, x, t, \beta)$ and referred to as the *substitution predicate*. It reads:

- "the formula α yields by substituting the term t for the variable x the formula β", or
- "the formula α yields by replacing the variable x with the term t the formula β".

Again, we shall prefer the smooth, second wording. Our example above said that $Subst(Px, x, b, Pb)$. Another example is $Subst(Px \lor Qy, y, a, Px \lor Qa)$. In the next definition, the predicate $Subst$ is introduced for our basic formulas, i.e., for atomic formulas, negations, disjunctions, and existential quantifications. It can, but need not, be extended to explicitly cover the remaining formulas defined thereby, i.e., conjunctions, conditionals, biconditionals, and universal quantifications.

Definition 214 (Substitution of terms in formulas).

1. $Subst(t_1 = t_2, x, t, \beta)$ *iff* $\beta \equiv \hat{s}(t_1, x, t) = \hat{s}(t_2, x, t)$;

2. $Subst(Pt_1 \ldots t_n, x, t, \beta)$ *iff* $\beta \equiv P\hat{s}(t_1, x, t) \ldots \hat{s}(t_n, x, t)$;

3. $Subst(\neg\alpha, x, t, \beta)$ *iff*   *There is a γ such that $Subst(\alpha, x, t, \gamma)$ and $\beta \equiv \neg\gamma$;*

4. $Subst(\alpha_1 \lor \alpha_2, x, t, \beta)$ *iff*   *There are γ_1 and γ_2 such that $Subst(\alpha_1, x, t, \gamma_1)$ and $Subst(\alpha_2, x, t, \gamma_2)$ and $\beta \equiv \gamma_1 \lor \gamma_2$;*

5. $Subst(\exists y\alpha, x, t, \beta)$ *iff*   *(i) x is not free in $\exists y\alpha$ and $\beta \equiv \exists y\alpha$; or (ii) x is free in $\exists y\alpha$ and t does not contain y and there is a γ such that $Subst(\alpha, x, t, \gamma)$ and $\beta \equiv \exists y\gamma$.*

The first four parts of this definition are self-contained. The essence of part 5 is that (i) bound variables must not be touched; and (ii) the new term that is to replace a free variable within the scope of a quantifier must not contain a variable that is bound by that quantifier. A few examples may illustrate. In the formula $\exists y(\neg Pyx \lor fx = y)$ the variable y is to be replaced with the term x. We obtain:

$$Subst\big(\exists y(\neg Pyx \lor fx = y), y, x, \exists y(\neg Pyx \lor fx = y)\big).$$

The initial formula remains unchanged because its variable y is not free, and according to Definition 214.5-(i), must not be replaced by any other term. Now, we try to replace x with the term y:

$$Subst\big(\exists y(\neg Pyx \lor fx = y), x, y, \exists y(\neg Pyx \lor fx = y)\big).$$

Again, nothing changes because the term x cannot be replaced. The reason is that it resides within the scope of $\exists$ and the new term y contains a variable that is bound by $\exists$. Definition 214.5-(ii) prohibits such a substitution. But the substitution of the term z for x is permitted:

$$Subst\big(\exists y(\neg Pyx \lor fx = y), x, z, \exists y(\neg Pyz \lor fz = y)\big).$$

A final example demonstrates the substitution of the term $g(a, b, fc)$ for the variable x in the formula $\neg \exists y Pyx$:

$$Subst\big(\neg \exists y Pyx, x, g(a, b, fc), \neg \exists y Pyg(a, b, fc)\big).$$

The name of the logic

We are now able to explain the name of the logic we are studying, i.e., *classical predicate logic of the first order with identity*. First, the qualification "classical" refers to the circumstance that our logic is based on some principles originating with the ancient Greeks. This feature will become clear on page 874. Second, our logic is a theory of inference in a *first-order language*, $\mathcal{L}_1$, whose sentences are composed of *predicates* and *identities*, i.e., P, Q, R, etc., and $t_1 = t_2$.

What is a first-order language? A first-order language like our $\mathcal{L}_1$ is one in which quantifiers bind only individual variables, e.g., $\forall x$ and $\exists y$. Quantification over functions and predicates, such as $\forall P$ or $\exists f$, is neither possible nor allowed simply on the grounds that the alphabet of a first-order language does not include predicate variables and function variables to be bound by quantifiers. The predicate symbols P, Q, R, ... and the function symbols f, g, h, ... that we have assembled in the alphabet of our $\mathcal{L}_1$ are not variables. As was emphasized on page 860, they are predicate constants and function constants such as "is a diabetic", "is greater than", "loves", "the father of", "the sum of", etc.

Thus, in $\mathcal{L}_1$ it does not make sense to say that "there is a P such that ..." or "there is an f such that ...", e.g., "there is a color such that it is nicer than red". We have already pointed out previously that in the language $\mathcal{L}_1$ predicates and function symbols, Ps and fs, are interpreted extensionally and denote sets. Quantification over such entities by a quantifier such as $\exists$ would mean, for example, that "there is a set P such that ..." or "there is a function f such that ...". We shall not be concerned with quantifications of this type. This is the task of languages and logics of higher order, i.e., second order, third order, etc. See Section 26.2.5 on page 904.

26.2.2 The Semantics of the Language $\mathcal{L}_1$

Although it could have been otherwise, historically, human beings have been fundamentally concerned with truth. It will also concern us on many occasions in the present book. To begin with, we shall inquire into the notion of *truth in $\mathcal{L}_1$* because the classical predicate logic that we are studying in this chapter is an *extensional logic*. That means that in reasoning processes it only considers the truth values of the statements used, but not their contents. As was briefly outlined on page 823, the extension of a statement is its truth value. Its content is its intension.[162]

It was already emphasized that one of the achievements of formal logic consists in replacing the semantic concept and technique of inference with syntactic ones. To appreciate the equivalence between both concepts and techniques, we must first provide the language $\mathcal{L}_1$ with a semantics. To this end, we shall introduce the notions of *interpretation, tautology,* and *validity,* and the basic notions of *elementary formula* and *structure,* on which they depend. These tools will enable us to understand what it means to say that a statement is *true in* $\mathcal{L}_1$, and that from a particular set of premises a particular consequence follows. We start by studying three basic semantic features of the language $\mathcal{L}_1$. They will also be relevant to our discussions on the general concept of truth in Section 11.1.1. Our considerations here divide into the following four sections:

▶ Three semantic principles
▶ The truth of formulas
▶ Tautology and validity
▶ The classical concept of inference.

Three semantic principles

Part V is concerned with the logic of medicine. There, different systems of logic are examined to assess whether any of them may be viewed, or even serve, as a 'logic of medicine'. Each of these logics is characterized by some philosophical-ontological peculiarities and commitments which may or may not qualify it for a logic of medicine. The logic we are currently studying is no exception. It also has its philosophical-ontological peculiarities that one should be aware of from the outset. Three of these are sketched in this section because they will play an important role in our analyses throughout.

In natural languages and everyday life, statements are qualified as true, false, verifiable, unverifiable, justified, unjustified, believable, unbelievable, plausible, implausible, etc. All these features are semantic or pragmatic ones. Therefore, in order for the language $\mathcal{L}_1$ and its logic, which is predicate logic, to be applicable to reasoning in natural languages, some sort of semantic or pragmatic adaptation is necessary. To this end, $\mathcal{L}_1$ and its logic incorporate

---

[162] The extensional semantics of predicate logic sketched in this section goes partly back to the Polish-American logician Alfred Tarski and is therefore called *Tarski semantics*. Tarski (1901–1983) was born in Warsaw and lectured there until 1939, emigrated to the USA, and taught at the University of California in Berkeley (1942–1968). He contributed extensively to the foundations of logic and mathematics. Among his important achievements is the analysis of the notion of a *true sentence*. His first, systematic papers on this issue, published in Polish and German in the 1930s, gave rise to the fields of semantics and model theory (see Tarski, 1933, 1983). His concept of truth will be discussed below and on page 462.

two of the above-mentioned features, i.e., the semantic features *true* and *false*. These two possible semantic properties of a sentence are called its *truth values*. If a sentence α such as "Elroy Fox is ill" is true or false, it is said to have the truth value *true* or *false,* respectively. $\mathcal{L}_1$ and its logic are based on the following three ancient, semantic principles, postulates, or dogmas:

    a. Principle of Two-Valuedness,
    b. Principle of Excluded Middle,
    c. Principle of Non-Contradiction.

The *Principle of Two-Valuedness,* or Bivalence, says that a statement such as "it is raining", "Elroy Fox is ill", or "AIDS is a viral disease" is either true or false even if we don't know whether it is actually true or false. Otherwise put, a statement is said to have one of the two truth values {true, false}. There is no other, intermediate truth value in $\mathcal{L}_1$ between these two extremes, e.g., 'probable', 'indeterminate', or 'unknown'. No statement takes a third truth value of this or another type. Tertium non datur. This is the *Principle of Excluded Middle,* or Excluded Third. The *Principle of Non-Contradiction* holds that a statement has only one of the two truth values {true, false}, but not both. No proposition can be true and false at the same time. For example, it cannot be reasonably asserted that "Elroy Fox is ill and he is not ill".

    The three basic principles above will determine the semantics, and thus the nature, of $\mathcal{L}_1$ and its logic. They originate from the ancient Greeks, especially Aristotle. Since they belong to the fundamentals of the worldview that we have inherited from him, they are qualified as *classical* and *Aristotelean.* This is why the logic we are studying, i.e., the *first-order predicate logic with identity,* is referred to both as classical and Aristotelean, also called Aristotelic. In later chapters, we shall also consider non-classical, non-Aristotelean logics.[163]

The truth values of formulas

After constructing the syntactic concept of inference below, we shall demonstrate that it is equivalent to the semantic one and enables us to reason without regard to problematic, semantic, and philosophical issues associated with the truth or untruth of premises and conclusions. To this end, the semantic concept of inference will be made precise first. Its preliminary version presented

---

[163] The three semantic principles mentioned in the body text are interrelated, even though not identical. They are basic constituents of the *Aristotelean worldview* that we have inherited from the ancient Greeks. Strictly speaking, the advocate of bivalence was the Megarian, Stoic philosopher Chrysippus (280–207 BC). Aristotle was a skeptic in this respect. In his famous sea battle argument in chapter 9 of his *De Interpretaione,* he has contemplated a third truth value (see footnote 181 on page 964). Nevertheless, he has vehemently propagated the Principle of Bivalence in his writings. See, for example, his *Metaphysics,* Book III, 996 b 25: "Everything must be either affirmed or denied".

in Definition 202 on page 851 shows that it is based on the notion of a true sentence. Sentences are represented in our language $\mathcal{L}_1$ by formulas. We must therefore inquire into what it means to say that a formula in $\mathcal{L}_1$ is true or false. To answer this question, we need some basic notions which will now be introduced in the following paragraphs:

▷ Elementary formulas
▷ Structures
▷ Interpretation of formulas
▷ Models for formulas.

Elementary formulas

Prime or elementary formulas are the smallest units of which every formula is a combination to the effect that the truth value of a formula depends on the truth values of its elementary formulas ('compositionality of truth'). To determine the truth value of a formula, we must therefore know of which elementary formulas it consists and what their truth values are. We have only the following three types of elementary formulas:

Formula:	Name:	Examples:	
$t_1 = t_2$	equality	$fa = b$	(Elroy Fox's pulse rate is 76)
$Pt_1 \ldots t_n$	predication	Pxy	(x loves y)
$\exists x \alpha$	existential quanti-fication	$\exists x P x a$	(someone loves Elroy Fox)

As the smallest units of all formulas they yield, with the aid of sentential connectives, compound formulas of arbitrary complexity in the following way:

$\neg \alpha$	negation	e.g.:	$\neg Pxy, \ \neg \exists x Qx, \ \neg \exists x \neg Pxy, \ \neg fa = b$
$\alpha \vee \beta$	disjunction		$fa = b \vee \neg Pxy$
$\alpha \wedge \beta$	cojunction		$(fa = b \vee \neg Pxy) \wedge Qz$
$\alpha \rightarrow \beta$	conditional		$Pxy \rightarrow fa = b$
$\alpha \leftrightarrow \beta$	biconditional		$Pxy \leftrightarrow \neg \exists z \neg Qz$

Negations as compound formulas also include formulas of the form $\neg \exists x \neg \alpha$. That is, according to the definition of the universal quantifier $\forall$ in Definition 206.4 on page 865, they include:

$\forall x \alpha$ universal quantification as a shorthand for $\neg \exists x \neg \alpha$.

The notion of an elementary formula can easily be put into an exact definition to prevent misunderstandings. Thus, we present a method to determine the *set of elementary formulas* of which a formula is composed. A phrase of the form "$el(\alpha)$", with "el" as a set-valued function, reads "elementary formulas of the formula α".

Definition 215 (Elementary formulas of a formula)**.**

1. $el(t_1 = t_2) = \{t_1 = t_2\}$
2. $el(Pt_1 \ldots t_n) = \{Pt_1 \ldots t_n\}$
3. $el(\neg\alpha) = \{\alpha\}$
4. $el(\alpha \vee \beta) = el(\alpha) \cup el(\beta)$
5. $el(\exists x\alpha) = \{\exists x\alpha\}.$

Conjunctions, conditionals, biconditionals, and universal quantifications need not be included in the definition because they are defined by negations, disjunctions, and existential quantifications. Accordingly, we can obtain the following:

$$el(\alpha \wedge \beta) = el\big(\neg(\neg\alpha \vee \neg\beta)\big)$$
$$el(\alpha \rightarrow \beta) = el(\neg\alpha \vee \beta)$$
$$el(\alpha \leftrightarrow \beta) = el(\alpha \rightarrow \beta \wedge \beta \rightarrow \alpha)$$
$$el(\forall x\alpha) = el(\neg\exists x\,\neg\alpha).$$

For example, the set of elementary formulas of $\forall x Px \rightarrow (\exists y \neg Qxy \wedge \neg Ry)$ may be determined thus:

$$
\begin{aligned}
el\big(\forall x Px \rightarrow (\exists y \neg Qxy \wedge \neg Ry)\big) &= el\big(\neg\forall x Px \vee (\exists y \neg Qxy \wedge \neg Ry)\big) \\
&= el(\neg\forall x Px) \cup el(\exists y \neg Qxy \wedge \neg Ry) \\
&= el(\forall x Px) \cup el\big(\neg(\neg\exists y \neg Qxy \vee \neg\neg Ry)\big) \\
&= el(\neg\exists x \neg Px) \cup el(\neg\exists y \neg Qxy \vee Ry) \\
&= el(\exists x \neg Px) \cup el(\neg\exists y \neg Qxy) \cup el(Ry) \\
&= el(\exists x \neg Px) \cup el(\exists y \neg Qxy) \cup el(Ry) \\
&= \{\exists x \neg Px, \exists y \neg Qxy, Ry\}.
\end{aligned}
$$

The truth value of a formula, e.g., of the example formula above, depends on the truth values of its elementary formulas and on the logical signs it contains. Therefore, we start by inquiring into the truth values of elementary formulas to explore how they bring about the truth value of a compound. To this end, and for later purposes, we need the notion of a *structure*.

Structures

Let there be any elementary formula, e.g., the predication Rab or the equality $fa = b$. It does not make sense to ask what the truth value of such a formula is. To determine its truth value, one must know what its constituent signs mean, i.e., the predicate R, the function symbol f, and the individual symbols a and b in the present two examples. The required knowledge may be acquired by *interpreting* the signs in a suitable structure. This will be explained in the current section and the next. First, what is a structure?

A set with one or more relations thereon we call a relational system, a relational structure, or a *structure* for short. That means that a $(1+w)$-tuple of the form $\langle \Omega, R_1, \ldots, R_w \rangle$ is a structure iff:

- Ω is a non-empty set of objects termed the domain, the base set, or the universe of the structure. Its elements are called the individuals of the structure,
- $R_1, \ldots, R_w$ are $w \geq 1$ n-place relations on Ω.

The name "structure" is due to the fact that the base set Ω is structured in a particular fashion by any relation $R_i \in \{R_1, \ldots, R_w\}$ that holds between its members. A simple example is the following tuple:

$$\langle \{x \mid x \text{ is a human being}\}; \{\langle x, y \rangle \mid x \text{ loves } y\} \rangle$$

with the set of human beings as its universe and the binary relation of loving thereon, i.e., $\langle \Omega, R \rangle$ where $\Omega = \{x \mid x \text{ is a human being}\}$ and $R = \{\langle x, y \rangle \mid x \text{ loves } y\}$. This relation of loving that holds between pairs of human individuals, *structures* the set of human beings. For some human being there is another human being whom she loves.

A relation $R_i \in \{R_1, \ldots, R_w\}$ of the structure may also be a function since a function is a single-valued relation. If we indicate the functions separately, we obtain a $(1+q+r)$-tuple of the form $\langle \Omega, R_1, \ldots, R_q; f_1, \ldots, f_r \rangle$ with $q + r \geq 1$. Moreover, a structure may contain $s \geq 0$ specified elements, $a_1, \ldots, a_s$, of its universe. We have thus, in general, a $(1+q+r+s)$-tuple of the following form:

$$\langle \Omega, R_1, \ldots, R_q; f_1, \ldots, f_r; a_1, \ldots, a_s \rangle.$$

An example is the quadruple $\langle \{x \mid x \text{ is a human being}\}; \{\langle x, y \rangle \mid x \text{ loves } y\};$ *Barack Obama, Michelle Obama*$\rangle$. It contains, in addition to the relation of loving, two specified individuals of its universe, i.e., Barack Obama and Michelle Obama. A structure may even contain $p \geq 1$ universes $\Omega_1, \ldots, \Omega_p$ such that $R_1, \ldots, R_q$ and $f_1, \ldots, f_r$ are relations and functions on them or on any Cartesian products of them. Then an entity of the form:

$$\langle \Omega_1, \ldots, \Omega_p; R_1, \ldots, R_q; f_1, \ldots, f_r; a_1, \ldots, a_s \rangle \qquad (228)$$

with $p, q + r \geq 1$ and $s \geq 0$ is referred to as a generalized relational system, generalized relational structure, or *structure* for short. Note that a relation $R_i \in \{R_1, \ldots, R_q\}$ in the structure above may also be a one-place relation, i.e., a simple set, a subset of a domain Ω_i. The term "relation" is general enough to cover all of the possibilities mentioned.

Interpretation of formulas

As was pointed out above, we do not know what a formula such as *Rab* means and whether it is true or false because the information is missing about what its constituents, *R*, *a*, and *b*, mean or represent. But we may *interpret* these signs by assigning to them any particular objects or relations 'in the world out there' to handle the formula and to analyze its truth value. For example, we may say or decide that *"a"* stands for "Romeo", *"b"* stands for "Juliet", and *"R"* stand for "loves". Under this interpretation, the formula *Rab* obviously means *"Romeo loves Juliet"*, and may be a true or false statement. This specific concept of interpretation will be studied in the current section.

Structures are formal representers of worlds. Formulas may be *interpreted* in structures to analyze their truth values as if they were interpreted in 'a real world out there'. But a formula cannot be adequately interpreted in every structure. The structure needs to be suitable to its language, or *suitable to the formula* for short. A structure is suitable to a formula α if it contains the following objects:

- a non-empty universe Ω;
- for each m-ary predicate of α other than "=" with $m > 1$, an m-ary relation $\boldsymbol{R}$ on Ω. This includes for each unary predicate of α, a unary relation $\boldsymbol{R}$ on Ω, i.e., a subset of Ω;
- for each n-ary function symbol of α, an n-ary function $\boldsymbol{f}$ from Ω to Ω, i.e., an $(n+1)$-ary single-valued relation on Ω;
- for each individual constant of α, a specified element $\boldsymbol{a}$ of Ω.[164]

---

[164] Concisely stated, a structure is suitable to a formula if it contains (i) as many relations of the same arities as the predicates contained in the formula; (ii) as many functions of the same arities as the function symbols contained in the formula; and (iii) as many specified individuals as individual constants contained in the formula. This relation of suitability between structures and formulas may be precisely defined as follows. On page 73, we sketched the term *"the type of a structure"*. This term will now be generalized. Given a structure $\mathcal{A}$ of the form (228) above, the set $\{\boldsymbol{R_1}, \ldots, \boldsymbol{R_q}; \boldsymbol{f_1}, \ldots, \boldsymbol{f_r}; \boldsymbol{a_1}, \ldots, \boldsymbol{a_s}\}$ of its relations, functions, and specified individuals is referred to as its *constants*, $\mathcal{C}(\mathcal{A})$ for short. On the one hand, an ordered sequence $\langle r_1, \ldots, r_q; r'_1, \ldots, r'_r; s \rangle$ of integers is said to be the type of the structure $\mathcal{A}$, written $type(\mathcal{A})$, if an r_i is the arity of the relation $\boldsymbol{R_i}$; an r'_j is the arity of the function $\boldsymbol{f_j}$; and s is the number of the specified individuals $\boldsymbol{a_1}, \ldots, \boldsymbol{a_s}$ in the structure. For example, if our structure $\mathcal{A}$ is $\langle \{x \mid x$ is a human being$\}; \{\langle x, y \rangle \mid x$ loves $y\}; Barack\ Obama,\ Michelle\ Obama \rangle$ with $\mathcal{C}(\mathcal{A}) = \langle$loves; Barack Obama, Michelle Obama$\rangle$, then $type(\mathcal{A}) = \langle 2; \varnothing; 2 \rangle$. On the other hand, if $\mathcal{C}(\alpha)$ signifies the set of *constants* of the formula α comprising its predicates, function symbols, and individual constants, then $type(\alpha)$ is a sequence of integers as above. We can now easily define a structure $\mathcal{A}$ to be suitable to a formula α if and only if $type(\mathcal{A}) = type(\alpha)$.

To dertermine the truth value of any formula, we must first determine the truth values of its elementary formulas. Elementary formulas are predications, identities, i.e., equalities, and existential quantifications:

- $P(t_1, \ldots, t_n)$ $\quad\quad$ ≡ predication,
- $t_1 = t_2$ $\quad\quad\quad\quad$ ≡ identity,
- $\exists x \alpha$ $\quad\quad\quad\quad\quad$ ≡ existential quantification.

We shall first explain the notion of *interpretation of atomic formulas,* i.e., predications and identities. For example, our above-mentioned structure $\langle \{x \mid x$ is a human being$\}$; $\{\langle x, y \rangle \mid x$ loves $y\}$; *Barack Obama, Michelle Obama*$\rangle$ is suitable to the predication *Rab*. Thus, this formula may be interpreted in that structure. Assign to its binary predicate R the two-place relation $\{\langle x, y \rangle \mid x$ loves $y\}$ of the structure; to its individual constant a the specified individual *Barack Obama;* and to its individual constant b the specified individual *Michelle Obama.* Under this interpretation, the formula *Rab* yields the statement "Barack Obama loves Michelle Obama". To judge from the media reports on the current U.S. president and his private life, the statement is true. However, another interpretation of the formula in the same structure as above or in another one may render the formula false. This may be illustrated by the identity $fa = b$ and the structure $\langle \{x \mid x$ is an integer$\}$; $\{\langle x, y \rangle \mid x$ squared is $y\}$; $4, 16 \rangle$. If we interpret the binary function symbol f of our formula by the binary function $\{\langle x, y \rangle \mid x$ squared is $y\}$, and its individual constants a and b by 4 and 16, respectively, we obtain the true statement "4 squared is 16", i.e., $squared(4) = 16$. By interpreting its individual constants other way, the false statement "$squared(16) = 4$" will emerge.

A suitable interpretation, or *interpretation* for short, of an atomic formula in a structure, then, is the act of assigning to each *descriptive sign* of the formula a suitable object in the structure. Specifically, we assign an m-place relation to an m-place predicate R_i; an n-place function to an n-place function symbol f_j; a particular, specified individual object in the structure to an individual constant a_k; and an individual object of the universe Ω to an individual variable x of the formula where $i + j, m, n \geq 1$ and $k \geq 0$. Thus, given a structure:

$$\langle \Omega_1, \ldots, \Omega_p; R_1, \ldots, R_q; f_1, \ldots, f_r; a_1, \ldots, a_s \rangle \tag{229}$$

the interpretation of an atomic formula in this structure may be viewed as a *function,* denoted $\Im$, such that:

- the interpretation of an R_i, written $\Im(R_i)$, is a suitable relation,
- $\Im(f_j)$ is a suitable function,
- $\Im(a_k)$ is a particular individual object, and
- $\Im(x)$ is an individual object of the universe of the structure.

We may now straightforwardly form a precise concept of interpretaion. To this end, we need the term "the set of *descriptive,* i.e., non-logical, *signs* of a formula α", symbolized by $\mathcal{S}(\alpha)$. This set, $\mathcal{S}(\alpha)$, contains the set of all constants of the formula, written $\mathcal{C}(\alpha)$ and comprising the predicates, function symbols and individual constants of the formula, togetehr with the set of its variables. That is, $\mathcal{S}(\alpha) = \mathcal{C}(\alpha) \cup \mathcal{V}(\alpha)$.

Definition 216 (Interpretation of atomic formulas). *If α is an atomic formula, $\mathcal{S}(\alpha)$ is the set of its descriptive signs, and $\mathcal{A}$ is a structure such as (229) above, then the interpretation of α in $\mathcal{A}$ is a function $\mathfrak{I}$ such that:*

$$\mathfrak{I}(\alpha) \colon \mathcal{S}(\alpha) \mapsto \mathcal{A}$$

with:

    1. $\mathfrak{I}\big(R_i \in \mathcal{S}(\alpha)\big) = \boldsymbol{R} \in \{\boldsymbol{R_1}, \ldots, \boldsymbol{R_q}\}$ *of the structure*
    2. $\mathfrak{I}\big(f_j \in \mathcal{S}(\alpha)\big) = \boldsymbol{f} \in \{\boldsymbol{f_1}, \ldots, \boldsymbol{f_r}\}$ *of the structure*
    3. $\mathfrak{I}\big(a_k \in \mathcal{S}(\alpha)\big) = \boldsymbol{a} \in \{\boldsymbol{a_1}, \ldots, \boldsymbol{a_s}\}$ *of the structure*
    4. $\mathfrak{I}\big(x \in \mathcal{S}(\alpha)\big) = \boldsymbol{x} \in \Omega$ *of the structure, where $\Omega \in \{\Omega_1, \ldots, \Omega_p\}$.*

For instance, in our last example above with the false result $16^2 = 4$, the identity $fa = b$ was suitably interpreted in the structure $\langle\{x \mid x$ is an integer$\}$; $\{\langle x, y\rangle \mid x$ squared is $y\}$; $4, 16\rangle$ thus:

$$\mathfrak{I}(f) = \{\langle x, y\rangle \mid x \text{ squared is } y\} \subseteq \langle\{x \mid x \text{ is an integer}\} \times \langle\{x \mid x \text{ is an integer}\}$$
$$\mathfrak{I}(a) = 16$$
$$\mathfrak{I}(b) = 4.$$

Clauses 2–4, of Definition 216 above, for the interpretation of function symbols and atomic terms also recursively enable the interpretation of compound terms of a formula, such as $ft_1 \ldots t_n$, in the following way: The interpretation of a compound term of the form $ft_1 \ldots t_n$ is the act of applying the interpretation of the function symbol f to the interpretations of the constituent terms $t_1, \ldots, t_n$. That is:

Definition 217 (Interpretation of atomic formulas continued: 1). *If the atomic formula α used in Definition 216 contains a compound term of the form $ft_1 \ldots t_n$, then the interpretation of this compound term is:*

    5. $\mathfrak{I}(ft_1 \ldots t_n) = \mathfrak{I}(f)\big(\mathfrak{I}(t_1), \ldots, \mathfrak{I}(t_n)\big)$.

For example, the compound term fab of a formula may in a particular, suitable structure be interpreted by $\mathfrak{I}(fab) = $ 'sum of 4 and 16', i.e., $4 + 16$, where "f" stands for "$+$".

    The substantial contribution of Alfred Tarski to semantics is his concept of truth in formal languages (Tarski, 1933). After the preliminaries above we may outline a Tarski semantics for the language $\mathcal{L}_1$ by introducing a concept of *truth* for formulas. We start with atomic formulas as they are the most basic formulas and constitute the interface between language and knowledge, on the one hand; and 'the word out there', on the other. Their yield is *material truth*, as compared to formal truth. For the distinction between these two types of truth, see Section 26.1.5 on page 855. In what follows, the truth values *true* and *false* are symbolized by "W" and "F", respectively.

Thus far the interpretation function $\mathfrak{I}$ had the descriptive signs of terms and atomic formulas as its domain, and the objects of structures as its range. It will now be *extended* in such a way that its domain will also include the set of all formulas, and its range will also include the two truth values $\{T, F\}$. We shall thus become able to state in addition that (for the notion of 'extension of a function', see Section 25.4.3 on page 843):

$$\mathfrak{I}(\alpha) = T \qquad (\equiv \alpha \text{ is true})$$
$$\mathfrak{I}(\alpha) = F \qquad (\equiv \alpha \text{ is false})$$

if the interpretation $\mathfrak{I}$ of descriptive signs of the formula α, as demonstrated above, renders it true or false, respectively.

Definition 218 (Interpretation of atomic formulas continued: 2). *Let $Pt_1 \ldots t_n$ be any predication; $t_1 = t_2$ any identity; and $\mathfrak{I}$ an interpretation of them in a suitable structure. Then in this structure we have:*

1. $\mathfrak{I}(Pt_1 \ldots t_n) = W$ *iff* $\mathfrak{I}(P)$ *applies to* $(\mathfrak{I}(t_1), \ldots, \mathfrak{I}(t_n))$
2. $\mathfrak{I}(t_1 = t_2) = W$ *iff* $\mathfrak{I}(t_1) = \mathfrak{I}(t_2)$.

For instance, let "Elroy Fox has diabetes" be a sentence of which we want to know whether it is true or false. To this end, we need a suitable structure of the type $\langle \{x \mid x \text{ is a human being}\}, \{x \mid x \text{ has diabetes}\}, \text{Elroy Fox} \rangle$ such that the set of diabetics, i.e., $\langle \{x \mid x \text{ has diabetes}\} \rangle$, is a subset of the universe of discourse, $\langle \{x \mid x \text{ is a human being}\} \rangle$. Our atomic sentence "Elroy Fox has diabetes" is true in that structure if and only if $\mathfrak{I}(\text{"has diabetes"})$, i.e., $\langle \{x \mid x \text{ has diabetes}\} \rangle$, applies to $\mathfrak{I}(\text{"Elroy Fox"})$, i.e., Elroy Fox.

Tarski's semantic theory of truth is in essence an *explication* of the term "is true" by providing a recursive definition of it with respect to a particular language and with Definitions 216–218 above being its basis. For a generalization of the theory, see (Mikenberg et al., 1986; da Costa, 1989; da Costa and Bueno, 1998; da Costa and French, 2003).

Until now we have dealt with the interpretation of predications and identities. A final example deals with the third type of elementary formulas, i.e., existential quantifications. Let $\exists x \exists y Rxy$ be such a formula which says that there are x and y such that x stands in the relation R to y. And let $\langle \{z \mid z \text{ is a human being}\}, \{\langle x, y \rangle \mid x \text{ loves } y\} \rangle$ be a structure without specified, particular individuals. We can interpret our formula in this structure in a way that it becomes true, for example, thus:

$$\mathfrak{I}(R) = \{\langle x, y \rangle \mid x \text{ loves } y\}$$
$$\mathfrak{I}(x) = \boldsymbol{x} \in \{z \mid z \text{ is a human being}\}, \quad \text{for instance: } \boldsymbol{x} = \text{Barack Obama}$$
$$\mathfrak{I}(y) = \boldsymbol{y} \in \{z \mid z \text{ is a human being}\}, \quad \text{for instance: } \boldsymbol{y} = \text{Michelle Obama}.$$

This interpretation of "Rxy" by "*Barack Obama loves Michelle Obama*" makes the formula $\exists x \exists y Rxy$ true in the structure $\langle \{z \mid z$ is a human being$\}$, $\{\langle x, y \rangle \mid x$ loves $y\}\rangle$ because there are obviously an $\boldsymbol{x}$ and a $\boldsymbol{y}$ in its universe such that $\boldsymbol{x}$ loves $\boldsymbol{y}$. However, another interpretation in the same structure or in another one may render our formula false, for example, "4 is greater than 16" in the structure $\langle \{x \mid x$ is an integer$\}; \{\langle x, y \rangle \mid x$ is greater than $y\}; 4, 16\rangle$.

The considerations above demonstrate that a suitable interpretation of an elementary formula α in a suitable structure is a function, $\mathfrak{I}$, that assigns to the *descriptive signs* of the formula suitable objects of the structure. By virtue of such an interpretation, the formula receives one of the truth values $\{$true, false$\}$. From now on, this bivalent set $\{$true, false$\}$ will conveniently be written $\{T, F\}$. For instance, in our final example above, the formula $\exists x \exists y Rxy$ turned out true in the structure $\langle \{z \mid z$ is a human being$\}, \{\langle x, y \rangle \mid x$ loves $y\}\rangle$. This means that we had $\mathfrak{I}(\exists x \exists y Rxy) = T$.

With the terminology above at our disposal, we will now study the interpretation of compound formulas and thereby provide a semantics for the basic *logical signs* of $\mathcal{L}_1$. Our goal is to come to grips with the notion of *formal truth* that we briefly sketched in Section 26.1.5 on page 855.

Definition 219 (Interpretation of negations, disjunctions, and existential quantifications)**.** *Let α and β be any formulas, and let $\mathfrak{I}$ be an interpretation of them in a suitable structure $\mathcal{A}$. Then in this structure we have:*

1. $\mathfrak{I}(\neg \alpha) = W$ *iff* $\mathfrak{I}(\alpha) = F$
2. $\mathfrak{I}(\alpha \vee \beta) = W$ *iff* $\mathfrak{I}(\alpha) = W$ *or* $\mathfrak{I}(\beta) = W$
3. $\mathfrak{I}(\exists x \alpha) = W$ *iff*   *there is an individual $\boldsymbol{x}$ in the universe Ω of the structure $\mathcal{A}$ such that $\mathfrak{I}(\alpha) = T$ when in α we set $\mathfrak{I}(x) = \boldsymbol{x} \in \Omega$.*

This semantics must be termed a *classical* one because it reflects the three classical, Aristotelean principles mentioned on page 874. As we shall see later, there are also non-classical semantics deviating from the present one which give rise to logics of a completely different type. We shall have to study, then, which one of these logics is appropriate for use in medicine. To begin with, note that according to part 1 of the definition, a negation $\neg \alpha$ is true if and only if α is false. That means that:

- $\neg \alpha$ has the value T if α has the value F,
- $\neg \alpha$ has the value F if α has the value T.

Consider a simple example: The statement "Elroy Fox has diabetes" is true if "Elroy Fox does not have diabetes" is false, and "Elroy Fox has diabetes" is false if "Elroy Fox does not have diabetes" is true.

The truth conditions above are depicted in the *truth table* of the negation sign $\neg$ in Table 29. The table shows that if α has the truth value indicated in the column below the header α, then $\neg \alpha$ has the corresponding truth value to its right. These truth conditions imitate our natural understanding of negation phrases such as "not", "it is not the case that . . .", and "it is not true that . . .".

Part 2 of Definition 219 says that a disjunction $\alpha \lor \beta$ is true if and only if at least one of its disjuncts, either α or β, is true. That means that:

- $\alpha \lor \beta$ has the value T if at least one of α and β has the value T,
- $\alpha \lor \beta$ has the value F if both of α and β has the value F.

For instance, the statement "Elroy Fox has diabetes or Elroy Fox has hepatitis" has the truth value T if at least one of its constituents, "Elroy Fox has diabetes" *or* "Elroy Fox has hepatitis", has the value T. It has the truth value F if both of its constituents have the value F. These truth conditions are illustrated by the truth table of disjunction in Table 30. In this table, each row below the headers in the first and second column displays the possible combination of the truth values of α and β. There are 2 truth values times 2 formulas = 4 such combinations. For each combination, the resulting truth value of $\alpha \lor \beta$ is recorded in the third column. Obviously, the truth of one part of the statement $\alpha \lor \beta$ does not preclude the truth of the other part. In this *inclusive* Or, both components of the disjunction may be true at the same time.

Table 29. The truth table of negation

α	$\neg\alpha$
T	F
F	T

Table 30. The truth table of disjunction. This definition imitates our natural understanding of the inclusive "or"

α	β	$\alpha \lor \beta$
T	T	T
T	F	T
F	T	T
F	F	F

Table 31. This classical semantics of the conjunction "$\land$" imitates our natural understanding of the phrase "and"

α	β	$\alpha \land \beta$
T	T	T
T	F	F
F	T	F
F	F	F

By contrast, in the *exclusive* OR that is usually expressed by *either-or-but-not-both,* this is not possible. For instance, "we shall either read the present handbook or Harry Potter, but not both". If we symbolize the exclusive OR by "OR", it may be defined by the inclusive Or, i.e. $\lor$, in the following way to the effect that exclusive OR is not needed in $\mathcal{L}_1$ as a special logical sign:

$$\alpha \text{ OR } \beta \quad \textit{iff} \quad (\alpha \lor \beta) \land \neg(\alpha \land \beta) \qquad \text{(Exclusive OR)}$$

According to part 3 of Definition 219, an existential quantification $\exists x \alpha$ is true if and only if the universe of the structure, i.e., set Ω, includes an individual object x such that in α the individual variable x can be interpreted thereby to make α true. We have already considered an example above. Since the remaining logical signs of $\mathcal{L}_1$, i.e., $\wedge$, $\rightarrow$, $\leftrightarrow$, and $\forall$, have been defined, in Definition 206 on page 865, by the three basic logical signs $\neg$, $\vee$, and $\exists$, we obtain from their definitions the following Corollary 10 which demonstrates the semantics for conjunctions, conditionals, biconditionals, and universal quantifications:

Corollary 10 (Interpretation of conjunctions, conditionals, biconditionals, and universal quantifications). *In a suitable structure* $\mathcal{A}$,

1. $\mathfrak{I}(\alpha \wedge \beta) = \mathrm{W}$ *iff* $\mathfrak{I}(\alpha) = \mathrm{W}$ *and* $\mathfrak{I}(\beta) = \mathrm{W}$
2. $\mathfrak{I}(\alpha \rightarrow \beta) = \mathrm{F}$ *iff*   *if* $\mathfrak{I}(\alpha) = \mathrm{W}$, *then* $\mathfrak{I}(\beta) = \mathrm{F}$
3. $\mathfrak{I}(\alpha \leftrightarrow \beta) = \mathrm{W}$ *iff* $\mathfrak{I}(\alpha \rightarrow \beta) = \mathrm{W}$ *and* $\mathfrak{I}(\beta \rightarrow \alpha) = \mathrm{W}$
4. $\mathfrak{I}(\forall x \alpha) = \mathrm{W}$ *iff*   *for every individual* $\boldsymbol{x}$ *in the universe* Ω *of the structure* $\mathcal{A}$, $\mathfrak{I}(\alpha) = \mathrm{T}$ *whenever, in* α, $\mathfrak{I}(x) = \boldsymbol{x} \in \Omega$.

According to part 1 of this corollary, a conjunction $\alpha \wedge \beta$ is true if and only if both of the conjuncts, α and β, are true; and false, otherwise. That means that:

- $\alpha \wedge \beta$ has the value T if both α and β have the value T,
- $\alpha \wedge \beta$ has the value F if at least one of α and β has the value F.

For instance, "Elroy Fox has diabetes and Elroy Fox has hepatitis" is true iff "Elroy Fox has diabetes" is true and "Elroy Fox has hepatitis" is true. In all other cases it is false. These truth conditions are illustrated by the truth table of conjunction in Table 31 on page 884.

Part 2 of Corollary 10 above shows that due to its definition by $\neg$ and $\vee$, a conditional $\alpha \rightarrow \beta$ turns out false only when its antecedent α is true and its consequent β is false. In all other cases it is true. These truth conditions yield the truth table of the conditional in Table 32 on page 886. Consider as a simple example the following conditional: "If Elroy Fox has bronchitis, then he coughs". This conditional is *true* if:

- "Elroy Fox has bronchitis" is true and "Elroy Fox coughs" is true,
- "Elroy Fox has bronchitis" is false and "Elroy Fox coughs" is true,
- "Elroy Fox has bronchitis" is false and "Elroy Fox coughs" is false.

It is false only if:

- "Elroy Fox has bronchitis" is true and "Elroy Fox coughs" is false.

According to part 3 of Corollary 10, a biconditional $\alpha \leftrightarrow \beta$ is true whenever its constituent formulas, α and β, have the same truth value, and false, otherwise. That means that:

- $\alpha \leftrightarrow \beta$ has the value T if both of α and β have the value T or F,
- $\alpha \leftrightarrow \beta$ has the value F if the values of α and β are different.

Table 32. This classical semantics of the sign of conditional → does not completely accord with our natural understanding of if-then (see the final row). It only follows from the definition of $\alpha \to \beta$ by $\neg \alpha \vee \beta$

Table 33. Consider as an example the statement "AIDS is curable if and only if it is a viral disease". This statement is true if AIDS is curable as well as a viral disease, or it is neither curable nor a viral disease. Otherwise, it is false

α	β	$\alpha \to \beta$
T	T	T
T	F	F
F	T	T
F	F	T

α	β	$\alpha \leftrightarrow \beta$
T	T	T
T	F	F
F	T	F
F	F	T

The truth conditions of the biconditional are illustrated in its truth table in Table 33.

Finally, part 4 of Corollary 10 says that a universal quantification $\forall x \alpha$ is true if and only if in α, the interpretation of the individual variable x by every individual of the universe Ω of the structure renders α true. Take as an example the formula "For all x, if x is P, then x is Q", i.e., $\forall x(Px \to Qx)$. It is true in the structure $\langle \{y \mid y$ is a living thing$\}, \{y \mid y$ is a human being$\}, \{y \mid y$ is mortal$\} \rangle$ if under the interpretation of P by "is a human being", and of Q by "is mortal", the conditional "if x is a human being, then x is mortal" is true for every living thing.

Models for formulas

Although we have committed ourselves to exercise conceptual parsimony in this book, sometimes it is unavoidable to touch upon important concepts that simplify our analyses, forge links to other fields, and enhance our understanding. The term "model" belongs to this category. The role it plays in logic will be briefly explained in what follows.

Like many other phrases, the word "model" suffers from confusing polysemy. Except logic and mathematics, in all other sciences and in everyday life as well a *model* is either (i) a miniature material object that stands for something similar, or (ii) a linguistic, abstract idea that represents something in the 'real world out there'. For example, wooden models of ships, and Watson and Crick's double helix are material models, while the Bohr model of the atom and the computer model of the mind are abstract ideas. Also empirical scientists call their hypotheses and theories "models of reality".

We do not subscribe to the above-mentioned usages of the term "model". In logic and mathematical model theory, a model is an entity of another type sketched in the definition below, although this concept too is not good enough. Considering the vagueness of all human knowledge, it is in need of revision to capture models of fuzzy empirical theories (see Section 9.4.6 on page 439).

Definition 220 (Model for, or of, a formula). *A structure:*

$$\langle \Omega_1, \ldots, \Omega_p; R_1, \ldots, R_q; f_1, \ldots, f_r; a_1, \ldots, a_s \rangle$$

with $p, q + r \geq 1$ and $s \geq 0$, as decribed on page 877 f., is a model for a *formula α iff there is an interpretation $\mathfrak{I}$ that renders α true in it.*

For example, the structure $\langle \{x \mid x$ is a human being$\}; \{x \mid x$ is a diabetic$\};$ Elroy Fox$\rangle$ is a model for the formula *"Pa"* where P is a unary predicate and a is an individual constant. Interpret P by "is a diabetic" and a by "Elroy Fox". Since Elroy Fox is a diabetic, the structure turns out a model for Pa.

If $\mathfrak{F}$ is a set of formulas, a structure is a model for $\mathfrak{F}$ if it is a model for each formula in $\mathfrak{F}$. For instance, the structure $\langle \{x \mid x$ is a human being$\}; \{x \mid x$ is a diabetic$\}; \{x \mid x$ is healthy$\};$ Elroy Fox, Amy Fox$\rangle$ is a model for the set $\{Pa, Qb\}$ of two formulas, e.g., {Elroy Fox is a diabetic, Amy Fox is healthy}, and also for their conjunction $Pa \wedge Qb$.

Tautology and validity

We have sketched the notion of formal truth already in Section 26.1.5 on page 855. The preliminaries above enable us to precisely define it to obtain the two fundamental semantic notions of predicate logic, *tautology* and *validity*. They will directly lead us to the concept of predicate-logical inference.

The truth tables of sentential connectives on pages 884–886 clearly demonstrate that these logical signs, not the quantifiers, operate as functions on truth values of formulas and transform them into other truth values. They are therefore said to be *truth-functional* and are called truth functions or truth operators. For example, the negation sign $\neg$ is a *unary* function, $f_\neg$, from $\{T, F\}$ to $\{T, F\}$:

$$f_\neg : \{T, F\} \mapsto \{T, F\}.$$

It takes the truth value of a formula as preimage and returns the opposite truth value as image such that $f_\neg(T) = F$ and $f_\neg(F) = T$. The other four sentential connectives are *binary* truth functions:

$$\nabla : \{T, F\} \times \{T, F\} \mapsto \{T, F\}$$

where ∇ represents each of the truth functions $f_\vee, f_\wedge, f_\rightarrow$, and $f_\leftrightarrow$. For instance, we have $f_\wedge(T, T) = T$, whereas $f_\wedge(T, F) = f_\wedge(F, T) = f_\wedge(F, F) = F$. See the truth table of conjunction in Table 31 on page 884. On this basis, the truth value of every compound formula of arbitrary complexity, ϕ, is truth-functionally computable. To demonstrate this, assign in a truth table to the elementary formulas $\alpha_1, \ldots, \alpha_n$ of ϕ their interpretations $\mathfrak{I}(\alpha_1), \ldots, \mathfrak{I}(\alpha_n)$, and calculate the interpretation $\mathfrak{I}(\phi)$ of the compound. We will now do so for following two sentences:

- If Elroy Fox has bronchitis, then he coughs and has fever,
- If Elroy Fox has bronchitis, then he coughs or he does not cough.

If we write $\alpha \equiv$ Elroy Fox has bronchitis; $\beta \equiv$ Elroy Fox coughs; and $\gamma \equiv$ Elroy Fox has fever, then the first sentence is of the form $\alpha \to \beta \wedge \gamma$, whereas the second sentence has the structure $\alpha \to \beta \vee \neg\beta$. Their truth tables are depicted in Table 34. The truth table of the first compound formula $\alpha \to \beta \wedge \gamma$ shows that among the eight possible combinations of the truth values of its elementary formulas α, β, and γ there are three which make the compound false. By contrast, there are no such combinations in the truth table of the second compound formula $\alpha \to \beta \vee \neg\beta$. Independently of the specific truth values of its constituent formulas, the formula receives the interpretation:

$$\Im(\alpha \to \beta \vee \neg\beta) = \mathrm{T}.$$

This example demonstrates that there are formulas whose interpretation renders them true in all circumstances. This is due to their syntactic *form* and not to any facts in 'the world out there' they would describe. A formula of this type that can be demonstrated by a truth table alone to be true in all circumstances, is said to be *tautological* or a tautology. Every suitable structure is a model for a tautology. Otherwise put, *a tautology is true everywhere.*

There is also another type of formulas whose interpretation renders them true in all circumstances, for example, the formula $\forall x(Px \vee \neg Px)$, whereas their universal truth cannot be demonstrated by a truth table. That means that they are not tautological. They all are quantified formulas. For instance, regarding our example formula given above, there is no truth table which would show that:

Table 34. The truth tables of the formulas $\alpha \to \beta \wedge \gamma$ (top) and $\alpha \to \beta \vee \neg\beta$ (bottom)

α	β	γ	$\beta \wedge \gamma$	$\alpha \to \beta \wedge \gamma$
T	T	T	T	T
T	T	F	F	F
T	F	T	F	F
T	F	F	F	F
F	T	T	T	T
F	T	F	F	T
F	F	T	F	T
F	F	F	F	T

α	β	$\neg\beta$	$\beta \vee \neg\beta$	$\alpha \to \beta \vee \neg\beta$
T	T	F	T	T
T	F	T	T	T
F	T	F	T	T
F	F	T	T	T

$$\Im\big(\forall x(Px \vee \neg Px)\big) = \mathrm{T}$$

holds in all circumstances. But it holds in all circumstances nonetheless. Independently of how the unary predicate P and by which individual the variable x is interpreted, the subformula $Px \vee \neg Px$ is true of *all* individuals of the universe Ω of all *suitable structures*. Such a formula is said to be universally valid, or *valid* for short. This term precisely captures what we have called "formal truth" on page 855. It is introduced by the following definition.

Definition 221 (Satisfiability and validity of formulas).

1. *A formula α is satisfiable in a suitable structure iff there is an interpretation $\mathfrak{I}$ of α in this structure such that $\mathfrak{I}(\alpha) = T$. That is, iff under this interpretation the structure is a model for the formula.*
2. *A formula α is satisfiable iff there is a suitable structure such that it is satisfiable in this structure. That is, iff there is a model for the formula.*
3. *A formula α is valid in a suitable structure iff for all interpretations $\mathfrak{I}$ in this structure, $\mathfrak{I}(\alpha) = T$. That is, iff under all interpretations the structure is a model for the formula.*
4. *A formula α is valid iff it is valid in every suitable structure. That is, iff every suitable structure is a model for the formula.*

Tautologies are valid, but not vice versa. Here are a few examples:

Satisfiable:	**tautological:**	**valid:**
$\alpha \wedge \beta$	$\alpha \vee \neg\alpha$	$\alpha \vee \neg\alpha$
$\alpha \to \beta \wedge \gamma$	$\alpha \to \alpha \vee \neg\alpha$	$\alpha \to \alpha \vee \neg\alpha$
$\forall x(Px \to Qx)$		$\forall x(Px \to Px), \quad \forall x(Px \to Px \vee Qx)$
$\forall x \exists y(Pxy \to Qyx)$		$\forall x \neg \exists y \neg(Pxy \wedge Qyx \to Pxy).$

A notion of unsatisfiability may easily be introduced in the following way: A formula is *unsatisfiable* if and only if it is not satisfiable (according to Definition 221.2). That is, if there exists no suitable structure in which it is true. For instance, $\alpha \wedge \neg\alpha$ is unsatisfiable and thus false in all structures.

The classical concept of inference

As we now have additional tools available, the provisional definition of the classical concept of inference presented in Definition 202 on page 851 may be updated in the following way to enable deeper insights into its structure. The symbol $\mathfrak{F}$ conveniently represents a set of $n \geq 0$ formulas.

Definition 222 (The classical concept of inference or implication).

1. *$\mathfrak{F} \vDash \beta$ iff for all interpretations $\mathfrak{I}$ in all suitable structures, if $\mathfrak{I}(\alpha_i) = T$ for all $\alpha_i \in \mathfrak{F}$, then $\mathfrak{I}(\beta) = T$. That is, iff every model for $\mathfrak{F}$ is a model for β.*
2. *$\alpha_1, \ldots, \alpha_n \vDash \beta$ iff $\{\alpha_1, \ldots, \alpha_n\} \vDash \beta$.*
3. *$\vDash \beta$ iff $\mathfrak{F} \vDash \beta$ and $\mathfrak{F} = \varnothing$.*

According to this definition we have, for instance, $\alpha \vDash \alpha \vee \beta$. Claims of this type which do not contain quantifiers, can easily be tested by a truth table. In the present example, a truth table will prove that whenever $\mathfrak{I}(\alpha) = T$, then $\mathfrak{I}(\alpha \vee \beta) = T$. As a simple example, consider the following inference which explains why the patient Elroy Fox coughs:

If someone has bronchitis, then she coughs
Elroy Fox has bronchitis

Elroy Fox coughs.

This argument is of the following form: $\forall x(Px \rightarrow Qx), Pa \vDash Qa$. It is a correct argument. However, no truth table can justify it. It needs to be justified by a semantic proof which demonstrates that, according to Definition 222, for all interpretations $\mathfrak{I}$ in all suitable structures, whenever $\mathfrak{I}\big(\forall x(Px \rightarrow Qx)\big) =$ T and $\mathfrak{I}(Pa) =$ T, then $\mathfrak{I}(Qa) =$ T. Semantic proofs of this type are often cumbersome and sometimes even practically impossible when premises get too complicated. A syntactic calculus is presented in the following section which demonstrates how to overcome such semantic difficulties.

We have in this section described a semantics for the language $\mathcal{L}_1$ to introduce a concept of inference for this language. This was made possible by introducing the terms *interpretation, tautology,* and *validity*. Note, however, that the meaning of these notions is relative to $\mathcal{L}_1$. In other languages they may be, and are in fact, defined otherwise. Their proper use is therefore 'interpretation in $\mathcal{L}_1$', '$\mathcal{L}_1$-tautology', and '$\mathcal{L}_1$-valid'.

26.2.3 A Predicate-Logical Calculus

We have reached the goal of our preceding conceptual constructions. The core of the logic we have been pursuing is presented in what follows. It is the calculus of a first-order predicate logic with identity.

In general, a calculus is a formal theory developed to guide the process of transforming a physical configuration of some particular objects, 'calculi', into another configuration. This process of transformation is a purely mechanical one that is usually called *calculation*. For example, the calculus of arithmetic enables us to perform arithmetical calculations by transforming a particular configuration of numbers such as '5 + 7' into the configuration '12' or something like that. Additional examples are the integral calculus and the probability calculus. Likewise, the calculus of the first-order predicate logic with identity, or *predicate calculus* for short, is a framework consisting of a couple of rules for writing down arrays of signs on a sheet of paper. An array written down and treated as 'calculi' according to those rules is called a *predicate-logical deduction,* derivation, or proof. Deduction as a purely syntactic operation accomplishes what the semantic concept of inference accomplishes, i.e., the drawing of a conclusion from some premises. We shall see, for instance, that writing down the following formulas (as 'premise' and 'conclusion'):

$\forall x(Px \rightarrow Qx)$

$Pa \rightarrow Qa$

is such a deduction. It represents the syntactic pattern of all arguments of the form "All men are mortal. So, if Socrates is a man, then Socrates is mortal".

Thus, predicate-logical deductions are syntactic calculations according to the principles of a predicate calculus. The indefinite article 'a' in the last sentence betrays that there are various predicate calculuses. Each one of them is a particular system of syntactic rules to formalize the semantic concept of inference introduced in Definition 222 above. All of them are of course equivalent. The calculus presented below is the most economic, elegant, and simple one. The history of its development goes back to the legendary *Principia Mathematica* mentioned in footnote 155 on page 845. Our study of the calculus divides into the following five parts:

▶ The calculus
▶ Deduction and deducibility
▶ Derived rules
▶ Predicate-logical equivalence
▶ Sentential logic.

The calculus

The calculus consists of only 10 sentences. Seven sentences are called *axioms*. They are valid formulas. The remaining three sentences are valid *rules* of deduction having a premise and a conclusion. They show how to transform a formula written down as a premise into another formula written down as its conclusion. An axiom may be considered a rule without premises, i.e., a rule that produces a true conclusion ex nihilo. Thus, the calculus consists of 10 rules. Each rule has a proper name by which we shall refer to it. See Table 35 on page 892.

We have presented the calculus, especially the rules, in a very simple and illustrative form to avoid complex definitions.[165] This is the reason why a rule is usually presented as an inference schema bearing a horizontal line. The line means that after writing down the formula(s) above it, it is permitted to write down the formula below it as well. For example, line 3 of the following argument emerges from the application of Modus ponens to its lines 1 and 2:

Formal:	A possible interpretation:
1. Pa	Elroy Fox has bronchitis
2. $Pa \rightarrow Qa$	if Elroy Fox has bronchitis, then Elroy Fox coughs
3. Qa	Elroy Fox coughs.

---

[165] Each axiom and each rule can be formulated as a definition. Here are two examples. We *could* define the term "Axiom 1" as follows: A formula α *is an Axiom 1* iff there is a formula β such that $\alpha \equiv \beta \vee \beta \rightarrow \beta$. Likewise, the rule Modus ponens could be put in the following way: A formula α_3 emerges from the *application of Modus ponens* to the formulas α_1 and α_2 iff there are formulas α and β such that $\alpha_1 \equiv \alpha$ and $\alpha_2 \equiv \alpha \rightarrow \beta$ and $\alpha_3 \equiv \beta$. Thus, the application of the calculus would consist in the application of ten definitions. A far-reaching philosophical consequence of this recognition is that *logic is a particular language put forth by definitions*. It has no other, profound source.

Table 35. A classical, predicate-logical calculus of the first order with identity. The term "axiom" originates from the Greek $\alpha\xi\iota\omega\mu\alpha$, meaning "the required" or "requirement". An axiom is a claim which is deemed to be true without explicit proof. But of course, all axioms of logic are provably true. They are *valid* formulas

Axioms:	Their names:

Every formula of the following form is an axiom:

$\alpha \vee \alpha \rightarrow \alpha$	Axiom 1
$\alpha \rightarrow \alpha \vee \beta$	Axiom 2
$\alpha \vee \beta \rightarrow \beta \vee \alpha$	Axiom 3
$(\alpha \rightarrow \beta) \rightarrow (\gamma \vee \alpha \rightarrow \gamma \vee \beta)$	Axiom 4
$x = x$	Identity Axiom 1
$t = x \rightarrow (\alpha \rightarrow \beta)$ $\big[$if $\mathrm{Subst}(\alpha,\, x,\, t,\, \beta)\big]$	Identity Axiom 2
$\alpha \rightarrow \exists x \alpha$	$\exists$-Introduction Axiom

Rules:

Every transformation of the following form is a rule:

α $\dfrac{\alpha \rightarrow \beta}{\beta}$	Modus (ponendo) ponens ($\equiv$ MP) ($\equiv$ Detachment Rule)
$\dfrac{\alpha \rightarrow \beta}{\exists x \alpha \rightarrow \beta}$ $\big[$if $\mathrm{Subst}(\alpha,\, x,\, t,\, \beta)\big]$	$\exists$-Introduction Rule
$\dfrac{\alpha}{\beta}$ $\big[$if $\mathrm{Subst}(\alpha,\, x,\, t,\, \beta)\big]$	Substitution Rule

The rule Modus ponens thus enables an operation of detachment, i.e., detaching the consequent Qa from the antecedent Pa in line 2, without which the inference of line 3 from the preceding lines 1 and 2 would not occur.

Deduction and deducibility

We are now in a position to introduce a syntactic concept that may replace the semantic concept of inference. In order to be distinguishable from its semantic counterpart, it is called *deduction, derivation,* or *proof*. We will show below that both concepts are indeed equivalent.

Definition 223 (Deduction, derivation, proof). *Let $\mathfrak{F}$ be a set of $m \geq 0$ formulas. A finite sequence $\alpha_1, \ldots, \alpha_n$ of $n \geq 1$ formulas listed horizontally or vertically:*

α_1

α_2

$\vdots$

α_n

is a deduction *or* derivation *from* $\mathfrak{F}$, *or* a proof, *iff each formula α_i of the sequence is an element of $\mathfrak{F}$, called a* premise, *or an axiom of the calculus, or emerges from applying some rules of the calculus to some preceding formulas.*

We shall represent a deduction as a vertical list like the one above. Members of the formula set $\mathfrak{F}$ mentioned in the definition are called *premises*. Note that $\mathfrak{F}$ is allowed to be empty. In such a case the deduction has no premises.

To keep a deduction easily understandable, it is recommended to number its formulas consecutively on the left and to briefly comment on the right-hand side to make clear where they come from. For example, the comment on the right-hand side of line 3 in the following deduction indicates that this line has emerged from applying Modus ponens to lines 1 and 2:

1. Pa Premise (i.e., $\in \mathfrak{F}$)
2. $Pa \rightarrow Pa \vee Qa$ Axiom 2
3. $Pa \vee Qa$ Modus ponens: 1, 2.

Definition 224 (Deducibility, derivability, provability). *Let $\mathfrak{F}$ be a set of $m \geq 0$ formulas. A formula α is* deducible *or* derivable *from $\mathfrak{F}$ iff:*

1. *there is a deduction $\alpha_1, \ldots, \alpha_n$ from $\mathfrak{F}$ such that*
2. *α is its final formula, i.e., $\alpha \equiv \alpha_n$.*

The clause $\alpha \equiv \alpha_n$ of this definition means that the final formula of a deduction is said to be *deducible from $\mathfrak{F}$*. For instance, from the deduction above we may say that $Pa \vee Qa$ is deducible from $\{Pa\}$. Deducible from $\mathfrak{F}$ is what we have, semantically, called the conclusion or consequence of an inference. An additional example may illustrate:

Assertion 7. *$\exists x Px$ is deducible from $\{Pa\}$. (A possible interpretation of this assertion is: From the statement "Elroy Fox has bronchitis" it is deducible that "there is someone who has bronchitis".)*

Proof 7:

1. Pa Premise
2. $Px \rightarrow \exists x Px$ $\exists$-Introduction Axiom
3. $Pa \rightarrow \exists x Px$ Substitution Rule: 2
4. $\exists x Px$ Modus ponens: 1, 3. QED

Note that in this deduction the set of premises, $\mathfrak{F}$, is $\{Pa\}$. The acronym "QED" at the end of the proof abbreviates the scholastic dictum "quod erat demonstrandum" meaning "the thing that was to prove". Traditionally, it marks the end of a proof.

To simplify the representation of assertions, proofs, and other technicalities, we shall symbolize the term "is deducible from" by "⊢". Thus, the expression "$\mathfrak{F} \vdash \alpha$" says that α is deducible from $\mathfrak{F}$. If $\mathfrak{F}$ is empty, we write $\varnothing \vdash \alpha$ instead of $\mathfrak{F} \vdash \alpha$. Such a deducibility claim means that the deduction of α does not require any premises; α is deducible simply from 'nothingness'.

Definition 225 (Deducibility is symbolized by "⊢").

1. $\mathfrak{F} \vdash \alpha$ iff α is deducible from $\mathfrak{F}$. (*See Definition 224.*)
2. $\alpha_1, \ldots, \alpha_n \vdash \alpha$ iff $\{\alpha_1, \ldots, \alpha_n\} \vdash \alpha$.
3. $\varnothing \vdash \alpha$ iff $\mathfrak{F} \vdash \alpha$ and $\mathfrak{F} = \varnothing$.
4. $\vdash \alpha$ iff $\varnothing \vdash \alpha$.

Assertion 8 (Deducibility of Axiom 1). $\vdash \alpha \vee \alpha \to \alpha$

Proof 8:

1. $\alpha \vee \alpha \to \alpha$ \qquad\qquad Axiom 1. QED

In this example, set $\mathfrak{F}$ is empty. It shows that an axiom of the calculus is, according to Definition 224, deducible ex nihilo. A formula that is deducible from the empty set is simply called a deducible, derivable, or provable formula. We shall encounter additional examples below.

Derived rules

Sometimes deductions may become too extensive, cumbersome, and tedious. But they can be shortened and simplified by employing so-called derived rules. A *derived rule* is a rule that has already been proven by a previous deduction. This may be illustrated by an example. We shall first prove a derived rule and shall then demonstrate how to use it. It is referred to as the *Chain Rule* because it chains conditionals to each other and belongs to a large class of such chain rules. A number of important derived rules are listed in Table 36.

Assertion 9 (Chain Rule). $\alpha \to \beta, \beta \to \gamma \vdash \alpha \to \gamma$

Proof 9:

1. $\alpha \to \beta$ \qquad\qquad Premise
2. $\beta \to \gamma$ \qquad\qquad Premise
3. $(\beta \to \gamma) \to (\neg\alpha \vee \beta \to \neg\alpha \vee \gamma)$ \qquad Axiom 4
4. $(\neg\alpha \vee \beta \to \neg\alpha \vee \gamma)$ \qquad MP: 2, 3
   $\equiv (\alpha \to \beta) \to (\alpha \to \gamma)$ \qquad (by definition of $\to$ in Definition 206)
5. $\alpha \to \gamma$ \qquad\qquad Modus ponens: 1, 4. QED

Table 36. Some derived predicate-logical rules and their names

Derived rules, theorems:	Their names:
1. $\vdash \alpha \vee \neg\alpha$	Principle of Excluded Middle
2. $\vdash \neg(\alpha \wedge \neg\alpha)$	Principle of Non-Contradiction
3. $\vdash \alpha \rightarrow \alpha$	Autoconditionalization
4. $\alpha \vdash \neg\neg\alpha$	Double Negation
5. $\neg\neg\alpha \vdash \alpha$	Double Negation
6. $\alpha \rightarrow \beta \vdash \neg\beta \rightarrow \neg\alpha$	Contraposition Rule
7. $\alpha, \neg\alpha \vdash \beta$	Ex Contradictione Quodlibet,
	($\equiv$ Ex Falso Quodlibet),
	($\equiv$ Principle of Explosion)
8. $\alpha \wedge \beta \vdash \alpha$	$\wedge$-Elimination
9. $\alpha \wedge \beta \vdash \beta$	$\wedge$-Elimination
10. $\alpha, \beta \vdash \alpha \wedge \beta$	$\wedge$-Introduction
11. $\alpha \vdash \alpha \vee \beta$	$\vee$-Introduction
12. $\alpha \rightarrow \beta, \neg\beta \vdash \neg\alpha$	Modus (tollendo) tollens
13. $(\alpha \rightarrow \beta \wedge \neg\beta) \vdash \neg\alpha$	Reductio ad absurdum
14. $\alpha \wedge \beta \rightarrow \gamma \vdash \alpha \rightarrow (\beta \rightarrow \gamma)$	Exportation Rule
15. $\alpha \rightarrow (\beta \rightarrow \gamma) \vdash \alpha \wedge \beta \rightarrow \gamma$	Importation Rule
16. $\alpha \rightarrow (\beta \rightarrow \gamma) \vdash \beta \rightarrow (\alpha \rightarrow \gamma)$	Permutation of Antecedents
17. $\alpha \rightarrow \beta, \beta \rightarrow \gamma \vdash \alpha \rightarrow \gamma$	Chain Rule
18. $\alpha_1 \rightarrow \alpha_2, \alpha_2 \rightarrow \alpha_3, \ldots, \alpha_{n-1} \rightarrow \alpha_n \vdash \alpha_1 \rightarrow \alpha_n$	Chain Rule
19. $\alpha \leftrightarrow \beta \vdash (\alpha \rightarrow \beta) \wedge (\beta \rightarrow \alpha)$	$\leftrightarrow$-Elimination
20. $\alpha \leftrightarrow \beta \vdash \alpha \rightarrow \beta$	$\leftrightarrow$-Elimination
21. $\alpha \leftrightarrow \beta \vdash \beta \rightarrow \alpha$	$\leftrightarrow$-Elimination
22. $(\alpha \rightarrow \beta) \wedge (\beta \rightarrow \alpha) \vdash \alpha \leftrightarrow \beta$	$\leftrightarrow$-Introduction
23. $\vdash t = t$	Reflexivity of Identity
24. $\vdash t_1 = t_2 \rightarrow t_2 = t_1$	Symmetry of Identity
25. $\vdash t_1 = t_2 \wedge t_2 = t_3 \rightarrow t_1 = t_3$	Transitivity of Identity
26. $\alpha \vdash \forall x \alpha$	$\forall$-Introduction
27. $\alpha \vdash \forall x_1 \ldots \forall x_n \alpha$	Iterated $\forall$-Introduction
28. $\forall x \alpha \vdash \alpha$	$\forall$-Elimination
29. $\forall x_1 \ldots \forall x_n \alpha \vdash \alpha$	Iterated $\forall$-Elimination

Whenever needed in the course of a deduction, one may use the Chain Rule in order not to repeat the Proof 9 within that deduction. A derived rule is used like any other rule of the calculus. For example, using the Chain Rule we will now explain why Elroy Fox does not sleep well when he has a bad cold. To this end, we assemble our vocabulary:

α	$\equiv$	Elroy Fox has a bad cold
β	$\equiv$	Elroy Fox has fever
γ	$\equiv$	Elroy Fox sleeps well
$\alpha \rightarrow \beta$	$\equiv$	If Elroy Fox has a bad cold, then Elroy Fox has fever
$\beta \rightarrow \neg\gamma$	$\equiv$	If Elroy Fox has fever, then Elroy Fox does not sleep well
$\alpha \rightarrow \neg\gamma$	$\equiv$	If Elroy Fox has a bad cold, then he does not sleep well.

Assertion 10 (Why is Elroy Fox sleepless?). $\alpha \rightarrow \beta, \beta \rightarrow \neg\gamma \vdash \alpha \rightarrow \neg\gamma$

Proof 10:

1. $\alpha \rightarrow \beta$ Premise
2. $\beta \rightarrow \neg\gamma$ Premise
3. $\alpha \rightarrow \neg\gamma$ Chain Rule: 1, 2. QED

Derived rules of the type above may be added to the calculus to enlarge its tools and to facilitate deductions. There is a variety of such derived rules a few of which may be found in Table 36 on page 895. A derived rule is also called a *theorem*. In general, a formula is said to be a theorem of the calculus if it is provable by means of the calculus.

To give a second example, by using the penultimate rule mentioned in Table 36, i.e., the rule of ∀-Elimination, we will prove a historically famous assertion originating with Aristotle. He himself was unable to prove his assertion because, as we pointed out in footnote 155 on page 845, he didn't have a genuine logic at his disposal. Consider the following: Why is Socrates mortal? Because all human beings are mortal, and Socrates is a human being; So, Socrates is mortal. We read: $Px \equiv x$ is a human being; $Qx \equiv x$ is mortal; $a \equiv$ Socrates.

Assertion 11 (Socrates is mortal). $\forall x(Px \rightarrow Qx), Pa \vdash Qa$

Proof 11:

1. $\forall x(Px \rightarrow Qx)$ Premise
2. Pa Premise
3. $Px \rightarrow Qx$ ∀-Elimination: 1
4. $Pa \rightarrow Qa$ Substitution Rule: 3
5. Qa Modus ponens: 2, 4. QED

A premise may be introduced at any point in a deduction when it is needed. For example, the above proof may be rewritten as follows:

1. $\forall x(Px \rightarrow Qx)$ Premise
2. $Px \rightarrow Qx$ ∀-Elimination: 1
3. $Pa \rightarrow Qa$ Substitution Rule: 2
4. Pa Premise
5. Qa Modus ponens: 3, 4. QED

In closing this section, an example may demonstrate that the logic we have sketched thus far is indeed also a logic of identities, i.e., identity logic. The example deals with Anna Freud and her father Sigmund Freud. Someone may assert: From the statement "Sigmund Freud is a psychoanalyst and the father of Anna Freud is Sigmund Freud" it is deducible that "the father of Anna Freud is a psychoanalyst". We read: $a \equiv$ Sigmund Freud; $b \equiv$ Anna Freud; $P \equiv$ is a psychoanalyst; $f \equiv$ father of.

Assertion 12 (Anna Freud's father is a psychoanalyst). $Pa \wedge fb = a \vdash Pfb$

Proof 12:

1. $Pa \wedge fb = a$	Premise
2. Pa	$\wedge$-Elimination: 1
3. $fb = a$	$\wedge$-Elimination: 1
4. $fb = x \rightarrow (Px \rightarrow Pfb)$	Identity Axiom 2
5. $fb = a \rightarrow (Pa \rightarrow Pfb)$	Substitution Rule: 4
6. $Pa \rightarrow Pfb$	Modus ponens: 3, 5
7. Pfb	Modus ponens: 2, 6. QED

Predicate-logical equivalence

While interviewing Elroy Fox, his family doctor asserts the diagnostic hypothesis that "Elroy Fox has hepatitis or he has gallstones". His student has a different opinion and suggests that "If Elroy Fox does not have hepatitis, then he has gallstones". The doctor counters: "That is exactly what I said. Your opinion is not different from mine. Our diagnoses are predicate-logically equivalent". What does he mean?

Two formulas are predicate-logically equivalent if and only if they always have the same truth values. That is the case if the biconditional that carries them on its left and right side is derivable, i.e., a theorem.

Definition 226 (Predicate-logical equivalence). α *is* equivalent *to* β *iff* $\vdash \alpha \leftrightarrow \beta$.

Due to this relationship, two equivalent formulas may be exchanged for each other in every context. A few derived rules of this type are listed in Table 37 on page 898. The ninth theorem demonstrates that the doctor above was right. His diagnostic hypothesis and that of his student are equivalent, and thus, interchangeable in every context.

Sentential logic

A minor subset of the predicate calculus introduced in preceding sections is separable from the remainder and constitutes an elementary, weak, independent logic that has come to be known as "the logic of sentences", *sentential logic,* sentence logic, or propositional logic. Its language, referred to as the *sentential language* $\mathcal{L}_0$, is based on the miniature alphabet (230):

$$\text{The alphabet of } \mathcal{L}_0 = \{\neg, \vee, \alpha, \beta, \gamma, \ldots, \alpha_1, \alpha_2, \ldots\} \tag{230}$$

being a subset of the alphabet of the language $\mathcal{L}_1$ such that the connectives $\neg$ and $\vee$ are its only logical signs, and $\alpha, \beta, \gamma, \ldots, \alpha_1, \alpha_2, \ldots$ are sentence variables. Formulas in $\mathcal{L}_0$ are defined as follows:

Table 37. Some predicate-logical equivalences and their names

Theorems:	Their names:
1. $\vdash \alpha \leftrightarrow \alpha$	Autobiconditionalization
2. $\vdash \alpha \leftrightarrow \neg\neg\alpha$	Double Negation
3. $\vdash (\alpha \rightarrow \beta) \leftrightarrow (\neg\beta \rightarrow \neg\alpha)$	Contraposition Rule
4. $\vdash (\alpha \wedge \beta \rightarrow \gamma) \leftrightarrow (\alpha \rightarrow (\beta \rightarrow \gamma))$	Exportation / Importaion
5. $\vdash (\alpha \wedge \beta \rightarrow \gamma) \leftrightarrow (\alpha \rightarrow \gamma) \vee (\beta \rightarrow \gamma)$	Antecedent Split
6. $\vdash (\alpha \vee \beta \rightarrow \gamma) \leftrightarrow (\alpha \rightarrow \gamma) \wedge (\beta \rightarrow \gamma)$	Antecedent Split
7. $\vdash (\alpha \rightarrow \beta \wedge \gamma) \leftrightarrow (\alpha \rightarrow \beta) \wedge (\alpha \rightarrow \gamma)$	Consequent Split
8. $\vdash (\neg\alpha \vee \beta) \leftrightarrow (\alpha \rightarrow \beta)$	Equivalence of $\neg\vee$ and $\rightarrow$
9. $\vdash (\alpha \vee \beta) \leftrightarrow (\neg\alpha \rightarrow \beta)$	Equivalence of $\vee$ and $\neg \rightarrow$
10. $\vdash \neg(\alpha \wedge \beta) \leftrightarrow (\neg\alpha \vee \neg\beta)$	De Morgan's Law
11. $\vdash \neg(\alpha \vee \beta) \leftrightarrow (\neg\alpha \wedge \neg\beta)$	De Morgan's Law
12. $\vdash (\alpha \wedge \beta) \leftrightarrow (\beta \wedge \alpha)$	Commutative Law ($\wedge$)
13. $\vdash (\alpha \vee \beta) \leftrightarrow (\beta \vee \alpha)$	Commutative Law ($\vee$)
14. $\vdash (\alpha \wedge \beta) \wedge \gamma \leftrightarrow \alpha \wedge (\beta \wedge \gamma)$	Associative Law ($\wedge$)
15. $\vdash (\alpha \vee \beta) \vee \gamma \leftrightarrow \alpha \vee (\beta \vee \gamma)$	Associative Law ($\vee$)
16. $\vdash \alpha \wedge (\beta \vee \gamma) \leftrightarrow (\alpha \wedge \beta) \vee (\alpha \wedge \gamma)$	Distributive Law
17. $\vdash \alpha \vee (\beta \wedge \gamma) \leftrightarrow (\alpha \vee \beta) \wedge (\alpha \vee \gamma)$	Distributive Law
18. $\vdash \forall x \alpha \leftrightarrow \neg \exists x \neg\alpha$	Equivalence of $\forall$ and $\neg\exists\neg$
19. $\vdash \exists x \alpha \leftrightarrow \neg \forall x \neg\alpha$	Equivalence of $\exists$ and $\neg\forall\neg$

Definition 227 (Formulas in the sentential language $\mathcal{L}_0$).

  1. Every variable α is a formula.
  2. If α is a formula, then $\neg\alpha$ is a formula.
  3. If α and β are formulas, then $\alpha \vee \beta$ is a formula.

The connectives $\wedge$, $\rightarrow$, and $\leftrightarrow$ are defined by $\neg$ and $\vee$ as in Definition 206 on page 865. The calculus consists of Axioms 1–4 and Modus ponens mentioned in the predicate calculus (Table 38).

As its syntax demonstrates, it is a logic of sentential connectives $\neg, \vee, \wedge, \rightarrow$, and $\leftrightarrow$. Its language *does not contain* the equality sign and quantifiers. Thus, it does not deal with identities and quantificational formulas. For example, those proofs in the foregoing sections in which quantifiers or identities are syntactically manipulated, require the entire predicate calculus. It is impossible to carry out such proofs by using the sentential logic alone. See, for example, Proofs 11–12. But Proofs 8–10 are purely sentential-logical ones.

26.2.4 Metalogic

Part V of this handbook is devoted to the question of whether there is a 'logic of medicine' and what kind of logic is the most appropriate one for use in medicine. To this end, we need to know something about the properties of the logics we are studying in the present Part VIII. A preliminary, important note may be in order. Always distinguish clearly the following three concepts:

Table 38. Classical Sentential Calculus. This logic is a subset of the classical predicate logic displayed in Table 35 on page 892

Axioms:	Their names:
Every formula of the following form is an axiom:	
$\alpha \vee \alpha \rightarrow \alpha$	Axiom 1
$\alpha \rightarrow \alpha \vee \beta$	Axiom 2
$\alpha \vee \beta \rightarrow \beta \vee \alpha$	Axiom 3
$(\alpha \rightarrow \beta) \rightarrow (\gamma \vee \alpha \rightarrow \gamma \vee \beta)$	Axiom 4

Rule:

The only rule of this logic is:

$$\frac{\begin{array}{l}\alpha \\ \alpha \rightarrow \beta\end{array}}{\beta}$$

Modus (ponendo) ponens
($\equiv$ MP)
($\equiv$ Detachment rule)

a. inference or implication: $\vDash$
b. provability, derivability, or deduction: $\vdash$
c. conditional: $\rightarrow$.

The first one is a semantic-metalinguistic concept; the second one is a syntactic-metalinguistic concept; and the third one is the object-linguistic *if-then* relation. To prevent confusion of object-level with meta-level, never call the if-then relation an "implication", and avoid reading "$\alpha \rightarrow \beta$" as "α implies β".

A logic may constitute the subject of investigation by an inquiry into its properties, virtues, and shortcomings. Both the investigation as well as the metatheory it yields about that logic have come to be termed "metalogic". For example, regarding the predicate calculus sketched above one may ask whether it is *sound, complete, decidable, consistent,* etc. Metalogical assertions about such features are usually referred to as metatheorems. We shall briefly mention a few useful metatheorems about our predicate calculus in the following sections:

▶ Soundness and completeness
▶ Deduction and Validity Theorems
▶ Decidability
▶ Consistency.

Their proofs will be omitted because they are too technical. For details and proofs, see (Barwise, 1977, Hermes, 1995; Shoenfield, 2001).

Soundness and completeness

The question whether the calculus is sound and complete asks whether the calculus emulates the semantic concept of inference correctly and completely. The following two metatheorems show that the answer is Yes.

Metatheorem 1 (Soundness). *Let $\mathfrak{F}$ be a set of closed formulas and α be any formula. Then:*

$$\text{If } \mathfrak{F} \vdash \alpha, \text{ then } \mathfrak{F} \vDash \alpha.$$

Note that this metatheorem, as well as the following one, applies to closed formulas, i.e., to formulas without free variables, and thus 'sentences' in terms of natural language. It states that whenever a formula is deducible from some closed formulas, it follows therefrom. Otherwise put, in the set of closed formulas, the syntactic relation $\vdash$ imitates the semantic relation $\vDash$ soundly.

Metatheorem 2 (Completeness). *Let $\mathfrak{F}$ be a set of closed formulas and α be any formula. Then:*

$$\text{If } \mathfrak{F} \vDash \alpha, \text{ then } \mathfrak{F} \vdash \alpha.$$

This metatheorem says that our predicate calculus presented above is a complete system in that every sentence that semantically *follows* from some premises, can be *deduced* therefrom syntactically.[166] The two Metatheorems 1 and 2 above yield the following biconditional:

$$\mathfrak{F} \vdash \alpha \text{ iff } \mathfrak{F} \vDash \alpha \qquad \text{(Soundness and completeness)} \qquad (231)$$

That means that in the set of closed formulas of the first-order language $\mathcal{L}_1$, syntactic deduction $\vdash$ is equivalent to semantic inference $\vDash$ and may thus replace it.

---

[166] The proof of completeness of a logic system was carried out for the first time by the Austrian-born mathematician and logician Kurt Gödel (Gödel, 1930). Gödel was born in 1906 in what is now Brno in the Czech Republic. He went through Czech, Austrian, German, and U.S.-American citizenships until he died in Princeton in 1978. Some people consider him 'one of the three greatest logicians of all times with Aristotle and Gottlob Frege'. Among his achievements is his legendary proof of his incompleteness theorems (Gödel, 1931; Nagel and Newman, 1958) according to which arithmetic, and a fortiori mathematics, cannot be made part of logic. This was a refutation of Bertrand Russell and Whitehead's logicist claim in their *Principia Mathematica* that "all pure mathematics follows from purely logical premises and uses only concepts definable in logical terms" (Russell, 1969, 74).

Deduction and Validity Theorems

The following is an additional metatheorem that establishes a very useful relationship:

Metatheorem 3 (Deduction Theorem 1). *Let $\mathfrak{F} \cup \alpha$ be a set of closed formulas and β be any formula. Then:*

$$\mathfrak{F} \cup \alpha \vdash \beta \text{ iff } \mathfrak{F} \vdash \alpha \rightarrow \beta.$$

This central metatheorem of predicate logic says that whenever a formula β is deducible from some set $\mathfrak{F} \cup \alpha$ of formulas, then the conditional $\alpha \rightarrow \beta$ is deducible from the reduced set $\mathfrak{F}$ of formulas alone. For instance, it is true that:

{If someone has bronchitis, then she coughs; Elroy Fox has bronchitis} $\vdash$ Elroy Fox coughs.

Now, by Deduction Theorem 1 we can justifiably assert that:

{If someone has bronchitis, then she coughs} $\vdash$ Elroy Fox has bronchitis → he coughs.

That is, the statement that whenever someone has bronchitis, then she coughs, implies that if Elroy Fox has bronchitis, then he coughs. Deduction Theorem 1 is in essence the conditionalization of the consequence of an argument with *any* of the premises of the argument as antecedent. A second, interesting, and more general metatheorem can easily be obtained therefrom:

Metatheorem 4 (Deduction Theorem 2). *Let $\alpha_1, \ldots, \alpha_n$ be closed formulas and β be any formula. Then:*

$$\alpha_1, \ldots, \alpha_n \vdash \beta \text{ iff } \vdash \alpha_1 \wedge \ldots \wedge \alpha_n \rightarrow \beta.$$

To illustrate, from the above example we can conclude:

$\vdash$ (If someone has bronchitis, then she coughs) $\wedge$ Elroy Fox has bronchitis → Elroy Fox coughs.

That is, a deduction from something is equivalent to the deduction of its conditionalized consequence from nothing. The significance of the Deduction Theorems 1–2 will become clear after considering the following metatheorem that establishes a relationship between semantic inference and validity.

Metatheorem 5 (Validity Theorem 1). $\models \alpha$ *iff α is valid.*

That means that a sentence that follows from nothingness is valid, e.g., "if Elroy Fox has bronchitis, then he has bronchitis". From all metatheorems above we obtain this important metatheorem:

Metatheorem 6 (Validity Theorem 2).

1. $\alpha_1, \ldots, \alpha_n \vdash \beta$ iff $\alpha_1 \wedge \ldots \wedge \alpha_n \to \beta$ is valid.
2. $\alpha_1, \ldots, \alpha_n \vDash \beta$ iff $\alpha_1 \wedge \ldots \wedge \alpha_n \to \beta$ is valid.
3. $\vdash \alpha$ iff α is valid.

Part 3 of this metatheorem says that what is deducible is universally valid. That is, deducibility (derivability, provability) is equivalent to universal validity. Otherwise put, the predicate calculus produces syntactically what is semantically valid. It identifies formal or *logical truths*. As we have already pointed out previously, however, "valid" and "logical truth" are always relative to a particular logic. In different logics they may look different. On this account, we can more correctly state that the first-order predicate logic identifies predicate-logical truths, i.e., truths in the language $\mathcal{L}_1$.

Decidability

The metatheorems above enable us to assess the significance of the decidability problem. A logic is said to be *decidable* if and only if there exists an algorithm such that for every formula of that logic the algorithm is capable of deciding in a finite number of steps whether or not the formula is a theorem of the calculus, i.e., deducible therefrom. In this case, the formula would be, according to Metatheorem 6.3, semantically valid and thus a *logical truth*. Unfortunately, the first-order predicate logic as a whole is not decidable. That means a fortiori that due to the Deduction Theorems above there is no *algorithm* by means of which one could decide whether from a particular set of premises a particular formula is deducible or not. However, considered separately, some parts of the calculus are decidable. Three such parts are briefly mentioned below. (For the term "algorithm", see footnote 9 on page 47.)

a. As was mentioned on page 897, a subset of the calculus comprising Axioms 1–4 and Modus ponens constitutes a minor, independent logic called *sentential logic* and displayed in Table 38 on page 899. This minor logic is decidable because the truth table construction provides such a decision algorithm. Valid formulas in sentential logic are just tautologies. To find out whether a formula is a tautology, examine it by a truth table.

b. The so-called *monadic first-order logic* is decidable. This is that subset of the first-order predicate calculus whose language contains only unary predicates. By adding a single many-place predicate, e.g., "loves", it becomes undecidable.

c. If all predicates are eliminated from the language $\mathcal{L}_1$ except the equality sign, the remaining logic, i.e., the *identity logic*, is decidable. It constitutes *the* logic of classical mathematics.

Consistency

An additional metalogical concern is the question whether the predicate calculus is consistent. As it turns out, the answer is Yes. From the perspective of classical logic, nothing in the world is more catastrophic than inconsistency. On that account, therefore, inconsistency is to be strictly avoided. However, a brief explanation will show that this long-standing inconsistency phobia is self-made, is of an Aristotelean origin, and is something that we could in principle live without.

Two sentences are said to *contradict* each other, or to be *contradictory,* if one is the negation of the other, e.g., α and $\neg\alpha$. A conjunction of two contradictory sentences of the form $\alpha \wedge \neg\alpha$ is referred to as a *contradiction.* An example is the statement "Elroy Fox has diabetes and he does not have diabetes". Due to the meaning of the particles "and" and "not" in natural languages, a contradiction is commonly considered not to be true. This is also reflected in the semantics of the languages $\mathcal{L}_0$ and $\mathcal{L}_1$, and the definitions of $\neg$ and $\wedge$. See pages 883–885. Accordingly, a truth table will easily verify that a contradiction:

$$\alpha \wedge \neg\alpha \hspace{6cm} \text{(Contradiction)}$$

is unsatisfiable because it is false in all circumstances. Advising against such vain falsehoods, Aristotle states in his *Metaphysics* "It is impossible at once to be and not to be" (ibid., Book III, 996 b 27–30), and further, "It is impossible for the same attribute at once to belong and not to belong to the same thing and in the same relation" (ibid., Book IV, 1005 b 19–23). Both statements are alternative formulations of the Aristotelean Principle of Non-Contradiction:

$$\neg(\alpha \wedge \neg\alpha) \hspace{4cm} \text{(Principle of Non-Contradiction)}$$

to prohibit contradictions. This principle has entered the predicate logic in that it is a predicate-logical theorem, i.e., $\vdash \neg(\alpha \wedge \neg\alpha)$ and as such, is valid. The same applies to his Principle of Excluded Middle:

$$\alpha \vee \neg\alpha \hspace{5cm} \text{(Principle of Excluded Middle)}$$

It is a predicate-logical theorem, i.e., $\vdash \alpha \vee \neg\alpha$. These considerations together with the Aristotelean bivalence of classical predicate logic justify its characterization as a logic of Aristotelean type. Note that the two principles above are equivalent: $\vdash \neg(\alpha \wedge \neg\alpha) \leftrightarrow (\alpha \vee \neg\alpha)$. They have already been mentioned on pages 831, 875, and in Table 36 on page 895.

A set of $n \geq 1$ formulas, $\mathfrak{F}$, is said to be inconsistent if and only if there exists a contradiction $\alpha \wedge \neg\alpha$ that is derivable therefrom, or equivalently, if and only if there are two contradictory formulas, α and $\neg\alpha$, which are derivable therefrom. An example is the following set of sentences: {All diabetics have hyperglycemia; Elroy Fox is a diabetic and does not have hyperglycemia}. This is an inconsistent set of sentences because it implies a contradiction: "Elroy

Fox has hyperglycemia and he does not have hyperglycemia". To prove this, we read: $P \equiv$ is a diabetic; $Q \equiv$ has hyperglycemia; and $a \equiv$ Elroy Fox.

Assertion 13 (An inconsistency). $\{\forall x(Px \rightarrow Qx), Pa \wedge \neg Qa\}$ *is inconsistent. That is, it implies a contradiction.*

Proof 13:

1.	$\forall x(Px \rightarrow Qx)$	Premise
2.	$Pa \wedge \neg Qa$	Premise
3.	Pa	$\wedge$-Elimination: 2
4.	$Px \rightarrow Qx$	$\forall$-Elimination: 1
5.	$Pa \rightarrow Qa$	Substitution Rule: 4
6.	Qa	Modus ponens: 3, 5
7.	$\neg Qa$	$\wedge$-Elimination: 2
8.	$Qa \wedge \neg Qa$	$\wedge$-Introduction: 6, 7. QED

By implying contradictions, inconsistent premises imply *everything,* be they true, false, reasonable, unreasonable, or even non-sensical. To demonstrate, the proof above will be continued. Let the numbers "2" and "33" be symbolized by the individual constants "b" and "c", respectively; and let the function symbol "f" designate the binary summation operation "+". Then $f(b, b) = c$ stands for $2 + 2 = 33$. This wrong assertion is implied by the above premises in the following way:

9.	$f(b, b) = c$	Ex Contradictione Quodlibet: 6, 7. QED

This fact trivializes inconsistent premises. It demonstrates that they say 'all and nothing'. Thus, in the realm of classical logic the inconsistency of a system leads to its breakdown. This is why classical logic is inconsistency intolerant and highly values consistency. The following definition implies that a system is *consistent* if there is at least one formula that is not deducible therefrom:

Definition 228 (Consistency and inconsistency).

1. *A set of formulas, $\mathfrak{F}$, is inconsistent iff every formula α is a theorem of $\mathfrak{F}$, i.e., iff $\mathfrak{F} \vdash \alpha$ for $\forall \alpha$.*
2. *A set of formulas, $\mathfrak{F}$, is consistent iff it is not inconsistent. That is, iff there is a formula α such that $\mathfrak{F} \nvdash \alpha$, where "$\nvdash$" is the negation of "$\vdash$".*

To prevent inconsistency, one only needs to use logic systems which are immune against rules of the type 'Ex Contradictione Quodlibet'. There are indeed such logics that we shall study in Section 28.3 on page 961.

26.2.5 Summary

In preceding sections we have provided an overview of classical first-order predicate logic with identity and some of its metalogical properties. Although it is a powerful logic, it is not powerful enough to satisfy all logical needs in science. A simple example may demonstrate how challenging the situation is. In natural languages we not only talk about individuals in that we say, for example, that a particular patient has endemic thalassemia, but also about groups of people. We say, for instance:

> There is a Mediterranean population whose members have en-
> demic thalassemia. $\qquad$ (232)

We can easily show why even this simple sentence goes beyond the first-order predicate logic. We may recall that this logic is a theory of deduction in the first-order language $\mathcal{L}_1$. As was emphasized on page 873, the only variables in $\mathcal{L}_1$ are individual variables such as x, y, z, etc. They range over individual objects and are therefore called first-order variables. Thus, the quantifiers $\exists$ and $\forall$ in $\mathcal{L}_1$ bind only first-order variables, for instance, $\forall x Q x$. Predicates and function symbols take terms as arguments like in Qx and $f(x) = y$.

A language may also contain second-order variables, third-order variables, and so on. When it does, it is called a second-order language, a third-order language, and so on. The example sentence (232) above belongs to a second-order language, $\mathcal{L}_2$, because it contains a second-order variable. It says:

> There is a P such that P is a Mediterranean population and its mem-
> bers have endemic thalassemia.

The second-order variable it contains, is the predicate variable P. As variables of the second order, predicate variables range over *sets* of individual objects, including *relations* between them. As our example above demonstrates, in a language of the second order or higher, (i) quantifiers bind predicate variables or function variables such as in the statement "$\exists P$ such that P is a Mediterranean population and its members have endemic thalassemia" that contains the bound predicate variable P; and (ii) predicates can also take such higher-order variables as arguments. This will be revealed by formalizing our example sentence to show that it is an $\mathcal{L}_2$ sentence:

> $\exists P(P$ is a Mediterranean population $\land \exists x(x$ is a member of $P \land x$ has endemic thalassemia$))$.

Let us write $M \equiv$ is a Mediterranean population; and $ET \equiv$ has endemic thalassemia. Thus we obtain:

> $\exists P(M(P) \land \exists x(Px \land ETx))$.

This string deviates from the syntax of $\mathcal{L}_1$ that we have fixed in Section 26.2.1, and is thus not a formula in $\mathcal{L}_1$. So, the predicate calculus we have studied cannot deal with strings of this type.

A logic of the language $\mathcal{L}_2$ is a second-order logic. A logic is higher-order if it is at least second-order. Unfortunately, however, a higher-order logic *cannot* be cast in a calculus. Gödel's incompleteness theorems referred to in footnote

166 on page 900 have demonstrated that a higher-order calculus is incomplete. That is, unlike a first-order logic, a higher-order logic cannot be axiomatized by a finite set of sentences. Thus, in higher-order languages the semantic inference ⊨ has no syntactic counterpart. Deduction and derivation in higher-order languages is impossible (see, e.g., van Benthem and Doets, 1983).

27

Modal Extensions of Classical Logic

27.0 Introduction

The classical first-order logic that we briefly covered in Chapter 26, is not a sufficient tool for use in medicine and also has some other shortcomings. Consequently, it must be extended, changed, amended, or abandoned. In this section, we shall address some of these concerns.

Classical first-order logic has emerged as the first system of modern logic, and as such, it has enjoyed extensive study and development. It is therefore usually identified with logic itself. Its principles, theorems, and laws are believed to be irrefutable and eternal truths. There are those who even maintain that "Dictators may be powerful today, but they cannot alter the laws of logic, nor indeed can God even do so" (Ewing, 1940, 217). This claim reflects a widespread error that we encounter not only in everyday life, but also in most scientific disciplines. However, in what follows we shall show that classical logic and its laws are not the final word.

As was pointed out previously, classical first-order logic has been constructed and extensively studied by mathematicians, and has been applied primarily in formalized areas such as mathematics. So, in addition to its characterization as 'modern', 'formal', and 'symbolic', it has come to be termed 'mathematical logic'. Due to its early development in mathematic departments, the main subjects of its concern have been metamathematical topics such as the soundness of mathematical reasoning, the concepts and methods of proof and deduction in mathematical sciences, axiomatizability and decidability of mathematical theories, computable functions, and the like. As a theory of the minor language $\mathcal{L}_1$ and a technique of reasoning in such confined languages, it has a limited scope, and thus, it is an insufficient logic for use in medical practice and research. We shall see below that the language of medicine is a powerful natural language and goes far beyond $\mathcal{L}_1$. Since it is much richer than $\mathcal{L}_1$, the inferences conducted in its non-$\mathcal{L}_1$ parts are not covered by classical predicate logic (see Figure 96).

K. Sadegh-Zadeh, *Handbook of Analytic Philosophy of Medicine*,
Philosophy and Medicine 113, DOI 10.1007/978-94-007-2260-6_27,
© Springer Science+Business Media B.V. 2012

Fig. 96. Only a minor subset of medical language is representable as an $\mathcal{L}_1$. The remainder extends far beyond $\mathcal{L}_1$, e.g., in diagnostics. Thus the question arises whether we should alter medical language and argumentation to fit classical logic, or change classical logic to fit medical language and argumentation. We prefer the latter alternative. No logic is sacrosanct

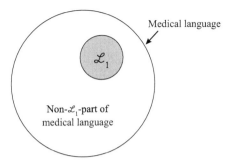

In the course of our study, we shall examine several reasons why we should either alter classical logic or replace it with another one. Here we will look at two specific reasons to do so. First, there are many valid arguments in medicine and everyday life which are not covered by classical logic. Suppose, for example, that in a particular clinical setting, a physician arrives at the following diagnostic conjecture:

- It is possible that the patient Elroy Fox has hepatitis, although I do not yet believe that he has. Rather, I am convinced that he has gallstones.

What can the physician predicate-logically infer from this diagnostic conjecture? The sobering answer is: nothing. The conjecture contains the following three expressions that are alien to the language $\mathcal{L}_1$ of predicate logic: "it is *possible* that", "I do not yet *believe* that", and "I am *convinced* that". These expressions are logical operators of a completely different type than the operators of predicate logic, i.e., connectives, universal quantifier, and existential quantifier. Consequently, predicate logic will not help. Thus it cannot serve as a sufficient diagnostic logic. For this purpose, it would need to be *extended* to include many additional operators.

Second, we have also emphasized on page 874 that first-order predicate logic is based on some classical, Aristotelean principles, e.g., Principles of Bivalence, Excluded Middle, and Non-Contradiction. In Chapters 28–30, we shall demonstrate that these age-old principles are objectionable and ought to be abandoned. Their abandonment, however, amounts to searching for an alternative, *non-classical* logic.

Both options are discussed in this chapter and the next. Several extensions of classical predicate logic are briefly introduced below, and we shall return to them in all other, seven parts of the book, I-VII. The extensions are newer systems of logic, called *modal logics,* that may be employed in medicine. Since they have originally been conceived by philosophers for philosophical purposes, and are intertwined with many philosophical problems, they have also been called *philosophical logics.* See (Gabbay and Guenthner, 1984; Gabbay and Woods, 2006; Goble, 2002; Jacquette, 2002).

Modal logics are increasingly becoming important as theoretical and practical tools in mathematics, computer science, artificial intelligence, linguistics, law, and other areas. They provide formal methods of reasoning about possibility and necessity, obligation and permission, knowledge and belief, and many other subjects. We will here outline a few representatives that are needed in Parts I–VII. To this end, we shall first explain the nature of these logics, and familiarize ourselves with some basic terminology. Consider the following example:

The patient Elroy Fox is icteric and does not feel well. He therefore consults his family physician. The doctor thinks that maybe Elroy Fox has hepatitis. Such a state of affairs may be qualified in a variety of ways. For instance, Elroy Fox's physician may utter *"possibly,* Elroy Fox has hepatitis", or equivalently *"it is possible that* Elroy Fox has hepatitis", while his wife may deplore *"regrettably,* Elroy has hepatitis", or equivalently *"it is regrettable that* Elroy has hepatitis". Such qualifications play a major role both in medical reasoning and in everyday life. To handle them adequately, they are conceived as *operations on sentences.* That is, instead of considering states of affairs themselves, we consider the sentences that represent them. Thus, let α be any sentence, e.g., the sentence "Elroy Fox has hepatitis" that denotes the state of affairs that Elroy Fox has hepatitis. It may be differently qualified by prefixing it with any particular word or phrase ∇, for example, the phrase "it is possible that" or "it is regrettable that" to obtain new sentences such as:

$$\text{it is possible that Elroy Fox has hepatitis,} \tag{233}$$

$$\text{it is regrettable that Elroy Fox has hepatitis,}$$

or in general:

$$\text{it is possible that } \alpha, \tag{234}$$

$$\text{it is regrettable that } \alpha.$$

The symbol "α" written above stands for any declarative sentence describing a state of affairs, while the state of affairs itself is outside of, or beyond, the written words. If the result of prefixing a sentence α with such a phrase ∇ *is itself a sentence* like (233) that talks about the *mode* of truth of the core sentence α, i.e., about how, when, where, under what circumstances, or with what effects α is true, then the phrase ∇ is said to represent a *modality,* and is therefore referred to as a *modal operator.* In the above-mentioned examples (233–234), the two italicized phrases are modal operators. The first one represents the modality of *possibility,* while the second one represents the modality of *regrettability.*

Let a modal operator such as "it is possible that" or "it is regrettable that" or any other one be symbolized by "∇". Its application to a sentence α yields a new sentence, $\nabla\alpha$, that is referred to as a *modal sentence.* Examples are the two modal sentences in (233) above. Modal operators generating such modal sentences are pervasive in highly developed natural languages such as English, German, French, and others. We shall look at the specifics below.

A *modal language* is a language whose vocabulary contains modal operators to enable the formation of modal sentences. Statements such as "it is possible that Elroy Fox has hepatitis" demonstrate that the language of medicine is a modal language, whereas the language $\mathcal{L}_1$ that underlies predicate logic is not. In a modal language, there exist many different relationships between its modal operators. Consider, for example, the following three examples:

It is actually true that Elroy Fox has hepatitis,	symbolized by: $AT\alpha$
it is possible that Elroy Fox has hepatitis,	$\Diamond\alpha$
it is necessary that Elroy Fox has hepatitis,	$\Box\alpha$.

The three operators used in these sentences express the modalities of *actuality, possibility,* and *necessity.* They have come to be termed *alethic modalities,* from the ancient Greek ἀλήθεια (aletheia) meaning "truth". The following and many other relationships hold between them:

$\Box\alpha \rightarrow AT\alpha$	(what is necessarily true is also actually true)
$AT\alpha \rightarrow \Diamond\alpha$	(what is actually true is also possibly true)
$\Box\alpha \rightarrow \Diamond\alpha$	(what is necessarily true is also possibly true)
$\neg\Diamond\alpha \rightarrow \neg AT\alpha$	(what is impossible is also not actually true)
$\Box\alpha \rightarrow \neg\Diamond\neg\alpha$	(what is necessarily true cannot be false).

A *modal logic* studies the relationships between modal sentences of a particular type. It provides a logic of specific modal operators, and thus a method of reasoning in modal contexts. Otherwise put, modal logics are theories of modal languages. They analyze different types of modal operators, and due to the resemblance between the behavior of these distinct types, they have more or less similar axioms and rules. In this chapter, we shall discuss a few such logics that are relevant in medical reasoning. Besides the alethic modal operators mentioned above, listed below are some other groups of modal operators, a few of which we shall cover in more detail:[167]

---

[167] For a detailed analysis of this terminology, see (Rescher, 1968, 24 f.). The vague term "modality" has different meanings in different disciplines. In logic and philosophy, it means the manner of being and doing. It derives from the Latin terms "modalitas" and "modus" that originate from the traditional metaphysics to express the ways ('modes') in which something is true or false. The study of modalities dates back to Aristotle and the Stoic philosopher Diodorus Cronus (4th century BC). In his syllogistic logic, Aristotle also tried to develop modal syllogisms in his books *De Interpretatione* and *Analytica Priora.* However, his analysis was confined to alethic modalities only, i.e., possibility and necessity. Other types of modalities were unknown at that time. For historical details, see (Bochenski, 1961; Kneale and Kneale, 1968). Medieval philosophers continued Aristotle's tradition (Knuuttila, 1981, 1988, 1993). But it was not until the twentieth century that

DEONTIC MODALITIES (from the Greek term δέον (deon, deont-) meaning "what is binding" and "duty"):
>   It is obligatory that ...
>   it is forbidden that ...
>   it is permitted that ...

EPISTEMIC MODALITIES (from the Greek term ἐπιστήμη (epistēmē) meaning "knowledge"):
>   It is known that ...

DOXASTIC MODALITIES (from the Greek term δόξα (doxa) meaning "belief" and "opinion"):
>   It is believed that ...
>   it is convincing that ...
>   it is plausible that ...

TEMPORAL MODALITIES (from *tempus*, Latin for "time"):
>   It has always been the case that ...
>   it will always be the case that ...
>   it has at some time been the case that ...
>   it will at some time be the case that ...

PROBABILITY MODALITY:
>   It is probable that ...
>   it is likely that ...

ASSERTION MODALITY:
>   It is asserted that ...

EVALUATIVE MODALITIES:
>   It is good that ...
>   it is bad that ...

BOULOMAIC MODALITIES (from the Greek verb βούλομαι (boulomai) meaning "to wish", "to desire", and "to will"):
>   It is desired that ...
>   It is hoped that ...
>   It is feared that ...
>   It is regretted that ...

---

various systems of modal logic emerged. Their origins lie in the work of the U.S.-American philosopher Clarence Irving Lewis (1883–1964) (Lewis, 1912; Lewis and Langford, 1932). The need for this innovation was felt by some philosophers after the appearance of predicate logic that was exaggeratedly identified with logic itself during the twentieth century. They discovered additional modalities and constructed modal logics to overcome the limitations of predicate logic.

There exist many more modalities that will not be mentioned here. For the sake of simplicity, epistemic and doxastic modalities will be grouped under the umbrella name "*epistemic* modalities". Likewise, epistemic and doxastic notions will be called *epistemic* notions.

In the present chapter, only the following four modal logics will be outlined: alethic modal logic, deontic logic, epistemic logic, and temporal logic. Each of them is a modal extension of a non-modal base logic, e.g., classical sentential logic, first-order classical predicate logic without identity, first-order classical predicate logic with identity, or some other logic. In each case, modal operators are added to the language of the base logic, and accordingly, extra axioms and rules of inference are added to the base logic to regulate the behavior of the new operators.

Modal operators are the logical signs of modal logics just as the sentential connectives $\neg, \vee, \wedge, \rightarrow$, and $\leftrightarrow$ are the logical signs of sentential logic. Recall that the sentential connectives are sentential operators that are so called because they are applied to sentences to produce new sentences. Negation $\neg$, for example, is a unary sentential operator that is applied to a single sentence α to obtain a compound sentence $\neg\alpha$; conjunction $\wedge$ is a binary operator applied to two sentences α and β to obtain a compound sentence $\alpha \wedge \beta$; and so on. Likewise, a modal operator *is a sentential operator* and may have an arbitrary arity of $n \geq 1$. We shall first consider unary modal operators such as $\Box$, "it is necessary that". As a modal sentential connective, it is applied to a single sentence α to create a single compound sentence $\Box\alpha$. Other modal operators may be binary, or ternary, or otherwise. But all of them have a characteristic semantic feature that clearly distinguishes them from the connectives $\neg, \vee, \wedge, \rightarrow$, and $\leftrightarrow$. In a nutshell, modal operators are *intensional* operators. This may be explained by using the modality of necessity as an example.

We have seen on page 887 that the sentential-logical connectives $\neg, \vee, \wedge, \rightarrow$, and $\leftrightarrow$ are truth-functional, and as such, extensional operators. That is, the truth value of a compound sentence depends only on the truth values of its constituent sentences, but not on their contents. Consider, for instance, a conjunction such as $\alpha \wedge \beta$ with a definite truth value, e.g., *true*. This value is invariant with respect to the replacement of the conjuncts, α or β or both, by equivalent sentences. If we replace α or β or both with any other sentence that has the same truth value, the original truth value of the conjunction will remain unchanged. For example, the conjunction "2 = 2 $\wedge$ the father of Jesus is Joseph" is true. Let us now replace its true constituent sentence "2 = 2" with the true sentence "the USA consists of 50 states". We obtain the conjunction "the USA consists of 50 states $\wedge$ the father of Jesus is Joseph" that again is true. That means that the truth function "$\wedge$" operates only on the truth values of its arguments, but not on their contents, so that $\wedge(T, T) = T$ independently of what specific sentences the bearers of Ts within the brackets are. Otherwise put, the truth value of a sentential-logical compound does not depend on the intension, i.e., content, of its components, but on their extension, i.e., their truth value.

Modal operators behave differently. To demonstrate their distinctive behavior, recall that a modal operator, say $\Box$, operates on a sentence α in that
it is attached to α to form a modal sentence, i.e., $\Box\alpha$. For instance, if we
prefix the sentence "$2 = 2$" with the modal operator "it is necessary that",
then we obtain the modal sentence "it is necessary that $2 = 2$", i.e., "'$2 = 2$'
is necessarily true". Now, substitute for its true constituent sentence "$2 = 2$"
the true sentence "the USA consists of 50 states" as we did before. The result is the new modal sentence "it is necessary that the USA consists of 50
states". This, however, is a false assertion. For it is not necessary that the
USA consists of 50 states. It could be otherwise. Our example demonstrates
that this time the replacement of truth with truth produced something false.
Obviously, the intensions of the constituents of a modal sentence are essential
for its truth value. Thus, a modal operator is an *intensional* operator. It operates on the intension, not on the extension, of sentences. The result is that
modal logics are *intensional* logics, in contrast to predicate logic, that is an
extensional one. We shall see in our study below that this has consequences in
both constructing and using modal logics. Our study will be concerned with
four different modal logics in the following four sections:

27.1   Alethic Modal Logic
27.2   Deontic Logic
27.3   Epistemic Logic
27.4   Temporal Logic.

27.1 Alethic Modal Logic

The alethic modalities of *possibility* and *necessity* constitute the subject of
alethic modal logic. They were the first modalities to be discovered in the
ancient Greek philosophy. Modal logic was initially developed to deal with
them, and has been extended into the logic of additional modalities during
the Middle Ages. Since alethic modalities play an important role in medical
reasoning, an elementary system of alethic modal logic will be introduced in
the following five sections:

27.1.1   Alethic Modalities and Operators
27.1.2   A First-Order Alethic Modal Logic
27.1.3   Metalogic
27.1.4   Necessary *vs.* Contingent Identity
27.1.5   *De re* and *de dicto*.

27.1.1 Alethic Modalities and Operators

As was mentioned previously, an alethic modality is the mode of truth of a
sentence. In natural languages, including the language of medicine, there are
a variety of phrases to represent alethic modalities, for instance:

For *possibility:*
  can; could; may; might; possibly; it is possible that; and the suffixes -able and -ible.
Examples:

- He may recover soon;
- Helicobacter pylori gastritis is easily treatable;
- possibly, Elroy Fox has hepatitis;
- it is possible that he has hepatitis.

For *necessity:*
  necessarily; it is necessary that; must; has to; needs to.
Examples:

- necessarily, $2 = 2$;
- it is necessary that $2 = 2$;
- Elroy Fox has to go to the hospital.[168]

We shall use only the phrases "it is possible that" and "it is necessary that" as our operators and shall symbolize them, respectively, by a diamond and a box, as follows:

$\Diamond$ $\equiv$ it is possible that;
$\Box$ $\equiv$ it is necessary that.

Let α be a sentence. By attaching any of these two operators to α, we obtain an alethic-modal sentence such as:

$\Diamond\alpha$ $\equiv$ "it is possible that α"   e.g.: it is possible that he has hepatitis;
$\Box\alpha$ $\equiv$ "it is necessary that α"   it is necessary that $2 = 2$.

The diamond operator and the box operator are obviously unary sentential operators. They are interdefinable. To say that something is possibly true is to say that it is not necessarily false. Thus, we define the possibility operator by necessity operator because we shall base our system on the latter:[169]

Definition 229 (The alethic possibility operator). *For all* $\alpha(\Diamond\alpha \leftrightarrow \neg\Box\neg\alpha)$.

---

[168] Expressions such as "has to", "must", and "needs to" are ambiguous. They play primarily a deontic role and mean *should* and *ought to*. We do not consider them as genuine alethic-modal expressions. See Section 27.2.1 on page 928.

[169] The modality of possibility covers all kinds of possibility, and can thus be understood as *logical possibility*, i.e., consistency with 'logical laws'; *nomological possibility*, i.e., consistency with scientific laws; *physical possibility*, i.e., the ease of doing something such as "you can eat ten eggs for breakfast, but you cannot carry this automobile"; *epistemic possibility*, i.e., consistency with what is known; *temporal possibility*, i.e., consistency with the order of time; and *metaphysical possibility*, i.e., consistency with metaphysical knowledge. The same obtains for the modality of necessity.

Another option would be the other way around: To say that something is necessarily true is to say that it cannot be false, i.e., $\Box\alpha \leftrightarrow \neg\Diamond\neg\alpha$. This shows that the two operators are dual to each other. There are also two additional alethic modalities:

Impossibility:
it is impossible that; cannot; could not; may not; might not.
Examples:
- it is impossible that Elroy Fox has gallstones;
- he cannot be treated.

Contingency:
maybe and maybe not; might have been and might not have been.
Examples:
- maybe and maybe not that he has liver cancer.

Both modalities are derived ones. They may be defined by the two operators above in the following fashion:

Definition 230 (Impossibility and contingency).
1. It is impossible that α *iff* $\neg\Diamond\alpha$.
2. It is contingent that α *iff* α *is neither necessary nor impossible, i.e.,* $\neg\Box\alpha \wedge \neg\neg\Diamond\alpha$.

From Definitions 229–230 it follows that α is impossible if and only if $\Box\neg\alpha$, and that α is contingent iff $\neg\Box\alpha \wedge \neg\Box\neg\alpha$. All empirical statements are contingent. What they report are neither necessary truths nor impossibilities. Thus, we have the following five alethic modalities, all of which are representable by $\Box$:

$$
\begin{aligned}
\text{It is necessary that } \alpha \quad &\equiv\quad \Box\alpha & (235)\\
\text{it is non-necessary that } \alpha \quad &\equiv\quad \neg\Box\alpha\\
\text{it is possible that } \alpha \quad &\equiv\quad \neg\Box\neg\alpha\\
\text{it is impossible that } \alpha \quad &\equiv\quad \Box\neg\alpha\\
\text{it is contingent that } \alpha \quad &\equiv\quad \neg\Box\alpha \wedge \neg\Box\neg\alpha.
\end{aligned}
$$

This central role the operator $\Box$ plays is the reason why we will choose it as our basic operator on which to ground our alethic modal logic. The relationships sketched above between the five modalities are diagrammed in Figure 97.

27.1.2 A First-Order Alethic Modal Logic

There are a large number of alethic modal-logic systems with different scopes, virtues, and limitations. In this section, the classical first-order predicate logic *without* identity, introduced *with* identity in Chapter 26, will be expanded into an alethic modal logic that we shall refer to as the first-order alethic modal

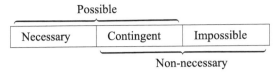

Fig. 97. Five alethic modalities. According to this folk logic, the three rectangular cells are jointly exhaustive and mutually exclusive sets. That is, a sentence is either necessary, contingent, or impossible, but never more than one of these. A possible sentence is either necessary or contingent. A non-necessary one is either impossible or contingent

logic S5 without identity, or the *first-order S5* for short. It is a predicate-logical version of the modal sentential-logical system S5. For details on these systems and their classification, see (Bull and Segerberg, 1984; Fitting and Mendelsohn, 1998; Goldblatt, 2006; Hughes and Cresswell, 2005).

We shall first briefly describe the syntax of the language of our logic and its semantics before we present its calculus. Thus, our discussion consists of the following three sections:

▶ The syntax of the first-order alethic modal language
▶ The semantics of the first-order alethic modal language
▶ The first-order alethic modal logic S5 without identity.

In Section 27.1.3 below, we shall explain why we have chosen a logic without the identity sign "=".

The syntax of the first-order alethic modal language

In this section, a modal language for our intended modal logic will be constructed. To this end, we will adopt the first-order language $\mathcal{L}_1$ – minus the identity sign – characterized in Table 28 on page 860, and will extend it to obtain a first-order *alethic modal language* without identity, or $\mathcal{AML}_1$ for short,

1. by adding to its logical signs the operator $\Box$, and accordingly,
2. by changing parts 1 and 3 of Definition 205 on page 862 as follows:
3. **Definition 205.1′:** Remove 205.1;
4. **Definition 205.3′:** If α is a formula, then $\neg\alpha$ and $\Box\alpha$ are formulas.

The possibility operator $\Diamond$ is used as a dual of $\Box$, i.e., according to Definition 229 as a shorthand for the complex operator $\neg\Box\neg$. Formulas are also called sentences because they represent natural language sentences. Note that according to Definition 205 and its updated clause 205.3′, all kinds of modalized formulas, except for identities, are formulas. For example, let the individual constant "a" denote the patient Elroy Fox, and "Pa" and "Qa" be the sentences "Elroy Fox has hepatitis" and "Elroy Fox is icteric", respectively. The following strings are formulas in $\mathcal{AML}_1$:

Pa	$\equiv$	Elroy Fox has hepatitis;
$\Diamond Pa$	$\equiv$	it is possible that Elroy Fox has hepatitis;
$Pa \rightarrow \neg \Box Qa$	$\equiv$	if Elroy Fox has hepatitis, then he need not be icteric;
$\exists x(Px \wedge \Diamond \neg Qx)$	$\equiv$	there are people with hepatitis who may be non-icteric;
$\Box(Pa \rightarrow \Diamond Qa)$	$\equiv$	necessarily, if Elroy Fox has hepatitis, then possibly he is icteric;
$\Box \Diamond \forall x(Px \rightarrow Qx)$	$\equiv$	necessarily, it is possible that whoever has hepatitis is icteric.

However, none of these sequences is a formula in $\mathcal{AML}_1$:

$\Box a Pa$

$\Diamond Pa \rightarrow Qa \neg \Box$

$\Diamond 2$

$2 = 2$

$(\Box 2) = 2.$

As to the binding strength of modal operators, note that $\Box$ and $\Diamond$ dominate, i.e., bind more strongly than, other logical signs. For example, $\Box \alpha \rightarrow \beta$ is the formula $(\Box \alpha) \rightarrow \beta$, but not $\Box(\alpha \rightarrow \beta)$. Additionally, we shall need for our purposes below the notion of a *free variable* occurrence in a modal formula. The notion of a free variable in a classical-logical formula was defined in Definitions 208–211 on pages 868–869. It may now be extended to include our modal sentences:

The free variables in $\Box \alpha$ as well as $\Diamond \alpha$ are those of α. That is, $\mathcal{F}(\Box \alpha) = \mathcal{F}(\Diamond \alpha) = \mathcal{F}(\alpha)$. For example, $\mathcal{F}(\Diamond \exists x(Px \wedge \Box Qy)) = \{y\}$, whereas $\mathcal{F}(\Diamond \exists x(Px \wedge \Box Qx)) = \varnothing$.

The semantics of the first-order alethic modal language

In the next section, the calculus of our modal logic will use a syntactic concept of inference, again symbolized by $\vdash$, for modal sentences. Recall that the semantic concept of inference, $\vDash$, introduced in Definitions 202 and 222 on pages 851 and 889, respectively, could be replaced with the syntactic one. That classical concept of inference is still valid for alethic modal logic. That is, a set of closed premises imply a particular conclusion if and only if it is the case that whenever all premises are true, the conclusion is true. For this reason, we need a semantics for operators and sentences of the modal language $\mathcal{AML}_1$, in order to understand what it means to say, for example, that a premise or conclusion of the form $\Box(Pa \rightarrow \Diamond Qa)$ is true.

Necessity and possibility are not features of the real world out there. We are therefore unable to empirically test modal claims. However, if they are untestable, why should we make and accept modal statements, e.g., the statement "it is possible that Elroy Fox has hepatitis" or "it is necessary that he has hepatitis"? What do the phrases "it is possible that" and "it is necessary that" mean in such sentences, and to what in the experiential world do they refer? The standard method used today to answer such semantic questions about possibility and necessity has come to be termed *possible-worlds seman-tics*. This important device will be explained here in order to refer to it in later contexts. Our explanations will be simple and brief. For details, see (Fitting and Mendelsohn, 1998; Hughes and Cresswell, 2005; Kripke, 1963; Popkorn, 2003).[170]

Without going into philosophical details, in the present context we naively call the actual state of the world the *actual world*. The actual world is the way things are. For example, in our actual world things are such that there is an Eiffel Tower in Paris; you are now reading this line; multiple sclerosis is still incurable; a mad German chancellor started Word War II; AIDS is caused by HIV; man has evolved from apes; there are billions of Milky Ways in the universe; Barack Obama is the current president of the USA; and so on. However, it is conceivable that things might have been otherwise. Any such alternative we call a *possible world*. In one of these possible worlds, for instance, there is no Eiffel Tower in Paris; you are reading this line; multiple sclerosis is curable; there has been no World War II; AIDS is caused by HIV; man has not evolved from apes; there is only one Milky Way consisting of two solar systems; the current president of the USA is Hillary Clinton; and so on. Thus, a possible world is not meant to be another planet in the universe. Rather, it is a collection of any conceivable objects and states of affairs, say an alternative scenario or situation, i.e., an alternative history of the world in the past, present, and future. Obviously, there are infinitely many such possible worlds. The actual world is only one of them. For a reconstruction of possible worlds as *situations,* see (Perry, 1986).

To examine whether or not a modal formula such as "it is possible that Elroy Fox has hepatitis" is true or false in the actual world, the formula must be *interpreted* as we did regarding $\mathcal{L}_1$ formulas on pages 879–886. The question arises, in what kind of structure are we to interpret a modal formula, e.g., $\lozenge Pa$, or $\lozenge Pa \rightarrow \square Qa$? The general consensus since Saul Kripke's proposal is that a set of *possible worlds* should serve as the frame of interpretation. We will briefly explain this idea (Kripke, 1963, 1980).

---

[170] The phrase "possible world" is usually credited to the German philosopher Gott-fried Wilhelm Leibniz (1646–1716). He meant that our world was the best of the infinitely many possible worlds, and said of necessary truths that "not only will they hold as long as the world exists, but also they would have held if God had created the world according to a different plan" (see Mates, 1989, 72–73, 106–107). Possible-worlds semantics proper, however, goes back to Rudolf Carnap (1947), Stig Kanger (1957), Jaakko Hintikka (1957), and especially the U.S.-American logician and philosopher Saul Aaron Kripke (born in 1940), after whom it is usually called *Kripke semantics*. Kripke initiated this formal semantics for modal logics, also called relational semantics, in 1956 when he was only 16 years old and still at high-school. It was first published in his early works (1959, 1963).

A *Kripke frame* is an ordered pair $\langle W, R \rangle$ such that W is a non-empty set of possible worlds $w_1, w_2, w_3, \ldots$; and R is a binary relation on W, i.e., $R \subseteq W \times W$, referred to as the relation of alternativeness or *accessibility*. Rw_iw_j with $i, j \geq 1$ says that world w_j is an alternative to, or accessible from, world w_i. The accessibility relation R is a general relation covering relationships such as logical accessibility, nomological accessibility, epistemic accessibility, technological accessibility, etc. For instance, X-logical accessibility between world w_i and world w_j means that the states of affairs at w_j are compatible with the laws of logic X at world w_i; nomological accessibility between world w_i and world w_j means that the states of affairs at w_j are compatible with scientific laws of the world w_i; and so on. Some algebraic properties are also usually required of the accessibility relation, e.g., the property of reflexivity which says that a world is accessible from itself, i.e., Rw_iw_i. We will not here discuss these specific features. Overly simplified, Kripke frames are used to define necessary and possible truth, i.e., the operators $\Box$ and $\Diamond$, and to interpret alethic modal sentences in the following way:

Definition 231 (Truth of alethic-modal sentences). *Let $\langle W, R \rangle$ be a Kripke frame with W being the set of all possible worlds. If w_i is a world in W, then:*

1. *A necessity sentence $\Box\alpha$ is true at w_i iff α is true at every world $w_j \in W$ that is accessible from w_i.*
2. *A possibility sentence $\Diamond\alpha$ is true at w_i iff α is true at some world $w_j \in W$ that is accessible from w_i.*

For example, the sentence "it is necessary that Elroy Fox has hepatitis" is true at the actual world if its non-modal kernel "Elroy Fox has hepatitis" is true at all possible worlds accessible from the actual one. And the sentence "it is possible that Elroy Fox has hepatitis" is true at the actual world if there is a possible world accessible from the actual one, such that its non-modal kernel "Elroy Fox has hepatitis" is true at that world. In a nutshell, necessity means *truth in all possible worlds*, while possibility means *truth in at least one of them*. This definition suggests that the operators $\Box$ and $\Diamond$ may be regarded as special quantifiers that range over the set of possible worlds. "$\Box$" is defined by "all accessible possible worlds" and is a formal analog of $\forall$, whereas "$\Diamond$" is defined by "at least one accessible possible world" and is a formal analog of $\exists$. Otherwise put, a sentence of the form $\Box\alpha$ says that "if ..., then $\forall w\alpha$", whereas the sentence $\Diamond\alpha$ says that "if ..., then $\exists w\alpha$". Here, *"w"* is a variable ranging over possible worlds.

On the basis of these considerations and analogous to what we have stated in Definition 219 on page 883 regarding classical logic, a notion of truth can be defined for compund alethic modal sentences, and a notion of validity can be introduced to elucidate the semantic notion of inference in modal contexts. But we will not go into these details here.[171]

---

[171] A concise reconstruction of the diverse ideas in the literature up to now may suffice. But a minor modification will be introduced because the formalism used

First-order alethic modal logic S5 without identity

This logical system, referred to as *first-order S5 without identity,* is an alethic modal extension of classical first-order predicate logic without identity introduced, with identity, in Table 35 on page 892. It is shown in Table 39.

Deduction and deducibility are defined in the same manner as in predicate logic on page 892. When a sentence α is deducible from a set of formulas, $\mathfrak{F}$, we write $\mathfrak{F} \vdash \alpha$. This may be exemplified by a few simple modal-logical proofs:

---

in Kripke semantics is objectionable (see Sadegh-Zadeh, Forthcoming). What we now need is an interpretation function, $\mathfrak{I}$, that assigns particular entities to modal formulas and returns their truth values. To this end, a Kripke frame $\langle W, R \rangle$ is extended into a *Kripke structure* $\langle W, R, \Omega_w, \mathcal{R} \rangle$ by adding the two components Ω_w and $\mathcal{R}$ such that Ω_w is a non-empty set of objects that may exist at world $w \in W$, i.e., its domain or universe; and $\mathcal{R}$ is a non-empty set of n-place relations and functions on that domain Ω_w. $\mathcal{R}$ may also contain $m \geq 0$ specified individuals $a_1, a_2, \ldots, a_m$ of Ω_w such as 'Elroy Fox', 'Eiffel Tower', etc. We say that the structure $\langle W, R, \Omega_w, \mathcal{R} \rangle$ is based on the frame $\langle W, R \rangle$. The terminal pair in a Kripke structure, i.e., the ordered pair $\langle \Omega_w, \mathcal{R} \rangle$, is exactly a *relational structure* of the sort we have used in the interpretation of first-order formulas of the non-modal language $\mathcal{L}_1$. In order for a modal formula to be interpretable on a Kripke structure $\langle W, R, \Omega_w, \mathcal{R} \rangle$, the structure must be a suitable one. It is a suitable one if its terminal pair $\langle \Omega_w, \mathcal{R} \rangle$ is a structure suitable to the language of the formula. For details, see the interpretation of formulas on pages 879–886. Now, a suitable interpretation function $\mathfrak{I}$ interprets a modal formula, e.g., $\Box \alpha$, at world $w \in W$ of a Kripke structure $\langle W, R, \Omega_w, \mathcal{R} \rangle$ just in the same way as we have done in the non-modal case. To interpret a formula at world $w \in W$ of a Kripke structure $\langle W, R, \Omega_w, \mathcal{R} \rangle$ means that the interpretation function $\mathfrak{I}$ assigns to a free individual variable of the formula an object from Ω_w; to an m-place predicate of the formula an m-place relation from $\mathcal{R}$; to an n-place function symbol of the formula an n-place function from $\mathcal{R}$; to an individual constant of the formula a specified individual from $\mathcal{R}$; and to the interpreted formula itself a truth value. The remainder of this procedure resembles the one described in Section "Interpretation of formulas" on pages 879–886. When under such an interpretation $\mathfrak{I}$ of a formula α at a world $w \in W$ the formula turns out true, we say that α is true at world $w \in W$ and write $\mathfrak{I}(\alpha, w) = \mathrm{T}$. Let $\langle W, R, \Omega_w, \mathcal{R} \rangle$ be a Kripke structure and $\mathfrak{I}$ an interpretation that interprets the necessity formula $\Box \alpha$ at world $w_i \in W$; then $\Box \alpha$ is true at world $w_i \in W$, i.e., $\mathfrak{I}(\Box \alpha, w_i) = \mathrm{T}$, iff for all $w \in W$, whenever w is accessible from w_i then $\mathfrak{I}(\alpha, w) = \mathrm{T}$. And analogously, a possibility formula $\Diamond \alpha$ is true at w_i iff there is a $w \in W$ such that w is accessible from w_i and α is true at w. Formula α is said to be satisfiable on a Kripke structure $\langle W, R, \Omega_w, \mathcal{R} \rangle$ iff there is an interpretation $\mathfrak{I}$ such that $\mathfrak{I}(\alpha, w) = \mathrm{T}$. Formula α is valid on a Kripke frame $\langle W, R \rangle$ iff α is satisfiable on *all* Kripke structures $\langle W, R, \Omega_w, \mathcal{R} \rangle$ based on $\langle W, R \rangle$. Finally, formula α is *valid* iff α is valid on *all* Kripke frames $\langle W, R \rangle$. Now, a formula β follows from a set $\{\alpha_1, \ldots, \alpha_n\}$ of premises, written $\{\alpha_1, \ldots, \alpha_n\} \vDash \beta$, iff for every interpretation $\mathfrak{I}$ on every Kripke structure $\langle W, R, \Omega_w, \mathcal{R} \rangle$, whenever $\mathfrak{I}(\alpha_i, w) = \mathrm{T}$ for all $\alpha_i \in \{\alpha_1, \ldots, \alpha_n\}$, then $\mathfrak{I}(\beta, w) = \mathrm{T}$.

Table 39. A first-order alethic-modal calculus without identity: S5

---

0. Include the first-order predicate calculus without identity, i.e., all of its non-identity axioms and rules introduced in Table 35 on page 892, taking into account Definitions 205.1′ and 205.3′ on page 916 above;

Additional axioms:	**Their names:**
1. $\Box(\alpha \to \beta) \to (\Box\alpha \to \Box\beta)$	Axiom K
2. $\Box\alpha \to \alpha$	Axiom T
3. $\Diamond\alpha \to \Box\Diamond\alpha$	Axiom E

Additional rule:

$$\frac{\vdash \alpha}{\Box\alpha}$$ Rule N ($\equiv$ Necessitation)

Assertion 14. *The diagnosis "Elroy Fox has hepatitis" implies "it is possible that Elroy Fox has hepatitis". That is, $Pa \vdash \Diamond Pa$.*

Proof 14:

1. Pa	Premise
2. $\Box\neg Pa \to \neg Pa$	Axiom T
3. $\neg\neg Pa \to \neg\Box\neg Pa$	Contraposition Rule: 2
4. $\neg\neg Pa$	Double Negation: 1
5. $\neg\Box\neg Pa$	Modus ponens: 3, 4
6. $\Diamond Pa$	Definition 229: 5. QED

In an analogous fashion, we may prove a derived rule called alethic Modus ponens:

Assertion 15. $\Box(\alpha \to \beta), \Box\alpha \vdash \Box\beta$

Proof 15:

1. $\Box(\alpha \to \beta)$	Premise
2. $\Box\alpha$	Premise
3. $\Box(\alpha \to \beta) \to (\Box\alpha \to \Box\beta)$	Axiom K
4. $\Box\alpha \to \Box\beta$	Modus ponens: 1, 3
5. $\Box\beta$	Modus ponens: 2, 4. QED

These examples demonstrate that alethic modal inferences may be performed syntactically, and need not ask whether the premises or the conclusion are true. A number of additional derived rules and theorems are listed in Table 40, that are provable in the same fashion as above and may be used in proofs. Theorems 7–10 show that in first-order S5 without identity, one may delete all but the last modal operator in any sequence of iterated and nested modal operators.

Table 40. Some derived rules and theorems of the alethic-modal logic S5

1. $\Box\alpha \to \Box\beta, \Box\alpha \vdash \Box\beta$	(alethic) Modus ponens
2. $\Box(\alpha \to \beta), \Diamond\alpha \vdash \Diamond\beta$	
3. $\vdash \alpha \to \Box\Diamond\alpha$	11. $\vdash \Box(\alpha \land \beta) \leftrightarrow \Box\alpha \land \Box\beta$
4. $\vdash \Box\alpha \to \Diamond\beta$	12. $\vdash (\Box\alpha \lor \Box\beta) \to \Box(\alpha \lor \beta)$
5. $\vdash \Box\alpha \to \Box\Box\alpha$	13. $\vdash \Box(\alpha \lor \beta) \to \Box\alpha \lor \Diamond\beta$
6. $\vdash \Box\Box\alpha \to \Box\alpha$	14. $\vdash \Diamond(\alpha \land \beta) \to \Diamond\alpha \land \Diamond\beta$
7. $\vdash \Diamond\alpha \leftrightarrow \Box\Diamond\alpha$	15. $\vdash \Diamond(\alpha \lor \beta) \leftrightarrow \Diamond\alpha \lor \Diamond\beta$
8. $\vdash \Box\alpha \leftrightarrow \Diamond\Box\alpha$	16. $\vdash \Box\forall x\alpha \leftrightarrow \forall x\Box\alpha$
9. $\vdash \Diamond\alpha \leftrightarrow \Diamond\Diamond\alpha$	17. $\vdash \Diamond\forall x\alpha \to \forall x\Diamond\alpha$
10. $\vdash \Box\alpha \leftrightarrow \Box\Box\alpha$	18. $\vdash \Diamond\exists x\alpha \leftrightarrow \exists x\Diamond\alpha$

27.1.3 Metalogic

Since antiquity, alethic modal logic has faced stubborn technical and philosophical problems, many of which remain without solution. The exemplar
sketched above, however, is relatively trouble-free. It is sound and complete,
i.e., $\mathfrak{F} \vdash \alpha$ iff $\mathfrak{F} \vDash \alpha$. For details, see (Hughes and Cresswell, 2005, 249 ff.).

The first-order S5 without identity "=" sketched above is only one of the
many systems of alethic modal logic, possibly the best one. Its only limitation
is that it is incapable of dealing with equalities. But the price for including the
identity sign would be the soundness of our logic. That is, the alethic modal
extension of predicate logic *with* identity does not yield a sound logic. In the
next section, we shall illustrate this by showing that an alethic modal logic
with identity allows dubious inferences.

27.1.4 Necessary *vs.* Contingent Identity

The question "what is identity?" is not only a fundamental issue in mathematics and logic. As a metaphysical problem, it is also an equally important issue
in medical disciplines, especially in psychiatry, where the concept of personal
identity plays significant roles in theories of depersonalization, schizophrenia,
and dissociative identity disorder. An intricate problem pertaining to this
topic is the metaphysical question of whether identity is a necessary or a contingent relation. To correctly understand the question, we must be aware that
identity is indeed a binary relation between two objects. This was represented
by an atomic formula of the form $t_1 = t_2$ in Definition 205.1 on page 862.
Each of the two terms $t_1 = t_2$ denoting the arguments, or the relata, of the
relation may be an atomic term such as x or y, or a compound term such
as $f(x_1, \ldots, x_n)$. See Definition 204 on page 861. For example, consider the
following sentences:

Sigmund Freud = Sigmund Freud
Sigmund Freud = the creator of psychoanalysis
Sigmund Freud = father of Anna Freud.

These examples may be formalized as follows:

1. $a = a$ where   "a" designates the individual Sigmund Freud,
2. $a = b$ "b" designates the creator of psychoanalysis,
3. $a = f(c)$ "f" designates the function *father_of*,
             "c" designates the individual Anna Freud.

Pick any of these identities and ask: Is this identity a necessary or a contingent relation? Otherwise put, is each of the three identities necessarily true, or could it be the case that:

1'. $a \neq a$ or
2'. $a \neq b$ or
3'. $a \neq f(c)$?

The answer to this question depends on the logic that one uses in justifying the answer. According to the first Identity Axiom of predicate logic, i.e., $x = x$, the relation $a \neq a$ does not hold since due to that axiom every object is identical with itself. But any of the other two relations, 2 and 3, might not have been the case in this world. It could have been otherwise. For example, psychoanalysis might have been created by a person different than Sigmund Freud and thereby justifying the relation 2' above. Likewise, the female individual who has come to be known as Anna Freud, might not have been generated by Sigmund Freud, but by someone else, thereby verifying the relation 3' above. That is, according to our common-sense judgment, identities 2 and 3 above are contingent. In what follows, we shall see that this common sense is violated by alethic modal logic *with* identity, which implies that contingent identity does not exist, and identity is a necessary relation. The primary advocate of this thesis is Saul Kripke (1980).

Suppose that in constructing our first-order alethic modal logic S5, we had used the first-order predicate logic *with* identity as our base logic. In this case, our alethic modal logic would be one with identity. It would then imply a theorem which states that whenever two objects are identical, they are necessarily so, i.e., $\vdash x = y \rightarrow \Box x = y$. This amounts to the postulate that the identity between two things is a necessary relation between them, and it might not have been otherwise. Here, we must distinguish between different cases:

For example, it is clear that $2 = 2$ is 'necessarily so'. For the predicate-logical Identity Axiom 1 requires that everything be identical with itself, $x = x$. And this implies, according to the alethic modal Rule N, that $\Box x = x$. Problems arise as soon as the identity is not the logical identity $x = x$, but the empirical identity between an object x and another object y such that their names, "x" and "y", have different senses. For instance, see examples 2 and 3 above. The name "Sigmund Freud" means an individual born on May 6, 1856 in Freiberg, now part of the Czech Republic. But "the creator of psychoanalysis" means a person who has invented the theory of psychoanalysis. An identity such as example 2 above would in alethic-modal logic with identity imply that it is 'necessarily so', i.e., $\Box$(Sigmund Freud = the creator of psychoanalysis). However, necessity claims of this sort are counter-intuitive and sometimes even falsifiable.

The following illustrates how the trouble arises. First-order predicate logic with identity contains two axioms of identity, presented in Table 35 on page 892. These two axioms are thus also included in our hypothetical first-order S5 with identity. They imply the following metatheorem on the substitution of variables. For the proof of the metatheorem, see (Monk, 1976, 178):

Metatheorem 7 (Substitution of identicals for identicals). *If α and β are formulas, and β is obtained from α if zero or more free occurrences of the individual variable x in α are replaced with free occurrences of the individual variable y, then $\vdash x = y \rightarrow (\alpha \rightarrow \beta)$.*

A simple example is: $\vdash x = a \rightarrow (Px \rightarrow Pa)$. For instance, $\vdash$ If $x =$ Elroy Fox, then, if x has diabetes, then Elroy Fox has diabetes. By means of the Metatheorem 7 we can, in S5 *with* identity, prove the following assertion of the necessity of identity which says that our hypothetical first-order S5 *with* identity implies "whenever two things are identical, then necessarily so".

Assertion 16. $\vdash x = y \rightarrow \Box x = y$

Proof 16:

1.	$x = y \rightarrow (\Box x = x \rightarrow \Box x = y)$	Metatheorem 7
2.	$\Box x = x \rightarrow (x = y \rightarrow \Box x = y)$	Permutation of Antecedents: 1
3.	$x = x$	Identity Axiom 1
4.	$\Box x = x$	Rule N: 3
5.	$x = y \rightarrow \Box x = y$	Modus ponens: 2, 4. QED

The sentence in line 1 of this proof starts with the antecedent $x = y$. By Metatheorem 7, we may therefore replace in the consequent $(\Box x = x \rightarrow \ldots)$ one free occurrence of the variable x in its antecedent $\Box x = x$ with a free occurrence of the variable y to obtain its consequent $\Box x = y$. The last line of the proof, i.e., the consequence of the argument, shows that according to our hypothetical first-order S5 *with* identity "two identical objects are necessarily identical. It could not be otherwise". But we have seen above that this is counter-intuitive. The individual *The creator of psychoanalyis* might have been someone different than *Sigmund Freud*.

The above considerations demonstrate that the alethic modal extension of the classical first-order predicate logic *with* identity fails. The only conclusion to draw from this result is that we ought not to include the identity sign "=" in the alphabet of our alethic modal language. We did so already in constructing the first-order S5 without identity in Section 27.1.2.[172]

---

[172] Saul Kripke, the main inventor of the possible-worlds semantics, takes another viewpoint. He not only accepts the necessity of identity, but also many more metaphysical consequences that a modal logic with identity carries with it, e.g.,

27.1.5 *De re* and *de dicto*

Part VI of this book, devoted to medical metaphysics, is concerned, among other things, with medical ontology pertaining to questions of the type whether medically relevant entities such as diseases, minds, and mental illness "really" exist or are merely imaginary and fictitious, as some scholars maintain. To this end, a modal assertion operator is introduced that clearly distinguishes between *what is* and *what is supposed to be*. This distinction needed in Part VI is best achieved by differentiating between two types of modalities:

- modality *de re,*   i.e., "of the thing"
- modality *de dicto,*   "of what is said".

To understand the nature of these two types and the difference between them, we should be aware of a particular ambiguity in modal contexts that may lead to misunderstandings and errors. This ambiguity troubled medieval logicians since its discovery by the French scholastic philosopher Pierre Abélard (1079–1142), and was not understood until the emergence of formal modal logic in the twentieth century. Consider as an example the following two sentences:

a.   There is someone who possibly has hepatitis,
b.   Possibly there is someone who has hepatitis.

These two sentences deal with two possibilities of a completely different type. The distinction between them is shown by their formalization below, where "Hx" means "x has hepatitis":

a'. $\exists x \Diamond (x \text{ has hepatitis})$ $\equiv \exists x \Diamond Hx$ (*de re*)
b'. $\Diamond \exists x (x \text{ has hepatitis})$ $\equiv \Diamond \exists x Hx$ (*de dicto*)

The first sentence says that there exists a thing (Latin: *res*), and about that thing (*de re*) it makes a possibility claim, namely that "possibly *the thing has hepatitis*". Such a possibility claim is therefore referred to as a *possibility de re*. The existence of the thing is independent of the possibility statement about its properties. In the second sentence, however, the modality of possibility precedes the whole statement, to yield a possibility assertion about what is said (Latin: *de dicto*), i.e., "possibly *there exists a thing that has hepatitis*". The subject of possibility consideration in this case is the very existence of the thing with all its properties. This is a *possibility de dicto*. Analogously, there are de re and de dicto necessities. Note, for instance, the difference between these two necessity statements:

---

necessary truths a posteriori, some sort of essentialism, and the transworld rigidity of designators. The latter, amazing doctrine says that a proper name, such as "Sigmund Freud" or "The Eiffel Tower", is a *rigid designator*. That means that it designates one and the same object in all possible worlds. The interested reader is directed to further readings (Kripke, 1980; Soames, 2002).

$$\forall x \Box (\text{man is mortal}) \qquad \equiv \forall x \Box (Px \to Qx) \qquad (de\ re)$$
$$\Box \forall x (\text{man is mortal}) \qquad \equiv \Box \forall x (Px \to Qx) \qquad (de\ dicto)$$

The first example says that man is necessarily mortal, and is thus stating a *necessity de re*. By contrast, the second example represents a *necessity de dicto* asserting that necessarily man is mortal. The difference between de re and de dicto is semantically highly relevant and important. Fortunately, as the above formalizations clearly show, it can be syntactically characterized to prevent fruitless metaphysical speculations and debates:

Concisely, *de re* and *de dicto* are discernible from the order of modal operators and quantifiers in a sentence:

In a *de re* sentence such as $\exists x \Diamond Hx$, the quantifier precedes the modal operator. The latter one lies in the scope of the quantifier that binds a variable, x, which is free in the scope of the modal operator, i.e., in Hx. This issue is referred to as quantifying into an intensional context, or *quantifying in* for short. In the present example, $\exists$ quantifies into the context of $\Diamond$.

In a *de dicto* sentence such as $\Diamond \exists x Hx$, however, the modal operator precedes the quantifier to the effect that no quantifying in occurs because the modal operator does not lie in the scope of the quantifier and bears no free variable in its scope, i.e., in $\exists x Hx$. For this reason, a *de re* statement and a *de dicto* statement are not, in general, equivalent and must not be confused. As was listed in Table 40 on page 922, in first-order S5 we have the equivalence $\vdash \Box \forall x \alpha \leftrightarrow \forall x \Box \alpha$. It consists of the two theorems:

$$\vdash \forall x \Box \alpha \to \Box \forall x \alpha \qquad \qquad \text{(Barcan Formula)}$$
$$\vdash \Box \forall x \alpha \to \forall x \Box \alpha \qquad \qquad \text{(Converse Barcan Formula)}$$

However, only the conditionals:

$$\Diamond \forall x \alpha \to \forall x \Diamond \alpha$$
$$\exists x \Box \alpha \to \Box \exists x \alpha$$

are valid, but not their converses:

$$\forall x \Diamond \alpha \to \Diamond \forall x \alpha$$
$$\Box \exists x \alpha \to \exists x \Box \alpha$$

to the effect that neither $\vdash \Diamond \forall x \alpha \leftrightarrow \forall x \Diamond \alpha$ nor $\exists x \Box \alpha \leftrightarrow \Box \exists x \alpha$ is a theorem. For details on *de re* and *de dicto,* see (Forbes, 1985; Garson, 2006; Hughes and Cresswell, 2005; Knuuttila, 1993).[173]

---

[173] The influential U.S.-American philosopher and logician Willard Van Orman Quine (1908–2000) was a vehement critic of quantificational modal logic and quantifying in (see Quine, 1943, 1947, 1963). The Barcan Formula and its converse mentioned above are important principles named in honor of Ruth Barcan Marcus, a U.S.-

27.1.6 Summary

As a highly-developed natural language, medical language is a multi-modal one. We have presented several groups of modal operators to demonstrate what types of modal logic medicine needs for using its language logically. These operators are intensional ones, in contrast to the sentential connectives $\neg, \vee, \wedge, \rightarrow$, and $\leftrightarrow$. Two historically well-known modal operators are the possibility and necessity operators, symbolized by $\Diamond$ and $\Box$, respectively, and referred to as alethic modal operators. They are interpreted as intensional analogs of the classical, extensional quantifiers, $\exists$ and $\forall$, ranging over possible worlds such that a possibility sentence $\Diamond\alpha$ is true if α is true at some possible world, while a necessity sentence $\Box\alpha$ is true if α is true at all possible worlds. Using these two operators, we have briefly sketched an alethic modal predicate logic without identity, the well-known system S5. We have also shown that by adding the identity sign "=" to the alphabet of this logic, an objectionable, counter-intuitive system emerges. Additionally, we discussed an important logical and metaphysical distinction between *de re* and *de dicto* applications of modal operators. We shall make use of this distinction when analyzing the ontological problems of medicine in Part VI as well as when constructing a concept of perspectivism in Section 23.2 on page 810.

27.2 Deontic Logic

When a physician knows that in a patient with acute myocardial infarction, immediate thrombolysis is indicated to remove coronary blockage, how does she know what is contra-indicated in this situation? The answer is deducible from the physician's knowledge that "in a patient with acute myocardial infarction, immediate thrombolysis is indicated". To conduct the deduction, however, the physician needs to have some knowledge of *deontic logic*.

As extensively discussed in Parts I–VII, successful reasoning in medical research and practice requires several types of logic. Of these several types, deontic logic is the most crucial, though this fact is absolutely unknown in medicine. In the current section, the nature of deontic logic is discussed in order to prepare its application in medicine and philosophy of medicine. Our discussion consists of the following five sections:

27.2.1 Deontic Modalities and Operators
27.2.2 The Standard System of Deontic Logic
27.2.3 Metalogic
27.2.4 Deontic Conditionals
27.2.5 *De re* and *de dicto*.

American logician and philosopher born in 1921. She is a pioneer in the quantification of modal logic. She discovered those principles and showed, contrary to Quine's view, that it was indeed possible to do sensible and metaphysically illuminating *quantifying in* (see Barcan Marcus, 1946, 1947, 1993).

27.2.1 Deontic Modalities and Operators

As was mentioned on page 911, the adjective "deontic" derives from the Greek term δέον (deon) that means "what is binding" and "duty". Accordingly, deontic logic is a branch of modal logic that studies a variety of normative concepts and their use in normative reasoning. It is therefore not only relevant to ethics, metaethics, law, authorities, and organizations, but also to medicine, for clinical reasoning is in fact normative reasoning. This special issue is analyzed in Parts II, V, and VI.

We will begin our discussion with normative or *deontic modalities*. They play a central role in normative reasoning. Five such modalities are known, i.e., obligation, prohibition, permission, optionality, and gratuitousness. In natural languages, they are represented by *deontic* phrases such as the following ones:

> For *obligation*:
> obligatory; ought to; required; should; must; obliged; duty;
> for *prohibition*:
> forbidden; prohibited; impermissible; must not; wrong; unacceptable; immoral;
> for *permission*:
> permitted; permissible; allowed; allowable; may;
> for *optionality*:
> optional;
> for *gratuitousness*:
> gratuitous; non-obligatory.

Some examples are:

- the physician *ought to* tell the patient the truth;
- providing assistance with suicide is *forbidden*;
- you are *permitted* to take aspirin;
- marriage is *optional* for everyone;
- antimicrobial therapy in a patient with acute appendicitis is *gratuitous*.

All of them are intensional operators. We shall use only the following ones as their representatives:

- it is obligatory that ...   symbolized by: OB
- it is forbidden that ... FO
- it is permitted that ... PE
- it is optional that ... OP
- it is gratuitous that ... GR.

They may be unambiguously used as unary sentential operators by prefixing them to sentences. Let α be any sentence, we shall write:

$OB\alpha$ $\equiv$ it is obligatory that α
$FO\alpha$ $\equiv$ it is forbidden that α
$PE\alpha$ $\equiv$ it is permitted that α
$OP\alpha$ $\equiv$ it is optional that α
$GR\alpha$ $\equiv$ it is gratuitous that α.

The above examples can be rewritten as the following:

- *it is obligatory that* the physician tells the patient the truth;
- *it is forbidden that* the physician provides assistance with suicide;
- *it is permitted that* you take aspirin;
- *it is optional that* one marries;
- *it is gratuitous that* a patient with acute appendicitis receives antimicrobial therapy.

That means semiformally:

OB(the physician tells the patient the truth),
FO(the physician provides assistance with suicide),
PE(you take aspirin),
OP(one marries),
GR(a patient with acute appendicitis receives antimicrobial therapy).

The five deontic operators sketched above are interdefinable. Like the necessity operator $\square$ in alethic modal logic, the obligation operator OB may serve as the undefined, basic operator from which the other four operators can be derived. Consider the following, multiple definition:

Definition 232 (Deontic operators).

1. $FO\alpha$ *iff* $OB\neg\alpha$
2. $PE\alpha$ *iff* $\neg FO\alpha$ and thus, $PE\alpha$ *iff* $\neg OB\neg\alpha$
3. $GR\alpha$ *iff* $\neg OB\alpha$
4. $OP\alpha$ *iff* $\neg OB\alpha \wedge \neg OB\neg\alpha$.

Due to the central role that the obligation operator OB plays, we shall use it as our basic concept on which to ground our deontic logic. The remaining operators are used as shorthands according to Definition 232. The relationships sketched above between the five deontic modalities may be diagrammed as shown in Figure 98.

27.2.2 The Standard System of Deontic Logic

The founder of modern deontic logic was the Austrian philosopher Ernst Mally (1879–1944). Due to some shortcomings, however, his work languished (Mally, 1926). Independently, the area was rediscovered and re-founded by the Finnish philosopher and logician Georg Henrik von Wright (1916–2003), who gave rise to deontic logic as a full-fledged branch of formal logic (von Wright, 1951b,

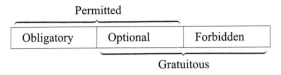

Fig. 98. The three rectangular cells are jointly exhaustive and mutually exclusive sets. That is, something is either obligatory, optional or forbidden, but never more than one of these. Something permitted is either obligatory or optional, while something gratuitous is either forbidden or optional. Notice the analogy with alethic modal operators in Figure 97 on page 916

1968, 1971, 1994).[174] Von Wright's system had its flaws as well, and consequently, has been modified and refined extensively. From these, a minor deontic logic has emerged that has come to be termed *Standard Deontic Logic,* SDL for short. It is the most studied system of deontic logic, but is also problematic. Over time, many competing systems have been put forward and analyzed. Nevertheless, there are still obstacles to constructing a vigorous deontic logic that is consistent and fit. However, as SDL is the simplest exemplar of deontic logic and less objectionable than the current alternatives, we shall use it here. For details, see (McNamara, 2006).

The awkward situation mentioned above is the main reason why deontic logic investigations are still undertaken within the confines of sentential logic. An acceptable quantificational deontic logic does not yet exist. Also, SDL is a deontic-modal extension of sentential logic. Our presentation of this miniature logic consists of the following three sections:

▶ The syntax of the deontic language $\mathcal{DL}_0$
▶ The semantics of the deontic language $\mathcal{DL}_0$
▶ The Standard Deontic Logic: SDL.

The syntax of the deontic language $\mathcal{DL}_0$

The syntax of SDL is based on the language $\mathcal{L}_0$ of sentential logic, introduced on page 898. We employ this basic language to construct a deontic language, $\mathcal{DL}_0$ for short. To this end, we extend the sentential language $\mathcal{L}_0$:

---

[174] Rudiments of deontic logic began as a branch of modal logic in the 14th century, when some scholastic philosophers observed analogies between alethic modalities ('possible', 'necessary') and deontic modalities, and studied the normative interpretation of laws of alethic modal logic (Hilpinen, 1981; Knuuttila, 1981, 1988, 1993). Later, the German philosopher Gottfried W. Freiherr von Leibniz (1646–1716) called the deontic modalities of the obligatory, forbidden, and permitted 'legal modalities', and also observed analogies between them and alethic modalities. He suggested that the obligatory is "what is *necessary* for a good man to do" and the permitted is "what is *possible* for a good man to do" (Hilpinen, 2002, 500).

1. by adding to its connectives the deontic operator OB, and accordingly,
2. by adding to Definition 227 on page 898 the following clause:
3. **Definition 227.4:** If α is a formula, then $OB\alpha$ is a formula.

The other four deontic operators PE, FO, OP, and GR for permission, prohibition, optionality, and gratuitousness, respectively, are used as shorthands according to Definition 232 above. The resulting language is the deontic language $\mathcal{DL}_0$. Formulas are also called sentences because they may be interpreted by natural language sentences. A sentence that contains at least one deontic operator, is referred to as a *deontic sentence*.

Note that according to Definition 227.4 above, all kinds of deontically modalized formulas of $\mathcal{L}_0$ turn out formulas in the language $\mathcal{DL}_0$, i.e., deontic sentences. For example, let:

$\alpha \quad \equiv$ the physician tells the patient the truth,
$\beta \quad \equiv$ the patient has acute myocardial infarction,
$\gamma \quad \equiv$ the physician administers thrombolysis to the patient,
$\delta \quad \equiv$ the physician administers oxygen to the patient

be formulas. Then the following compounds are also formulas:

$OB\alpha \qquad\qquad \equiv$ it is *obligatory* that the physician tells the patient the truth;

$\beta \rightarrow OB\gamma \qquad \equiv$ if the patient has acute myocardial infarction, then it is *obligatory* that the physician administers thrombolysis to the patient;

$\beta \rightarrow FO\neg\gamma \qquad \equiv$ if the patient has acute myocardial infarction, then it is *forbidden* that the physician omits administering thrombolysis to the patient;

$\beta \rightarrow PE\delta \qquad \equiv$ if the patient has acute myocardial infarction, then it is *permitted* that the physician administers oxygen to the patient;

$\beta \rightarrow OB\gamma \wedge PE\delta \quad \equiv$ if the patient has acute myocardial infarction, then it is *obligatory* that the physician administers thrombolysis to the patient, and it is *permitted* that she administers oxygen to the patient.

However, none of these strings is a formula:

$OB\alpha\neg$

$\beta \rightarrow \delta PE$

$\alpha \rightarrow FO\beta\gamma\delta.$

As to the binding strength of deontic operators, note that OB and the other operators bind more strongly than $\neg, \vee, \wedge, \rightarrow$, and $\leftrightarrow$. For example, $OB\alpha \rightarrow \beta$ is is the formula $(OB\alpha) \rightarrow \beta$, but not the formula $OB(\alpha \rightarrow \beta)$.

The semantics of the deontic language $\mathcal{DL}_0$

Analogous to alethic modal logic, it has become customary to interpret deontic sentences by possible-worlds semantics. However, the situation here is much more complicated and presents difficult technical and metaphysical problems some of which appear to be unsolvable. We shall circumvent these problems and simplify the issue. For details, see (Åqvist, 1984; McNamara, 2006).

Let $\langle W, R \rangle$ be a Kripke frame with W being a set of possible worlds. An obligation sentence $OB\alpha$ is true at a world $w_i \in W$ if and only if α is true at every world $w_j \in W$ that is accessible from w_i. And a permission sentence $PE\alpha$ is true at $w_i \in W$ if and only if α is true at some world $w_j \in W$ that is accessible from w_i. For example, the sentence "it is *obligatory* that the physician tells the patient the truth" is true at the actual world if at all possible worlds accessible from the actual one its non-deontic kernel "the physician tells the patient the truth" is true. And the sentence "it is *permitted* that the physician administers oxygen to a patient with acute myocardial infarction" is true at the actual world if there is a possible world accessible from the actual one, such that its non-deontic kernel "the physician administers oxygen to a patient with acute myocardial infarction" is true at that world. Thus, *obligation* is interpreted as truth in all possible worlds, whereas *permission* is interpreted as truth in at least one of them. Compare the analogies with the semantics of alethic modal operators on page 917 ff.

The customary semantics above is metaphysically problematic, however. On the one hand, obligations and permissions are human norms instituted by human beings themselves to regulate their social life, and are thus subject to change over time. They are not statements that assert facts. Therefore, it does not seem meaningful to speculate about their truth, untruth, satisfiability, or validity at any actual, possible, or impossible world. They are obeyed or violated. That is all. On the other hand, it is obvious that there is some relation of entailment, for example, between the obligations $OB(\alpha \wedge \beta)$ and $OB\alpha$. Whoever ought to tell the truth and not to kill, ought therefore to tell the truth. The former obligation implies the latter. For this reason, deontic logic seeks to find out in deontic contexts what follows from what. To this end, semantic experiments such as above are undertaken to establish a concept of deontic inference, that according to Aristotelean tradition requires a concept of deontic truth. As in the logics that we have considered up to now, also in deontic logic the relation of implication between a set $\{\alpha_1, \ldots, \alpha_n\}$ of premises and a conclusion β, i.e., $\{\alpha_1, \ldots, \alpha_n\} \vDash \beta$, is conceived as a truth preserving relation between sentences. This semantic relation is snytactically imitated by the following deontic calculus.

The Standard Deontic Logic: SDL

SDL is a deontic extension of classical sentential logic that was presented in Table 38 on page 899. It is displayed in Table 41.

Table 41. The Standard Deontic Logic: SDL

Axioms:

0. All axioms of classical sentential logic introduced in Table 38 on page 899, taking into account Definition 227.4 on page 930 which said that if α is a formula, then $OB\alpha$ is a formula;

1. $OB(\alpha \rightarrow \beta) \rightarrow (OB\alpha \rightarrow OB\beta)$ Axiom K
2. $OB\alpha \rightarrow \neg OB\neg\alpha$ Axiom D

Rules:

$\dfrac{\begin{array}{c}\alpha \\ \alpha \rightarrow \beta\end{array}}{\beta}$ Modus ponens (MP)

$\dfrac{\vdash \alpha}{OB\alpha}$ Rule N

The SDL calculus introduced in Table 41 may be strengthened into an SDL$^+$ by including the following formula as an additional axiom, which states that obligations must be fulfilled:

AXIOM 3: $OB(OB\alpha \rightarrow \alpha)$.

Deduction and deducibility are defined in the usual way. When a sentence α is SDL deducible from a set of premises, $\mathfrak{F}$, we write $\mathfrak{F} \vdash \alpha$. Presented below is an example which proves the following theorem: It is provable that if it is obligatory that α be obligatory, then α is in fact obligatory.

Theorem 7 (Double obligation implies obligation). $\vdash OB\,OB\alpha \rightarrow OB\alpha$.

Proof 7:

1. $OB(OB\alpha \rightarrow \alpha) \rightarrow (OB\,OB\alpha \rightarrow OB\alpha)$ Axiom 1 (K)
2. $OB(OB\alpha \rightarrow \alpha)$ Axiom 3
3. $(OB\,OB\alpha \rightarrow OB\alpha)$ Modus ponens: 1, 2. QED

A few additional derived rules and theorems of SDL are listed in Table 42.

27.2.3 Metalogic

The deontic logic SDL is sound and complete with respect to a particular class of Kripke frames that will not be discussed here (see McNamara, 2006, 213). Soundness and completeness, however, are mere formal properties, and

Table 42. Some derived rules and theorems of the Standard Deontic Logic

1. $OB\alpha \to OB\beta,\ OB\alpha \vdash OB\beta$	(deontic) Modus ponens
2. If $\vdash \alpha \to \beta$, then $OB\alpha \to OB\beta$	
3. $\vdash OB\alpha \to PE\alpha$	(what is required is permitted)
4. $\vdash OB(\alpha \wedge \beta) \leftrightarrow (OB\alpha \wedge OB\beta)$	
5. $\vdash OB\alpha \to OB(\alpha \vee \beta)$	
6. $\vdash OB(\alpha \to \beta) \to (PE\alpha \to PE\beta)$	
7. $\vdash PE\alpha \to PE(\alpha \vee \beta)$	
8. $\vdash PE(\alpha \vee \beta) \to PE\alpha \vee PE\beta$	
9. $\vdash PE(\alpha \wedge \beta) \to PE\alpha$	
10. $\vdash PE(\alpha \wedge \beta) \to PE\beta$	

not sufficient to render a logic useful and acceptable. Practical adequacy and applicability to real-life issues and situations are important requirements as well. SDL has some problems in this respect, even though it is the most robust deontic logic. Here we will cover only one such problem, the so-called Ross's paradox, that originates with the Danish philosopher Alf Ross (Ross, 1941).

The SDL theorems listed in Table 42 also include the following theorem that is derivable from the sentential-logical axiom $\alpha \to \alpha \vee \beta$, Rule N, and Axiom K:

$$\vdash OB\alpha \to OB(\alpha \vee \beta)$$

An example is this:

> If it is obligatory that the physician administers thrombolysis to a patient with acute myocardial infarction, then the physician ought either to administer thrombolysis to the patient or terminate her life. $\hfill (236)$

Suppose now that the following clinical obligation exists, as indeed it does:

> It is obligatory that the physician administers thrombolysis to a patient with acute myocardial infarction. $\hfill (237)$

Both sentences, (236) and (237), jointly imply that the physician ought either to administer thrombolysis to the patient or terminate her life. This either-or obligation is satisfiable by terminating the patient's life. It is obvious that a logic with such strange consequences may not be very useful in real-life situations. There are additional paradoxes and dilemmas with SDL and other deontic-logical systems, one of which is of a particular practical relevance to medicine. We shall briefly explain this special issue in the next section to refer to it later in our discussion.

27.2.4 Deontic Conditionals

Commitments play an important role in medicine. As extensively analyzed in Parts II, V, and VI, clinical practice and research are based on commitments. A commitment is a deontic sentence that demands or forces a course of action in a specified situation. A simple example is this: "It is obligatory that you visit your patient if you promise her to do so". This example gives the impression that the notion of a commitment is something trivial. Yet there is no agreement about how to formalize commitments to render them amenable to deontic logic. To clarify the issue, let us first distinguish between an absolute norm and a conditional norm. An *absolute norm* is an absolute deontic sentence, i.e., an obligation, permission, or prohibition without any precondition on which it depends. Examples are:

It is obligatory that you tell the truth $\equiv OB\alpha$
It is permitted that you take aspirin $\equiv PE\beta$
It is forbidden that you smoke $\equiv FO\gamma$

Thus, an absolute norm binds independently of the factual circumstances, because no such circumstances are specified therein. By contrast, a *conditional norm* has a precondition such that when it is fulfilled, some action is obligatory, permitted, or forbidden. An example was given above. It says:

If you promise your patient to visit her, *then* it is obligatory that you do so.   (238)

Its precondition is "if you promise your patient to visit her". Thus, it seems to be a conditional of the following form:

$$\alpha \rightarrow OB\beta \qquad (239)$$

with:

$\alpha \equiv$ you promise your patient to visit her,

$\beta \equiv$ you visit your patient.

The disagreement about how to formalize the commitment (238) above is this. It is not yet clear whether the commitment (238) is adequately represented by sentence (239) above or by the following sentence (240):

$$OB(\alpha \rightarrow \beta). \qquad (240)$$

Both formalizations give rise to problems in deontic contexts. However, for the sake of brevity, we will not go into details here. Readers interested in the issue may refer to the literature on the debate about Chisholm's *contrary-to-duty paradox* (Chisholm, 1963; Åqvist, 1984; McNamara, 2006).

For two reasons, the alternative (240) cannot be viewed as an adequate formalization of the commitment under discussion. First, its verbatim translation says "it is obligatory that if you promise your patient to visit her, you do so". Thus, it deviates from the original "if you promise your patient to visit her, then it is obligatory that you do so". Second, obviously it says that the conditional $\alpha \rightarrow \beta$ is an obligation. But it does not say what we are to do *when* the antecedent α is true. As an adequate formalization of conditional norms we therefore consider conditionals of the following form like in (239):

$$\alpha \rightarrow OB\beta \qquad \text{conditional obligation,}$$
$$\beta \rightarrow PE\gamma \qquad \text{conditional permission,}$$
$$\beta \rightarrow FO\delta \qquad \text{conditional prohibition,}$$

which we call *deontic conditionals*. The first one is a conditional obligation, the second one is a conditional permission, and the third one is a conditional prohibition. A commitment is a conditional obligation, i.e., an obligation such as $OB\beta$, on the condition that something specified, α, is the case: $\alpha \rightarrow OB\beta$. The clinical-practical significance of this issue is extensively discussed in Parts II, V, and VI.

27.2.5 *De re* and *de dicto*

The *de re* versus *de dicto* distinction discussed in alethic modal logic in Section 27.1 is relevant in every modal logic, and as well in deontic logic. For example, obviously there is an important difference between the following two obligations: (i) there is someone who ought to be hospitalized; (ii) it ought to be the case that there is someone who is hospitalized. The difference is pointed up by the following two formal representations:

$$\exists x OB\alpha \qquad (de \ re)$$
$$OB\exists x\alpha \qquad (de \ dicto).$$

In the first sentence, the operator OB is attached to the sentence α, whereas in the second one the operand of α is the existential quantification $\exists x$. To understand what this means, we must consider the order of quantifiers and deontic operators in a deontic sentence. In other words, we need to understand quantificational deontic sentences. In order to do so, we will expand the first-order language $\mathcal{L}_1$ into a deontic-modal language:

1. by adding to its logical signs the operator OB, and accordingly,
2. by changing part 3 of Definition 205 on page 862 as follows:
3. **Definition 205.3'**: If α is a formula, then $\neg\alpha$ and $OB\alpha$ are formulas.

The other four deontic operators PE, FO, OP, and GR for permission, prohibition, optionality, and gratuitousness, respectively, are introduced as short-hands by Definition 232 on page 929. The resulting language is referred to as the first-order deontic language, $\mathcal{DL}_1$. In this language, it is possible to form quantificational deontic sentences. Examples are:

$$\forall x(Px \rightarrow OBQx) \qquad \text{e.g.:} \quad \text{all humans ought to tell the truth} \qquad (de\ re)$$
$$OB\forall x(Px \rightarrow Qx) \qquad\qquad \text{it ought to be the case that all} \qquad (de\ dicto)$$
$$\qquad\qquad\qquad\qquad\qquad\qquad \text{humans tell the truth}$$

where Px means "x is a human" and Qx means "x tells the truth". Additional uses will be made of $\mathcal{DL}_1$ in Parts II, V, and VI.

27.2.6 Summary

Clinical reasoning requires deontic logic, because diagnostic-therapeutic decisions are based on normative judgment. These issues are addressed in several chapters of this handbook. For this purpose, we have introduced a minor system of deontic logic that has come to be known as the *Standard Deontic Logic,* SDL. It is a sentential logic. We have extended the expressive power of our modal language to also include quantificational deontic sentences, which are needed in our analyses of the deontic character of medical practice and research. We have demonstrated that by means of such sentences, an important distinction can be made between *de re* and *de dicto* deonticity. In addition, we have fixed the syntax of deontic conditionals, which is used in reconstructing medical knowledge and clinical judgment in Parts II, V, and VI.

27.3 Epistemic Logic

The patient Elroy Fox's family physician is searching for a diagnosis to explain and manage his health problems. While interviewing and examining the patient, she has arrived at the following intermediate judgment:

1. *I believe that* Elroy Fox has hepatitis,
2. If Elroy Fox has hepatitis, then he does not have gallstones.

A few minutes later, X-ray images are taken of the patient's abdomen. They clearly show several stones in his gallbladder. Based upon this evidence, the physician asserts:

3. *I know that* Elroy Fox has gallstones.

The question arises whether this last statement logically affects the physician's diagnostic opinion that now consists of all three statements. Is it a coherent set of statements, or is it now inconsistent and therefore requires revision? Her own common-sense impression is that it has become inconsistent. Specifically, she thinks that she cannot uphold assertion 1 any more, and should abandon it. Is she right? How can she justify her suspicion so as to logically manage her diagnostic judgment that contains phrases such as "I know that ..." and "I believe that ..."? *Epistemic logic*, from the Greek term ἐπιστήμη (epistēmē) for "knowledge", addresses questions of this type. It seeks to formalize the discourse and reasoning about knowledge and belief. That part of it concerned solely with conviction, belief, conjecturing, and possibility considerations, is also termed *doxastic logic,* from the Greek word δόξα (doxa) for "opinion" and "belief". But as mentioned previously, we shall use the more general term "epistemic logic" covering both epistemic logic proper and doxastic logic.

Rudiments of epistemic logic grew in the Middle Ages in philosophical works by Pierre Abélard (1079–1142) and William of Ockham (1280/85–1347/50). The most prolific period was during the fifteenth century. For historical details, see (Boh, 1993; Knuuttila, 1988, 1993). As a branch of formal modal logic, it goes back to the work of a few analytic philosophers in the twentieth century such as the German-American philosopher of science and logician Rudolf Carnap (1891–1970), the Finnish philosopher and logician Georg Henrik von Wright (1916–2003), and particularly his compatriot Jaakko Hintikka (born 1929) (Carnap, 1947; von Wright, 1951a; Hintikka, 1962). However, one should be aware that there are no sharp boundaries between epistemic logic, epistemology, and metaphysics (see Rescher, 2005). The current section provides only a brief introduction. For details, see (Gochet and Gribomont, 2006; Lenzen, 1978, 1980, 2004; Meyer and van der Hoek, 2004; van Ditmarsch et al., 2008). Our discussion divides into the following six sections:

27.3.1 Epistemic Modalities and Operators
27.3.2 A First-Order Epistemic Logic
27.3.3 Metalogic
27.3.4 Opaque Epistemic Contexts
27.3.5 *De re* and *de dicto*
27.3.6 Dynamic Epistemic Logic.

27.3.1 Epistemic Modalities and Operators

Epistemic logic deals with epistemic and doxastic operators. These operators represent epistemic and doxastic modalities, respectively. There are a large variety of such modalities of which we list the following main representatives in the order of their decreasing strength. The first one is the only epistemic modality, while (b–e) are doxastic modalities:

a. knowing, knowledge,
b. conviction, certainty,
c. believing,
d. conjecturing, guessing,
e. considering possible.

We shall use the adjective "epistemic" throughout to denote both groups. An epistemic modality is usually considered a mental attitude of an epistemic subject or *agent* such as a particular human being *a,* say Elroy Fox, toward a state of affairs. Examples are Elroy Fox's knowing or believing that he has hepatitis. The above-mentioned modalities will be uniformly represented by the following operators, respectively, where *a* is an epistemic agent:

1. a knows that ...
2. a is convinced that ...   (strong belief)
3. a believes that ...   (weak belief)
4. a conjectures that ...
5. a considers it possible that ...

They are sentential operators. That is, an operator is applied to a sentence to yield a new sentence. The yield is an epistemic-modal sentence. A few examples may illustrate. In these examples, a sentence to which an operator is attached, is written in bold face, while the operator itself is italicized:

- Elroy Fox *knows that* **he is icteric**,
- His wife *is convinced that* **Elroy Fox has hepatitis**,
- Dr. Smith *believes that* **Elroy Fox has gallstones**,
- Amy *conjectures that* **she is pregnant**,
- Beth *considers it possible that* **AIDS will become curable soon**.

Such sentences describe or represent epistemic attitudes as mental states of individual agents x, y, and z like Elroy Fox, his wife, Dr. Smith, and so on. We will not go into the details of epistemic logic here, but confine ourselves to the study of two main operators only, i.e., x *knows that* and y *believes that*. They are applied to a sentence such as α or β as above:

x knows that α,   e.g.,   Elroy Fox knows that he is icteric,
y believes that β,   Dr. Smith believes that Elroy Fox has gallstones.

They are obviously two-place operators. For simplicity's sake, we shall symbolize them as follows:

$$K(x, \alpha) \quad \equiv \quad x \text{ knows that } \alpha$$
$$B(y, \beta) \quad \quad \quad y \text{ believes that } \beta$$

where α and β are any sentences. Since our epistemic sentences will grow increasingly complex and may thus become difficult to read, we introduce a slightly simplified notational convention. The two-place operators $K(x, \alpha)$ and $B(y, \beta)$ above will be represented as pseudo-unary ones in the following manner:

$$K_x \alpha \quad \equiv \quad x \text{ knows that } \alpha$$
$$B_y \beta \quad \quad \quad y \text{ believes that } \beta$$

such as, for example:

$$K_{Elroy\_Fox} \alpha \quad \equiv \quad \text{Elroy Fox knows that } \alpha$$
$$B_{Dr\_Smith} \beta \quad \quad \quad \text{Dr. Smith believes that } \beta.$$

A subscript such as x or y is the name of the individual knower or believer. Thus, K and B are treated as individualized epistemic operators of particular agents x and y, respectively.

27.3.2 A First-Order Epistemic Logic

The purpose of epistemic logic is to analyze the properties of and the interaction between epistemic operators, the relationships between epistemic sentences, and to construct a method of reasoning with such sentences. This task requires an *epistemic language* with a specified syntax and semantics. Such an epistemic language will be constructed in the next section. In the subsequent three sections we shall briefly sketch an epistemic logic of knowledge *without* identity and shall indicate some interesting relationships between knowledge and belief. The reason why we waive identity, will be explained in Section 27.3.4 below. Thus, our discussion consists of the following three parts:

▶ The syntax and semantics of the epistemic language $\mathcal{EL}_1$
▶ A logic of knowledge: System S5
▶ Knowledge and belief.

The syntax and semantics of the epistemic language $\mathcal{EL}_1$

The first-order language $\mathcal{L}_1$ without identity is extended to an epistemic language without identity, denoted $\mathcal{EL}_1$:

1. by adding to its logical signs the operators K_x and B_x, and accordingly,
2. by changing parts 1 and 3 of Definition 205 on page 862 as follows:
3. **Definition 205.1′:** Remove 205.1;
4. **Definition 205.3′:** If α is a formula and x is an atomic term, then $\neg\alpha$, $K_x\alpha$, and $B_x\alpha$ are formulas.

For example, let the individual constants "a" and "b" denote, respectively, the patient Elroy Fox and his family physician Dr. Smith. And let "Ix", "Hx", and "Gx" stand for the sentences "x is icteric", "x has hepatitis", and "x has gallstones", respectively. The following strings are formulas in the first-order epistemic language $\mathcal{EL}_1$ without identity:

K_aIa	$\equiv$	Elroy Fox knows that he is icteric;
$K_aIa \wedge \neg B_aGa$	$\equiv$	Elroy Fox knows that he is icteric, but he does not believe that he has gallstones;
$K_aIa \wedge B_a\neg Ga$	$\equiv$	Elroy Fox knows that he is icteric and he believes that he does not have gallstones;
$K_aB_b(Ga \wedge \neg Ha)$	$\equiv$	Elroy Fox knows that Dr. Smith believes that he has gallstones, but not hepatitis;
$\exists x(Hx \wedge \neg K_xHx)$	$\equiv$	there are people with hepatitis who don't know it;
$K_b\neg B_a\neg Ha$	$\equiv$	Dr. Smith knows that Elroy Fox does not believe that he doesn't have hepatitis.

However, none of the sequences $IaK_a \wedge Ha$ and $\exists x(B_b(x) \wedge Gx\neg K_a)$ is a formula.

As regards the semantics of our epistemic language $\mathcal{EL}_1$, again the situation is analogous to other modal languages we covered previously. Kripke semantics is used to interpret its sentences. Roughly, a knowledge sentence of the form $K_x\alpha$ is true in a world w, if in every possible world w' compatible with what x knows in w, it is the case that α. And a belief sentence of the form $B_x\alpha$ is true in a world w, if in every possible world w' compatible with what x believes in w, it is the case that α. Finally, the relation of inference is the familiar truth preserving relation $\models$ between premises and conclusion.

A logic of knowledge: System S5

To understand the motivation for doing and employing epistemic logic, suppose that someone utters either of the following two sentences: (i) I know that I have diabetes, but I don't have diabetes; (ii) I know that I have diabetes, but I do not believe that I have diabetes. No doubt, we would consider such a person to be either unreasonable or unaware of the meaning of the terms "knowing" and "believing". This example demonstrates that knowing and believing have particular properties that cannot be sensibly ignored. These properties include the following:

Minimum criteria of knowledge: (241)

1. $K_x\alpha \rightarrow \alpha$
2. $K_x\alpha \rightarrow B_x\alpha$.

The classical concept of knowledge put forward by Plato (428–347 BC), considered in Definition 116 on page 385, entails the two minimum criteria above. Epistemic logic systematically studies such relationships. In the present section, we will briefly outline a first-order logic of knowledge without identity, referred to as system S5, to familiarize ourselves with a minimum set of principles and rules of epistemic-logical reasoning. It is displayed in Table 43. Deduction and deducibility are defined in the usual way as outlined previously. When a sentence α is deducible from a set of premises, $\mathfrak{F}$, we write $\mathfrak{F} \vdash \alpha$. The example below demonstrates an epistemic-logical proof in system S5.

Assertion 17 (Knowledge of untruth is impossible). $\vdash \neg(K_x\alpha \wedge \neg\alpha)$. *That is, it cannot be the case that one knows something that is not true, e.g., "it cannot be the case that Dr. Smith knows that Elroy Fox has hepatitis, whereas Elroy Fox doesn't have hepatitis".*

Proof 17:

1. $K_x\alpha \rightarrow \alpha$	Axiom T
2. $\neg K_x\alpha \vee \alpha$	Equivalence of $\neg\vee$ and $\rightarrow$: 1
3. $\neg\neg(\neg K_x\alpha \vee \alpha)$	Double Negation: 2
4. $\neg(K_x\alpha \wedge \neg\alpha)$	De Morgan's Law: 3. QED

Table 43. A first-order epistemic logic without identity: The system S5

---

0. Include the first-order predicate calculus without identity, i.e., all of its non-identity axioms and rules introduced in Table 35 on page 892, taking into account Definitions 205.1′ and 205.3′ on page 940 above;

Additional axioms: **Their names:**

1. $K_x(\alpha \to \beta) \to (K_x\alpha \to K_x\beta)$ Axiom K
2. $K_x\alpha \to \alpha$ Axiom T
3. $K_x\alpha \to K_xK_x\alpha$ KK Axiom (or Axiom of positive introspection)
4. $\neg K_x\alpha \to K_x\neg K_x\alpha$ Axiom of wisdom (or negative introspection)

Additional rule:

$$\frac{\vdash \alpha}{K_x\alpha} \qquad \text{Rule N}$$

A few additional epistemic-logical theorems which are provable in the calculus above, are listed in Table 44. They may be used as derived rules.

Table 44. Some epistemic-logical theorems in system S5

---

1. $\vdash \alpha \to \neg K_x\neg\alpha$	7. $\vdash K_x\alpha \to K_x(\alpha \vee \beta)$
2. $\vdash K_x\alpha \to \neg K_x\neg\alpha$	8. $\vdash K_x(\alpha \wedge \beta) \leftrightarrow K_x\alpha \wedge K_x\beta$
3. $\vdash K_x\neg K_x\neg\alpha \leftrightarrow \neg K_x\neg\alpha$	9. $\vdash K_x\alpha \vee K_x\beta \to K_x(\alpha \vee \beta)$
4. $\vdash \neg K_x\alpha \leftrightarrow K_x\neg K_x\alpha$	10. $\vdash K_x\alpha \wedge K_x(\alpha \to \beta) \to K_x\beta$
5. $\vdash \neg K_x\neg K_x\alpha \leftrightarrow K_x\alpha$	11. $\vdash (\alpha \to \beta) \to (K_x\alpha \to K_x\beta)$
6. $\vdash K_x\alpha \leftrightarrow K_xK_x\alpha$	12. $\vdash \forall y K_x\alpha \leftrightarrow K_x\forall y\alpha$

Knowledge and belief

There are also axiomatic calculuses for reasoning with the remaining epistemic operators. However, we will not go into details here. A few brief remarks on the interaction between knowledge and belief may suffice. For further study, refer to (Gochet and Gribomont, 2006; Lenzen, 1980, 2004).

There are many interesting principles on the relationships between the operators K_x and B_x. But they also have some counter-intuitive consequences. There is as yet no general agreement as to which one of those principles to reject in order to prevent such consequences. Listed in Table 45 below are four principles whose addition as axioms to the knowledge calculus S5 above would yield a combined *logic of knowledge and belief*:

Table 45. Knowledge and belief in S5

1. $B_x(\alpha \to \beta) \to (B_x\alpha \to B_x\beta)$	(Axiom K for Belief)
2. $B_x\alpha \to \neg B_x\neg\alpha$	(Axiom D for Belief)
3. $K_x\alpha \to B_x\alpha$	(Axiom KB 1)
4. $B_x\alpha \to K_x B_x\alpha$	(Axiom KB 2)

Some useful consequences of these principles are:

$$\vdash B_x\alpha \to B_x B_x\alpha$$
$$\vdash \neg B_x\alpha \to K_x\neg B_x\alpha$$
$$\vdash \neg B_x\alpha \to B_x\neg B_x\alpha$$
$$\vdash K_x(\alpha \to \beta) \to (B_x\alpha \to B_x\beta)$$
$$\vdash (\alpha \to \beta) \to (B_x\alpha \to B_x\beta)$$
$$\vdash B_x\alpha \land K_x\beta \to B_x(\alpha \land \beta)$$
$$\vdash B_x\alpha \lor K_x\beta \to B_x(\alpha \lor \beta).$$

27.3.3 Metalogic

The epistemic logic S5 discussed above is sound and complete (Meyer and van der Hoek, 2004, 228). However, as we have emphasized previously and shall encounter once more in the next chapter, completeness and soundness are merely formal properties with respect to a formal language. They are not sufficient to qualify a logic as an acceptable one. The currently available epistemic logics, including those sketched above, have unrealistic properties and consequences. Among them are (i) their axioms of positive and negative introspection mentioned above:

$\vdash K_x\alpha \to K_x K_x\alpha$	(everybody is aware of her own knowledge)
$\vdash \neg K_x\alpha \to K_x\neg K_x\alpha$	(everybody is aware of her own ignorance)
$\vdash B_x\alpha \to B_x B_x\alpha$	(everybody believes her own beliefs)
$\vdash \neg B_x\alpha \to K_x\neg B_x\alpha$	(everybody is aware of her own disbeliefs).

They allow the iteration and embedding of operators. This peculiarity may be referred to as the property of *personal omniscience*. It says that the bearer of an operator such as K_x and B_x, be it a human or artificial agent, is always aware of what she knows and believes. (ii) The unpleasant consequences also include another property called *logical omniscience* according to which an epistemic agent is aware of all classical-logical truths. That is, if a sentence is classical-logically valid, e.g., $\alpha \to \alpha \lor \beta$ or $(\alpha \land \beta \to \gamma) \to ((\alpha \to \gamma) \lor (\beta \to \gamma))$, then the agent both knows and believes it. This is an effect of the epistemic Rule N. There is, however, no human being in the real world out there who satisfies this postulate. Nobody knows or believes all classical-logical truths. In addition, the property of logical omniscience also entails that one knows and believes the logical consequences of one's knowledge and belief. For example, in virtue of Theorem 10 mentioned in Table 44 on page 942, i.e., $\vdash K_x\alpha \wedge K_x(\alpha \to \beta) \to K_x\beta$, the truth of the premise $K_x\alpha \wedge K_x(\alpha \to \beta)$ brings with it that the agent x knows that β is the case. It is unrealistic to suppose that anyone of us is capable of such logical omniscience. In a nutshell, real-world human beings' epistemic behavior does not accord with what the epistemic extension of classical logic suggests. This is so because epistemic logic is not a descriptive system of human beings' factual knowing and believing, but a normative system to enable 'rational' knowing and believing.

There is no doubt that the problems mentioned above originate with the very concepts of knowledge and belief. They have particular, more or less psychological meanings in natural languages and epistemology. In epistemic logic, however, they are axiomatically characterized and are interpreted by possible-worlds semantics that deviates considerably from natural language usage. So, the question arises, what is logic at all and of what use is it? These issues are discussed in Parts V and VI.

We have deliberately introduced an epistemic logic *without* identity. The reason is that modal logics with identity, based on classical logic, are highly problematic. We touched on this issue already when evaluating alethic modal logic in Section 27.1. Like alethic modal and deontic logics, the epistemic extension of the first-order classical predicate logic *with identity* does not yield a sound epistemic logic. In an epistemic logic with identity, we would have to accept, for example, the following absurd consequence that if two things y and z are identical, then everybody knows that they are identical, i.e., $y = z \to K_x y = z$ for $\forall x$. The proof is analogous to that given of the necessity of identity in Proof 16 on page 924. In the next section, we shall look at another hotly debated subject in the metaphysics of epistemic modalities that will demonstrate why epistemic logics with identity ought to be avoided in medicine and philosophy of medicine. It is the so-called *referential opacity* of some epistemic contexts generated by epistemic operators.

27.3.4 Opaque Epistemic Contexts

A logic is expected to provide support for sound reasoning. An epistemic logic with identity, however, provides confusion rather than support. Suppose that we had used the first-order predicate logic with identity as the base logic of our epistemic logic, and had introduced an epistemic logic *with* identity. In that case we would have quickly run into the problems discussed in this section.

Let there be any sentence that contains a term t ("term" in logical sense), e.g., "the heart rate of Elroy Fox is 76". In this sentence, there are three terms: (i) the individual constant "Elroy Fox"; (ii) the compound term "the heart rate of Elroy Fox", or $hr(Elroy\ Fox)$ for short; and (iii) the number 76 as a second individual constant. Thus we have the equality $hr(Elroy\ Fox) = 76$.

Two terms are said to be coextensive or *coreferential* if and only if they have the same extension, i.e., refer to the same object. Examples are "Cicero" and "Marcus Tullius" as well as "the morning star" and "the evening star". The first two terms co-refer to the Roman philosopher and statesman (106–43 BC); the second ones co-refer to the planet Venus. If a term x is an identical of another term y, i.e., if $x = y$, then they are of course coreferential.

A context containing a sentence α with a term t is said to be *referentially transparent* with respect to t if t may be replaced with any of its identicals without affecting the truth value of α. For example, every context containing the sentence "$hr(Elroy\ Fox) = 76$" is referentially transparent with respect to the term "76", for without affecting the truth value of our assertion we can replace 76 with any other number that equals it. For instance: $hr(Elroy\ Fox) = 38 + 38$. Thus, in Elroy Fox's patient history his doctor may write either one of the two equivalent sentences. Nothing will be lost. But consider now another example that will immediately lead to a surprise. Let α be the following true sentence that contains the individual constant "Jocasta" as a term:

1. Oedipus is married to Jocasta $\equiv Mab$

where:

$M \equiv$ is married to
$a \equiv$ Oedipus
$b \equiv$ Jocasta.

We know that Jocasta is Oedipus' mother such that we have the identity $Jocasta = Oedipus'\ mother$, i.e.:

$$b = f(a)$$

where the function symbol "f" represents the unary function "*mother_of*". Thus, Oedipus' mother is an identical of Jocasta to the effect that both terms, "*Jocasta*" and "*Oedipus' mother*", are coreferential. By replacing the term "*Jocasta*" in the sentence (1) above with its identical "*Oedipus' mother*", $f(a)$, we obtain the following true sentence:

2. Oedipus is married to his mother $\equiv Maf(a)$.

In this sentence we have written "*his mother*" instead of "*Oedipus' mother*" for stylistic reasons. Both sentences still refer to the same state of affairs. The substitution of a term for a coreferential term has not changed the content of the context. Thus, according to the definition above, the context is referentially transparent. The transformation of the first sentence above to the second sentence is an implicit, non-modal, predicate-logical inference of the form:

Oedipus is married to Jocasta
Jocasta = Oedipus' mother
Therefore: Oedipus is married to his mother.

It may be reconstructed by an explicit, predicate-logical proof of the following form that clearly demonstrates its referential transparency:

Assertion 18 (Oedipus is married to his mother). $Mab,\ b = f(a) \vdash Maf(a)$

Proof 18:

1.	Mab	Premise
2.	$x = f(a) \rightarrow \big(Max \rightarrow Maf(a)\big)$	Identity Axiom 2
3.	$b = f(a) \rightarrow \big(Mab \rightarrow Maf(a)\big)$	Substitution Rule: 2, i.e., $\big[Subst(2, x, b, 3)\big]$
4.	$b = f(a)$	Premise
5.	$Mab \rightarrow Maf(a)$	Modus ponens: 3, 4
6.	$Maf(a)$	Modus ponens: 1, 5. QED

By contrast, a context is said to be *referentially opaque* if the substitution of identicals fails in that the replacement of a term with a coreferential term affects the content and truth value of the context. Consider the following example which, in contrast to the non-modal argument above, is an epistemic argument, and thus, a modal argument. It leads from the two true premises (i) and (ii) to the false conclusion (iii):

(i)   Oedipus knows that he is married to Jocasta
(ii)   Jocasta = Oedipus' mother
(iii)   Therefore: Oedipus knows that he is married to his mother.

Again, this intuitive argument is reconstructible by an explicit, allegedly 'epistemic-logical' proof like the purely predicate-logical one above:

Assertion 19 (Oedipus knows that . . .). $K_a Mab,\ b = f(a) \vdash K_a Maf(a)$

Proof 19:

1.	Mab	Premise
2.	$x = f(a) \rightarrow \big(K_a Max \rightarrow K_a Maf(a)\big)$	Identity Axiom 2
3.	$b = f(a) \rightarrow \big(K_a Mab \rightarrow K_a Maf(a)\big)$	Substitution Rule: 2
4.	$b = f(a)$	Premise
5.	$K_a Mab \rightarrow K_a Maf(a)$	Modus ponens: 3, 4
6.	$K_a Maf(a)$	Modus ponens: 1, 5. QED

In this argument, however, true premises have led to the false conclusion $K_a Maf(a)$ which says that Oedipus knows that he is married to his mother. For he is in fact not aware of that. How did the fallacy occur? The sobering answer is that the epistemic-logical extension of first-order classical predicate logic *with identity* irremediably fails.[175]

---

[175] The notion of referential opacity has been introduced by Willard Van Orman Quine in 1953 who has argued that modal contexts are, in general, referentially

27.3.5 *De re* and *de dicto*

The problem of *de re* and *de dicto* distinction also affects epistemic contexts. However, we will not concern ourselves further with this issue. Suffice it to note that the statement "I know that there is someone who is married to his mother" is not synonymous with the statement "there is someone of whom I know that he is married to his mother". This is so because the following formulas representing them are not equivalent:

$K_i \exists x (x$ is married to his mother),

$\exists x K_i (x$ is married to his mother).

Notice it is the order of the epistemic operator and the existential quantifier in the sentences above that causes the distinction. In some other cases, however, epistemic *de re* and *de dicto* sentences are indeed equivalent. See, for example, Theorem 12 in Table 44 on page 942 which entails the Barcan Formula and its converse. For Barcan Formula and its converse, see page 926. See also footnote 173 on page 926.

27.3.6 Dynamic Epistemic Logic

So far, we have focused on *static* epistemic logic only. Our epistemic attitudes, however, are dynamic. In everyday life as well as in medical practice, they change constantly. At time t_1, we doubt that the patient has hepatitis; an hour later, at time t_2, we consider it possible that she has; still half an hour later, at time t_3, we know that she does not have hepatitis, but gallstones instead; and so on. This enduring flux of our epistemic attitudes toward states of affairs is usually referred to as belief change. Since it is not confined to belief, however, it has elsewhere been termed *epistemic kinematics,* embracing the change of all types of epistemic-doxastic attitudes (Sadegh-Zadeh, 1982b, 109).

To make epistemic kinematics logically systematic and coherent, all epistemic operators ought to be taken into account. In order not to complicate our discussions, we have until now considered two main epistemic operators only, i.e., *to know that* and *to believe that,* and have left out the following three operators:

---

opaque (Quine, 1953a, [1963] p. 142). His supposition and the issues related to the distinction between *de re* and *de dicto* have been the reasons of his opposition against *quantifying in* and modal logics in general. See page 926. Jaakko Hinktikka, however, has argued that Quine's supposition may not be quite correct and suggests solutions to the problem (see Hintikka, 1962, 1972). At this juncture, we can only briefly remark that not everything needs to be possible in this world. It is impossible to construct epistemic and deontic logics *with identity* for use by human beings on the basis of classical logic. The present author presumes that the failure is caused by the simplicity of the classical concept of inference. It should be constrained. But this is not the appropriate place to continue this discussion. See (Sadegh-Zadeh, Forthcoming).

x is convinced that α	$\equiv$	$C_x\alpha$	(strong belief)
x conjectures that α	$\equiv$	$CJ_x\alpha$	(conjecturing, guessing)
x considers it possible that α	$\equiv$	$CP_x\alpha$	(possibility consideration).

The following chain of relationships holds between the descending strengths of all five operators:

$$K_x\alpha \to C_x\alpha \qquad \text{(knowledge entails conviction)} \tag{242}$$

$$C_x\alpha \to B_x\alpha \qquad \text{(conviction entails belief)}$$

$$B_x\alpha \to CJ_x\alpha \qquad \text{(believing entails conjecturing)}$$

$$CJ_x\alpha \to CP_x\alpha \qquad \text{(conjecturing entails possibility consideration).}$$

This chain implies, by the Chain Rule in Table 36 on page 895, sentences such as $K_x\alpha \to CJ_x\alpha$; $C_x\alpha \to CP_x\alpha$; and so on. Now, consider a diagnostic process in the cᴄurse of which a physician, x, is collecting data about the patient Elroy Fox's health condition, and successively forms diagnostic judgments. For instance, she says:

at time t_1: C_x(Elroy Fox does not have hepatitis) $\wedge$
B_x(Elroy Fox has gallstones)

at time t_2: CP_x(Elroy Fox has hepatitis) $\wedge$
C_x(Elroy Fox has gallstones) $\wedge$
CJ_x(Elroy Fox has gastritis)

at time t_3: K_x(Elroy Fox does not have hepatitis) $\wedge$
K_x(Elroy Fox has gallstones) $\wedge$
C_x(Elroy Fox does not have gastritis) $\wedge$
CJ_x(Elroy Fox has duodenal ulcers).

Summarizing, we have the following epistemic sentences:

at time t_1: $C_x\neg\alpha \wedge B_x\beta$ or: $\{C_x\neg\alpha, B_x\beta\}$

at time t_2: $CP_x\alpha \wedge C_x\beta \wedge CJ_x\gamma$ $\{CP_x\alpha, C_x\beta, CJ_x\gamma\}$

at time t_3: $K_x\neg\alpha \wedge K_x\beta \wedge C_x\neg\gamma \wedge CJ_x\delta$ $\{K_x\neg\alpha, K_x\beta, C_x\neg\gamma, CJ_x\delta\}$.

Apparently, the doctor's epistemic attitudes toward the patient's state of health change over time. Unfortunately, however, there is as yet no logic that enables us to analyze and understand this epistemic kinematics in relation to the evidence the physician obtains in the process of clinical decision-making. Only recently have first attempts been made to construct *dynamic epistemic logics* that promise to shed some light on these and related issues. They clearly underline the point made above that no sharp boundaries exist among epistemic logic, epistemology, and metaphysics. But we cannot here go into the details of these demanding issues (see van Ditmarsch et al., 2008).

27.3.7 Summary

In clinical decision-making the physician's beliefs, convictions, and knowledge about a patient's health condition characterize the outcome of her clinical judgment. She *believes* that the patient has disease *A,* is *convinced* that she does not have disease *B,* and *knows* that she has disease *C.* The process of acquiring such epistemic attitudes may at first glance appear as something exclusively psychological. But a closer look reveals that at least partially it is something epistemic-logical, for in many situations we attain our epistemic attitudes by revising preceding ones in the light of new evidence. Questions arise about how we may logically manage this epistemic kinematics and how we may derive conclusions from premises which contain at least one epistemic sentence. Epistemic logic is concerned with problems of this type. We have briefly outlined an epistemic logic of the first order without identity, the so-called *system S5,* that may support epistemic reasoning in medical decision-making. We have described the circumstances under which epistemic contexts become referentially opaque. And we have shown that the *de re* and *de dicto* distinction also holds in epistemic discourse and may be syntactically recognized.

27.4 Temporal Logic

Medical knowledge and reasoning is primarily concerned with statements about processes, i.e., about phenomena that change over time. Examples are pathophysiological and biochemical processes, disease histories, recovering, and so on. Temporal logic, from the Latin term "tempus" meaning *time,* is the logic of reasoning with such time-dependent statements, and is therefore needed in all medical domains. Consider the following example adapted from a formally similar one by Burgess (Burgess, 2002, 1):

Example 11.
    Dr. A: We shall operate on Elroy Fox's gallbladder shortly;
    Dr. B: He ought to receive a blood transfusion before the operation;
    Dr. A: I have not yet administered him a blood transfusion;
    Dr. B: Then you will have to do so soon.

This is a simple example of temporal reasoning leading to the conclusion "then you will have to do so soon". It demonstrates that even our most elementary conversations and arguments involve issues of temporal order. In natural languages, this order is expressed by changes in verb forms, such as *I do, I did, I shall do;* by terms referring to explicit instants, periods, dates, and so on, such as *right now, yesterday, today,* and *tomorrow;* or by terms such as *now, before, after, later, earlier, always, never, since, until,* etc. This rich terminology may be grouped into the three general categories *past, present,* and *future* referred to as tenses. Temporal logic studies the role the tenses play in sound reasoning.

Therefore, it is also called *tense logic*. Tense logic is increasingly becoming an important tool in knowledge engineering to enable the automated processing of temporal relationships used in knowlege bases and data. For this reason, temporal logic today is, like epistemic logic, extensively investigated and used in computer sciences, artificial intelligence, and expert systems research (see Fisher et al., 2005; Galton, 1987; Kröger and Merz, 2008).

There are two different approaches to temporal logic, a modal one and a non-modal one. In what follows, we shall briefly consider both of them. A logic in the proper sense of this term provides only the modal approach. It goes exclusively back to the pioneering work of the New Zealandian logician and philosopher Arthur Norman Prior (Prior, 1955, 1957, 1967, 1968).[176]

Modal temporal logic is the most complex, problematic, and disputed one among modal logics. Moreover, it lacks any sharp demarcation from the philosophy, protophysics, and mathematics of time. Therefore, we will here confine ourselves to a minimal system of temporal logic that is not susceptible to these problems. Our discussion is divided into the following six sections:

27.4.1 Temporal Modalities and Operators
27.4.2 A Minimal System of Temporal Logic
27.4.3 Metalogic
27.4.4 Since and Until
27.4.5 Metric Temporal Logic
27.4.6 Alternative Approaches.

For those interested in the intricacies of the subject, see (Gabbay and Guenthner, 2002; Øhrstrøm and Hasle, 1995, 2006; van Benthem, 1991).

27.4.1 Temporal Modalities and Operators

Example 11 above shows that drawing conclusions from tensed statements requires knowledge of how to logically treat tenses. For instance, its first premise says *it will at some time be the case that* we operate on Elroy Fox's gallbladder. Arthur Prior, the inventor of modal temporal logic, conceived tenses as modalities and represented them by modal operators like the italicized phrase in the preceding sentence. There are four such Priorian temporal modalities expressed by four *unary* sentential operators, two for the past tense and two for the future tense:

P	$\equiv$ It has at some time been the case that ...	(weak past)
F	$\equiv$ It will at some time be the case that ...	(weak future)
H	$\equiv$ It has always been the case that ...	(strong past)
G	$\equiv$ It will always be the case that ...	(strong future).

---

[176] Arthur Prior (1914–1969) taught philosophy and logic at Canterbury University College in New Zealand, and philosophy at the University of Manchester (1959–1966) and at Balliol College in Oxford (1966–1969).

P and F are called weak tense operators, while H and G are known as strong tense operators. A tense operator is prefixed to a sentence α to generate a new, tensed sentence of the form $P\alpha, F\alpha, H\alpha$, and $G\alpha$. For example, let α be the sentence "Elroy Fox has gallbladder colic", then we have:

$P\alpha$ ≡ It has at some time been the case that Elroy Fox has gallbladder colic;
$F\alpha$ ≡ It will at some time be the case that Elroy Fox has gallbladder colic;
$H\alpha$ ≡ It has always been the case that Elroy Fox has gallbladder colic;
$G\alpha$ ≡ It will always be the case that Elroy Fox has gallbladder colic.[177]

These sentences formally represent natural-language statements of the form: Elroy Fox had gallbladder colic; he will have gallbladder colic; he always had gallbladder colic; he will always have gallbladder colic.

Weak and strong tense operators are dual to each other and thus inter-definable to the effect that only two tense operators suffice to axiomatize temporal logic. We thus define P by H, and F by G:

Definition 233 (Tense operators or temporal operators).

1. $P\alpha$ *iff* $\neg H\neg\alpha$
2. $F\alpha$ *iff* $\neg G\neg\alpha$.

27.4.2 A Minimal System of Temporal Logic

Like other logics, temporal logic requires a particular language with a specified syntax and semantics. Such a language of temporal logic will be introduced first by extending the language $\mathcal{L}_0$ of sentential logic described on page 897, and will be referred to here as $\mathcal{TL}_0$. Following this, a minimal system of temporal logic, called K_t, will be introduced which is a temporalized variant of classical sentential logic. Our discussion divides into these three sections:

▶   The syntax of the temporal language $\mathcal{TL}_0$
▶   The semantics of the temporal language $\mathcal{TL}_0$
▶   The minimal temporal logic K_t.

Because of immense technical and metaphysical problems of quantificational temporal logic, no such system will be discussed here. For details, see (Gabbay et al., 1994a, 2000; van Benthem, 1991).

---

[177] Arthur Prior believed that all tensed statements could be expressed by the four tense modalities $PFHG$. But his belief has turned out to be wrong. His inspiration for conceiving tenses as modalities came from Diodorus Cronus. Diodorus Cronus, also called Diodorus Chronus, Diodoros Chronos, or Diodoros Kronos, was a Greek logician and philosopher of the Stoic School and lived in the fourth century BC. He tried to reduce alethic modalities to temporal ones by defining them in the following way: *possible* is what is or will be, while *necessary* is what is and always will be. That is, $\Diamond\alpha \equiv \alpha \vee F\alpha$; and $\Box\alpha \equiv \alpha \wedge G\alpha$. Aristotle added to the Diodorean modalities the past as part of what is possible or necessary, respectively. That is, in our present terminology: $\Diamond\alpha \equiv P\alpha \vee \alpha \vee F\alpha$; and $\Box\alpha \equiv H\alpha \wedge \alpha \wedge G\alpha$. See (Prior, 1967; Kneale and Kneale, 1968; Hintikka,1973; Øhrstrøm and Hasle, 1995).

The syntax of the temporal language $\mathcal{TL}_0$

The temporal extension of the sentential language $\mathcal{L}_0$ we call the temporal language $\mathcal{TL}_0$. This temporal language, $\mathcal{TL}_0$, is the object language of the minimal temporal logic K_t and is obtained from $\mathcal{L}_0$:

1. by adding to its connectives the tense operators H and G, and
2. by adding to Definition 227 on page 898 the following clause:
3. **Definition 227.4:** If α is a formula, then $H\alpha$ and $G\alpha$ are formulas.

The weak tense operators P and F for past and future are introduced as shorthands by Definition 233 above. The resulting language is the temporal language $\mathcal{TL}_0$. Formulas are also called sentences because they may be interpreted by natural language sentences. A sentence that contains at least one tense operator, is referred to as a tensed or *temporal sentence*.

Note that according to Definition 227.4 above, all formulas of $\mathcal{L}_0$ temporalized by $PFHG$ turn out formulas in the language $\mathcal{TL}_0$, i.e., temporal sentences. For example, let:

$$
\begin{aligned}
\alpha &\equiv \text{Elroy Fox has gallbladder colic,} \\
\beta &\equiv \text{we operate on Elroy Fox's gallbladder,} \\
\gamma &\equiv \text{we administer Elroy Fox a blood transfusion,} \\
\delta &\equiv \text{Elroy Fox is discharged from the hospital}
\end{aligned}
$$

be formulas. Then the following compounds are also formulas:

$P\alpha$	$\equiv$	it has at some time been the case that Elroy Fox has gallbladder colic;
$P\alpha \to F\beta$	$\equiv$	if it has at some time been the case that Elroy Fox has gallbladder colic, then it will at some time be the case that we operate on his gallbladder;
$P\alpha \to F\gamma \wedge F\beta$	$\equiv$	if Elroy Fox did have gallbladder colic, then we will administer him a blood transfusion and will operate on him;
$FP\beta \to F\delta$	$\equiv$	after we will have operated on Elroy Fox's gallbladder, he will be discharged from the hospital;
$FP\beta \to G\neg\alpha$	$\equiv$	after having been operated on, Elroy Fox will never again have gallbladder colic.
$FP\beta \to \neg F\alpha$		

However, none of these strings is a formula: $\beta \to H\delta\neg G$, $P\alpha \to F\beta\neg\gamma\delta$, $\alpha F\wedge$.

As to the binding strength of tense operators, note that they bind stronger than $\neg, \vee, \wedge, \to$, and $\leftrightarrow$. For example, $P\alpha \to \beta$ is the formula $(P\alpha) \to \beta$, but not the formula $P(\alpha \to \beta)$.

The semantics of the temporal language $\mathcal{TL}_0$

The tense operators are interpreted over a *flow of time,* referred to as a temporal frame. A temporal frame is an ordered pair of the form $\langle T, < \rangle$ such that T is a set of time instants or periods, and $<$ is the binary earlier-later relation on T. If t_1 and t_2 are two elements of T, then "$t_1 < t_2$" means that t_1 is earlier than t_2, i.e., t_2 is later than t_1. Now, the semantics of the language $\mathcal{TL}_0$ is based on the following interpretation of the atomic formulas over a temporal frame $\langle T, < \rangle$:

- $H\alpha$ is true at $t \in T$ iff α is true at all times $t' \in T$ such that $t' < t$
- $G\alpha$ is true at $t \in T$ iff α is true at all times $t' \in T$ such that $t < t'$.

These definitions and Definition 233 above imply:

- $P\alpha$ is true at $t \in T$ iff α is true at some time $t' \in T$ such that $t' < t$
- $F\alpha$ is true at $t \in T$ iff α is true at some time $t' \in T$ such that $t < t'$.

The truth, satisfiability, and validity of compound formulas are defined in the usual way. Also the concept of semantic inference is the usual, classical one, i.e., the truth preserving relation of implication $\{\alpha_1, \ldots, \alpha_n\} \vDash \beta$ between the premises $\{\alpha_1, \ldots, \alpha_n\}$ and a conclusion β. This semantic relation is snytactically imitated by the following calculus.

The minimal temporal logic K_t

There are dozens of temporal-logical calculi of different size and quality of which we will here introduce only the basic one called the minimal temporal logic K_t. It is a temporalization of classical sentential logic without quantificational capabilities and is displayed in Table 46. Deduction and deducibility are defined in the usual way as outlined previously. When a sentence α is deducible from a set of premises, $\mathfrak{F}$, we write $\mathfrak{F} \vdash \alpha$. Two simple examples may demonstrate a temporal-logical proof in the system K_t.

Metatheorem 8 (Enduring future truth). $\vdash \alpha \rightarrow \beta$, then $G\alpha \rightarrow G\beta$. (*That is, if $\alpha \rightarrow \beta$ is a tautology, then, if it will always be the case that α, then it will always be the case that β.*)

Proof of Metatheorem 8:

1. $\alpha \rightarrow \beta$		Supposed tautology (e.g., $\alpha \rightarrow \alpha \vee \neg\alpha$)
2. $G(\alpha \rightarrow \beta)$		Rule G: 1
3. $G(\alpha \rightarrow \beta) \rightarrow (G\alpha \rightarrow G\beta)$		Axiom 1
4. $G\alpha \rightarrow G\beta$		Modus ponens: 2, 3. QED

A proved metatheorem such as above may be added to the calculus as a derived rule to be employed in future proofs. Thus we will use the above metatheorem to prove the following theorem.

Table 46. The minimal temporal logic K_t

Axioms:

0. Include all axioms of classical sentential logic introduced in Table 38 on page 899, taking into account Definition 227.4 on page 952 above which said that if α is a formula, then $H\alpha$ and $G\alpha$ are formulas;
1. $G(\alpha \to \beta) \to (G\alpha \to G\beta)$
2. $H(\alpha \to \beta) \to (H\alpha \to H\beta)$
3. $\alpha \to GP\alpha$
4. $\alpha \to HF\alpha$.

Rules:

$$\frac{\begin{array}{c}\alpha \\ \alpha \to \beta\end{array}}{\beta} \qquad \text{Modus ponens (MP)}$$

$$\frac{\vdash \alpha}{G\alpha} \qquad \text{Rule G}$$

$$\frac{\vdash \alpha}{H\alpha} \qquad \text{Rule H}$$

Theorem 8. $\vdash G(\alpha \to \beta) \to (F\alpha \to F\beta)$

Proof of Theorem 8:

1. $(\alpha \to \beta) \to (\neg\beta \to \neg\alpha)$		Tautology (Contraposition Rule)
2. $G(\alpha \to \beta) \to G(\neg\beta \to \neg\alpha)$		Metatheorem 8: 1
3. $G(\neg\beta \to \neg\alpha) \to (G\neg\beta \to G\neg\alpha)$		Axiom 1
4. $G(\alpha \to \beta) \to (G\neg\beta \to G\neg\alpha)$		Chain Rule: 2, 3
5. $G(\alpha \to \beta) \to (\neg G\neg\alpha \to \neg G\neg\beta)$		Contraposition of Consequent: 4
6. $G(\alpha \to \beta) \to (F\alpha \to F\beta)$		Definition 233.2: 5. QED

A few additional theorems that are provable in the above calculus are listed in Table 47. They may be used as derived rules.

27.4.3 Metalogic

The calculus K_t is sound and complete for all temporal frames $\langle T, < \rangle$ and is decidable. It can even be enlarged by including additional axioms to increase its scope and potential. However, this is beyond the scope of our current project. For details, see (Burgess, 2002).

Table 47. Some temporal-logical theorems in the system K_t

1. $\vdash G\alpha \rightarrow F\alpha$	7. $\vdash G\alpha \vee G\beta \rightarrow G(\alpha \vee \beta)$
2. $\vdash H\alpha \rightarrow P\alpha$	8. $\vdash H\alpha \vee H\beta \rightarrow H(\alpha \vee \beta)$
3. $\vdash G\alpha \rightarrow G(\alpha \vee \beta)$	9. $\vdash P(\alpha \wedge \beta) \leftrightarrow P\alpha \wedge P\beta$
4. $\vdash H\alpha \rightarrow H(\alpha \vee \beta)$	10. $\vdash F(\alpha \wedge \beta) \leftrightarrow F\alpha \wedge F\beta$
5. $\vdash G(\alpha \wedge \beta) \leftrightarrow G\alpha \wedge G\beta$	11. $\vdash G(\alpha \rightarrow \alpha \wedge \beta) \rightarrow (F\alpha \rightarrow F(\alpha \wedge \beta))$
6. $\vdash H(\alpha \wedge \beta) \leftrightarrow H\alpha \wedge H\beta$	12. $\vdash PG\alpha \rightarrow \alpha$

Like other modal logics, the modal-temporal logic K_t has problems. For example, consider theorem 12 in Table 47. It says that if at some time in the past it has been true that in the future α will always be true, then α is true. The problematic consequence of this theorem is that everybody who makes a true utterance about the entire future, e.g., the utterance $G\alpha$ in the very theorem, must be supposed to be absolutely infallible.

We have deliberately avoided quantificational tense logic on the grounds that it has not yet matured. The unsolvable problems it generates include an analog of the necessity of identity that we have already encountered previously on pages 922–924. It postulates the eternity of identity that amounts to the implausible claim that the identity between two objects is an eternal property. It says: $x = y \rightarrow H(x = y) \wedge G(x = y)$. But the following counterexample falsifies this claim: The time-honored identity 'the number of planets = 9' ceased to exist on August 24, 2006 when the International Astronomical Union, IAU, defined the term "planet" anew and thereby stripped Pluto of its planetary status to the effect that the number of planets became 8.

It is worth noting that the *de re* and *de dicto* problem recurs in quantificational temporal logic. For instance, the natural language statement "a physician will be the president" may be construed in the following two ways:

- $\exists x \big(physician(x) \wedge Fpresident(x)\big)$
- $F\exists x \big(physician(x) \wedge president(x)\big)$.

The first sentence is *de re*, the second one is *de dicto*. Their vague, natural language version does not betray this significant difference. As emphasized previously, they are not equivalent.

27.4.4 Since and Until

An important question to ask about any logic is whether and to what extent it is applicable to human reasoning in natural languages. In this regard, the Priorian temporal logic with its two operator pairs *PF* and *HG* is not sufficient to manage the wide range of natural temporal reasoning in medicine. The reason is that it does not cover essential temporal modalities which play central roles in medical language and clinical decision-making, e.g., *now, then, before, after,* and most importantly, *since* and *until.* A valuable contribution to this issue was made by Hans Kamp in his doctoral dissertation (Kamp, 1968).

Kamp analyzed a host of temporal terms including "now", "since", and "until". He demonstrated that the latter two denote two basic temporal modalities, and are thus two basic operators by means of which all other ones, including the Priorian tense operators P, F, H, and G, are definable. The converse does not hold. Thus, a temporal logic could be based upon *since* and *until* as well. We therefore introduce into our discussion these two operators and symbolize them by S and U, respectively:

$$S \quad \equiv \quad \text{since}$$
$$U \quad \equiv \quad \text{until.}$$

Each of them is a binary sentential connective and is applied to two sentences, α and β, to yield a new sentence of the form:

$S(\alpha, \beta)$ reads: β since α
$U(\alpha, \beta)$ β until α.

Consider these two examples:

- Ever since Elroy Fox has married he has gallbladder pain,
- he will suffer until he is operated on.

They say:

- S(Elroy Fox has married, he has gallbladder pain),
- U(Elroy Fox is operated on, he will suffer).

The intended meanings of S and U are:

$S(\alpha, \beta)$ $\equiv$ β has been true *since* a time when α was true
$U(\alpha, \beta)$ $\equiv$ β will be true *until* a time when α is true.

Thus, the S and U operators are definable as follows:

$S(\alpha, \beta)$ is true now   *iff* α has been true at some past time and β has been true ever since then;
$U(\alpha, \beta)$ is true now   *iff* α will be true at some future time and β will be true up to then.

This yields, over a temporal frame $\langle T, < \rangle$, the following more precise definitions:[178]

---

[178] One may define the Priorian tense operators P and F by means of S and U as follows. Let there be any tautology, e.g., $\alpha \lor \neg \alpha$. Then we have $P\alpha \equiv S(\alpha, \alpha \lor \neg \alpha)$ and $F\alpha \equiv U(\alpha, \alpha \lor \neg \alpha)$. The other two Priorian operators, H and G, may be conceived as $H\alpha \equiv \neg P \neg \alpha$ and $G\alpha \equiv \neg F \neg \alpha$. For details, see (Kamp, 1968).

$S(\alpha, \beta)$ is true at t *iff* $\exists t_1$ such that $t_1 < t \wedge \alpha$ is true at $t_1 \wedge$
                                      $\forall t_2$(if $t_1 < t_2 < t$, then β is true at t_2);

$U(\alpha, \beta)$ is true at t *iff* $\exists t_1$ such that $t < t_1 \wedge \alpha$ is true at $t_1 \wedge$
                                      $\forall t_2$(if $t_1 < t_2 < t$, then β is true at t_2).

There are a number of additional tense operators which ought to be taken into account in constructing a temporal logic, e.g., "when", "while", "recently", "uninterruptedly", "henceforth", "soon", "next", "eventually", etc. But we will not go into details here (see Burgess, 2002; Øhrstrøm and Hasle, 2006; van Benthem, 1991).

27.4.5 Metric Temporal Logic

Many temporal statements in medicine and everyday life as well are quantitative in character. They talk about definite lengths of time flows. For instance, in the statement "the survival time for this patient is *five years from now*", the italicized phrase is a quantitative time expression. Other examples are "tomorrow at 4 p.m."; "in about two hours"; "ten years ago"; and the like. There are a variety of temporal operators that regulate the use and logical handling of such quantitative expressions, and may therefore be referred to as quantitative or metric temporal operators. Two prominent and pivotal examples are the operators "hence" and "ago" in time expressions such as "a week hence" and "three years ago". They are briefly introduced below.

    The future and past tense operators *hence* and *ago* are written, respectively, $\mathcal{F}$ and $\mathcal{P}$. They are binary operators. Joining them with a time duration yields the following formulas:

$\mathcal{F}(x, \alpha)$ means: it will be the case x time units hence that α
$\mathcal{P}(y, \beta)$ it has been the case y time units ago that β.

Examples are:

$\mathcal{F}(2 \text{ weeks, Elroy Fox recovers})$ $\equiv$ Elroy Fox will recover in two weeks
$\mathcal{P}(3 \text{ days, he is hospitalized})$ $\equiv$ he was hospitalized three days ago.

The ago operator $\mathcal{P}$ can be defined by the hence operator $\mathcal{F}$ since $\mathcal{P}(x, \alpha)$ is equivalent to $\mathcal{F}(-x, \alpha)$. The Priorian operators P, F, H, and G are also definable in terms of $\mathcal{F}$:

$P\alpha$ $\equiv$ there is an x such that $x < 0$ and $\mathcal{F}(x, \alpha)$;
$F\alpha$ $\equiv$ there is an x such that $x > 0$ and $\mathcal{F}(x, \alpha)$;
$H\alpha$ $\equiv$ for all x, if $x < 0$, then $\mathcal{F}(x, \alpha)$;
$G\alpha$ $\equiv$ for all x, if $x > 0$, then $\mathcal{F}(x, \alpha)$.

In the discussion above, the hence operator $\mathcal{F}$ is conceived as instant-based in that its time argument is an instant. It may also be conceived as interval-based such that $\mathcal{F}([x, y], \alpha)$ reads "it will be the case within x to y time units hence that α". For example, "Elroy Fox will recover within the next two weeks". In any case, the metric hence operator $\mathcal{F}$ may serve both as the base operator of a qualitative, Priorian temporal logic as well as a metric temporal logic. A temporal logic of the latter type is better suited for practical application in medicine because many medical-temporal statements deal with time intervals such as acuteness, chronicity, incubation period, and survival time. However, the creation of a metric temporal logic is not an easy task. It involves issues in the mathematics and philosophy of time, for it raises the question whether 'the time' should be viewed, or conceived, as something discrete or continuous, linear or branching, and so on. For details on metric temporal logic, see, for example (Koymans, 1990; Alur and Henzinger, 1993).

27.4.6 Alternative Approaches

Temporal statements, i.e., statements which refer to time instants, periods, dates, or tenses such as "Elroy Fox will be hospitalized at some time in the future", may also be formulated in a non-modal language, for example, in the language $\mathcal{L}_1$ of the first-order predicate logic. To this end, $\mathcal{L}_1$ needs to be extended by adding time variables $t_1, t_2, t_3, \ldots$, time constants $t'_1, t'_2, t'_3, \ldots$, and the binary predicate constant "<" denoting the earlier-later relation. For instance, "now" is a time constant. In this extended language, say $\mathcal{TL}_1$, the example sentence above reads:

$\exists t(now < t$ and Elroy Fox is hospitalized at $t)$.

That is, there is some time t that is later than now, and Elroy Fox will be hospitalized at that time. But the host of modal-temporal operators discussed in the preceding sections are not translatable into the simple relation '<' of a first-order language. From this we can conclude that there is no genuine alternative to modal-temporal logic. This fact is demonstrated by extensive temporal logic research and application in artificial intelligence and knowledge engineering (Fisher et al., 2005; Gabbay et al., 1994a, 2000).

27.4.7 Summary

A developed natural language such as English or German has a far-ranging temporal vocabulary, including a large number of temporal modal operators. The task of temporal logic is, among other things, to construct an appropriate calculus for dealing with these operators that enables viable temporal reasoning. Due to its extraordinary complexity, this task has been fulfilled only partially until now. We have therefore introduced here a minimal system of sentential, temporal-modal logic known as the system K_t. This system may be of some assistance in medical-temporal research and reasoning. But it is still an insufficient tool because it lacks quantification over time. A quantificational temporal logic has not yet emerged. However, attempts are being made to develop alternative, non-modal temporal logics based on predicate logic.

Non-Classical Logics

28.0 Introduction

Classical logic is usually viewed as a masterpiece of the human mind. It serves as the basic logic of classical mathematics and almost all other sciences. However, despite its long history and venerable reputation, it is not an ideal logic. It faces serious objections which demonstrate that as a practical tool, it is inadequate. A logic is an inadequate tool if its practical use generates counter-intuitive and absurd situations that are highly incompatible with common sense and natural language. Classical logic and its modal extensions that we studied in the preceding chapter are just such logics. A few examples will suffice to prove the point. Consider the following three derived rules each of which is a valid classical-logical deduction (for additional examples, see Priest, 2008):

- $\neg(\alpha \rightarrow \beta) \vdash \alpha$
- $\alpha \wedge \beta \rightarrow \gamma \vdash (\alpha \rightarrow \gamma) \vee (\beta \rightarrow \gamma)$
- $(\alpha \rightarrow \beta) \wedge (\gamma \rightarrow \delta) \vdash (\alpha \rightarrow \delta) \vee (\gamma \rightarrow \beta).$[179]

Below, each of these rules is restated, in the same order as above, in its natural language equivalent instances in turn. Thus, the resulting statements represent valid classical-logical arguments. Note, however, that they are obviously absurd, as they generate false conclusions from true premises:

1. It is not the case that if the present reader of this book has no lungs, then she will live over 500 years. So, the present reader of this book has no lungs.

---

[179] Check the validity of these rules simply by truth-table tests. To this end, transform each of them by means of Deduction Theorem 2, given on page 901, into a conditional and observe by means of a truth table that the conditional is a tautology. For instance, the first rule is the derivable conditional $\neg(\alpha \rightarrow \beta) \rightarrow \alpha$. That is, $\vdash \neg(\alpha \rightarrow \beta) \rightarrow \alpha$.

K. Sadegh-Zadeh, *Handbook of Analytic Philosophy of Medicine*,
Philosophy and Medicine 113, DOI 10.1007/978-94-007-2260-6_28,
© Springer Science+Business Media B.V. 2012

2. If the right half of the present reader's heart functions well and the left half of her heart functions well, then she will be OK. So, it is the case either that if the right half of the present reader's heart functions well she will be OK, or that if the left half of her heart functions well she will be OK.

3. If a patient has enteritis she has an intestinal disease, and if she has Alzheimer's disease she has a brain disease. So, it is the case either that if a patient has enteritis she has a brain disease, or that if she has Alzheimer's disease she has an intestinal disease.

Note that the second example will do even with only one of the two conjuncts, say $\alpha \rightarrow \gamma \vdash (\alpha \rightarrow \gamma) \vee (\beta \rightarrow \gamma)$. There are many more instances of the type above which demonstrate that something must be wrong with classical logic. This inevitable, lethal conclusion has caused unorthodox logicians and philosophers in the twentieth century to search for alternative logics. Consequently, a large number of such *non-classical logics* have developed. We shall briefly mention only a few exemplars in what follows. Each of them effectively dismantles the classical logic in a particular way. Our outline divides into the following five sections:

28.1 Relevance Logic
28.2 Intuitionistic Logic
28.3 Paraconsistent Logic
28.4 Non-Monotonic Logic
28.5 Many-Valued Logic.

It is not our aim here to give an introduction to these technically demanding topics. We shall only cursorily touch upon them to show how they challenge the classical logic and its modal extensions, and to stimulate interest in novel logical tools which might be useful in medicine and its philosophy. The five exemplars of non-classical logics sketched below destroy five main pillars of classical logic, including the three Aristotelean principles we discussed on page 874: The Principle of Excluded Middle, the Principle of Non-Contradiction, and the Principle of Two-Valuedness.

28.1 Relevance Logic

The target of this non-classical logic is the classical conditional sign, $\rightarrow$. In classical logic, this sign is supposed to represent the *if-then* relation of our natural languages. According to its semantics in the language $\mathcal{L}_1$, a conditional $\alpha \rightarrow \beta$, such as "if someone has bronchitis, then she coughs", is false only whenever its antecedent is true and its consequent is false. In all other circumstances it is true. This odd semantics is considered one of the main reasons for the failure of classical logic. Due to this semantics, only a *formal* relationship exists between the antecedent and the consequent of a conditional.

The antecedent need not bear any *material,* i.e., content-based, relevance to the consequent. An example is the statement "if the moon consists of green cheese, then AIDS is caused by HIV". The absence of a content-based connection between the antecedent and the consequent directly affects the classical concept of inference, ⊨, for it is defined by means of a conditional. According to that concept of inference, the premises and the conclusion of an argument are tied together only by a truth preserving relationship between them. There need not be any relationship of whatsoever between their contents. That is, the content of the premises of a valid argument in classical logic need not be in any sense relevant to the content of the conclusion. See the Deduction Theorem 2 on page 901 that transforms the relationship of inference into a formal conditional.

In order to prevent the classical breakdown demonstrated above, it has been suggested that a conditional $\alpha \rightarrow \beta$ be a *relevant* one, i.e., that its antecedent α be required to have content-based relevance to its consequent β. Considerable effort has been taken to define such a concept of relevance. The result is the so-called relevant or *relevance logic* put forward by Anderson and Belnap (see Anderson and Belnap, 1975, 1992; Bimbó, 2007; Dunn and Restall, 2002).

28.2 Intuitionistic Logic

The target of *intuitionistic logic* is the Principle of Excluded Middle, $\alpha \vee \neg \alpha$. The Dutch mathematician Luitzen Egbertus Jan Brouwer (1881–1966), the founder of intuitionism in mathematics and logic, analyzed in his doctoral dissertation "On the Foundations of Mathematics" (1907) some concepts and features of modern mathematics and logic. His analysis included the criticism that the Principle of Excluded Middle cannot be accepted over infinite domains. According to him, we have no general method to decide whether a disjunction such as "all integers either have the property P or they don't have it" is true or false. A statement of this form, i.e., $\alpha \vee \neg \alpha$, is meaningful only if we can prove at least one of its constituents, α or $\neg \alpha$. On this account, intuitionistic logic counters the general validity of the Principle of Excluded Middle (see Brouwer, 1907; Heyting, 1971, 1975; Van Dalen, 1986).

28.3 Paraconsistent Logic

The *paraconsistent logic* considers the requirement of consistency to be both unrealistic and practically unsatisfiable. For this reason, it does not condemn inconsistency. Its target is thus the Principle of Non-Contradiction, $\neg(\alpha \wedge \neg \alpha)$.

Suppose we are using a set of premises, e.g., an item of clinical knowledge and some patient data, say about Elroy Fox, to arrive at a diagnosis. As usual, the patient data originate from different sources, for example, from different physicians, laboratories, family members, etc. Therefore, it is likely that they will contain contradictory information about the patient, e.g., a sentence α such as "Elroy Fox has hyperglycemia", and its opposite, $\neg\alpha$. Thus, our premises may consist of a dozen of any formulas, $\mathfrak{F}$, and the contradiction $\{\alpha, \neg\alpha\}$. We know that in this situation the application of classical logic to our premises simply will not work, for its concept of inference is explosive. This is briefly explained below.

Definition 234 (Inferential explosion). *A concept of inference, "$\vdash$", be it a semantic or syntactic one, is explosive iff for all formulas α and β we have that $\{\alpha, \neg\alpha\} \vdash \beta$.*

Such a concept of inference leads from a contradiction to the explosion of the set of its consequences in that *every* sentence is derivable from the premises, be it something true, false, irrelevant, or nonsensical. According to this peculiarity, the classical-logical inference rule *Ex Contradictione Quodlibet* that we have used in Proof 13 on page 904, will produce all true and false, plausible and implausible diagnostic judgments about the patient Elroy Fox above:

Explosion: $\mathfrak{F} \cup \{\alpha, \neg\alpha\} \vdash \beta$ as well as $\mathfrak{F} \cup \{\alpha, \neg\alpha\} \vdash \neg\beta$

since β is *any* statement. We shall obtain, for example, the diagnosis that Elroy Fox has diabetes, and also the diagnosis that he does not have diabetes. In classical logic, then, inconsistent premises, $\mathfrak{F} \cup \{\alpha, \neg\alpha\}$, become trivial. To prevent this, classical logic requires that we eliminate inconsistencies from our premises. However, this is easier said than done. The identification and elimination of inconsistency is a very difficult, and sometimes unfeasible, task. For example, try to find out whether the theory of autoimmune pathology or psychoanalysis is consistent or inconsistent. It is well-nigh impossible to do so. The alternative, therefore, is to tolerate possible inconsistencies and to make sure, by preventing explosion, that they will not harm allowing us to draw reasonable conclusions. To this end, the logic must be *altered* by excluding the rule of Ex Contradictione Quodlibet and analogous rules of explosive inference. Paraconsistent logic has been devised for exactly this purpose.

A logic is said to be *paraconsistent* if and only if its concept of inference is not explosive. It thereby becomes an inconsistency tolerant system and allows for contradictions which we, as imperfect human beings, are unable to prevent or eliminate. This feature qualifies paraconsistent logic as a suitable tool in clinical decision-making. Details may be found in (da Costa, 1974; da Costa et al., 2007; Priest et al., 1989; Bremer, 2005).[180]

---

[180] Paraconsistent logic research originated around 1910 with the Russian physician Nikolaj Alexandrovic Vasiliev (1880–1940) who at the beginning of the 20th century taught philosophy at the University of Kazan, Russia. Inspired by Nikolaj Lobachevski's non-Euclidean geometries in which the Euclidean parallel postulate is not valid, he attempted to construct new, 'Imaginary Logics' by discarding

28.4 Non-Monotonic Logic

In classical logic, the set of conclusions derivable from a set of premises grows when the premises grow. For example, two premises have a larger set of consequences than only one premise has. Three premises have more consequences than two premises, and so on. This property of increasing consequences is *monotonic*, i.e., the more premises the more consequences: If β is a consequence of a set of formulas, $\mathfrak{F}$, then β is also a consequence of the enlarged set $\mathfrak{F} \cup \{\alpha\}$ where α is any additional sentence. That means that a conclusion once drawn from a set of premises, will be preserved as a conclusion even if the set of premises increases.

Some important human common-sense reasoning is *non-monotonic*, however. In our everyday life we draw conclusions from certain premises that we would not draw if we had more information available. *Non-monotonic logics* are formal frameworks concerned with just this type of defeasible reasoning, i.e., a manner of reasoning that does not share the monotonicity property above. Conclusions are always drawn tentatively. They may be retracted in the light of new information. Thus, in these logics the set of conclusions warranted on the basis of some given knowledge, does not necessarily grow if new knowledge is added. It may even shrink by withdrawing some of the previous conclusions. As an example, consider the infelicitous, epistemic-logical argument about Oedipus given in Proof 19 on page 946. It concluded from true premises that:

Oedipus knows that he is married to his mother $\equiv K_a Maf(a)$

while Oedipus does not know that. Now, add the latter statement:

Oedipus does not know that he is married to his mother $\equiv \neg K_a Maf(a)$

as a true premise to those already used in the argument. The false conclusion will still be derivable. And thus, we have the contradiction $\{K_a Maf(a),$

---

some basic laws of classical logic (Arruda, 1977; da Costa et al., 1995). These logics would enable us to study a large class of 'imaginary worlds', he said, which are impossible to classical logic, but nevertheless quite well imaginable. Independently, also the Polish logician Jan Lukasiewicz suggested at the same time that 'non-Aristotelean' logics could be obtained by rejecting the Principle of Non-Contradiction (cf. Arruda, 1977, 1980, 1989). His idea inspired his student Stanislaw Jaśkowski to construct a 'discussive logic' (Jaśkowski, 1948). After these forerunners, specific research in this new field of non-classical logics was initiated by the Brazilian logician and philosopher Newton C.A. da Costa in 1958 (da Costa, 1958, 1963), followed by the Argentinian logician Asenjo and the British-born Australian logician Graham Priest (Asenjo, 1966; Priest, 1987). The term 'paraconsistent logic' was coined by the Peruvian philosopher F. Miro Quesada in 1976 in a letter to da Costa (da Costa et al., 2007, 793). For a comprehensive account of the subject, see (da Costa et al., 2007; Priest, 1989, 2002).

$\neg K_a M a f(a)\}$. This renders the epistemic-logical system presented in Section 27.3.2 inconsistent, and thus useless, because it is a monotonic logic. A non-monotonic epistemic logic would make it impossible to draw the same false conclusion after adding the premise $\neg K_a M a f(a)$. For details on non-monotonic logic, see (Bochman, 2005; Gabbay et al., 1994b; Marek and Truszcyński, 1993).

28.5 Many-Valued Logic

The target of *many-valued logic* is the Principle of Bivalence. The term "many-valued" or "multivalued" means *more than two* truth values on which the semantics of a logic is based. All logics outlined previously are two-valued logics confined to the two truth values *true* and *false*. The many-valued logic, however, uses in addition to these two truth values many other ones. It was created by the Polish logician Jan Łukasiewicz in 1920 (Łukasiewicz, 1970).

Łukasiewicz rejected the Aristotelean two-valuedness on philosophical-speculative grounds. He supposed that it would lead to determinism and fatalism. Although this assumption is erroneous, to resist fatalism Łukasiewicz concluded that there must be statements which are neither true nor false. For example, suppose that someone says "you will send an email to the author of the present book on January 1 next year". We can reasonably assume that the mode of your behavior on January 1 next year is neither positively nor negatively determined now. So, it is possible, but not necessary, that you will send an email to the author of this book on January 1 next year. Accordingly, the statement that you will send such an email is currently neither true nor false. If it were true now, your sending of the email on January 1 next year would have to be necessary. If it were false now, your sending of the email on January 1 next year would have to be impossible. Thus the statement that you will send an email to the author of the present book on January 1 next year, is at the moment neither true nor false. It must have a third truth value different from *true* and *false*.[181]

---

[181] This is a modified version of Łukasiewicz' example in (Łukasiewicz, 1930). The problem concerning the current truth state of statements about the future, known as the problem of *future contingency* (Aristotle's "sea battle tomorrow"), has already been addressed by Aristotle himself in his work *De Interpretatione,* chapter 9 (Kneale and Kneale, 1968, 45 ff.). He has propagated two-valuedness nonetheless. Anticipations of many-valuedness prior to Łukasiewicz' work in 1920 may be found in the works of the Scottish philosopher and logician Hugh MacColl (1837–1909)[see Cavaliere, 1996], the U.S.-American philosopher Charles Sanders Peirce (1839–1914), and the Russian physician and philosopher Nikolaj Alexandrovic Vasiliev (1880–1940). However, many-valued logic research proper originated with Łukasiewicz in 1920. Independently, the Polish-born U.S.-American mathematician and logician Emil Leon Post (1897–1954) also contributed a pioneering system in some six pages of his 1921 paper (Post, 1921). Other systems were added later, e.g., by Stephen Cole Kleene (1952, § 64).

Statements with problematic truth values need not only concern the future. For example, according to the Heisenberg's Principle of Uncertainty, there are statements about elementary particles whose truth value is inherently unknowable due to inevitable limitations of measurement. Many-valued logic enables us to deal with statements of this type with a 'third' truth value. What this new, third truth value is called, is of no consequence. Call it, for instance, 'unknown', 'indeterminate', 'intermediate', 'neutral', or something else. It has become customary to denote 'true' by '1' and 'false' by '0'. So, one may symbolize the third truth value by '$\frac{1}{2}$'.

Based on the line of argumentation above and the expanded truth value set $\{0, \frac{1}{2}, 1\}$, Łukasiewicz initially constructed a 3-valued logic, called L$_3$. But it was not long before he realized that there was no need to stop at three truth values, and generalized his approach to infinite-valued systems. Without going into details, we shall give here only a brief sketch of L$_3$.[182]

Table 48. Definition of the connectives $\neg$ and $\rightarrow$ by the truth tables of negation (top) and conditional (bottom), respectively

α	$\neg\alpha$
0	0
$\frac{1}{2}$	$\frac{1}{2}$
1	0

$\rightarrow$	0	$\frac{1}{2}$	1
0	1	1	1
$\frac{1}{2}$	$\frac{1}{2}$	1	1
1	0	$\frac{1}{2}$	1

The *syntax* of L$_3$ may be the same as that of classical sentential logic sketched on page 897. Łukasiewicz used the negation and conditional signs, $\neg$ and $\rightarrow$, as the basic logical signs and extended their classical *semantics* according to the truth tables given in Table 48.

For example, if we have a sentence such as "coronary heart disease is caused by Chlamydophila pneumoniae infection" with a truth value $\frac{1}{2}$, also its negation which says that coronary heart disease is not caused by Chlamydophila pneumoniae infection, has the truth value $\frac{1}{2}$. Further, the truth value of the following conditional is 1: "if coronary heart disease is caused by Chlamydophila pneumoniae infection, then the Eiffel Tower is in Paris". Additional connectives are introduced by following definitions:

$$\alpha \vee \beta \quad \equiv \quad (\alpha \rightarrow \beta) \rightarrow \beta$$
$$\alpha \wedge \beta \quad \equiv \quad \neg(\neg\alpha \vee \neg\beta)$$
$$\alpha \leftrightarrow \beta \quad \equiv \quad (\alpha \rightarrow \beta) \wedge (\beta \rightarrow \alpha).$$

Due to the semantics depicted in Table 48, their truth tables turn out as shown in Tables 49–51.

As in classical sentential logic, a formula is a *tautology* in L$_3$ if it takes the truth value 1 in all circumstances; and it is contradictory (inconsistent) if

---

[182] The introduction of many-valued logic by Łukasiewicz was motivated by his desire to understand the notion of possibility, i.e., alethic modal logic, in a 3-valued way (see Section 27.1 on page 913).

Table 49. The truth table of disjunction in L₃

∨	0	$\frac{1}{2}$	1
0	0	$\frac{1}{2}$	1
$\frac{1}{2}$	$\frac{1}{2}$	$\frac{1}{2}$	1
1	1	1	1

Table 50. The truth table of conjunction in L₃

∧	0	$\frac{1}{2}$	1
0	0	0	0
$\frac{1}{2}$	0	$\frac{1}{2}$	$\frac{1}{2}$
1	0	$\frac{1}{2}$	1

Table 51. The truth table of biconditional in L₃

↔	0	$\frac{1}{2}$	1
0	1	$\frac{1}{2}$	0
$\frac{1}{2}$	$\frac{1}{2}$	1	$\frac{1}{2}$
1	0	$\frac{1}{2}$	1

it takes the truth value 0 in all circumstances. An example is a tautological statement of the form $\alpha \to (\beta \to \alpha)$. It is no surprise that due to the third truth value, $\frac{1}{2}$, the set of tautologies in L₃ differs from the set of two-valued, classical tautologies. Interestingly, none of the following, classical-logical pillars is valid in L₃:

$\alpha \vee \neg\alpha$ (Principle of Excluded Middle)

$\neg(\alpha \wedge \neg\alpha)$ (Principle of Non-Contradiction)

To confirm this, assign $\frac{1}{2}$ to sentence α, then the truth value of $\neg\alpha$ is also $\frac{1}{2}$. So, both classical principles above obtain the truth value $\frac{1}{2}$ and are thus not tautological in L₃. Likewise, not all classical-logically inconsistent formulas are inconsistent in L₃. For example, the age-old *Liar paradox* "I am now not speaking truly" is no longer a paradox in L₃ because its pathology, i.e., the classical-logically inconsistent formula $\alpha \leftrightarrow \neg\alpha$, is not L₃-inconsistent.[183]

Łukasiewicz generalized his 3-valued logic L₃ in 1922 and introduced a family of n-valued logics with $n \geq 2$, both finite-valued and infinite-valued. Since then, a variety of similar logics have been developed. We will not go into details about them here. For our future purposes, however, a few general remarks on the endeavor are in order. For details, see (Łukasiewicz, 1970; Gottwald, 2001, 2007; Rescher, 1969).

For any $n \geq 2$, the truth values in an n-valued Łukasiewicz logic, L$_n$, is usually represented by rational numbers in the unit interval $[0, 1]$. They evenly subdivide the interval into equal parts. Thus, the truth value set of an n-valued logic, denoted T$_n$, is defined as follows:

$$T_n = \{0, \frac{1}{n-1}, \frac{2}{n-1}, \frac{3}{n-1}, \dots, \frac{n-2}{n-1}, \frac{n-1}{n-1} = 1\}.$$

---

[183] Epimenides the Cretan, a Greek philosopher-poet in the 6th century BC, is supposed to have said "I am now not speaking truly". If he didn't speak truly, then what he said was true, and if he spoke truly, then what he said was false. Thus, his statement is true if and only if it is false: $\alpha \leftrightarrow \neg\alpha$. There are a number of paradoxes of the Liar family. All of them owe their paradoxical character to the inconsistency of $\alpha \leftrightarrow \neg\alpha$ in classical logic. A well-known, simple instance is the statement "this sentence is false". It is false if and only if it is true. However, if we do not use the semantics of classical logic, all of these inconsistencies disappear. Such is the case in L₃ and other many-valued logics. See also the semantic theory of truth on page 462.

They are called degrees of truth. To understand how such a logic works, we shall use three auxiliary notions, i.e., the absolute value of a real number r, written $|r|$; the minimum of two real numbers m and n, written $min(m,n)$; and their maximum, written $max(m,n)$. They are precisely defined in Definitions 18 and 33 on pages 94 and 172, respectively.[184]

As an example logic, consider an n-valued sentential logic with the unit interval $[0,1]$ as its truth value set. It may have the following connectives: $\neg, \vee, \wedge, \rightarrow$, and $\leftrightarrow$. Its syntax may be the same as that of classical sentential logic. Its semantics may be given by an interpretation function $\Im$ that maps the formulas to $[0,1]$ such that for any two formulas α and β we have the following truth values:

$$\Im(\neg\alpha) = 1 - \Im(\alpha)$$
$$\Im(\alpha \wedge \beta) = min\big(\Im(\alpha), \Im(\beta)\big)$$
$$\Im(\alpha \vee \beta) = max\big(\Im(\alpha), \Im(\beta)\big)$$
$$\Im(\alpha \rightarrow \beta) = min\big(1, 1 - \Im(\alpha) + \Im(\beta)\big)$$
$$\Im(\alpha \leftrightarrow \beta) = 1 - |\Im(\alpha) - \Im(\beta)|.$$

We use as an example an 8-valued logic with the following truth value set: $T_8 = \{0, \frac{1}{7}, \frac{2}{7}, \frac{3}{7}, \frac{4}{7}, \frac{5}{7}, \frac{6}{7}, 1\}$. The elementary sentences "Elroy Fox has diabetes" and "he has hepatitis" may be briefly represented as follows:

$\alpha \quad \equiv$ Elroy Fox has diabetes

$\beta \quad \equiv$ Elroy Fox has hepatitis.

They may have, respectively, the truth values $\frac{4}{7}$ and $\frac{2}{7}$. According to the above semantics, we may now calculate:

$$\Im(\neg\alpha) = 1 - \frac{4}{7} = \frac{3}{7}$$
$$\Im(\neg\beta) = 1 - \frac{2}{7} = \frac{5}{7}$$
$$\Im(\alpha \wedge \beta) = min(\frac{4}{7}, \frac{2}{7}) = \frac{2}{7}$$
$$\Im(\alpha \vee \beta) = max(\frac{4}{7}, \frac{2}{7}) = \frac{4}{7}$$
$$\Im(\alpha \rightarrow \neg\beta) = min(1, 1 - \frac{4}{7} + \frac{5}{7}) = 1$$
$$\Im(\alpha \leftrightarrow \neg\beta) = 1 - |\frac{4}{7} - \frac{5}{7}| = 1 - \frac{1}{7} = \frac{6}{7}.$$

The sequence $L_2, L_3, \ldots, L_\infty$ of n-valued Łukasiewicz logics contains the two extremes L_2 and L_∞. The first one is the classical two-valued logic. The latter

---

[184] For the notion of real number, see footnote 12 on page 74.

one is an infinite-valued logic. If the truth value set T_∞ of this infinite-valued logic is the uncountable set of real numbers in $[0, 1]$, it is called the *standard Łukasiewicz logic* L_1, denoted $L_{\aleph_1}$. The symbol '$\aleph_1$' reads 'aleph 1' and signifies the cardinality of the continuum. Reference is made to this non-classical logic in other chapters of the book.

28.6 Summary

In the preceding sections, we briefly sketched a few systems of non-classical logic. There are many additional ones that for the sake of brevity are not mentioned here. The important point is this: All these logics demonstrate that classical logic by no means represents 'the' logic as it is commonly believed. It is merely the simplest and best developed one. We had deliberately emphasized on page 874 that the Aristotelean Principles of Bivalence, Non-Contradiction, and Excluded Middle are basic to classical logic. We have seen above that none of these principles is secure. As a result, classical logic has lost its basis. What remains untouched, is the classical concept of inference, i.e., the truth preserving relationship between premises and conclusion. This relationship characterizes all logics that we have considered thus far as deductive logics. In the next section, we shall look at an additional, non-classical logic whose target is the truth preserving relation of deductive inference itself. Since it is a *non-deductive* logic, it is outlined in a separate section. The system we envisage is the so-called *inductive logic* discussed in Section 29.2. It requires familiarity with the concept of probability. Our discussion will therefore be preceded by a brief introduction to the basic notions of probability, which are used throughout.[185]

---

[185] Like the modal extensions of classical logic that we studied in Chapter 27, non-classical logics may also be extended. There are indeed a variety of such non-classical modal logics. See, for example (da Costa,, N.C.A., 1988; Grana, 1990; Stalanker, 1993; Wolter and Zakharyaschev, 1998).

Probability Logic

29.0 Introduction

A valid argument, via any of the deductive logics above, is considered sound because it is allegedly truth preserving. However, the limited scope of the syntax of these logics does not cover the wide variety and expressiveness of natural language sentences. For instance, none of them is adequate to infer a conclusion from the following premises:

- 30% of patients with coronary heart disease suffer myocardial infarction;
- Elroy Fox has coronary heart disease.

Should we conclude from these premises that Elroy Fox will suffer myocardial infarction or should we conclude that he will not? In either case, the conclusion does not follow from the premises. We are therefore uncertain about what to conclude. The concept of *probability* is a tool to manage, among other things, uncertainties of this type; with it, we may now ask two different questions:

1. What is the probability that Elroy Fox will suffer myocardial infarction?
2. What is the probability that the statement "Elroy Fox will suffer myocardial infarction" is true?

The first question asks about the probability of an *event* that might occur 'in the world out there', i.e., the probability of the individual Elroy Fox's suffering myocardial infarction. The second question, however, concerns the probability of a *statement*. Thus the latter notion of probability concerning an element of language is a metalinguistic notion, whereas the former one is an object-linguistic notion. Although the two notions are expressed by the same word, they are not synonymous. Thus, the natural language phrase "probability" is ambiguous. It does not distinguish between events, on the one hand, and statements describing them, on the other.

The object-linguistic notion of probability pertaining to events is the basic concept of the standard *probability theory* upon which statistics is also based.

K. Sadegh-Zadeh, *Handbook of Analytic Philosophy of Medicine*,
Philosophy and Medicine 113, DOI 10.1007/978-94-007-2260-6_29,
© Springer Science+Business Media B.V. 2012

By contrast, *inductive logic* is a theory of the metalinguistic probability. They are two completely different theories whose aim is to enable probability logic, i.e., logical reasoning in probabilistic contexts. In the present chapter, we shall briefly introduce their building blocks and shall also sketch a third method of probabilistic reasoning, the so-called *Bayesian logic*. Our discussion thus divides into the following three sections:

29.1   Probability Theory
29.2   Inductive Logic
29.3   Bayesian Logic.

Over the last two centuries, medicine has undergone an increasing 'probabilization'. As a result, probability and statistics now play a predominant role in medical research and practice. Our aim is to understand the philosophical, methodological, and practical consequences of this process. The probabilistic approach is extensively used and referred to in our medical-philosophical and methodological inquiries in other chapters of this book, particularly in our theory of medical etiology in Section 6.5.3, of clinical practice in Chapter 8, and of medical logic in Section 16.4.

29.1 Probability Theory

To express our uncertainty over whether a particular event will occur, we often use the term "probable" in that we say, for example, "it is probable that Elroy Fox will suffer myocardial infarction", or "probably he will suffer myocardial infarction". Our uncertainty in this example is an epistemic uncertainty, i.e., a state of partial ignorance. We do not *know* whether Elroy Fox will suffer myocardial infarction or not. We consider the event *probable* in that we say "it is probable that …". As indicated on page 911, this phrase is a modal operator. The vast theory of probability is a mathematical theory of this tiny operator. It introduces a quantitative function, denoted "the degree of probability of" or simply "the probability of", called *probability*. This enables us to talk about the probability of events, for instance, "the probability that Elroy Fox will suffer myocardial infarction, is 0.3", and to calculate such probabilities. We shall sketch the formal system of probability theory only to the extent that we need it in this book. For details, see (Gut, 2007; Jaynes, 2003; Ross, 2008).[186]

---

[186] The terms "chance", "probable", and their derivatives have been around in many languages for a long time. However, the theory of probability as a framework for the mathematical treatment of these notions emerged in the mid-seventeenth century. A few works dealing with 'games of chance' had appeared before in France and Italy. A French courtier, Chevalier de Méré (1607–1648), gambled frequently to increase his wealth. In 1654, he posed to the mathematician and philosopher Blaise Pascal (1623–1662) two gambling questions. Pascal initiated a correspon-

Before presenting the core concept of probability theory in the next section, let us look at a few preliminaries. To begin with, note that *probability theory* does not inform us about whether or not a particular event will occur, for instance, whether Elroy Fox will suffer myocardial infarction, or what will occur tomorrow in the White House and with what probability. It is not an empirical theory about objects or processes in the real world such as trees, climates, or autoimmune diseases. It provides a formal framework for dealing with the notion of probability only. The framework starts with a calculus involving a quantitative function referred to as the *probability measure*. This lays the foundations of a logic for managing subjective *uncertainty,* on the one hand; and objective *randomness,* on the other. While subjective uncertainty is an inner, psychic feature of human beings, randomness or chance is taken to be the irregularity in the occurrence of events outside of the realm of human power (see also Section 16.4.1).

Although probability theory is a highly abstract system, a quick look at its core will convince us how simple a framework it really is. It rests on the following three axioms, which originated with the Russian mathematician Andrey Nikolaevich Kolmogorov (1903–1987):

1. The probability of an event equals or is greater than 0,
2. The probability of the sure event is 1,
3. The probabilities of mutually exclusive events add up.

These basic principles have come to be known as the *Kolmogorov Axioms.* They determine the meaning of the basic concept of the theory, i.e., "the probability of". A few examples are given below to illustrate. In order not to complicate the subject, we shall use simple examples throughout. The most instructive one is to produce random events by *tossing a dice.*[187]

Suppose we have an unbiased, fair dice with six faces numbered 1 through 6. Suppose further that when we roll the dice, it will fall with only one of these six numbers up. We want to roll it once to see what will happen. We

---

dence thereon with his colleague Pierre de Fermat (1601–1665) which eventually led to the theory of probability. The mathematician Jacob Bernoulli (1654–1705) put the theory on a real theoretical basis. His *Ars conjectandi* (1713) is considered the first substantial treatise on probability. Since then, many scientists have contributed to the theory, e.g., Pierre de Laplace, Augustus De Morgan, George Boole, John Venn, Andrey Markov, Richard von Mises, and others. However, its axiomatization had to wait until Andrey Nikolaevich Kolmogorov (Kolmogorov, 1933). For details of the history of probability theory, see (David, 1998).

[187] Since probability theory is concerned with the logic of dealing with randomness, it is also called *stochastics*. The Greek term στόχος (stochos) means "guess, conjecture, pertaining to chance". In compounds such as "stochastic processes", the adjective "stochastic" is often used as an antonym of the word "deterministic" that means that indeterministic, random events are not involved (see Section 6.5.2).

don't know in advance which one of its six faces will fall up. However, the following premises characterize the space of our reasoning:

- There are six possible events: the dice will fall 1, 2, 3, 4, 5, or 6,
- the dice is fair, i.e., all the six events are equally probable, and
- the sure event is: one of the six events will occur.

From these premises and the above three Kolmogorov Axioms we may derive a large number of conclusions in advance. Thus, we already know quite a lot about the possible behavior of the dice before tossing it. To demonstrate this, let us introduce some event names:

Ω $\equiv$ the dice falls '1, 2, 3, 4, 5 or 6'. This is the sure event and says that the dice falls with at least one of its six faces up,

One $\equiv$ the dice falls 1,

Four $\equiv$ the dice falls 4.

If A is any event, we will conveniently symbolize the sentence that "the probability of A is r" by "$p(A) = r$" where r is a real number in the unit interval $[0, 1]$. This one-place function p is "the probability of" and takes events, like A, as its arguments. For example, "$p(\text{Four}) = \frac{1}{6}$" means "the probability of the event *the dice falls 4* is $\frac{1}{6}$".

Now, what is the probability of the event Ω above? Since Ω is the sure event, according to the above-mentioned Kolmogorov Axiom 2, $p(\Omega) = 1$. Likewise, according to our premise of equal chance above we have $p(\text{One}) = \frac{1}{6}$ and $p(\text{Four}) = \frac{1}{6}$. What is the probability of the event 'One or Four'? Note that this event says 'the dice falls 1 or 4'. Since One and Four are mutually exclusive events, we have according to Kolmogorov Axiom 3 above $p(\text{One or Four}) = p(\text{One}) + p(\text{Four}) = \frac{1}{6} + \frac{1}{6} = \frac{1}{3}$. What is the probability of the dice falling with an odd number up? This is the event 'One or Three or Five'. It consists of three mutually exclusive events, i.e., One, Three, and Five. Again, according to Kolmogorov Axiom 3 above, their probabilities add up such that we have $p(\text{One or Three or Five}) = \frac{1}{6} + \frac{1}{6} + \frac{1}{6} = \frac{1}{2} = 0.5$.

We may further complicate our experiment to deal with even more intricate questions. For example, we may toss the dice two or more times and ask what the probability of a complex event such as the following is: 'Four occurs in the first toss, Six occurs in the second toss, and Two occurs in the third toss'. Or we may toss three dice once and ask for the probability of getting the following outcome: 'All three dice fall an even number'. No matter how complex our experiments and questions are, the three simple axioms above enable us to calculate in advance all of the probabilities we want to know.

When one replaces the dice with something medical, for example, with individual diseases such as diabetes, AIDS, or influenza which by their random incidence affect some members of the population, or with an epidemic or with other medical events and processes, one understands how useful probability calculations in medicine may be. In order to be generally applicable in all domains and situations, however, probability theory must provide a framework independently of specific settings like tossing a dice, disease processes, epidemics, and others. To this end, it must fix a syntax and suggest a general calculus that does not refer to particular situations. Such a 'randomness logic' will be briefly outlined below. Our discussion divides into the following six sections:

29.1.1 Probability Space
29.1.2 Probability Distribution
29.1.3 Probabilistic Independence
29.1.4 Conditional Probability
29.1.5 Bayes's Theorem
29.1.6 What Does "Probability" Mean.[188]

29.1.1 Probability Space

We shall first look at some auxiliary notions, which will be used in presenting the probability calculus below. We begin by introducing the notion of sample space.

It is worth noting that the probability calculus is based on classical set theory and logic. As was emphasized above, it is not an empirical, but a formal, mathematical theory that is meant to be applicable to real-world situations, e.g., observations, analyses, experiments, and the like. Any such inquiry may be viewed as an experiment in randomness, referred to as a 'random experiment', because its results depend on things that are not knowable in advance. For example, we would want to find out whether a particular patient is suffering from diabetes, or we would want to toss a dice twice to see what the sum of two subsequent faces will be. Such an experiment's being a random experiment means that the experiment has more than one possible outcome, and we cannot anticipate what the result will be. But we do know what the possible results are. For relative to a particular logic L, we can L-logically calculate the set of *all* possible outcomes of our experiment. Regarding our patient, for example, and relative to classical logic, the set of all possible outcomes is {the patient has diabetes, the patient does not have diabetes}. Such an exhaustive set of all classical-logically possible outcomes is referred to as the *sample space* and will be symbolized by Ω. For instance, in flipping a coin once, the sample space is $\Omega = $ {heads, tails}. In tossing a single dice, the sample space is $\Omega = \{1, 2, 3, 4, 5, 6\}$. In flipping a coin twice the sample space is $\Omega = $ {heads

---

[188] We shall concern ourselves with some basic notions of the traditional probability theory. This theory is said to be 'Kolmogorovian' because its axioms originated with Kolmogorov (see footnote 186 on page 970). There are also attempts to construct Non-Kolmogorovian theories of probability. They are not yet well-developed, however. Among them are also fuzzy probability theories (see, e.g., Ross et al., 2002; Zadeh, 1976a).

heads, heads tails, tails heads, tails tails} where "heads heads" means that *heads* is the outcome in both flips; "heads tails" means that the outcome in the first flip is *heads* and in the second flip is *tails;* and so on.

The entities to which probabilities are assigned, are referred to as events. An event is construed as a *set* so that we may use set theory and logic. Below, we shall define more precisely the notion of an event. First, we need the notion of an *event algebra*, introduced in the following two definitions.

Definition 235 (Algebra of sets). *Y is a field or* algebra of sets *on a set X iff Y is a non-empty family of subsets of X and closed under complementation and union. That is, for every A and B in Y:*

1. $\overline{A} \in Y$,
2. $A \cup B \in Y$.

From this definition it follows that also:

- the base set $X \in Y$ because with any element A of Y also its complement $\overline{A}$ is in Y and the union $A \cup \overline{A}$ is in Y. This union is just X.
- $\varnothing \in Y$ because $\varnothing = \overline{X}$ that is also in Y.
- $A \cap B \in Y$ due to $A \cap B = \overline{(\overline{A} \cup \overline{B})}$. See page 830.

Definition 236 (Event algebra). *If Ω is the sample space of a random experiment, an algebra of sets on Ω is referred to as the* event algebra, *denoted by the mnemonic $\mathcal{E}$.*

Elements of the event algebra $\mathcal{E}$ are called *events* and represented by Roman capitals A, B, C, etc. Consider the following simple example. Suppose we want to know what will happen when we flip a coin once. The coin has two sides, heads and tails. Thus, there are two possible outcomes. Either "the coin falls heads" or "the coin falls tails". They will be represented by "h" and "t", respectively. Only one of these outcomes can occur. Therefore, we have the following sample space and event algebra, Ω and $\mathcal{E}$:

$$\Omega = \{h, t\}$$
$$\mathcal{E} = \{\{h\}, \{t\}, \{h, t\}, \overline{\{h, t\}}\}$$
$$= \{\{h\}, \{t\}, \Omega, \varnothing\}.$$

Note that in the present event algebra $\mathcal{E}$, the complement of the possible outcome $\{h\}$ is $\{t\}$ and vice versa because heads and tails are mutually exclusive. Their union $\{h\} \cup \{t\}$ is $\{h, t\}$ and thus Ω. And the complement of their union, $\overline{\{h\} \cup \{t\}}$, is $\overline{\{h\}} \cap \overline{\{t\}} = \{t\} \cap \{h\} = \varnothing$. Now, events as elements of the event algebra $\mathcal{E} = \{\{h\}, \{t\}, \Omega, \varnothing\}$ may be conveniently symbolized by $A, B, C, \ldots$ to simplify our work:

$$A = \{t\}$$
$$B = \{h\}$$
$$C = \{h, t\} \quad \text{(i.e., "at least } h \text{ or } t \text{ occurs")}$$
$$D = \varnothing \quad \text{(i.e., "nothing occurs").}$$

Before we proceed to construct the concept of probability, we assemble in Table 52 the notation introduced above.

Table 52. Set-theoretical notation in probability

Ω	Sample space
$\mathcal{E}$	Event algebra, an algebra of sets on Ω,
$A \in \mathcal{E}$	A is an event,
$A \cap B = \varnothing$	Events A and B are disjoint, and thus incompatible,
$A \cap B = C$	C is the event which occurs when events A and B both occur,
$A \cup B = C$	C is the event which occurs when at least one of the events A, B occurs,
$A = \overline{B}$	A is the event which occurs when event B does not occur,
$A = \varnothing$	Event A is impossible,
$A = \Omega$	Event A is certain,
$A \subseteq B$	If event A ocurs, then even B also occurs.

Thus far we have introduced a mere frame consisting of $\langle \Omega, \mathcal{E} \rangle$. We will now add in this frame a function p which maps the event algebra $\mathcal{E}$ to the unit interval $[0, 1]$. That is, a number from the interval $[0, 1]$ is assigned to each member of $\mathcal{E}$, and thus to each event. The emerging triple, $\langle \Omega, \mathcal{E}, p \rangle$, is the basic structure of the probability calculus and yields its basic concept introduced in the following definition.

Definition 237 (Probability space). *A triple $\langle \Omega, \mathcal{E}, p \rangle$ is a (finitely additive) probability space iff:*

1. *Ω is a non-empty set referred to as the sample space;*
2. *$\mathcal{E}$ is an algebra of sets on Ω referred to as the event algebra;*
3. *p is a function such that $p: \mathcal{E} \mapsto [0, 1]$;*
4. *For every $A, B \in \mathcal{E}$:*
    - *4.1. $p(A) \geq 0$*
    - *4.2. $p(\Omega) = 1$*
    - *4.3. If $A \cap B = \varnothing$, then $p(A \cup B) = p(A) + p(B)$.[189]*

The clauses 4.1–4.3 represent, respectively, Kolmogorov Axioms 1, 2, and 3 that we had noted in an intuitive fashion previously on page 971. They are referred to, respectively, as Axiom of non-negativity, Axiom of normalization, and Axiom of finite additivity. There is also an infinitely additive probability space for infinite sample spaces in which the third axiom pertains to an infinite number of events. We shall not be concerned with such infinite cases, however.

---

[189] For a representation of the concept of probability space by a set-theoretical predicate, see Definition 26 on page 101.

To illustrate by a simple example, consider flipping the coin above twice and speculating about the probability of getting at least one heads. Supposing that the coin is fair, we have the following sample space:

$$\Omega = \{\langle h, h \rangle, \langle h, t \rangle, \langle t, h \rangle, \langle t, t \rangle\}$$

such that $\langle h, h \rangle$ stands for the outcome *heads* in both flips; $\langle h, t \rangle$ stands for the outcome *heads* in the first and *tails* in the second flip; and so on. The event algebra $\mathcal{E}$ on Ω is large and will therefore be only partially displayed:

$$\mathcal{E} = \{\{\langle h, h \rangle\}, \{\langle h, t \rangle\}, \{\langle t, h \rangle\}, \{\langle t, t \rangle\}, \ldots, \{\langle h, h \rangle, \langle h, t \rangle, \langle t, h \rangle, \langle t, t \rangle\}\}.$$

It contains as events, according to Definition 236, all subsets of the sample space Ω above and their complements and unions. So, it also contains the following events:

$$A = \{\langle h, h \rangle, \langle h, t \rangle, \langle t, h \rangle\}$$
$$B = \langle h, t \rangle, \langle t, h \rangle\}.$$

A is the event of getting at least one heads, while B is the event of getting exactly one heads. Since according to Kolmogorov Axiom 2 we have:

$$p(\Omega) = p(\{\langle h, h \rangle, \langle h, t \rangle, \langle t, h \rangle, \langle t, t \rangle\}) = 1,$$

for each event $X \in \Omega$ we obtain:

$$p(X) = \frac{1}{4}.$$

Thus, according to Kolmogorov Axiom 3, the probability of getting at least one heads in two flips, $p(A)$, is:

$$
\begin{aligned}
p(A) &= p(\{\langle h, h \rangle, \langle h, t \rangle, \langle t, h \rangle\}) \\
&= p(\{\langle h, h \rangle\}) + p(\{\langle h, t \rangle\}) + p(\{\langle t, h \rangle\}) \\
&= \frac{1}{4} + \frac{1}{4} + \frac{1}{4} \\
&= \frac{3}{4} \\
&= 0.75.
\end{aligned}
$$

29.1.2 Probability Distribution

In dealing with probability spaces and probabilities, the notion of a *probability distribution* plays an important role. This is a complex technical term and will be only briefly sketched here.

It was pointed out above that if $\langle \Omega, \mathcal{E}, p \rangle$ is a finitely additive probability space, then its sample space Ω contains all possible outcomes. They are always

$n > 1$ exhaustive and mutually exclusive events and may be symbolized by $A_1, A_2, \ldots, A_n$. It is natural to assume that any of these possible outcomes, A_i, has a particular probability $p(A_i)$ such that for the entire sample space we shall have:

$$p(A_1) = r_1 \tag{243}$$
$$p(A_2) = r_2$$
$$\vdots$$
$$p(A_n) = r_n$$

and, in addition, according to Kolmogorov Axioms 1 and 3 it will be the case that $r_1 + r_2 + \cdots + r_n = 1$. The reason is that the events $A_1, A_2, \ldots, A_n$ are mutually exclusive and jointly exhaustive. That is, for any two distinct events A_i and A_j we have $A_i \cap A_j = \varnothing$ such that $A_1 \cup A_2 \cup \ldots \cup A_n = \Omega$ and $p(\Omega) = 1$. The set of all probabilities listed in (243) reflects the distribution over Ω of the total probability 1 and is therefore referred to as a *probability distribution*. It need not be stressed that two random experiments of the same type may, and will, in general have different probability distributions.[190]

---

[190] Stated a little bit more precise, a probability distribution is actually a distribution function of a so-called *random variable*. (Although the phrase "random variable" is a well-established, central, and technical term in the theory of probability, it is in fact a misnomer that was coined long ago by people who lacked knowledge of logic and its terminology. It may cause confusion since what it denotes is not a variable, but a *function*, specifically, a function that is not random, but well known and even computable. The term "randomness function" would have been a better choice. What is called a random variable is simply a particular *function* of the following type *whose arguments* are randomly occurring events.) Let $\langle \Omega, \mathcal{E}, p \rangle$ be a probability space. A so-called random variable v on this probability space is a function from the sample space Ω to the set $\mathbb{R}$ of real numbers, i.e., $v \colon \Omega \mapsto \mathbb{R}$. It assigns numbers to possible, random outcomes of an experiment (inquiry, observation, and the like). Thus, its arguments are single, possible, unknown, i.e., random outcomes, and its values are known numbers. For example, let $\Omega = \{\langle h, h \rangle, \langle h, t \rangle, \langle t, h \rangle, \langle t, t \rangle\}$ be the set of all possible outcomes of flipping a coin twice such that $\langle h, h \rangle$ stands for the outcome *heads* in both flips; $\langle h, t \rangle$ stands for the outcome *heads* in the first and *tails* in the second flip; and so on. Then the following function v is a 'random variable':

$$v(\langle h, h \rangle) = 0, \quad v(\langle h, t \rangle) = 1, \quad v(\langle t, h \rangle) = 2, \quad v(\langle t, t \rangle) = 3.$$

Random variables are usually represented by upper-case letters such as X and Y. Here we deviate from this tradition because functions are symbolized by lower case letters such as $f, g, \ldots, v$, etc. Using the badly named random variables, the terminology of events is translated into the terminology of functions and numbers. For instance, event $\langle t, h \rangle$ in our present example is 2. In a quite sloppy fashion, a statement of the form "event $\langle t, h \rangle$ occurs" is usually written "$v = 2$" to express that the random variable v takes outcome No. 2 as its value. Accordingly, $p(v = 2) = 0.25$ says that "the probability that event $\langle t, h \rangle$ occurs, is 0.25".

29.1.3 Probabilistic Independence

A famous philosophical question about causality asks whether the growth of a stork population in an area increases the human birthrate in that area, or vice versa. This question also lies at the heart of medical etiology. We shall have to answer it in our theory of etiology in Section 6.5. To prepare our analyses, we here familiarize ourselves with the basic issue of dependence of events by asking the question what it means to say that two events are dependent, or independent, of one another. They are simply independent of one another if the occurrence of one of them does not influence the occurrence of the other. To put it into precise words, we use the well-founded independence concept of probability theory:

Definition 238 (Probabilistic independence of events). *Two events A and B are stochastically or probabilistically independent of one another if and only if $p(A \cap B) = p(A) \cdot p(B)$, i.e., if the probability of their joint occurrence equals the product of the probabilities of their individual occurrence.*

To give an example, suppose that we flip a fair coin twice. The event of getting heads on the first flip, i.e., $\langle heads, X \rangle$, may be written H_1, and the event of getting heads on the second flip, i.e., $\langle X, heads \rangle$, may be written H_2. We know that:

$$p(H_1) = 0.5$$
$$p(H_2) = 0.5.$$

The joint occurrence of both events, $H_1 \cap H_2$, is the event of getting heads in two successive flips of the coin. If it turns out that this joint event has a probability of 0.25, then we may say that the two single events H_1 and H_2 are probabilistically independent of one another because:

$$p(H_1 \cap H_2) = 0.25 = 0.5 \cdot 0.5 = p(H_1) \cdot p(H_2).$$

29.1.4 Conditional Probability

The probability that a newborn baby in Berlin will be female, is 0.51. Thus we are in a position to speculate about the gender of the Berlin resident Mrs. Carla Fox's next baby. The probability that her next baby will be female, is

---

Now, the *probability distribution* function of a random variable v is a function f_v such that for every event A and every value x of the random variable v we have $f_v(x) = p(v = x)$ iff $v(A) = x$. What all these mathematical contraptions accomplish is, first, to translate the probabilities of outcomes into probabilities of numbers so as to free talk about probabilities from specific events, and second, to treat a probability space in a variety of ways by using various random variables. Note that a random variable v is a point function, whereas the probability p is a set function. For the difference, see Section 25.4.4 on page 843.

0.51. If the event that Carla Fox's next baby will be female is represented by A, then we may write $p(A) = 0.51$. This is the unconditional or *absolute probability* of the event A. It is so called because it is not considered in relationship to another event. Now, consider the following information: The probability that a pregnant Berlin resident's next baby will be female if her last two babies have been daughters, is 0.1. We now have a new hypothesis about Carla Fox's next baby that we can formulate thus: "The probability that Carla Fox's next baby will be female *on the condition that* her last two babies are daughters, is 0.1". Carla Fox's last two babies have in fact been daughters. If we symbolize this event by B, then our new statement says $p(A, B) = 0.1$. A probability of this type is called a *conditional probability*. The probability of the event A is conditional based on another event B. This is summarized in Table 53:

Table 53. Conditional probability vs. absolute probability

Absolute probability:	$p(A)$
Conditional probability:	$p(A, B)$
Example (absolute probability):	The probability that Carla Fox's next baby will be female, is 0.51
Example (conditional probability):	The probability that Carla Fox's next baby will be female on the condition that her last two babies have been female, is 0.1
Absolute probability:	$p(A) = 0.51$
Conditional probability:	$p(A, B) = 0.1$.

Note that absolute probability is a probability expressed by a *unary* probability function, whereas the conditional probability is a probability expressed by a *binary* probability function. This is the primary difference between both types of probability. Due to logical carelessness in probability theory these two logically different functions are represented by the same symbol "p". We cannot change this established bad habit. The conditional probability is usually written:

$$p(A \mid B) = r$$

instead of $p(A, B) = r$ and reads: "The probability of event A on the condition that event B has already occurred", or "the probability of A conditional on B", or simply "the probability of A given B". We shall use all these conventions. The conditional probability $p(A \mid B)$ is defined in terms of absolute probability in the following way:

Definition 239 (Conditional probability). *If A and B are two events and $p(B) > 0$, then*

$$p(A \mid B) = \frac{p(A \cap B)}{p(A)}. \tag{244}$$

The probability $p(B)$ in the denominator must be greater than zero because we cannot divide by zero. There are also attempts to introduce the concept of conditional probability directly by axiomatizing a conditional probability space. We shall not be concerned with this approach (see, e.g., Roeper and Leblanc, 1999).

29.1.5 Bayes's Theorem

Sketched below is an interesting application of conditional probability. Consider the following situation. Suppose that in the population of people over 60 years of age 15% of those who have coronary heart disease show ST segment depression in their resting ECG. We may thus state that in the population mentioned, the probability of ST depression occurring in resting ECG on the condition that coronary heart disease is present, is 0.15. That is:[191]

$$p(ST \mid CHD) = 0.15. \tag{245}$$

The shorthands used in this sentence mean:

ST   ≡ ST depression in resting ECG is present,
CHD   ≡ coronary heart disease is present.

The patient Elroy Fox is 70 years old. In a checkup, his family physician has recorded a resting ECG and is surprised at observing ST depression therein. She is wondering whether Elroy Fox has coronary heart disease. She knows a theorem which relates a conditional probability of the form $p(A \mid B)$ with the inverted conditional probability $p(B \mid A)$. It enables her to conclude from (245) above that:

$$p(CHD \mid ST) = 0.93. \tag{246}$$

This conclusion says that the probability that a patient older than 60 years has coronary heart disease conditional on ST depression in his resting ECG, is 0.93. Thus the physician has strong reason to believe that Elroy Fox has coronary heart disease and to act accordingly. The theorem by which she was able to conclude (246) from (245), has come to be known as *Bayes's Theorem*. It was discovered by the eighteenth century English clergyman Thomas Bayes (1702–1761), and published posthumously in 1763, before probability theory had even been explicitly formulated (Bayes, 1763). (Usually, the term "Bayes's Theorem" is incorrectly written "Bayes' Theorem".)

Bayes's Theorem is directly derivable from the concept of probability space introduced in Definition 237 on page 975. It exists in a variety of versions. We shall here demonstrate its elementary version that only covers two events

---

[191] The ST segment in ECG connects the S wave and the T wave of ECG. When it is below the baseline, it is said to be depressed. ST depression is indicative of myocardial ischemia that may cause myocardial infarction.

A and *B*, and shall not consider the general version covering an arbitrary number of events. This simple version can be derived from the definition of conditional probability above. From Definition 239 it follows that:

$$p(A \cap B) = p(A \mid B) \cdot p(B).$$

If we divide both sides by $p(A)$ and substitute using formula (244), we obtain:

Theorem 9 (Bayes's Theorem).

$$p(B \mid A) = \frac{p(A \mid B) \cdot p(B)}{p(A)}.$$

To illustrate, let us refer to the events CHD and ST depression in the example above. Suppose that in the population of people over 60 years of age we have:

$p(CHD) = 0.01$

$p(ST) = 0.0016$

Given the basic information (245) above, i.e., $p(ST \mid CHD) = 0.15$, we can now use Bayes's Theorem to understand how Elroy Fox's physician concluded the high probability 0.93 that the patient has coronary heart disease on the evidence that he has ST depression in his resting ECG:

$$
\begin{aligned}
p(CHD \mid ST) &= \frac{p(ST \mid CHD) \cdot p(CHD)}{p(ST)} \\
&= \frac{0.15 \cdot 0.01}{0.0016} \\
&= \frac{0.0015}{0.0016} \\
&= 0.9375.
\end{aligned}
$$

By using Bayes's Theorem we have computed the conditional probability $p(CHD \mid ST)$ on the basis of $p(CHD)$. The absolute probability $p(CHD)$ that is needed on the right hand-side of the theorem is called the *prior probability*, or simply the prior, of the event CHD, i.e., its probability known before ST depression occurring. After the event ST has occurred, the conditional probability of CHD, i.e., $p(CHD \mid ST)$, is referred to as its *posterior probability*, or just the posterior. The strength of Bayes's Theorem, then, is that given some evidence, it allows one to conclude from the prior the posterior probability of an event. Thus, it is often used in clinical diagnostics and other areas where the prior probability of an event supposed before an observation is made, is changed by the observation.

The simplest form of Bayes's Theorem presented above is confined to two events only. It may be generalized to cover any number of mutually exclusive and jointly exhaustive events. We will not go into details here because the generalization brings additional problems with it. For details, see (Jaynes, 2003).

29.1.6 What Does "Probability" Mean?

In practical applications, it is useful to know what the term "probability" means. The notion of probability introduced in Definition 237 on page 975 and represented by the function symbol "p", is an uninterpreted term. Thus far it plays only a formal role in the probability theory because like other mathematical theories, this theory itself as a whole is an empirically uninterpreted framework. According to its formal role fixed by the three Kolmogorov Axioms, the function p can only be characterized as a *normalized additive measure*. It is a *set function* that assigns to subsets of its domain real numbers from the unit interval $[0, 1]$. That is all that we can say about it. (For the notion of a set function, see Section 25.4.4 on page 843.)[192]

The theory of probability goes no further in answering the question, "what is probability?". The formal notion of probability, p, may of course be semantically *interpreted* in a variety of ways to obtain different meanings and applications. There are at least four such interpretations: frequency interpretation, propensity interpretation, subjective probability, and logical probability. We shall consider them briefly in turn to motivate our discussion of inductive logic in Section 29.2 and Bayesian logic in Section 29.3 below. For details, see (Gillies, 2000; Suppes, 2002, 129–263).

Frequency interpretation or objective probability

Frequentists hold the view that probability is a feature of the objective world. They are therefore called objectivists. They consider the probability of an event to be its relative frequency in a reference class. For example, the probability of getting heads in a coin toss is identified with the frequency of getting heads in a suitable sequence of flips divided by the total number of flips. In finite frequentism, this sequence is finite. In infinite frequentism, it is infinite. In this latter view, probability is the limiting relative frequency in the long run. The main long run frequentists were Hans Reichenbach and Richard von Mises (Reichenbach, 1935; von Mises, 1939).

Propensity interpretation

This physical interpretation is due to the Austrian-born British philosopher of science Karl Raimund Popper (1957, 1959). Like the preceding one, it is an objectivist interpretation in that it considers probability as a physical property of a chance set-up, say experiment, specifically as its disposition, tendency,

---

[192] A measure is a function that assigns a *non-negative* real number to members of a given set, e.g., height, volume, and age. It starts with the value 0, so it is non-negative; and is said to be a normalized one if its maximum value is 1. Thus the probability function p is in fact a probability *measure* satisfying both of these conditions because $p(\Omega) = 1$ and, as a result, $p(\varnothing) = 0$. Further, its *additivity* is expressed in Kolmogorov Axiom 3 (see Definition 237 on page 975).

or *propensity* to produce outcomes of a certain, stable long run frequency (Popper, 1957, 67). In this sense, probability as propensity is comparable to length and density of an object, and is measured by the function p. For example, the statement that the probability of tossing heads with a particular coin is 0.499, is interpreted as a statement about the physical propensity of an experimental set-up, part of which is that coin. See also (Mellor, 1971; Salmon, 1979).

Subjectivist interpretation or subjective probability

In contrast to both types of objectivism above, probabilistic subjectivism is the doctrine that probability is something psychological, personal, and subjective such that the function p is always the measure of belief of a particular person. When an individual x says that $p(A) = r$, for example, $p(Elroy\ Fox\ has\ coronary\ heart\ disease) = 0.7$, this number r is the degree of her own belief in A that may be indicated by $p_x(A)$. The belief of another person y is $p_y(A)$ such that the inequality $p_x(A) \neq p_y(A)$ is not excluded. An individual's degree of belief that event A will occur, may be measured by her betting quotient, i.e., the rate at which she is prepared to bet on A. If you are prepared to pay \$$a$ for the right to receive \$$b$ provided that event A occurs, then that means that you are prepared to bet on A with a betting quotient of $\frac{a}{b}$. This ratio represents the subjective probability that you assign to A, i.e., $p_{you}(A) = \frac{a}{b}$. The early advocates of probabilistic subjectivism were the British philosopher Frank Plumpton Ramsey, the Italian mathematician Bruno de Finetti, and the U.S.-American Statistician Leonard Jimmie Savage (Ramsey, 1926; de Finetti, 1937; Savage, 1954).

Logical probability

There is also a view of probability as an extension of logic. This view was adopted by the famous British economist John Maynard Keynes (1883–1946) who argued that probability was a logical relation between evidence and belief (Keynes, 1921; Jeffreys, 1939). He found a few followers the most imaginative and influential one among them being the German-born U.S.-American philosopher of science Rudolf Carnap (1891–1970). Carnap held the view that there are two concepts of probability. The first one, he said, means limiting relative frequency referred to above, whereas the second one denotes a logical relationship between statements (Carnap, 1962, 23 f.). He presented an extensive theory of the latter concept, which he called *inductive logic,* giving rise thereby to a new branch of logic research under this label. We shall sketch this perspective in the next section.[193]

---

[193] Keynes credits the German philosopher Gottfried Wilhelm Leibniz (1646–1716) for first conceiving the idea that probability was a branch of logic. For historical details, see (Hacking, 1975a, ch. 10).

The proponents of the interpretations sketched above, except for Carnap, consider only their own interpretation to be the right one and reject the others, as if the semantic *interpretation* of a blank word could be right or wrong. This erroneous view reflects an archaic philosophy that allows a word to bear only one, 'god-given' meaning in all contexts and languages, referred to as *word magic* by Ogden and Richards (1989).

29.2 Inductive Logic

In the early twentieth century, after modern deductive logic was well established, philosophers of science made the shocking discovery that scientific knowledge could not be logically deduced from observations, and therefore could not be true. And if it could not be true, why should we consider scientific knowledge to be trustworthy or taken seriously? In analyzing this issue, inductive logic emerged as an attempt to search for methods of reasoning that would justify human belief in a *statement* that does not deductively follow from other statements. The aim was to develop a concept of *degree of confirmation* of a hypothesis with respect to a given body of evidence. To clearly understand this idea, we must carefully distinguish between deduction and induction. All of the systems of logic we considered in previous sections are specific theories of deduction. But what is induction? We shall briefly answer this basic question of sciences in the following two subsections concerned with Hume's problem of induction and Carnap's degree of confirmation. See also our analysis of the concept of confirmation on pages 470–475.

Hume's problem of induction

Medicine as well as other empirical disciplines could not make any progress if their reasoning techniques only consisted of deductive-logical systems. For a deductive-logical argument is truth preserving and does not produce new knowledge. What its conclusion asserts, is completely entailed by its premise. Thus, in pursuing new knowledge in medicine, we need non-deductive reasoning. This can be demonstrated by a simple argument that is deductively invalid:

Every raven that has been observed until now was black

All ravens are black.

Although every raven that human beings have ever encountered may have been black, the next raven could nonetheless be white or red. That is, the conclusion of the above argument does not deductively follow from its premise. In spite of this deductive-logical gap, acquisition and accumulation of knowledge in medicine and other areas proceed by employing deductively invalid arguments similar to the one above. For example, from observations about *some* patients presenting a particular symptom, it is concluded that *all* patients will exhibit that symptom. For instance, it is argued that:

Every patient with pneumonia observed until now had a fever

All patients with pneumonia have a fever.

The conclusion of this deductively invalid argument is an assertion about a potentially infinite number of patients. It has been formed by an *inductive generalization* of what its premise reports on a finite number of observations. Medical knowledge emerges on the basis of such inductive generalizations. When in a clinical textbook we find the statement that "all pneumonia patients have elevated body temperature, usually 101–103 °F", we may ask the author, "how do you know that?". She will reply with an argument like the one above. In contrast to deductive arguments, however, the argument above is not truth preserving. It is possible for its premise to be true and its conclusion false because its conclusion asserts more than is entailed by the premise. An ampliative inference of this type is called *inductive*. Thus, "inductive" means *non-deductive and ampliative*. Accordingly, "induction" means "inductive inference" by taking an inductive step from some premises to a conclusion.[194]

Most of our reasoning in both science and everyday life is inductive. Yet there is no logic to guide this reasoning, i.e., an *inductive logic* that might parallel deductive logic. The obvious question is, why not? The not so obvious answer is that it's not even possible in principle.

In traditional philosophy since Aristotle, the term "induction" meant to infer 'general statements' from 'statements on particulars' like in our two inductive generalizations above. However, the following example shows that this Aristotelean doctrine, still widely held today, is wrong. In this example, just the opposite is the case; a statement about a particular is inductively inferred from a general statement:

Every patient with pneumonia observed until now had a fever

The next patient with pneumonia will have a fever.

In 1748, the Scottish philosopher David Hume (1711–1776) identified what has come to be known as Hume's problem or *the problem of induction*. He discovered that a logic of inductive inference is impossible on the grounds that any attempt to justify an inductive inference requires another inductive inference, and yet another to justify that, and so on in an infinite regress (Hume,

---

[194] To be distinguished from induction and inductive inference is the so-called *mathematical induction*. Mathematical induction is a special method of deductive proof used in mathematical sciences. Although it represents a well-established technique of deductive reasoning, the term is a misnomer nonetheless. The same applies to the notion of "inductive definition" studied in Section 5.3.5 on page 96. It has nothing to do with induction and inductive methods in the above sense.

1748).[195] Therefore, no inductive inference can be justified. To elucidate, consider the inductive inferences in the three inductive arguments above. We had the inference from the black color of ravens *up to now* to the black color of other ravens *in the future;* from fever in pneumonia patients observed *up to now* to fever in other pneumonia patients *in the future;* and again, from fever in pneumonia patients observed *up to now* to fever in another pneumonia patient *in the future.* All these inferences, like any other inductive inference, presuppose that the world is uniform in that it does not change its structure over time. It continues to behave in the future as it has behaved in the past. From the past we can infer the future. But how do we know that this assumption of the uniformity of the world is true? As a statement about the *experiential* world, it cannot be proven *logically.* Many worlds are imaginable that lack a uniform structure and change their behavior from day to day or from year to year. Maybe the assumption can be supported by recourse to our evidence up to now? This, however, would be an inductive argument itself, Hume says. So induction cannot be reasonably justified.

Degree of confirmation

Rudolf Carnap tackled the problem of induction anew to show that it was not unsolvable, as it had been believed to be since Hume (Carnap, 1945, 1952, 1962; Carnap and Jeffrey, 1971; Jeffrey, 1980). Following John Maynard Keynes, his plan was to extend the relation of total implication, $\models$, by introducing a more general concept of partial implication for cases where the conclusion of an argument does not deductively follow from its premises. We will try to explain this idea to understand why Carnap's famous program failed and to shed further light on why inductive logic is still lacking. He conceived of a partial implication as a two-place function of the following form between *statements:*

To the extent *r,* evidence *e* partially implies hypothesis *h,*

or equivalently:

---

[195] The philosopher, historian, and essayist David Hume was born, and died, in Edinburgh. He lived for a time in France (1734–37) where he wrote his first philosophical work, *A Treatise of Human Nature,* published in 1739–40. Hume is generally regarded as the most important philosopher ever to write in English. His major philosophical works also include (Hume, 1748, 1998a, 1998b). He was the last of the founders of British empiricism (Francis Bacon, John Locke, and George Berkeley), advocating the thesis that human knowledge arises only from sense experience. His skeptical arguments concerning induction, causality, knowledge, and religion shaped 19th- and 20th-century empiricist philosophy. Even the great German philosopher Immanuel Kant (1724–1804) developed his critical philosophy in direct reaction to Hume.

to the extent r, hypothesis h partially follows from evidence e.

Here the variables "h" and "e" denote statements, and r is a real number in the unit interval $[0, 1]$. The supposed quantitative relation of implication above between statements, Carnap expressed in terms of a *probability* relationship between them, i.e., as a metalinguistic probability that he called logical or inductive probability:

The inductive probability of hypothesis h relative to evidence e is r.

For example, the patient Elroy Fox's doctor may suppose that in light of the evidence "Elroy Fox has angina pectoris", the inductive probability of the hypothesis "he has coronary heart disease" is 0.4.

Recall that the "probability" as the basic concept of probability theory introduced in Section 29.1 is a set function. However, inductive probability is, according to Carnap's terminology, a two-place, quantitative, sentential, or propositional function. He identified it with the degree of confirmation that a single statement h receives from a set of $n \geq 1$ statements of evidence, denoted e. This may be written:

$$c(h, e) = r$$

and read "evidence e confirms hypothesis h to the extent r". Thus, in Carnap's system these three notions are synonyms: inductive probability, partial implication, and degree of confirmation. He constructed his inductive logic as a theory of this degree of confirmation. For instance, it may be that in a particular context we obtain the following inductive argument:

1. 93 percent of patients with ST depression in their resting ECG have coronary heart disease,
2. Elroy Fox has ST depression in his resting ECG,

$$\text{\rule{8cm}{0.4pt}} \quad [0.93]$$

3. Elroy Fox has coronary heart disease.

The bracketed real number 0.93 indicates the extent to which the two premises confirm the conclusion. If we symbolize the first premise by e_1, the second premise by e_2, and the concluded hypothesis 3 by h, the inductive argument above means: $c(h, e_1 \wedge e_2) = 0.93$.

As outlined in Section 11.5.1 on page 499, Carnap was a logical empiricist. He had conceived his inductive logic as a theory of quantitative confirmation in the hope that it could be used in grounding scientific knowledge on empirical evidence. In spite of the immense efforts invested in this project, it has yielded no acceptable inductive logic. In fact, in Carnap's inductive logic, the degree of confirmation that a universal hypothesis such as "all ravens are black" receives from all available empirical evidence is always 0. We may conclude from this tragic failure that Carnap's initial intuition has not been a fruitful one. What remains uncontroversial, is merely a couple of axioms that regulate the basic meaning of the confirmation function $c(h, e) = r$. In effect, these axioms are an adjustment of Kolmogorov Axioms of probability and use *sentences* instead of *events*. We will list a few of them to understand why axioms alone do not provide an inductive logic. The symbol "$\vdash$" represents the classical-logical relation of deduction, and h, h_1, h_2, e, e_1, and e_2, are first-order sentences.

Axiom 1.   If $e \vdash h$, then $c(h, e) = 1$,

Axiom 2.   If $\vdash e_1 \leftrightarrow e_2$, then $c(h, e_1) = c(h, e_2)$,

Axiom 3. $c(h_1 \wedge h_2, e) = c(h_1, h_2 \wedge e) \cdot c(h_2, e)$,

Axiom 4.   If $\vdash h$, then $c(h, e) = 1$ for all e,

Axiom 5.   If $\vdash \neg(h_1 \wedge h_2)$, then $c(h_1 \vee h_2, e) = c(h_1, e) + c(h_2, e)$.

Axiom 5 is the only interesting one. It says that when evidence entails the incompatibility of two hypotheses h_1 and h_2, i.e., when only one of these hypotheses can be true, then the degrees of their confirmation by evidence e add up. For example, with regard to our above example $c(h, e_1 \wedge e_2) = 0.93$ about ST depression in ECG and coronary heart disease, Axioms 1 and 5 jointly imply that $c(\neg h, e_1 \wedge e_2) = 0.07$. That means that the evidence "93 percent of patients with ST depression in their resting ECG have coronary heart disease and Elroy Fox has ST depression in his resting ECG" supports the hypothesis "Elroy Fox does not have coronary heart disease" to the extent 0.07. The crucial problem is how to obtain degrees of confirmation such as 0.93 that we need to justify inductive inferences of this type. Inductive logic was designed to provide us with such data. Without a viable system of inductive logic, no such data exist.

29.3 Bayesian Logic

As outlined in Section 27.3.6 on page 947, the physician's attitudes toward states of affairs is characterized by epistemic kinematics, usually referred to as belief change or *belief revision*, while unfortunately there exists no logic to manage this process. For instance, consider a doctor who seeks a diagnosis for a patient, Elroy Fox. At the beginning of the patient interview she does not believe that Elroy Fox has coronary heart disease. But two hours later she strongly believes in this hypothesis because she has obtained new evidence by recording and interpreting an ECG in the meantime. This is an example of the continuous change of our beliefs, or *belief revision*. The aim of inductive logic has been to assist us in managing the change of our beliefs in the light of new evidence and to serve as a logic of belief revision. However, as we have seen above, it has not succeeded. There are scholars, called Bayesians, who favor the use of Bayes's Theorem as an alternative method that is usually referred to as Bayesian reasoning, Bayesian inference, Bayesian logic, or simply Bayesianism.

To give a brief outline of Bayesian logic, it is preferable to consider statements and not events to be the subject of our beliefs. When you believe that it will rain tomorrow, you believe that the hypothesis "it will rain tomorrow" will turn out true. If we interpret the term "belief" as subjective probability, then the process of our belief revision may be conceived of as the kinematics of our subjective probabilities, i.e., the temporal dynamics of the degrees of probabilities that we ascribe to hypotheses in the course of time. Suppose that the strength of your belief in a hypothesis h is 0.2 at time t_1 and 0.8 at time t_2. Obviously, during the time interval $[t_1, t_2]$ the degree of your subjective probability, $p(h)$, has changed from 0.2 to 0.8. It may even change from 0.8 to 0.4 in the next hour. For this dynamics to be reasonable, requires that our subjective probabilities obey at least some minimum criteria of probability calculus. But the standard concept of probability introduced in preceding sections operates on events and not on statements. A reformulation of that concept for application to statements is necessary. The domain of the probability function p would then consist of statements. Accordingly, the set-theoretical operations such as union and intersection that are used in the standard probability calculus, would then need to be replaced by logical connectives. Essentially, this means that while the standard probability theory is formulated in object language, subjective probability theory, like the confirmation theory above, will be a metalinguistic framework. This fact we shall have to bear in mind throughout. To this end, we shall briefly sketch a concept of metalinguistic probability to be used below. An elaborate exposition like Definition 237 on page 975 will be omitted. We shall only present the Kolmogorov Axioms from which everything else follows. Classical logic will serve as the underlying logic.

Let $\mathcal{L}$ be a language and let Ω be a set of sentences of this language, e.g., Ω = {Elroy Fox has diabetes, he coughs}. An algebra of sentences on Ω, denoted $\mathcal{A}$, is a set of sentences such that (1) it contains every element of Ω; (2) if a sentence α is an element of $\mathcal{A}$, then its negation $\neg\alpha$ is also an element of $\mathcal{A}$; and (3) if sentences α and β are elements of $\mathcal{A}$, then their disjunction $\alpha \vee \beta$ is also an element of $\mathcal{A}$.

Definition 240 (Probability space for sentences). *A triple $\langle \Omega, \mathcal{A}, p \rangle$ is a (finitely additive) probability space iff:*

1. *Ω is a non-empty set of sentences over a language $\mathcal{L}$;*
2. *$\mathcal{A}$ is an algebra of sentences on Ω;*
3. *p is a function such that $p \colon \mathcal{A} \mapsto [0,1]$;*
4. *For all sentences α and β in $\mathcal{A}$:*

    4.1. $p(\alpha) \geq 0$
    4.2. If α is a valid sentence, then $p(\alpha) = 1$
    4.3. If $\{\alpha, \beta\}$ is inconsistent, then $p(\alpha \vee \beta) = p(\alpha) + p(\beta)$.

For instance, $p(\text{Elroy Fox has diabetes}) \geq 0$; $p(\text{Elroy Fox has diabetes or Elroy Fox does not have diabetes}) = 1$; $p(\text{Elroy Fox has diabetes or Elroy Fox does}$

not have diabetes) = p(Elroy Fox has diabetes) + p(Elroy Fox does not have diabetes).

The probability that a person assigns to a statement, is not something objective that she might obtain by a statistical frequency analysis. It is the degree of her belief that the statement is or will turn out true. Thus, it is subjective probability. An important application of this subjective probability is Bayesian logic which will be briefly discussed below. It is worth mentioning that from the concept of sentence probability above we can infer the following metalinguistic form of Bayes's Theorem for sentence probability. Let α and β be any statements of a language $\mathcal{L}$, then:[196]

$$p(\beta \mid \alpha) = \frac{p(\alpha \mid \beta) \cdot p(\beta)}{p(\alpha)} \qquad \text{(Bayes's Theorem)}$$

Recall the health condition of our now 70-year-old patient Elroy Fox on page 980 above. When entering the office of his family physician, the doctor notes that Elroy Fox is short of breath. This symptom is indicative of a large number of disorders each of which may be present in the patient. One of them is, for example, coronary heart disease. The doctor knows that in the age group of this patient, the probability of coronary heart disease is about 0.01. So her first diagnostic conjecture is:

"the patient has coronary *heart disease*" $\equiv$ *chd*

On the basis of her experience and expert knowledge she believes to the extent 0.01 that the hypothesis *chd* is true. Thus, we have the following prior subjective probability that the doctor assigns to her diagnostic hypothesis:

$$p(chd) = 0.01. \tag{247}$$

While recording a resting ECG of the patient, she observes ST depression in the ECG. The evidence:

"the patient has ST depression in his resting ECG" $\equiv$ *st*

increases the strength of her prior belief in the hypothesis *chd*. To update her prior belief (247), she is contemplating the degree of this posterior probability:

$$p(chd \mid st) = ? \tag{248}$$

The move from the absolute degree of belief, $p(chd)$, to the conditional degree of belief $p(chd \mid st)$ is called Bayesian conditioanlization. The belief revision the doctor seeks is provided by Bayes's Theorem that relates prior and posterior probabilities, (247) and (248), in the following fashion:

---

[196] Analogous to the standard conditional probability, the conditional probability of statements is defined as follows: $p(\beta \mid \alpha) = \frac{p(\beta \wedge \alpha)}{p(\alpha)}$ when $p(\alpha) > 0$. The expression $p(\beta \mid \alpha)$ reads "the probability of β on the condition that α obtains".

$$p(chd \mid st) = \frac{p(st \mid chd) \cdot p(chd)}{p(st)}.$$

On the basis of personal experience and literature studies the physician may form the probabilities:

$$p(st \mid chd) = 0.15$$
$$p(st) = 0.0016.$$

With the aid of this data she is able to infer from Bayes's Theorem above the posterior probability $p(chd \mid st) = 0.93$. Upon any additional evidence, α, the physician may of course proceed in a similar fashion by iterative conditionalization of the form $p(chd \mid st \wedge \alpha)$ to apply Bayes's Theorem as above and to successively revise her diagnostic belief.

Many Bayesians believe that Bayesian logic is the only appropriate method of reasoning both in science and everyday life. This is an exaggeration, however. First, the probabilities that are required on the right hand side of Bayes's Theorem above, are not objective probabilities to be elicited by empirical analyses. They are the physician's subjective probabilities. Where do they come from? Second, the theorem is not applicable to universal hypotheses, e.g., "All humans are mortal". No rational human being would be prepared to bet on a universal hypothesis with a betting quotient greater than 0. Therefore, the degree of her rational belief in such a hypothesis will never exceed 0. Thus, regardless of the amount of evidence that supports a general statement, the statement has a subjective probability of 0. Bayesian logic will help just as little as inductive logic was able to. It does not resolve David Hume's problem of induction. Rather, it evades the problem by assisting us in learning from experience and revising our beliefs. "On pain of incoherence, we should always have a belief structure that satisfies the probability axioms" (Hacking, 2001, 256–257).

29.4 Summary

The theory of probability is a vast, axiomatic-deductive system to assist us in managing randomness and uncertainty. A brief introduction has been given to some of its basic concepts that we shall employ in this book. Specifically, the concepts of probability space, absolute probability, conditional probability, and probabilistic independence as well as Bayes's Theorem have been discussed. Also a sketch has been given of inductive logic that its creator, Rudolf Carnap, had envisioned as some sort of non-classical and non-deductive logic. However, we have seen that the endeavor has not yet succeeded. Also Bayesian logic, based on Bayes's Theorem, turns out insufficient because, as in inductive logic, general hypotheses get assigned a probability of 0. However, there is an alternative, recent approach to non-deductive reasoning, i.e., *fuzzy logic*. Fuzzy logic is a non-classical and non-probabilistic system. It represents a promising novel methodology that is likely to revolutionize all scientific disciplines, technology, culture, and civilization. We shall briefly introduce its basic notions in the next chapter.

Fuzzy Logic

30.0 Introduction

Medical knowledge as well as clinical practice are characterized by inescapable uncertainty. There are many reasons this is the case, but foremost among them is that almost everything in medicine is inevitably vague, be it something linguistic such as the term "illness", or something extra-linguistic such as the condition referred to as *illness*. If we ask ourselves, then, what the term "illness" means exactly, on the one hand; and how we may precisely delimit the condition *illness*, on the other; we shall recognize that to answer these and similar questions requires specific methods that enable us to adequately cope with vagueness. As we shall see below, fuzzy logic provides us with just such methods.

The term "fuzzy" is an adjective that means *vague, imprecise, unsharp, blurred, cloudy*. A salient feature of medical language as a natural language is the vagueness of its terms. Familiar examples are terms such as *pain, fever, sleep disorder, icterus, cyanosis, headache, psychosis, acute, chronic, few, much, most, many, rapid heart beat, slow breathing*, etc. Their vagueness makes it more difficult to acquire reliable knowledge about medical subjects. It infects medical knowledge with imprecision and thereby introduces into medicine a considerable amount of uncertainty to the effect that much of medical reasoning in practice and research is approximate rather than exact. By approximate reasoning, or *fuzzy reasoning*, we mean a process of inference by which a fuzzy conclusion is drawn from a collection of fuzzy premises. Consider, for example, the following two statements. The first one contains the fuzzy quantifier "many" and is therefore fuzzy ('how many' things are 'many' things?):

1. Many diabetics are at risk of suffering coronary heart disease,
2. The patient Elroy Fox is a diabetic.

From these premises, we can loosely infer the rather unhelpful statement "it is likely that Elroy Fox will suffer coronary heart disease". None of the logical

K. Sadegh-Zadeh, *Handbook of Analytic Philosophy of Medicine*,
Philosophy and Medicine 113, DOI 10.1007/978-94-007-2260-6_30,
© Springer Science+Business Media B.V. 2012

systems we have studied thus far will be of much use to us here because they cannot handle the fuzzy quantifier "many". An additional logic is needed to manage this type of problem and other, similar problems arising from the ubiquitous vagueness in medicine. In this chapter, we shall briefly introduce a powerful tool for this task: *fuzzy logic*.

Fuzzy logic came into being in 1973–74 as a novel theory of inference. Although it has been extensively used in technology since then, e.g., in cameras, washing machines, televisions, automobiles, trains, computers, software, etc., it remains largely unknown in many scientific disciplines. Even many logicians are not acquainted with, or ignore, this fascinating logic. Some are even vituperatively hostile toward it, e.g., Susan Haack (1996, 229–258), because it deviates from their out-dated understanding of logic. As we shall see later, however, it is for several reasons the best logic for use in medicine.

"Fuzzy logic has a much broader scope and a much higher level of generality than traditional logical systems, among them the classical bivalent logic, multivalued logics, modal logics, probabilistic logics, etc. The principal objective of fuzzy logic is formalization – and eventual mechanization – of two remarkable human capabilities. First, the capability to converse, communicate, reason, and make decisions in an environment of imprecision, uncertainty, incompleteness of information, partiality of truth, and partiality of possibility. And second, the capability to perform a wide variety of physical and mental tasks – such as driving a car in city traffic and summarizing a book – without any measurement and any computation" (Zadeh, 2009, 3985 f.).

It is based on its precursor, i.e., *fuzzy set theory*. Fuzzy set theory emerged in 1965. It is the theory of *fuzzy sets* and represents an extension, or generalization, of classical set theory. Informally, a fuzzy set is a vague class as defined in Definition 1 on page 39. It lacks sharp boundaries to the effect that there is no clear dividing line between its members and non-members. Fuzzy set theory provides an outstanding tool for dealing with this type of class. As such, it provides an ideal method of reasoning about complex systems, e.g., cells, organisms, patients, diseases, therapies, and similar objects and processes that are not amenable to precise analyses, and are preferably described by vague terms such as "is *very* ill", "has *severe* headache", "has *acute* pneumonia", "is *highly* efficacious", and the like. The approach thus focuses on building methods of analysis, reasoning, and decision-making that are more efficient in managing imprecision and uncertainty.

The logics we have considered thus far, whether they be classical or nonclassical, are based on concepts of classical set theory and the seemingly plausible notions of truth and inference. Fuzzy logic, however, departs entirely from traditional logics, systems, and concepts. Its basis, fuzzy set theory, as well as its concepts of truth and inference are *non-classical*, novel creations in light of which previous systems of logic and mathematics appear either implausible or incomplete. Indeed, it is better capable than alternative logics of resolving many of medicine's theoretical and practical problems. Below, we briefly introduce its essentials in order to prepare our analyses and discussions in other parts of the book, Parts I–VII. Details may be found in (Dubois et al., 1993, Dubois and Prade, 1998; Klir and Yuan, 1995; Mordeson and Nair, 2001; Zadeh, 2009).

Note that the term "fuzzy logic" has two different meanings, a narrow and a wider one. Fuzzy logic in the narrow sense, or FLn for short, is a logical system dealing with inexact, vague, or approximate *reasoning*. In this sense, FLn is an extension of the many-valued logic we outlined in Section 28.5 on pages 964–968. But its agenda is quite different both in spirit and in substance. FLn is one of the branches of fuzzy logic in the wide sense of the term, or FLw for short. The core of FLw comprises, in addition to FLn, (i) fuzzy set theory; (ii) the theory of linguistic variables, (iii) the theory of fuzzy if-then rules; (iv) possibility theory; and (v) the theory of computing with words (Zadeh, 1996b, 2).

Fuzzy logic in the wide sense, FLw, is in predominant use. Depending on the context, we shall use the term in either of its two meanings. One should be aware, however, that fuzzy logic itself is not fuzzy, but the subjects it deals with. Fuzzy logic is a precise *theory of fuzziness* and imprecision. It helps us understand the thesis that almost everything in the world is inherently and without remedy vague and uncertain. Our discussion of FLw consists of the following four parts:

30.1 Fuzzy Sets
30.2 Operations on Fuzzy Sets
30.3 Fuzzy Relations
30.4 Fuzzy Logic Proper, i.e., FLn.

Our aim is to outline only some elementary notions of the theory. Technical details will be omitted. We start by introducing the basic idea of the theory, i.e., the concept of a fuzzy set, presented by Lotfi Zadeh in his seminal twin papers (Zadeh, 1965a, 1965b).[197]

30.1 Fuzzy Sets

The theory of fuzzy sets is a rapidly growing body of concepts, principles, methods, and subtheories for dealing in a systematic way with the vagueness

---

[197] Fuzzy set theory was developed in 1965 by the U.S.-American computer scientist and system theorist Lotfi A. Zadeh at the University of California at Berkeley. Zadeh was born on February 4, 1921 in Baku, the capital of the then Soviet Republic Azerbaijan, to a Russian mother and an Azeri father of Iranian descent. He is an alumnus of the University of Teheran, MIT, and Columbia University. Most of his own contributions to fuzzy logic, from 1965 to 1995, are available in two collected volumes (Yager et al., 1987; Klir and Yuan, 1996). For the history of fuzzy set theory and logic, see (McNeill and Freiberger, 1993; Seising, 2007a). Additional information and medical applications may be found in the companion website http://www.philmed-online.net.

that arises when a class of objects lacks sharp boundaries. Simple examples are the classes of *young people, bald men, suffering human beings, large cells, patients with high blood pressure, patients with headache, beautiful women, warm days, red roses, small numbers, trees, bushes,* and many others. We call a class of this type a vague class or *fuzzy set.*

In a fuzzy set, there is no dividing line between those objects that are its members and those that are not. For example, it is not clear and will remain so forever whether a 42-year-old individual belongs to the set of *young* people or not. Such a fuzzy set differs from ordinary or classical sets in that it does not require that an object be either fully a member or fully a non-member of the set.

Consider, for instance, the set of integers, i.e., the number sequence $\{\ldots, -4, -3, -2, -1, 0, 1, 2, 3, 4, \ldots\}$ extending on both sides of zero into infinity. Some of these numbers are *even.* An even number is an integer of the form $2n$ for some integer n. Thus, even numbers are elements of the set $\{\ldots, -4, -2, 0, 2, 4, \ldots\}$ that are divisible by 2. The remaining integers, i.e., $\{\ldots, -5, -3, -1, 1, 3, 5, \ldots\}$, are not even. They are referred to as *odd* numbers. Both of these two sets, the set of even numbers and the set of odd numbers, are classical sets. They have sharp boundaries between their members and non-members. Take, for instance, the set of even numbers, $\{x \mid x$ is an even number$\}$. Every number is clearly either a member of this set or not. For instance, while 6 is definitely an even number such that $6 \in \{x \mid x$ is an even number$\}$, 7 is definitely an odd number to the effect that $7 \notin \{x \mid x$ is an even number$\}$. Thus, the set of even numbers has sharp boundaries. There are no borderline cases between $\in$ and $\notin$ of which it would be unclear whether they are members of the set or not. As was emphasized on page 826, such sets with sharp boundaries are referred to as ordinary, classical, or *crisp* sets.

Contrary to crisp sets such as *even numbers,* consider the set of *healthy* people. It is impossible to sharply separate those people who definitely belong to it, i.e., are healthy, from those who definitely do not belong to it, i.e., are not healthy. That means that the set of healthy people is not crisp, but fuzzy. There are some borderline cases of which we cannot decide with certainty whether they are its members or not, that is, whether they are healthy or not healthy. Thus, the membership in a fuzzy set such as the set of healthy people is not a matter of affirmation or denial as in classical, crisp sets. Rather, it is a matter of degree. It does not make sense to say of a crisp set, such as that of even numbers, that:

18 is fairly even,
332 is very even,
123456 is extremely even,
1200 is more even than 10,
6 is hardly even.

However, since the typical characteristic of a fuzzy set, such as that of *healthy* people, is the gradedness of membership, it makes sense to say, for example, that:

> Amy is fairly healthy,
> Beth is very healthy,
> Carla is extremely healthy,
> Dirk is healthier than Elroy,
> Elroy is hardly healthy.

The presence of varying strengths of membership in a set is indicative of the granular constitution of the set. A granule comprises an imprecisely delimited group of more or less similar members in a set, such as a group of 'very young' people in the set of *young* people. For instance, the granules of the set of *healthy* people are its blurred subsets that include groups of people who are, respectively, *fairly healthy, very healthy, extremely healthy, hardly healthy,* and so on. Classical set theory is incapable of dealing with such granular sets and their granules. Fuzzy set theory is a clearly superior alternative.

The concept of a fuzzy set is profoundly changing science and technology. As the basis of fuzzy logic, it is an important source of innovative ideas, frameworks, and methods that may be useful in medical research, practice, and philosophy. The concept was conceived by Lotfi Zadeh a few years before he published it in 1965. He extended classical set theory to fuzzy set theory by making the sharp set membership, $\in$, a matter of degree. He did so because as an experienced system theorist, he had come to the conclusion that the conceptual apparatus of the received sciences was unable to cope with complex systems:

In fact, there is a fairly wide gap between what might be regarded as 'animate' system theorists and 'inanimate' system theorists at the present time, and it is not at all certain that this gap will be narrowed, much less closed, in the near future. There are some who feel this gap reflects the fundamental inadequacy of the conventional mathematics – the mathematics of precisely-defined points, functions, sets, probability measures, etc. – for coping with the analysis of biological systems, and that to deal effectively with such systems, which are generally orders of magnitudes more complex than man-made systems, we need a radically different kind of mathematics, the mathematics of fuzzy or cloudy quantities which are not described in terms of probability distributions ... (Zadeh, 1962, 857).

Such 'fuzzy or cloudy' objects and processes in medicine are, for example, patient complaints, symptoms, states of the organism, diseases, therapies, and recoveries. The concept of a fuzzy set provides a powerful tool for dealing with them. But it completely contravenes the traditional canons of Western thought. Recall from page 874 the three ancient Principles of Two-Valuedness, Excluded Middle, and Non-Contradiction. They are the underlying principles of Western thought, both in everyday life and in science. As essential ingredients of the Aristotelean worldview, they have in common an *only-two-options,* black-or-white, either-or, yes-no, all-or-nothing perspective.[198] Correspondingly, in the history of the Western culture a manner of perceiving, categorizing, and thinking has predominated that causes almost all of us to dichotomize any domain of our perception and discourse. No matter how complex such a domain may be, we look at it from the only-two-options perspective and categorize its objects as true or false, good or bad, even or odd, near or far, normal or abnormal, large or small, thin or thick, and so on. It is no surprise that Georg Cantor's classical set theory, discussed in Chapter 25, also reflects this tradition. We have seen that in this theory a set A is conceived of as a collection of objects such that an object x either is a member of the set, $x \in A$; or it is not a member of the set, $x \notin A$. No third option exists. Thus, a classical set is crisp in that it includes only full members, excludes non-members, and has sharp boundaries between these two categories to disallow borderline cases such as quasi members and quasi non-members. This trait is exactly the yes-no and all-or-nothing doctrine of the classical or crisp set theory (see Figures 88–93 in Chapter 25, pp. 826–838).

To assess the limitations of crisp set theory for use in medicine and to elucidate the superiority of fuzzy set theory, the notion of the *characteristic function* of a set will be introduced first. Let "Ω" denote a collection of any objects that we may be talking about in a particular context. That is, Ω is our universe of discourse, or simply the universe. The universe Ω will always have a number of subsets. For instance, if Ω is the set of integers, we may distinguish its many subsets such as even numbers, odd numbers, prime numbers, negative integers, positive integers, and so on. To delimit any such subset of Ω, call it A, we differentiate those elements of Ω that belong to A from those that do not belong to A by the so-called indicator function or *characteristic function of set A,* symbolized by "f_A". This function assigns the number 1 to each element of Ω that is a member of A, and the number 0, otherwise. Thus, it is defined as follows.

Definition 241 (The characteristic function of a set). *If Ω is a universe of discourse and A is a subset of Ω, then for each object $x \in \Omega$:*

$$f_A(x) = \begin{cases} 1 & \text{if } x \in A \\ 0 & \text{if } x \notin A. \end{cases}$$

For simplicity's sake, let Ω be the set of integers and its subset A be the set of even numbers, i.e., $\Omega = \{x \mid x \text{ is an integer}\}$ and $A = \{x \mid x \text{ is an even number}\}$. Then the question of whether a particular integer $y \in \Omega$ is an even number or not, reduces to the question whether $f_{even\_number}(y) = 1$ or $f_{even\_number}(y) = 0$, where "f_{even_number}" is the characteristic function of the set of even numbers. We have, for example:

---

[198] See also footnote 163 on page 875.

$$f_{even\_number}(6) = 1$$
$$f_{even\_number}(7) = 0.$$

Another example is:

$$f_{odd\_number}(6) = 0$$
$$f_{odd\_number}(7) = 1.$$

These statements mean that 6 is an even number, whereas 7 is not an even number; 6 is not an odd number, whereas 7 is an odd number. They show that crisp, yes-no membership is representable by the assignment of the binary digits 1 and 0, which are utterly separate from one another. The characteristic function of a crisp subset A in Ω is thus a function, f_A, that maps Ω to the two-valued set $\{0, 1\}$:

$$f_A : \Omega \mapsto \{0, 1\}$$

to the effect that the transition from membership, 1, to non-membership, 0, is abrupt. This is demonstrated by the graph of the characteristic function of the crisp set of the even numbers 6, 8, and 10 in Figure 99.

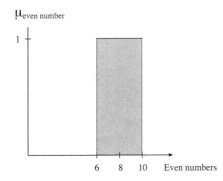

Fuzzy set theory breaks with this Aristotelean, only-two-options tradition by graduating the characteristic function f_A of a set A, and increasing the number of degrees that members of A can take, to infinity. The motivation for this departure is that classes in the real world are not crisp, and consequently, the crisp set theory with its only-two-options perspective cannot deal with them appropriately. It is only the formal world of mathematics where some or many sets of mathematical objects obey the bivalent yes-no, $\{0, 1\}$, criterion for membership, e.g., the sets of even and odd numbers above. The innumerable real-world classes resist this confined, bivalent criterion because they are classes of completely different type lacking sharp boundaries. Consider, for instance, the set of those people who are *young*. Suppose that someone, say Amy, is 17 years

Fig. 99. The characteristic function of the crisp set of even numbers 6, 8, 10. The figure shows that it is a step function. By contrast, the characteristic function of a fuzzy set is a continuous function. See Figure 100 on page 1002

old. Without doubt she is young. We are thus justified to state that she is a member of that set, i.e., Amy $\in \{x \mid x$ is young$\}$, or equivalently, $f_{young}(\text{Amy})$ $= 1$. However, each day Amy grows a little bit older such that on one fine day, for instance, when she becomes 87 years old, we shall have to state that she is not young any more, i.e., Amy $\notin \{x \mid x$ is young$\}$, or equivalently, $f_{young}(\text{Amy}) = 0$. Now, the question arises, when during Amy's life between ages 17 and 87 does our predication change from Amy $\in \{x \mid x$ is young$\}$ to Amy $\notin \{x \mid x$ is young$\}$, and thus, from $f_{young}(\text{Amy}) = 1$ to $f_{young}(\text{Amy}) = 0$? Otherwise put, what age constitutes the boundary between the set of young people and its complement set of non-young people? Is it age 20, 31.8, 41, 55, or another age, say X? What is the exact value of this age X? Does the set of young people have a sharp borderline at all between those individuals who are in the set, and those who are not? These questions express the basic problem the founder of fuzzy set theory observed when initiating his *Fuzzy Revolution* in 1965. Illuminating and still unsurpassed are his introductory notes in his seminal paper on Fuzzy Sets (Zadeh, 1965a):

More often than not, the classes of objects encountered in the real physical world do not have precisely defined criteria of membership. For example, the class of animals clearly includes dogs, horses, birds, etc. as its members, and clearly excludes such objects as rocks, fluids, plants, etc. However, such objects as starfish, bacteria, etc. have an ambiguous status with respect to the class of animals. The same kind of ambiguity arises in the case of a number such as 10 in relation to the "class" of all real numbers which are much greater than 1.

Clearly, the "class of all real numbers which are much greater than 1", or "the class of beautiful women", or "the class of tall men" do not constitute classes or sets in the usual mathematical sense of these terms. Yet, the fact remains that such imprecisely defined "classes" play an important role in human thinking, particularly in the domains of pattern recognition, communication of information, and abstraction.

The purpose of this note is to explore in a preliminary way some of the basic properties and consequences of a concept which may be of use in dealing with "classes" of the type cited above. The concept in question is that of a *fuzzy set*, that is, a "class" with a continuum of grades of membership (Zadeh, 1965a, 338–339).

It is to our advantage to construe and reconstruct almost all classes as fuzzy sets because real-world classes in general have no sharp boundaries between their full members and definite non-members. To give a few examples, consider the sets of objects that are *red, green, human beings, persons, young, old, human beings suffering from pneumonia, children, ill children, trees, bushes, fruits, warm days, large numbers, alive, dead, heavy, ripe tomatoes, criminals,* or *proficient physicians*. A simple answer of the yes-no type is not always a sensible reaction to the question whether a particular object is a member of such a fuzzy set or not, for example, whether it is red or not. With the intuitive ideas above thoroughly in mind, we are now in a position to discuss the technical concept of a fuzzy set.

A *fuzzy* set is a collection of objects with a *continuum of grades*, or *degrees, of membership*. The greater the grade of membership of an object in the set, the more it belongs to the set, and vice versa. To elaborate on this basic idea, we shall conceive a fuzzy set, A, as the product of a *function*, μ, that associates with each object x a real number in the closed, unit interval $[0, 1]$ called the degree of membership of x in A, i.e., $\mu(x, A)$. Thus, we may conveniently write:

$$\mu(x, A) = r$$

and read "the degree of membership of x in A is r". For example, consider the family Fox in Table 54 consisting of the five persons {Amy, Beth, Carla, Dirk, Elroy}. It may be that the degree of membership of Amy in the set *young* is 1, i.e., $\mu(Amy, young) = 1$, whereas $\mu(Carla, young) = 0.5$. The nearer the value of $\mu(x, A)$ to unity, the higher the degree of membership of x in A. The binary function μ that measures the membership degrees of a fuzzy set A, is referred to as the *membership function* of A. Since unary functions are easier to manage, we will artificially represent μ in the form of a pseudo-unary function as follows:

Table 54. Ages of members of the Fox family and their degrees of membership in the fuzzy set *young*

Person:	age:	degree of youth: i.e., $\mu(x, young)$
Amy	17	1
Beth	25	0.9
Carla	33	0.5
Dirk	42	0.1
Elroy	70	0

$$\mu_A(x) \quad \text{is a shorthand for:} \quad \mu(x, A).$$

The subscript A in μ_A indicates the fuzzy set of which μ_A is the membership function. Analogously, μ_B and μ_C are the membership functions of the fuzzy sets B and C, respectively, and so on. For instance, μ_{young} is the membership function of the fuzzy set *young*. Thus, Table 54 may be listed this way:

$\mu_{young}(Amy) = 1 \qquad \equiv$ Amy is young to the extent 1
$\mu_{young}(Beth) = 0.9 \qquad \equiv$ Beth is young to the extent 0.9
$\mu_{young}(Carla) = 0.5 \qquad \equiv$ Carla is young to the extent 0.5
$\mu_{young}(Dirk) = 0.1 \qquad \equiv$ Dirk is young to the extent 0.1
$\mu_{young}(Elroy) = 0 \qquad \equiv$ Elroy is young to the extent 0.

Individuals in this family are obviously to different degrees members of the same set of young people. Otherwise put, the set of young people contains its members to different degrees between 1 and 0 inclusive. As a result, the transition from membership, 1, to non-membership, 0, is not abrupt, but continuous such that there is no sharp dividing line between members and non-members of the set (see Figure 100).

The considerations above demonstrate that the membership function μ_A of a fuzzy set A maps a universe of discourse Ω, e.g., the family Fox above, to the infinite unit interval $[0, 1]$. We thus arrive at the formal concept of a fuzzy set introduced in the following two definitions.

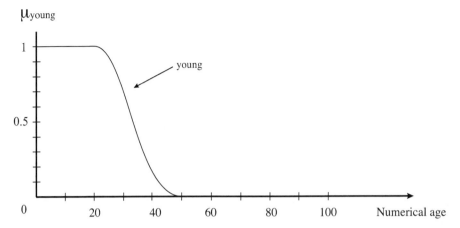

Fig. 100. The membership function of the fuzzy set *young*. In contrast to the characteristic function of a crisp set as depicted in Figure 99 on page 999, the membership function of a fuzzy set is continuous. Membership degrees smoothly decrease in the direction of zero, i.e., non-membership. Young people and non-young people are not sharply separable from one another. See Figure 101

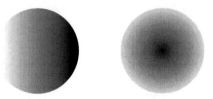

Fig. 101. Grey, fog, and cloud as symbols of a fuzzy set. The more a member of the set is in the grey area the lesser is the degree of its membership in the set

Definition 242 (Fuzzy subset of a base set). *If Ω is any collection of objects, then A is a* fuzzy subset *of, or over, Ω iff there is a function μ_A such that:*

  1. $\mu_A : \Omega \mapsto [0,1]$
  2. $A = \big\{ \big(x, \mu_A(x) \big) \mid x \in \Omega \big\}$

Clause 2 means that A is the set of all pairs $\big(x, \mu_A(x) \big)$ such that x is a member of the base set Ω and $\mu_A(x)$ is the degree of its membership in A. On the basis of Definition 242, we obtain from the binary term "is a fuzzy subset of" a handy, unary concept of fuzzy set in the following fashion:

Definition 243 (Fuzzy set). *A is a* fuzzy set *iff there is a collection Ω such that A is a fuzzy subset of Ω. The collection Ω is referred to as the universe of discourse or the base set.*[199]

For example, let our base set be the above-mentioned family {Amy, Beth, Carla, Dirk, Elroy} conveniently represented by their initials $\{a, b, c, d, e\}$;

---

[199] In the literature on fuzzy set theory and logic, a fuzzy set is often identified with its membership function. Such an identification is formally, methodologically, and philosophically objectionable.

and let μ_{young} be the membership function of the fuzzy set *young* over this base set. Then we have:

$$\mu_{young}(a) = 1$$
$$\mu_{young}(b) = 0.9$$
$$\mu_{young}(c) = 0.5$$
$$\mu_{young}(d) = 0.1$$
$$\mu_{young}(e) = 0$$

such that the fuzzy set *young* over the universe $\{a, b, c, d, e\}$ is the following set of pairs:

$$Young = \{(a, 1), (b, 0.9), (c, 0.5), (d, 0.1), (e, 0)\}.$$

We are now in a position to recognize the limitations of classical set theory. As we have seen above, the characteristic function f_A of a crisp set ranges over the two-valued set $\{0, 1\}$. Thus, the membership function μ_A of a fuzzy set A with the unit interval $[0, 1]$ as its range is the generalization of the classical characteristic function, or its extension from $\{0, 1\}$ to $[0, 1]$, because the infinite set $[0, 1]$ includes the finite set $\{0, 1\}$. While a classical set is only two-valued, $\{0, 1\}$, a fuzzy set is a many-valued set whose members may take infinitely many values from $[0, 1]$. Otherwise put, since $\{0, 1\} \subset [0, 1]$, a classical characteristic function f_A also maps the underlying base set Ω to $[0, 1]$. Hence, the characteristic function f_A of a classical set A is the membership function of the set. A classical set turns out a two-valued fuzzy set. For example, in our base set $\{\text{Amy, Beth, Carla, Dirk, Elroy}\}$ we have the following two classical subsets:

$$\begin{aligned} Female &= \{a, b, c\} \\ Male &= \{d, e\}. \end{aligned}$$

They are the following fuzzy sets:

$$\begin{aligned} Female &= \{(a, 1), (b, 1), (c, 1), (d, 0), (e, 0)\} \\ Male &= \{(a, 0), (b, 0), (c, 0), (d, 1), (e, 1)\}. \end{aligned}$$

Thus, the concept of a fuzzy set is the more general one and also includes the classical sets. The latter ones, viewed from this perspective as special fuzzy sets with the extreme membership values 1 and 0, are referred to as *crisp* sets. Fuzzy set theory is a many-valued, non-classical extension of classical set theory. The reason why it is qualified as a non-classical system, will become clear in the next section.

The question of where the membership degrees of a fuzzy set come from, may be answered right now to prevent misunderstandings: They come simply from the *definition* of the membership function for that set. The definiens of such a definition may be provided in different ways, e.g., (i) stipulatively by personal decision; (ii) by an assessment on the scale $[0, 1]$ as it is usual in psychology and in quality of life and quality of health care research; (iii) by a measurement on the scale $[0, 1]$; or (iv) by the transformation of a measurement result to the unit interval $[0, 1]$ if the measurement scale is a different one. As an example, a stipulative definition is given below of the membership function μ_{young} to construct the fuzzy set *young* thereby.

Definition 244 (The membership function μ_{young}). *If the set of numerical ages of human beings is* $\{0, 1, 2, 3, \ldots, 100, \ldots\}$, *then:*

$$\mu_{young}(x) = \begin{cases} 1 & \text{if } 0 \leq x < 20 \\ \frac{1}{30}(50 - x) & \text{if } 20 \leq x < 50 \\ 0 & \text{if } 50 \leq x. \end{cases}$$

This definition yields a graph of the fuzzy set *young* as depicted in Figure 102. The figure differs from Figure 100 because the latter one was drawn without reference to formal definitions. For simplicity's sake, we shall keep this policy also in what follows.

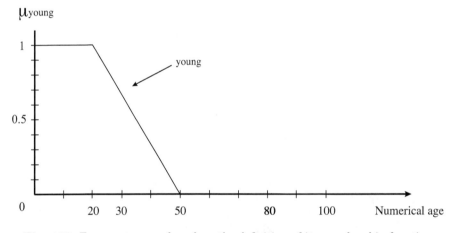

Fig. 102. Fuzzy set *young* based on the definition of its membership function

It is worth noting that the unit interval $[0, 1]$ used as the range of fuzzy set membership functions is a powerful device and provides a universally applicable numerical reference space. All real numbers, and thus all kinds of assessment and measurement scales, can easily be transformed to this space. For a proof of this thesis, see (Kosko, 1997).

30.2 Operations on Fuzzy Sets

Since the interval $[0, 1]$ is uncountably infinite, a base set Ω may be mapped to $[0, 1]$ in innumerably different ways. There is thus an uncountably infinite number of fuzzy sets A, B, C, ... in a base set Ω. In this section, a few basic types of them will be introduced for use throughout our discussion.

A variety of operations may be carried out on fuzzy sets, e.g., the operations of complementation, intersection, and union to emulate the natural language connectives "not", "and", and "or". Contrary to the classical case, however, these operations on fuzzy sets are not unique. This is due to the circumstance that natural language connectives have different meanings in different contexts and when they are applied by different individuals. Therefore, there is a wide range of semantics for connectives in fuzzy set theory. We will here present and use only the *standard fuzzy operations*, introduced in turn in the following three sections:

    30.2.1 Fuzzy Complement
    30.2.2 Fuzzy Intersection and Union
    30.2.3 Empty Fuzzy Set and Fuzzy Powerset.

In addition, in the following two sections degrees of fuzziness and clarity will be introduced and it will be shown that the fuzzy logic is a non-classical system:

    30.2.4 Degrees of Fuzziness and Clarity
    30.2.5 Fuzzy Logic is a Non-Classical System.

In Chapter 25 we introduced several symbols for classical set operations. They include the symbol $\overline{A}$ for complementation, $\cap$ for intersection, and $\cup$ for union. In order to prevent a plethora of symbols, from now on we shall use these symbols primarily in the context of fuzzy sets and will avoid introducing new, special symbols for fuzzy set operations. Misunderstandings will not arise.

30.2.1 Fuzzy Complement

Given any fuzzy set A in a base set Ω, the *complement* of A in Ω, called its negation and denoted by *Not A* or $\overline{A}$, is a fuzzy set that is defined by the following membership function $\mu_{\overline{A}}$:

$$\mu_{\overline{A}}(x) = 1 - \mu_A(x).$$

Put into a precise definition, that means:

Definition 245 (Fuzzy complement).

$$\overline{A} = \left\{ \left(x, \mu_{\overline{A}}(x)\right) \mid x \in \Omega \ \ and \ \ \mu_{\overline{A}}(x) = 1 - \mu_A(x) \right\}.$$

The fuzzy complement $\overline{A}$ represents a fuzzy negation ('Not A'). For instance, let $\Omega = \{a, b, c, d\}$ be a set of four male doctors such that each one of them is proficient to a particular extent and we have the following fuzzy set of proficient doctors in Ω:

$Proficient\ doctor = \{(a, 0), (b, 0.4), (c, 0.8), (d, 1)\}$.

Then the complement of this set in Ω is:

$Not\ proficient\ doctor = \{(a, 1), (b, 0.6), (c, 0.2), (d, 0)\}$.

30.2.2 Fuzzy Intersection and Union

Two fuzzy sets A and B in a universe of discourse, Ω, may have any relationships with one another. For example, their *intersection,* denoted by $A \cap B$, is a fuzzy set that is defined by the minima of their joint membership degrees, i.e., by the following membership function $\mu_{A \cap B}$ (for the definition of the functions $min(x, y)$ and $max(x, y)$ used in this section, see Definition 18 on page 94):

$$\mu_{A \cap B}(x) = min(\mu_A(x),\ \mu_B(x)).$$

That is:

Definition 246 (Fuzzy intersection).
$A \cap B = \{(x, \mu_{A \cap B}(x)) \mid x \in \Omega \ and \ \mu_{A \cap B}(x) = min(\mu_A(x),\ \mu_B(x))\}$.

And the union of two fuzzy sets A and B, denoted by $A \cup B$, is a fuzzy set that is defined by the maxima of their joint membership degrees, i.e., by the following membership function $\mu_{A \cup B}$:

$$\mu_{A \cup B}(x) = max(\mu_A(x),\ \mu_B(x)).$$

That is:

Definition 247 (Fuzzy union).
$A \cup B = \{(x, \mu_{A \cup B}(x)) \mid x \in \Omega \ and \ \mu_{A \cup B}(x) = max(\mu_A(x),\ \mu_B(x))\}$.

A few examples will illustrate this terminology. We shall not explain them, as they are self-explanatory.

$\Omega = \{a, b, c, d\}$

$Proficient\ doctor = \{(a, 0), (b, 0.4), (c, 0.8), (d, 1)\}$ (249)

$Young = \{(a, 0.9), (b, 0.5), (c, 0.3), (d, 0.7)\}$

$Proficient\ doctor \cap Young = \{(a, 0), (b, 0.4), (c, 0.3), (d, 0.7)\}$

$Proficient\ doctor \cup Young = \{(a, 0.9), (b, 0.5), (c, 0.8), (d, 1)\}$.

The fuzzy intersection $A \cap B$ represents a fuzzy conjunction ('A and B'). The fuzzy union $A \cup B$ represents a fuzzy disjunction ('A or B').[200]

---

[200] As emphasized above, the definitions of fuzzy intersection and fuzzy union provided here are the standard ones. A more general method of defining them that

30.2.3 Empty Fuzzy Set and Fuzzy Powerset

A base set Ω itself is the fuzzy set $\{(x, \mu_\Omega(x) = 1) \mid x \in \Omega\}$. All of its members have the membership degree 1. On the other hand, the empty fuzzy set, written $\varnothing$, is $\{(x, \mu_\varnothing(x) = 0) \mid x \in \Omega\}$. The degree of membership of every object in this set is 0. Both fuzzy sets are crisp. For instance, regarding the base set $\Omega = \{a, b, c, d\}$ of our four male doctors above we have:

$$\Omega = \{a, b, c, d\}$$
$$Male = \{(a, 1), (b, 1), (c, 1), (d, 1)\} = \Omega$$
$$Female = \{(a, 0), (b, 0), (c, 0), (d, 0)\} = \varnothing.$$

The fuzzy set *Female* in Ω above is empty because Ω consists of male doctors only. Recall that the classical powerset of the base set Ω is denoted by 2^Ω. Its *fuzzy powerset*, mnemonically written $F(2^\Omega)$, is the set of *all* fuzzy subsets of Ω.

Definition 248 (Fuzzy powerset of a collection Ω). $F(2^\Omega) = \{A \mid A \text{ is a fuzzy subset of } \Omega\}$.

While a crisp powerset 2^Ω of a finite base set Ω is finite and contains 2^n elements, its fuzzy powerset $F(2^\Omega)$ is uncountably infinite because every base set Ω may be mapped to $[0, 1]$ in infinitely different ways to generate infinitely many fuzzy sets. The fuzzy powerset $F(2^\Omega)$ forms a unit hypercube that is extensively used in Parts II and V. See page 207.

30.2.4 Degrees of Fuzziness and Clarity

In the current section, some interesting concepts are introduced that are useful in assessing the vagueness of a disease. For applications, see page 216. Our discussions will presuppose knowledge of the concept of fuzzy hypercube that has been presented and extensively explained on pages 207–216.

The amount of vagueness and indeterminacy a set carries within itself, is referred to as its *fuzziness* or *fuzzy entropy*. It is measured with a fuzzy entropy measure, denoted by *ent*, that maps the fuzzy hypercube to $[0, 1]$:

$$ent \colon F(2^\Omega) \longmapsto [0, 1].$$

The definition of this function *ent* will be based upon the notions of *nearest* and *farthest* ordinary set to be understood in the following way (cf. Kaufmann, 1975, 22; Kosko, 1986; Sadegh-Zadeh, 1999):

---

yields an infinite number of fuzzy conjunction and disjunction types is based on the so-called triangular norms and conorms, generally known as *t*-norms and *t*-conorms. However, we must refrain from going into details here (see, e.g., Klir and Yuan, 1995).

In a fuzzy hypercube, i.e., the fuzzy powerset $F(2^\Omega)$ of a base set Ω, there is always an ordinary set which is the nearest one to a fuzzy set $A \in F(2^\Omega)$, denoted A_{near}; and another one that is the farthest one to A, denoted A_{far}. They will be defined informally. For simplicity's sake, we shall make use of the vector notation, that is, a fuzzy set $\{(x_1, a_1), \ldots, (x_n, a_n)\}$ is briefly represented by the vector $(a_1, \ldots, a_n)$ of its membership degrees (see p. 210).

Given a fuzzy set A in a fuzzy hypercube $F(2^\Omega)$, A_{near} is a set with the vector $(b_1, \ldots, b_n)$ such that if $A = (a_1, \ldots, a_n)$, then:

$$
\begin{aligned}
b_i &= 1 && \text{if } a_i > 0.5, \\
&= 0 && \text{if } a_i < 0.5, \\
&= 0 \text{ or } 1 && \text{if } a_i = 0.5.
\end{aligned}
$$

And A_{far} is a set with the vector $(b_1, \ldots, b_n)$ such that if $A = (a_1, \ldots, a_n)$, then:

$$
\begin{aligned}
b_i &= 0 && \text{if } a_i > 0.5, \\
&= 1 && \text{if } a_i < 0.5, \\
&= 1 \text{ or } 0 && \text{if } a_i = 0.5.
\end{aligned}
$$

For example, if $A = (0.2, 0.8, 0.6)$, we have $A_{near} = (0, 1, 1)$ and $A_{far} = (1, 0, 0)$. Let $A = (a_1, \ldots, a_n)$ be any fuzzy set in a fuzzy hypercube. Taking into account that ordinary sets reside at the cube's 2^n vertices, there is among them a vertex nearest to A in the cube called A_{near}; and another one farthest to A referred to as A_{far}. The *fuzzy entropy* of set A is defined as the ratio of the Hamming distance, denoted $dist^1$, from vertex A_{near} to vertex A_{far}:

Definition 249 (Fuzzy entropy of a set A).

$$
ent(A) = \frac{dist^1(A, A_{near})}{dist^1(A, A_{far})}.
$$

The two-dimensional hypercube in Figure 103 provides a geometrical illustration. It shows that the entropy of a set that resides at the vertices of the hypercube, equals 0 because at a vertex the numerator of the ratio at the right-hand side of the equation in Definition 249 is 0. Hence, there is no fuzzy entropy at a vertex. This reflects the fact that the inhabitants of the cube vertices are members of the classical set 2^Ω. Any component of a set membership vector $(a_1, \ldots, a_n)$ at a vertex is either 1 or 0 that amounts to the nonfuzzy information that an object x_i definitely is, or is not, a member of the set. By contrast, if a fuzzy set $X = (a_1, \ldots, a_n)$ is the hypercube midpoint, we obtain according to Definition 249 $ent(X) = 1$ because X at the midpoint is equidistant from all 2^n vertices. In addition, due to $a_1 = \cdots = a_n = 0.5$, we have $X = \overline{X}$ where $\overline{X}$ is the fuzzy complement of X. That means that the complement $\overline{X}$ also resides at the cube midpoint. Set X is maximally fuzzy because it cannot be distinguished from its own complement. Fuzzy entropy

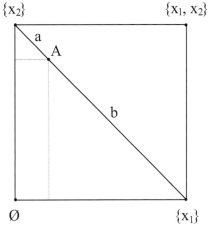

Fig. 103. The farthest vertex A_{far} resides opposite the long diagonal from the nearest vertex A_{near}. For fuzzy set $A = \{(x_1, 02), (x_2, 0.8)\}$, we have $ent(A) = \frac{a}{b}$ where $a = dist^1(A, A_{near})$ and $b = dist^1(A, A_{far})$. For any set X, $ent(X) = 0$ at a vertex and $ent(X) = 1$ at the center of the hypercube. Since $A = (0.2, 0.8)$, we have $ent(A) = (|0.2 - 0|) + |0.8 - 1|)/(|0.2 - 1|) + |0.8 - 0|) = 0.4/1.6 = 0.25$. See Figure 104

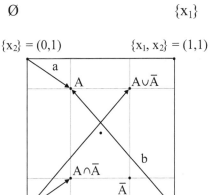

Fig. 104. Symmetrical position of the four fuzzy sets A, $\overline{A}$, $A \cap \overline{A}$, and $A \cup \overline{A}$ in the hypercube. They are therefore equidistant from their $vertex_{near}$ and $vertex_{far}$. This is due to how complement, intersection, and union are defined in fuzzy set theory. As these four set points move from periphery toward the center of the cube, they become more and more similar to one another until they equalize at the midpoint. See body text

smoothly increases as a set point moves from any vertex toward the midpoint of the hypercube, and thus, its distance to its complement decreases.

The opposite of fuzzy entropy is the *clarity* of a set. The clarity of a set A, denoted by $clar(A)$, is the additive inverse of its entropy:

Definition 250 (Fuzzy clarity of a set A). $clar(A) = 1 - ent(A)$.

We have therefore $clar(A) = 1$ at all vertices, whereas $clar(A) = 0$ at the center of the hypercube. The clarity of a set A grows as the distance increases between A and its complement $\overline{A}$, and thus, A moves from midpoint to any vertex of the hypercube. As Figure 104 demonstrates, the four fuzzy sets A, $\overline{A}$, $A \cap \overline{A}$, and $A \cup \overline{A}$ have equal distance both from their $vertex_{near}$ and their $vertex_{far}$. The more they move toward the midpoint, the more similar to one another they become, until they equalize at the midpoint: $A = (0.5, \ldots, 0.5)$

$= \overline{A} = (0.5, \ldots, 0.5) = A \cap \overline{A} = (0.5, \ldots, 0.5) = A \cup \overline{A}$. Thus, at the midpoint we have $ent(A) = ent(\overline{A}) = ent(A \cap \overline{A}) = ent(A) \cup \overline{A}) = 1$. Likewise, $clar(A) = clar(\overline{A}) = clar(A \cap \overline{A}) = clar(A \cup \overline{A}) = 0$. For instance, regarding the fuzzy set $A = (0.2, 0.8)$ we have $ent(A) = 0.25$ and $clar(A) = 1 - 0.25 = 0.75$. Due to the equal distance of the four fuzzy sets A, $\overline{A}$, $A \cap \overline{A}$, and $A \cup \overline{A}$ from their $vertex_{near}$ and $vertex_{far}$, Definitions 249–250 together with a theorem that cannot be discussed here, imply the following *Fuzzy Entropy Theorem*. It relates fuzzy entropy with set size (for proof, see Kosko, 1992, 277):

Theorem 10 (Fuzzy Entropy Theorem: Entropy of a fuzzy set A).

$$ent(A) = \frac{c(A \cap \overline{A})}{c(A \cup \overline{A})}.$$

For instance, for fuzzy set $A = (0.2, 0.8)$ used in Figures 103–104, we have:

$$A = (0.2, 0.8)$$
$$\overline{A} = (0.8, 0.2)$$
$$A \cap \overline{A} = (0.2, 0.2)$$
$$A \cup \overline{A} = (0.8, 0.8)$$

$$ent(A) = \frac{c(0.2, 0.2)}{c(0.8, 0.8)} = 0.25.$$

For an application to the entropy and clarity of diseases, see page 216.

30.2.5 Fuzzy Logic is a Non-Classical System

Fuzzy logic is a non-classical system because fuzzy sets as its basis are non-classical sets. They do not accord with the classical, Aristotelean Principles of Excluded Middle and Non-Contradiction that we have outlined on page 831. This is easily seen from the evidence that (i) the union of a fuzzy set A and its complement $\overline{A}$ need not necessarily be the base set; and (ii) their intersection need not necessarily be empty:

$A \cap \overline{A} \neq \varnothing$ 　　　　　　violation of the Principle of Non-Contradiction

$A \cup \overline{A} \neq \Omega$ 　　　　　　violation of the Principle of Excluded Middle.

For instance, regarding our example fuzzy set 'proficient doctor' in (249) above we have:

$$\textit{Proficient doctor} \cup \textit{Not proficient doctor} = \{(a, 1), (b, 0.6), (c, 0.8), (d, 1)\} \quad (250)$$
$$\neq \Omega$$

$$\textit{Proficient doctor} \cap \textit{Not proficient doctor} = \{(a, 0), (b, 0.4), (c, 0.2), (d, 0)\} \quad (251)$$
$$\neq \varnothing.$$

The union in (250) falls short of the base set, 'the middle is not excluded'; and the intersection in (251) exceeds emptiness, 'A does not contradict not A'. See the contrasting laws for classical sets (221–222) on page 831.

30.3 Fuzzy Relations

The classical concept of relation outlined in Section 25.3 captures the mere presence of an association between members of given sets, for example, 'Amy is *younger than* Carla'. Fuzzy set theory enables us in addition to represent the strength of the association, e.g., 'Amy is *much younger than* Carla' or '*to the extent 0.5* Amy is younger than Carla'. That is, relations are treated as fuzzy relations.

Predicates denoting fuzzy sets we call vague or *fuzzy predicates*. Examples are the predicates "is young", "is a child", "is red", "has bronchitis", and the like. A one-place fuzzy predicate denotes a fuzzy set. A many-place fuzzy predicate denotes a fuzzy relation, for example, "is much younger than" and "is more ill than". The concept of fuzzy relation constitutes an essential and powerful part of fuzzy logic and plays a central role in all areas of its application, especially in fuzzy diagnosis, fuzzy therapy, fuzzy control, medical expert systems, and fuzzy technology in general. We shall try to utilize it in the philosophy of these and other medical subjects as well. For this purpose, we shall here very briefly introduce the concept and shall illustrate some of its basic properties in the following two sections:

  30.3.1 The Concept of a Fuzzy Relation
  30.3.2 Composition of Fuzzy Relations.

30.3.1 The Concept of a Fuzzy Relation

First consider a simple example that may help us understand the abstract issue at hand. That Amy is younger than Beth to the extent 0.1, and is younger than Carla to the extent 0.5, is representable as a fuzzy set:

$$Younger\_than = \big\{ \big((Amy, Beth), 0.1\big), \big((Amy, Carla), 0.5\big) \big\}. \tag{252}$$

That means that to the extent 0.1 Amy and Beth stand in the relation Younger_than, and to the extent 0.5 Amy and Carla stand in the relation Younger_than. Obviously, a *fuzzy relation* R is, in general, a fuzzy set of the following form:

$$R = \big\{ \big(\langle x_1, \ldots, x_n \rangle, a\big), \big(\langle y_1, \ldots, y_n \rangle, b\big), \big(\langle z_1, \ldots, z_n \rangle, c\big), \ldots \big\}$$

with $a, b, c \in [0, 1]$, where the first element of each pair in the set is an ordered n-tuple such as $\langle x_1, \ldots, x_n \rangle$ with $n \geq 2$; and the second element of each pair is the degree of membership of the n-tuple in the fuzzy set R. In our example (252) above, the n-tuple in the first pair is the 2-tuple (Amy, Beth), and the degree of its membership in the fuzzy set *Younger_than* is 0.1. In the second pair, the n-tuple is the 2-tuple (Amy, Carla), and the degree of its membership in the fuzzy set *Younger_than* is 0.5. Our discussion below will prepare us for a more precise definition of the concept.

We have seen previously that a crisp relation is a subset of a Cartesian product $A_1 \times \cdots \times A_n$, and as such, represents an association between members of two or more not necessarily distinct sets $A_1, \ldots, A_n$. For example, if A is the set of human beings, then the binary relation of someone's being *younger than* someone else is a subset of $A \times A$:

Younger_than $\subseteq A \times A$

such that the following three statements are equivalent:

Amy is *younger than* Beth
$\langle$Amy, Beth$\rangle$ stands in the relation *Younger_than*
$\langle$Amy, Beth$\rangle \in$ *Younger_than*.

This crisp concept of a relation can be generalized to allow for degrees of strength of association between the elements of a Cartesian product. To do this, note that by Definition 241 on page 998, an n-ary crisp relation R, as a set, has the following characteristic function, denoted f_R. If the universe of discourse is $\Omega = A_1 \times \cdots \times A_n$ and $R \subseteq A_1 \times \cdots \times A_n$, then for every $\langle x_1, \ldots, x_n \rangle \in \Omega$:

$$f_R(x_1, \ldots, x_n) = \begin{cases} 1 & \text{if } (x_1, \ldots, x_n) \in R \\ 0 & \text{if } (x_1, \ldots, x_n) \notin R. \end{cases}$$

Thus, if R is the relation of someone's being *younger than* someone else, we may say that $f_{younger\_than}(Amy, Beth) = 1$ instead of "Amy is younger than Beth". Since the characteristic function $f_{younger\_than}$ establishes a mapping from $A \times A$ to the bivalent set $\{0, 1\}$, we may easily generalize it to obtain a fuzzy *membership function*, $\mu_{younger\_than}$, in the following way:

$\mu_{younger\_than} : A \times A \mapsto [0, 1]$.

This would enable us to state *to what extent* a pair $\langle x, y \rangle$ is a member of the set *Younger_than*, that is, to what extent the individual x is younger than another individual y. For instance, in our example family Fox {Amy, Beth, Carla, Dirk, Elroy} listed in Table 54 on page 1001, we may observe that:

$\mu_{younger\_than}(\text{Amy, Beth}) = 0.1$
$\mu_{younger\_than}(\text{Amy, Carla}) = 0.5$
$\mu_{younger\_than}(\text{Amy, Dirk}) = 0.9$
$\mu_{younger\_than}(\text{Amy, Elroy}) = 1$
$\mu_{younger\_than}(\text{Beth, Carla}) = 0.4$
$\mu_{younger\_than}(\text{Beth, Dirk}) = 0.8$
$\mu_{younger\_than}(\text{Beth, Elroy}) = 0.9$
$\mu_{younger\_than}(\text{Carla, Dirk}) = 0.4$
$\mu_{younger\_than}(\text{Carla, Elroy}) = 0.5$
$\mu_{younger\_than}(\text{Dirk, Elroy}) = 0.1$.

These ten statements describe a fuzzy relation in the family, that is, the following fuzzy set in which each first element of a pair is an ordered pair:

$$\Big\{ \big((Amy, Beth), 0.1\big), \big((Amy, Carla), 0.5\big), \ldots, \big((Beth, Elroy), 0.9.\big), \ldots \Big\}.$$

With the above in mind, we may now succinctly state that a fuzzy relation R is a *fuzzy set* in a Cartesian product $A_1 \times \cdots \times A_n$. That is, if the base set Ω is a Cartesian product of the form $\Omega = A_1 \times \cdots \times A_n$, a membership function μ_R that maps it to $[0, 1]$ yields a fuzzy relation R on Ω. The function μ_R assigns a number $r \in [0, 1]$ to an n-tuple $(x_1, \ldots, x_n)$ such that $\mu_R(x_1, \ldots, x_n) = r$ is the membership degree of the tuple in the n-ary fuzzy set R.

Definition 251 (Fuzzy relation). *If $\Omega = A_1 \times \cdots \times A_n$ is a base set, then R is an n-ary fuzzy relation on $A_1, \ldots, A_n$ iff there is a membership function μ_R such that:*

1. *$\mu_R : A_1 \times \cdots \times A_n \mapsto [0, 1]$*
2. *$\big\{ \big((x_1, \ldots, x_n), \mu_R(x_1, \ldots, x_n)\big) \mid x_1 \in A_1 \text{ and } \ldots \text{ and } x_n \in A_n \big\}$.*

This definition is an analog of Definition 242 on page 1002 expressed in other words. It may be illustrated by a fuzzy binary relation. Let $X = \{a, b\}$ and $Y = \{c, d\}$ be two sets of human individuals. Their Cartesian product is $X \times Y = \{\langle a, c\rangle, \langle a, d\rangle, \langle b, c\rangle, \langle b, d\rangle\}$. Now, construct a fuzzy relation of loving on $X \times Y$ referred to as *loves*. Table 55 shows a matrix, called a membership or *fuzzy matrix*, that indicates to what extent the first element of a pair in $X \times Y$ loves its second element. The fuzzy matrix displays the following membership function:

Table 55. A fuzzy matrix of the relation *'loves'* between two groups of people

$$\begin{bmatrix} & c & d \\ a & 0.2 & 1 \\ b & 0.7 & 0 \end{bmatrix}$$

$$\mu_{loves} : X \times Y \mapsto [0, 1]$$

with the membership degrees:

$$\mu_{loves}(a, c) = 0.2$$
$$\mu_{loves}(a, d) = 1$$
$$\mu_{loves}(b, c) = 0.7$$
$$\mu_{loves}(b, d) = 0$$

which yield the following binary fuzzy relation:

$$Loves = \big\{ \big((a, c), 0.2\big), \big((a, d), 1\big), \big((b, c), 0.7\big), \big((b, d), 0\big) \big\}.$$

One may think of a membership degree in a fuzzy relation as representing the strength of relationship between the elements of the respective n-tuple, i.e., between the *relata* of the relation. The closer the membership degree to 1, the stronger the relationship between them. In the example above, a loves d to the extent 1, whereas b does not love d at all.

Since a fuzzy relation is a fuzzy set, all operations on fuzzy sets sketched in the preceding section are applicable to them as well. Basic operations on relations are also applicable, for example, the operation of composition that we introduced for functions on page 841. There are different types of composition of fuzzy relations. The standard composition called *max-min composition* will be outlined in the next section to be used in our fuzzy logic below.

30.3.2 Composition of Fuzzy Relations

As in other places in this book, we will have a preliminary discussion to make way for the abstract concept and its definition. Consider two binary fuzzy relations, A and B, such that A is a fuzzy relation on $X \times Y$ and B is a fuzzy relation on $Y \times Z$. The relation A fuzzily associates members of set X with those of set Y; and the relation B fuzzily associates members of set Y with those of set Z. Apparently, members of X and Z are not associated with one another. However, the two relations A and B share set Y that is the range of the first and the domain of the second relation. Using this shared set Y as a bridge between the two separated sets X and Z, the method of *max-min composition* enables us to compose of the relations A and B their composition, written $A \circ B$, as a new, fuzzy relation on $X \times Z$. The definition will be presented after the following example.

The three sets X, Y, and Z referred to may be three families. Suppose there is some similarity between members of X and Y, on the one hand; and between members of Y and Z, on the other. We may now ask the question whether there is any similarity between members of the families X and Z, and if so, how similar they are to each other. To answer this question, let us take a closer look at the families and the similarities between their members. The families are:

$$X = \{Amy, Ada\}$$
$$Y = \{Beth, Bernd, Beryl\}$$
$$Z = \{Carla, Cecil\}$$

which may be conveniently symbolized by:

$$X = \{x_1, x_2\}$$
$$Y = \{y_1, y_2, y_3\}$$
$$Z = \{z_1, z_2\}.$$

As stated above, there exists a fuzzy similarity relation A from set X to set Y; and a fuzzy similarity relation B from set Y to set Z. These relations are displayed in two fuzzy matrixes given in Tables 56–57. The matrixes may also be written in fuzzy set notation as follows:

$$A = \big\{\big((x_1, y_1), 1\big), \big((x_1, y_2), 0.8\big), \big((x_1, y_3), 0.2\big), \big((x_2, y_1), 0.1\big),$$
$$\big((x_2, y_2), 0\big), \big((x_2, y_3), 0.3\big)\big\}$$
$$B = \big\{\big((y_1, z_1), 0.7\big), \big((y_1, z_2), 0.6\big), \big((y_2, z_1), 0\big), \big((y_2, z_2), 0.1\big),$$
$$\big((y_3, z_1), 0.5\big), \big((y_3, z_2), 0.4\big)\big\}.$$

Table 56. The fuzzy matrix of the relation of similarity between members of the families X and Y

$$A = \begin{bmatrix} & y_1 & y_2 & y_3 \\ x_1 & 1 & 0.8 & 0.2 \\ x_2 & 0.1 & 0 & 0.3 \end{bmatrix}$$

Table 57. The fuzzy matrix of similarity between families Y and Z

$$B = \begin{bmatrix} & z_1 & z_2 \\ y_1 & 0.7 & 0.6 \\ y_2 & 0 & 0.1 \\ y_3 & 0.5 & 0.4 \end{bmatrix}$$

To explain, observe that in the relation A person x_1 resembles person y_2 to the extent 0.8; and in the relation B person y_3 resembles person z_2 to the extent 0.4. That is, $\mu_A(x_1, y_2) = 0.8$; and $\mu_B(y_3, z_2) = 0.4$. However, no similarity is indicated between a person x_i in family X and a person z_j in family Z. A relationship between them may be *composed* in the following way by using the y members of family Y as mediators because they are present in both relations, A and B. The procedure will be explained by showing how an association may be established between member x_1 and member z_2. Associations between other x and z members are established in the same fashion.

A pair of the form $\langle \mu_A(x_i, y_j), \mu_B(y_j, z_k) \rangle$ is a number pair such as (0.2, 0.5) and consists of A and B membership degrees, respectively, of the member pairs (x_i, y_j) and (y_j, z_k) that have the member y_j in common. For instance, in the above matrices we have $\big(\mu_A(x_1, y_3), \mu_B(y_3, z_1)\big) = (0.2, 0.5)$. As an *example*, we list the A-B membership degree pairs $\big(\mu_A(x_1, y_i), \mu_B(y_i, z_2)\big)$ for *all* y_i with $i = 1, 2, 3$ in the present families:

$$\big(\mu_A(x_1, y_1), \mu_B(y_1, z_2)\big) = (1, 0.6)$$
$$\big(\mu_A(x_1, y_2), \mu_B(y_2, z_2)\big) = (0.8, 0.1)$$
$$\big(\mu_A(x_1, y_3), \mu_B(y_3, z_2)\big) = (0.2, 0.4).$$

We take from each number pair the minimum degree, $min(-, -)$, and put it on a list. We obtain:

$$(0.6, 0.1, 0.2).$$

We then determine the maximum element of this list, $max(-, -, -)$:

$$= 0.6.$$

Summarizing the above steps, this result was attained by using the procedure:

$$max\Big(min\big(\mu_A(x_1,y_1),\ \mu_B(y_1,z_2)\big),$$
$$min\big(\mu_A(x_1,y_2),\ \mu_B(y_2,z_2)\big),$$
$$min\big(\mu_A(x_1,y_3),\ \mu_B(y_3,z_2)\big)\Big).$$

That is:

$$max\big(min(1,0.6),\ min(0.8,0.1),\ min(0.2,0.4)\big)=max(0.6,0.1,0.2)$$
$$=0.6$$

The complex procedure *above* may be formally simplified thus:

$$max_{y\in Y}min\big(\mu_A(x_1,y),\ \mu_B(y,z_2)\big)\qquad\text{for all } y\in Y.$$

That means: For *all* members y of set Y, *max* of $min\big(\mu_A(x_1,y),\mu_B(y,z_2)\big)$. This is just the (x_1,z_2) membership degree that we are seeking for the composition $\mu_{A\circ B}(x_1,z_2)$ of the two relations A and B. We are now prepared to define the concept.

Definition 252 (Max-min composition of fuzzy relations). *If A is a fuzzy relation on $X\times Y$, and B is a fuzzy relation on $Y\times Z$, then their* max-min composition, *denoted $A\circ B$, is a fuzzy relation on $X\times Z$ defined by the membership function:*

$$\mu_{A\circ B}(x,z)=max_{y\in Y}min\big(\mu_A(x,y),\ \mu_B(y,z)\big)\qquad\begin{array}{l}\textit{for all } x\in X,\ y\in Y,\\ \textit{and}\ \ (x,z)\in X\times Z.\end{array}$$

Regarding our example above, the max-min composition of the similarity relations between the families X and Y, on the one hand; and Y and Z, on the other, yields the similarity relation $A\circ B$ between the two remote families X and Z shown by its fuzzy matrix in Table 58:

Table 58. The max-min composition $A\circ B$ of the binary fuzzy relations A and B

$$A\circ B=\begin{bmatrix} & y_1 & y_2 & y_3\\ x_1 & 1 & 0.8 & 0.2\\ x_2 & 0.1 & 0 & 0.3\end{bmatrix}\circ\begin{bmatrix} & z_1 & z_2\\ y_1 & 0.7 & 0.6\\ y_2 & 0 & 0.1\\ y_3 & 0.5 & 0.4\end{bmatrix}=\begin{bmatrix} & z_1 & z_2\\ x_1 & 0.7 & 0.6\\ x_2 & 0.3 & 0.3\end{bmatrix}$$

The composed fuzzy relation $A\circ B$ may be represented in fuzzy set notation as follows:

$$A\circ B=\big\{\big((x_1,z_1),0.7\big),\big((x_1,z_2),0.6\big),\big((x_2,z_1),0.3\big),\big((x_2,z_2),0.3\big)\big\}.$$

We have thus been able to construct a completely new fuzzy relation on $X\times Z$ that represents the similarity between members of family X and family Z. For instance, person x_1, Amy, resembles person z_2, Cecil, to the extent 0.6.

30.4 Fuzzy Logic Proper

Fuzzy logic is a novel, non-classical logic. It emerged in the early development of fuzzy set theory. Zadeh introduced it in 1974 after supplementing his fuzzy set theory in 1973 with the *theory of linguistic variables,* which made this revolutionary logic possible (Zadeh, 1973, 1974a, 1975a, 1975b).[201]

The aim of fuzzy logic is to enable reasoning and decision-making in fuzzy environments including natural languages that are known to be inexact. It came into being as a method of approximate reasoning, a term which means drawing fuzzy conclusions from fuzzy premises. For example, at the beginning of this chapter it was pointed out that traditional logics cannot draw any conclusion from premises of the following type:

1. Many diabetics are at risk of suffering coronary heart disease,
2. The patient Elroy Fox is a diabetic.

Here is another example: A village in Mexico has about 1000 inhabitants. Most are infected with Mexican Swine Flu (MSF). What is the number of non-infected inhabitants? And yet another: Usually, most patients recover from MSF if they take Tamiflu. What is the probability that the patient Elroy Fox who is infected with MSF will recover if he takes Tamiflu?

The 'secret' of the examples above lies in the fuzzy terms such as "many", "most", and "usually" that characterize natural languages. Fuzzy logic provides intelligent methods for precisely dealing with them. It enables us to draw conclusions from the imprecise natural language sentences that all other logics are unable to deal with because these sentences do not fulfill their syntactic and semantic requirements. Unlike other systems of logic, fuzzy logic has no agreed-upon syntax and semantics yet, and therefore, it lacks an explicit and closed calculus of axioms and rules. In its current state, it is an open, both semiformal and formal system consisting of many conceptual tools, principles, methods, and frameworks, any of which may be applied pragmatically like different mathematical tools used for solving a particular problem. Although fuzzy logic has developed independently of many-valued logics, it may be viewed as an extension of infinite-valued logic by incorporating fuzzy sets

---

[201] The term "fuzzy logic" has received three different meanings since its inception. In its original, narrow sense, that we called FLn, it refers to a semiformal theory of approximate reasoning introduced by Zadeh (1974a, 1975a). In a wider sense, that we termed FLw, it denotes FLn, fuzzy set theory, the theory of linguistic variables, the theory of fuzzy if-then rules, possibility theory, and the theory of computing with words. But there is a very recent addition to this family, i.e., a third use of the term in its narrowest sense signifying a mathematical, multiple-valued logic that refers to infinite-valued, formal logics with truth values in the real, unit interval (see, e.g., Cignoli et al., 2000; Gottwald, 2005; Hajek, 2000, 2002; Novak et al., 2000; Turunen, 1999). The father of the whole movement, Lotfi Zadeh, does not consider this latter approach to be a fuzzy logic (personal communication, 2005).

and linguistic variables into the system of standard Łukasiewicz logic $L_{\aleph_1}$ discussed in Section 28.5 on page 964. See Figure 105.

Fig. 105. The relationship between classical logic and fuzzy logic. A double arrow symbolizes correspondence, a simple arrow symbolizes extension. There is a conceptual correspondence between classical logic and classical set theory, on the one hand; and infinite-valued logic and fuzzy set theory, on the other. The latter two systems in conjunction with Zadeh's theory of linguistic variables provide the conceptual basis of fuzzy logic

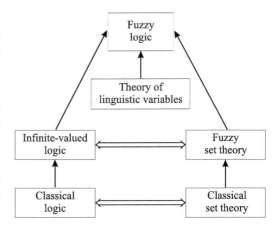

Because of the immense complexity of the subject, it is impossible to go into details. In the present section, only a few elementary ideas of fuzzy logic will be introduced. To this end, we must first familiarize ourselves with some basic notions. Our study divides into the following four parts:

30.4.1   Linguistic and Numerical Variables
30.4.2   Fuzzy Quantifiers
30.4.3   Fuzzy Sentences
30.4.4   Fuzzy Reasoning.

30.4.1 Linguistic and Numerical Variables

"All that can be measured, all that can be known". This is a widespread dogma in natural sciences and medicine, and has been so ever since Francis Bacon (1561–1626) and Galileo Galilei (1564–1642) philosophized on knowledge. In the scientific areas just mentioned, it is usually believed that qualitative terms and so-called soft labels such as "red", "fast", and "warm" are not useful elements of a scientific language on the grounds that they are imprecise. We are therefore recommended to replace them with quantitative terms like "wave length", "speed per hour" and "temperature", respectively. In contrast to this precisionism, however, we learn from Zadeh's theory of linguistic variables that this age-old view is inadequate because soft concepts are not only powerful tools, but also indispensable in science, technology, and everyday life. One of Zadeh's main motives for constructing his fuzzy logic has been to do justice to the significance and indispensability of qualitative terms and to exploit their unique strength in human cognition, reasoning, and decision-making. To this end, he has introduced the ingenious concept of a *linguistic variable*. As a prerequisite for understanding fuzzy logic, we shall therefore briefly sketch this concept in the following five sections:

► Linguistic variables
► Linguistic modifiers
► Graphs of linguistic variables
► Fuzzy truth values
► Fuzzy probabilities.

The outline will be instrumental throughout and will be employed especially in our philosophy of disease, diagnosis, medical knowledge, and fuzzy control in medicine. Details of the theory may be found in Zadeh's original contributions (Zadeh, 1973, 1975a–b, 1976a–b, 1979, 2009).

Linguistic variables

For the notion of a variable, see footnote 10 on page 58. In fuzzy logic, we distinguish between *numerical variables* and *linguistic variables*. They are briefly discussed in turn below.

(i) A numerical, or quantitative, variable (from the Latin word "numerus" for *number*) is exactly what a quantitative concept denotes (see p. 70). Examples are *heigth, length, weigth, speed,* or *temperature*. This type of concept is thoroughly studied on pages 70–76. A numerical variable is represented by a quantitative *function f*, such as "the temperature of", and usually assumes single numbers as values. It thus belongs to the class of point-valued functions discussed in Section 25.4.4 on page 843. A simple example is the statement "the temperature of this room is 23 °C" that may be rewritten as:

$$temperature(\text{this\_room}) = 23 \text{ °C} \tag{253}$$

with the syntax:

$$f(x) = y.$$

Here, "*f*" stands for the quantitative function "temperature". In this statement, the numerical variable *temperature* has taken the value '23 °C'. But it may take another value an hour from now, for it is a *variable*.

(ii) In contrast to point-valued numerical variables above, a *linguistic variable* resembles set-valued functions, discussed in Section 25.4.4 on page 843. It is a set-valued, or granular, variable that assumes granules as its values whose names are linguistic entities instead of numerals, such as atomic or composite words. It is therefore commonly, and mistakenly, said that a linguistic variable assumes words as its values. It doesn't do so. For example, *color* in the statement "the color of this page is white", rewritten as:

$$color(\text{this\_page}) = \text{white} \tag{254}$$

is a linguistic variable that takes granular values such as *white, yellow, red, green,* etc. In the present example (254), it has taken the granule *white* as its value. But this specific color, *white,* is not a word. It is an attribute of objects in the world out there. Be that as it may, the possible values of a linguistic variable are commonly called its *linguistic values* or *linguistic terms*. Let v be a linguistic variable. The user-defined set of all of its linguistic terms is referred to as its *term set* and written $T(v)$. In the present example, we have $T(color) = \{white, yellow, red, green, blue, orange, brown, \ldots\}$.

The concept of a linguistic variable plays a central role in the theory and practice of fuzzy logic. In other parts of this book, I-VII, it is shown to be a powerful tool for use in both medicine and philosophy. The term set of a linguistic variable may be viewed as a microlanguage by means of which the variable is able to approximately characterize a complex, vague, and ill-defined system or phenomenon, e.g., an organism, organ, disease, physiological, or pathological process, etc. For example, the high blood pressure may be characterized using the term set {mild, moderate, severe, very severe} of the linguistic variable *high blood pressure*. To prevent misunderstandings, however, note that both terms, "linguistic variable" and "linguistic value", are misnomers for the following reason. As mentioned above, an entity such as *white* or *yellow* that a linguistic variable may assume as its value, is in fact nothing linguistic. Viewed from the intensional perspective, it is an attribute, i.e., a property, feature, or quality of an object in the world out there. Viewed from the extensional perspective, it is a granule and indicates the belonging of that object to a particular clump or class of colored objects. For instance, the statement "the color of this page is white" means that this page belongs to the vague class of white objects. Thus, the variable *color* assigns to this page the quality *white* as its value. On this account, a better choice would be:

- to refer to a linguistic variable intensionally as a qualitative, classificatory, or taxonomic variable; and extensionally as a granular variable;
- to refer to a linguistic value intensionally as a qualitative, classificatory, or taxonomic value; and extensionally as a granule.

However, these initial labels that belong to the congenital vocabulary of fuzzy logic are well-established in the literature and impossible to change. Highly important for our purposes is the interesting relationship between linguistic and numerical variables that will play a central role in fuzzy logic and its application to our problems in this book. For our explanation of this relationship, we will use the variable *age,* as it is a simple, well-structured, and instructive variable. Typically, it demonstrates that unfortunately, in natural languages the syntactic make-up of a variable does not betray whether it is a numerical or a linguistic one. For instance, when asked about the *age* of a particular individual, we may respond in two different ways. We may either reply that she is, for example, young (linguistic) or that she is 17 years old (numerical). That means that the age of people may be described by two types of statements. First, by qualitative statements such as:

Amy is young, (255)

Teresa is quite old,

and second, by quantitative statements such as:

Amy is 17 years old, (256)

Teresa is 87 years old.

Relationships of this type may be differentiated and more adequately conceptualized by introducing two syntactically distinct variables, a linguistic variable *Age* and a numerical variable *age* in the present example. We shall always write linguistic variables with upper-case initial letters, and numerical variables with lower-case ones. While the linguistic variable *Age* assigns to an individual a linguistic term like in (255):

Age of Amy is *young*   i.e., Age(Amy) = young
Age of Teresa is *quite old*   Age(Teresa) = quite old,

the numerical variable *age* assigns a numerical age like in (256):

age of Amy is 17 years   i.e., age(Amy) = 17
age of Teresa is 87 years   age(Teresa) = 87.

The range of a linguistic variable such as *Age* is a term set, i.e., a set of linguistic terms denoting granules such as:

$T(Age) = \{$very young, young, not young, old, fairly old, quite old, ...$\}$,

whereas the range of a numerical variable such as *age* is a set of numbers, e.g., $\{0, 1, 2, \ldots, 100, \ldots\}$. The relationship between these two types of variables can be illustrated in the following way (Figure 106).

The numerical variable *age* with its possible values $0, 1, 2, 3, \ldots$ constitutes what may be called the *base variable* for the linguistic variable *Age*. The latter one operates on the base variable as its domain or universe of discourse, and assigns to its points fuzzy sets labeled "very young", "young", "old", "quite old", etc. Thus, the linguistic variable *Age* is a fuzzy set-valued variable that for any individual x with the numerical value $age(x)$ returns a fuzzy set such as *very young, young,* or *old* as its linguistic value. For example:

Age(Amy) = Age(age(Amy)) = Age(17) = young.

Since *young* is a fuzzy set without sharp boundaries, the statement that an individual x is young imposes a *fuzzy restriction* on the possible values that the base variable *age* may assume for this individual x. For example, age(x) cannot be 87, 65, or 50. It may be 28 rather than 45. The fuzzy restriction is

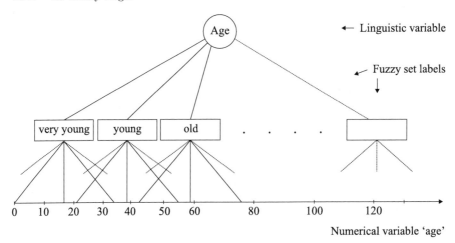

Fig. 106. The hierarchical structure of the linguistic variable 'Age' and its terms *young, not young, old,* etc. Each of the latter ones is a label for a granule, i.e., an entire fuzzy set of numerical ages. See body text

characterized by a *compatibility function* that associates with each value of the base variable, e.g., 17 years, a number in the unit interval $[0,1]$ as the degree of its compatibility with the concept of *young*. For instance, the compatibility of the numerical ages 17, 30, and 50 with *young* might be 1, 0.7, and 0, respectively. The compatibility function may be regarded as the membership function μ_{young} of a fuzzy set called "young" in the present example:

$$\{\ldots, (17 \text{ years}, 1), (30 \text{ years}, 0.7), (50 \text{ years}, 0), \ldots\}.$$

This fuzzy set is what we take to be the meaning of the linguistic term "young". In general, any term τ_i of the term set $T(Age)$ is *the name of a fuzzy set* over the set of numerical ages. A name τ_i such as "young" or "old" subsumes an entire set of different numerical ages under a single fuzzy set label. It is therefore quite reasonable to ask of any particular numerical age such as 17 or 87 to what extent it is a member of that fuzzy set τ_i, e.g., of the fuzzy set *young*. How *young* is a person aged 17 years? How old is she? See Figure 107.

Note that the *compatibility* referred to above must not be confused with probability. That the compatibility of an age of 35 years with the concept of *young* is 0.4, does not mean that the probability of someone's being young is 0.4 provided that she is 35 years old. It indicates only one's judgment on the extent to which the age value 35 fits her conception of the label "young". Thus, degree of probability and fuzzy set membership degree are by no means identical.

The term set of the variable age, $T(Age)$, was only partially displayed above. Actually, it is a large set of linguistic terms like the following one:

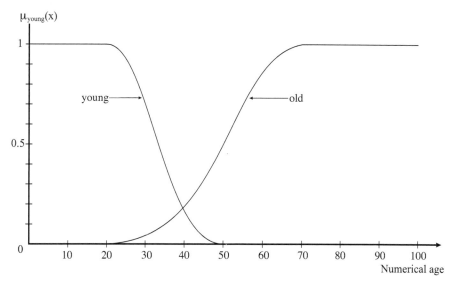

Fig. 107. The meaning of *young* and *old* as fuzzy sets tentatively represented as graphs over the base set of the numerical ages. The x-coordinate axis represents the set of numerical ages $\Omega = \{0, 1, 2, \ldots, 100, \ldots\}$ as our universe of discourse. The y-coordinate axis displays the degrees of membership, $\mu_{\tau_i}(x)$, of numerical ages in any of the fuzzy sets *young* and *old*. The graphs visualize these two fuzzy sets by depicting their membership functions. For instance, a newborn is *young* to the extent 1 and old to the extent 0. The same holds true for numerical ages 10 and 20. But a 35-year-old individual is *young* only to the extent 0.4 and *old* to the extent 0.1. Thus, the membership functions μ_{young} and μ_{old}, represented by μ_{τ_i}, map the set of numerical ages $\{0, 1, 2, \ldots\} = \Omega$ to the closed interval $[0, 1]$ generating two fuzzy subsets of the base set Ω that we call *young* and *old*, respectively. The assertion that a 35-year-old individual is *young* to the extent 0.4, then, means $\mu_{young}(35) = 0.4$. And analogously, $\mu_{old}(35) = 0.1$ says that she is old to the extent 0.1

$$T(Age) = \{young, \text{ very young, not young, very very young,}$$
$$\text{fairly young, quite young, middle-aged, old, fairly old,}$$
$$\text{quite old, very old, not young and not old, very very old,}$$
$$\text{more or less old, extremely old, } \ldots\}.$$

The concept of linguistic variable informally introduced above, may now be defined in the following way.

Definition 253 (Linguistic variable). *ξ is a linguistic variable* iff *there are v, $T(v)$, Ω, and M such that:*

1. *$\xi = \langle v, T(v), \Omega, M \rangle$,*
2. *v is the name of the variable, e.g., "Age";*
3. *$T(v)$ is its term set, e.g., $\{young, \text{ very young, old, quite old, } \ldots\}$;*
4. *Ω is a universe of discourse on which the elements of the term set $T(v)$ are fuzzy sets, e.g., $\Omega = \{0, 1, 2, \ldots, 100, \ldots\}$ that we have used as*

numerical ages to interpret $T(v)$. The universe Ω is usually provided by a numerical variable, e.g., the base variable age *in Figure 107 above;*

5. *M is a method that associates with each linguistic value $\tau_i \in T(v)$ its meaning, i.e., a fuzzy set of the universe Ω denoted by τ_i. See Figure 107 above; Figures 110–111 on pages 1029 and 1029; and Figures 31–32 on page 190.*[202]

The term set $T(Age)$ listed above is obviously based upon only a few primitives such as "young" and "old" which we may call the *primary terms* of the variable. Its remaining elements are composite terms such as "very young", "not young", "not young and not old", "quite old", and others. They are composed of primary terms to which semantic operators such as *very, not,* and *quite* have been applied to modify their meaning. A subset of $T(Age)$, e.g., the minimum term set {young, old}, may therefore be used as a set of primary terms from which the remainder of $T(Age)$ may be obtained by definition. In this process of constructing a term set such as $T(Age)$ from a few primary terms, semantic operators of the following type are employed:

- Logical operators: Fuzzy connectives "not", "or", and "and";
- linguistic modifiers: "very", "fairly", "quite", etc. (Zadeh, 1972a; Lakoff, 1973).

Logical operators have already been dealt with previously. We will now discuss Zadeh's discovery of linguistic modifiers with a view to making use of them in other chapters of the book.

Linguistic modifiers

A linguistic term may be an atomic one such as "young", or a compound one such as "very young" and "more or less young". Compound linguistic terms emerge from attaching semantic operators to other linguistic terms. Semantic operators of particular significance are linguistic modifiers, also called *linguistic hedges*. Examples are phrases such as "very", "quite", and "extremely". Like fuzzy connectives "not", "or", and "and", they act as nonlinear operators and modify the meaning of a term when attached to it. For instance, in the statement "Elroy Fox is very ill", the linguistic modifier "very" strengthens the meaning of the term "ill". Other examples are modifiers such as *more or less, highly, fairly, weakly, typically, essentially, slightly,* etc. A linguistic term denotes a fuzzy set as a fuzzy restriction on the values of a universe of discourse Ω, be it an atomic or a compound one (see Figure 106 on page 1022).

A linguistic modifier can only be attached to a fuzzy term to modify its meaning, be it a fuzzy predicate, a fuzzy truth value, or a fuzzy probability,

---

[202] Our definition of the term "linguistic variable" is a simplified version of its original conception by Zadeh (1975c, 199 f.).

e.g., *"very* young", *"quite* true", and *"highly* probable". It cannot be attached to crisp terms. Otherwise put, a reliable criterion for differentiating a crisp term from a fuzzy term is whether linguistic modifiers can sensibly be attached to the term. For instance, phrases such as "very brother", "more or less pregnant", and "fairly $p(X) = 0.8$" are meaningless.

It is obvious that linguistic modifiers cannot be dealt with in classical and other bivalent logics, and are therefore not considered in their syntax and semantics. That is, they do not exist in those logics. This is additional evidence that classical and other bivalent logics are too weak to sufficiently cover natural languages and fully emulate human reasoning capabilities.

When a linguistic modifier such as "very" is attached to a fuzzy phrase "A" to form the expression "very A", e.g., *very young,* it functions as a unary operator with fuzzy set A as its argument that it transforms, by modifying A's membership function, into the new fuzzy set *very A* as its value. It is thus an operator, OP, on the unit interval $[0, 1]$:

$$OP: [0, 1] \mapsto [0, 1]$$

such that membership degrees of the first set, A, are transformed to new membership degrees to form a new fuzzy set, $Op(A)$. For example, the modifier "very" strengthens or *concentrates,* whereas the modifier "fairly" weakens or *dilates* the set. To illustrate, let A be a fuzzy set over a base set Ω. Then we have:

$$\text{concentration of } A \quad \text{is:} \quad A^2 = \left(\mu_A(x)\right)^2 \quad \text{for all } x \in \Omega \quad (257)$$

$$\text{dilation of } A \quad \text{is:} \quad \sqrt{\mu_A(x)} \quad \text{for all } x \in \Omega.$$

That means that if A is a fuzzy set with the membership function μ_A, then:

a. very A is a fuzzy set with: $\mu_{very(A)}(x) = \left(\mu_A(x)\right)^2$

b. fairly A is a fuzzy set with: $\mu_{fairly(A)}(x) = \sqrt{\mu_A(x)}.$

(a) is a concentration and (b) is a dilation. For instance, consider our example family Fox already mentioned in Table 54 on page 1001, i.e., the universe of discourse $\Omega = \{$Amy, Beth, Carla, Dirk, Elroy$\}$ that we want to symbolize by $\{$a, b, c, d, e$\}$. The fuzzy set *young* over this universe listed in the table is:

$$Young = \{(a, 1), (b, 0.9), (c, 0.5), (d, 0.1), (e, 0)\}.$$

The concentration ('very') and dilation ('fairly') of this fuzzy set yield:

$$Very\ young = \{(a, 1), (b, 0.81), (c, 0.25), (d, 0.01), (e, 0)\}$$
$$Fairly\ young = \{(a, 1), (b, 0.95), (c, 0.7), (d, 0.3), (e, 0)\}.$$

The individual c, for example, who is *young* to the extent 0.5, turns out *very young* to the extent $0.5^2 = 0.25$ and fairly young to the extent $\sqrt{0.5} = 0.7$. These standard approximations are illustrated in Figure 108.

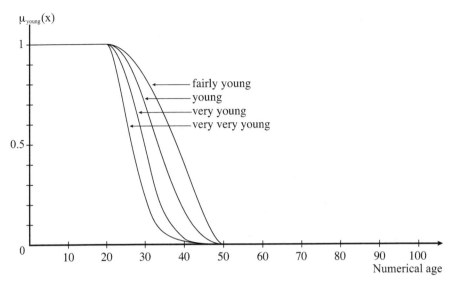

Fig. 108. The illustration of standard concentration and dilation

Accordingly, by employing linguistic modifiers we obtain from the primary term set {young, old} a wide range of derived terms for $T(Age)$ like the following ones:

$$very\ young = very(young) = young^2$$
$$fairly\ young = fairly(young) = \sqrt{young}$$
$$very\ old = very(old) = old^2$$
$$not\ very\ old = not\big(very(old)\big) = \overline{(old^2)} = 1 - old^2$$
$$very\ very\ old = very\big(very(old)\big) = (old^2)^2 = old^4$$
$$not\ young\ and\ not\ old = not(young)\ and\ not(old)$$
$$= (1 - young) \cap (1 - old)$$

by:

$$\mu_{very\_young}(x) = \big(\mu_{young}(x)\big)^2$$
$$\mu_{fairly\_young}(x) = \sqrt{\big(\mu_{young}(x)\big)}$$
$$\mu_{very\_old}(x) = \big(\mu_{old}(x)\big)^2$$
$$\mu_{not\_very\_old}(x) = 1 - \big(\mu_{old}(x)\big)^2$$
$$\mu_{very(very(old))}(x) = \big(\mu_{old}(x)\big)^4$$
$$\mu_{not(young) \cap not(old)}(x) = \big(1 - \mu_{young}(x)\big) \cap \big(1 - \mu_{old}(x)\big)$$
$$= min\big(1 - \mu_{young}(x),\ 1 - \mu_{old}(x)\big).$$

The last term, "not young and not old", may be illustrated by a simple example. To this end, we supplement the above fuzzy set "young" by the dimension "old" in the same family $\Omega = \{a, b, c, d, e\}$:

$Young = \{(a, 1), (b, 0.9), (c, 0.5), (d, 0.1), (e, 0)\},$

$Not\ young = \{(a, 0), (b, 0.1), (c, 0.5), (d, 0.9), (e, 1)\},$

$Old = \{(a, 0), (b, 0), (c, 0.1), (d, 0.25), (e, 1)\},$

$Not\ old = \{(a, 1), (b, 1), (c, 0.9), (d, 0.75), (e, 0)\},$

$Not\ young\ and\ not\ old = \{(a, 0), (b, 0.1), (c, 0.5), (d, 0.75), (e, 0)\}.$

The 42-year-old individual d, i.e., Dirk Fox, is *not young and not old* to the extent 0.75. Additional examples and details are studied in other chapters of the book when the theory of linguistic variables is applied to our philosophy, methodology and logic of medicine. Figures 108–109 and Table 59 illustrate the above considerations.

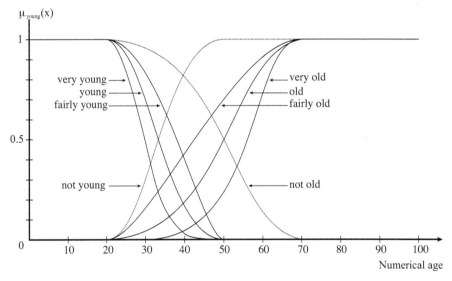

Fig. 109. This figure visualizes the impact of different semantic operators on fuzzy sets. Particular attention is to be paid to the fuzzy set "not young and not old". Its membership function is represented by the dotted sides of the quasi-triangle that constitutes the intersection $\overline{young} \cap \overline{old}$. The 42-year-old Dirk Fox is a member of this fuzzy set to the extent 0.75. Again, note that *young* and *old* are not mutual complements. Rather, they are independent of one another. The complement of *young* is *not young*; and that of *old* is *not old*

Table 59. Membership degrees in the fuzzy sets *young* and *old* of ages 10 through 100, and their concentrations and dilations. Note that *old* is not the complement of *young*

	Years of age									
	10	20	30	40	50	60	70	80	90	100
$\mu_{young}(x)$	1	1	0.7	0.17	0	0	0	0	0	0
$\mu_{fairly\_young}(x)$	1	1	0.83	0.41	0	0	0	0	0	0
$\mu_{very\_young}(x)$	1	1	0.49	0.02	0	0	0	0	0	0
$\mu_{old}(x)$	0	0	0.03	0.19	0.5	0.85	1	1	1	1
$\mu_{fairly\_old}(x)$	0	0	0.17	0.43	0.7	0.92	1	1	1	1
$\mu_{very\_old}(x)$	0	0	0.0009	0.03	0.25	0.72	1	1	1	1

Graphs of linguistic variables

As depicted in Figure 99 (p. 999), the characteristic function of an ordinary set is a step function. By contrast, membership functions of fuzzy sets are continuous and may have different shapes. They may be triangular, trapezoidal, bell-shaped, sinusoidal, etc. Since the linguistic values of linguistic variables are fuzzy sets, linguistic variables may be graphically represented by depicting their linguistic values. The graphical representation of linguistic variables is of great heuristic, methodological, philosophical, and practical significance. This can be illustrated with a few simple examples.

Let there be a linguistic variable over a particular universe of discourse, e.g., the linguistic variable *Body_Temperature*. For simplicity's sake, let us assume that this variable has the following small term set: T(Body_Temperature) = {very low, low, normal, slightly high, fairly high, extremely high}. It may operate on the Celsius scale 0, 1, 2, 3, ..., i.e., on the range of the numerical variable *body_temperature*. This range usually extends from 34 °C to 42 °C. What the linguistic variable Body_Temperature accomplishes, is a fuzzy partitioning of the universe of discourse {34, 35, ..., 42} into six fuzzy sets whose membership functions may be visualized by triangular and trapezoidal graphs as shown in Figure 110.

Linguistic values of other variables may have other shapes. In most applications of *fuzzy control* in medicine, discussed in Section 16.5.1, the membership functions of linguistic values are conceived as triangular, trapezoidal, sinusoidal, bell-shaped, S-shaped, or Z-shaped (see Figures 111–112, 107, and 113–114).

In practice, the number of linguistic values of a linguistic variable is usually in the range of three to seven. Linguistic values are used to simplify both the handling of the numerical base variables and communication about them. For example, in cardiology the information that the patient has a *rapid heart rate*, i.e., tachycardia, is more useful than a numerical value such as 140. For the soft label "tachycardia" represents a choice out of three possible values (bradycardia, normal, tachycardia), whereas "140" is a choice out of, say, 350 values. This simple example demonstrates that linguistic values accomplish data compression. This type of data compression is referred to as granulation of information (Zadeh, 1994, 193; 2009).

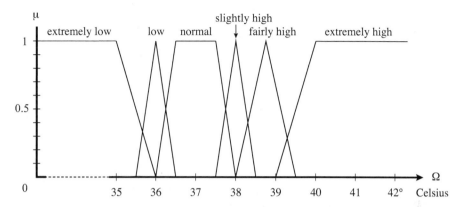

Fig. 110. The linguistic variable Body_Temperature has 3 triangular and 3 trapezoidal linguistic values. It acts on the numerical variable *body_temperature* as our universe of discourse $\Omega = \{34, 35, \ldots, 42\}$ °C. A body temperature of 37 °C, for example, is *normal* to the extent 1. A body temperature of 39,1 °C is *fairly high* to the extent 0.4 and *extremely high* to the extent 0.1. Note that a *slightly high, fairly high,* and *extremely high* body temperature is what is usually referred to as *fever,* i.e., *slight fever, high fever,* and *extremely high fever,* respectively, whereas the linguistic values *low* and *extremely low* represent hypothermia

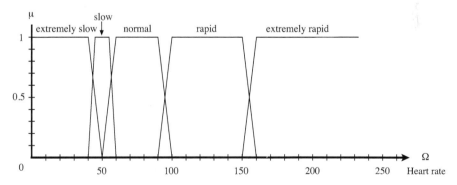

Fig. 111. The linguistic variable Heart_Rate in adults. It has trapezoidal linguistic values and acts on the numerical variable *heart_rate*. In clinical terminology, *extremely slow* and *slow* constitute *bradycardia*, whereas *rapid* and *extremely rapid* are subsumed under *tachycardia*. See also Figures 107 and 113–114

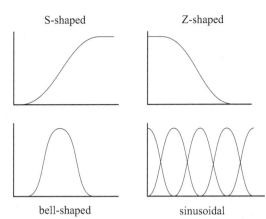

Fig. 112. S-shaped, Z-shaped, bell-shaped, and sinusoidal linguistic values

Granulation of information by linguistic values manages a peculiar property of classes mentioned on page 997, i.e., their being granuled. Informally, a *granule* in a universe of discourse Ω is a clump of elements of Ω which are drawn together by similarity, indistinguishability, and other properties that render the class *granular*. For example, *young* and *old* people form granules in the class of human beings; people with *moderate hypertension* form a granule in the class of those who suffer from hypertension; etc. A linguistic variable such as *Age* or *Hypertension* is a granular variable (Zadeh, 2009).

Fuzzy truth values

What philosophers have not noticed during the last 50 years, is the revolution in the concepts of truth and logic that has occurred in Western philosophy some 2,300 years after Aristotle's *Metaphysics* and *Organon*: Zadeh's conception of truth as a linguistic variable. By this construction, Zadeh has fuzzified the concept of truth and has thereby invented a novel type of logic, *fuzzy logic*, that is well-suited to dislodge the Aristotelean tradition of reasoning and worldview (Sadegh-Zadeh, 2001a; Forthcoming).[203] As he has observed, in contrast to the scholarly and sterile world of philosophy, in everyday discourse our characterization of the truth state of a proposition is not confined to the bivalent expressions "true" and "false". Rather, we use a variety of terms such as *true, fairly true, very true, quite true, not true, false, fairly false, very false, completely false,* etc. We say, for example:

- The statement "Elroy Fox has angina pectoris" is quite true,
- the statement "AIDS is incurable" is completely false.

---

[203] The revolution is strengthened by an additional, mathematical invention, which is in fact the most important invention to have occurred in mathematics since the invention of Arabic numerals, i.e., Zadeh's invention of fuzzy numbers. See page 1035.

By attaching to the naked terms "true" and "false" linguistic modifiers such as "quite" and "completely", we enhance our expressive power enormously. To do justice to, and exploit, this unrivaled facility of everyday language in comparison to the poor, two-valued language of philosophy and other sciences, Zadeh treated *truth* as a linguistic variable that he called a *linguistic truth variable*. Its possible values he called *linguistic truth values* or *fuzzy truth values* (Zadeh, 1973, 1975c–d, 1976a–b).

Let the linguistic truth variable be denoted by "Truth". Its term set, i.e., $T(Truth)$, contains in addition to the traditional two truth values, *true* and *false,* a myriad of other ones and may be conceived of as something like the following set of fuzzy, linguistic truth values:

$$T(Truth) \;=\; \{\text{true, not true, fairly true, very true, very very true,}$$
$$\text{completely true, essentially true, not very true,}$$
$$\text{not completely true, essentially not true, false, very false,}$$
$$\text{very very false, completely false, } \ldots \}.$$

We have seen in Section 28.5 on page 964 that the truth values of statements in an n-valued logic are represented by rational or real numbers in the unit interval $[0, 1]$. This concept of truth is a *numerical truth variable* and may be denoted by "truth" in order to differentiate it from the linguistic truth variable "Truth" above. Its values are points in the interval $[0, 1]$, e.g., 0.7, and will be referred to as *numerical truth values*.

We have thus the linguistic truth variable *Truth* with its linguistic truth values, on the one hand; and the numerical truth variable *truth* with its numerical truth values, on the other. The numerical truth variable *truth* plays the role of a base variable for the linguistic truth variable *Truth* providing the unit interval $[0, 1]$ as a universe of discourse, Ω. In this way, a linguistic truth value such as *true, very true, false, not very true,* and the like may be interpreted as a fuzzy subset of the interval $[0, 1]$. It is characterized by an S-shaped, Z-shaped, and bell-shaped membership function and may therefore be referred to as a *fuzzy truth value*. See Figure 113.

The linguistic truth value *true* may serve as the primary term of $T(\text{Truth})$ to introduce all other terms by definition. Its negation is the term "not true" that is defined as its fuzzy complement:

$$\mu_{not\_true}(x) = 1 - \mu_{true}(x).$$

For instance, $\mu_{not\_true}(0.8) = 1 - \mu_{true}(0.8) = 1 - 0.5 = 0.5$. In contrast to everyday language and traditional logics, however, the term "false" is defined not as the negation of *true,* but as its dual, i.e., its mirror image with respect to the point 0.5 of the base variable $[0, 1]$ thus:

$$\mu_{false}(x) = \mu_{true}(1 - x).$$

For example, $\mu_{false}(0.8) = \mu_{true}(1 - 0.8) = \mu_{true}(0.2) = 0$. Thus we have:

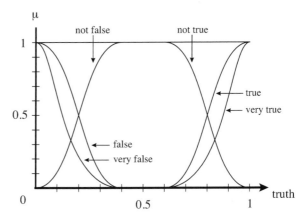

Fig. 113. Compatibility functions of some fuzzy truth values. Fuzzy truth values must not be confused with fuzzy probabilities such as "likely", "very likely", "unlikely", etc. See next section

$$\mu_{not\_true}(0.8) = 0.5$$
$$\mu_{false}(0.8) = 0.$$

Or we can simply state that:

$$not\ true = \overline{true} \qquad (\text{"}\overline{true}\text{" means "the complement of true"}),$$
$$false = 1 - true.$$

That is, *false* ≠ *not true*. Other linguistic truth values may be obtained by applying linguistic modifiers to *true* and *false*. For example, *very true* is $true^2$. For details of this truth theory, see (Zadeh, 1975a, 1975d).

Fuzzy truth values in the term set T(Truth) enable us to assess the truth value of a statement in more than the traditional two fashions. For instance, consider the statement "Elroy Fox has angina pectoris". The assignment of a fuzzy truth value such as *very true* to the statement in question yields: "Elroy Fox has angina pectoris" is very true. Suppose now that we have three different statements of this type about the same patient from which we want to draw a conclusion. Each of them may bear a fuzzy truth value. The first statement may be *very true*, the second one may be *fairly true*, and the third one may be *more or less false*. When drawing a conclusion from them, what truth value does the conclusion bear? That is, what truth value does the truth value combination {very true, fairly true, more or less false} in the premises propagate to the conclusion? This question leads us directly to fuzzy reasoning that we shall discuss in Section 30.4.4 below.

Fuzzy probabilities

It was already emphasized that *randomness* of events is a feature of the objective world out there, whereas *uncertainty* pertains to the inner, subjective world of human agents and refers to their ability or inability to say whether a statement is true or not. The concept of probability enables us to handle both aspects, randomness and uncertainty, in three different ways:

1. *quantitatively:* the probability that Elroy Fox has diabetes, is 0.7;
2. *comparatively:* it is more probable than not that Elroy Fox has diabetes;
3. *qualitatively:* that Elroy Fox has diabetes, is quite probable.

The quantitative concept of probability represented by the function p with the syntax $p(X) = r$ constitutes the central notion of probability theory and was discussed in Chapter 29. In our present terminology, p represents a numerical variable and assigns to an event X a real number r from the unit interval $[0, 1]$ as its degree of probability, for example, "the probability that Elroy Fox has diabetes, is 0.7". In the history of science prior to Lotfi A. Zadeh, it was only this quantitative concept of probability that received attention. The result is the well-known and highly influential theory of probability and statistics that led to the "probabilization" of science and is used in all scientific disciplines. Consider, however, an instance when we do not have numerical information on an event at our disposal and can only qualitatively say that the event is more or less probable. For example, what is the probability that the Mexican Influenza that broke out in Mexico recently, will lead to a pandemic during the next three months? Without background information, we are unable to give precise numerical answers to such questions, e.g., 0.8 or the like. A vague response such as "it is fairly probable" appears to be more reasonable.

To handle the issue of *qualitative* probabilities, Lotfi Zadeh introduced a qualitative concept of probability as a linguistic variable. Based on this novel concept, he constructed a theory of qualitative, *fuzzy probability* as a counterpart of the traditional theory of quantitative probability. Roughly, his theory is capable of answering questions about the probability of an event based on vague information, such as that represented in Example 12 below by the italicized, fuzzy words "approximately", "several", and "ill":

Example 12.

A city is inhabited by *approximately* n people of whom *several* are *ill*. What is the probability that an individual selected at random is *ill?*

Problems of this type are not unique. In fact, they constitute the vast majority of the problems we face in medicine. It is for this reason that fuzzy probability is so important. However, for our purposes, a brief sketch will be given here of the linguistic variable only. For details of the elegant and powerful theory itself, see (Zadeh, 1976a, 1984a).

Let the expression "*The_Probability_Of*", written $\mathcal{P}(\ )$, be a linguistic variable such that $\mathcal{P}(x)$ reads "The_Probability_Of x". Its term set, $T(\mathcal{P})$, may be conceived of as something like the following:

$$T(\mathcal{P}) = \{\text{likely, fairly likely, more or less likely, very likely, not likely,}$$
$$\text{unlikely, very unlikely, more or less unlikely, neither very}$$
$$\text{likely nor very unlikely, probable, close to 1, close to 0, } \ldots \}.$$

The linguistic variable $\mathcal{P}$, 'The_Probability_Of', operates on the numerical probability function p as the base variable such that the unit interval $[0, 1]$ constitutes the universe of discourse, Ω. Each term $\tau_i \in T(\mathcal{P})$ is the label of an S-shaped, Z-shaped, or bell-shaped fuzzy set over the base variable p, and thus, represents a fuzzy probability. Some of these fuzzy probabilities are depicted in Figure 114.

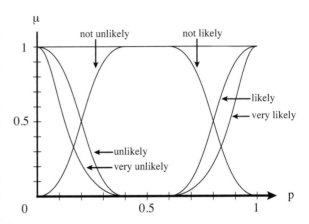

Fig. 114. Compatibility functions of some qualitative, linguistic, or *fuzzy probabilities*. (All these three terms are synonymous.) The linguistic variable is the qualitative notion of probability, $\mathcal{P}$, with its compatibility or membership function μ_{τ_i}. The probability measure p discussed in Chapter 29 is the base variable

The phrase "likely" may serve as the primary term. The term "probable" is taken as synonymous with "likely" and "close to 1", while "improbable" may be introduced as synonymous with "unlikely" and "close to 0". Many other terms may be introduced by definition. The linguistic term "not likely" is the negation of "likely" and defined as its fuzzy complement:

$$\mu_{not\_likely}(x) = 1 - \mu_{likely}(x).$$

For example, $\mu_{not\_likely}(0.7) = 1 - \mu_{likely}(0.7) = 1 - 0.1 = 0.9$. The term "unlikely" is defined not as the negation of "likely", but as its dual, i.e., its mirror image with respect to the point 0.5 of the base variable in $[0, 1]$. That is:

$$\mu_{unlikely}(x) = \mu_{likely}(1 - x).$$

For instance, $\mu_{unlikely}(0.7) = \mu_{likely}(1 - 0.7) = \mu_{likely}(0.3) = 0$. And we have:

$$\mu_{not\_likely}(0.7) = 0.9$$
$$\mu_{unlikely}(0.7) = 0.$$

Simplistically, we can state that:

$$not\ likely = \overline{likely} \qquad (\text{"}\overline{likely}\text{" means "the complement of likely"}),$$
$$unlikely = 1 - likely.$$

That is, *unlikely* ≠ *not likely*. Other fuzzy probability values may be obtained by applying linguistic modifiers to *likely, unlikely, not likely*, etc. For example, *very likely* is *likely*². For methods of computation with fuzzy probabilities and for other details of this qualitative probability theory, see (Zadeh, 1976a).

30.4.2 Fuzzy Quantifiers

The only quantifiers known and used in traditional logics are the existential quantifier "there is" (∃) and the universal quantifier "all" (∀). As Lotfi Zadeh discovered, however, there are a variety of additional, intermediate quantifiers between these two classical extremes such as, for instance, "a few", "several", "many", "about half", "a great deal of", "a large part of", "most", "almost all", and many more. They are called *fuzzy quantifiers* because the domains over which they range, are vague. For instance, in sentences of the form:

- *many* patients with high blood pressure suffer apoplexia,
- *about half* of these apoplexia patients recover completely,
- *a few* of them die,

it is not known how many patients constitute a set of *many* patients, or *about half of them*, or only *a few* of them. Traditional logics cannot deal with fuzzily quantified statements of this type because the alphabets of their languages do not contain such quantifiers. Fuzzy logic provides an interesting framework for the interpretation and treatment of fuzzy quantifiers as *fuzzy numbers*. Thus, with the aid of fuzzy arithmetic, it enables approximate reasoning with fuzzily quantified sentences. See (Zadeh, 1975a, 1983, 1984b, 1985).

Because of its complexity, the notion of a fuzzy number cannot be addressed here adequately. Roughly, a fuzzy number is a number *close* to a given real number such as 5. Fuzzy numbers, as the basic objects of fuzzy arithmetic, are triangular, trapezoidal, or bell-shaped fuzzy sets of real numbers. They are thus *approximate numbers or intervals* such as, for example, "close to 5", "about 12", "approximately 450", and the like. Analogously, a fuzzy interval is an interval around a given interval such as, for example, "approximately in the range of 5 to 10". See Figure 115. For details, see (Kaufmann and Gupta, 1991; Klir and Yuan, 1995).

There are two types of fuzzy quantifiers. Fuzzy quantifiers of the first type refer to absolute counts and are defined on the real line, ℝ. They are denoted by terms such as *a few, several, at least about 10, about 25, much more than 500*, and so on. Fuzzy quantifiers of the second type refer to relative counts and are defined on the unit interval [0, 1]. They are represented by terms such as *almost all, most, many, about half*, and so on. See Figure 116.

30.4.3 Fuzzy Sentences

As pointed out on page 1017, fuzzy logic in the wide sense of this term does not have an agreed-upon syntax and semantics yet. Nevertheless, four types of

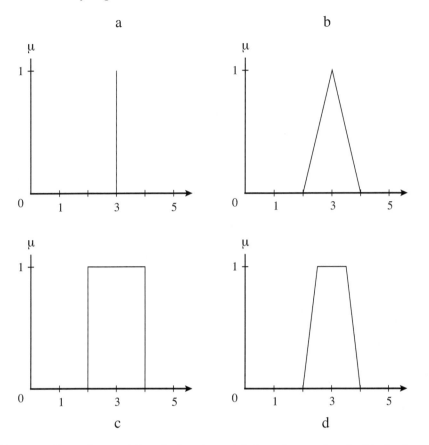

Fig. 115. Some fuzzy-arithmetical notions: (a) the crisp number *3*; (b) the fuzzy number *about 3;* (c) the crisp interval [2, 4]; (d) the fuzzy interval *roughly in the range of 2 to 4*

Fig. 116. Fuzzy quantifiers, as fuzzy numbers, are fuzzy sets of real numbers with triangular, trapezoidal, S-shaped or Z-shaped membership functions. As fuzzy sets, fuzzy quantifiers are computable operators. See (Zadeh, 1985)

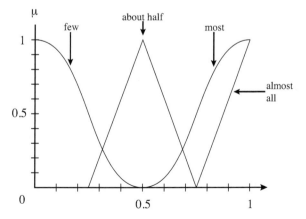

fuzzy sentences may be distinguished that are dealt with in fuzzy reasoning. They are informally outlined by simple examples in what follows.

A sentence is said to be fuzzy if it contains at least one fuzzy word. Elementary examples are sentences such as the following ones: Mr. Elroy Fox is very icteric; many icteric patients have severe hepatitis; tomorrow will be a warm day. For additional types of fuzzy sentences, see page 391. It need not be stressed that most natural language sentences are fuzzy sentences.

A fuzzy sentence such as "Elroy Fox is very icteric" cannot be said to be *true* or *false* because we do not know how to draw the dividing line between 'very icteric' and 'not very icteric' sets of patients in order to find out to which one of these categories the patient definitely belongs. Since an individual may be a member of a fuzzy set to a lesser degree than 1 or to a greater degree than 0, Mr. Elroy Fox may be a member of 'very icteric' patients to the extent 0.6. On this account, he will be also a member of 'not very icteric' patients to the extent $1-0.6 = 0.4$. Now, what should it mean to say that the sentence "Elroy Fox is very icteric" is true or that it is false? Fuzzy sentences assume more than only the two classical truth values true and false. The truth or falsity of a fuzzy sentence is a matter of degree. It may be expressed as a numerical truth value, i.e., a number in the unit interval $[0, 1]$, or as a linguistic truth value such as *true, fairly true, very true, false, fairly false, quite false,* and so on as was discussed previously.

A sentence may be (i) *categorical* such as "Elroy Fox has diabetes"; or (ii) it may be *qualified* by a truth value, probability value, usuality or otherwise, e.g., "Elroy Fox has diabetes is *fairly true*"; "Elroy Fox has hepatitis is *unlikely*"; "*usually,* diabetics have hyperglycemia". We call sentences of this type truth-qualified, probability-qualified, and usuality-qualified, respectively. A qualified sentence may be an unconditional or a conditional one. Thus we have four types of sentences:

- Unconditional and categorical sentences such as "Elroy Fox's blood sugar level is *extremely high*". In this sentence, a linguistic variable ('Blood_Sugar_Level') takes a value from its term set, i.e., *extremely high;*
- Unconditional and qualified sentences such as "Elroy Fox's blood sugar level is extremely high is *very true*";
- Conditional and categorical sentences such as "If Elroy Fox's blood sugar level is *extremely high,* then he will have *strong* glucosuria". This is a fuzzy conditional of the form $\alpha \to \beta$ with categorical fuzzy antecedent and consequent;
- Conditional and qualified sentences such as "If Elroy Fox's blood sugar level is extremely high, then *probably* he will have strong glucosuria".

Conditional fuzzy sentences play a central role in fuzzy knowledge-based systems and in fuzzy control. A conditional fuzzy sentence, or a *fuzzy conditional* for short, is a conditional $\alpha \to \beta$ with any fuzzy terms in its antecedent, consequent, or both. This subject is extensively utilized in Section 16.5. A particular and very important class of fuzzy sentences is composed of *fuzzily quantified* sentences such as "*many* icteric patients have severe hepatitis" which contain at least one fuzzy quantifier of the first or second type discussed in the previous section.

30.4.4 Fuzzy Reasoning

According to the traditional concept of inference first introduced in Definition 202 on page 851 and made precise in Definition 222 on page 889, the relation of inference between premises and conclusion is a truth preserving one. Such is the case, for instance, in the following argument (258) in which x and y are real numbers:

x is small	Premise 1	(258)
x and y are equal	Premise 2	
_____		
y is small	Conclusion.	

Fuzzy logic is not based on this traditional, truth preserving concept of inference. In fuzzy logic, the relationship between premises and conclusion, and thus, the rules of inference are approximate rather than truth preserving. A simple example of such fuzzy inference is the following argument:

x is small	Premise 1	(259)
x and y are approximately equal	Premise 2	
_____		
y is more or less small	Conclusion.	

While this latter example is a valid argument in fuzzy logic, it is invalid in all the other logics that we considered previously. The terms "small" and "approximately equal" in the premises denote values of two linguistic variables. The modified value "more or less small" in the conclusion is a linguistic approximation to them. There is no deductive relationship any more between the premises and the conclusion of this approximate argument. Many inferences in both everyday life and science are of this approximate type because the notions used in them, e.g., "small", "approximately equal", and "more or less small", denote fuzzy sets and are vague. Since rules of fuzzy inference are too complex, not all of them can be discussed here. As an example we will only present the basic rule that underlies the argument (259) above, i.e., *the compositional rule of inference*. In a simplified form, it may be stated as follows (Zadeh, 1974b, 33 f.).

Let the first premise of the argument (259) above be symbolized by "x is P" where "P" stands for the fuzzy predicate "small" or any other unary predicate. And let its second premise be symbolized by "(x, y) is Q" where

"Q" represents the binary fuzzy predicate "approximately equal" or any other binary predicate. "(x, y) is Q" says that the pair (x, y) stands in the relation "approximately equal". Thus, the argument may be formalized this way:

x is P	Premise 1
(x, y) is Q	Premise 2
————————	
y is $P \circ Q$	Conclusion

where $P \circ Q$ in the conclusion is the max-min composition of the unary relation P with the binary relation Q, i.e., *small* $\circ$ *approximately equal*. The concept of max-min composition of fuzzy relations was introduced in Definition 252 on page 1016. To illustrate how the composition $P \circ Q$ emerges and functions, suppose our base set Ω consists of the numbers $\{1, 2, 3, 4\}$ such that the fuzzy set P, i.e., *small*, over this base set is given by Table 60.

x	1	2	3	4
$\mu_{small}(x)$	1	0.6	0.2	0

Table 60. The fuzzy set of small numbers in the base set $\Omega = \{1, 2, 3, 4\}$

Thus, we have the following fuzzy set:

$$small = \{(1, 1), (2, 0.6), (3, 0.2), (4, 0)\}.$$

Analogously, the binary fuzzy relation Q, i.e., *approximately equal*, may be defined by:

$$
\begin{aligned}
approximately\ equal = \ & \{((1,1), 1), ((2,2), 1), ((3,3), 1), ((4,4), 1), \\
& ((1,2), 0.5), ((2,1), 0.5), ((2,3), 0.5), \\
& ((3,2), 0.5), ((3,4), 0.5), ((4,3), 0.5), \\
& ((1,3), 0), ((1,4), 0), ((2,4), 0), \ldots\}.
\end{aligned}
$$

We thus obtain the max-min composition $P \circ Q$ given in Table 61:

Table 61. The fuzzy matrix of max-min composition $P \circ Q$

$$
P \circ Q = \begin{bmatrix} 1 & 0.6 & 0.2 & 0 \end{bmatrix} \circ \begin{bmatrix} 1 & 0.5 & 0 & 0 \\ 0.5 & 1 & 0.5 & 0 \\ 0 & 0.5 & 1 & 0.5 \\ 0 & 0 & 0.5 & 1 \end{bmatrix} = \begin{bmatrix} 1 & 0.6 & 0.5 & 0.2 \end{bmatrix}
$$

It yields the fuzzy set:

$$small \circ approximately\ equal = \big\{(1,1),(2,0.6),(3,0.5),(4,0.2)\big\}$$

that may be linguistically approximated as *more or less small*. This approximation has been used in the verbal argument above. Without further explanation, an important special case of the compositional rule of inference will be mentioned below. Due to its similarity with the classical inference:

> x is P
> If x is P, then y is Q
>
> ---
>
> y is Q

which is based on Modus ponens, Lotfi Zadeh has called it the *generalized Modus ponens*. We shall retain this well-established name and will here only present the rule to stimulate the reader to further inquiries. Because of their intricacy the introduction of the concepts involved is omitted. First consider a simple illustration:

> Elroy Fox's body temperature is *very high*
> If Elroy Fox's body temperature is *high*, then he is *ill*
>
> ---
>
> Elroy Fox is *very ill*.

In any other logic, such an argument is impossible and does not exist. It becomes possible by employing the generalized Modus ponens:

> x is P
> If x is R, then y is Q
>
> ---
>
> y is Q'.

The modified value Q' in the conclusion represents the composition $P \circ (\overline{R}^* \oplus Q^*)$ in which $\overline{R}^*$ is the cylindric extension of the complement of R; the operator $\oplus$ denotes the bounded sum; and Q^* is the cylindric extension of Q. For details, see (Bellman and Zadeh, 1977, 147 ff.).[204]

If in a fuzzy argument of the structure above $P = R$, the rule of generalized Modus ponens reduces to the classical Modus ponens. There are also a number of other fuzzy inference rules that cannot be touched upon here. For brevity, we cannot concern ourselves with other useful facilities of this logic either. Additional aspects are discussed in the context of our inquiries in other chapters of this book.

---

[204] The *bounded sum* of two fuzzy sets A and B is $A \oplus B = \big\{(x, \mu_{A \oplus B}(x)) \mid \mu_{A \oplus B}(x) = min(1, \mu_A(x) + \mu_B(x))\big\}$. For instance, if $A = \{(a, 0.5), (b, 0.2)\}$ and $B = \{(a, 0.9), (b, 0.6)\}$, then $A \oplus B = \{(a, 1), (b, 0.8)\}$. For the notion of cylindric extension of a fuzzy relation, see (Klir and Yuan, 1995, 122 f.).

30.5 Summary

The mathematization of scientific research during the last few centuries has been advanced in most areas at the expense of the significance of the yield. As Zadeh observed, a variety of important issues in which the data, the objectives, and the constraints are too complex or too ill-defined to admit of mathematical analysis, have been and are still being neglected because of their mathematical intractability (Zadeh, 1972b, 3). To enhance the significance of inquiries into such complex and ill-defined systems, e.g., human beings in medicine or sociology and psychology, he provided by his fuzzy logic a basis for qualitative approaches and thereby marked the beginning of a novel direction and era of research. In the current chapter, some elementary notions of this logic were briefly outlined in order that they can be employed in other chapters of the book. Details may be found in standard works, e.g., (Dubois and Prade, 1998; Klir and Yuan, 1995, 1996; Ruspini et al., 1998; Yager et al., 1987).

We have emphasized on several occasions that fuzzy set theory is a non-classical system in which the Aristotelean Principles of Bivalence, Excluded Middle, and Non-Contradiction are not valid. It constitutes the foundation of a new, non-Aristotelean, fuzzy logic, on the one hand; and of a many-valued, fuzzy mathematics, on the other. Both are novel systems deviating from all traditional ones. Since its inception, the fuzzy approach is steadily changing all sciences and technology. It can be predicted that no theory and technology will survive that is not based on this approach. The reasons for this successful, all-embracing revolution are manifold. Two of them may be mentioned briefly. The first one is expressed by Zadeh's Principle of Fuzzifiability. It says, in essence, that everything is fuzzy because everything is *fuzzifiable*:

Principle of Fuzzifiability: Any crisp theory can be fuzzified by replacing the concept of a set in that theory by the concept of a fuzzy set (Zadeh, 1994, 192; 1996a, 816; 1996b, 3).

Once a subject has been successfully fuzzified, it becomes, as a fuzzy set, amenable to the entire corpus of fuzzy logic. This principle is extensively used in the book.

The second reason is Zadeh's *linguistic approach* by his powerful theory of linguistic variables. In this way, the behavior and performance of all systems, be they inanimate or animate ones, may be described by linguistic variables. Thanks to this advantage, fuzzy logic has found many real-world applications ranging from engineering to natural sciences to medicine to social and behavioral sciences. Also this approach constitutes one of the main methods applied in our philosophy of medicine.

References

[Ackrill, 1963] Ackrill JL. *Aristotles's Categories and De Interpretaione*. Oxford: Clarendon Press, 1963.

[Adams, 1955] Adams EW. *Axiomatic Foundations of Rigid Body Mechanics*. Ph.D. Dissertation, Stanford University, 1955.

[Ader, 2007] Ader R (ed.). *Psychoneuroimmunology*. Burlington, MA: Elsevier Academic Press, 2007.

[Adlassnig, 1980] Adlassnig K-P. A fuzzy logical model of computer-assisted medical diagnosis. *Methods Inform Med* 1980; 19:141–148.

[Adlassnig, 1986] Adlassnig K-P. Fuzzy set theory in medical diagnosis. *IEEE Trans Syst Man Cybernet* 1986; 16:260–265.

[Adlassnig and Akhavan-Heidari, 1989] Adlassnig K-P, and Akhavan-Heidari M. CADIAG-2/GALL: An experimental diagnostic expert system for gallbladder and biliary tract diseases. *Artif Intell Med* 1989; 1:71–77.

[Alexander, 1934] Alexander F. The influence of psychologic factors upon gastrointestinal disturbances: A symposium. General principles, objectives and preliminary results. *Psychoanalytic Quarterly* 1934; 3:501–539.

[Alexander, 1939] Alexander F. Psychoanalytic study of a case of essential hypertension. *Psychosomatic Medicine* 1939; 1:139–152.

[Alexander, 1950] Alexander F. *Psychosomatic Medicine: Its Principles and Applications*. New York: W.W. Norton & Company, 1950.

[Alston, 1989] Alston W. *Epistemic Justification*. Ithaca: Cornell University Press, 1989.

[Alur and Henzinger, 1993] Alur R, and Henzinger TA. Real-time logics: Complexity and expressiveness. *Information and Computation* 1993; 104:35–77.

[Andersen, 2000] Andersen H. Kuhn's account of family resemblance: A solution to the problem of wide-open texture. *Erkenntnis* 2000; 52:313–337.

[Anderson, 2006] Anderson JA. *Automata Theory with Modern Applications*. Cambridge: Cambridge University Press, 2006.

[Anderson and Belnap, 1975] Anderson AR, Belnap ND, Jr. *Entailment. The Logic of Relevance and Necessity. Vol. I*. Princeton: Princeton University Press, 1975.

[Anderson and Belnap, 1992] Anderson AR, Belnap ND, Jr., and Dunn JM. *Entailment. The Logic of Relevance and Necessity. Vol. II*. Princeton: Princeton University Press, 1992.

K. Sadegh-Zadeh, *Handbook of Analytic Philosophy of Medicine*,
Philosophy and Medicine 113, DOI 10.1007/978-94-007-2260-6,
© Springer Science+Business Media B.V. 2012

[Åqvist, 1984] Åqvist L. Deontic Logic. In: DM Gabbay and F Guenthner (eds.), *Handbook of Philosophical Logic, Volume II,* pp. 605–714. Dordrecht: D. Reidel Publishing Company, 1984.

[Aquinas, 1994] Aquinas T. *Truth. Three volumes.* A reprint of the critical Leonine edition. Indianapolis, IN: Hackett Publishing Company, 1994.

[Aristotle, 1963] Aristotle. *Categories.* Translated with notes by J. L. Ackrill. Oxford: Clarendon Press, 1963.

[Aristotle, 1999] Aristotle. *The Metaphysics.* Translated by Hugh Lawson-Tancred. New York: Penguin Group, 1999.

[Aristotle, 2009] Aristotle. *Politics.* Oxford: Oxford University Press, 2009.

[Armour-Garb and Beall, 2005] Armour-Garb BP, Beall JC (eds.). *Deflationary Truth.* Chicago: Open Court Publishing Company, 2005.

[Armstrong, 1993a] Armstrong DM. *Belief, Truth, and Knowledge.* Cambridge: Cambridge University Press, 1973.

[Armstrong, 1993b] Armstrong DM. *A Materialist Theory of the Mind.* London: Routledge, 1993.

[Armstrong, 1997] Armstrong DM. *A World of States of Affairs.* Cambridge: Cambridge University Press, 1997.

[Armstrong, 1999] Armstrong DM. *The Mind-Body Problem: An Opinionated Introduction.* Boulder, CO: Westview Press, 1999.

[Armstrong, 2004] Armstrong DM. *Truth and Truthmakers.* Cambridge: Cambridge University Press, 2004.

[Aronson, 1999] Aronson J. When I use a word... Please please me. *British Medical Journal* 1999; 318:716.

[Arruda, 1977] Arruda AI. On the imaginary logic of N.A. Vasil'év. In: Arruda AI, da Costa NCA, and Chuaqui R (eds.), *Non-Classical Logic, Model Theory and Computability,* pp. 3–24. Amsterdam: North-Holland Publishing Company, 1977.

[Arruda, 1980] Arruda AI. A survey of paraconsistent logic. In: Arruda AI, Chuaqui R, and da Costa NCA (eds.), *Mathematical Logic in Latin America,* pp. 3–41. Amsterdam: North-Holland Publishing Company, 1980.

[Arruda, 1989] Arruda AI. Aspects of the historical development of paraconsistent logic. In: Priest G, Routley R, and Norman J (eds.), *Paraconsistent Logic. Essays on the Inconsistent,* pp. 99–130. München: Philosophia Verlag, 1989.

[Asenjo, 1966] Asenjo FG. A calculus of antinomies. *Notre Dame Journal of Formal Logic* 1966; 7:103–105.

[Audi, 2003] Audi R. *Epistemology. A Contemporary Introduction to the Theory of Knowledge.* New York: Routledge, 2003.

[Aumann, 1976] Aumann R. Agreeing to disagree. *Annals of Statistics* 1976; 4:1236–1239.

[Austin, 1946] Austin JL. Other minds. *Proceedings of the Aristotelean Society* 1946; Suppl. Vol. 20, pp. 148–187. Reprinted in [Austin, 1979], pp. 76–116.

[Austin, 1956] Austin JL. Performative utterances. Talk delivered in the Third Programme of the B.B.C. in 1956. Published in [Austin, 1979], pp. 233–252.

[Austin, 1962] Austin JL. *How To Do Things With Words.* Cambridge, MA: Harvard University Press, 1962.

[Austin, 1979] Austin JL. *Philosophical Papers.* Edited by JO Urmson and GJ Warnock. Oxford: Oxford University Press, 1979.

[Awodey, 2006] Awodey S. *Category Theory.* Oxford: Oxford University Press, 2006.

[Ayer, 1959] Ayer AJ (ed.). *Logical Positivism.* New York: The Free Press, 1959.

[Baars, 1988] Baars BJ. *A Cognitive Theory of Consciousness*. Cambridge: Cambridge University Press, 1988.

[Bacon, 1620] Bacon F. *Novum Organum*. See [Verulam, 1893].

[Baghramian, 2004] Baghramian M. *Relativism*. London: Routledge, 2004.

[Balzer, 1978] Balzer W. *Empirische Geometrie und Raum-Zeit-Theorie in mengentheoretischer Darstellung*. Kronberg: Scriptor-Verlag, 1978.

[Balzer and Moulines, 1996] Balzer W, and Moulines CU (eds.). *Structuralist Theory of Science. Focal Issues, New Results*. Berlin: De Gruyter, 1996.

[Balzer and Sneed, 1977] Balzer W, and Sneed JD. Generalized net structures of empirical theories: I. *Studia Logica* 1977; 36:195–211.

[Balzer and Sneed, 1978] Balzer W, and Sneed JD. Generalized net structures of empirical theories: II. *Studia Logica* 1978; 37:167–194.

[Barcan Marcus, 1946] Barcan Marcus RC. A functional calculus of first order based on strict implication. *The Journal of Symbolic Logic* 1946; 11:1–16.

[Barcan Marcus, 1947] Barcan Marcus RC. The identity of individuals in a strict functional calculus of second order. *The Journal of Symbolic Logic* 1947; 12:12–15.

[Barcan Marcus, 1993] Barcan Marcus RC. *Modalities: Philosophical Essays*. New York: University of Oxford Press, 1993.

[Bareiss and Porter, 1987] Bareiss E, and Porter P. Protos: An exemplar-based learning apprentice. In: *Proceedings of the Fourth International Workshop on Machine Learning*, pp. 12–23, 1987.

[Barnes et al., 1996] Barnes B, Bloor D, and Henry J. *Scientific Knowledge: A Sociological Analysis*. Chicago: The University of Chicago Press, 1996.

[Barré-Sinoussi et al., 1983] Barré-Sinoussi F, Montagnier L, et al. Isolation of a T-lymphotropic retrovirus from a patient at risk for acquired immune deficiency syndrome (AIDS). *Science* 1983; 220:868–671.

[Barro and Marin, 2002] Barro S & Marin R (eds.). *Fuzzy Logic in Medicine*. Heidelberg: Physika-Verlag, 2002.

[Barwise, 1977] Barwise J (ed.). *Handbook of Mathematical Logic*. Amsterdam: North-Holland Publishing Company, 1977.

[Baumes, 1798] Baumes JBT. *Essai d'un système chimique de la science de l'homme*. Nîmes, 1798.

[Baumes, 1801] Baumes JBT. *Traité élémentaire de nosologie, contenant une classification de toutes les maladies. 4 volumes*. Paris, 1801–1802.

[Baumes, 1806] Baumes JBT. *Traité de l'Ictère ou Jaunisse des Enfans des Naissance* (English translation: Treatise on Icterus or Jaundice of Newborn Infants). 2nd edition, Paris: Méquignon, 1806.

[Bayes, 1763] Bayes T. An essay toward solving a problem in the doctrine of chances. *Transactions of the Royal Society of London* 1763; 53:370–418.

[Beakley, 2006] Beakley B, Ludlow P (eds.). *Philosophy of Mind: Classical Problems - Contemporary Issues*. Cambridge, MA: MIT Press, 2006.

[Beauchamp and Childress, 2001] Beauchamp TL, and Childress JF. *Principles of Biomedical Ethics*. Fifth edition. Oxford: Oxford University Press, 2001.

[Beauchamp and DeGrazia, 2004] Beauchamp TL, DeGrazia D. Principles and principlism. In: Khushf G (ed.), *Handbook of Bioethics*, pp. 55–74. Dordrecht: Kluwer Academic Publishers, 2004.

[Bell and Slomson, 2006] Bell JL, and Slomson AB. *Models and Ultraproducts: An Introduction*. New York: Dover Publications, 2006.

[Bellman and Zadeh, 1970] Bellman RE, and Zadeh LA. Decision-making in a fuzzy environment. *Management Science* 1970; 17:141–164.

[Bellman and Zadeh, 1977] Bellman RE, and Zadeh LA. *Local and fuzzy logics.* In: Dunn JM, and Epstein E (eds.), *Modern Uses of Multiple-Valued Logic*, pp. 105–151. Dordrecht: D. Reidel Publishing Company, 1977.

[Bender, 1989] Bender J (ed.). *The Current State of the Coherence Theory.* Dordrecht: Kluwer Academic Publishers, 1989.

[Berger and Luckmann, 1966] Berger P, and Luckmann T. *The Social Construction of Reality.* New York: Doubleday, 1966.

[Bezdek, 1981] Bezdek JC. *Pattern Recognition with Fuzzy Objective Function Algorithms.* New York: Plenum 1981.

[Bezdek et al., 1999] Bezdek JC, Keller J, Krisnapuram R, and Pal NR. *Fuzzy Models and Algorithms for Pattern Recognition and Image Processing.* Boston: Kluwer Academic Publishers, 1999. Volume 4 of [Dubois and Prade 1998–2000].

[Bieganski, 1909] Bieganski W. *Medizinische Logik. Kritik der ärztlichen Erkenntnis.* Würzburg: Kabitzsch, 1909.

[Bijker et al., 1999] Bijker WE, Hughes TP, and Pinch T (eds.). *The Social Construction of Technological Systems. New Directions in the Sociology and History of Technology.* Cambridge, MA: MIT Press, 1999.

[Bimbó, 2007] Bimbó K. Relevance Logic. In: Jacquette D (ed.), *Philosophy of Logic*, pp. 723–789. Amsterdam: Elsevier, 2007.

[Birkhoff and Neumann, 1936] Birkhoff G, and von Neumann J. The logic of quantum mechanics. *Annals of Mathematics* 1936; 37:823–843.

[Bittner and Donnelly, 2007] Bittner T, and Donnelly M. Logical properties of foundational relations in bio-ontologies. *Artificial Intelligence in Medicine* 2007; 39:197–216.

[Black, 1937] Black M. Vagueness. An exercise in logical analysis. *Philosophy of Science* 1937; 4: 427–455.

[Black, 1963] Black M. Reasoning with loose concepts. *Dialogue* 1963; 2:1–12.

[Blair and Subrahmanian, 1987] Blair HA, and Subrahmanian VS. Paraconsistent logic programming. In: *Proceedings of the Seventh Conference on Foundations of Software Technology and Theoretical Computer Science in Pune, India*, pp. 340–360. London: Springer-Verlag, 1987.

[Blair and Subrahmanian, 1989] Blair HA, and Subrahmanian VS. Paraconsistent logic programming. *Theoretical Computer Science* 1989; 68:135–154.

[Blancard, 1756] Blancard S. *Lexicon medicum renovatum.* Leiden: Luchtmans, 1756.

[Blane, 1819] Blane G. *Elements of Medical Logick.* London: Thomas & George Underwood, 1819.

[Blanshard, 1939] Blanshard B. *The Nature of Thought.* London: George Allen and Unwin, 1939.

[Blaser, 2005] Blaser MJ. An endangered species in the stomach. Is the decline of Helicobacter pylori, a bacterium living in the human stomach since time immemorial, good or bad for public health? *Scientific American* 2005; 292(2):38–45.

[Bliss, 2007] Bliss M. *The Discovery of the Insulin.* Chicago: The University of Chicago Press, 2007.

[Block, 1997] Block N. *Consciousness.* In: Guttenplan S (ed.), *A Companion to the Philosophy of Mind*, pp. 210–219. Oxford: Blackwell Publishers Ltd., 1997.

[Bloor, 1983] Bloor D. *Wittgenstein: A Social Theory of Knowledge.* London: The Macmillan Press Ltd., 1983.

[Bloor, 1991] Bloor D. *Knowledge and Social Imagery*. Chicago: The University of Chicago Press, 1991.

[Bochenski, 1961] Bochenski IM. *A History of Formal Logic*. Notre Dame: The University of Notre Dame Press, 1961.

[Bochman, 2005] Bochman A. *Explanatory Nonmonotonic Reasoning*. Singapore: World Scientific Publishing Company 2005.

[Boegl et al., 2004] Boegl K, Adlassnig K-P, Hayashi Y, Rothenfluh T, and Leitich H. Knowledge acquisition in the fuzzy knowledge representation framework of a medical consultation system. *Artif Intell Med* 2004; 30:1–26.

[Boh, 1993] Boh I. *Epistemic Logic in the Later Middle Ages*. London: Routledge, 1993.

[Bok, 2002] Bok S. *Common Values*. Columbia: University of Missouri Press, 2002.

[Bolzano, 1837] Bolzano B. *Wissenschaftslehre. Versuch einer ausführlichen und grösstentheils neuen Darstellung der Logik mit steter Rücksicht auf deren bisherige Bearbeiter*. 4 vols. Sulzbach: J.E. von Seidelsche Buchhandlung, 1837.

[Boole, 1847] Boole G. *The Mathematical Analysis of Logic, Being an Essay Toward a Calculus of Deductive Reasoning*. Cambridge: Barclay & Macmillan, 1847.

[Boole, 1848] Boole G. The calculus of logic. *The Cambridge and Dublin Mathematical Journal* 1848; 3:183–198.

[Boole, 1854] Boole G. *An Investigation of the Laws of Thought on which are Founded the Mathematical Theories of Logic and Probabilities*. Cambridge: Macmillan, 1854.

[Boorse, 1975] Boorse C. On the distinction between disease and illness. *Philosophy and Public Affairs* 1975; 5:49–68.

[Boorse , 1977] Boorse C. Health as a theoretical concept. *Philosophy of Science* 1977; 44:542–573.

[Boorse, 1997] Boorse. A rebuttal on health. In: Humber JM, and Almeder RF (eds.), *What Is Disease?* pp. 3–134. Totowa, NJ: Humana Press, 1997.

[Borst, 1970] Borst CV (ed.). *The Mind-Body Identity Theory*. London: Macmillan, 1970.

[Bourbaki, 1950] Bourbaki N. The architecture of mathematics. *American Mathematical Monthly* 1950; 57:231–232.

[Bourbaki, 1968] Bourbaki N. *Theory of Sets*. Boston, MA: Herman and Addison-Wesley, 1968.

[Boyle, 2004] Boyle J. Casuistry. In Khushf G (ed.), *Handbook of Bioethics. Taking Stock of the Field From A Philosophical Perspective*, pp. 75–88. Dordrecht: Kluwer Academic Publishers, 2004.

[Braddon-Mitchell and Jackson, 2007] Braddon-Mitchell D, and Jackson F. *Philosophy of Mind: An Introduction*. Malden, MA: Blackwell Publishing, 2007.

[Bramer, 2005] Bramer M. *Logic Programming with Prolog*. London: Springer, 2005.

[Bremer, 2005] Bremer M. *An Introduction to Paraconsistent Logics*. Frankfurt: Peter Lang, 2005.

[Brentano, 1874] Brentano FC. *Psychologie vom empirischen Standpunkt*. Berlin: Duncker & Humblot, 1874. (English translation by AC Rancurello, DB Terrell, and L McAlister: *Psychology From An Empirical Standpoint*. London: Routledge, 1973.)

[Bridgman, 1927] Bridgman, PW. *The Logic of Modern Physics*. New York: Macmillan, 1927.

[Bridgman, 1936] Bridgman, PW. *The Nature of Physical Theory*. New York: Dover Publications, 1936.

[Brinck, 1997] Brinck I. *The Indexical 'I'. The First Person in Thought and Language*. Dordrecht: Kluwer Academic Publishers, 1997.

[Broad, 1925] Broad CD. *The Mind and its Place in Nature*. London: Kegan Paul, 1925.

[Brock, 1988] Brock TD. *Robert Koch: A Life in Medicine and Bacteriology*. Madison, WI: Science Tech Publishers, 1988.

[Brody, 1980] Brody H. *Placebos and the Philosophy of Medicine*. Chicago: The University of Chicago Press, 1980.

[Brouwer, 1907] Brouwer LEJ. *On the Foundations of Mathematics*. Thesis, Amsterdam; English translation in [Heyting, 1975], pp. 11–101.

[Brown, 2003] Brown FM. *Boolean Reasoning: The Logic of Boolean Equations*. New York: Dover Publications, 2003.

[Buber, 1958] Buber, M. *I and Thou*. Translated by Ronald Gregor Smith. New York: Charles Scribner's Sons, 1958.

[Buchanan and Shortliffe, 1984] Buchanan B, and Shortliffe EH (eds.), *Rule-Based Expert Systems. The MYCIN Experiments of the Stanford Heuristic Programming Project*. Reading, MA: Addison-Wesley, 1984.

[Buckley, 2006] Buckley JJ. *Fuzzy Probability and Statistics*. Berlin: Springer-Verlag, 2006.

[Buja, 1996] Buja LM. Does atherosclerosis have an infectious etiology? Circulation 1996; 94:872–873.

[Bull and Segerberg, 1984] Bull R, and Segerberg K. Basic modal logic. In: Gabbay DM, and Guenthner F, *Handbook of Philosophical Logic*, Volume II, pp. 1–88. Dordrecht: D. Reidel Publishing Company, 1984.

[Bunge, 1967] Bunge M. *Scientific Research. Vol. II: The Search for Truth*. Berlin: Springer-Verlag, 1967.

[Bunge, 1983] Bunge M. *Treatise on Basic Philosophy, Volume 6. Epistemology & Methodology II: Understanding the World*. Dordrecht: D. Reidel Publishing Company, 1983.

[Burger et al., 2008] Burger A, Davidson D, and Baldock R (eds.). *Anatomy Ontologies for Bioinformatics*. Berlin: Springer-Verlag, 2008.

[Burgess, 2002] Burgess JP. Basic tense logic. In: Gabbay DM, and Guenthner F, *Handbook of Philosophical Logic*, 2nd Edition, Volume 7, pp. 1–42. Dordrecht: Kluwer Academic Publishers, 2002.

[Burkhardt and Smith, 2002] Burkhardt H, and Smith B (eds.). *Handbook of Metaphysics and Ontology*. Two Volumes. München: Philosophia Verlag, 2002.

[Calero et al., 2006] Calero C, Ruiz F, and Piattini M (eds.). *Ontologies for Software Engineering and Software Technology*. Berlin: Springer-Verlag, 2006.

[Campbell, 1984] Campbell K. *Body and Mind*. Notre Dame, IN: University of Notre Dame Press, 1984.

[Campbell, 1990] Campbell K. *Abstract Particulars*. Oxford: Basil Blackwell, 1990.

[Caplan et al., 1981] Caplan AL, Engelhardt HT Jr., McCartney JJ (eds.). *Concepts of Health and Disease. Interdisciplinary Perspectives*. London: Addison-Wesley, 1981.

[Caplan et al., 2004] Caplan AL, McCartney JJ, and Sisti DA (eds.). *Health, Disease, and Illness. Concepts in Medicine*. Washington, D.C.: Georgetown University Press, 2004.

[Carnap, 1928] Carnap R. *Der Logische Aufbau der Welt*. Berlin: Weltkreis-Verlag, 1928. (English translation: *The Logical Structure of the World*. Berkeley: University of California Press, 1967.)

[Carnap, 1931] Carnap R. Die physikalische Sprache als Universalsprache der Wissenschaft. *Erkenntnis* 1931; 2:432–465.

[Carnap, 1932] Carnap R. Überwindung der Metaphysik durch logische Analyse der Sprache. *Erkenntnis* 1932; 2:219–241.

[Carnap, 1936] Carnap R. Testability and meaning. *Philosophy of Science* 1936; 3:419–471 and 1937; 4:1–40.

[Carnap, 1945] Carnap R. On inductive logic. *Philosophy of Science* 1945; 12:72–97.

[Carnap, 1947] Carnap R. *Meaning and Necessity.* Chicago: The University of Chicago Press, 1947.

[Carnap, 1952] Carnap R. *The Continuum of Inductive Methods.* Chicago: The University of Chicago Press, 1952.

[Carnap, 1954] Carnap R. *Introduction to Symbolic Logic and Its Applications.* New York: Dover Publications, 1954.

[Carnap, 1962] Carnap R. *Logical Foundations of Probability.* Chicago: The University of Chicago Press, 1962.

[Carnap, 1966] Carnap R. *Philosophical Foundations of Physics.* New York: Basic Books, 1966.

[Carnap and Jeffrey, 1971] Carnap R, Jeffrey RC (eds.). *Studies in Inductive Logic and Probability, Vol. 1.* Berkeley: University of California Press, 1971.

[Cartwright, 2004] Cartwright SA. Report on the diseases and physical peculiarities of the Negro Race. (Originally published in 1851.) Reprinted in: Caplan AL, McCartney JJ, and Sisti DA (eds.). *Health, Disease, and Illness. Concepts in Medicine,* pp. 28–39. Washington, D.C.: Georgetown University Press, 2004.

[Casati and Varzi, 1999] Casati R, and Varzi AC. *Parts and Places: The Structures of Spatial Representation.* Cambridge, MA: MIT Press, 1999.

[Cassell, 2004] Cassell, EJ. *The Nature of Suffering and the Goals of Medicine.* New York: Oxford University Press, 2004.

[Cavaliere, 1996] Cavaliere F. L'Opera Di Hugh MacColl Alle Origini Delle Logiche Non-Classiche. *Modern Logic* 1996; 6:373–402.

[Chalmers, 2002] Chalmers DJ (ed.). *Philosophy of Mind: Classical and Contemporary Readings.* Oxford: Oxford University Press, 2002.

[Chandrasekaran et al., 1989] Chandrasekaran B, Smith JW, and Sticklen J. Deep models and their relation to diagnosis. *Artif Intell Med* 1989; 1:29–40.

[Chisholm, 1963] Chisholm RM. Contrary-to-duty imperatives and deontic logic. *Analysis* 1963; 24:33–36.

[Chisholm, 1996] Chisholm RM. *A Realistic Theory of Categories.* Cambridge: Cambridge University Press, 1996.

[Church, 1956] Church A. *Introduction to Mathematical Logic.* Princeton: Princeton University Press, 1956.

[Churchland, 1981] Churchland Paul M. Eliminative materialism and the propositional attitudes. *Journal of Philosophy* 1981; 78:67–90.

[Churchland, 1988] Churchland Paul M. *Matter and Consciousness.* Cambridge, MA: MIT Press, 1988.

[Churchland, 1986] Churchland Patricia S. *Neurophilosophy: Toward a Unified Science of the Mind/Brain.* Cambridge, MA: MIT Press, 1986.

[Cignoli et al., 2000] Cignoli R, D'Ottaviano I, and Mundici D. *Algebraic Foundations of Many-Valued Reasoning.* Dordrecht: Kluwer Academic Publishers, 2000.

[Cios, et al., 2007] Cios KJ, Pedrycz W, Swiniarski RW, and Kurgan LA. *Data Mining: A Knowledge Discovery Approach.* New York: Springer Science and Business Media, 2007.

[Clarke, 1981] Clarke B. A calculus of individuals based on "connection". *Notre Dame Journal of Formal Logic* 1981; 22:204–218.

[Clarke, 1985] Clarke B. Individuals and points. *Notre Dame Journal of Formal Logic* 1985; 26:61–75.

[Clocksin and Mellish, 2003] Clocksin F, and Mellish CS. *Programming in Prolog: Using the ISO Standard.* Berlin: Springer-Verlag, 2003.

[Clouser and Gert, 1990] Clouser KD, and Gert B. A critique of principlism. *The Journal of Medicine and Philosophy* 1990; 15:219–236.

[Clouser et al., 1997] Clouser KD, Culver CM, Gert B. Malady. In: Humber JM, and Almeder RF (eds.), *What Is Disease?* pp. 175–217. Totowa, NJ: Humana Press, 1997.

[Cohen and Schnelle, 1986] Cohen RS, and Schnelle T (eds.). *Cognition and Fact. Materials on Ludwik Fleck.* Dordrecht: D. Reidel Publishing Company, 1986.

[Cohn and Varzi, 2003] Cohn AG, and Varzi AC. Mereotopological connection. *Journal of Philosophical Logic* 2003; 32:357–390.

[Collins, 2007] Collins J. Counterfactuals, causation, and preemption. In: Jacquette D (ed.), *Philosophy of Logic,* pp. 1127–1143. Amsterdam: Elsevier, 2007.

[Cooper, 1988] Cooper GF. Computer-based medical diagnosis using belief networks and bounded probabilities. In: Miller PL (ed.), *Selected Topics in Medical Artificial Intelligence,* pp. 85–98. New York: Springer-Verlag, 1988.

[Cooper R, 2005] Cooper R. *Classifying Madness. A Philosophical Examination of the Diagnostic and Statistical Manual of Mental Disorders.* Dordrecht: Springer, 2005.

[Cooper SB, 2003] Cooper SB. *Computability Theory.* Boca Raton, FL: Chapman & Hall/CRC, 2003.

[Cox, 2006] Cox DR. *Principles of Statistical Inference.* Cambridge, UK: Cambridge University Press, 2006.

[Coyne, 2009] Coyne JA. *Why Evolution is True.* New York: Penguin Group Inc., 2009.

[Cuneo, 2010] Cuneo T. *The Normative Web: An Argument for Moral Realism.* Oxford: Oxford University Press, 2010.

[Cunningham and Williams, 2002] Cunningham W, Williams P (eds.). *The Laboratory Revolution in Medicine.* Cambridge: Cambridge University Press, 2002.

[Cutler, 1998] Cutler P. *Problem Solving in Clinical Medicine. From Data to Diagnosis.* Third Edition. Baltimore: Williams & Wilkins, 1998.

[da Costa, 1958] da Costa NCA. Nota sobre o conceito de contradio. *Anuário da Sociedade Paranaense de Mathemática* 1958; 1:6–8.

[da Costa, 1963] da Costa NCA. *Sistemas Formais Inconsistentes.* Curitiba, Brazil: Universidade Federal do Parana, 1963.

[da Costa, 1974] da Costa NCA. On the theory of inconsistent formal systems. *Notre Dame Journal of Formal Logic* 1974; 15:497–510.

[da Costa, 1982] da Costa NCA. Logic and ontology. Campinas, SP: Universidade Estadual de Campinas, 1982.

[da Costa, 1988] da Costa NCA. New systems of predicate deontic logic. *The Journal of Non-Classical Logic* 1988; 5(2):75–80.

[da Costa, 1989] da Costa NCA. Logic and pragmatic truth. In: Fenstad J. et al. (eds.), *Logic, Methodology and Philosophy of Science VIII,* pp. 247–261. Amsterdam: Elsevier, 1989.

[da Costa and Bueno, 1998] da Costa NCA, and Bueno O. The logic of pragmatic truth. *Journal of Philosophical Logic* 1998; 27:603–620.

[da Costa and Carnielli, 1986] da Costa NCA, and Carnielli WA. On paraconsistent deontic logic. *Philosophia* 1986; 16:293–305.

[da Costa and French, 2003] da Costa NCA, and French S. *Science and Partial Truth. A Unitary Approach to Models and Scientific Reasoning.* Oxford: Oxford University Press, 2003.

[da Costa and Subrahmanian, 1989] da Costa NCA, and Subrahmanian VS. Paraconsistent logics as a formalism for reasoning about inconsistent knowledge bases. *Artif Intell Med* 1989; 1:167–174.

[da Costa et al., 1991] da Costa NCA, Doria FA, and Papavero N. Meinong's theory of objects and Hilbert's ε-symbol. Reports on Mathematical Logic 1991; 25:119–132.

[da Costa et al., 1995] da Costa NCA, Béziau JY, Bueno O. Paraconsistent logic in a historical perspective. *Logique & Analyse* 1995; 150/151/152: 111–125.

[da Costa et al., 1998] da Costa NCA, Bueno O, and French S. Is there a Zande Logic? *History and Philosophy of Logic* 1998; 19:41–54.

[da Costa et al., 2007] da Costa NCA, Krause D, and Bueno O. Paraconsistent logics and paraconsistency. In: Jacquette D (ed.), *Philosophy of Logic*, pp. 791–911. Amsterdam: Elsevier, 2007.

[Dalla Chiara and Giuntini, 2002] Dalla Chiara ML, and Giuntini R. Quantum logics. In: Gabbay DM, and Guenthner F (eds.), *Handbook of Philosophical Logic*, 2nd Edition, Volume 6, pp. 129–228. Dordrecht: Kluwer Academic Publishers, 2002.

[Danesi, 1994] Danesi M. *Messages and Meanings: An Introduction to Semiotics.* Toronto: Canadian Scholars' Press, 1994.

[Dauben, 1990] Dauben JW. *Georg Cantor. His Mathematics and Philosophy of the Infinite.* Princeton: Princeton University Press, 1990.

[David, 1998] David FN. *Games, Gods, and Gambling. A History of Probability and Statistical Ideas.* New York: Dover Publications, 1998.

[Davidson, 1970] Davidson D. Mental events. In: Foster L, and Swanson JW (eds.), *Experience and Theory*, pp. 79–101. Amherst, MA: The University of Massachusetts Press and Duckworth, 1970.

[de Finetti, 1937] de Finetti B. La prévision: Ses lois logiques, ses sources subjectives". *Annales de l'Institut Henri Poincaré* 1937; 7:1–68. Translated as "Foresight. Its Logical Laws, Its Subjective Sources", in Kyburg HE, Jr., and Smokler HE (eds.), *Studies in Subjective Probability*, pp. 53–118. Huntington, NY: Robert E. Krieger Publishing Company, 1980.

[de Kleer et al., 1992] de Kleer J, Mackworth AK, and Reiter R. Characterizing diagnoses and systems. *Artificial Intelligence* 1992; 56:197–222.

[Dennett, 1987] Dennett DC. *The Intentional Stance.* Cambridge, MA: MIT Press, 1987.

[Dennett, 1991] Dennett DC. *Consciousness Explained.* Boston: Little Brown & Company, 1991.

[DePaul, 2000] DePaul M (ed.). *Resurrecting Old-Fashioned Foundationalism.* Lanham, MA: Rowman and Littlefield, 2000.

[DeRose, 2009] DeRose K. *The Case for Contextualism.* Oxford: Oxford University Press, 2009.

[Descartes, 1986] Descartes R. *Meditationes de prima philosophia. Meditationen über die erste Philosophie.* Lateinisch-Deutsch. Übersetzt und herausgegeben von Gerhart Schmidt. Stuttgart: Reclam, 1986.

[Dingler, 1928] Dingler H. *Das Experiment: Sein Wesen und seine Geschichte.* München: Verlag Ernst Reinhardt, 1928.

[Dompere, 2010] Dompere KK. *Cost-Benefit Analysis and the Theory of Fuzzy Decisions: Fuzzy Value Theory.* Berlin: Springer-Verlag, 2010.

[Donnelly et al., 2006] Donnelly M, Bittner T, and Rosse C. A formal theory of spatial representation and reasoning in biomedical ontologies. *Artif Intell Med* 2006; 36:1–27.

[Dragulinescu, 2010] Dragulinescu S. Diseases as natural kinds. *Theoretical Medicine and Bioethics,* 2010; 31:347–369.

[Dubois and Prade, 1988] Dubois D, and Prade H. *Possibility Theory. An Approach to Computerized Processing of Uncertainty.* New York: Plenum Press, 1988.

[Dubois and Prade, 1998] Dubois D, and Prade H (eds.). *The Handbook of Fuzzy Sets Series.* 7 volumes. Boston: Kluwer Academic Publishers, 1998–2000.

[Dubois et al., 1993] Dubois D, Prade H, and Yager RR. *Readings in Fuzzy Sets for Intelligent Systems.* San Mateo, CA: Morgan Kaufmann Publishers, 1993.

[Dubois et al., 2000] Dubois D, Nguyen HT, and Prade H. Possibility theory, probability and fuzzy sets. In: Dubois D, and Prade H (eds.), *The Handbook of Fuzzy Sets Series. 7 volumes. Vol 1: Fundamentals of Fuzzy Sets,* pp. 343–438. Boston: Kluwer Academic Publishers, 2000.

[Duhem, 1954] Duhem P. *The Aim and Structure of Physical Theories.* Translated by P Wiener and foreworded by PL de Broglie (French original published 1906). Princeton: Princeton University Press, 1954.

[Dummett, 1993] Dummett M. *The Seas of Lanaguage.* Oxford: Oxford University Press, 1993.

[Dunn and Restall, 2002] Dunn JM, and Restall G. *Relevance Logic.* In: Gabbay DM, and Guenthner F (eds.), *Handbook of Philosophical Logic,* 2nd Edition, Vol. 6, pp. 1–128. Dordrecht: Kluwer Academic Publishers, 2002.

[Durkheim, 1965] Durkheim E. *The Elementary Forms of the Religious Life.* English translation by Joseph Swain. New York: The Free Press, 1965. (First published 1912.)

[Dyson et al., 1920] Dyson FW, Eddington AS, and Davidson CR. A determination of the deflection of light by the sun's gravitational field, from observations made at the solar eclipse of May 29, 1919. *Phil. Trans. Roy. Soc.* 1920; A 220:291–333.

[Eells, 2008] Eells E. *Probabilistic Causality.* Cambridge: Cambridge University Press, 2008.

[Ehrlich, 1891] Ehrlich P. Experimentelle Untersuchungen über Immunität. I. Über Ricin. *Deutsche Medicinische Wochenschrift* 1891; 17:976–979. Experimentelle Untersuchungen über Immunität. II. Über Albrin. *Deutsche Medicinische Wochenschrift* 1891; 17:1218–1219.

[Elstein et al., 1978] Elstein AS, Shulman LS, and Sprafka SA. *Medical Problem Solving. An Analysis of Clinical Reasoning.* Cambridge, MA: Harvard University Press, 1978.

[Engel, 1977] Engel GL. The need for a medical model: A challenge for biomedicine. *Science* 1977; 196:129–136.

[Engelberg, 2005] Engelberg S. *A Mathematical Introduction to Control Theory.* Singapore: World Scientific Publishing Company, 2005.

[Engelhardt, 1975] Engelhardt HT Jr (1975). The concepts of health and disease. In: Engelhardt HT, Jr., and Spicker SF (eds.), *Evaluation and Explanation in the Biomedical Sciences,* pp. 125–141. Dordrecht: D. Reidel Publishing Company, 1975.

[Engelhardt, 1976] Engelhardt HT, Jr. Ideology and etiology. *The Journal of Medicine and Philosophy* 1976; 1:256–268.

[Engelhardt, 1980] Engelhardt HT, Jr. Ethical issues in diagnosis. *Metamedicine* 1980; 1:39–50.

[Engelhardt, 1986] Engelhardt HT, Jr. *The Foundations of Bioethics.* New York: Oxford University Press, 1986.

[Engelhardt, 2000] Engelhardt HT, Jr. The philosophy of medicine and bioethics: An introduction to the framing of a field. In: Engelhardt HT, Jr. (ed.), *The Philosophy of Medicine,* pp. 1–15. Dordrecht: Kluwer Academic Publishers, 2000.

[Engelhardt, 2006] Engelhardt HT, Jr. 'Global bioethics: An introduction to the collapse of consensus'. In: Engelhardt HT, Jr. (ed.), *Global Bioethics. The Collapse of Consensus,* pp. 1–17. Salem, MA: M&M Scrivener Press, 2006.

[EUROGAST, 1993] EUROGAST Study Group. An international association between Helicobacter pylori infection and gastric cancer. *Lancet* 1993; 341:1359–1362.

[Everett and Hofweber, 2000] Everett A, and Hofweber T (eds.). *Empty Names, Fiction and the Puzzles of Non-Existence.* Stanford, CA: Center for the Study of Language and Information, 2000.

[Ewing, 1940] Ewing AC. The linguistic theory of a priori propositions. *Proceedings of the Aristotelean Society* 1940; 40:207–244.

[FCAT, 1998] FCAT (Federative Committee on Anatomical Terminology). *Terminologia Anatomica: International Anatomical Terminology.* Stuttgart: Thieme, 1998.

[Feigl, 1958] Feigl H. The "Mental" and the "Physical" '. In: Feigl H, Scriven M, and Maxwell G (eds.), *Concepts, Theories, and the Mind-Body Problem. Minnesota Studies in the Philosophy of Science,* Vol. 2, pp. 370–497. Minneapolis: University of Minnesota Press, 1958.

[Feyerabend, 1960] Feyerabend PK. Das Problem der Existenz theoretischer Entitäten. In: Topitsch E (ed.), *Probleme der Wissenschaftstheorie. Festschrift für Victor Kraft.* Vienna: Springer-Verlag, 1960.

[Fibiger, 1898] Fibiger JAG. Om Serumbehandling af Difteri. *Hospitalstidende* 1898; 6:309–25, 337–50.

[Field and Lohr, 1990] Field MJ, and Lohr KN. *Guidelines for Clinical Practice: Directions for a New Program.* Washington, DC: Institute of Medicine, National Academic Press, 1990.

[Fischer and Kirchin, 2006] Fischer A, and Kirchin S (eds.). *Arguing About Metaethics.* Abingdon, UK: Routledge, 2006.

[Fisher et al., 2005] Fisher M, Gabbay DM, and Vila L (eds.). *Handbook of Temporal Reasoning in Artificial Intelligence.* Amsterdam: Elsevier, 2005

[Fitting and Mendelsohn, 1998] Fitting MC, and Mendelsohn R. *First-Order Modal Logic.* Dordrecht: Kluwer Academic Publishers, 1998.

[Fleck, 1979] Fleck L. *Genesis and Development of a Scientific Fact.* Edited by Trenn TJ, and Merton RK. Chicago: The University of Chicago Press, 1979. (First published in German 1935 by Benno Schwabe in Basel, Switzerland.)

[Fleck, 1983] Fleck L. *Erfahrung und Tatsache. Gesammelte Aufsätze mit einer Einleitung herausgegeben von Lothar Schäfer und Thomas Schnelle.* Frankfurt: Suhrkamp, 1983.

[Fodor, 1968] Fodor JA. *Psychological Explanation.* New York: Random House, 1968.

[Forbes, 1985] Forbes G. *The Metaphysics of Modality.* Oxford: Clarendon Press, 1985.

[Foucault, 1994] Foucault M. *The Birth of the Clinic. An Archaeology of Medical Perception* New York: Vintage Books, 1994.

[Frank, 1997] Frank AW. *The Wounded Storyteller. Body, Illness, and Ethics.* Chicago: The University of Chicago Press, 1997.

[Frankfurt, 1971] Frankfurt HG. Freedom of the will and the concept of a person. *The Journal of Philosophy* 1971; 68:5–20.

[Frege, 1879] Frege G. Begriffsschrift. *Eine der arithmetischen nachgebildete Formelsprache des reinen Denkens.* Halle, Germany: L. Nebert, 1879. Translated into English as "Begriffsschrift, A formula language, modeled upon that of arithmetic, for pure thought" in van Heijenoort J (ed.), *From Frege to Gödel. A Source Book in Mathematical Logic,* pp. 1-82. Cambridge, MA: Harvard University Press, 1971.

[Frege, 1884] Frege G. *The Foundations of Arithmetic. A Logico-Mathematical Enquiry Into the Concept of Number* (in German). Breslau: W. Koebner, 1884.

[Frege, 1891] Frege G. *Funktion und Begriff.* Jena, Germany: Verlag von Hermann Pohle. (A lecture held on January 9, 1891 in Jena, Germany, at a meeting of the "Jenaische Gesellschaft für Medizin und Naturwissenschaft".) Translated as 'Function and Concept' by P. Geach in [Geach and Black, 1952].

[Frege, 1892a] Frege G. Über Sinn und Bedeutung. *Zeitschrift für Philosophie und philosophische Kritik, Neue Folge* 1892; 100:25–50. Translated as "On Sense and Reference" in [Geach and Black, 1952], pp. 56–78.

[Frege, 1892b] Frege G. Über Begriff und Gegenstand. *Vierteljahresschrift für wissenschaftliche Philosophie* 1892; 16:192–205. Translated as "Concept and Object" in [Geach and Black, 1952].

[Frege, 1893] Frege G. *The Basic Laws of Arithmetic: Exposition of the System. Volume I* (in German). Jena: H. Pohle, 1893.

[Frege, 1904] Frege G. Was ist eine Funktion? In: Meyer S (ed.), *Festschrift Ludwig Boltzmann gewidmet zum sechzigsten Geburtstage, 20. Februar 1904,* pp. 656–666. Leipzig: Johann Ambrosius Barth, 1904. Translated as "What is a Function?" in [Geach and Black, 1952].

[Freud and Breuer, 1895] Freud S, and Breuer J. *Studien über Hysterie.* Leipzig and Wien: Franz Deuticke, 1895.

[Friedman et al., 1998] Friedman LM, Furberg CD, and DeMets, DL. *Fundamentals of Clinical Trials.* Third Edition. New York: Springer-Verlag, 1998.

[Friedman et al., 2004] Friedman H, Yamamoto Y, and Bendinelli M (eds.). Chlamydia pneumoniae: Infection and Disease. New York: Kluwer Academic / Plenum Publishers, 2004.

[Fullér, 2000] Fullér R. *Introduction to Neuro-Fuzzy Systems.* Heidelberg: Physica-Verlag, 2000.

[Gabbay and Guenthner, 1984] Gabbay DM, and Guenthner F (eds.). *Handbook of Philosophical Logic,* Volume II. Dordrecht: D. Reidel Publishing Company, 1984.

[Gabbay and Guenthner, 2002] Gabbay DM, and Guenthner F (eds.). *Handbook of Philosophical Logic.* 2nd Edition, Volume 7. Dordrecht: Kluwer Academic Publishers, 2002.

[Gabbay and Woods, 2006] Gabbay DM, and Woods J (eds.). *Handbook of the History of Logic, Volume 7, Logic and the Modalities in the Twentieth Century.* Amsterdam: Elsevier, 2006.

[Gabbay et al., 1994a] Gabbay DM, Hodkinson I, and Reynolds M. *Temporal Logic: Mathematical Foundations and Computational Aspects, Volumes 1*. Oxford: Oxford University Press, 1994.

[Gabbay et al., 1994b] Gabbay DM, Hogger C, and Robinson J (eds.). *Handbook of Logic in Artificial Intelligence and Logic Programming, Vol. 3*. Oxford: Oxford University Press, 1994.

[Gabbay et al., 2000] Gabbay DM, Hodkinson I, and Reynolds M. *Temporal Logic: Mathematical Foundations and Computational Aspects, Volumes 2*. Oxford: Oxford University Press, 2000.

[Galen, 1985] Galen. *Three Treatises on the Nature of Science: On the Sects for Beginners, An Outline of Empiricism, On Medical Experience*. Translated by Walzer R, and Frede M. Indianapolis: Hackett Publishing Company, 1985.

[Gallin and Ognibene, 2007] Gallin JI, and Ognibene FP (eds.). *Principles and Practices of Clinical Research*. Burlington, MA: Academic Press, 2007.

[Galton, 1987] Galton A (ed.). *Temporal Logics and Their Applications*. London: Academic Press, 1987.

[Garson, 2006] Garson JW. *Modal Logic for Philosophers*. Cambridge: Cambridge University Press, 2006.

[Geach and Black, 1952] Geach P, and Black M (eds.). *Translations from the Philosophical Writings of Gottlob Frege*. Oxford: Blackwell, 1952.

[Georgiou et al., 2008] Georgiou DN, Karakasidis TE, Nieto JJ, and Torres A. A study of genetic sequences using metric spaces and fuzzy sets. Manuscript, 2008.

[Gert, 2004] Gert B. *Common Morality: Deciding What To Do*. New York: Oxford University Press, 2004.

[Gert et al., 2006] Gert B, Culver CM, and Clouser KD (2006). *Bioethics: A Systematic Approach*. Oxford: Oxford University Press.

[Gettier, 1963] Gettier E, Jr. Is justified true belief knowledge? *Analysis* 1963; 23:121–123.

[Ghaemi, 2007] Ghaemi SN. *The Concepts of Psychiatry. A Pluralistic Approach to the Mind and Mental Illness*. Baltimore: The Johns Hopkins University Press, 2007.

[Giarratano and Riley, 2004] Giarratano J, and Riley G. *Expert Systems: Principles and Programming*. Boston: WPS Publishing Company 2004.

[Giere, 2006] Giere RN. *Scientific Perspectivism*. Chicago: The University of Chicago Press, 2006.

[Gillies, 2000] Gillies D. *Philosophical Theories of Probability*. London: Routledge, 2000.

[Givant and Halmos, 2009] Givant S, and Halmos P. *Introduction to Boolean Algebras*. New York: Springer Science and Business Media, 2009.

[Glass, 1976] Glass GV. Primary, secondaray, and meta-analysis of research. *Education Research* 1976; 5:3–8.

[Goble, 2002] Goble L (ed.). *The Blackwell Guide to Philosophical Logic*. Oxford: Blackwell Publishers, 2002.

[Gochet and Gribomont, 2006] Gochet P, and Gribomont P. Epistemic logic. In: Gabbay DM, and Woods J (eds.), *Handbook of the History of Logic, Volume 7, Logic and the Modalities in the Twentieth Century*, pp. 99–195. Amsterdam: Elsevier, 2006.

[Goclenius, 1613] Goclenius R. *Lexicon Philosophicum, quo tanquam clave Philosophiae fores aperiuntur*. Frankfurt a.M.: Musculus, 1613.

[Gödel, 1930] Gödel K. Die Vollständigkeit der Axiome des logischen Funktionenkalküls. *Monatshefte für Mathematik und Physik* 1930; 37:349–360. (English translation in [van Heijenoort, 1971], pp. 582–591.)

[Gödel, 1931] Gödel K. Über formal unentscheidbare Sätze der Principia mathematica und verwandter Systeme I. *Monatshefte für Mathematik und Physik* 1931; 38:173–198. (English translation in [van Heijenoort, 1971], pp. 596–616.)

[Gofman, 1992] Gofman JW. Bio-medical "un-knowledge" and nuclear pollution: A common-sense proposal. On the occasion of the Right Livelihood Award, Stockholm, December 9, 1992. http://www.ratical.org/radiation/CNR/BioMedUnknow.html. Last accessed on December 20, 2009.

[Goldblatt, 2006] Goldblatt R. Mathematical modal logic: A view of its evolution. In: Gabbay DM and Woods J (eds.), *Handbook of the History of Logic. Volume 7, Logic and the Modalities in the Twentieth Century,* pp. 1–98. Amsterdam: Elsevier, 2006.

[Goldman, 1979] Goldman AI. What is justified belief? In: Pappas G (ed.), *Justification and Knowledge,* pp. 1–23. Dordrecht: D. Reidel Publishing Company, 1979.

[Goldman, 1986] Goldman AI. *Epistemology and Cognition.* Cambridge, MA: Harvard University Press, 1986.

[Goldman, 1993] Goldman AI (ed.). *Readings in Philosophy and Cognitive Science.* Cambridge, MA: MIT Press, 1993.

[Goldman, 2003] Goldman AI. *Knowledge in a Social World.* Oxford: Oxford University Press, 2003.

[Goldman, 2004] Goldman AI. Reliabilism. In: Dancy J, and Sosa E (eds.), *A Companion to Epistemology,* pp. 433–436. Malden, MA: Blackwell Publishing, 2004.

[Gómez-Pérez et al, 2004] Gómez-Pérez A, Fernández-López, and Corcho O. *Ontological Engineering.* London: Springer, 2004.

[Goodman, 1975] Goodman N. Words, works, worlds. *Erkenntnis* 1975; 9:57–73.

[Goodwin et al., 1989] Goodwin CS, Armstrong JA, Chilvers T, Peters M, Collins MD, Sly L, McConnell W, and Harper WES. Transfer of Cympylobacter pylori and Campylobacter mustelae gen. nov. as Helicobacter pylori comb. nov. and Helicobacter mustelae comb. nov., respectively. *International Journal of Systematic Bacteriology* 1989; 39:397–405.

[Gorovitz and MacIntyre, 1976] Gorovitz S, and MacIntyre A. Toward a theory of medical fallibility. *The Journal of Medicine and Philosophy* 1976; 1:51–71.

[Gottwald, 2001] Gottwald S. *A Treatise on Many-Valued Logics.* Baldock: Research Studies Press Ltd., 2001.

[Gottwald, 2005] Gottwald S. Mathematical fuzzy logic as a tool for the treatment of vague information. *Information Sciences* 2005; 172:41–71.

[Gottwald, 2007] Gottwald S. Many-Valued Logics. In: Jacquette D (ed.), *Philosophy of Logic,* pp. 675–722. Amsterdam: Elsevier, 2007.

[Graff and Williamson, 2002] Graff D, and Williamson T (eds.). *Vagueness.* Hampshire, UK: Ashgate Publishing 2002.

[Grana, 1990] Grana N. *Logica deontica paraconsistente.* Naples: Liguori Editore, 1990.

[Grant and Subrahmanian, 1995] Grant J, and Subrahmanian VS. Reasoning in inconsistent knowledge bases. *IEEE Transactions on Knowledge and Data Engineering* 1995; 7:177–189.

[Grayling, 2004] Grayling AC. *An Introduction to Philosophical Logic.* Malden, MA: Blackwell Publishing, 2004.

[Grayston, 1965] Grayston JT. Immunisation against trachoma. *Pan American Health Organization Scientific Publications* 1965; 147:549.

[Grayston et al., 1989] Grayston JT, Kuo CC, Campbell LA, and Wang SP. Chlamydia pneumoniae, specia nova for Chlamydia sp. strain TWAR. *International Journal of Systematic Bacteriology* 1989; 39:88–90.

[Grenon et al., 2008] Grenon P, Smith B, and Goldberg L. Biodynamic ontology: Applying BFO in the biomedical domain. In: Burger A, Davidson D, and Baldock R (eds.), *Anatomy Ontologies for Bioinformatics,* pp. 20–38. Berlin: Springer-Verlag, 2008.

[Grewendorf and Meggle, 2002] Grewendorf G, and Meggle G (eds.). *Speech Acts, Mind, and Social Reality. Discussions with John R. Searle.* Dordrecht: Kluwer Academic Publishers, 2002.

[Grice, 1989] Grice HP. *Studies in the Ways of Words.* Cambridge, MA: Harvard University Press, 1989.

[Griesinger, 1845] Griesinger W. *Die Pathologie und Therapie der psychischen Krankheiten.* Stuttgart: A. Krabbe, 1845.

[Groopman, 2007] Groopman J. *How Doctors Think.* Boston: Houghton Mifflin Company, 2007.

[Gross and Löffler, 1997] Gross R, Löffler M. *Prinzipien der Medizin. Eine Übersicht ihrer Grundlagen und Methoden.* Berlin: Springer-Verlag, 1997.

[Grossmann, 1983] Grossmann R. *The Categorial Structure of the World.* Bloomington, Indiana: Indiana University Press, 1983.

[Grover, 1992] Grover D. *A Prosentential Theory of Truth.* Princeton: Princeton University Press, 1992.

[Grover et al., 1975] Grover D, Camp J, and Belnap N. A prosentential theory of truth. *Philosophical Studies* 1975; 27:73–125.

[Gruber, 1993] Gruber TR. A translation approach to portable ontology specifications. Knowledge Acquisition 1993; 5:199–220.

[Guarino and Musen, 2009] Guarino N, and Musen MA (eds.). *Applied Ontology. An Interdisciplinary Journal of Ontological Analysis and Conceptual Modeling.* http://www.iospress.nl/loadtop/load.php?isbn=15705838. Last accessed December 3, 2010.

[Gut, 2007] Gut A. *Probability: A Graduate Course.* New York: Springer-Verlag, 2007.

[Guyatt et al., 1992] Guyatt G, and 40 co-authors ('The Evidence-Based Medicine Working Group'). Evidence-based medicine: A new approach to teaching the practice of medicine. *JAMA* 1992; 268:2420–2425.

[Guyatt et al., 2008a] Guyatt G, Rennie D, Meade MO, and Cook DJ. *Users' Guides to the Medical Literature. A Manual for Evidence-Based Clinical Practice.* American Medical Association and McGraw-Hill Companies, 2008.

[Guyatt et al., 2008b] Guyatt G, Rennie D, Meade MO, and Cook DJ. *Users' Guides to the Medical Literature. Essentials of Evidence-Based Clinical Practice.* American Medical Association and McGraw-Hill Companies, 2008.

[Haack, 1996] Haack S. *Deviant Logic, Fuzzy Logic. Beyond the Formalism.* Chicago: The University of Chicago Press, 1996.

[Habermas, 1968a] Habermas J. *Technik und Wissenschaft als Ideologie.* Frankfurt: Suhrkamp, 1968.

[Habermas, 1968b] Habermas J. *Erkenntnis und Interesse*. Frankfurt: Suhrkamp, 1968. (English edition, trans. by Shapiro JJ: Knowledge and Human Interests. Boston: Beacon Press, 1971.)

[Habermas, 1973] Habermas J. Wahrheitstheorien. In: H. Fahrenbach (ed.), *Wirklichkeit und Reflexion,* pp. 211–265. Pfullingen: Verlag Günter Neske, 1973.

[Habermas, 2003] Habermas J. *Truth and Justification*. Translated by Barbara Fultner. Cambridge, MA: MIT Press, 2003.

[Hackett et al., 2007] Hackett EJ, Amsterdamska O, Lynch M, and Wajcman J (eds.). *The Handbook of Science and Technology Studies*. Cambridge, MA: The MIT Press, 2007.

[Hacking, 1965] Hacking I. *Logic of Statistical Inference*. Cambridge, UK: Cambridge University Press, 1965.

[Hacking, 1975a] Hacking I. *The Emergence of Probability: A Philosophical Study of Early Ideas About Probability, Induction and Statistical Inference*. Cambridge, UK: Cambridge University Press, 1975.

[Hacking, 1975b] Hacking I. All kinds of possibility. *Philosophical Review* 1975; 84: 321–347.

[Hacking, 2001] Hacking I. *An Introduction to Probability and Inductive Logic*. Cambridge, UK: Cambridge University Press, 2001.

[Hacking, 2003] Hacking I. *The Social Construction of What?* Cambridge, MA: Harvard University Press, 2003.

[Hackshaw, 2009] Hackshaw A. *A Concise Guide to Clinical Trials*. Hoboken, NJ: Wiley-Blackwell, 2009.

[Hage, 2005] Hage J. *Studies in Legal Logic*. Dordrecht: Springer, 2005

[Hajek, 2000] Hajek P. Fuzzy predicate calculus and fuzzy rules. In: Ruan D, and Kerre EE (eds.), *Fuzzy IF-THEN Rules in Computational Intelligence: Theory and Applications,* pp. 27–36. Dordrecht: Kluwer Academic Publishers, 2000.

[Hajek, 2002] Hajek P. *Metamathematics of Fuzzy Logic*. Dordrecht: Kluwer Academic Publishers, 2002.

[Hales and Welshon, 2000] Hales SD, and Welshon R. *Nietzsche's Perspectivism*. Urbana: University of Illinois Press, 2000.

[Halpern, 2009] Halpern P. Collider: *The Search for the World's Smallest Particles*. Hobken, NJ: John Wiley & Sons, Inc., 2009.

[Hampel et al., 2000] Hampel R, Wagenknecht M, and Chaker N (eds.). *Fuzzy Control: Theory and Practice*. Heidelberg: Physica-Verlag, 2000.

[Han and Kamber, 2005] Han J, and Kamber M. *Data Maining. Concepts and Techniques*. San Francisco: Morgan Kaufmann, 2005.

[Hanfling, 1981] Hanfling O. *Logical Positivism*. New York: Columbia University Press, 1981.

[Hanson, 1958] Hanson NR. *Patterns of Discovery*. Cambridge: Cambridge University Press, 1958.

[Hanson, 2009] Hanson SS. *Moral Acquaintances and Moral Decisions: Solving Moral Conflicts in Medical Ethics*. Dordrecht: Springer-Verlag, 2009.

[Hardwig, 1985] Hardwig J. Epistemic dependence. *The Journal of Philosophy* 1985; 82:335–349.

[Hartmann, 1977] Hartmann F. Wandlungen im Stellenwert von Diagnose und Prognose im ärztlichen Denken. *Metamed* 1977; 1:139–160.

[Hawkes, 2003] Hawkes T. *Structuralism and Semiotics*. London: Routledge, 2003.

[Heidegger, 1927] Heidegger M. *Sein und Zeit*. First published in Edmund Husserl's journal *Jahrbuch für Philosophie und phänomenologische Forschung*, Vol. VIII, Halle 1927. (Engl. transl. by John Macquarrie and Edward Robinson: *Being and Time*. New York: Harper & Row, 1962.)

[Heidegger, 1929] Heidegger M. Was ist Metaphysik? An inaugural lecture held at the University of Freiburg, Germany, 1929. See [Heidegger 1965].

[Heidegger, 1965] Heidegger M. *Was ist Metaphysik?* Frankfurt a.M.: Vittorio Klostermann, 1965 (9th edition).

[Heinroth, 1818] Heinroth JCA. *Lehrbuch der Störungen des Seelenlebens oder der Seelenstörungen und ihrer Behandlung*. Two volumes. Leipzig: F.C.W. Vogel, 1818.

[Heinroth, 1823] Heinroth JCA. *Lehrbuch der Seelengesundheitskunde*. Two volumes. Leipzig: F.C.W. Vogel, 1823–24.

[Heisenberg, 1958] Heisenberg W. *Die physikalischen Prinzipien der Quantentheorie*. Mannheim: Bibliographisches Institut, 1958.

[Hempel, 1943] Hempel CG. A purely syntactical definition of confirmation. *Journal of Symbolic Logic* 1943; 8:122–143.

[Hempel, 1945] Hempel CG. Studies in the logic of confirmation. *Mind* 1945; 54:1–26 and 97–121. Reprinted in [Hempel, 1965], pp. 3–51.

[Hempel, 1952] Hempel CG. *Fundamentals of Concept Formation in Empirical Science*. Chicago: The University of Chicago Press, 1952.

[Hempel, 1954] Hempel CG. A logical appraisal of operationism. *Scientific Monthly* 1954; 79:215–220. Reprinted in [Hempel 1965], pp. 123–133.

[Hempel, 1965] Hempel CG. *Aspects of Scientific Explanation and other Essays in the Philosophy of Science*. New York: Free Press, 1965.

[Hempel and Oppenheim, 1948] Hempel CG, and Oppenheim P. Studies in the logic of explanation. *Philosophy of Science* 1948; 15:135–175.

[Hermes, 1971] Hermes H. *Aufzählbarkeit, Entscheidbarkeit, Berechenbarkeit. Einführung in die Theorie der rekursiven Funktionen*. Heidelber: Springer-Verlag, 1971.

[Hermes, 1995] Hermes H. *Einführung in die Mathematische Logik*. Stuttgart: B.G. Teubner, 1995.

[Hesiod, 2007] Hesiod. *Works and Days*. Translated by Hugh G. Evelyn-White. First published 1914. Republished by Forgotten Books AG in www.forgottenbooks.org, 2007.

[Hesslow, 1976] Hesslow G. Two notes on the probabilistic approach to causality, *Philosophy of Science* 1976; 43:290–292.

[Hesslow, 1993] Hesslow G. Do we need a concept of disease? *Theoretical Medicine* 1993; 14:1–14.

[Heyting, 1971] Heyting A. *Intuitionism: An Introduction. Third Revised Edition*. Amsterdam: North-Holland Publishing Company, 1971.

[Heyting, 1975] Heyting A (ed.). *L.E.J. Brouwer: Collected Works 1: Philosophy and Foundations of Mathematics*. Amsterdam: Elsevier, 1975.

[Hilpinen, 1981] Hilpinen R (ed.). *New Studies in Deontic Logic: Norms, Actions and the Foundations of Ethics*. Dordrecht: D. Reidel Publishing Company 1981.

[Hilpinen, 2002] Hilpinen R. Deontic, Epistemic, and Temporal Modal Logics. In: Jacquette D (ed.), *A Companion to Philosophical Logic*, pp. 491–509. Oxford, UK: Blackwell Publishers, 2002.

[Hinkley, 2008] Hinkley AE. Metaphysical problems in the philosophy of medicine and bioethics. *The Journal of Medicine and Philosophy* 2008; 33:101–105.

[Hintikka, 1957] Hintikka J. Quantifiers in deontic logic. *Societas Scientiarum Fennica, Commentationes Humanarum Litterarum* 1957; 23(4):1–23.

[Hintikka, 1962] Hintikka J. *Knowledge and Belief: An Introduction to the Logic of the Two Notions.* Ithaca: Cornell University Press, 1962.

[Hintikka, 1972] Hintikka J. The semantics of modal notions and the indeterminacy of ontology. In: Davidson D, and Harman G (eds.), *Semantics of Natural Language,* pp. 398–414. Dordrecht: D. Reidel Publishing Company, 1972.

[Hintikka, 1973] Hintikka J. *Time and Necessity: Studies in Aristotles's Theory of Modality.* Oxford: Clarendon Press, 1973.

[Hodges, 2008] Hodges W. *Model Theory.* Cambridge: Cambridge University Press, 2008.

[Holzkamp, 1968] Holzkamp K. *Wissenschaft als Handlung.* Berlin: de Gruyter, 1968.

[Höppner et al., 2000] Höppner F, Klawonn F, Kruse R, and Runkler T. *Fuzzy Cluster Analysis: Methods for Classification, Data Analysis and Image Recognition.* New York: John Wiley & Sons, 2000.

[Horgan and Timmons, 2006] Horgan T, and Timmons M (eds.). *Metaethics After Moore.* Oxford: Oxford University Press, 2006.

[Hovda, 2009] Hovda P. What is classical mereology? *Journal of Philosophical Logic* 2009; 38:55–82.

[Hsu, 2004] Hsu CH. Fuzzy logic automatic control of the Phoenix-7 total artificial heart. *Journal of Artificial Organs* 2004; 7:69–76.

[Huang et al., 1999] Huang JW, Held CM, and Roy RJ. Hemodynamic management with multiple drugs using fuzzy logic. In: Teodorescu HN , Kandel A, and Jain LC (eds.), *Fuzzy and Neuro-Fuzzy Systems in Medicine,* pp. 320–340. Boca Raton: CRC Press, 1999.

[Hüllermeier, 2007] Hüllermeier E. *Case-Based Approximate Reasoning.* Dordrecht: Springer, 2007.

[Hughes and Cresswell, 2005] Hughes GE, and Cresswell MJ. *A New Introduction to Modal Logic.* London: Routledge, 2005.

[Humber and Almeder, 1997] Humber JM, Almeder RF (eds.). *What Is Disease?* Totowa, NJ: Humana Press, 1997.

[Hume, 1748] Hume D. *An Enquiry Concerning Human Understanding.* Modern Edition by LA Selby-Bigge. Oxford: The Clarendon Press, 1894.

[Hume, 1998a] Hume D. *Enquiry Concerning the Principles of Morals* (1751). Edited by TL Beauchamp. Oxford: Oxford University Press, 1998.

[Hume, 1998b] Hume D. *Dialogues Concerning Natural Religion* (1779). Edited by RH Popkin. Indianapolis, IN: Hackett Publishing Company, 1998.

[Hume, 2000] Hume D. *A Treatise of Human Nature* (1739–40). Edited by DF Norton and MJ Norton, Oxford: Oxford University Press, 2000.

[Husserl, 2001] Husserl E. *Logical Investigations.* Two volumes. London: Routledge, 2001. (First published in German. Halle: Max Niemeyer, 1900–1901.)

[Huxley, 1904] Huxley TH. On the Hypothesis that Animals are Automata. First published in 1874. Reprinted in: Huxley TH, *Collected Essays, Vol. 1, Method and Results,* 4th edition, pp. 199–250. London: Macmillan, 1904.

[Hyde, 2008] Hyde D. *Vagueness, Logic and Ontology.* Hampshire, UK: Ashgate Publishing 2008.

[Ibbeken, 2008] Ibbeken C. *Konkurrenzkampf der Perspektiven: Nietzsches Interpretation des Perspektivismus.* Würzburg: Verlag Königshausen & Neumann, 2008.

[ICDL, 2000] ICDL. *Clinical Practice Guidelines: Redefining the Standards of Care for Infants, Children and Families with Special Needs*. Bethesda, MD: The Interdisciplinary Council on Developmental and Learning Disorders, 2000.

[Jacquette, 1996] Jacquette D. *Meinongian Logic: The Semantics of Existence and Nonexistence*. Berlin: Walter de Gruyter, 1996.

[Jacquette, 2002] Jacquette D (ed.). *A Companion to Philosophical Logic*. Oxford: Blackwell Publishers Ltd., 2002.

[Jacquette, 2007] Jacquette D (ed.). *Philosophy of Logic*. Amsterdam: Elsevier, 2007.

[James, 1907] James W. *Pragmatism: A New Name for Some Old Ways of Thinking*. New York: Longmans, Green and Company, 1907.

[Jamison, 1956] Jamison BN. *An Axiomatic Treatment of Langrange's Equations*. M.S. Thesis. Stanford: Stanford University, 1956.

[Jansen and Smith, 2008] Jansen L, and Smith B (eds.). *Biomedizinische Ontologie: Wissen strukturieren für den Informatik-Einsatz*. Zürich: vdf Hochschulverlag AG, 2008.

[Jantzen, 2007] Jantzen J. *Foundations of Fuzzy Control*. Chichester: John Wiley and Sons Ltd., 2007.

[Jaśkowski, 1948] Jaśkowski S. Propositional calculus for contradictory deductive systems. *Studia Logica* 1969; 24:143–157. Originally published in Polish, in: *Studia Societatis Scientiarum Torunensis* 1948; Sectio A, Vol. I, Issue No. 5, pp. 55–77.

[Jaynes, 2003] Jaynes ET. *Probability Theory: The Logic of Science*. Cambridge, UK: Cambridge University Press 2003.

[Jecker et al., 2007] Jecker NS, Jonsen AR, and Pearlman RA. *Bioethics: An Introduction to the History, Methods, and Practice*. Sudbury, MA: 2007.

[Jeffrey, 1980] Jeffrey RC (ed.). *Studies in Inductive logic and Probability, Vol. 2*. Berkeley: University of California Press, 1980

[Jeffrey, 1990] Jeffrey RC. *The Logic of Decision*. Chicago: The University of Chicago Press, 1990.

[Jeffreys, 1939] Jeffreys H. *Theory of Probability*. Oxford: Oxford University Press, 1939.

[Jenicek, 1995] Jenicek M. *Epidemiology. The Logic of Modern Medicine*. Montreal: Epimed International, 1995.

[Jenicek, 2003] Jenicek M. *Foundations of Evidence-Based Medicine*. New York: The Parthenon Publishing Group, 2003.

[Jennings, 1989] Jennings RC. Zande logic and Western logic. *Brit. J. Phil. Sci.* 1989; 40:275–285.

[Jonsen, 1998] Jonsen AR. *The Birth of Bioethics*. Oxford: Oxford University Press, 1998.

[Jonsen and Toulmin, 1988] Jonsen AR, and Toulmin S. *The Abuse of Casuistry. A History of Moral Reasoning*. Berkeley: University of California Press, 1988.

[Josephson and Josephson, 1996] Josephson JR, and Josephson SG (eds.). *Abductive Inference: Computation, Philosophy, Technology*. Cambridge: Cambridge University Press, 1996.

[Jurisica et al., 1998] Jurisica I, Mylopoulos J, Glasgow J, Shapiro H, and Casper RF. Case-based reasoning in IVF: prediction and knowledge mining, *Artif Intell Med* 1998; 12:1–24.

[Jütte, 1996] Jütte R. *Geschichte der Alternativen Medizin. Von der Volksmedizin zu den unkonventionellen Therapien von heute*. München: Verlag C.H. Beck, 1996.

1062   References

[Kamp, 1968] Kamp H. *Tense Logic and the Theory of Linear Order*. PhD Thesis, University of California at Los Angeles, 1968.

[Kane, 2002] Kane R (ed.). *The Oxford Handbook of Free Will*. New York: Oxford University Press, 2002.

[Kane, 2003] Kane R (ed.). *Free Will*. Malden, MA: Blackwell Publishing Ltd., 2003.

[Kanger, 1957] Kanger S. *New Foundations for Ethical Theory*. Stockholm: Almqvist & Wiksell, 1957.

[Kant, 2003] Kant I. *Critique of Pure Reason*. Translated by Norman Kemp Smith. With a new preface by Howard Caygill. New York: Palgrave Macmillan, 2003. (First published 1781.)

[Kaufmann, 1975] Kaufmann A. *Introduction to the Theory of Fuzzy Subsets. Volume I: Fundamental Theoretical Elements*. New York: Academic Press, 1975.

[Kaufmann and Gupta, 1991] Kaufmann A, and Gupta MM. *Introduction to Fuzzy Arithmetic. Theory and Applications*. London: International Thomson Computer Press, 1991.

[Kaulbach, 1990] Kaulbach F. *Philosophie des Perspektivismus*. Tübingen: Mohr Siebeck, 1990.

[Keck, 2007] Keck FS. Wer hat vor die Therapie die Diagnose gesetzt? *Hessisches Ärzteblatt* 2007; 6: 388.

[Keefe, 2007] Keefe R. *Theories of Vagueness*. Cambridge: Cambridge University Press, 2007.

[Keefe and Smith, 1999] Keefe R, and Smith P (eds.). *Vagueness: A Reader*. Cambridge, MA: MIT Press, 1999.

[Keenan and Shannon, 1995] Keenan JF, and Shannon TA. *The Context of Casuistry*. Washington, DC: Georgetown University Press, 1995.

[Kendal and Creen, 2007] Kendal S, and Creen M. *An Introduction to Knowledge Engineering*. London: Springer-Verlag, 2007.

[Kenny, 2000] Kenny A. *Frege: An Introduction to the Founder of Modern Analytic Philosophy*. Oxford: Blackwell Publishers, 2000.

[Keravnou and Washbrook, 1989] Keravnou ET, and Washbrook J. Deep and shallow models in medical expert systems. *Artif Intell Med* 1989; 1:11–28.

[Keynes, 1921] Keynes JM. *A Treatise on Probability*. London: Macmillan, 1921.

[Kidd and Modlin, 1998] Kidd M, and Modlin I. A century of helicobacter pylori. Paradigms lost - Paradigms regained. *Digestion* 1998; 59:1–15.

[Kim, 2006] Kim J. *Philosophy of Mind*. Boulder: Westview Press, 2006.

[Kirkham, 1995] Kirkham RL. *Theories of Truth. A Critical Introduction*. Cambridge, MA: MIT Press, 1995.

[Kitchen, 2001] Kitchen M. *Kaspar Hauser: Europe's Child*. Houndmills, UK: Palgrave, 2001.

[Kleene, 1952] Kleene SC. *Introduction to Metamathematics*. Groningen: Wolters-Noordhoff Publishing, 1952.

[Kleinman, 1981] Kleinman A. *Patients and Healers in the Context of Culture. An Exploratin of the Borderland between Anthropology, Medicine, and Psychiatry*. Berkeley: University of California Press, 1981.

[Kleinman, 1988] Kleinman A. *The Illness Narratives. Suffering, Healing, and the Human Condition*. New York: Basic Books, 1988.

[Kleinman, 2006] Kleinman A. *What Really Matters. Living a Moral Life Admidst Uncertainty and Danger*. Oxford: Oxford University Press, 2006.

[Klir and Yuan, 1995] Klir GJ, and Yuan B. *Fuzzy Sets and Fuzzy Logic. Theory and Applications*. Upper Saddle River, NJ: Prentice Hall, 1995.

[Klir and Yuan, 1996] Klir GJ, and Yuan B (eds.). *Fuzzy Sets, Fuzzy Logic, and Fuzzy Systems. Selected Papers by Lotfi A. Zadeh.* Singapore: World Scientific, 1996.

[Kneale and Kneale, 1968] Kneale W, and Kneale M. *The Development of Logic.* Oxford: The Clarendon Press, 1968.

[Knorr Cetina, 1981] Knorr Cetina K. *The Manufacture of knowledge. An Essay on the Construction and Contextual Nature of Science.* Oxford: Pergamon Press, 1981.

[Knorr Cetina, 2003] Knorr Cetina K. *Epistemic Cultures. How Sciences Make Knowledge.* Cambridge, MA: Harvard University Press, 2003.

[Knuuttila, 1981] Knuuttila S. The emergence of deontic logic in the fourteenth century. In: Hilpinen R (ed.), *New Studies in Deontic Logic,* pp. 225–248. Dordrecht: D. Reidel Publishing Company, 1981.

[Knuuttila, 1988] Knuuttila S (ed.). *Modern Modalities. Studies of the History of Modal Theories from Medieval Nominalism to Logical Positivism.* Dordrecht: Kluwer Academic Publishers, 1988.

[Knuuttila, 1993] Knuuttila S. *Modalities in Medieval Philosophy.* Routledge: London, 1993.

[Koch, 1920] Koch, Richard. *Die ärztliche Diagnose. Beitrag zur Kenntnis des ärztlichen Denkens.* Wiesbaden: Verlag J.F. Bergmann, 1920.

[Kolmogorov, 1933] Kolmogorov AN. *Grundbegriffe der Wahrscheinlichkeitsrechnung.* Berlin: Springer-Verlag 1933.

[Kolodner, 1993] Kolodner JL. *Case-Based Reasoning.* San Mateo, CA: Morgan Kaufmann Publishers, 1993.

[Kolodner and Kolodner, 1987] Kolodner JL, and Kolodner RM. Using experience in clinical problem solving: Introduction and framework. *IEE Trans Syst Man Cybern* 1987; 17:420 and 431.

[Konturek et al., 1996] Konturek PC, Konturek JW, and Konturek SJ. Gastric secretion and the pathogenesis of peptic ulcer in Helicobacter pylori infection: Historical Background - Polish link to the discovery of spiral bacteria in the stomach. *J. Physiol.. Pharmacol* 1996; 47:5–19.

[Kosko, 1986] Kosko B. Fuzzy entropy and conditioning. *Information Sciences* 1986; 40:165-174.

[Kosko, 1992] Kosko B. *Neural Networks and Fuzzy Systems. A Dynamical Systems Approach to Machine Intelligence.* Englewood Cliffs, NJ: Prentice Hall, 1992.

[Kosko, 1997] Kosko, B. *Fuzzy Engineering.* Upper Saddle River, NJ: Prentice Hall, 1997.

[Koslicki, 2008] Koslicki K. *The Structure of Objects.* Oxford: Oxford University Press, 2008.

[Koton, 1988] Koton P. Reasoning about evidence in causal explanation. *Proceedings AAAI-88,* 1988; pp. 256–261.

[Koymans, 1990] Koymans R. Specifying real-time properties with metric temporal logic. *Real-Time Systems* 1990; 2:255–299.

[Kraft, 1953] Kraft V. *The Vienna Circle.* Translated by Arthur Pap. New York: Philosophical Library,1953.

[Kramer, 2009] Kramer MH. *Moral Realism as a Moral Doctrine.* Chichester: John Wiley & Sons Ltd., 2009.

[Krantz et al., 2007] Krantz DH, Luce RD, Suppes P, and Tversky A. *Foundations of Measurement, Volume I: Additive and Polynomial Representation.* Mineola, NY: Dover Publications Inc., 2007. (First published 1971 by Academic Press.)

[Kripke, 1959] Kripke SA. Semantical analysis of modal logic (abstract). *The Journal of Symbolic Logic* 1959; 24:1-14.

[Kripke, 1963] Kripke SA. Semantical analysis of modal logic I. Normal modal propositional calculi. *Zeitschrift für Mathematische Logik und Grundlagen der Mathematik* 1963; 9:67–96.

[Kripke, 1980] Kripke SA. *Naming and Necessity.* Oxford: Basil Blackwell, 1980.

[Kripke, 1982] Kripke SA. *Wittgenstein on Rules and Private Language.* Cambridge, MA: Harvard University Press, 1982.

[Kröger and Merz, 2008] Kröger F, and Merz S. *Temporal Logic and State Systems.* Berlin: Springer-Verlag, 2008.

[Kuhn, 1977] Kuhn TS. Second thoughts on paradigms. In: Suppe F (ed.), *The Structure of Scientific Theories,* second edition, pp. 459–482. Urbana: University of Illinois Press, 1977.

[Kuhn, 1996] Kuhn TS. *The Structure of Scientific Revolutions.* Chicago: The University of Chicago Press, 1996. (First published 1962.)

[Künne, 2003] Künne W. *Conceptions of Truth.* Oxford: Clarendon Press, 2003.

[Kusch, 2004] Kusch M. *Knowledge By Agreement.* Oxford: Clarendon Press, 2004.

[Lackey, 2010] Lackey J. *Learning from Words: Testimony as a Source of Knowledge.* Oxford: Oxford University Press, 2010.

[Lakatos, 1978] Lakatos I. *The Methodology of Scientific Research Programmes: Philosophical Papers Volume 1.* Cambridge: Cambridge University Press, 1978.

[Lakoff, 1973] Lakoff G. Hedges: A study in meaning criteria and the logic of fuzzy concepts. *Journal of Philosophical Logic* 1973; 2:458–508.

[Lakoff, 1987] Lakoff G. *Women, Fire, and Dangerous Things.* Chicago: The University of Chicago Press 1987.

[Lam et al., 1997] Lam SK, Ching CK, Lai KC, Chan CK, and Ong L. Does treatment of Helicobacter pylori with antibiotics alone heal duodenal ulcer? A randomised double blind placebo controlled study. *Gut* 1997; 41:43–48.

[Latour, 1987] Latour B. *Science in Action. How to ollow scientists and engineers through society.* Cambridge, MA: Harvard University Press, 1987.

[Latour and Woolgar, 1986] Latour B, and Woolgar S. *Laboratory Life. The Construction of Scientific Facts.* Princeton: Princeton University Press, 1986.

[Ledley and Lusted, 1959] Ledley RS, and Lusted LB. Reasoning foundations of medical diagnosis. *Science* 1959; 130:9–21.

[Leeland, 2010] Leeland AM. *Case-Based Reasoning: Processes, Suitability and Aplications.* Hauppauge NY: Nova Science Publishers, 2010.

[Lehrer, 2000] Lehrer K. *Theory of Knowledge.* Boulder: Westview Press, 2000.

[Leibniz, 2006] Leibniz GW. *Discourse on Metaphysics and the Monadology.* Translated by George R. Montgomery. Mineola, NY: Dover Publications, 2006.

[Lenzen, 1978] Lenzen W. Recent work in epistemic logic. *Acta Philosophica Fennica* 1978; 30: 5–219.

[Lenzen, 1980] Lenzen W. *Glauben, Wissen und Wahrscheinlichkeit.* Systeme der epistemischen Logik. Wien: Springer-Verlag, 1980.

[Lenzen, 2004] Lenzen W. Epistemic logic. In: Niiniluoto I, Sintonen M, and Woleński J (eds.), *Handbook of Epistemology,* pp. 963–983. Dordrecht: Kluwer Academic Publishers, 2004.

[Lewes, 1874] Lewes GH. *Problems of Life and Mind.* Five volumes. London: Trübner & Co., 1874–1879.

[Lewis, 1912] Lewis CI. Implication and the algebra of logic. *Mind* 1912; 21:522–531.

[Lewis, 1966] Lewis DK. An argument for the identity theory. *Journal of Philosophy* 1966; 63:17–25.

[Lewis, 1969] Lewis DK. *Convention*. Cambridge: Cambridge University Press, 1969.

[Lewis, 1973a] Lewis DK. Causation. *Journal of Philosophy* 1973; 70:556–567.

[Lewis, 1973b] Lewis DK. *Counterfactuals*. Oxford: Blackwell, 1973.

[Lewis, 2000] Lewis DK. Causation as influence. *The Journal of Philosophy* 2000; 97 (4):182–197.

[Lewis and Langford, 1932] Lewis CI, and Langford CH. *Symbolic Logic*. New York: The Century Co., 1932.

[Libet, 1985] Libet B. Unconscious cerebral initiative and the role of conscious will in voluntary action. *Behavioral and Brain Sciences* 1985; 8:529–566.

[Libet, 1999] Libet B. Do we have free will? *Journal of Consciousness Studies* 1999; 6/8–9:47–57.

[Libet, 2004] Libet B. *Mind Time: The Temporal Factor in Consciousness*. Cambridge, MA: Harvard University Press, 2004.

[Libet et al., 1982] Libet B, Wright EW, and Gleason CA. Readiness-potentials preceding unrestricted 'spontaneous' vs. pre-planned voluntary acts. *Electroencephalography and Clinical Neurophysiology* 1982; 54:322–35.

[Libet et al., 1983] Libet B, Gleason CA, Wright EW, and Pearl DK. Time of conscious intention to act in relation to onset of cerebral activity (readiness-potential). The unconscious initiation of a freely voluntary act. *Brain* 1983; 106:623–42.

[Libet et al., 1999] Libet B, Freeman A, and Sutherland K (eds.). *The Volitional Brain: Toward a Neuroscience of Free Will*. Exeter, UK: Imprint Academic, 1999.

[Ligeza, 2006] Ligeza A. *Logical Foundations for Rule-Based Systems*. Berlin: Springer-Verlag, 2006.

[Lin, 1997] Lin, CT. Adaptive subsethood for radial basis fuzzy systems. In [Kosko, 1997], Chapter 13, pp. 429–464.

[Lincoln, 2009] Lincoln D. *The Quantum Frontier: The Large Hadron Collider*. Baltimore: The Johns Hopkins University Press, 2009.

[Lind, 1753] Lind J. *A Treatise on the Scurvy. In Three Parts. Containing an Inquiry into the Nature, Causes and Cure of that Disease. Together with a Critical and Chronological View of what has been published on the Subject*. London: A. Millar, 1753.

[Lindahl and Lindwall, 1982] Lindahl O, Lindwall L. Is all therapy just a placebo effect? *Metamedicine* 1982; 3:255–259.

[Locke, 2008] Locke J. *An Essay Concerning Human Understanding*. Oxford: Oxford University Press, 2008. (Reprint. First published in 1690.)

[Lorhardus, 1606] Lorhardus J. *Ogdoas scholastica*. Sangalli (St. Gallen): Georgium Straub, 1606.

[Loux and Zimmermann, 2005] Loux NJ, and Zimmermann DW (eds.). *The Oxford Handbook of Metaphysics*. Oxford: Oxford University Press, 2005.

[Luce and Raiffa, 1989] Luce RD, Raiffa H. *Games and Decisions: Introduction and Critical Survey*. New York: Dover Publications, 1989.

[Luce et al., 2007] Luce RD, Krantz DH, Suppes P, and Tversky A. *Foundations of Measurement, Volume III: Representation, Axiomatization, and Invariance*. Mineola, NY: Dover Publications Inc., 2007. (First published 1990 by Academic Press.)

[Łukasiewicz, 1930] Łukasiewicz J. Philosophische Bemerkungen zu mehrwertigen Systemen des Aussagenkalküls. *Comptes Rendus des Séances de la Société de Sciences et des Lettres de Varsovie, Classe III* 1930; 23:51–77. (English translation in: McCall S (ed.), *Polish Logic 1920–1939*. With an Introduction by Tadeusz Kotarbinski, pp. 40–65. Oxford: Oxford University Press, 2005.)

[Łukasiewicz, 1970] Lukasiewicz J (1970). *Selected Works,* edited by L Borkowski. Amsterdam: North-Holland Publishing Company, 1970.

[Lusted, 1968] Lusted LB. *Introduction to Medical Decision Making.* Springfield: Charles C. Thomas, 1968.

[Lynch, 1985] Lynch M. *Art and Artifact in Laboratory Science: A Study of Shop Work and Shop Talk in a Research Laboratory.* London: Routledge and Kegan Paul, 1985.

[Lynch, 2001] Lynch MP (ed.). *The Nature of Truth. Classic and Contemporary Perspectives.* Cambridge, MA: MIT Press, 2001.

[Lyon, 1967] Lyon A. Causality. *Brit. J. Phil. Sci.,* 1967; 18:1–20.

[MacKenzie and Wajcman, 1999] MacKenzie D, and Wajcman J (eds.). *The Social Shaping of Technology.* Buckingham: Open University Press, 1999.

[Mackie, 1974] Mackie JL. *The Cement of the Universe. A Study of Causation.* Oxford: The Clarendon Press, 1974.

[Mahfouf et al., 2001] Mahfouf M, Abbod MF, and Linkens DA. A survey of fuzzy logic monitoring and control utilisation in medicine. *Artif Intell Med* 2001; 21:27–42.

[Maimon and Rokach, 2005] Maimon O, and Rokach R (eds.). *The Data Maining and Knowledge Discovery Handbook.* Berlin: Springer-Verlag, 2005.

[Mally, 1926] Mally E. *Grundgesetze des Sollens. Elemente der Logik des Willens.* Graz: Leuschner & Lubensky, 1926.

[Mandelbaum, 1963] Mandelbaum DG (ed.). *Selected Writings of Edward Sapir in Language, Culture, and Personality.* Berkeley: University of California Press, 1963.

[Mannheim, 1925] Mannheim K. Das Problem einer Soziologie des Wissens. *Archiv für Sozialwissenschaft und Sozialpolitik* 1925; 53: 577–652.

[Mannheim, 1929] Mannheim K. *Ideologie und Utopie.* Bonn: Friedrich Cohen, 1929. All page references are to the English edition in [Mannheim, 1985].

[Mannheim, 1985] Mannheim K. *Ideology and Utopia. An Introduction to the Sociology of Knowledge.* Translated from German by Louis Wirth and Edwards Shils. San Diego: Harcourt Inc., 1985.

[Marcum, 2008] Marcum JA. *An Introductory Philosophy of Medicine: Humanizing Modern Medicine.* Dordrecht: Springer-Verlag, 2008.

[Marek and Truszcyński, 1993] Marek VW, and Truszcyński M. *Nonmonotonic Logic: Context-Depedent Reasoning.* Berlin: Springer-Verlag 1993.

[Margolis, 1969] Margolis J. Illness and medical values. *Philosophy Forum* 1969; 8:55–76.

[Margolis, 1976] Margolis J. The concept of disease. *The Journal of Medicine and Philosophy* 1976; 1:238–255.

[Marshall, 1994] Marshall BJ. Helicobacter pylori. *American Journal of Gastroenerology* 1994; 89 (Suppl. 8), S116–S128.

[Marshall, 2002a] Marshall BJ. The discovery that Helicobacter pylori, a spiral bacterium, caused peptic ulcer disease. In [Marshall, 2002b], pp. 165–202.

[Marshall, 2002b] Marshall BJ (ed.) *Helicobacter Pioneers. Firsthand accounts from the scientists who discovered helicobacters, 1892–1982.* Singapore: Blackwell Science Asia Pry Ltd., 2002.

[Marshall and Warren, 1984] Marshall BJ, and Warren JR. Unidentified curved bacilli in the stomach of patients with gastritis and peptic ulceration. *Lancet* 1984; Vol. 1, 1311–1315.

[Marshall et al., 1985] Marshall BJ, Armstrong JA, McGechie DB, and Clancy RJ. Attempt to fulfil Koch's postulates for pyloric campbylobacter. *Medical Journal of Australia* 1985; 142:436–439.

[Marx and Engels, 1975] Marx K, and Engels F. *Collected Works.* New York and London: International Publishers, 1975.

[Massad et al., 2008] Massad E, Ortega NRS, de Barros LC, and Struchiner CJ. *Fuzzy Logic in Action: Applications in Epidemiology and Beyond.* Berlin: Springer-Verlag, 2008.

[Masterman, 1970] Masterman M. The nature of a paradigm. In: Lakatos I, and Musgrave A (eds.), *Criticism and the Growth of Knowledge,* pp. 59–90. Cambridge: Cambridge University Press, 1970.

[Mates, 1989] Mates B. *The Philosophy of Leibniz: Metaphysics and Language.* Oxford: Oxford University Press, 1989.

[Matthews, 2006] Matthews JNS. *Introduction to Randomized Controlled Clinical Trials.* Second Edition. Boca Raton, FL: Chapman & Hall / CRC, 2006.

[Maurin, 2002] Maurin A-S. *If Tropes.* Dordrecht: Kluwer Academic Publishers, 2002.

[Mauris et al., 1996] Mauris G, Benoit E, and Foulloy L. Fuzzy sensors: An overview. In: Dubois D, Prade H, and Yager RR (eds.), *Fuzzy Information Engineering,* pp. 13–30. New York: John Wiley and Sons, 1996.

[McCall, 2005] McCall S (ed.). *Polish Logic 1920–1939. With an Introduction by Tadeusz Kotarbinski.* Oxford: Oxford University Press, 2005.

[McCulloch and Pitts, 1943] McCulloch MS, and Pitts WA. A logical calculus of the ideas immanent in nervous activity. *Bulletin of Mathematical Biophysics* 1943; 5:115–133.

[McKinsey et al., 1953] McKinsey JCC, Sugar AC, and Suppes P. Axiomatic foundations of classical particle mechanics. *Journal of Rational Mechanics and Analysis* 1953; 2:253–272.

[McKinsey and Suppes, 1955] McKinsey JCC, and Suppes P. On the notion of invariance in classical mechanics. *Brit. J. Phil. Sci.* 1955; 5:290–302.

[McNamara, 2006] McNamara P. Deontic Logic. In: Gabbay DM, and Woods J (eds.), *Handbook of the History of Logic, Volume 7, Logic and the Modalities in the Twentieth Century,* pp. 197–288. Amsterdam: Elsevier, 2006.

[McNeill and Freiberger, 1993] McNeill D, Freiberger P. *Fuzzy Logic. The Revolutionary Computer Technology That is Changing Our World.* New York: Simon and Schuster, 1993.

[Meggle, 2002a] Meggle G. Common belief and common knowledge. In: Sintonen M, Ylikoski P, and Miller K (eds.), *Realism in Action,* pp. 244–251. Dordrecht: Kluwer Academic Publishers, 2002.

[Meggle, 2002b] Meggle G. Mutual knowledge and belief. In: Meggle G (ed.), *Social Facts and Collective Intentionality,* pp. 205–223. Frankfurt: Dr. Hänsel-Hohenhausen AG.

[Meinong, 1904] Meinong A. Über Gegenstandstheorie. In: A Meinong (ed.), *Untersuchungen zur Gegenstanstheorie und Psychologie*, pp. 1–50. Leipzig: Verlag von Johann Ambrosius Barth, 1904. Translated as 'The theory of objects' in Chisholm RM (ed.), *Realism and the Background of Phenomenology*, pp. 76–117. New York: Free Press, 1960.

[Meja and Stehr, 1999] Meja V, and Stehr N (eds.). *The Sociology of Knowledge*. (The International Library of Critical Writings in Sociology, Volume 12.) Cheltenham, UK: Edward Elgar Publishing, 1999.

[Mellor, 1971] Mellor DH. *The Matter of Chance*. Cambridge: Cambridge University Press, 1971.

[Mendall et al., 1995] Mendall MA, Carrington D, Strachan D, et al. Chlamydia pneumoniae: risk factors for seropositivity and association with coronary heart disease. *J. Infect.* 1995; 30:121–128.

[Meyer and van der Hoek, 2004] Meyer JJC, and van der Hoek W. *Epistemic Logic for AI and Computer Science*. Cambridge: Cambridge University Press, 2004.

[Miamoto, 2008] Miamoto S, Ichihashi H, and Honda K. *Algorithms for Fuzzy Clustering: Methods in c-Means Clustering with Applications*. Berlin: Springer-Verlag 2008.

[Michels et al., 2006] Michels K, Klawonn F, Kruse R, and Nürnberger A. *Fuzzy Control: Fundamentals, Stability and Design of Fuzzy Controllers*. Berlin: Springer-Verlag, 2006.

[Miettinen et al., 1996] Miettinen H, Lehto S, Saikku P, et al. Association of Chlamydia pneumoniae and acute coronary heart disease events in non-insulin dependent diabetic and non-diabetic subjects in Finland. *European Heart Journal* 1996; 17:682–688.

[Mikenberg et al., 1986] Mikenberg IF, da Costa NCA, and Chuaqui R. Pragmatic truth and approximation to truth. *Journal of Symbolic Logic* 1986; 51:201–221.

[Mill, 1843] Mill JS. *A System of Logic*. London: John W. Parker, 1843.

[Miller, 1974] Miller D. Poppers's qualitative theory of verisimilitude. *Brit. J. Phil. Sci.* 1974; 25:155–160.

[Miller, 2003] Miller A. *An Introduction to Contemporary Metaethics*. Cambridge, UK: Polity Press, 2003.

[Money, 1992] Money J. *The Kaspar Hauser Syndrome of "Psychological Dwarfism": Deficient Statural, Intellectual, and Social Growth Induced by Child Abuse*. Amherst, NY: Prometheus Books, 1992.

[Monk, 1976] Monk JD. *Mathematical Logic*. New York: Springer-Verlag, 1976.

[Montgomery, 2006] Montgomery K. *How Doctors Think. Clinical Judgment and the Practice of Medicine*. New York: Oxford University Press, 2006.

[Moore, 1936] Moore GE. Is existence a predicate? *Aristotelean Society Supplementary* 1936; 15:154–188.

[Moore and Hutchins, 1980] Moore GW, and Hutchins GM. Effort and demand logic in medical decision making. *Metamedicine* 1980; 1:277–303.

[Moore and Hutchins, 1981] Moore GW, and Hutchins GM. A Hintikka possible world model for certainty levels in medical decision making. *Synthese* 1981; 48:87–119.

[Mordeson et al., 2000] Mordeson JN, Malik DS, and Cheng SC. Fuzzy Mathematics in Medicine. Heidelberg: Physika-Verlag, 2000.

[Mordeson and Malik, 2002] Mordeson JN, and Malik DS. *Fuzzy Automata and Languages: Theory and Applications*. Boca Raton, FL: Chapman & Hall/CRC 2002.

[Mordeson and Nair, 2001] Mordeson JN, and Nair PS. *Fuzzy Mathematics.* Heidelberg: Physica-Verlag, 2001.

[Morgan, 1923] Morgan CL. *Emergent Evolution.* London: Williams & Norgate, 1923.

[Morgagni, 1761] Morgagni GB. *De Sedibus et Causis Morborum per Anatomen Indagatis.* Venice: Remondini, 1761.

[Morris, 1938] Morris CW. *Foundations of the Theory of Signs.* Chicago: The University of Chicago Press, 1938.

[Moulines, 1975] Moulines CU. A logical reconstruction of simple equilibrium thermodynamics. *Erkenntnis* 1975; 9:101–130.

[Moulines, 2008] Moulines CU. *Die Entwicklung der modernen Wissenschaftstheorie (1890–2000). Eine historische Einführung.* Münster: Lit Verlag, 2008.

[Mueller-Kolck, 2010] Mueller-Kolck U. *The Logical Structure of Clinical Medicine.* Norderstedt, Germany: Books on Demand, 2010.

[Muhlestein et al., 1996] Muhlestein JB, Hammond EH, Carlquist JF, et al. Increased incidence of Chlamydia species within coronary arteries of patients with symptomatic atherosclerosis versus other forms of cardiovascular disease. *J. Amer. College of Cardiol.* 1996; 27:1555–1561.

[Müller, 1985] Müller U. *Die Struktur der Ionentheorie der Erregung von A.L. Hodgkin, A.F. Huxley und B. Katz.* Tecklenburg: Burgverlag, 1985.

[Müller and Pilatus, 1982] Müller U, and Pilatus S. On Hodgkin and Huxley's theory of excitable membranes. *Metamedicine* 1982; 3:193–208.

[Munson, 1981] Munson R. Why medicine cannot be a science. *The Journal of Medicine and Philosophy* 1981; 6:183–208.

[Murphy, 1997] Murphy EA. *The Logic of Medicine.* Baltimore: The Johns Hopkins University Press, 1997.

[Naegeli, 1937] Naegeli O. *Differentialdiagnose in der inneren Medizin,* Leipzig: Thieme, 1937.

[Nagel and Newman, 1958] Nagel E, and Newman JR. *Gödel's Proof.* New York: New York University Press, 1958.

[Naunyn, 1909] Naunyn B. "Physicians and laymen" (in German, 1900). Reprinted in: *Gesammelte Abhandlungen 1862–1909, Vol. 2,* pp. 1327–1355. Würzburg: Stürtz, 1909.

[Neapolitan, 1990] Neapolitan RE. *Probabilistic Reasoning in Expert Systems: Theory and Algorithms.* New York: John Wiley & Sons, 1990.

[Nietzsche, 1955] Nietzsche F. *Beyond Good and Evil: Prelude to a Philosophy of the Future.* (In German.) In: *Werke in drei Bänden. Vol. 2,* pp. 563–759. München: Carl Hanser Verlag, 1954 (1), 1955 (2), 1966 (3).

[NIH, 1994] NIH 1994. Helicobacter pylori in peptic ulcer disease. *NIH Consensus Statement* 1994 Jan 7–9; 12(1) 1–23.

[Niiniluoto et al., 2004] Niiniluoto I, Sintonen M, and Woleński J (eds.). *Handbook of Epistemology.* Dordrecht: Kluwer Academic Publishers, 2004.

[Novak et al., 2000] Novak V, Perfilieva I, and Mockor J. *Mathematical Principles of Fuzzy Logic.* Dordrecht: Kluwer Academic Publishers, 2000.

[O'Connor, 1975] O'Connor DJ. *The Correspondence Theory of Truth.* London: Hutchinson, 1975.

[O'Connor, 2000] O'Connor T. *Persons and Causes: The Metaphysics of Free Will.* New York: Oxford University Press, 2000.

[Oehler, 1961] Oehler K. Der consensus omnium als Kriterium der Wahrheit in der antiken Philosophie und Patristik. *Antike und Abendland* 1961; 10:103–129.

[Oesterlen, 1852] Oesterlen F. *Medizinische Logik.* Tübingen: Verlag der H. Laupp'schen Buchhandlung, 1852.

[Ogden and Richards, 1989] Ogden CK, and Richards IA. *The Meaning of Meaning.* San Diego: Harcourt Brace Jovanovich Publishers, 1989. (First published 1923.)

[Øhrstrøm and Hasle, 1995] Øhrstrøm P, and Hasle P. *Temporal Logic: From Ancient Ideas to Artificial Intelligence.* Dordrecht: Kluwer Acedemic Publishers, 1995.

[Øhrstrøm and Hasle, 2006] Øhrstrøm P, and Hasle P. Modern temporal logic. In: Gabbay DM, and Woods J (eds.), *Handbook of the History of Logic, Volume 7, Logic and the Modalities in the Twentieth Century,* pp. 447–498. Amsterdam: Elsevier, 2006.

[Osborne, 2004] Osborne MJ. *An Introduction to Game Theory.* New York: Oxford University Press, 2004.

[Ouellette and Byrne, 2004] Ouellette SP, and Byrne GI. Chlamydia pneumoniae: Prospects and predictions for an emerging pathogen. In: Friedman H, Yamamoto Y, and Bendinelli M (eds.), *Chlamydia pneumoniae: Infection and Disease,* pp. 1–9. New York: Kluwer Academic / Plenum Publishers, 2004.

[Pal et al., 2001] Pal SK, Dillon TS, and Yeung DS (eds.). *Soft Computing in Case-Based Reasoning.* London: Springer, 2001.

[Pal and Shiu, 2004] Pal SK, and Shiu SCK. *Foundations of Soft Case-Based Reasoning.* Hoboken, NJ: John Wiley & Sons, 2004.

[Parsons, 1951] Parsons T (Talcott). *The Social System.* Glencoe, IL: The Free Press, 1951.

[Parsons, 1980] Parsons T (Terence). *Nonexistent Objects.* New Haven, CT: Yale University Press, 1980

[Pass, 2004] Pass S. *Parallel Paths to Constructivism.* Jean Piaget and Lev Vygotsky. Charlotte, NC: Information Age Publishing, 2004.

[Passmore and Robson, 1975] Passmore R, and Robson JS. *A Companion to Medical Studies, Vol. 3, Part I.* Oxford: Blackwell, 1975.

[Pauker and Kassirer, 1980] Pauker SG, and Kassirer JP. The threshold approach to clinical decision making. *N. Engl. J. Med.* 1980; 302:1109–1117.

[Pearl, 2001] Pearl J. *Causality: Models, Reasoning, and Inference.* Cambridge: Cambridge University Press, 2001.

[Peirce, 1902] Peirce CS. Vague. In: Baldwin JM (ed.), *Dictionary of Philosophy and Psychology,* p. 748. New York: Macmillan, 1902.

[Peirce, 1931] Peirce CS. *Collected Papers* (8 vols.). Edited by Charles Hartshorne and Paul Weiss (vols. 1–6) and Arthur W Burks (vols. 7–8). Cambridge, MA: Harvard University Press, 1931–1958.

[Peleg, 2008] Peleg R. Is truth a supreme value? *Journal of Medical Ethics* 2008; 34:325–326.

[Pellegrino, 2008] Pellegrino ED. *The Philosophy of Medicine Reborn: A Pellegrino Reader.* Edited by HT Engelhardt, Jr., and F Jotterand. Notre Dame: University of Notre Dame Press, 2008.

[Pellegrino and Thomasma, 1981] Pellegrino ED, and Thomasma DC. *A Philosophical Basis for Medical Practice: Toward a Philosophy and Ethics of the Healing Profession.* New York: Oxford University Press, 1981.

[Penfield and Jasper, 1954] Penfield WG, and Jasper HH. *Epilepsy and the functional Anatomy of the Human Brain.* Boston: Little Brown, 1954.

[Penner and Hull, 2008] Penner PS, and Hull RT. The beginning of individual human personhood. *The Journal of Medicine and Philosophy* 2008; 33:174–182.

[Penrose, 1996] Penrose R. *Shadows of Mind: A Search for the Missing Science of Consciousness.* Oxford: Oxford University Press, 1996.

[Penrose, 2002] Penrose R. *The Emperor's New Mind: Concerning Computers, Minds, and the Laws of Physics.* Oxford: Oxford University Press, 2002.

[Perry, 1986] Perry J. From worlds to situations. *Journal of Philosophical Logic* 1986; 15:83–107.

[Perry, 2000] Perry J. *The Problem of the Essential Indexical and Other Essays, Expanded Edition.* Stanford, CA: Center for the Study of Language and Information, 2000.

[Perszyk, 1993] Perszyk, KJ. *Nonexistent Objects. Meinong and Contemporary Philosophy.* Dordrecht: Kluwer Academic Publishers, 1993.

[Petitti, 2000] Petitti DB. *Meta-Analysis, Decision Analysis, and Cost-Effectiveness Analysis. Methods for Quantitative Synthesis in Medicine.* New York: Oxford University Press, 2000.

[Piaget, 1937] Piaget J. *La construction du réel che l' enfant.* Neuchatel: Delacheaux, 1937.

[Piantadosi, 2005] Piantadosi S. *Clinical Trials: A Methodological Perspective.* Hoboken, NJ: John Wiley & Sons, 2005.

[Pickering, 1984] cit: Pickering1984 Pickering A. *Constructing Quarks: A Sociological History of Particle Physics.* Edinburgh: Edinburgh University Press, 1984.

[Pickering, 1992] Pickering A (ed.). *Science as Practice and Culture.* Chicago: The University of Chicago Press, 1992.

[Pickering, 1995] Pickering A. *The Mangle of Practice. Time, Agency, and Science.* Chicago: The University of Chicago Press, 1995.

[Pilatus, 1985] Pilatus S. *Die Struktur der Assoziations-Induktions-Theorie von Gilbert Ning Ling.* Burgverlag: Tecklenburg, 1985.

[Pinel, 1798] Pinel P. *Nosographie philosophique, ou la méthode de l'analyse appliquée à la médecine.* Paris: Mardan, 1798.

[Pinel, 1801] Pinel P. *Traité médico-philosophique sur l'aliénation mentale, ou la manie.* Paris: Richard, Caille et Ravier, 1801.

[Pisanelli, 2007] Pisanelli DM (ed.). *Ontologies in Medicine.* Amsterdam: IOS Press, 2007.

[Pitcher, 1964] Pitcher G (ed.). *Truth.* Englewood Cliffs: Prentice Hall, 1964.

[Place, 1956] Place UT. Is consciousness a brain process? *British Journal of Psychology* 1956; 47:44–50.

[Place, 2004] Place, UT. *Identifying the Mind. Selected Papers of UT Place. Edited by G. Graham and E.R. Valentine.* Oxford: Oxford University Press, 2004.

[Planck, 1949] Planck M. *Scientific Autobiography and Other Papers. Translated by Frank Gaynor.* New York: Philosophical Library Inc., 1949.

[Plato, 1973] Plato. *Theaetetus. Translated by John McDowell.* Oxford: Oxford University Press, 1973.

[Plato, 1993] Plato. *Sophist. Translated by NP White.* Indianapolis, IN: Hackett Publishing Company, 1993.

[Plato, 1998] Plato. *Cratylus. Translated by CDC Reeve.* Indianapolis, IN: Hackett Publishing Company, 1998.

[Plato, 2008] Plato. Meno. *Translated   by   Benjamin   Jowett.* www.forgottenbooks.org, 2008.

[Pollock, 1986] Pollock J. *Contemporary Theories of Knowledge.* Totowa: Rowman and Littlefield, 1986.

[Pontow and Schubert, 2006] Pontow C, and Schubert R. A mathematical analysis of theories of parthood. *Data and Knowledge Engineering* 2006; 59:107–138.

[Popkorn, 2003] Popkorn S. *First Steps in Modal Logic.* Cambridge: Cambridge University Press, 2003.

[Popper, 1945] Popper, Karl Raimund. *The Open Society and Its Enemies.* London: Routledge and Kegan Paul, 1945.

[Popper, 1957] Popper, Karl Raimund. The propensity interpretation of the calculus of probability, and the quantum theory. In Körner S (ed.), *Observation and Interpretation,* pp. 65–70. London: Butterworths Scientific Publications, 1957.

[Popper, 1959] Popper, Karl Raimund. The Propensity Interpretation of Probability. *Brit. J. Phil. Sci.* 1959; 10:25–42.

[Popper, 1963] Popper, Karl Raimund. *Conjectures and Refutations.* London: Routledge and Kegan Paul, 1963.

[Popper, 1972] Popper, Karl Raimund. *Objective Knowledge.* Oxford: The Clarendon Press, 1972.

[Popper, 1978] Popper, Karl Raimund. Natural selection and the emergence of mind. *Dialectica* 1978; 32:339–355.

[Popper, 2004] Popper, Karl Raimund. *The Logic of Scientific Discovery.* London: Routledge, 2004. (First published 1935 in German by Julius Springer, Vienna.)

[Popper and Eccles, 1985] Popper, Karl Raimund, and Eccles JC. *The Self and Its Brain.* Heidelberg: Springer-Verlag, 1985.

[Post, 1921] Post EL. Introduction to a general theory of elementary propositions. *American Journal of Mathematics* 1921; 43:163–185.

[Priest, 1987] Priest G. *In Contradiction.* Dordrecht: Nijhoff, 1987.

[Priest, 2002] Priest G. 'Paraconsistent logic'. In: Gabbay DM, and Guenthner F (eds.), *Handbook of Philosophical Logic, 2nd edition, Vol. 6,* pp. 287–393. Dordrecht: Kluwer Academic Publishers, 2002.

[Priest, 2007] Priest G. *Toward Non-Being: The Logic and Metaphysics of Intentionality.* Oxford: Clarendon Press, 2007.

[Priest, 2008] Priest G. *An Introduction to Non-Classical Logic.* Cambridge, UK: Cambridge University Press, 2008.

[Priest et al., 1989] Priest G, Routley R, and Norman J (eds.). *Paraconsistent Logics. Essays on the Inconsistent.* München: Philosophia Verlag, 1989.

[Prior, 1955] Prior AN. Diodoran modalities. *Philosophical Quarterly* 1955; 5:205–213.

[Prior, 1957] Prior AN. *Time and Modality.* Oxford: Clarendon Press, 1957.

[Prior, 1967] Prior AN. *Past, Present and Future.* Oxford: Clarendon Press, 1967.

[Prior, 1968] Prior AN. *Papers on Time and Tense.* Oxford: Clarendon Press, 1968.

[Putnam, 1960] Putnam HW. Minds and Machines. In: Hook S (ed.), *Dimensions of Mind,* pp. 138–164. New York: Collier Books, 1960.

[Putnam, 1962] Putnam HW. What theories are not. In: Nagel E, Suppes P, and Tarski A (eds.), *Logic, Methodology and Philosophy of Science,* pp. 240–251. Stanford, CA: Stanford University Press, 1962.

[Quine, 1943] Quine WVO. Notes on existence and necessity. *Journal of Philosophy* 1943; 40:113–127.

[Quine, 1947] Quine WVO. The problem of interpreting modal logic. *The Journal of Symbolic Logic* 1947; 12:43–48.

[Quine, 1948] Quine WVO. On what there is. *Review of Metaphysics* 1948; 5:21–38. Reprinted in [Quine, 1963], pp. 1–19. All page references are to the reprinted version.

[Quine, 1951] Quine WVO. Two dogmas of empiricism. *The Philosophical Review* 1951; 60:20–43. Reprinted in [Quine, 1963], pp. 20–46. All page references are to the reprinted version.

[Quine, 1953a] Quine WVO. Reference and modality (grown out of a fusion of [Quine, 1943] with [Quine, 1947]). Reprinted in [Quine, 1963], pp. 139–159. All page references are to the reprinted version.

[Quine, 1953b] Quine WVO. On mental entities. *Proceedings of the American Academy of Arts and Sciences* 1953; 80:198–203.

[Quine, 1960] Quine WVO. *Word and Object*. Cambridge, MA: MIT Press, 1960.

[Quine, 1963] Quine WVO. *From A Logical Point of View*. New York: Harper and Row, 1963.

[Quine, 1966] Quine WVO. *Methods of Logic*. London: Routledge and Kegan Paul, 1966.

[Quine, 1969a] Quine WVO. Ontological Relativity. In [Quine, 1969c], pp. 26–68.

[Quine, 1969b] Quine WVO. Epistemology naturalized. In [Quine, 1969c], pp. 69–90

[Quine, 1969c] Quine WVO. *Ontological Relativity and other Essays*. New York: Columbia University Press, 1969.

[Quine, 1970] Quine WVO. *Philosophy of Logic*. Englewood Cliffs, NJ: Prentice Hall Inc., 1970.

[Quine, 1973] Quine WVO. *Philosophie der Logik*. Stuttgart: Verlag W. Kohlhammer, 1973. (German edition of [Quine, 1970].)

[Quine, 1992] Quine WVO. *Pursuit of Truth*. Cambridge, MA: Harvard University Press, 1992.

[Quine, 1995] Quine WVO. *Unterwegs zur Wahrheit*. Paderborn: Ferdinand Schöningh, 1995 (German edition of [Quine, 1992].)

[Ramsey, 1922] Ramsey FP. The nature of truth. Posthumusly published in: *Episteme* 1990; 16:6–16. Originally written in 1922.

[Ramsey, 1926] Ramsey FP. Truth and probability (written in 1926). Reprinted in Ramsey 1931, pp. 156–198. All page references are to the reprint in [Ramsey, 1931].

[Ramsey, 1927] Ramsey FP. Facts and propositions. *Proceedings of the Aristotelean Society* 1927; Suppl. Vol. 7, pp. 153–170. All page references are to the reprint in [Ramsey, 1931].

[Ramsey, 1931] Ramsey FP. *The Foundations of Mathematics and other Logical Essays*. Edited by RB Braithwaite. London: Routledge & Kegan Paul Ltd., 1931.

[Reed, 1972] Reed SK. Pattern recognition and categorization. *Cognitive Psychology* 1972; 3:382–407.

[Reichenbach, 1935] Reichenbach H. *Wahrscheinlichkeitslehre. Eine Untersuchung über die logischen und mathematischen Grundlagen der Wahrscheinlichkeitsrechnung*. Leiden: A.W. Sijthoff's Uitgeversmij N.V., 1935. (English translation: The Theory of Probability. Berkeley: University of California Press, 1949.)

[Reichenbach, 1938] Reichenbach H. *Experience and Prediction. An Analysis of the Foundations and the Structure of Knowledge*. Chicago: The University of Chicago Press, 1938

[Reichenbach, 1944] Reichenbach H. *Philosophical Foundations of Quantum Mechanics*. Berkeley: University of California Press, 1944.

[Reichenbach, 1956] Reichenbach H. *The Direction of Time*. Berkeley: University of California Press, 1956.

[Reisner, 1982] Reisner TA. De Quincey's palimpsest reconsidered. *Modern Language Studies* 1982; 12:93–95.

[Reiter, 1987] Reiter R. A theory of diagnosis from first principles. *Artificial Intelligence* 1987; 32: 57–95.

[Rescher, 1968] Rescher N. *Topics in Philosophical Logic*. Dordrecht: D. Reidel Publishing Company, 1968.

[Rescher, 1969] Rescher N. *Many-Valued Logic*. New York: McGraw-Hill, 1969.

[Rescher, 1973] Rescher N. *The Coherence Theory of Truth*. Oxford: Oxford University Press, 1973.

[Rescher, 2005] Rescher N. *Epistemic Logic. A Survey of the Logic of Knowledge*. Pittsburgh: University of Pittsburgh Press, 2005.

[Reznek, 1987] Reznek L. *The Nature of Disease*. London: Routledge and Kegan Paul, 1987.

[Reznek, 1991] Reznek L. *The Philosophical Defence of Psychiatry*. London: Routledge, 1991.

[Richman, 1962] Richman RJ. Something common. *The Journal of Philosophy* 1962; 59:821–830.

[Rickey and Srzednicki, 1986] Rickey VF, and Srzednicki JT (eds.). *Leśniewski's Systems: Ontology and Mereology*. Heidelberg: Springer-Verlag, 1986.

[Ridker et al., 1997] Ridker PM, Cushman M, Stampfer M, et al. Inflammation, aspirin, and the risk of cardiovascular disease in apparently healthy men, *N. Engl. J. Med.* 1997; 336:973–979.

[Roeper and Leblanc, 1999] Roeper P, and Leblanc H. *Probability Theory and Probability Logic*. Toronto: University of Toronto Press, 1999.

[Rogers, 1987] Rogers H, Jr. *Theory of Recursive Functions and Effective Computability*. Cambridge, MA: MIT Press, 1987.

[Rorty, 1965] Rorty R. Mind-body identity, privacy, and categories. *Review of Metaphysics* 1965; 19:24–54.

[Rosch, 1973] Rosch EH. Natural categories. *Cognitive Psychology* 1973; 4:328–350.

[Rosch, 1975] Rosch E. Cognitive representations of semantic categories. *Journal of Experimental Psychology: General* 1975; 104:192–233.

[Rosch, 1978] Rosch E. Principles of categorization. In: Rosch E, and Lloyd BB (eds.), *Cognition and Categorization*, pp. 27–48. Hillsdale, NJ: Lawrence Erlbaum Associates, 1978.

[Rosch, 1988] Rosch E. Principles of Categorization. In: Collins A, and Smith EE (eds.), *Readings in Cognitive Science: A Perspective from Psychology and Artificial Intelligence*, pp. 312–322. San Mateo: Morgan Kaufmann, 1988.

[Rosch and Mervis, 1975] Rosch E, and Mervis CB. Family resemblances: Studies in the internal structure of categories. *Cognitive Psychology* 1975; 7:573–605.

[Rosenthal, 1991] Rosenthal DM (ed.). *The Nature of Mind*. Oxford: Oxford University Press, 1991.

[Ross, 1941] Ross A. Imperatives and logic. Theoria 1941; 7:53–71.

[Ross, 2008] Ross S. *A First Course in Probability*. Upper Saddle River: Pearson Higher Education, 2008.

[Ross et al., 2002] Ross TJ, Booker JM, and Parkinson JW (eds.). *Fuzzy Logic and Probability Applications: A Practical Guide*. Philadelphia: SIAM Publishers, 2002.

[Rosse and Mejino, 2003] Rosse C, and Mejino JL, Jr. A reference ontology for biomedical informatics: the Foundational Model of Anatomy. *Journal of Biomedical Informatics* 2003; 36:478–500.

[Rosse and Mejino, 2008] Rosse C, and Mejino JL, Jr. The foundational model of anatomy ontology. In: Burger A, Davidson D, and Baldock R (eds.), *Anatomy Ontologies for Bioinformatics*, pp. 59–117. Berlin: Springer-Verlag, 2008.

[Roth, 2003] Roth G. *Fühlen, Denken, Handeln*. Frankfurt: Suhrkamp, 2003.

[Roth and Vollmer, 2002] Roth G, and Vollmer G. Es geht ans Eingemachte. *Spektrum der Wissenschaft* 2002, Issue No. 2, pp. 60–63.

[Rothschuh, 1963] Rothschuh KE. *Theorie des Organismus. Bios, Psyche, Pathos*. München: Urban & Schwarzenberg, 1963. (First published 1958.)

[Rothschuh, 1975] Rothschuh KE (ed.). *Was ist Krankheit? Erscheinung, Erklärung, Sinngebung*. Darmstadt: Wissenschaftliche Buchgesellschaft, 1975.

[Rothschuh, 1978] Rothschuh KE. Iatrologie. Zum Stand der klinisch-theoretischen Grundlagendiskussion. Eine Übersicht. *Hippokrates* 1978; 49:3–21.

[Routley, 1981] Routley R. *Exploring Meinong's Jungle and Beyond*. Canberra: Australian National University, 1981.

[Royakkers , 1998] Royakkers LL. *Extending Deontic Logic for the Formalisation of Legal Rules*. Dordrecht: Kluwer Academic Publishers Group, 1998.

[Ruspini et al., 1998] Ruspini EH, Bonissone PP, and Pedrycz W. *Handbook of Fuzzy Computation*. Bristol: Institute of Physics Publishing, 1998.

[Russell, 1903] Russell, Bertrand. *Principles of Mathematics*. London: George Allen and Unwin Ltd., 1903.

[Russell, 1905] Russell, Bertrand. On denoting. *Mind* 1905; 14:479–493.

[Russell, 1912] Russell, Bertrand. *The Problems of Philosophy*. London: Williams & Norgate, 1912.

[Russell, 1914] Russell, Bertrand. *Our Knowledge of the External World*. London: Open Court, 1914.

[Russell, 1918] Russell, Bertrand. The philosophy of logical atomism. *The Monist* 1918; 28: 495–527.

[Russell, 1919] Russell, Bertrand. *Introduction to Mathematical Philosophy*. London: Allen & Unwin, 1919.

[Russell, 1923] Russell, Bertrand. Vagueness. *Australasian Journal of Psychology and Philosophy* 1923; 1:84–92.

[Russell, 1924] Russell, Bertrand. Logical Atomism. In: Muirhead JH (ed.), *Contemporary British Philosophy* (first series), pp. 359–383. London: Allen & Unwin, 1924.

[Russell, 1969] Russell, Bertrand. *My Philosophical Development*. London: George Allen & Unwin Ltd., 1969.

[Ryle, 1949] Ryle G. *The Concept of Mind*. London: Hutchinson, 1949.

[Sackett et al., 1996] Sackett DL, Rosenberg WMC, Muir Gray JA, et al. Evidence based medicine: what it is and what it isn't. *British Medical Journal* 1996; 312:71–72.

[Sadegh-Zadeh, 1970a] Sadegh-Zadeh K. The organism as a cyclic-causal system. *Ärztekolloquium* 1970; No. 1, pp. 26–39, edited by Duensing F. Department of Clinical Neurophysiology, University of Göttingen. (In German.)

[Sadegh-Zadeh, 1970b] Sadegh-Zadeh K. Psyche and self-consciousness by cerebral representation and metarepresentation of the organism. *Ärztekolloquium* 1970; No. 3, pp. 11–18, edited by Duensing F. Department of Clinical Neurophysiology, University of Göttingen. (In German.)

[Sadegh-Zadeh, 1970c] Sadegh-Zadeh K. Is psychiatry a science? *Ärztekolloquium* 1970; No. 4, pp. 22–33, edited by Duensing F. Department of Clinical Neurophysiology, University of Göttingen. (In German.)

[Sadegh-Zadeh, 1974] Sadegh-Zadeh K. Zur Erkenntnismethodologie der modernen Medizin. *Mitteilungen der Gesellschaft für Wissenschaftsgeschichte* 1974; 12:51–52.

[Sadegh-Zadeh, 1976] Sadegh-Zadeh K. Clinical judgments as performatives. Paper delivered at the Deutsch-Niederländische Medizinhistorikertreffen. Haus Wellbergen, in Wellbergen near Münster, 24 July 1976. (Unpublished manuscript.)

[Sadegh-Zadeh, 1977a] Sadegh-Zadeh K. Concepts of disease and nosological systems. *Metamed* 1977; 1:4–41. (In German.)

[Sadegh-Zadeh, 1977b] Sadegh-Zadeh K. Basic problems in the theory of clinical practice. Part 1: Explication of the concept of medical diagnosis. *Metamed* 1977; 1:76–102. (In German.)

[Sadegh-Zadeh, 1977c] Sadegh-Zadeh K. What is clinical methodology and why do we need it? Inaugural paper presented at the first meeting of the Arbeitskreis für Methodologie der klinischen Medizin, Herzog August Bibliothek Wolfenbüttel, Germany, March 23, 1977. (In German.)

[Sadegh-Zadeh, 1978a] Sadegh-Zadeh K. On the limits of the statistical-causal analysis as a diagnostic procedure. *Theory and Decision* 1978; 9:93–107.

[Sadegh-Zadeh, 1978b] Sadegh-Zadeh K. Clinical medicine as a utilitarian technology. Paper presented at the second meeting of the Arbeitskreis für Methodologie der klinischen Medizin, University of Münster, Germany, July 6, 1978. (Unpublished manuscript, in German.)

[Sadegh-Zadeh, 1979] Sadegh-Zadeh K. *Problems of Causality in Clinical Practice.* University of Münster Clinicum, 1979. (In German.)

[Sadegh-Zadeh, 1980a] Sadegh-Zadeh K. Toward metamedicine. *Metamedicine* 1980; 1:3–10.

[Sadegh-Zadeh, 1980b] Sadegh-Zadeh K. Bayesian diagnostics. A bibliography: Part 1. *Metamedicine* 1980; 1:107–124.

[Sadegh-Zadeh, 1980c] Sadegh-Zadeh K. Wissenschaftstheoretische Probleme der Medizin. In: Speck J (ed.), *Handbuch wissenschaftstheoretischer Begriffe,* pp. 406–411. Göttingen: Vandenhoeck & Ruprecht, 1980.

[Sadegh-Zadeh, 1981a] Sadegh-Zadeh K. Normative systems and medical metaethics. Part 1: Value kinematics, health, and disease. *Metamedicine* 1981; 2:75–119.

[Sadegh-Zadeh, 1981b] Sadegh-Zadeh K. Normative systems and medical metaethics. Part 2: Health-maximizing and persons. *Metamedicine* 1981; 2:343–359.

[Sadegh-Zadeh, 1981c] Sadegh-Zadeh K. Über die relative Vermeidbarkeit und absolute Unvermeidbarkeit von Fehldiagnosen. In: *Wissenschaftliche Information* 1981; 7(4), pp. 33–43. (Proceedings of the 17th Annual Conference of the Society of Pediatric Radiology, Münster 1980. Edited by H.-J. von Lengerke.)

[Sadegh-Zadeh, 1981d] Sadegh-Zadeh K. Foundations of clinical praxiology. Part I: The relativity of medical diagnosis. *Metamedicine* 1981; 2:183–296.

[Sadegh-Zadeh 1981e] Sadegh-Zadeh K. On the concept of multifactorial genesis. *Pathology Research and Practice* 1981; 171:50–58.

[Sadegh-Zadeh, 1982a] Sadegh-Zadeh K. Perception, illusion, and hallucination. *Metamedicine* 1982; 3:159–191.

[Sadegh-Zadeh, 1982b] Sadegh-Zadeh K. Foundations of clinical praxiology. Part II: Categorical and conjectural diagnoses. *Metamedicine* 1982; 3:101–114.

[Sadegh-Zadeh, 1982c] Sadegh-Zadeh K. Therapeuticum and therapy: A commentary on Lindahl and Lindwall's skepticism. *Metamedicine* 1982; 3:261–262.

[Sadegh-Zadeh, 1982d] Sadegh-Zadeh K. Organism and disease as fuzzy categories. Paper presented at the conference on Medicine and Philosophy, Humboldt University of Berlin, 21 July 1982, Berlin.

[Sadegh-Zadeh, 1983] Sadegh-Zadeh K. *Medicine as Ethics and Constructive Utopia: 1.* Tecklenburg: Burgverlag, 1983. (In German.)

[Sadegh-Zadeh, 1990] Sadegh-Zadeh K. In dubio pro aegro. *Artif Intell Med* 1990; 2:1–3.

[Sadegh-Zadeh, 1994] Sadegh-Zadeh K. Fundamentals of clinical methodology: 1. Differential indication, *Artif Intell Med* 1994; 6:83–102.

[Sadegh-Zadeh, 1998] Sadegh-Zadeh K. Fundamentals of clinical methodology: 2. Etiology. *Artif Intell Med* 1998; 12:227–270.

[Sadegh-Zadeh, 1999] Sadegh-Zadeh K. Advances in fuzzy theory. *Artif Intell Med* 1999; 15:309–323.

[Sadegh-Zadeh, 2000a] Sadegh-Zadeh K. Fundamentals of clinical methodology: 4. Diagnosis. *Artif Intell Med* 2000; 20:227–241.

[Sadegh-Zadeh, 2000b] Sadegh-Zadeh K. Fuzzy genomes. *Artif Intell Med* 2000; 18:1–28.

[Sadegh-Zadeh, 2000c] Sadegh-Zadeh K. Fuzzy health, illness, and disease. *The Journal of Medicine and Philosophy* 2000; 25:605–638.

[Sadegh-Zadeh, 2000d] Sadegh-Zadeh K. *When Man Forgot How to Think. The Emergence of Machina Sapiens.* (In German.) Tecklenburg, Germany: Burgverlag, 2000.

[Sadegh-Zadeh, 2001a] Sadegh-Zadeh K. The Fuzzy Revolution: Goodbye to the Aristotelean Weltanschauung. *Artif Intell Med* 2001; 21:1–25.

[Sadegh-Zadeh, 2001b] Sadegh-Zadeh K. Foreword: Intelligent Systems in Patient Care. In: Adlassnig KP (ed.), *Intelligent Systems in Patient Care,* pp. IX–X. Austrian Computer Society, 2001.

[Sadegh-Zadeh, 2001c] Sadegh-Zadeh K. Forschungsfreiheit: Schuldig ist der Staat. *Laborjournal* 2001; Issue No. 7–8, pp. 32–33

[Sadegh-Zadeh, 2002] Sadegh-Zadeh K. Fuzzy Deontik: 1. Der Grundgedanke. *Bioethica* 2002; 1:4–22.

[Sadegh-Zadeh, 2007] Sadegh-Zadeh K. The fuzzy polynucleotide space revisited. *Artif Intell Med* 2007; 41:69–80.

[Sadegh-Zadeh, 2008] Sadegh-Zadeh K. The prototype resemblance theory of disease. *The Journal of Medicine and Philosophy* 2008; 33:106–139.

[Sadegh-Zadeh, Forthcoming] Sadegh-Zadeh K. *Fuzzy Metaphysics.* In preparation.

[Saikku, 1992] Saikku P, Leinonen M, Tenkanen L, et al. Chronic Chalamydia pneumoniae infection as a risk factor for coronary heart disease in the Helsinki Heart Study. *Ann. Intern. Med.* 1992; 116:273–278.

[Saikku et al., 1988] Saikku P, Leinonen M, Matilla K, et al. Serologic evidence of an association of a novel Chlamydia, TWAR, with chronic coronary heart disease and acute myocardial infarction. *Lancet* 1988; 2:983–986.

[Sainsbury, 2010] Sainsbury RM. *Fiction and Fictionalism.* London: Routledge, 2010.

[Salmon, 1971] Salmon WC (ed.). *Statistical Explanation and Statistical Relevance.* Pittsburgh: University of Pittsburgh Press, 1971.

[Salmon, 1979] Salmon WC. Propensities: A discussion review. *Erkenntnis* 1979; 14:183–216.

[Salmon, 1980] Salmon WC. Probabilistic Causality. *Pacific Philosophical Quarterly* 1980; 61:50–74.

[Sanchez and Pierre, 2000] Sanchez E, and Pierre P. Intelligent decision making systems: From medical diagnosis to vocational guidance. In: Szczepaniak PS, Lisboa PJG , and Kacprzyk J (eds.), *Fuzzy Systems in Medicine*, pp. 204–223. Heidelberg: Physika-Verlag, 2000.

[Santayana, 1937] Santayana G. The Realm of Matter. In: *Works, Vol. 14,* pp. 288–304. New York: Scribners, 1937.

[Saussure, 1916] Saussure F de. *Course in General Linguistics* (translated by Roy Harris). London: Duckworth, 1983. (First published 1916.)

[Savage, 1954] Savage LJ. *The Foundations of Statistics.* New York: John Wiley and Sons, 1954.

[Scheff, 1966] Scheff TJ. *Being Mentally Ill: A Sociological Theory.* Piscataway, NJ: Aldine Transaction, 1966.

[Scheff, 1999] Scheff TJ. *Being Mentally Ill: A Sociological Theory.* Third Edition. Piscataway, NJ: Aldine Transaction, 1999.

[Scheler, 1924] Scheler M (ed.). *Versuche zu einer Soziologie des Wissens.* München and Leipzig: Duncker & Humblot, 1924.

[Schiener, 2010] Schiener A. *Der Fall Kaspar Hauser.* Regensburg: Verlag Friedrich Pustet, 2010.

[Schofield et al., 2008] Schofield PN, Rozell B, and Gkoutos GV. Toward a disease ontology. In: Burger A, Davidson D, and Baldock R (eds.), *Anatomy Ontologies for Bioinformatics,* pp. 119–130. Berlin: Springer-Verlag, 2008.

[Schüffel and von Uexküll, 1995] Schüffel W, and von Uexküll T. Ulcus duodeni. In: von Uexküll T (ed.), *Psychosomatische Medizin,* pp. 825–838. Fifth edition. München: Urban und Schwarzenberg, 1995.

[Schulz and Hahn, 2005] Schulz S, and Hahn U. Part-whole representation and reasoning in formal biomedical ontologies. *Artif Intell Med* 2005; 34:179–200.

[Schwann, 1839] Schwann T. *Mikroskopische Untersuchungen ueber die Uebereinstimmung in der Struktur und dem Wachsthum der Thiere und Pflanzen.* Berlin: Sander, 1839. (Engl. transl. by Henry Smith: Microscopic Researches into the Accordance in the Structure and Growth of Animals and Plants. London: Printed for the Sydenham Society, 1847.)

[Schwarz, 1993] Schwarz MKL. *Strukturelle und dynamische Aspekte klinischer Indikation,* Med. Diss., Universität Münster, 1993.

[Searle, 1969] Searle JR. *Speech Acts.* New York: Cambridge University Press, 1969.

[Searle, 1980] Searle JR. Minds, brains, and programs. *Behavioral and Brain Sciences* 1980; 3:417–424.

[Searle, 1992] Searle JR. *The Rediscovery of the Mind.* Cambridge, MA: MIT Press, 1992.

[Searle, 1995] Searle JR. *The Construction of Social Reality.* New York: The Free Press, 1995.

[Seising, 2007a] Seising R. *The Fuzzification of Systems: The Genesis of Fuzzy Set Theory and its Initial Applications - Developments up to the 1970s.* Berlin: Springer-Verlag, 2007.

[Seising, 2007b] Seising R. Between empiricism and rationalism: A layer of perception modeling fuzzy sets as intermediary in philosophy of science. In: Melin P, Castillo O, Aguilar LT, Kacprzyk J, and Pedrycz W (eds.), *IFSA 2007. LNCS, Vol. 4529,* pp. 101–108. Heidelberg: Springer, 2007.

[Seising, 2007c] Seising R. Scientific theories and the computational theory of perceptions: A structuralist view including fuzzy sets. In: Štepnika M, Novák V, and

Bodenhofer U (eds.), *New Dimensions in Fuzzy Logic and Related Technologies. Proceedings of the 5th EUSFLAT Conference* (European Society for Fuzzy Logic and Technology). Ostrava, Czech Republic. Vol. 1, pp. 401–408.

[Seising, 2009] Seising R. Fuzzy sets and systems and philosophy of science. In: Seising R (ed.), *Views on Fuzzy Sets and Systems*, pp. 1–35. Berlin: Springer, 2009.

[Shafer-Landau, 2005] Shafer-Landau R. *Moral Realism: A Defence.* Oxford University Press: Oxford, 2005.

[Shoenfield, 2001] Shoenfield JR. *Mathematical Logic.* Wellesley, MA: A K Peters Ltd., 2001.

[Simon, 2010] Simon JR. Advertisement for the ontology for medicine. *Theoretical Medicine and Bioethics* 2010; 31:333–346.

[Simons, 2000a] Simons, PM. Identity through time and trope bundles. *Topoi* 2000; 14:147–155.

[Simons, 2000b] Simons PM. *Parts: A Study in Ontology.* New York: Oxford University Press, 2000.

[Simpson, 1951] Simpson EH. The interpretation of interaction in contingency tables. *Journal of the Royal Statistical Society, Series B,* 1951; 13:238–241.

[Singer, 2003] Singer W. *Ein neues Menschenbild?* Frankfurt: Suhrkamp, 2003.

[Singer and Metzinger, 2002] Singer W, and Metzinger T. Ein Frontalangriff auf unser Selbstverständnis und unsere Menschenwürde. *Gehirn und Geist* 2002, Issue No. 4, pp. 32–35.

[Sismondo, 2004] Sismondo S. *An Introduction to Science and Technology Studies.* Oxford: Blackwell Publishing Ltd., 2004.

[Skinner, 1938] Skinner BF. *The Behavior of Organisms: An Experimental Analysis.* New York: D. Appleton-Century Company, 1938.

[Skinner, 1953] Skinner BF. *Science and Human Behavior.* New York: The Macmillan Company, 1953.

[Skyrms, 2009] Skyrms B. *Choice and Chance.* Belmont, CA: Wadsworth Publishing Company, 2000.

[Smart, 1959] Smart, JJC. Sensations and brain processes. *Philosophical Review* 1959; 68:141–156.

[Smith, 2004] Smith B. Beyond concepts, or: Ontology as reality representation. In: Varzi A, and Vieu L (eds.), *Formal Ontology and Information Systems. Proceedings of the Third International Conference,* pp. 73–84. Amsterdam: IOS Press, 2004.

[Smith, 2008] Smith B. Realitätsrepräsentation: Das Ziel der Ontologie. In: Jansen L, and Smith B (eds.), *Biomedizinische Ontologie: Wissen strukturieren für den Informatik-Einsatz,* pp. 30–45. Zürich: vdf Hochschulverlag AG, 2008.

[Smith and Medin, 1981] Smith EE, and Medin DL. *Categories and Concepts.* Cambridge, MA: Harvard University Press, 1981.

[Sneed, 1971] Sneed JD. *The Logical Structure of Mathematical Physics.* Dordrecht: D. Reidel Publishing Company, 1971.

[Sneed, 1976] Sneed JD. Philosophical problems in the empirical science of science: A formal approach. *Erkenntnis* 1976; 10:115–146.

[Soames, 2002] Soames S. *Beyond Rigidity: The Unfinished Semantic Agenda of Naming and Necessity.* New York: Oxford University Press, 2002.

[Sommerhoff, 2000] Sommerhoff G. *Understanding Consciousness. Its Function and Brain Processes.* London: SAGE Publications, 2000.

[Sorensen, 2004] Sorensen R. *Vagueness and Contradiction*. Oxford: Oxford University Press, 2004.

[Sox et al., 2006] Sox HC, Blatt MA, Higgins MC, and Marton KI. *Medical Decision Making*. Philadelphia: American College of Physicians, 2006.

[Sperber and Wilson, 1995] Sperber D, Wilson D. *Relevance: Communication and Cognition*. Oxford: Basil Blackwell, 1995.

[Staab and Studer, 2004] Staab S, and Studer R (eds.). *Handbook on Ontologies*. Berlin: Springer-Verlag, 2004.

[Stalanker, 1993] Stalanker R. A note on non-monotonic modal logic. *Artificial Intelligence* 1993; 64:183–196.

[Standring, 2005] Standring S (ed.). *Gray's Anatomy: The Anatomical Basis of Clinical Practice*. Edinburgh: Churchill Livingstone, 2005.

[Stanley, 2007] Stanley J. *Knowledge and Practical Interests*. Oxford: Oxford University Press, 2007.

[Starbuck, 2006] Starbuck WH. *The Production of Knowledge: The Challenge of Social Science Research*. Oxford: Oxford University Press, 2006.

[Stegmüller, 1970] Stegmüller W. *Probleme und Resultate der Wissenschaftstheorie und Analytischen Philosophie. Band II: Theorie und Erfahrung*. Berlin: Springer-Verlag, 1970.

[Stegmüller, 1973a] Stegmüller W. *Probleme und Resultate der Wissenschaftstheorie und Analytischen Philosophie. Band II: Theorie und Erfahrung. Zweiter Halbband: Theorienstrukturen und Theoriendynamik*. Berlin: Springer-Verlag, 1973. (English translation in [Stegmüller, 1976].)

[Stegmüller, 1973b] Stegmüller W. *Probleme und Resultate der Wissenschaftstheorie und Analytischen Philosophie. Band IV: Personelle und Statistische Wahrscheinlichkeit. Zweiter Halbband: Statistisches Schließen, Statistische Begründung, Statistische Analyse*. Berlin: Springer-Verlag, 1973.

[Stegmüller, 1976] Stegmüller W. *The Structure and Dynamics of Theories*. New York: Springer-Verlag, 1976.

[Stegmüller, 1979] Stegmüller W. *The Structuralist View of Theories. A Possible Analogue of the Bourbaki Programme in Physical Science*. Berlin: Springer-Verlag, 1979.

[Stegmüller, 1980] Stegmüller W. *Neue Wege der Wissenschaftsphilosophie*. Berlin: Springer-Verlag, 1980.

[Stegmüller, 1983] Stegmüller W. *Probleme und Resultate der Wissenschaftstheorie und Analytischen Philosophie. Band I: Wissenschaftliche Erklärung und Begründung*, Second Edition. Berlin: Springer-Verlag, 1983. (First edition published in 1969.)

[Steimann, 1997] Steimann F. Fuzzy set theory in medicine. *Artif Intell Med* 1997; 11:1–7.

[Steimann, 2001a] Steimann F. On the use and usefulness of fuzzy sets in medical AI. *Artif Intell Med* 2001; 21:131–137.

[Steimann, 2001b] Steimann F (ed.). *Fuzzy Theory in Medicine*, Vol. 21 of the journal *Artificial Intelligence in Medicine*. Festschrift for Lotfi A. Zadeh on the occasion of his 80th birthday. Amsterdam: Elsevier, 2001.

[Steinberg, 2004] Steinberg H. The sin in the aetiological concept of Johann Christian August Heinroth (1773–1843). *History of Psychiatry* 2004; 15:437–454.

[Steinberg, 2005] Steinberg H. Johann Christian August Heinroth (1773–1843) - der erste Lehrstuhlinhaber für Psychiatrie und sein Krankheitskonzept. In: Angermeyer MC, and Steinberg H (eds.), *200 Jahre Psychiatrie an der Universität Leipzig*, pp. 1–80. Heidelberg: Springer-Verlag, 2005.

[Steinberg, 2007] Steinberg H. Die Geburt des Wortes "psychosomatisch" in der medizinischen Weltliteratur durch Johann Christian August Heinroth. *Fortschritte der Neurologie und Psychiatrie* 2007; 75:413–417.

[Stephan, 2007] Stephan A. *Emergenz: Von der Unvorhersagbarkeit zur Selbstorganisation*. Paderborn, Germany: Mentis, 2007.

[Sterling and Shapiro, 1994] Sterling L, and Shapiro E. *The Art of Prolog*. Cambridge: MIT Press, 1994.

[Strawson, 1949] Strawson PF. Truth. *Analysis* 1949; 9: 83–97.

[Strawson, 1950] Strawson PF. Truth. *Proceedings of the Aristotelean Society* 1950; Suppl. Vol. 24, pp. 129–156.

[Strawson, 1970] Strawson PF. 'Social morality and individual ideal'. In: Wallace G, and Walker ADM (eds.), *The Definition of Morality*, pp. 98–118. London: Methuen & Co. Ltd., 1970.

[Strong, 1999] Strong C. Critiques of casuistry and why they are mistaken, *Theoretical Medicine and Bioethics* 1999; 20:395–411.

[Sturrock, 2003] Sturrock J. *Structuralism*. London: Blackwell Publishing Ltd., 2003.

[Suppe, 1977] Suppe F. *The Structure of Scientific Theories*. Urbana: University of Illinois Press, 1977.

[Suppe, 1989] Suppe F. *The Semantic Conception of Theories and Scientific Realism*. Urbana: University of Illinois Press, 1989.

[Suppes, 1951] Suppes P. A set of independent axioms for extensive quantities. *Portugaliae Mathematica* 1951; 10:163–172.

[Suppes, 1957] Suppes P. *Introduction to Logic*. New York: Van Nostrand Reinhold Company, 1957.

[Suppes, 1959] Suppes P. Axioms for relativistic kinematics with or without identity. In: Henkin L, Suppes P, and Tarski A (eds.), *The Axiomatic Method,* pp. 291–307. Amsterdam: North-Holland Publ. Co., 1959.

[Suppes, 1960] Suppes P. A comparison of the meaning and uses of models in mathematics and the empirical sciences. *Synthese* 1960; 12:287–301.

[Suppes, 1962] Suppes P. Models of Data. In: Nagel E, Suppes P, and Tarski A (eds.), *Logic, Methodology and Philosophy of Science: Proceedings of the 1960 International Congress,* pp. 252–261. Stanford: Stanford University Press, 1962.

[Suppes, 1967] Suppes P. What is a scientific theory? In: Morgenbesser S (ed.), *Philosophy of Science Today,* pp. 55–67. New York: Basic Books, 1967.

[Suppes, 1970a] Suppes P. *A Probabilistic Theory of Causality*. North-Holland Publishing Company, Amsterdam, 1970.

[Suppes, 1970b] Suppes P. *Set-Theoretical Structures in Science*. Mimeogr. Stanford, CA: Institute for Mathematical Studies in the Social Sciences, January 1970.

[Suppes, 1984] Suppes P. *Probabilistic Metaphysics*. Oxford, UK: Basil Blackwell Publisher Ltd., 1984.

[Suppes, 2002] Suppes, P. *Representation and Invariance of Scientific Structures*. Stanford, CA: Center for the Study of Language and Information, 2002.

[Suppes et al., 1953] Suppes P, McKinsey JCC, and Sugar AC. Axiomatic foundations of classical particle mechanics. *Journal of Rational Mechanics and Analysis* 1953; 2:253–272.

[Suppes et al., 2007] Suppes P, Krantz DH, Luce RD, and Tversky A. *Foundations of Measurement. Volume II: Geometrical, Threshold, and Probabilistic Representations.* Mineola, NY: Dover Publications Inc., 2007. (First published 1989 by Academic Press.)

[Szasz, 1960] Szasz T. The myth of mental illness. *American Psychologist* 1960; 15:113–118.

[Szasz, 1970] Szasz T. *The Manufacture of Madness.* New York: Harper and Row, 1970.

[Szasz, 1984] Szasz T. *The Myth of Mental Illness: Foundations of a Theory of Personal Conduct.* New York: Harper Perennial, 1984.

[Szasz, 2007] Szasz T. *The Medicalization of Everyday Life: Selected Essays.* Syracuse, NY: Syracuse University Press, 2007.

[Szasz, 2008] Szasz T. *Psychiatry: The Science of Lies.* Syracuse, NY: Syracuse University Press, 2008.

[Szasz, 2009a] Szasz T. Psychiatry: The Shame of Medicine. *The Freeman* 2009; 59 (March), 12–13.

[Szasz, 2009b] Szasz T. The Shame of Medicine: The Case of Alan Turing. *The Freeman* 2009; 59 (May), 16–17.

[Szczepaniak et al., 2000] Szczepaniak PS, Lisboa PJG, and Kacprzyk J (eds.). *Fuzzy Systems in Medicine,* Heidelberg: Physika-Verlag, 2000.

[Tarski, 1927] Tarski A. Foundation of the geometry of solids. Reprinted in [Tarski, 1983], pp. 24–29.

[Tarski, 1933] Tarski A. The concept of truth in formalized languages. (Originally published in Polish: Prace Towarzystwa Naukowego Warszawskiego, Wydzial III Nauk Matematyczno-Fizycznych 34, Warsaw.) Expanded English translation in [Tarski, 1983], pp. 152–278.

[Tarski, 1983] Tarski A. *Logic, Semantics, Metamathematics. Papers from 1923 to 1938.* Edited by John Corcoran. Indianapolis, IN: Hackett Publishing Company, 1983.

[Teodorescu et al., 1999] Teodorescu HN, Kandel A, and Jain LC (eds.). *Fuzzy and Neuro-Fuzzy Systems in Medicine.* Boca Raton: CRC Press, 1999.

[Thagard, 1999] Thagard P. *How Scientists Explain Disease.* Princeton: Princeton University Press, 1999.

[Thom et al., 1992] Thom DH, Grayston JT, Siscovick DS, et al. Association of prior infection with Chlamydia pneumoniae and angiographically demonstrated coronary artery disease. *JAMA* 1992; 268:68–72.

[Thomasma and Pellegrino, 1981] Thomasma DC, and Pellegrino ED. Philosophy of Medicine as the Source for Medical Ethics. *Metamedicine* 1981; 2:5–11.

[Thomasson, 1999] Thomasson AL. *Fiction and Metaphysics.* Cambridge: Cambridge University Press, 1999.

[Thomson, 1891] Thomson W (Lord Kelvin). *Popular Lectures and Addresses,* 3 Volumes. London: McMillan, 1891.

[Thorburn, 1918] Thorburn WM. The myth of Occam's razor. *Mind* 1918; 27:345–353.

[Tichy, 1974] Tichy P. On Popper's definitions of verisimilitude. *Brit. J. Phil. Sci.* 1974; 25:155–188.

[Tierney et al., 2004] Tierney LM, McPhee SJ, and Papadakis MA (eds.). *Current Medical Diagnosis and Treatment.* New York: McGraw-Hill, 2004.

[Triplett, 1988] Triplett T. Azande logic versus Western logic. *Brit. J. Phil. of Sci.* 1988; 39:361–366.

[Tröhler, 2001] Tröhler U. *To Improve the Evidence of Medicine: The 18th Century British Origins of a Critical Approach.* Edinburgh: Royal College of Physicians of Edinburgh, 2001.

[Tuomela, 2002] Tuomela R. *The Philosophy of Social Practices. A Collective Acceptance View.* Cambridge: Cambridge University Press, 2002.

[Turing, 1936] Turing AM. On computable numbers, with an application to the Entscheidungsproblem. *Proceedings of the London Mathematical Society, Series 2,* 1936; 42:230–265 and 43:544–546.

[Turing, 1937] Turing AM. Computablity and -definability. *The Journal of Symbolic Logic* 1937; 2:153–163.

[Turner, 1997] Turner J. *The Institutional Order. Economy, Kinship, Religion, Polity, Law, and Education in Evolutionary and Comparative Perspective.* New York: Longman, 1997.

[Turner, 1989] Turner RM. Using schemas for diagnosis. *Computer Methods and Programs in Biomedicine* 1989; 30:199–208.

[Turunen, 1999] Turunen E. *Mathematics Behind Fuzzy Logic.* Heidelberg: Physica-Verlag, 1999.

[Tversky, 1977] Tversky A. Features of similarity, *Psychological Review* 1977; 84:327–352.

[van Benthem, 1991] van Benthem J. *The Logic of Time.* Dordrecht: Kluwer Academic Publishers, 1991.

[van Benthem and Doets, 1983] van Benthem J, and Doets K. Higher-Order Logics. In: Gabbay DM, and Guenthner F (eds.), *Handbook of Philosophical Logic, Vol. I,* pp. 275–329. Dordrecht: D. Reidel Publishing Company, 1983.

[Van Dalen, 1986] Van Dalen D. Intuitionistic Logic. In: Gabbay DM, and Guenthner F (eds.), *Handbook of Philosophical Logic, Vol. III,* pp. 225–339. Dordrecht: D. Reidel Publishing Company, 1986.

[van Ditmarsch et al., 2008] van Ditmarsch H, van der Hoek W, and Kooi B. *Dynamic Epistemic Logic.* Dordrecht: Sprineger, 2008.

[van Fraassen, 1980] van Fraassen B. *The Scientific Image.* Oxford: Clarendon Press, 1980.

[van Heijenoort, 1971] van Heijenoort J (ed.). *From Frege to Gödel. A Source Book in Mathematical Logic, 1879–1931.* Cambridge, MA: Harvard University Press, 1971.

[van Inwagen, 2005] van Inwagen P. Existence, ontological commitment, and fictional entities. In: Loux NJ, and Zimmermann DW (eds.), *The Oxford Handbook of Metaphysics,* pp. 131–157. Oxford: Oxford University Press, 2005.

[van Rootselaar, 1970] van Rootselaar B. Dictionary of Scientific Biography, Vol. 1, pp. 273–279 (Bernard Bolzano). New York: Charles Scribner's Sons, 1970.

[Verulam, 1893] Verulam, Lord Francis. *Novum Organum or True Suggestions for the Interpretation of Nature.* London: G. Routledge, 1893.

[Vesalius, 1543] Vesalius A. *De Humanis Corporis Fabrica.* Basilae: Ex Officina Ioannis Oporini, Mense Junio, 1543.

[Vico, 1710] Vico G. *De antiquissima Italorum sapientia ex linguae latinae originibus eruenda librir tres.* Naples 1710. (Translated to Engl. by LM Palmer: *On the Most Ancient Wisdom of the Italians Unearthed from the Origins of the Latin Language.* Ithaca, NY: Cornell University Press, 1988.)

[Virchow, 1855] Virchow R. Cellular-Pathologie. *Archiv für Pathologische Anatomie und Physiologie und für Klinische Medicin* 1855; 8:3–39.

[Virchow, 1858] Virchow R. *Die Cellularpathologie in ihrer Begründung auf physiologische und pathologische Gewebelehre.* Berlin: Verlag von August Hirschwald, 1858. (First Englisch edition: *Cellular Pathology as Based upon Physiological and Pathological Histology.* London: John Churchill, 1860.)

[Volhard, 1942] Volhard F. *Nierenerkrankungen und Hochdruck. Eine Sammlung klinischer Vorträge,* pp. 214–227. Leipzig: Johann Ambrosius Barth, 1942.

[Volhard, 1952] Volhard F. *In Memoriam. Vor die Therapie setzten die Götter die Diagnose.* Grenzach: Deutsche Hoffmann-La Roche AG, 1952.

[von Glasersfeld, 1987] von Glasersfeld E. *The Construction of Knowledge: Contributions to Conceptual Semantics.* Seaside, CA: Intersystems Publications, 1987.

[von Glasersfeld, 1995] von Glasersfeld E. *Radical Constructivism: A Way of Knowing and Learning.* London: The Falmer Press, 1995.

[von Mises, 1939] von Mises R. *Probability, Statistics, and Truth.* New York: Macmillan, 1939.

[von Uexküll, 1985] von Uexküll. *Grundfragen der psychosomatischen Medizin.* Reinbek bei Hamburg: Rowohlt, 1985. (First published in 1963.)

[von Wright, 1951a] von Wright GH. *An Essay in Modal Logic.* Amsterdam: North-Holland Publishing Company, 1951.

[von Wright, 1951b] von Wright GH. Deontic logic. *Mind* 1951; 60:1–25.

[von Wright, 1968] von Wright GH. *An Essay in Deontic Logic and the General Theory of Action.* Amsterdam: North-Holland Publishing Company, 1968.

[von Wright, 1971] von Wright GH. A new system of deontic logic. *Danish Yearbook of Philosophy* 1971; 1:173–182.

[von Wright, 1994] von Wright GH. *Normen, Werte und Handlungen.* Frankfurt: Suhrkamp Verlag, 1994.

[Vygotsky, 1986] Vygotsky LS. *Thought and Language.* Edited by Alex Kozulin. Cambridge, MA: MIT Press, 1986. (First published 1934 in Russian.)

[Walter, 2001] Walter H. *Neurophilosophy of Free Will: From Libertarian Illusions to a Concept of Natural Autonomy.* Translated by Cynthia Klohr. Cambridge, MA: MIT Press, 2001.

[Walton, 2005] Walton D. *Abductive Reasoning.* Birmingham, AL: University of Alabama Press, 2005.

[Warren, 2002] Warren JR. The discovery of Helicobacter pylori in Perth, Western Australia. In [Marshall, 2002b], pp. 151–164.

[Warren and Marshall, 1983] Warren JR, and Marshall BJ. Unidentified curved bacilli on gastric epithelium in active chronic gastritis. *Lancet* 1983; Vol. 1, pp. 1273–1275.

[Wartofsky, 1986] Wartofsky MW. Clinical judgment, expert programs, and cognitive style: A counter-essay in the logic of diagnosis. *The Journal of Medicine and Philosophy* 1986; 11:81–92.

[Washbrook and Keravnou, 1992] Washbrook J, and Keravnou E. Making deepness explicit. In E Keravnou (ed.), *Deep Models for Medical Knowledge Enginnering,* pp. 161–167. Amsterdam: Elsevier, 1992.

[Watson, 1919] Watson JB. *Psychology from the Standpoint of a Behaviorist.* Philadelphia: J.B. Lippincott Company, 1919.

[Watson, 2003] Watson G (ed.). *Free Will.* Oxford: Oxford University Press, 2003.

[Welbourne, 1993] Welbourne M. *The Community of Knowledge.* Aldershot, UK: Gregg Revivals, 1993.

[Welbourne, 1994] Welbourne M. Testimony, knowledge and belief. In: Matilal BK, and Chakrabarti (eds.), *Knowing from Words*, pp. 297–313. Dordrecht: Kluwer Academic Publishers, 1994.

[Westmeyer, 1972] Westmeyer H. *Logik der Diagnostik*. Stuttgart: W. Kohlhammer, 1972.

[Westmeyer, 1975] Westmeyer H. The diagnostic process as a statistical-causal analysis. *Theory and Decision* 1975; 6:57–86.

[Westmeyer, 1989] Westmeyer H (ed.). *Psychological Theories From A Structuralist Point of View*. New York: Springer-Verlag, 1989.

[Westmeyer, 1992] Westmeyer H (ed.). *The Structuralist Program in Psychology: Foundations and Applications*. Seatle: Hogrefe and Huber Publishers, 1992.

[Whitehead, 1929] Whitehead AN. *Process and Reality*. New York: Macmillan, 1929.

[Whitehead and Russell, 1910] Whitehead AN, and Russell B. *Principia Mathematica, 3 vols*. Cambridge: At the University Press, 1910–1913.

[WHO, 2004] WHO (World Health Organization). *ICD-10: International Statistical Classification of Diseases and Related Problems. Tenth Revision. Three Volumes*. WHO, 2004.

[Whorf, 1956] Whorf BL. *Language, Thought, and Reality: Selected Writings of Benjamin Lee Whorf*. Edited by John B. Carroll. Cambridge, MA: Technology Press of Massachusetts Institute of Technology, 1956.

[Wieland, 1975] Wieland W. *Diagnose. Überlegungen zur Medizintheorie*. Berlin: Walter de Gruyter, 1975.

[Wieland, 1986] Wieland W. *Strukturwandel der Medizin und ärztliche Ethik*. Heidelberg: Carl Winter Universitätsverlag, 1986.

[Willett and Manheim, 1987] Willett J, and Manheim R (eds.) with the cooperation of Erich Fried. *Bertolt Brecht Poems 1913–1956*. London: Eyre Methuen, 1987.

[Williams, 1953] Williams DCW. On the elements of being: I and II. *Review of Metaphysics* 1953; 7:3–18, 171–192.

[Williamson, 1994] Williamson T. *Vagueness*. London: Routledge, 1994.

[Williamson, 2005] Williamson T. Vagueness in Reality. In [Loux and Zimmermann, 2005], pp. 690–715.

[Winkler, 1954] Winkler WT. On the concept of ego anachoresis in schizophrenia (in German). *European Archives of Psychiatry and Clinical Neuroscience* 1954; 192:234–240.

[Wittgenstein, 1922] Wittgenstein L. *Tractatus Logico-Philosophicus*. London: Kegan Paul, 1922. (First published in German: Logisch-philosophische Abhandlung. In: *Annalen der Natur- und Kulturphilosophie* 1921; 14:184–262.)

[Wittgenstein, 1953] Wittgenstein L. *Philosophical Investigations*. Translated by GEM Anscombe and edited by GEM Anscombe and R Rhees. Oxford: Basil Blackwell, 1953.

[Wittgenstein, 1958] Wittgenstein L. *The Blue and Brown Book*. Oxford: Basil Blackwell, 1958.

[Wolff, 1730] Wolff C. *Philosophia Prima sive Ontologia*. Frankfurt: Libraria Rengeriana, 1730.

[Wolkowitz, 2003] Wolkowitz OM, and Rothschild AJ (eds.). *Psychoneuroendocrinology. The Scientific Basis of Clinical Practice*. Arlington, VA: American Psychiatric Publishing, Inc., 2003.

[Wolter and Zakharyaschev, 1998] Wolter F, and Zakharyaschev M. Intuitionistic modal logics as fragments of classical bimodal logics. In: Orlowska E (ed.), *Logic at Work, Essays in Honour of Helena Rasiowa*, pp. 168–186. Heidelberg: Physica-Verlag, 1998.

[Woods, 2007] Woods J. Fictions and Their Logic. In: Jacquette D (ed.), *Philosophy of Logic*, pp. 1061–1126. Amsterdam: Elsevier, 2007.

[Woolf, 1977] Woolf V. *The Waves*. London: Triad Grafton Books 1977. (First published 1931.)

[Worall and Worall, 2001] Worall J, and Worall JG. Defining disease: Much ado about nothing? In: Tymieniecka A-T, and Agazzi E (eds.), *Analecta Husserliana, Vol. LXXII: Life - Interpretation of the Sense of Illness within the Human Condition*, pp. 33–55. Dordrecht: Kluwer Academic Publishers, 2001.

[Wundt, 1874] Wundt WM. *Grundzüge der physiologischen Psychologie*. Leipzig: Wilhelm Engelmann, 1874. (Reprinted Bristol: Thoemmes Press, 1999.)

[Yager et al., 1987] Yager RR, Ovchinnikov S, Tong RM, and Nguyen HT (eds.). *Fuzzy Sets and Applications. Selected Papers by L.A. Zadeh*. New York: John Wiley and Sons, 1987.

[Zabczyk, 2007] Zabczyk J. *Mathematical Control Theory: An Introduction*. Boston: Birkhäuser, 2007.

[Zadeh, 1962] Zadeh LA. From circuit theory to systems theory. *Proc. IRE,* 1962; 50:856–865.

[Zadeh, 1965a] Zadeh LA. Fuzzy sets. *Information and Control* 1965; 8:338–353.

[Zadeh, 1965b] Zadeh LA. Fuzzy sets and systems. In Fox J (ed.), *System Theory*. Brooklyn, NY: Polytechnic Press, 1965, pp. 29–39.

[Zadeh, 1968a] Zadeh LA. Probability measures of fuzzy events. *Journal of Mathematical Analysis and Applications* 1968; 23:421–427.

[Zadeh, 1968b] Zadeh LA. Fuzzy algorithms. *Information and Control* 1968; 12:94–102.

[Zadeh, 1971] Zadeh LA. Toward a theory of fuzzy systems. In: Kalman RE, and DeClairis RN (eds.), *Aspects of Networks and Systems Theory*, pp. 469-490. New York: Holt, Rinehart & Winston, 1971.

[Zadeh, 1972a] Zadeh LA. A fuzzy-set-theoretical interpretation of linguistic hedges. *Journal of Cybernetics* 1972; 2:4–34.

[Zadeh, 1972b] Zadeh LA. A rationale for fuzzy control. *Journal of Dynamical Systems, Measurement, and Control* (Trans. ASME, Ser. G), 1972; 94(1):3–4.

[Zadeh, 1973] Zadeh LA. Outline of a new approach to the analysis of complex systems and decision processes. *IEEE Trans. Systems, Man and Cybernetics* 1973; 3:28–44.

[Zadeh, 1974a] Zadeh LA. Fuzzy logic and its application to approximate reasoning. *Information Processing 74, Proc. IFIP Congr.* 1974 (3), pp. 591–594.

[Zadeh, 1974b] Zadeh LA. On the analysis of large-scale systems. In: Göttinger H (ed.), *Systems Approaches and Environment Problems*, pp. 23–37. Göttingen, Germany: Vandenhoeck and Ruprecht, 1974.

[Zadeh, 1975a] Zadeh LA. Fuzzy logic and approximate reasoning. *Synthese* 1975; 30:407–428.

[Zadeh, 1975b] Zadeh LA. Calculus of fuzzy restrictions. In Zadeh LA, Fu KS, Tanaka K, and Shimura M (eds.), *Fuzzy Sets and their Applications to Cognitive and Decision Processes*, pp. 1–39. New York: Academic Press, 1975.

[Zadeh, 1975c] Zadeh LA. The concept of a linguistic variable and its application to approximate reasoning, I. *Information Sciences* 1975; 8:199–251.

[Zadeh, 1975d] Zadeh LA. The concept of a linguistic variable and its application to approximate reasoning, II. *Information Sciences* 1975; 8:301–357.

[Zadeh, 1976a] Zadeh LA. The concept of a linguistic variable and its application to approximate reasoning, III. *Information Sciences* 1976; 9:43–80.

[Zadeh, 1976b] Zadeh LA. A fuzzy-algorithmic approach to the definition of complex or imprecise concepts. *International Journal of Man-Machine Studies* 1976; 8:249–291.

[Zadeh, 1978a] Zadeh LA. Fuzzy sets as a basis for a theory of possibility. *Fuzzy Sets and Systems* 1978; 1:3–28.

[Zadeh, 1978b] Zadeh LA. PRUF A meaning representation language for natural languages. *Internatinal Journal of Man-Machine Studies* 1978; 10:395–460.

[Zadeh, 1979] Zadeh LA. A theory of approximate reasoning. In: Hayes J, Michie D, and Mikulich LI (eds.). *Machine Intelligence*, Vol. 9, pp. 149–194. New York: Halstead Press, 1979.

[Zadeh, 1981] Zadeh LA. Possibility theory and soft data analysis. In: Cobb L, and Thrall RM (eds.), *Mathematical Frontiers of the Social and Policy Sciences*, pp. 69–129. Boulder, Colorado: Westview Press, 1981.

[Zadeh, 1982] Zadeh LA. Test-score semantics for natural languages and meaning representation via PRUF. In: Rieger B (ed.), *Empirical Semantics*, pp. 281–349. Bochum: Brockmeyer, 1982.

[Zadeh, 1983] Zadeh LA. A computational approach to fuzzy quantifiers in natural languages. *Computers and Mathematics with Applications* 1983; 9:149–184.

[Zadeh, 1984a] Zadeh LA. Fuzzy probabilities. *Information Processing and Management* 1984; 20:363–372.

[Zadeh, 1984b] Zadeh LA. A Theory of commonsense knowledge. In: Skala HJ, Termini S, and Trillas E (eds.), *Aspects of Vagueness*. Dordrecht: D. Reidel, 1984, pp. 257–296.

[Zadeh, 1985] Zadeh LA. Syllogistic reasoning in fuzzy logic and its application to usuality and reasoning with dispositions. *IEEE Trans. Systems, Man, and Cybernetics* 1985; SMC-15, pp. 754–765.

[Zadeh, 1986] Zadeh LA. Test-score semantics as a basis for a computational approach to the representation of meaning. *Literary and Linguistic Computing* 1986; 1:24–35.

[Zadeh, 1994] Zadeh LA. The role of fuzzy logic in modeling, identification and control. *Modeling, Identification and Control* 1994; 15:191–203.

[Zadeh, 1996a] Zadeh LA. The birth and evolution of fuzzy logic, soft computing and computing with words: A personal perspective. In: Klir GJ, and Yuan B (eds.), *Fuzzy Sets, Fuzzy Logic, and Fuzzy Systems. Selected Papers by Lotfi A. Zadeh,* pp. 811–819. Singapore: World Scientific, 1996.

[Zadeh, 1996b] Zadeh LA. Fuzzy logic and the calculi of fuzzy rules and fuzzy graphs. A precis. *Multi. Val. Logic* 1996; 1:1–38.

[Zadeh, 2009] Zadeh LA. Fuzzy logic. In Meyers AR (ed.), *Encyclopedia of Complexity and Systems Science,* pp. 3985–4009. New York: Springer, 2009.

[Zaiß et al., 2005] Zaiß A, Graubner B, Ingenerf J, Leiner F, Lochmann U, Schopen M, Schrader U, and Schulz S. Medizinische Dokumentation, Terminologie und Linguistik. In Lehmann TM (ed.), *Handbuch der Medizinischen Informatik*, pp. 89–143. München: Carl Hanser Verlag, 2005.

[Zweig, 1993] Zweig S. The Eyes of the Eternal Brother. A Legend. (German title: Die Augen des ewigen Bruders. Eine Legende.) Frankfurt: Insel Verlag, 1993. (First published 1922.)

Index of Names

Subject Index